Clinical Hematology
Theory and Procedures

FIFTH EDITION

Mary L. Turgeon, EdD, MT(ASCP)

Clinical Laboratory Education Consultant
Mary L. Turgeon & Associates
Boston, Massachusetts & St. Petersburg, Florida

Clinical Adjunct Assistant Professor
Tufts University
School of Medicine
Boston, Massachusetts

Professor
College of Professional Studies
Northeastern University
Boston, Massachusetts

Professor
Physician Assistant Graduate Program
South University
Tampa, Florida

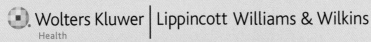
. Wolters Kluwer | Lippincott Williams & Wilkins
Health

Philadelphia · Baltimore · New York · London
Buenos Aires · Hong Kong · Sydney · Tokyo

Acquisitions Editor: Peter Sabatini
Product Manager: Meredith L. Brittain
Marketing Manager: Allison Powell
Designer: Stephen Druding
Production Services: SPi Technologies

Fifth Edition

Library of Congress Cataloging-in-Publication Data
Turgeon, Mary Louise.
   Clinical hematology : theory and procedures / Mary Louise Turgeon. — 5th ed.
      p. ; cm.
   Includes bibliographical references and index.
   ISBN 978-1-60831-076-0
 1. Hematology. I. Title.
   [DNLM: 1. Hematologic Diseases. 2. Hematology—methods. WH 100]
   RB145.T79   2010
   616.1'5—dc22
                                                                    2010031295

DISCLAIMER
Care has been taken to confirm the accuracy of the information present and to describe generally accepted practices. However, the authors, editors, and publisher are not responsible for errors or omissions or for any consequences from application of the information in this book and make no warranty, expressed or implied, with respect to the currency, completeness, or accuracy of the contents of the publication. Application of this information in a particular situation remains the professional responsibility of the practitioner; the clinical treatments described and recommended may not be considered absolute and universal recommendations.

   The authors, editors, and publisher have exerted every effort to ensure that drug selection and dosage set forth in this text are in accordance with the current recommendations and practice at the time of publication. However, in view of ongoing research, changes in government regulations, and the constant flow of information relating to drug therapy and drug reactions, the reader is urged to check the package insert for each drug for any change in indications and dosage and for added warnings and precautions. This is particularly important when the recommended agent is a new or infrequently employed drug.

Some drugs and medical devices presented in this publication have Food and Drug Administration (FDA) clearance for limited use in restricted research settings. It is the responsibility of the health care provider to ascertain the FDA status of each drug or device planned for use in their clinical practice.

Namaste
To my husband, Dick Mordaunt
May we continue to fulfill our dreams of
adventure and learning

PREFACE

It is a pleasure to author the 5th edition of *Clinical Hematology*. Since the 1st edition was published in 1988, each edition has included exciting changes in clinical hematology and posed challenges to learn more and teach more in a fixed time frame. The 5th edition retains the pedagogy that set the standard for clinical laboratory science textbooks since it was introduced in the 1st edition. *Clinical Hematology* now features integrated four-color images, tables, and boxes throughout the book for ease of learning. New online ancillaries include PowerPoint presentations, a quiz bank for students, and more than 800 unique test questions for instructors (see Additional Resources, below, for more information).

Each chapter in this edition capitalizes on the strengths of previous editions; up-to-date information presented at conferences and published in the professional literature; and comments received from students, faculty, faculty reviewers, and working professionals from around the globe. *Clinical Hematology* has been classroom and laboratory "field tested" by medical laboratory technician (MLT) and medical laboratory science (MLS) students, instructors, and the author. Hands-on presentation of the information and techniques discussed in *Clinical Hematology* underscores the importance of clarity, conciseness, and continuity of information for the entry-level student. Sole authorship of this textbook ensures a smooth transition from chapter to chapter without unnecessary redundancy or changes in writing style.

THE AUDIENCE

Clinical Hematology, 5th edition, is primarily intended to fulfill the needs of medical laboratory science (MLS) and medical laboratory technician (MLT) students and faculty as a time-tested book. MLT students may omit some portions of the book depending on the length of the curriculum. Other health professionals can use the book as an instructional or reference guide.

WHAT IS NEW IN THIS EDITION

The 5th edition continues with the innovative expansion of exciting molecular discoveries that assumed importance in the 4th edition—for example, p53 function in DNA repair and mechanisms of apoptosis. The book includes knowledge recognized by the Nobel Prize in Physiology or Medicine in 2009 for discoveries of telomere structure and maintenance and covers other genetic irregularities relevant to the pathophysiology and treatment of hematologic disease—for example, genetic abnormalities leading to ribosome dysfunction in Diamond-Blackfan anemia and genetic abnormalities in Fanconi anemia. The expansion of

classifications found in the recent World Health Organization Classifications appears in this edition. The treatment of many hematology disorders, particularly effective therapy for chronic myelogenous leukemia and chronic lymphocytic leukemia, clearly focuses research on understanding the molecular aspects of diagnosis and treatment of many other blood disorders.

Numerous new discoveries associated with red blood cells have been reported since the 4th edition. New discoveries are related to diagnosis and treatment of hemoglobin defects—that is, hemoglobinopathies. This information has a direct application to the laboratory, where the importance of global population migration creates new or an increased number of patients with disorders that were not commonly seen in clinical hematology before. In addition, this book describes exciting discoveries in iron metabolism and the relationship of iron physiology to anemia of chronic disorders.

Beginning with the 1st edition of *Clinical Hematology*, safety has been an important consideration. The 5th edition covers the latest safety information associated with the importance of immune status—that is, screening and recommended vaccinations of employees, and proper removal of disposable gloves. ISO 15189, quality and preanalytical error management issues, and a Spanish-English Phlebotomy guide (see Appendix D) are also included. The newest specimen-related information in this edition includes additional types of evacuated tubes, environmental factors that influence evacuated tubes, order of draw of multiple evacuated tubes collection, and order of draw of capillary specimens.

Hematology instrumentation continues to expand the menu of available assays. This edition presents the latest comparative instrument product information for cell counting and identification, and blood coagulation testing. The manual procedures chapter (Chapter 26) has been streamlined, with older techniques moved to a web-based repository. The format of the procedures continues to comply with Clinical Laboratory Standards Institute (CLSI) standards. The 1st edition of this book was the first clinical laboratory science textbook to institute standardization of procedures using the CLSI protocol.

ORGANIZATIONAL PHILOSOPHY

The six-part organization of *Clinical Hematology* follows the original profile for a logical combination of textbook, cellular morphology atlas, and procedure manual. Part 1, The Principles of Hematology, discusses the newest fundamental concepts including safety, quality assessment, and specimen collection. Chapter 3, Molecular Genetics and Cellular Morphology, continues to be of extreme importance in understanding the pathophysiology and diagnosis of many blood disorders and related therapy. The last chapter in this part, Chapter 4, presents the normal development of blood cells in humans. This is essential basic information.

Parts 2 and 3 of *Clinical Hematology* focus on erythrocytes and leukocytes, respectively. The content of the chapters in each of these parts progresses from normal structure and function to specific abnormalities in each grouping.

In Part 4, Additional Groups of Clonal Disorders, is in focus. Each of the two chapters investigates multiple disorders that share a common clonal origin.

Part 5, Principles and Disorders of Hemostasis and Thrombosis, presents a distinct specialty in hematology: blood coagulation. An abundance of new knowledge about platelets and coagulation factors continues to emerge.

The final part, Part 6, focuses on hematological analysis. This section includes diversified types of analysis including body fluid analysis, manual procedures, and instrumentation. This part is conveniently located at the end of the book for easy reference when reading other parts of the book.

Handy appendices include answers to review questions, medical terminology basics, SI units, a list of English-Spanish medical phrases for the phlebotomist, the newest evacuated tube pictorial directory, and a sample Material Safety Data Sheet (MSDS). A glossary at the end of the book defines all the key words bolded throughout the text.

CHAPTER STRUCTURE AND FEATURES

Each chapter of *Clinical Hematology* provides the following elements to enhance the usability of the text:

- **Learning objectives** provide a quick overview of the content to be covered.
- **Case studies** reinforce concepts with real-world applications.
- **Procedure boxes** provide step-by-step information for key processes.
- **Key terms** that emphasize important concepts are italicized and defined in the end-of-book glossary.
- **Review questions** reinforce the student's understanding of key concepts and aid in test preparation.
- **Chapter highlights** enable a quick review of material learned in each chapter.

ADDITIONAL RESOURCES

Clinical Hematology includes additional resources for both instructors and students that are available on the book's companion Web site at http://thePoint.lww.com/Turgeon5e.

Instructor Resources

Approved adopting instructors will be given access to the following additional resources:

- Two test banks—one contains more than 800 unique questions; the other contains all the review questions from the book
- PowerPoint slides for each chapter
- An image bank of all the figures and tables in the book

Student Resources

Students who have purchased *Clinical Hematology,* 5th edition have access to the following additional resources:

- A quiz bank of 270 questions
- A lab manual of additional procedures

In addition, purchasers of the text can access the searchable Full Text On-line by going to the *Clinical Hematology* Web site at http://thePoint.lww.com/Turgeon5e.

ACKNOWLEDGMENTS

My objective in writing *Clinical Hematology,* 5th edition, continues to be to share basic scientific concepts, procedural theory, and clinical applications with fellow teachers and students. Because the knowledge base and technology in hematology continues to expand, writing and revising a book that addresses the need of teachers and students at multiple levels in the clinical sciences continue to be a challenge. In addition, this book continues to provide me with the opportunity to learn and share my working and teaching experience, and insight as an educator, with others.

Special thanks to John Goucher for initiating the project and to Meredith Brittain for her organizational efforts in the process of turning the manuscript into a four-color book. An additional thank you is extended to Christine Selvan and her team at SPi for their excellent performance in the preparation of the manuscript for publication.

Comments from instructors and students are welcome at m.turgeon@neu.edu.

Mary L. Turgeon
Boston, Massachusetts
St. Petersburg, Florida

CONTENTS

PART ONE

The Principles of Hematology

CHAPTER 1

Safety and Quality in the Hematology Laboratory

OBJECTIVES

An overview of the hematology laboratory

- Explain the role of the hematology laboratory staff in providing quality patient care.
- List five basic functions of the hematology laboratory.

Safety in the hematology laboratory

- Explain the basic techniques in the prevention of disease transmission.
- Compare the features of general safety regulations governing the clinical laboratory, including components of the Occupational Safety and Health Administration (OSHA)-mandated plans for chemical hygiene and for occupational exposure to bloodborne pathogens, and the importance of the laboratory safety manual.
- List and describe the basic aspects of infection control policies and practices, including how and when to use personal protective equipment or devices (e.g., gowns, gloves, goggles), and the reasons for using standard precautions.

- Explain the purpose and correct procedure of handwashing.
- Describe the contents of the laboratory procedures manual.

Quality Assessment and quality control in the hematology laboratory

- Summarize the essential nonanalytical factors in quality assessment.
- Briefly describe computer-based control systems.
- Define terms used in quality control and basic statistical terms.
- Describe the basic terms and state the formulas for the standard deviation, coefficient of variation, and z score.
- Describe the use of a Levey-Jennings quality control chart.
- Compare three types of changes that can be observed in a quality control chart.
- Explain the most frequent application of a histogram.

AN OVERVIEW OF THE HEMATOLOGY LABORATORY

Hematology, the discipline that studies the development and diseases of blood, is an essential medical science. In this field, the fundamental concepts of biology and chemistry are applied to the medical diagnosis and treatment of various disorders or diseases related to or manifested in the blood and bone marrow.

The Study of Hematology

Basic procedures performed in the hematology laboratory, such as the complete blood cell count (CBC), which includes the measurement and examination of red blood cells (erythrocytes), white blood cells (leukocytes), and platelets (thrombocytes), and the erythrocyte sedimentation rate (ESR), frequently guide the primary care provider in establishing a

patient's differential diagnosis. Molecular diagnostics, flow cell cytometry, and digital imaging are modern techniques that have revolutionized the laboratory diagnosis and monitoring of many blood disorders, for example, acute leukemias and inherited blood disorders. The field of hematology encompasses the study of blood coagulation—hemostasis and thrombosis.

Functions of the Hematology Laboratory

Medical laboratory scientists, medical laboratory technicians, laboratory assistants, and phlebotomists employed in the hematology laboratory play a major role in patient care.

The assays and examinations that are performed in the laboratory can do the following:

- Establish a diagnosis or rule out a diagnosis
- Confirm a physician's clinical impression of a possible hematological disorder

- Detect an unsuspected disorder
- Monitor the effects of therapy
- Detect minimal residual disease following therapy

Although the CBC is the most frequently requested procedure, a laboratory professional must be familiar with the theory and practice of a wide variety of automated and manual tests performed in the laboratory to provide quality patient care. Continuing education is a necessity to keep up with continually changing knowledge and instrumentation in the field.

SAFETY IN THE HEMATOLOGY LABORATORY

The practice of safety should be uppermost in the mind of all persons working in a clinical hematology laboratory. Accidents do not just happen; they are caused by carelessness, lack of attention to detail, or lack of proper communication. Most laboratory accidents are preventable by exercising good technique, staying alert, and using common sense.

Safety standards for patients and clinical laboratories are initiated, governed, and reviewed by governmental agencies and professional organizations (see Box 1.1). The Joint Commission (www.jointcommission.org) has established National Patient Safety Goals. One of the goals of particular interest to laboratory professionals addresses the issue of critical laboratory assay values, the high and low boundaries of the life-threatening values of laboratory test results (see "Quality Assessment in the Hematology Laboratory"). Urgent clinician notification of critical results is the responsibility of the laboratory.

The Safety Officer

A designated safety officer is a critical part of a laboratory safety program. This individual has many duties affecting staff including compliance with existing regulations affecting the laboratory and staff, for example, labeling of chemicals and providing supplies for the proper handling and disposal of biohazardous materials.

BOX 1.1

Safety Agencies and Organizations

- U.S. Department of Labor's Occupational Safety and Health Administration (OSHA)
- Clinical and Laboratory Standards Institute (CLSI)
- CDC, part of the U.S. Department of Health and Human Services (DHHS), Public Health Service
- College of American Pathologists (CAP)
- The Joint Commission (The Joint Commission on Accreditation of Healthcare Organizations)

Occupational Safety and Health Administration Acts and Standards

To ensure safe and healthful working conditions for workers, the US federal government created a system of safeguards and regulations under the Occupational Safety and Health Act of 1970. In 1988, the Act expanded the Hazard Communication Standard to apply to hospital staff. The programs deal with many aspects of safety and health protection and places responsibility for compliance on management and employees.

The Occupational Safety and Health Administration (OSHA) standards include provisions for warning labels or other appropriate forms of warning to alert all workers to potential hazards, suitable protective equipment, exposure control procedures, and implementation of training and education programs. The primary purpose of OSHA standards is to ensure safe and healthful working conditions for every US worker.

OSHA and the Centers for Disease Control and Prevention (CDC) have published numerous safety standards and regulations that are applicable to clinical laboratories (e.g., 1988 OSHA Hazard Communication Standard). Ensuring safety in the clinical laboratory includes the following measures:

- A formal safety program
- Specifically mandated plans (e.g., chemical hygiene, bloodborne pathogens)
- Identification of various hazards (e.g., chemical, biological)

Chemical Hygiene Plan

In 1991, OSHA mandated that all clinical laboratories must implement a chemical hygiene plan (CHP) and an exposure control plan. As part of the CHP, a copy of the material safety data sheet (MSDS) must be readily accessible and available to all employees at all times. This document ensures that laboratory workers are fully aware of the hazards associated with chemicals in their workplaces. The MSDS describes hazards, safe handling, storage, and disposal of hazardous chemicals. The information is provided by chemical manufacturers and suppliers about each chemical and accompanies the shipment of each chemical.

On September 30, 2009, OSHA published the long-awaited Proposed Rule to modify the Hazard Communication Standard (HCS) to conform with the United Nations' (UN's) Globally Harmonized System (GHS) of Classification and Labeling of Chemicals. OSHA has made a preliminary determination that the proposed modifications will improve the quality and consistency of information provided to employers and employees regarding chemical hazards and associated protective measures.

The proposed modifications to the chemical hazard communication (HAZCOM) standard include:

- Revised criteria for classification of chemical hazards
- Revised labeling provisions that include requirements for use of standardized signal words, pictograms, hazard statements, and precautionary statements
- A specified format for safety data sheets (currently known as material safety data sheets)

■ Related revisions to definitions of terms used in the standard and requirements for employee training on labels and safety data sheets

OSHA is also proposing to modify provisions of a number of other standards, including standards for flammable and combustible liquids, process safety management, and most substance-specific health standards, to ensure consistency with the modified HCS requirements. OSHA currently anticipates a 2-year phase-in period for new hazard communication training requirements and a 3-year phase-in period for overall implementation once the Final Rule is published.

"Right to Know" Laws

Legislation on chemical hazard precautions, such as state "right to know" laws, and OSHA document 29 CFR 1910 set the standards for chemical hazard communication (HAZCOM) and determine the types of documents that must be on file in a laboratory. For example, a yearly physical inventory of all hazardous chemicals must be performed, and MSDSs should be made available in each department for use. Each institution should also have at least one centralized area where all MSDSs are stored.

Occupational Exposure to Bloodborne Pathogens

The OSHA-mandated program, Occupational Exposure to Bloodborne Pathogens, became law in March 1992. This regulation requires that laboratories develop, implement, and comply with a plan that ensures the protective safety of laboratory staff to potential infectious bloodborne pathogens, hepatitis B virus (HBV), and human immunodeficiency virus (HIV). The law further specifies the rules for managing and handling medical waste in a safe and effective manner.

The CDC also recommends safety precautions concerning the handling of all patient specimens, known as standard precautions. The CLSI has also issued guidelines for the laboratory worker in regard to protection from bloodborne diseases spread through contact with patient specimens. In addition, the CDC provides recommendations for treatment after occupational exposure to potentially infectious material.

Avoiding Transmission of Infectious Diseases

History of Infectious Disease Prevention

The recognition of HIV-1 generated new policies from the CDC and mandated regulations by the OSHA. Current safety guidelines for the control of infectious disease are based on the original CDC publication, "Recommendations for Prevention of HIV Transmission in Health-Care Settings" (*MMWR*, Suppl 2S, 1987). Clarifications of safety practices appear in the 1988 CDC clarifications of the original guidelines (*MMWR*, 37(24), 1988); in the Department of Labor, OSHA's "Occupational Exposure to Bloodborne Pathogens": Part 1910 to title 29 of the Code of Federal Regulations, 64175–64182, (Fed Reg, 56(235), 1991); and in the U.S. Department of Health and Human Services' "Regulations

for Implementing the Clinical Laboratory Improvement Amendments of 1988: A Summary" (*MMWR*, 41(RR-2), 1992). Laboratory personnel must remain alert to further updates of these policies.

The purpose of the standards for bloodborne pathogens and occupational exposure is to provide a safe work environment. OSHA mandates that an employer does the following:

■ Educate and train all healthcare workers in standard precautions and in preventing bloodborne infections
■ Provide proper equipment and supplies, for example, gloves
■ Monitor compliance with the protective biosafety policies

HIV has been isolated from blood and body fluids, for example, semen, vaginal secretions, saliva, tears, breast milk, cerebrospinal fluid (CSF), amniotic fluid, and urine, but only blood, semen, vaginal secretions, and breast milk have been implicated in transmission of HIV to date. Recently, sperm cells themselves have been discovered to be capable of transmitting HIV. Evidence for the role of saliva in the transmission of virus is unclear, but standard precautions do not apply to saliva uncontaminated with blood.

Preventing Occupational Transmission of HBV and HIV

Blood is the single most important source of HIV, HBV, and other bloodborne pathogens in the occupational setting.

Needlestick Prevention

The CDC estimates that more than 380,000 needlestick injuries occur in US hospitals each year; approximately 61% of these injuries are caused by hollow-bore devices. Blood is the most frequently implicated infected body fluid in HIV and HBV exposure in the workplace.

An occupational exposure is defined as a percutaneous injury, for example, needlestick or cut with a sharp object, or contact by mucous membranes or nonintact skin (especially when the skin is chapped, abraded, or affected with dermatitis), or the contact is prolonged or involves an extensive area with blood, tissues, blood-stained body fluids, body fluids to which standard precautions apply, or concentrated virus.

Among healthcare personnel with documented occupationally acquired HIV infection, prior percutaneous exposure is the most prevalent route of infection. Certain percutaneous injuries carry a higher risk of infection. Risk of infection is greater with:

■ A deep injury
■ Late-stage HIV disease in the source patient
■ Visible blood on the device that caused the injury
■ Injury with a needle that had been placed in a source patient's artery or vein

There are a small number of instances when HIV has been acquired through contact with nonintact skin or mucous membranes (i.e., splashes of infected blood in the eye or aerosols). The risk of infection not only varies with the type of exposure but also may be influenced by:

- Amount of infected blood in the exposure
- Length of contact with infectious material
- Amount of virus in the patient's blood or body fluid or tissue at the time of exposure

On November 6, 2000, the Needlestick Safety and Prevention Act became law. The provisions of the new law include:

- Requires healthcare employers to provide safety-engineered sharp devices and needleless system to employees to reduce the risk of occupational exposure to HIV, hepatitis C, and other bloodborne disease.
- Expands the definition of engineering controls to include devices with engineered sharps injury protection.
- Requires that exposure control plans document consideration and implementation of safer medical devices designed to eliminate or minimize occupational exposure. These plans must be reviewed and updated at least annually.
- Requires each healthcare facility to maintain a sharps injury log with detailed information regarding percutaneous injuries.
- Requires employers to solicit input from healthcare workers when identifying and selecting sharps and document process.

The good news is that most occupational exposures do not result in infection. The average risk for HIV transmission after exposure to infected blood is low—about 3 per 1,000 injuries.

Sharps Prevention

The most widespread control measure required by OSHA and CLSI is the use of puncture-resistant sharps containers. (Fig. 1.1). The primary purpose of using these containers is to eliminate the need for anyone to transport needles and other sharps while looking for a place to discard them. Sharps containers are to be located in the patient areas as well as conveniently placed in the laboratory.

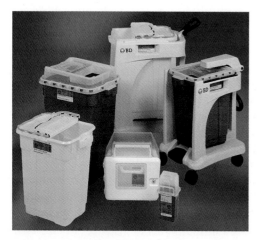

FIGURE 1.1 Puncture-resistant sharps containers. (Courtesy of Becton Dickinson, Franklin Lakes, New Jersey.)

Phlebotomists should carry these red, puncture-resistant containers in their collection trays. Needle containers should not project from the top of the container. Use of the special sharps container permits quick disposal of a needle without recapping as well as of other sharp devices that may be contaminated with blood. This supports the recommendation against recapping, bending, breaking, or otherwise manipulating any sharp needle or lancet device by hand. Most needlestick accidents have occurred during recapping of a needle after a phlebotomy. Injuries also can occur to housekeeping personnel when contaminated sharps are left on a bed, concealed in linen, or disposed of improperly in a waste receptacle. Most accidental disposal-related exposures can be eliminated by the use of sharps containers. To discard sharps, containers are closed and placed in the biohazard waste. A needlestick injury must be reported to the supervisor or other designated individual.

Issues Related to HBV, HIV, and HCV Transmission

Medical personnel must be aware that HBV and HIV are totally different viruses. Exposure to HIV is uncommon, but cases of occupational transmission to healthcare personnel with no other known high-risk factors have been documented. Although HIV is an unlikely work-related hazard, it cannot be underrated because it can be fatal. The most feared hazard of all, the transmission of HIV through occupational exposure, is among the least likely to occur, if proper safety practices are followed. The transmission of HBV can also be fatal and is more probable than transmission of HIV.

HBV can be present in extraordinarily high concentrations in blood, but HIV is usually found in lower concentrations. HBV may be stable in dried blood and blood products at 25°C for up to 7 days. HIV retains infectivity for more than 3 days in dried specimens at room temperature and for more than 1 week in an aqueous environment at room temperature.

HBV Vaccination

Before the advent of the hepatitis B vaccine, the leading occupationally acquired infection in healthcare workers was hepatitis B. Although the number of cases of hepatitis B in healthcare workers has sharply declined since hepatitis B vaccine became widely available in 1982, approximately 800 healthcare workers still become infected with HBV each year following occupational exposure. The likelihood of infection after exposure to blood infected with HBV or HIV depends on additional factors:

1. Concentration of HBV or HIV; viral concentration is higher for HBV than for HIV.
2. Presence of skin lesions or abrasions on the hands or exposed skin of the healthcare worker.
3. Immune status of the healthcare worker for HBV.

OSHA issued a federal standard in 1991 mandating employers to provide the hepatitis B vaccine to all employees who have or may have occupational exposure to blood or other potentially infective materials. The vaccine is to be offered at no expense to the employee, and if the employee refuses the vaccine, a declination form must be signed.

Vaccination against hepatitis B and compliance with precautions are the best prophylaxis against bloodborne pathogen exposure. If an individual has not been vaccinated, hepatitis B immune globulin (HBIG) is usually given concurrently with hepatitis B vaccine after exposure to penetrating injuries. If administered in accordance with the manufacturer's directions, both products are considered safe and have been proven free of any risk of infection with HBV or HIV.

Postexposure Issues

Although the most important strategy for reducing the risk of occupational HIV transmission is to prevent occupational exposures, plans for postexposure management of healthcare personnel should be in place. The CDC has issued guidelines for the management of healthcare personnel exposures to HIV and recommendations for PEP. (Updated U.S. Public Health Service Guidelines for the Management of Occupational Exposures to HBV, HCV, and HIV and Recommendations for Postexposure Prophylaxis, *MMWR*, 50[RR-11], 2001).

An occupational exposure should be considered to be an urgent medical concern to ensure timely postexposure management. If an accidental occupational exposure does occur, laboratory staff members should be informed of options for treatment. Because a needlestick can trigger an emotional response, it is wise to think about a course of action before the occurrence of an actual incident. If a "source patient" can be identified, part of the workup could involve testing the patient for various infectious diseases. Laws addressing the patient's rights in regard to testing of a source patient can vary from state to state.

After skin or mucosal exposure to blood, the ACIP recommends immunoprophylaxis, depending on several factors. If an individual has not been vaccinated, HBIG is usually given, within 24 hours if practical, concurrently with hepatitis B vaccine postexposure injuries. HBIG contains antibodies to HBV and offers prompt but short-lived protection.

An exposed worker should be advised of and alerted to the risks of infection and evaluated medically for any history, signs, or symptoms consistent with HIV infection. Serologic testing for HIV antibodies should be made available to all healthcare workers who are concerned that they may have been infected with HIV.

If a known or suspected parenteral exposure takes place, a laboratory professional may request follow-up monitoring for hepatitis or HIV antibodies. This monitoring and follow-up counseling must be provided free of charge. If voluntary informed consent is obtained, the source of the potentially infectious material and the technician/technologist should be tested immediately. The laboratory professional should also be tested at intervals after exposure. An injury report must be filed after parenteral exposure.

Immune globulin and antiviral agents (e.g., interferon with or without ribavirin) are not recommended for PEP of hepatitis C. For hepatitis C virus (HCV) postexposure management, the HCV status of the source and the exposed person should be determined. For healthcare personnel exposed to an HCV-positive source, follow-up HCV testing should be performed to determine if infection develops. After exposure to blood of a patient with (or with suspected) HCV infection, immune globulin should be given as soon as possible. No vaccine is currently available.

Immune Status: Screening and Vaccination

Screening of Employees

Screening is important for a variety of conditions. These include tuberculosis, rubella, and hepatitis B surface antigen.

Tuberculosis: Purified Protein Derivative (PPD, Mantoux) Skin Test

If healthcare workers have recently spent time with and been exposed to someone with active tuberculosis (TB), their TB skin test reaction may not yet be positive. They may need a second skin test 10 to 12 weeks after the last time they had contact with the infected person. It can take several weeks after infection for the immune system to react to the TB skin test. If the reaction to the second test is negative, the worker probably does not have latent TB infection. Workers who have strongly positive reactions, with a skin test diameter greater than 15 mm, and symptoms suggestive of TB should be evaluated clinically and microbiologically. Two sputum specimens collected on successive days should be investigated for TB by microscopy and culture.

Rubella

All phlebotomists and laboratory staff need to demonstrate immunity to rubella. If antibody is not demonstrable, vaccination is necessary.

Hepatitis B Surface Antigen

All phlebotomists and laboratory staff need to demonstrate immunity to hepatitis B. If antibodies are not demonstrable, vaccination is necessary.

Vaccination of Employees

Individuals are recognized for being at risk for exposure to, and possible transmission of, diseases that can be prevented by immunizations. A well-planned and properly implemented immunization program is an important component of a healthcare organization's infection prevention and control program. When planning these programs, valuable information is available from the Advisory Committee on Immunization Practices (ACIP), the Hospital Infection Control Practices Advisory Committee (HICPAC), and the CDC. Major considerations include the characteristics of the healthcare workers employed and the individuals served, as well as the requirements of regulatory agencies and local, state, and federal regulations. Preemployment health profiles with baseline screening of students and laboratory staff should include an immune status evaluation for hepatitis B, rubella, and measles at a minimum.

See Box 1.2 for vaccines recommended for teens and college students.

Vaccines Recommended for Teens and College Students

- Tetanus-Diphtheria-Pertussis vaccine
- Meningococcal vaccine
- HPV vaccine series
- Hepatitis B vaccine series
- Polio vaccine series
- Measles-Mumps-Rubella (MMR) vaccine series
- Varicella (chickenpox) vaccine series
- Influenza vaccine
- Pneumococcal polysaccharide vaccine (PPV)
- Hepatitis A vaccine series
- Annual Flu + H1N1 flu shot

Note: For complete statements by the Advisory Committee on Immunization Practices (ACIP), visit www.cdc.gov/vaccines/pubs/ACIP-list.htm.
Source: www.cdc.gov, retrieved January 5, 2010 (Vaccines Needed for Teens and College Students) and September 11, 2009 (H1N1 flu advisory, Recommended Vaccines).

SAFE WORK PRACTICES AND PROTECTIVE TECHNIQUES FOR INFECTION CONTROL

Safety Manual, Policies, and Practices

Each laboratory must have an up-to-date safety manual. This manual contains a comprehensive listing of approved policies, acceptable practices, and precautions including standard precautions. Specific regulations that conform to current state and federal requirements such as OSHA regulations must be included in the manual. Other sources of mandatory and voluntary standards include the Joint Commission on Accreditation of Healthcare Organizations (JCAHO), the College of American Pathologists (CAP), and the CDC.

Each laboratory is required to evaluate the effectiveness of its plan at least annually and to update it as necessary. The written plan must be available to employees. A laboratory's written plan must include the purpose and scope of the plan, references, definitions of terms and responsibilities, and detailed procedural steps to follow.

Because many hazards in the clinical laboratory are unique, a special term, biohazard, was devised. This word is posted throughout the laboratory to denote infectious materials or agents that present a risk or even a potential risk to the health of humans or animals in the laboratory. The potential risk can be either through direct infection or through the environment. Infection can occur during the process of specimen collection or from handling, transporting, or testing the specimen.

Laboratory policies are included in a laboratory reference manual that is available to all hospital personnel. Such

manuals that are frequently published online contain information regarding patient preparation for laboratory tests. Approved policies regarding the reporting of abnormal values are clearly stated in this document.

Standard Precautions

Standard precautions are intended to prevent occupational exposures to bloodborne pathogens. This approach eliminates the need for separate isolation procedures for patients known or suspected to be infectious. The application of standard precautions also eliminates the need for warning labels on specimens. According to the CDC concept of standard precautions, see CDC "Preventing Occupational HIV Transmission to Healthcare Personnel" (February 2002), all human blood and other body fluids are treated as potentially infectious for HIV, HBV, and other bloodborne microorganisms that can cause disease in humans.

The risk of nosocomial transmission of HBV, HIV, and other bloodborne pathogens can be minimized if laboratory personnel are aware of and adhere to essential safety guidelines. The National Nosocomial Infections Surveillance (NNIS) System of the CDC estimates that nosocomial infections occur in 5% of all acute-care hospitalizations. In the United States, the incidence of hospital-acquired infection (HAI) is more than 2 million cases per year. Nosocomial infections can be caused by viral, bacterial, and fungal pathogens.

Handwashing

Frequent handwashing is an important safety precaution. It must be performed after contact with patients and laboratory specimens. Gloves should be used as an adjunct to, not a substitute for, handwashing.

The efficacy of handwashing in reducing transmission of microbial organisms has been demonstrated. At the very minimum, hands should be washed with soap and water (if visibly soiled) or by hand antisepsis with an alcohol-based handrub (if hands are not visibly soiled) in the following cases:

1. After completing laboratory work and before leaving the laboratory.
2. After removing gloves. The Association for Professionals in Infection Control and Epidemiology reports extreme variability in the quality of gloves, with leakage in 4% to 63% of vinyl gloves and in 3% to 52% of latex gloves.
3. Before eating, drinking, applying makeup, and changing contact lenses as well as before and after using the lavatory.
4. Before all activities that involve hand contact with mucous membranes or breaks in the skin.
5. Immediately after accidental skin contact with blood, body fluids, or tissues. If the contact occurs through breaks in gloves, the gloves should be removed immediately and the hands thoroughly washed. If accidental contamination occurs to an exposed area of the skin or because of a break in gloves, one must wash first with a liquid soap,

rinse well with water, and apply a 1:10 dilution of bleach or 50% isopropyl or ethyl alcohol. The bleach or alcohol is left on the skin for at least 1 minute before final washing with liquid soap and water.

Two important points in the practice of hand hygiene technique are:

▪ When decontaminating hands with a waterless antiseptic agent (e.g., an alcohol-based handrub), apply product to the palm of one hand and rub hands together, covering all surfaces of hands and fingers, until hands are dry. Follow the manufacturer's recommendations on the volume of product to use. If an adequate volume of an alcohol-based handrub is used, it should take 15 to 25 seconds for hands to dry.
▪ When washing with a nonantimicrobial or antimicrobial soap, wet hands first with warm water, apply 3 to 5 mL of detergent to hands, and rub hands together vigorously for at least 15 seconds, covering all surfaces of the hands and fingers. Rinse hands with warm water and dry thoroughly with a disposable towel. Use the towel to turn off the faucet.

The Department of Health and Human Services (CDC) issued a draft guide in 2001 for Hand Hygiene in Healthcare Settings (see Box 1.3).

 BOX 1.3

Guidelines for Handwashing and Hand Antisepsis in Healthcare Settings

1. Wash hands with a nonantimicrobial soap and water or an antimicrobial soap and water when hands are visibly dirty or contaminated with proteinaceous material.
2. Use an alcohol-based waterless antiseptic agent for routine decontamination of hands, if not visibly soiled.
3. Waterless antiseptic agents are highly preferable, but hand antisepsis using antimicrobial soap may be considered in certain circumstances.
4. Decontaminate hands after contact with the patient's skin.
5. Decontaminate hands after contact with blood and body fluids.
6. Decontaminate hands if moving from a contaminated area to clean body site during patient care.
7. Decontaminate hands after contact with inanimate objects in the immediate vicinity of a patient.
8. Decontaminate hands after removing gloves.

Modified from Centers for Disease Control and Prevention, U.S. Department of Health and Human Services. Guideline for Hand Hygiene in Healthcare Settings, *Morb Mortal Wkly Rep*, 51(RR-16):1, 2002.

Personal Protective Equipment

OSHA requires laboratories to have a personal protective equipment (PPE) program. The components of this regulation include the following:

▪ A workplace hazard assessment with a written hazard certification
▪ Proper equipment selection
▪ Employee information and training, with written competency certification
▪ Regular reassessment of work hazards

Laboratory personnel should not rely solely on devices for PPE to protect themselves against hazards. They also should apply PPE standards when using various forms of safety protection. A clear policy on institutionally required standard precautions is needed. For usual laboratory activities, PPE consists of gloves and a laboratory coat or gown. In a hematology laboratory, splash shields are also used.

Selection and Use of Gloves

Gloves for phlebotomy and laboratory work are nonsterile and made of vinyl or latex. There are no reported differences in barrier effectiveness between intact latex and intact vinyl gloves. Either type is usually satisfactory for phlebotomy and as a protective barrier when performing technical procedures. Latex-free gloves should be available for personnel with sensitivity to the typical glove material. In some laboratories, latex-free gloves are available for everyone to use.

Care must be taken to avoid indirect contamination of work surfaces or objects in the work area. Gloves should be properly placed on the hands and removed (see Fig. 1.2). An uncontaminated glove or paper towel is required before answering the telephone, handling laboratory equipment, or touching doorknobs.

The guidelines for the use of gloves during phlebotomy procedures are the following:

▪ Must be worn when performing fingersticks or heelsticks on infants and children
▪ Must be worn when receiving phlebotomy training
▪ Should be changed between each patient contact
▪ Must be worn when processing specimens

Facial Barrier Protection and Occlusive Bandages

Facial barrier protection (shields) should be used if there is a potential for splashing or spraying of blood or certain body fluids. Masks and facial protection should be worn if mucous membrane contact with blood or certain body fluid is anticipated. All disruptions of exposed skin should be covered with a water-impermeable occlusive bandage. This includes defects on the arms, face, and neck.

Laboratory Coats or Gowns as Barrier Protection

A color-coded, two–laboratory coat or equivalent system should be used whenever laboratory personnel are working with potentially infectious specimens. The coat worn in the laboratory must be changed or covered with an

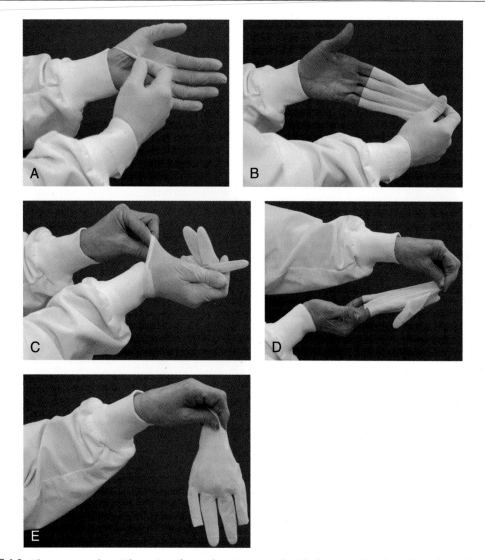

FIGURE 1.2 Glove removal. **A:** The wrist of one glove is grasped with the opposite gloved hand. **B:** The glove is pulled inside out, over, and off the hand. **C:** With the first glove held in the gloved hand, the fingers of the non-gloved hand are slipped under the wrist of the remaining glove without touching the exterior surfaces. **D:** The glove is then pulled inside out over the hand so that the first glove ends up inside the second glove, with no exterior glove surfaces exposed. **E:** Contaminated gloves ready to be dropped into the proper waste receptacle. (Reprinted with permission from McCall RE, Tankersley CM. *Phlebotomy Essentials*, 4th ed. Baltimore, MD: Lippincott Williams & Wilkins, 2008.)

uncontaminated coat when leaving the immediate work area. Coats should be changed immediately if grossly contaminated with blood or body fluids, to prevent seepage through street clothes to skin. Contaminated coats or gowns should be placed in an appropriately designated biohazard bag for laundering. Disposable plastic aprons are recommended if blood or certain body fluids may be splashed. Aprons should be discarded into a biohazard container.

Decontamination of Work Surfaces, Equipment, and Spills

All work surfaces are cleaned and sanitized at the beginning and end of the shift with a 1:10 dilution of household bleach (Table 1.1) or an EPA-registered disinfectant.

Disinfection describes a process that eliminates many or all pathogenic microorganisms, except bacterial spores, on inanimate objects. In healthcare settings, objects usually are disinfected by liquid chemicals or wet pasteurization. The effective use of disinfectants is part of a multibarrier strategy to prevent healthcare-associated infections. Surfaces are considered noncritical items because they contact intact skin. Use of noncritical items or contact with noncritical surfaces carries little risk of causing an infection in patients or staff.

Disinfecting Solutions

Hypochlorites are the most widely used of the chlorine disinfectants. The most prevalent chlorine products in the United States are aqueous solutions of 5.25% to 6.15% sodium

TABLE 1.1	Preparation of Diluted Household Bleach			
Volume of Bleach	Volume of H$_2$O	Ratio	% Sodium Hypochlorite	% Solution
1 mL	9 mL	1:10	0.5	10

Note: A 10% solution of bleach is stable for 1 week at room temperature when diluted with tap water.

hypochlorite, usually called household bleach. Bleach, a broad spectrum of antimicrobial activity, does not leave a toxic residue and is unaffected by water hardness. In addition, bleach is inexpensive and fast acting, removes dried or fixed microorganisms from surfaces, and has a low incidence of serious toxicity. A hazard is that sodium hypochlorite at the concentration used in household bleach can produce ocular irritation or oropharyngeal, esophageal, and gastric burns. The Environmental Protection Agency (EPA) has determined that the currently registered uses of hypochlorites will not result in unreasonable adverse effects to the environment.

Hypochlorites are widely used in healthcare facilities in a variety of settings. Inorganic chlorine solution is used for spot disinfection of countertops and floors. A 1:10 to 1:100 dilution of 5.25% to 6.15% sodium hypochlorite (i.e., household bleach) can be used.

For small spills of blood (i.e., drops of blood) on noncritical surfaces, the area can be disinfected with a 1:100 dilution of 5.25% to 6.15% sodium hypochlorite or an EPA-registered tuberculocidal disinfectant. Because hypochlorites and other germicides are substantially inactivated in the presence of blood, large spills of blood require that the surface be cleaned before an EPA-registered disinfectant or a 1:10 (final concentration) solution of household bleach is applied. If a sharps injury is possible, the surface initially should be decontaminated and then cleaned and disinfected (1:10 final concentration).

An important issue concerning use of disinfectants for noncritical surfaces in healthcare settings is that the contact time specified on the label of the product is often too long to be practically followed. The labels of most products registered by EPA for use against HBV, HIV, or *Mycobacterium tuberculosis* specify a contact time of 10 minutes. Such a long contact time is not practical for disinfection of environmental surfaces in a healthcare setting because most healthcare facilities apply a disinfectant and allow it to dry (~1 minute). Multiple scientific papers have demonstrated significant microbial reduction with contact times of 30 to 60 seconds.

Hypochlorite solutions in tap water at a pH > 8 stored at room temperature (23°C) in closed, opaque plastic containers can lose up to 40% to 50% of their free available chlorine level over 1 month. Sodium hypochlorite solution does not decompose after 30 days when stored in a closed brown bottle.

Disinfecting Procedure

While wearing gloves, employees should clean and sanitize all work surfaces at the beginning and end of their shift with a 1:10 dilution of household bleach. Instruments such as scissors or centrifuge carriages should be sanitized daily with a diluted solution of bleach. It is equally important to clean and disinfect work areas frequently during the workday as well as before and after the workday. Studies have demonstrated that HIV is inactivated rapidly after being exposed to common chemical germicides at concentrations that are much lower than those used in practice. Disposable materials contaminated with blood must be placed in containers marked "Biohazard" and properly discarded.

Neither HBV (or HCV) nor HIV has ever been documented as being transmitted from a housekeeping surface (e.g., countertops). However, an area contaminated by either blood or body fluids needs to be treated as potentially hazardous, with prompt removal and surface disinfection. Strategies differ for decontaminating spills of blood and other body fluids; the cleanup procedure depends on the setting (e.g., porosity of the surface) and volume of the spill. The following protocol is recommended for managing spills in a clinical laboratory:

1. Wear gloves and a laboratory coat.
2. Absorb the blood with disposable towels. Remove as much liquid blood or serum as possible before decontamination.
3. Using a diluted bleach (1:10) solution, clean the spill site of all visible blood.
4. Wipe down the spill site with paper towels soaked with diluted bleach.
5. Place all disposable materials used for decontamination into a biohazard container.
6. Decontaminate nondisposable equipment by soaking overnight in a dilute bleach (1:10) solution and rinsing with methyl alcohol and water before reuse. Disposable glassware or supplies that have come in contact with the blood should be autoclaved or incinerated.

General Infection Control Safety Practices

All laboratories need programs to minimize risks to the health and safety of employees, volunteers, and patients. Suitable physical arrangements, an acceptable work environment, and appropriate equipment need to be available to maintain safe operations.

A variety of other safety practices should be adhered to, to reduce the risk of inadvertent contamination with blood or certain body fluids. These practices include the following:

1. All devices in contact with blood that are capable of transmitting infection to the donor or recipient must be sterile and nonreusable.
2. Food and drinks should not be consumed in work areas or stored in the same area as specimens. Containers, refrigerators, or freezers used for specimens should be marked as containing a biohazard.
3. Specimens needing centrifugation should be capped and placed into a centrifuge with a sealed dome.
4. Rubber-stoppered test tubes are opened slowly and carefully with a gauze square over the stopper to minimize aerosol production (the introduction of substances into the air).
5. Autodilutors or safety bulbs are used for pipetting. Pipetting of any clinical material by mouth is strictly forbidden (see the following discussion).
6. No tobacco products can be used in the laboratory.
7. No manipulation of contact lenses or teeth-whitening strips should be done with gloved or potentially infectious hands.
8. Do not apply lipstick or makeup.
9. All personnel should be familiar with the location and use of eyewash stations and safety showers.

Pipetting Safeguards: Automatic Devices

Pipetting must be done by mechanical means. Such a device is a bottle top dispenser that can be used to deliver repetitive aliquots of reagents. It is designed as a bottle-mounted system that can dispense selected volumes in an easy, precise manner. It is usually trouble free and requires minimal maintenance.

Specimen-Processing Protection

Protective gloves should always be worn for handling any type of biological specimen.

Biohazards are generally treated with great respect in the clinical laboratory (see Fig. 1.3). The adverse effects of pathogenic substances on the body are well documented.

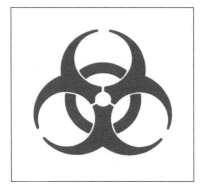

FIGURE 1.3 Biohazard symbol. (Reprinted with permission from McCall RE, Tankersley CM. *Phlebotomy Essentials*, 4th ed. Baltimore, MD: Lippincott Williams & Wilkins, 2008.)

The presence of pathogenic organisms is not limited to the culture plates in the microbiology laboratory. Airborne infectious particles, or aerosols, can be found in all areas of the laboratory where human specimens are used.

In the hematology laboratory, centrifuge accidents, or the improper removal of rubber stoppers from test tubes, produce airborne droplets (aerosols) that can result in an occupational exposure. If these aerosol products are infectious and come in direct contact with mucous membranes or nonintact skin, direct transmission of virus can potentially result.

When the cap is being removed from a specimen tube or a blood collection tube, the top should be covered with a disposable gauze pad or a special protective pad. Gauze pads with an impermeable plastic coating on one side can reduce contamination of gloves. The tube should be held away from the body and the cap gently twisted to remove it. Snapping off the cap or top can cause some of the contents to aerosolize. When not in place on the tube, the cap should still be kept in the gauze and not placed directly on the work surface or countertop.

When specimens are being centrifuged, the tube caps should always be kept on the tubes. Centrifuge covers must be used and left on until the centrifuge stops. The centrifuge should be allowed to stop by itself and should not be manually stopped by the worker.

Another step that should be taken to control the hazard from aerosols is to exercise caution in handling pipettes and other equipment used to transfer human specimens, especially pathogenic materials. These materials should be discarded properly and carefully.

Specially constructed plastic splash shields are used in many laboratories for the processing of blood specimens. The tube caps are removed behind or under the shield, which acts as a barrier between the person and the specimen tube. This is designed to prevent aerosols from entering the nose, eyes, or mouth. Laboratory safety boxes are commercially available and can be used to remove stoppers from tubes or perform other procedures that might cause spattering. Splash shields and safety boxes should be periodically decontaminated.

Specimen-Handling and Shipping Requirements

The proper handling of blood and body fluids is critical to the accuracy of laboratory test results, and the safety of all individuals who come in contact with specimens must be guaranteed. If a blood specimen is to be transported, the shipping container must meet OSHA requirements for shipping clinical specimens (Federal Register 29, CAR 1910.1030). Shipping containers must meet the packaging requirements of major couriers and Department of Transportation hazardous materials regulations. Approved reclosable plastic bags for handling biohazardous specimens and amber bags for specimens for analysis of light-sensitive drugs are available. These bags must meet the NCCLS M29-A3 specimen-handling guidelines. Approved bags have bright orange and black graphics that clearly identify bags as holding hazardous materials (Fig. 1.4).

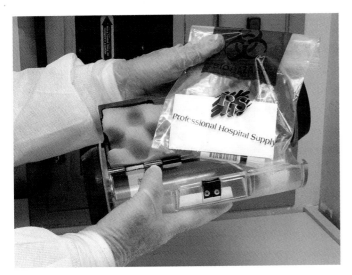

FIGURE 1.4 Approved plastic bags. (Reprinted with permission from McCall RE, Tankersley CM. *Phlebotomy Essentials*, 4th ed. Baltimore, MD: Lippincott Williams & Wilkins, 2008.)

Some products have an additional marking area that allows phlebotomists to identify contents that must be kept frozen, refrigerated, or at room temperature. Maintaining specimens at the correct preanalytical (preexamination) temperature is extremely important. Products such as the Insul-Tote (Palco Labs) are convenient for specimen transport from the field to the clinical laboratory. This particular product has a reusable cold gel pack that keeps temperatures below 70°F for 8 hours even if the exterior temperature is above 100°F. Many laboratory courier services use everyday household coolers.

Blood specimen collection and processing should conform with the current checklist requirements adopted by the CAPs (http://www.cap.org). Errors in specimen collection and handling, preanalytical (preexamination) errors, are a significant cause of erroneous results.

Storage of Processed Specimens

Some specimens must be analyzed immediately after they reach the laboratory. Blood specimens for hematology studies can be stored in the refrigerator for 2 hours before being used in testing. After storage, anticoagulated blood must be thoroughly mixed after it has reached room temperature.

Plasma and serum often can be frozen and preserved satisfactorily until a determination can be done. Whole blood cannot be frozen because RBCs rupture on freezing. Freezing preserves heat-sensitive coagulation factors. A laboratory determination is best done on a fresh specimen.

OSHA Medical Waste Standards

OSHA standards provide for the implementation of a waste disposal program (see Box 1.4). On the federal level, the storage and management of medical waste is primarily regulated by OSHA. Laws and statutes are defined by the Occupational Health and Safety Act and the Clean Air Act.

BOX 1.4

OSHA Regulation of Medical Waste

■ Contaminated reusable sharps must be placed in containers that are puncture resistant; labeled or color coded; and leakproof on the sides and bottom. Reusable sharps that are contaminated with blood or other potentially infectious materials must not be stored or processed in a manner that requires employees to reach by hand into the containers.

■ Specimens of blood or other potentially infectious material are required to be placed in a container that is labeled or color coded and closed prior to being stored, transported, or shipped. Contaminated sharps must be placed in containers that are closeable, puncture resistant, leakproof on sides and bottoms, and labeled or color coded.

■ Regulated wastes (liquid or semiliquid blood or other potentially infectious materials; contaminated items that would release blood or other potentially infectious materials in a liquid or semiliquid state if compressed; items that are caked with dried blood or other potentially infectious materials and are capable of releasing these materials during handling; contaminated sharps; and pathological and microbiological wastes containing blood or other potentially infectious materials) must be placed in containers that are closeable, constructed to contain all contents and prevent leakage of fluids, labeled or color coded, and closed prior to removal (see a full discussion below of biohazard containers and biohazard bag).

■ All bins, pails, cans, and similar receptacles intended for reuse, which have the likelihood of becoming contaminated with blood or other potentially infectious materials, are required to be inspected and decontaminated on a regularly scheduled basis. Waste containers must be easily accessible to personnel and must be located in the laboratory areas where they are typically used. Containers for waste should be constructed so that their contents will not be spilled if the container is tipped over accidentally.

■ Labels affixed to containers of regulated waste; refrigerators and freezers containing blood or other potentially infectious materials; and other containers used to store, transport, or ship blood or other potentially infectious materials must include the biohazard symbol; be fluorescent orange or orange-red or predominantly so, with lettering and symbols in contrasting color; and be affixed as closely as possible to the container by adhesive or wire to prevent loss or removal.

Source: www.fedcenter.gov

QUALITY ASSESSMENT IN THE HEMATOLOGY LABORATORY

The assessment of quality results for the various analyses is critical and is an important component of the operation of a high-quality laboratory. Quality assessment programs monitor the following:

- Test request procedures
- Patient identification
- Specimen procurement
- Specimen labeling
- Specimen transportation and processing procedures
- Laboratory personnel performance
- Laboratory instrumentation, reagents, and analytical (examination) test procedures
- Turnaround times
- Accuracy of the final result

Complete documentation of all procedures involved in obtaining the analytical (examination) result for the patient sample must be maintained and monitored in a systematic manner.

Regulations and Organizations Impacting Quality

Clinical Laboratory Improvement Amendments

In 1988, the U.S. Congress enacted the Clinical Laboratory Improvement Amendments of 1988 (CLIA'88) in response to the concerns about laboratory testing errors. The final CLIA rule, Laboratory Requirements Relating to Quality Systems and Certain Personnel Qualifications, was published in the Federal Register on January 24, 2003. Enactment of CLIA established a minimum threshold for all aspects of clinical laboratory testing. CLIA'88 also incorporates proficiency testing in the regulations.

Voluntary Accrediting Organizations

Voluntary accrediting agencies, for example, the Joint Commission on Accreditation of Healthcare Organization and the CAP, have set standards that include quality assessment programs.

ISO 15189

The International Organization for Standardization (ISO), a network of the national standards institutes of 159 countries, is the world's largest developer and publisher of international standards. ISO is a nongovernmental organization that forms a bridge between the public and private sectors. ISO standards and certification are widely used by industry but now ISO 15189 has been formulated for clinical laboratories. The standard, ISO 15189, is based on ISO/IEC 17025, the main standard used by testing and calibration laboratories, and ISO 9001. The 15189 standard was developed with the input of the CAP and has gained acceptance as a mandatory accreditation in Australia, the Canadian province of Ontario, and many European countries. In the United States, 15189 accreditation remains optional.

ISO 15189:2007 is for use by medical laboratories in developing their quality management systems and assessing their own competence and for use by accreditation bodies in confirming or recognizing the competence of medical laboratories.

Components of Quality Assessment

- A Quality Assessment system is divided into two major components: nonanalytical factors and the analysis of quantitative data (quality control [QC]).

Quality Assessment is used in the clinical hematology laboratory to ensure excellence in performance. A systematic approach to quality assures that correct laboratory results are obtained in the shortest possible time and at a reasonable cost.

The total testing process (TTP) serves as the primary point of reference for focusing on quality in the clinical laboratory. TTP is defined by activities in three distinct phases related to workflow outside and inside the laboratory:

1. Preanalytical (preexamination)
2. Analytical (examination)
3. Postanalytical (postexamination)

Nonanalytical Factors in Quality Assessment

To guarantee the highest quality patient care through laboratory testing, a variety of preanalytical (preexamination) and Postanalytical (postexamination) factors in addition to analytical (examination) data must be considered. For laboratories to comply with CLIA'88 and be certified to perform testing, they must meet minimum standards. In some cases, deficiencies are noted and must be corrected.

Nonanalytical factors that support quality testing include the following:

1. Qualified personnel
2. Laboratory policies
3. Laboratory procedure manual
4. Test requisitioning
5. Patient identification and specimen procurement and labeling
6. Specimen collection, transport, processing and storage
7. Preventive maintenance of equipment
8. Appropriate methodology
9. Accuracy in reporting results and documentation

Qualified Personnel

The entry-level examination competencies of all certified persons in hematology must be validated. Validation takes the form of both external certification and new employee orientation to the work environment.

Continuing competency is equally important. Participation in continuing education activities is essential to the maintenance of competency and is required in some instances to maintain professional certification. Personnel performance should be monitored with periodic evaluations and reports. Quality assessment demands that a supervisor monitors the results of daily work and that all analytical (examination) reports produced during a particular shift be evaluated for errors and omissions.

Laboratory Policies

Laboratory policies should be included in a laboratory reference manual that is available to all hospital personnel. Each laboratory must have an up-to-date safety manual. This manual contains a comprehensive listing of approved policies, acceptable practices, and precautions, including standard blood and body fluid precautions. Specific regulations that conform to current state and general requirement, such as OSHA regulations, must be included in the manual. Other sources of mandatory and voluntary standards include JCAHO, CAP, and the CDC.

Laboratory Procedure Manual

Laboratory procedures should be contained in a current and complete document of laboratory procedures, including approved policies for the reporting of results. The manual must be reviewed regularly, in some cases annually, by the supervisory staff and updated, as needed.

The laboratory procedure manual describes each procedure performed in the hematology laboratory. This manual must comply with the CLSI format standards for a procedure manual. CLSI is an internationally recognized group of laboratory professionals who lead Quality Assessment efforts. To support a QC program, methods for documenting laboratory results must be included in the procedure manual. Proper documentation ensures that control specimens have been properly monitored. The procedural format found in Chapter 26 of this book follows the CLSI guidelines.

The CLSI recommends that the procedure manual follows a specific pattern of organization. Each assay done in the hematology laboratory must be included in the manual. The minimal components are as follows:

- Title of the assay
- Principle of the procedure and statement of clinical applications
- Protocol for specimen collection and storage
- QC information
- Reagents, supplies, and equipment
- Procedural protocol
- Reference "normal" ranges
- Technical sources of error
- Limitations of the procedure
- Proper procedures for specimen collection and storage
- Approved policies for the reporting of results

Test Requisitioning

A laboratory test can be requested by a primary care provider or, in some states, the patient. The request, either hard copy or electronic, must include the patient identification data, the time and date of specimen collection, the source of the specimen, and the analyses to be performed. The information on the accompanying specimen container must match exactly the patient identification on the test request. The information needed by the physician to assist in ordering tests must be included in an online database or printed handbook.

Patient Identification, Specimen Procurement, and Labeling

Maintaining an electronic database or handbook of specimen requirement information is one of the first steps in establishing a quality assessment program for the clinical laboratory. Current information about obtaining appropriate specimens, special collection requirements for various types of tests, ordering tests correctly, and transporting and processing specimens appropriately should be included in the database.

Patients must be carefully identified. Preanalytical (preexamination) errors are the most common source of laboratory errors (see Box 1.5). For example, identification errors, either of the patient or of the specimen, are major potential sources of error. The use of computerized bar code identification of specimens is an asset to specimen identification. Using established specimen requirement information, the clinical specimens must be properly labeled once they have been obtained from the patient. Computer-generated bar code labels (Fig. 1.5) assist in making certain that proper patient identification is noted on each specimen container sent to the

BOX 1.5

Examples of Potential Preanalytical (preexamination)/Analytical (examination)/ Postanalytical (postexamination) Errors

PREANALYTICAL (PREEXAMINATION)
- Specimen obtained from the wrong patient
- Specimen procured at the wrong time
- Specimen collected in the wrong tube or container
- Blood specimens collected in the wrong order
- Incorrect labeling of specimen
- Improper processing of specimen

ANALYTICAL (EXAMINATION)
- Oversight of instrument flags
- Out-of-control QC results
- Wrong assay performed

POSTANALYTICAL (POSTEXAMINATION)
- Verbal reporting of results
- Instrument: Laboratory Information System (LIS) incompatibility error
- Confusion about reference ranges
- Failure to report critical values immediately

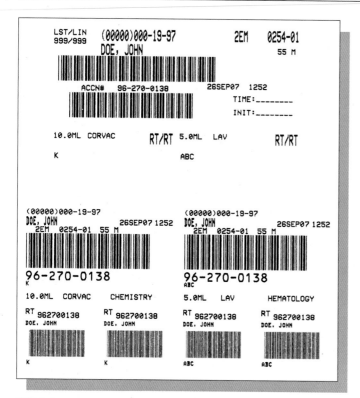

FIGURE 1.5 Bar code. (Reprinted with permission from McCall RE, Tankersley CM. *Phlebotomy Essentials*, 4th ed. Baltimore, MD: Lippincott Williams & Wilkins, 2008.)

laboratory. An important rule to remember is that the analytical result can only be as good as the received specimen.

Specimen Collection, Transporting, Processing and Storage

Strict adherence to correct procedures for specimen collection and storage is critical to the accuracy of any test.

Specimens must be efficiently transported to the laboratory. Some assays require special handling conditions, such as placing the specimen on ice immediately after collection. Specimens should be tested within 2 hours of collection to produce accurate results. The documentation of specimen arrival times in the laboratory as well as other specific test request data is an important aspect of the quality assessment process. It is important that the laboratory processing system is able to track a specimen.

Correct storage of specimens is critical to obtaining accurate results. Specimen integrity is an important issue when blood is collected at a site away from the testing facility. Samples may need to be drawn several hours before testing. In many cases, cooling of specimens on ice is critical. This is particularly true for coagulation testing (e.g., prothrombin time [PT] and activated partial thromboplastin time [aPTT]).

According to CLSI (*Collection, Transport, and Processing of Blood Specimens for Testing Plasma-Based Coagulation Assays*, 5th ed, Approved Guidelines, H21-A5, 2008), blood samples collected for PT and aPTT analysis in tubes with

sodium citrate should be handled using the following sample protocol when collected off-site. The sample tube should remain unopened before testing. Centrifugation and testing of such samples can be delayed for up to 2 hours at 22° to 24°C (71.6° to 75.2°F) or for up to 4 hours at 2° to 4°C (35.6° to 39.2°F). The sample must be kept in a well-chilled, properly insulated cooler or a refrigerated block. Either storage device must have a thermometer to monitor its temperature to prevent overheating or partial freezing of whole blood samples. Separation of the sample upon standing should not affect sample integrity. In addition, this method of storage should be confirmed for compatibility by contacting both the manufacturer of the evacuated tube collection system and the technical supervisor of coagulation testing.

Preventive Maintenance of Equipment

Monitoring of the temperatures of equipment and refrigerators is important to the quality of test performance. Microscopes, centrifuges, and other pieces of equipment need regularly to be cleaned and checked for accuracy. A preventive maintenance schedule should be followed for all automated equipment.

Equipment such as microscopes, centrifuges, and spectrophotometers should be cleaned and checked for accuracy on a regular schedule. A preventive maintenance schedule should be followed (refer to the section "Instrument Protocol," Chapter 27 for examples) for all pieces of automated equipment (e.g., cell-counting instruments). Failure to monitor equipment regularly can produce inaccurate test results and lead to expensive repairs.

Manufacturers will recommend a calibration frequency determined by measurement system stability and will communicate in product inserts the specific criteria for mandatory recalibration of instrument systems. These may include the following:

■ Instrument maintenance
■ Reagent lot change
■ Major component replacement
■ New software installation

Clinical laboratories must follow CLIA or the manufacturer's requirements for instrument calibration frequency, whichever is most stringent. CLIA requires that laboratories recalibrate an analytical (examination) method at least every 6 months.

Appropriate Methodology

When new methods are introduced, it is important to check the procedure for accuracy and variability. Replicate analyses using control specimens are recommended to check for accuracy and to eliminate factors such as day-to-day variability, reagent variability, and differences between technologists.

A template for a standard protocol for the introduction of new testing into a clinical laboratory is presented in Box 1.6.

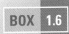

Seven Steps for New Assay Development

STEP 1: SELECT AN ASSAY
Determine the need for the assay, the volume of tests and cost-effectiveness, and site of testing.

STEP 2: RESEARCH ISSUES RELATED TO TESTING
Analyze physical and financial requirements, workflow analysis, and required approvals.

STEP 3: NEGOTIATE WITH VENDORS
Communicate with vendors to evaluate related equipment and supplies, validation panels, and related training and education.

STEP 4: MAKE A DECISION
"Which particular assay or multiple assays will optimally meet the specified needs of the laboratory?"
"Do the cost/benefit ratio, demand for the assay, and quality of available products meet the requirements established by due diligence (Step 2)?"
"Can special requirements for the performance of the assay be met?"

STEP 5: ESTABLISH SPECIFIC REQUIREMENTS
Determine FDA status of assay, the CLIA'88 level of complexity of the assay, parameters of validation study, and the method of documentation consistent with good laboratory practices (GLP).

STEP 6: DEVELOP DOCUMENTATION
Write a standard operating procedure (SOP) for the assay including the technical procedure and QC log, and monitor, assess, and correct problems. A quality assessment document should be included to designate responsible staff, verification of results, proficiency testing, and maintenance of all regulations. Other supplemental documents can include logs of patients, inventory, discrepant results, temperature log, and personnel training.

STEP 7: CONDUCT AND ASSESS TRAINING AND PROFICIENCY
After selection of personnel for training, the actual training is conducted. Competency evaluations should be conducted initially and periodically (after 6 months, after 1 year, and annually). Proficiency testing is conducted to verify accuracy and reliability of testing. The frequency of testing is determined by regulatory agencies.

Source: Lazzari MA. *LABMEDICINE*. 40(7):2009, 389–393.

Accuracy in Reporting Results and Documentation

Many laboratories have established critical values or the Delta check system to monitor individual patient results. The difference between a patient's present laboratory result and consecutive previous results that exceed a predefined limit is referred to as a Delta check. An abrupt change, high or low, can trigger this computer-based warning system and needs to be investigated before reporting a patient result. Delta checks are investigated by the laboratory internally to rule out errors, for example, mislabeling of a specimen.

Highly abnormal individual test values and significant differences from previous results in the Delta check system alert the technologist to a potential problem. At times, a phone call to the primary care provider may be made by the laboratory technologist to investigate possible preanalytical (preexamination) errors such as:

1. Obtaining specimens from IV lines
2. Specimen processing error
3. Actual changes in a patient's clinical condition

Other quantitative control systems (discussed later) are also used to ensure the quality of test results.

Reporting Results

The ongoing process of making certain that the correct laboratory result is reported for the right patient in a timely manner and at the correct cost is known as continuous quality improvement (CQI). This process assures the clinician ordering the test that the testing process has been done in the best possible way to provide the most useful information in diagnosing or managing the particular patient in question. Quality assessment indicators are evaluated as part of the CQI process. Each laboratory will set its own indicators, depending on the specific goals of the laboratory. Any quality assessment indicators should be appreciated as a tool to ensure that reported results are of the highest quality.

Documentation is an important aspect of quality assessment. CLIA regulations mandate that any problem or situation that might affect the outcome of a test result be recorded and reported. All such incidents must be documented in writing, including the changes proposed and their implementation, and follow-up monitored.

Another valuable quality assessment technique is to look at the data generated for each patient and inspect the relationships between them. These many relationships include the relationship between hemoglobin and hematocrit and the appearance of the blood smear on microscopic examination.

Documentation

The use of laboratory computer systems and information processing expedites record keeping. Quality assessment programs require documentation, and computer record–keeping capability assists in this effort. When control results are within the acceptable limits established by the laboratory, these data provide the necessary link between the control and patient data, thus giving reassurance that the patient results are reliable, valid, and reportable. This information is necessary to document that uniform protocols have been established and that they are being followed. The data can also support the proper functioning capabilities of test systems being used at the time patient results are produced.

QUALITY CONTROL IN THE HEMATOLOGY LABORATORY

QC monitors the accuracy and precision of test performance over time.

The purpose of QC is to detect errors that result from:

■ Test system failure
■ Adverse environmental conditions
■ Variance, a general term that describes the factors or fluctuations that affect the measurement, in operator performance

It is important for hematology technologists or technicians to understand basic statistical concepts used in QC. Knowledge of specific elements of statistics is important in hematology for two reasons:

1. Application of statistical analysis of results in Quality Assessment protocols
2. Instrumental applications of statistics to erythrocyte, leukocyte, and platelet reports

Accrediting agencies require monitoring and documentation of QC records. CLIA states, "The laboratory must establish and follow written quality control procedures for monitoring and evaluating the quality of the analytical (examination) testing process of each method to assure the accuracy and reliability of patient test results and reports." For tests of moderate complexity, CLIA states that laboratories comply with the more stringent of the following requirements:

■ Perform and document control procedures using at least two levels of control material each day of testing.
■ Follow the manufacturer's instructions for QC.

QC activities include monitoring the performance of laboratory instruments, reagents, other testing products, and equipment. A written record of QC activities for each procedure or function should include details of deviation from the usual results, problems, or failures in functioning or in the analytical (examination) procedure and any corrective action taken in response to these problems.

Documentation of QC includes preventive maintenance records, temperature charts, and QC charts for specific assays. All products and reagents used in the analytical (examination) procedures must be carefully checked before actual use in testing patient samples. Use of QC specimens, proficiency testing, and standards depends on the specific requirements of the accrediting agency.

Terms Used in Clinical Quality Control

In the clinical hematology laboratory, several terms are used to describe different aspects of Quality Assessment:

1. Accuracy (Fig. 1.6) describes how close a test result is to the true value. This term implies freedom from error. Reference samples and standards with known values are needed to check accuracy.
2. Calibration is the comparison of an instrument measurement or reading to a known physical constant.
3. Control (noun) represents a specimen that is similar in composition to the patient's whole blood or plasma. The value of a control specimen is known. A control specimen must be carried through the entire test procedure and treated in exactly the same way as any unknown specimen; it must be affected by all the variables that affect the unknown specimen. Control specimens are tested daily or in conjunction with the unknown (patient) specimen. Controls are the best measurements of precision and may represent normal or abnormal test values.
4. Precision (Fig. 1.6) describes how close the test results are to one another when repeated analyses of the same material are performed. Precision refers to the reproducibility of test results. It is important to make a distinction between precision and accuracy. The term accuracy implies freedom from error; the term precision implies freedom from variation.

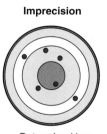 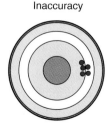

Imprecision   Inaccuracy

Determined by: Determined by:
Repeated analysis study   1) Recovery study
    2) Interference study
    3) Comparison of methods study

A   **B**

FIGURE 1.6 Precision accuracy. Graphic representation of (**A**) imprecision and (**B**) inaccuracy on a dartboard configuration with bull's-eye in the center. (Reprinted with permission from Bishop ML, Fody EP, Schoeff LE. *Clinical Chemistry*, 6th ed. Baltimore, MD: Lippincott Williams & Wilkins, 2010.)

5. Proficiency Testing is incorporated into the CLIA requirements with each laboratory participating in an external PT program as a means of verification of laboratory accuracy. Periodically, identical samples are sent to a group of laboratories participating in the PT program; each laboratory analyzes the specimen, reports the results to the agency, and is evaluated and graded on those results in comparison to results from other laboratories. In this way, QC between laboratories is monitored. Laboratory proficiency testing is required by federal CLIA regulations.

6. Standards are highly purified substances of a known composition. A standard may differ from a control in its overall composition and in the way it is handled in the test. Standards are the best way to measure accuracy. Standards are used to establish reference points in the construction of graphs (e.g., manual hemoglobin curve) or to calculate a test result.

7. QC is a process that monitors the accuracy and reproducibility of results through the use of control specimens.

Functions of a Quality Control Program

Assaying control specimens and standards along with patient specimens serves several major functions:

- Providing a guide to the functioning of equipment, reagents, and individual technique
- Confirming the accuracy of testing when compared with reference values
- Detecting an increase in the frequency of both high and low minimally acceptable values (dispersion)
- Detecting any progressive drift of values to one side of the average value for at least 3 days (trends)
- Demonstrating an abrupt shift or change from the established average value for 3 days in a row (shift)

If the value of the QC specimen for a particular method is not within the predetermined acceptable range, it must be assumed that the values obtained for the unknown specimens are also incorrect, and the results are not reported. After the procedure has been reviewed for any indication of error and the error has been found and corrected, testing must be repeated until the control value falls within the acceptable range.

Analysis of Quantitative Data

It is important for hematology technologists and technicians to understand basic statistical concepts used in QC. Knowledge of specific elements of statistics is important in hematology for two reasons:

1. Application of statistical analysis of results in Quality Assessment protocols
2. Instrumental applications of statistics to erythrocyte, leukocyte, and platelet reports

Terms and Definitions

Average equals the sum of the test results divided by the number of tests. The average is the arithmetic mean value.

Mean is the term used to express the average or arithmetic mean value. The mean value is 13.6 for the following series of values: 10, 11, 14, 16, and 17.

Median is the middle value of a set of numbers arranged according to their magnitude. If two middle values exist in an even number of mathematical observations, the median is the arithmetic mean of the two middle values. The median value is 14 if the following five test values are arranged in order of size: 10, 11, 14, 16, and 17.

Mode is the term used to indicate the number or value that occurs with the greatest frequency. The mode is 45 if the following values are obtained for a control blood test: 45, 48, 35, 39, 51, 42, 45, 39, 45, 44, and 45.

Measurements of Variation

In the laboratory, measures of variation can include the range, the variance, the standard deviation, the coefficient of variation, and the z score.

Range is the term used to express the difference between the highest and lowest measurements in a series. The range is expressed in the same units as the raw data. Therefore, if the value of the raw data is expressed as a percentage (%), the range is also expressed as a percentage. If the following values are obtained, the range can be determined. The range is 0.5% to 2.0% for the following values (expressed as percentages): 1, 1.5, 1, 0.5, 2.0, 1.5, and 1.0.

Variance is an expression of the position of each observation or test result in relationship to the mean of the values. The variance is determined by examining the deviation from the mean of each individual value. If the mean value for this series of assays is 8, the variance can be determined in this example. The following test results were obtained: 3, 4, 5, 6, 8, 9, 10, 12, and 15. The variance from the mean (deviance from the mean) of each individual result is $-5, -4, -3, -2, 0, 1, 2, 4$, and 7. To compute the variance, the squares of each deviation are used. The formula for computing a population variance is as follows:

$$\sigma^2 = \frac{\Sigma(X-\mu)^2}{N}$$

where σ^2 = the variance
X = the observation
μ = the mean
N = finite population size

Standard deviation (SD) expresses the degree to which the test data tend to vary about the average value (mean). To obtain a measure of variation expressed in the same units as the raw data, the square root of the variance or the SD is used.

SD, as a measure of variability, has meaning only when two or more sets of data having the same units of measurement are compared. However, the principle of SD can be used to describe the single-set measurement.

The traditional formula for calculating the SD is the square root of the sum of all the differences from the mean squared and subsequently divided by the number of determinations (tests) minus 1. The traditional formula is as follows:

$$SD = \sqrt{\frac{\Sigma(X - \bar{X})^2}{N-1}}$$

where Σ = sum
X = individual value
$\bar{X}$ = mean individual value
N = number of individual values

To calculate the SD of a laboratory test in the traditional manner, the following steps should be used:

1. A minimum of 20 results are needed. These results represent 20 consecutive days of testing of a control from the same pool sample.
2. Calculate the average (mean).
3. Determine the variance of each number from the mean.
4. Square each variance.
5. Add the squared variances.
6. Divide by the number of test results minus 1.
7. Find the square root of this number.

The value obtained represents 1 SD. In many cases, the traditional formula is not appropriate because the mean does not lend itself to easy manipulation and the sum of the differences does not add up to a sum of zero. In these cases, the alternate formula, which is also the formula programmed into a scientific calculator, should be used. This formula is:

$$s^2 = \frac{n\Sigma x^2 - (\Sigma x)^2}{n(n-1)}$$

The coefficient of variation (CV), or related standard deviation, is a statistical tool used to compare variability in nonidentical data sets. The CV of each data set allows comparison of two or more test methods, laboratories, or specimen sets. To do this, the variability in each data set must be expressed as a relative rather than an absolute measure. This is accomplished for each data set by expressing the SD as a percentage of the mean. The formula for this calculation is as follows:

$$\text{Coefficient of variation (\%)} = \frac{SD}{\bar{X}} \times 100$$

where SD = standard deviation
$\bar{X}$ = mean

The z score measures how many standard deviations a particular number is from the right or left of the mean (Fig. 1.7A). A positive z score measures the number of standard deviations an observation is above the mean, and a negative z score gives the number of standard deviations an observation is below the mean. The z score is a unitless measure.

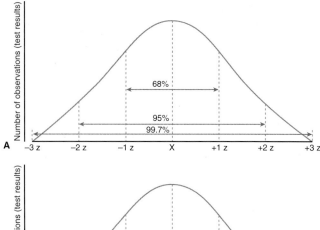

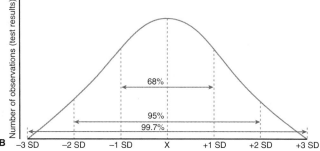

FIGURE 1.7 Frequency distribution. **A:** Z score. **B:** Gaussian distribution: normal frequency distribution curve.

To compare the ranking of two observations from two different populations, the ranking is converted into standard units referred to as z scores or z values. The formula to compute the z score is:

$$z = \frac{x - \mu}{\sigma}$$

where x = an observation from a population
μ = the mean
σ = standard deviation

Using Statistical Analysis of Results in Quality Assessment

Statistical analysis of results has been used in the clinical laboratory since the original introduction of the Levey-Jennings chart. With the advent of computer technology and computerized instrumentation in hematology, many additional systems have been introduced to monitor test results numerically.

In this section, the following methods will be presented:

1. The Levey-Jennings chart
2. The cumulative sum (Cusum) method
3. Trend line analysis
4. Power functions

The Levey-Jennings Chart

QC charts are used in the clinical laboratory to graphically display the assay values of controls versus time (e.g., day or specimen run). The Levey-Jennings chart is the traditional approach to monitoring QC (e.g., instrument calibration or lot-to-lot reagent changes).

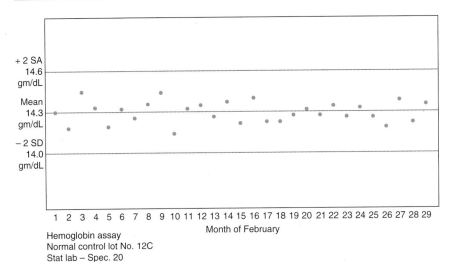

FIGURE 1.8 Levey-Jennings control chart. The normal or abnormal control value is plotted each day. This value must be within 2 standard deviations (SD) of the mean value.

Confidence or control limits are calculated from the mean and the SD. The confidence limits represent a set of mathematically established limits into which the majority of values (results) will fall. Within the confidence limits, the results are assumed to be accurate. It is common practice to use ±2 SD as the limit of confidence.

In the Levey-Jennings control chart (Fig. 1.8), the control results are plotted on the y-axis versus time on the x-axis. This chart shows the expected mean value by the solid line in the center and indicates the control limits or range of acceptable values by the dotted points. If the control assay value is outside the confidence limits, the control value and the patient's values are considered to be out of control and cannot be reported. If the control assay value falls within the confidence limits, the control value and patient specimens assayed at the same time are considered to be in control, and the results can be reported.

Types of Changes

The classification of changes in a QC system is important because different kinds of changes suggest different sources. Three types of changes are commonly observed in the Levey-Jennings QC approach (Fig. 1.9):

1. Systematic drift
2. Increased dispersion of results
3. Shift or abrupt change in results

Systematic drift or trend is displayed when the control value direction moves progressively in one direction from the mean for at least 3 days. Systematic drift or a trend in control values suggests that a problem is progressively developing. This problem may be because of the deterioration of a reagent or control. Diluent contamination affects erythrocyte and leukocyte controls with an upward trend as bacterial growth increases.

Dispersion is observed when random errors or the lack of precision increases. This type of pattern indicates inconsistency in technique or a stability problem (e.g., fluctuating electrical voltage or poor mixing of a cellular control specimen).

Shift or abrupt change is observed when a problem develops suddenly. This type of change can be associated with the malfunction of an instrument or an error in technique.

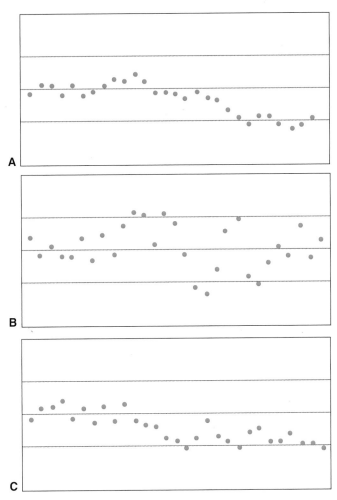

FIGURE 1.9 Types of QC changes. Three kinds of changes may be observed in QC results. **A:** Drift or trend. **B:** Dispersion. **C:** Shift or abrupt change. Each of these types of changes is indicative of a problem that must be corrected before patient results can be reported.

Computed-Based Control Systems

Cumulative Sum (Cusum) Method. This was an early supplementary control method. Decision limits can be manually calculated from the SD with this method; however, computer systems are more efficient. This method allows for the rapid detection of trends and shifts from the mean. Its major disadvantages are that too many out of control results are obtained, and it does not readily control for random error (precision). Cusum can be used as a supplement to the Levey-Jennings system.

Trend Line Analysis. Observed daily results of either the control value or the change in the SD introduced by the control value are tracked. The tracking value at each point is plotted and compared against known error limits for the control of both the mean (accuracy) and the SD (precision). If the value exceeds determined limits, a message is sent to the technologist.

Power Functions

These systems are a means of displaying the performance of a QC rule by plotting the probability for rejection versus the size of the analytical (examination) error. This computerized method can be used to determine what control rule is most useful in detecting an error of given magnitude when a specific number of controls is evaluated.

Other Statistical Applications in the Hematology Laboratory

Frequency Distribution

In any large series of measurements (test results) of a normal population, the results are evenly distributed about the average value. Grouping of data in classes and determining the number of observations that fall in each of the classes is a frequency distribution of grouped data (Table 1.2).

Histogram

Information regarding frequency distribution is easier to understand if presented graphically. A bar chart provides immediate information about a set of data in a condensed form; the related pictorial representation is a histogram.

Histograms can have almost any shape or form. The most frequently encountered type of distribution is the bell-shaped

histogram, which is symmetrical. The bell shape may vary, with some curves being flatter and wider than others; however, most values cluster about the mean, with a few values falling in the extreme tails of the curve. This normal curve is referred to as a gaussian distribution (see Fig. 1.7B).

In the bell-shaped normal curve, ±1 SD includes 68% of all of the values, ±2 SD includes 95% of the values, and ±3 SD includes 99.7% of the values. For biological studies, control confidence limits are usually established at ±2 SD. When values fall outside these limits, the procedure is considered out of control. In the establishment of reference values for a procedure, the reference range for a specific assay reflects the statistical processing of a large number of normal samples and represents the values found within 2 or 3 SDs.

In Chapter 27, histogram data generated by automated cell-counting systems are presented. The interpretation of patient histograms compared with histograms based on established normal values for erythrocytes, leukocytes, and platelets is presented in detail.

CHAPTER HIGHLIGHTS

Hematology is the discipline that studies the development and diseases of blood. Basic procedures performed in the hematology laboratory include the CBC. Molecular diagnostics, flow cell cytometry, and digital imaging are modern techniques that have revolutionized the laboratory diagnosis and monitoring of many blood disorders. The field of hematology encompasses the study of blood coagulation—hemostasis and thrombosis.

Medical laboratory professionals in the hematology laboratory and phlebotomists who are on the front lines play a major role in patient care. Although the CBC is the most frequently requested procedure, a laboratorian must be familiar with the theory and practice of a wide variety of automated and manual tests performed in the laboratory to provide quality patient care.

Safety in the Hematology Laboratory

The practice of safety should be uppermost in the mind of all persons working in a clinical hematology laboratory. Most laboratory accidents are preventable by exercising good technique, staying alert, and using common sense. One of the goals of particular interest to laboratory professionals addresses the issue of critical laboratory assay values because urgent notification of critical results to the primary healthcare provider is the responsibility of the laboratory.

A designated safety officer is a critical part of a laboratory safety program. OSHA Acts and Standards ensure that workers have safe and healthful working conditions. The "Right to Know" laws and the OSHA-mandated Occupational

TABLE 1.2	An Example of a Frequency Distribution of Grouped Data
Class Boundaries	**Frequency (f)**
0.5–35	3
3.5–6.5	8
6.5–9.5	10
9.5–12.5	7
12.5–15.5	4

Exposure to Bloodborne Pathogens regulation require that laboratories develop, implement, and comply with a plan that ensures the protective safety of laboratory staff to potential infectious bloodborne pathogens, HBV and HIV. The law further specifies the rules for managing and handling medical waste in a safe and effective manner.

Blood is the most frequently implicated infected body fluid in HIV and HBV exposure in the workplace. An occupational exposure is defined as a percutaneous injury, for example, needlestick or cut with a sharp object, or contact by mucous membranes or nonintact skin, or the contact is prolonged or involves an extensive area with blood, tissues, blood-stained body fluids, body fluids to which standard precautions apply, or concentrated virus. The most widespread control measure required by OSHA and CLSI is the use of puncture-resistant sharps containers. An occupational exposure should be considered to be an urgent medical concern to ensure timely postexposure management. After skin or mucosal exposure to blood, the ACIP recommends immunoprophylaxis, depending on several factors.

Safe Work Practices and Protective Techniques for Infection Control

Each laboratory must have an up-to-date safety manual. This manual contains a comprehensive listing of approved policies, acceptable practices, and precautions including standard precautions. Standard precautions represent an approach to infection control used to prevent occupational exposures to bloodborne pathogens.

Gloves should be used as an adjunct to, not a substitute for, handwashing. All work surfaces are cleaned and sanitized at the beginning and end of the shift with a 1:10 dilution of household bleach or an EPA-registered disinfectant. A variety of other safety practices should be adhered to, to reduce the risk of inadvertent contamination with blood or certain body fluids. Protective gloves should always be worn for handling any type of biological specimen.

Quality Assessment in the Hematology Laboratory

The assessment of quality results for the various analyses is critical and is an important component of the operation of a high-quality laboratory. Quality assessment is used in the clinical hematology laboratory to ensure excellence in performance. A systematic approach to quality assures that correct laboratory results are obtained in the shortest possible time and at a reasonable cost. A quality assessment system is divided into two major components: nonanalytical factors and the analysis of quantitative data (QC). Nonanalytical factors that support quality testing include qualified personnel, laboratory policies, laboratory procedure manual, test requisitioning, patient identification, and specimen procurement and labeling; specimen collection, transport, and processing and storage; and preventive maintenance of equipment, appropriate methodology, and accuracy in reporting results and documentation. Delta checks are particularly important to rule out mislabeling, clerical error, or possible an analytical (examination) error.

Quality Control in the Hematology Laboratory

QC monitors the accuracy and precision of test performance over time. The purpose of QC is to detect errors that result from test system failure, adverse environmental conditions, and variance.

It is important for hematology technologists and technicians to understand basic statistical concepts used in QC. Knowledge of specific elements of statistics is important in hematology in order to apply statistical analysis of results and in instrumental applications of statistics to erythrocyte, leukocyte, and platelet reports.

Statistical analysis of results has been used in the clinical laboratory since the original introduction of the Levey-Jennings chart. With the advent of computer technology and computerized instrumentation in hematology, many additional systems have been introduced to monitor test results numerically.

REVIEW QUESTIONS

1. The function (or functions) of a hematology laboratory is (are) to
   A. confirm the physician's impression of a possible hematological disorder
   B. establish or rule out a diagnosis
   C. screen for asymptomatic disorders
   D. all of the above
2. The major intended purpose of the laboratory safety manual is to
   A. protect the patient and laboratory personnel
   B. protect laboratory and other hospital personnel
   C. comply with local health and state regulatory requirements
   D. comply with OSHA regulations
3. Which of the following is *not* an appropriate safety practice?
   A. Disposing of needles in biohazard, puncture-proof containers
   B. Frequent handwashing
   C. Sterilizing lancets for reuse
   D. Keeping food out of the same areas as specimens

(continued)

4. If a blood specimen is spilled on a laboratory bench or floor area, the first step in cleanup should be
   A. wear gloves and a lab coat
   B. absorb blood with disposable towels
   C. clean with freshly prepared 1% chlorine solution
   D. wash with water

5. Which of the following procedures is the most basic and effective in preventing nosocomial infections?
   A. Washing hands between patient contacts
   B. Wearing laboratory coats
   C. Isolating infectious patients
   D. Isolating infectious specimens

6. The likelihood of infection after exposure to HBV-infected or HIV-infected blood or body fluids depends on all of the following factors except the
   A. source (anatomical site) of the blood or fluid
   B. concentration of the virus
   C. duration of the contact
   D. presence of nonintact skin

7. HBV and HIV may be directly transmitted in the occupational setting by all of the following except
   A. parenteral inoculation with contaminated blood
   B. exposure of intact skin to contaminated blood or certain body fluids
   C. exposure of intact mucous membranes to contaminated blood or certain body fluids
   D. sharing bathroom facilities with an HIV-positive person

8. Standard precautions have been instituted in clinical laboratories to prevent _____ exposures of healthcare workers to bloodborne pathogens such as HIV and HBV.
   A. parenteral
   B. nonintact mucous membrane
   C. nonintact skin
   D. all of the above

9. Exposure to _____ constitutes the major source of HIV and HBV infection in healthcare personnel.
   A. sputum
   B. blood
   C. urine
   D. semen

10. The transmission of HBV is _____ probable than transmission of HIV.
    A. less
    B. more

11. Gloves for medical use may be
    A. sterile or nonsterile
    B. latex or vinyl
    C. used only once
    D. all of the above

Questions 12 and 13: Diluted bleach for disinfecting work surfaces, equipment, and spills should be prepared daily by preparing a _____ (12) dilution of household bleach. This dilution requires _____ (13) mL of bleach diluted to 100 mL with H^2O.

12.
   A. 1:5
   B. 1:10
   C. 1:20
   D. 1:100

13.
   A. 1
   B. 10
   C. 25
   D. 50

14. The laboratory procedure manual does *not* need to include
    A. test method, principle of the test, and clinical applications
    B. specimen collection and storage procedures
    C. the name of the supplier of common laboratory chemicals
    D. QC techniques, procedures, normal values, and technical sources of error

15. Which of the following statements is *not* a nonanalytical factor in a Quality Assessment system?
    A. Qualified personnel and established laboratory policies
    B. Monitoring the standard deviation and reporting results of normal and abnormal controls
    C. Maintenance of a procedure manual and the use of appropriate methodology
    D. Preventive maintenance of equipment and correct specimen collection

16. In which of the following laboratory situations is a verbal report *permissible*?
    A. When the patient is going directly to the physician's office and would like to have the report available
    B. When the report cannot be found at the nurse's station
    C. When emergency test results are needed by a physician
    D. None of the above.

Questions 17 through 19: Match the following terms with the best description.

17. _____ Accuracy
18. _____ Calibration
19. _____ Control

   A. The value is known in a specimen similar to a patient's whole blood or serum.
   B. Closeness to the *true* value
   C. The process of monitoring accuracy
   D. Comparison to a known physical constant

(continued)

Questions 20 through 22: Match the following terms with the best description.

20. _____ Precision
21. _____ Standards
22. _____ Quality

A. How close test results are when repeated.
B. A purified substance of a known composition.
C. The process of monitoring accuracy and reproducibility of known control results.
D. The value is unknown.

23. Which of the following is *not* a function of a quantitative QC program?
 A. Monitors the correct functioning of equipment, reagents, and individual technique
 B. Confirms the correct identity of patient specimens
 C. Compares the accuracy of controls to reference values
 D. Detects shifts in control values

Questions 24 through 27: Match the following terms with the appropriate description.

24. _____ Mean
25. _____ Range
26. _____ Variance
27. _____ Standard deviation

A. The difference between the upper and lower measurements in a series of results
B. The expression of the position of each test result to the average
C. The arithmetic average
D. The degree to which test data vary about the average

28. The coefficient of variation is the
 A. sum of the squared differences from the mean
 B. square root of the variance from the mean
 C. standard deviation expressed as a percentage of the mean
 D. degree to which test data vary about the average

29. The z score measures
 A. how many standard deviations a particular number is from the right or left of the mean
 B. the sum of the squared differences from the mean
 C. the square root of the variance from the mean
 D. the expression of the position of each test result to the average

30. Acceptable limits of a control value must fall
 A. within ±1 standard deviation of the mean
 B. between 1 and 2 standard deviations of the mean
 C. within ±2 standard deviations of the mean
 D. within ±3 standard deviations of the mean

31. A trend change in QC data is
 A. a progressive change all in one direction away from the mean for at least 3 days
 B. an abrupt shift in the control values
 C. scattered variations from the mean
 D. a progressive change in various directions away from the mean for at least 1 week

32. A continuously increasing downward variation in a control sample in one direction from the mean can indicate
 A. deterioration of reagents used in the test
 B. deterioration of the control specimen
 C. deterioration of a component in an instrument
 D. all of the above

33. Which of the following statements is true of a gaussian curve?
 A. It represents the standard deviation.
 B. It represents the coefficient of variation.
 C. It represents variance of a population.
 D. It represents a normal bell-shaped distribution.

34. Two standard deviations (2 SD) from the mean in a normal distribution curve would include
 A. 99% of all values
 B. 95% of all values
 C. 75% of all values
 D. 68% of all values

BIBLIOGRAPHY

Clinical and Laboratory Standards Institute (CLSI). Clinical laboratory waste management: approved guideline, 2nd ed, Wayne, PA, GP5-A2, 2002.

Clinical Laboratory and Standards Institute (CLSI): Clinical laboratory safety: approved guideline, 2nd ed, Wayne, PA, GP17-A2, 2004.

CLSI Clinical and Laboratory Standards Institute (CLSI) Protection of laboratory workers from infectious disease transmitted by blood, body fluids, and tissue: tentative guideline, 3rd ed, Wayne, PA, M29-A3, 2005.

DeCraemer D. Postmortem viability of human immunodeficiency virus—implications for the tracking of anatomy, *N Engl J Med*, 33(19):1315, 1994.

Dunikoski LK. Take pride in SAFEty: A comprehensive lab-safety program, *Med Lab Observer*, 35(10):28–31, 2003.

Ferdinand M. OSHA's bloodborne pathogens standard: enforcement, compliance and comment, *J Healthc Mater Manag*, 11(8):12–14, 1993.

Gile TJ. Laboratory training: safety at any age, *Med Lab Observer*, 37(8):28, 2005.

Harty-Golder B. Prepare for occupational bloodborne pathogen exposure. *Med Lab Observer*, 41(4):40, 2009.

Kaplan LA, Pesce AJ. Clinical chemistry: theory, analysis, and correlation, 4th ed, St Louis, MO, Mosby, 2004.

Larson EL. APIC guideline for hand washing and hand antisepsis in health-care settings, *Am J Infect Control*, 23:251–269, 1995.

McPherson RA. Laboratory statistics, In: *Henry's Clinical Diagnosis and Management by Laboratory Methods*, 21st ed, Saunders, 2007, Chapter 9.

Rutala WA, Weber DJ, the Healthcare Infection Control Practices Advisory Committee (HICPAC). *Guideline for Disinfection and Sterilization in Healthcare Facilities*, 2008, www.cdc.gov (retrieved August 16, 2009).

Sebazcp S. Considerations for immunization programs, www.infectioncontroltoday.com/articles/0a1feat4.html (retrieved May 2005).

U.S. Department of Health and Human Services. Centers for Disease Control and Prevention. Preventing Occupational HIV Transmission to Healthcare Personnel, February 2002.

U.S. Department of Health and Human Services, Centers for Disease Control and Prevention (CDC). Hand Hygiene in Healthcare Settings, *MMWR*, 51(RR16):1–44, 10/25/ 2002.

U.S. Department of Health and Human Services: Centers for Disease Control and Prevention Guidelines for environmental infection control in health-care facilities, 2003.

U.S. Department of Health and Human Services, Centers for Disease Control and Prevention (CDC). Exposure to Blood: What Health-Care Workers Need to Know, Washington, DC, 2003.

U.S. Department of Health and Human Services Centers for Disease Control and Prevention, Hospital Infection Control Practices Advisory Committee (HICPAC): Guidelines for isolation precautions in hospitals, 1996.

U.S. Department of Health and Human Services Centers for Disease Control and Prevention, MMWR May 1, 2008/57 (Early Release);1–4 Measles — United States, January 1–April 25, 2008

Wians FH Jr. Clinical laboratory tests: which, why, and what do the results mean? *Lab Med*, 40(2):105–113, 2009.

Williams, D. Address deficiencies in bloodborne pathogens exposure management, Medical Laboratory Observer (MLO), vol 41, no. 7, July, 2009. 24, 26.

www.fedcenter.gov Summary of Regulations for Medical Waste, retrieved Oct. 20, 2009.

Yundt-Pacheco J, Parvin CA. The impact of QC frequency on patient results, *Med Lab Observ (MLO)*, 40(9):24–26, 2008.

CHAPTER 2

Principles of Blood Collection

Quality in phlebotomy

- Describe the importance of treating patients while using excellent interpersonal skills as well as the collection of a blood specimen.

Blood collection supplies and equipment

- Name the major potential type of error in specimen collection.
- Name the three anticoagulants most commonly used in hematology and briefly explain their modes of action.
- Compare the color codes of evacuated tubes with the additives contained in the tubes.
- Describe the equipment used for venous blood collection.
- Explain various considerations to meet specimen handling requirements.

Blood collection techniques

- Describe the proper technique for the collection of a venous blood specimen.
- Name and explain five specific venipuncture site selection situations.
- Name and describe the solutions to eight typical phlebotomy problems.
- Explain some techniques for obtaining blood from small or difficult veins.
- Describe special considerations for pediatric and geriatric patients in the collection of a blood specimen.

- Name the six categories of phlebotomy complications and describe the symptoms and treatment for each type of complication.
- Describe the proper technique for the collection of a capillary blood specimen.

Preparation of a blood smear

- Describe the procedure for preparing a push-wedge blood smear.
- List the characteristics of a good push-wedge blood smear.
- Explain the factors that influence the preparation of a high-quality push-wedge blood smear.
- Describe the coverslip method of blood film preparation.

Special collection procedures

- Name the appropriate sites for bone marrow aspiration in adults and children.
- Explain the proper technique for preparing bone marrow specimens.

Routine staining of peripheral blood films

- Explain the principle of the Wright stain.
- Cite the reasons Romanowsky-type stains produce too red or too blue an appearance on microscopic examination of blood cells.
- Describe the manual procedure of the Wright stain, including sources of error in the technique.

QUALITY IN PHLEBOTOMY

The role of the phlebotomist has never been more important. In the United States, it is estimated that more than 1 billion venipunctures are performed annually, and errors occurring within this process may cause serious harm to patients, either directly or indirectly. Critical areas include:

- Appropriateness of the test request
- Patient and sample identification
- Criteria for acceptance and rejection of specimens
- Communication and interpretation of results[1]

Quality Assessment

The accuracy of laboratory testing begins with the quality of the specimen received by the laboratory. This quality depends on how a specimen was collected, transported, and processed. The term quality assessment or the older term quality assurance is used to describe management of the treatment of the whole patient. As it applies to phlebotomy, quality assessment includes preparation of a patient for any specimens to be collected, collection of valid samples, and proper specimen transport.

Patient Care Partnership

The delivery of healthcare involves a partnership between patients and physicians and other healthcare professionals. When collecting blood specimens, it is important that the phlebotomist considers the rights of the patient at all times. The American Hospital Association has developed the Patient Care Partnership document, which replaces the former Patient's Bill of Rights. Patients themselves, or another person chosen by the patient, can exercise these patient rights. A proxy decision maker can act on the patient's behalf if the patient lacks decision-making ability, is legally incompetent, or is a minor.

The Phlebotomist as Laboratory Ambassador

A phlebotomist is frequently the only laboratory staff member that a patient sees. This means that the professional image of the laboratory is solely represented by the phlebotomist. The phlebotomist is expected to deliver unexcelled customer satisfaction. It is important to understand and know the patient's expectations, manage unrealistic expectations through patient education, and be diplomatic with customer complaints. If a patient is unhappy, sincerely apologize and listen to find out about the details of the problem. Be sure to understand and confirm the problem, act on the complaint, keep your promises, and follow-up on resolution of the problem.

PATIENTS WITH SPECIAL CONSIDERATIONS

Pediatric Patients

When working with children, it is important to be gentle and treat them with compassion, empathy, and kindness. Attempt to interact with the pediatric patient, realizing that both the patient and the parent (if present) may have anxiety about the procedure and be unfamiliar with the new settings. Acknowledge the parent and the child. Be friendly, courteous, and responsive. Allow enough time for the procedure.

Adolescent Patients

When obtaining a blood specimen from an adolescent, it is important to be relaxed and perceptive about any anxiety that he or she may have. General interaction techniques include allowing enough time for the procedure, establishing eye contact, and allowing the patient to maintain a sense of control.

Geriatric Patients

It is extremely important to treat geriatric patients with dignity and respect. Do not demean the patient. It is best to address the patient with a more formal title such as Mrs., Ms., or Mr. rather than by his or her first name.

Senior patients may enjoy a short conversation. Keep a flexible agenda so that enough time is allowed for the patient. Speak slowly because elderly patients are frequently hearing impaired. Allow enough time for questions. The elderly have the right of informed consent. Too many times this fact is lost in dealing with any patient, but it seems more prevalent in dealing with aging patients.

BLOOD COLLECTION SUPPLIES AND EQUIPMENT

To make the phlebotomy procedure easier for the technician, the following suggestions should be implemented:

- Prepare supplies and have them readily available.
- Review the minimally acceptable volume of blood for an individual assay or group of assays.
- Determine the minimally acceptable volume of blood for each type of collection tube.
- Develop a plan and an alternative plan each time a phlebotomy procedure is preformed.

A properly collected blood specimen is essential to a quality laboratory outcome. Strict adherence to the rules of specimen collection is critical to the accuracy of any test. Preanalytical (pre-examination) errors such as identification errors, either of the patient or of the specimen, are major potential sources of error.

For hematological studies, anticoagulated blood is the type of specimen most frequently used. When fresh whole blood is mixed with substances that prevent blood clotting, anticoagulants, the blood can be separated into plasma, a straw-colored fluid, and the cellular components: erythrocytes, leukocytes, and platelets (thrombocytes) (see Fig. 2.1). Whole blood that is allowed to clot normally produces the straw-colored fluid serum.

Anticoagulants

Three types of anticoagulants are commonly used in the hematology laboratory:

1. Dipotassium ethylenediaminetetraacetate (K_2 EDTA)
2. Sodium citrate
3. Heparin

Each of the anticoagulant types prevents the coagulation of whole blood in a specific manner. The proper proportion of anticoagulant to whole blood is important to avoid the introduction of errors into test results. The specific type of

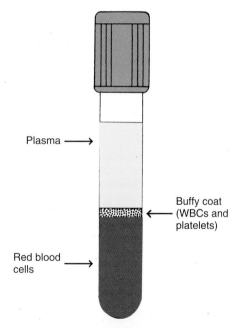

FIGURE 2.1 Separated whole blood specimen. (Reprinted with permission from McCall RE, Tankersley CM. *Phlebotomy Essentials*, 5th ed, Baltimore, MD: Lippincott Williams & Wilkins, 2012.)

anticoagulant needed for a procedure should be stated in the laboratory procedure manual.

Dipotassium EDTA

The salts of the chelating (calcium-binding) agent K_2 EDTA are recommended by the International Council for Standardization in Hematology (ICSH) and CLSI as the anticoagulant of choice for blood cell counting and sizing because they produce less shrinkage of RBCs and less of an increase in cell volume on standing. For hematology applications, EDTA is available in three forms, including dry additives (K_2 EDTA or Na2 EDTA) and a liquid additive (K_3 EDTA). EDTA prevents clotting by chelating calcium, an important cofactor in coagulation reactions. The amount of EDTA per milliliter of blood is essentially the same for all three forms of EDTA.

EDTA is spray-dried on the interior surface of evacuated plastic tubes. The proper ratio of EDTA to whole blood is important because some test results will be altered if the ratio is incorrect. Excessive EDTA produces shrinkage of erythrocytes, thus affecting tests such as the manually performed packed cell volume or microhematocrit.

EDTA is used in concentrations of 1.5 mg/1 mL of whole blood. The mode of action of this anticoagulant is that it removes ionized calcium (Ca^{2+}) through a process referred to as chelation. This process forms an insoluble calcium salt that prevents blood coagulation.

EDTA is the most commonly used anticoagulant in hematology for tests such as the complete blood cell count (CBC) or any of its component tests (hemoglobin, packed cell volume or microhematocrit, total leukocyte count, and leukocyte differential count) and platelet count.

Sodium Citrate

Sodium citrate removes calcium from the coagulation system by precipitating it into an unusable form. Sodium citrate is effective as an anticoagulant because of its mild calcium-chelating properties.

Sodium citrate in the concentration of a 3.2% solution has been adopted as the appropriate concentration by the ICSH and the International Society for Thrombosis and Hemostasis for coagulation studies. The College of American Pathologists (CAP) also recommends the use of 3.2% sodium citrate. The correct ratio of one part anticoagulant to nine parts of whole blood in blood collection tubes is critical. An excess of anticoagulant can alter the expected dilution of blood and produce errors in the results. The other available citrate concentration, 3.8% sodium citrate, is higher in concentration and its use may result in falsely lengthened clotting times with calcium-dependent coagulation tests (i.e., prothrombin time [PT] and activated prothrombin time [aPTT]), with slightly underfilled samples and with samples with high hematocrits.

Sodium citrate is used as an anticoagulant for aPTT and PT testing and for the Westergren erythrocyte sedimentation rate (ESR). Because of the dilution of anticoagulant to blood, sodium citrate is generally unacceptable for most other hematology tests.

Heparin

Heparin is used as an in vitro and in vivo anticoagulant. It acts as a substance that inactivates the blood-clotting factor thrombin. It anticoagulates blood by inhibiting thrombin and factor Xa.

Heparin is used to coat capillary blood collection tubes. Heparin is an inappropriate anticoagulant for many hematology tests, including Wright-stained blood smears.

Adverse Effects of Additives

■ *Alteration of constituents*: The additives chosen for specific determinations must not alter the blood components or affect the laboratory tests to be done. An additive may alter cellular constituents. An example would be the use of an older anticoagulant additive, oxalate, in hematology. Oxalate distorts the cell morphology; RBCs become crenated (shrunken), vacuoles appear in the granulocytes, and bizarre forms of lymphocytes and monocytes appear rapidly when oxalate is used as the anticoagulant. Another example is the use of heparin as an anticoagulant for blood to be used in the preparation of blood films that will be stained with Wright stain. Unless the blood films are stained within 2 hours, heparin gives a blue background with Wright stain.

■ *Incorrect amount of anticoagulant*: If too little additive is used, partial clotting of whole blood will occur. This interferes with cell counts. By comparison, if too much liquid anticoagulant is used, it dilutes the blood sample and thus interferes with certain quantitative measurements.

Safe Blood Collection

An increased emphasis on safety has led to new product development by various companies. Newer designs of this equipment are reducing the incidence of postphlebotomy needlesticks.

The standard needle for blood collection with a syringe or evacuated blood collection tubes is a 21-G needle. Butterfly needles are being used more frequently as the acuity of patients increases. The collecting needle is a double-pointed needle. The longer end is for insertion into the patient's vein, and the shorter end pierces the rubber stopper of the collection tube. Sterile needles that fit a standard holder are used. Various needle sizes are available. In addition to length, needles are classified by gauge size. The higher the gauge number, the smaller the inner diameter or bore. These double-pointed needles are either single-sample or multiple-sample types. The multiple-sample type has a short rubber sleeve on the short end of the needle, which punctures the rubber stopper. The rubber sleeve prevents blood from leaving the system when more than one evacuated tube is needed for testing.

The specially designed, single-use needle holder is used to secure the needle. It is no longer acceptable to wash and reuse this plastic needle holder device. The BD Vacutainer One-Use Holder is a clear plastic needle holder prominently marked with the words "Do Not Reuse" and "Single Use Only." Once a venipuncture is completed, the entire needle and holder assembly is disposed in a sharps container. The needle should not be removed from the holder. No change in venipuncture technique is required.

On October 15, 2003, the U.S. Occupational Safety and Health Administration (OSHA) posted a Safety and Health Information Bulletin (SHIB) (www.osha.gov) to clarify its position on reusing tube holders during blood collection procedures, a clarification of the OSHA Blood-borne Pathogens Standard [29 CFR 1910.1030 (d) (2) (vii) (A)]. The standard prohibits the removal of a contaminated needle from a medical device. Prohibition of needle removal from any device is addressed in the 1991 and 2001 standards, the OSHA compliance directive (CPL 2-2.69), and in a 2002 letter of interpretation. Blood collected into the syringe would then need to be transferred into a tube before disposing of the contaminated syringe. In these situations, a syringe with an engineered sharps injury-prevention feature and safe work practices should be used whenever possible. Transfer of the blood from the syringe to the test tube must be done using a needleless blood transfer device.

As with any OSHA rule or regulation, noncompliance may result in the issuance of citations by an OSHA compliance officer after the completion of a site inspection. It is the responsibility of each facility to evaluate their work practices, implement appropriate engineering controls, and institute all other applicable elements of exposure control to achieve compliance with current OSHA rules and regulations. The OSHA SHIB provides a step-by-step Evaluation Toolbox for a facility to follow (Box 2.1).

The BD Company (www.bd.com) is an example of a manufacturer who offers an extensive variety of safety-engineered, blood collection products. The BD blood collection products include:

1. BD Vacutainer Eclipse Blood Collection Needle
2. BD Blood Transfer Device
3. BD Vacutainer Safety-Lok Blood Collection Set
4. BD Vacutainer Plastic Tubes
5. BD Genie Safety Lancet
6. BD Quikheel Safety Lancet

BD Vacutainer Eclipse Blood Collection Needle

This is a safety-engineered multi-sample blood collection needle that reduces the possibility of needlestick injuries. It features a patented safety shield that allows for one-handed activation to cover the needle immediately upon withdrawal from the vein and confirms proper activation with an audible click.

BD Blood Transfer Device

The BD Blood Transfer Device is an easy-to-use, latex-free device used to facilitate safe and simple specimen transfers. It protects the health and safety of healthcare workers who draw and transfer bodily fluids by reducing the risk of spills and needlesticks.

BOX 2.1

OSHA Safety and Health Information Bulletin: Evaluation Toolbox

1. Employers must first evaluate, select, and use appropriate engineering controls (e.g., sharps with engineered sharps injury protection [SESIP]), which includes single-use blood tube holders with SESIP attached.
2. The use of engineering and work practice controls provides the highest degree of control in order to eliminate potential injuries after performing blood draws. Disposing of blood tube holders with contaminated needles attached after the activation of the safety feature affords the greatest hazard control.
3. In very rare situations, needle removal is acceptable.
   ■ If the employer can demonstrate that no feasible alternative to needle removal is available (e.g., inability to purchase single-use blood tube holders because of a supply shortage of these devices).
   ■ If the removal is necessary for a specific medical or dental procedure.
   ■ In these rare cases, the employer must ensure that the contaminated needle is protected by an SESIP before disposal. In addition, the employer must ensure that a proper sharps disposal container is located in the immediate area of sharps use and is easily accessible to employees. This information must be clearly detailed and documented in the employer's Exposure Control Plan.
4. If it is necessary to draw blood with a syringe, a syringe with engineered sharps injury protection must be used, in which the protected needle is removed using safe work practices, and transfer of blood from the syringe to the tube must be done using a needleless blood transfer device.

Reprinted from www.OSHA.gov (retrieved May 2005).

BD Vacutainer Safety-Lok Blood Collection Set

These are safety-engineered winged sets indicated for both infusion and blood collection. They feature a translucent, integrated protective shield that provides one-handed activation immediately after use to minimize the risk of needlestick injuries and that allows for clear visibility of blood flashback.

BD Vacutainer Plastic Tubes

BD Vacutainer Plastic Tubes offer a safe method for blood collection. Plastic tubes reduce the risk of tube breakage and specimen spillage. Disposal of plastic tubes is safe, simple, and in accordance with Environmental Protection Agency (EPA) guidelines.

BD Genie Safety Lancet

These are safety-engineered, single-use capillary blood sampling devices. They offer a permanently retractable blade or needle feature that minimizes the possibility of injury or reuse.

BD Quikheel Safety Lancet

The BD Quikheel Lancet is a safety-engineered product designed for heelsticks on infants and premature babies. It features a sweeping surgical blade that permanently retracts after creating an incision.

Laser Equipment

Laser technology is the first radical change in phlebotomy in more than 100 years. The risk of an accidental needlestick injury haunts every phlebotomist. Devices that can draw blood without the use of sharp objects received approval from the Food and Drug Administration (FDA) in 1997.

A laser device emits a pulse of light energy that lasts a minuscule fraction of a second. The laser concentrates on a very small portion of skin, literally vaporizing the tissue about 1 to 2 mm to the capillary bed. The device can draw a 100-μL blood sample, a sufficient amount for certain tests. The laser process is less painful and heals faster than when blood is drawn with traditional lancets. The patient feels a sensation similar to heat, as opposed to the prick of a sharp object.

Evacuated Blood Collection Tubes

Evacuated tubes are the most widely used system for collecting venous blood samples. This system (Fig. 2.2) consists of a collection needle, a nonreusable needle holder, and a tube containing enough vacuum to draw a specific amount of blood.

Evacuated tubes come in various (mL) sizes, including pediatric sizes, with color-coded stoppers. The stopper color denotes the type of anticoagulant or additive in the tube (Table 2.1). The use of plastic tubes is becoming more widespread. BD Vacutainer Systems recommends that all plastic blood collection tubes be stored at the proper temperature to ensure that they function properly. BD recommends that

storage temperature for all BD Vacutainer blood collection tubes not exceed 25°C or 77°F. If plastic tubes reach higher temperatures, a situation that can happen if the tubes are stored in a car trunk or on an automobile dashboard, the tubes may lose their vacuum or implode.

Evacuated tubes are intended for one-time use. Use of evacuated tubes with double-pointed collection needles makes possible a closed sterile system for specimen collection. This preserves the quality of the specimen during transport before testing and protects the patient from infection.

CLSI has set guidelines concerning the correct procedures for collecting and handling blood specimens. When collecting multiple tubes of blood, a specified "order of draw" of multiple evacuated tubes protocol (Table 2.2) needs to be followed to diminish the possibility of cross-contamination between tubes caused by the presence of different additives. Errors in the proper order of draw can produce an error in the laboratory test results.

Environmental Factors Associated with Evacuated Blood Collection Tubes

A variety of environment factors can impact the quality of evacuated tubes used to collect blood. These factors can then influence the published expiration dates of the evacuated tubes. Environmental factors affecting evacuated tubes include

■ Ambient temperature
■ Altitude
■ Humidity
■ Sunlight

Ambient Temperature

If evacuated tubes are stored at low temperature, the pressure of the gas inside the tube will decrease. This would lead to an increase in draw volume for the evacuated tube. Conversely, higher temperatures could cause reductions in draw volume.

Also, the stability of certain tube additives, for example, biochemicals or even gel, could be negatively impacted by increased temperature in evacuated tubes. Gel is a compound

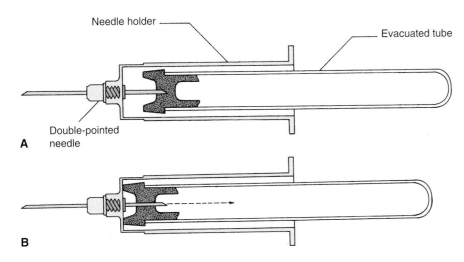

FIGURE 2.2 Evacuated tube system. **A:** The end of the doublepointed needle partially inserted into the rubber stopper. This is the preferred position of the needle before entering the blood vessel. **B:** After the opposite end of the needle successfully enters the blood vessel, the evacuated tube is gently pushed until the partially inserted needle fully pierces the rubber stopper. This allows the blood to enter the evacuated tube.

TABLE 2.1	Examples of Stopper Colors for Venous Blood Collection[a]
Color	**Anticoagulant**
Lavender	K_2 EDTA (spray-coated plastic tube) K_3 EDTA (liquid in glass tube)
Pink	K_2 EDTA (spray-coated plastic tube)
Green	Heparin
Light blue or clear (Hemogard closure)	Buffered Sodium citrate (0.105M in glass, 0.109M in plastic) Citrate, theophylline, adenosine, dipyridamole (CTAD)
White[b]	K_2 EDTA with gel
Red/light gray[c] or clear (Hemogard closure)	None (plastic)
Red	Silicone coated (glass) Clot activator, Silicone coated (plastic)

[a]See inside book cover for the comprehensive BD Vacutainer Venous Blood Collection Tube Guide.
[b]New tube for use in molecular diagnostic test methods.
[c]New red/light gray for use as a discard tube or secondary specimen tube.
Adapted with permission from BD Vacutainer Venous Blood Collection Tube Guide, 2010.

that could potentially degrade when exposed to high temperatures.

Altitude

In situations where blood is drawn at high altitudes (>5,000 ft), the draw volume may be affected. Because the ambient pressure at high altitude is lower than at sea level, the pressure of the residual gas inside the tube will reach this reduced ambient pressure during filling earlier than if the tube were drawn at sea level. The resulting draw volume will be lower.

Humidity

The impact of storage under different humidity conditions can impact only plastic evacuated tubes, due to the greater permeability of these materials to water vapor relative to glass. Conditions of very high humidity could lead to the migration of water vapor inside a tube that contains a moisture-sensitive material, such as a lyophilized additive. Conditions of very low humidity could hasten the escape of water vapor from a tube containing a wet additive. It is possible that such storage conditions could compromise the accuracy of clinical results.

Light

A special additive mixture for coagulation testing that is sensitive to light and found only in glass evacuated tubes is called CTAD (citric acid, theophylline, adenosine, and dipyridamole). The CTAD mixture minimizes platelet activation after blood collection. Normally, this additive has a slightly yellow appearance that becomes clear when no longer viable. These tubes are generally packaged in small quantities to minimize exposure to light.

Expiration Dates of Evacuated Tubes

Expiration dates are determined through shelf-life testing performed under known environmental conditions. Shelf life of an evacuated tube is defined by the stability of the additive, as well as vacuum retention. Most evacuated tubes on the market have at least a 12-month shelf life. It is important that tubes be stored under recommended conditions.

The expiration dates of glass tubes are generally limited by the shelf life of the additives because vacuum and water vapor losses are minimal over time. Exposure to irradiation during sterilization of tubes and to moisture or light during the shelf life of the product can limit the stability of biochemical additives. The expiration dates of evacuated plastic tubes are often also limited by the same factors that affect glass tubes. However, evacuated plastic tubes do sustain a measurable loss of vacuum over time, and some evacuated plastic blood collection tubes may have their expiration dates determined by their ability to assure a known draw volume.

It is important to understand that evacuated blood collection tubes are not completely evacuated. There is a small amount of gas (air) still residing in the tube, at low pressure. The higher the pressure of the gas inside the tube on the date of manufacture, the lower the intended draw volume will be for a tube of a given size. The draw volume specified for a given tube is achieved by manufacturing the tube at a designated evacuation pressure.

The dynamics of blood collection inside the tube are based on the ideal gas law: $PV = nRT$. In the equation, P is the pressure inside the tube, V is the volume that the gas occupies, n is the number of moles of gas inside the tube, R is the

TABLE 2.2	Order of Draw of Multiple Evacuated Tubes Collections[a]	
Order	**Closure Color Mix by Inverting**	**Type of Tube**
1	Yellow	Blood cultures-SPS—aerobic and anaerobic 8–10×
2	Light blue	Citrate tube[b] 3–4×
3	Gold or red/gray	BD Vacutainer SST gel separator Tube 5×
	Red	Serum tube (plastic) 5×
	Red	Serum tube (glass)
	Orange	BD vacutainer rapid serum tube (RST) 5–6×
4.	Light green or	BC vacutainer PST
	Green/gray	Gel separator tube with heparin 8–10×
	Green	Heparin 8–10×
5	Lavender	EDTA 8–10×
6	White	BD vacutainer PPT separator tube K₂ EDTA with gel 8–10×
7	Gray	Fluoride (glucose) Tube 8–10×

[a]The order of draw has been revised to reflect the increased use of plastic evacuated collection tubes. Plastic serum tubes containing a clot activator may cause interference in coagulation testing. Some facilities may continue using glass serum tubes without a clot activator as a waste tube before collecting special coagulation assays. reflects change in CLSI recommended Order of Draw (H3-A5, Vol 23, No 32, 8.10.2)

[b]If a winged blood collection set for venipuncture and a coagulation (citrate) tube is the first specimen tube to be drawn, a discard tube should be drawn first. To ensure a proper blood to citrate ratio, use the discard tube to fill the air space with blood. The discard tube does not need to be completely filled.

Reprinted with permission from Becton, Dickinson and Company, 2010.

universal gas constant, and T is the temperature inside the tube.

According to the equation, if the moles of gas and the temperature do not change, the product of pressure and volume is a constant. When blood starts filling the tube, the residual gas inside is confined into a decreasing volume, causing the pressure of the gas to increase. When the pressure of this gas reaches ambient pressure, the collection process is completed for that tube. The specially designed, single-use needle holder is used to secure the needle. It is no longer acceptable to wash and reuse this plastic needle holder device.

Anticoagulants and Additives in Evacuated Blood Tubes

Although there are evacuated tubes for venous blood collection without additives are used to yield serum (or used as discard tubes), all other evacuated tubes contain some type of anticoagulant or additive (see inside book cover). The additives range from those that promote faster clotting of the blood to those that preserve or stabilize certain analytes or cells. The inclusion of additives at the proper concentration in evacuated tubes greatly enhances the accuracy and consistency of test results and facilitates faster turnaround times in the laboratory.

Anticoagulants and additives may exist as either dry or liquid ("wet") in evacuated tubes depending on whether the tube is glass or plastic and depending on the stability of the solution. The CLSI and ISO Standards define the concentrations of these additives dispensed into tubes per milliliter of blood.

Capillary Blood

The order of draw for collection of capillary blood in BD Microtainer tubes differs from the collection of venous blood (Table 2.3). Several types of microcollection tubes are available for use in capillary blood collection.

Microhematocrit capillary tube collection is another method of blood collection. This small tube may be heparinized or plain. For special tests, a 100 or 200 lambda micropipette may be used. The BD Vacutainer plastic-clad

TABLE	2.3	**Bd Microtaine Tubes with BD Microgard Closure Order of Draw**		

Order	Closure Color	Additive	Mix by Inverting
1	Lavender	K_2 EDTA	10×
2	Green	Lithium heparin	10×
3	Mint green	Lithium heparin and gel	10×
4	Gray	NaFl/Na_2 EDTA	10×
5	Gold	Clot activator and gel	5×
6	Red	None	0×

Reprinted with permission from Becton, Dickinson and Company, LabNotes, Vol. 20, No. 1, 2009, p.7.

microhematocrit tubes are safety-engineered to help protect healthcare workers from accidental injury during some of the most common medical procedures. Each BD plastic-coated microhematocrit tube is encased in a film of mylar so thin that it does not interfere with the accuracy for the user's visual inspection of the sample. However, the mylar layer has a very high tensile strength along with remarkable flexibility that prevents it from breaking even if the underlying glass is cracked or shattered in the course of the work. The mylar film will keep the pieces intact and safely contained.

The order of draw with capillary specimens varies from other methods of collection (Table 2.4).

Specimen Handling Requirements

The proper handling of blood and body fluids is critical to the accuracy of laboratory test results. In addition, the safety of all individuals who come in contact with specimens must be guaranteed. If a blood specimen is to be transported, the shipping container must meet OSHA requirements for shipping clinical specimens (OSHA Fed. Reg. 29, CAR 1910.1030). Shipping containers must meet the packaging requirements of major couriers and Department of Transportation hazardous materials regulations. Approved reclosable plastic bags for handling biohazard specimens and amber bags for specimens for analysis of light-sensitive drugs are available. These bags must meet the CLSI M29-A3 specimen handling guidelines (M28 A3 Protection of Laboratory Workers from Infectious Disease Transmitted by Blood, Body Fluids and Tissue).

Approved bags such as LabGuard Reclosable Bags have bright orange and black graphics that clearly identify bags as holding hazardous materials. Some products have an additional marking area that allows phlebotomists to identify contents that must be kept frozen, refrigerated, or at room temperature.

Maintaining specimens at the correct preanalytical (preexamination) temperature is extremely important. Products such as the Insul-Tote (Palco Labs) are convenient for specimen transport from the field to the clinical laboratory. This particular product has a reusable cold gel pack that keeps temperatures below 70°F for 8 hours even if the exterior temperature is above 100°F. Many laboratory courier services use everyday household coolers.

Blood specimen collection and processing should conform with the current checklist requirements adopted by the CAP (http://www.cap.org). Errors in specimen collection and handling, preanalytical (preexamination) errors, are a significant cause of erroneous patient results.

TABLE	2.4	**Order of Draw for Capillary Specimens**[a]

Order	
1	Blood gases
2	EDTA tubes
3	Other additive minicontainers
4	Serum

[a]Order of draw for capillary blood collection is different from blood specimens drawn by venipuncture.
Adapted with permission from Becton, Dickinson and Company, Lab Notes, Vol. 20, No. 1, 2009, p. 2.
Note: If multiple specimens are collected by heel or fingerstick puncture (capillary blood collection), anticoagulant tubes must be collected first to avoid the formation of tiny clots due to prolonged collection time. Blood gases should be collected first, if the phlebotomy team is responsible for collection of these specimens.

BLOOD COLLECTION TECHNIQUES

The two sources of blood for examination in the hematology laboratory are venous blood and capillary blood. Although arterial blood may be needed to perform procedures such as blood gas analysis, this procedure is not usually performed in the hematology laboratory. To obtain quality specimens for assay, strict adherence to proper specimen collection is necessary.

GENERAL PROTOCOL

1. Phlebotomists should pleasantly introduce themselves to the patient and clearly explain the procedure that is to be performed. It is always a friendly courtesy to speak a few words in a patient's native language, if English is not his or her first language. Ethnic populations vary geographically but many patients are now Spanish speaking. Appendix C lists some English-Spanish medical phrases for the phlebotomist.
2. Patient identification is the critical first step in blood collection. In the 2007 Laboratory Services National Patient Safety Goals from the Joint Commission, goal 1 is accuracy in patient identification. Patient misidentification errors are potentially associated with the worst clinical outcomes because of the possibility of misdiagnosis and mishandled therapy.

   It is necessary both to ask the patient's name and to check the identification band that is physically attached to the patient. Wristbands with unique barcoded patient identifiers have great potential for reducing patient misidentification. Unfortunately, wristband errors do occur. A study conducted by the CAP identified six major types of wristband errors:
   - Absent or wrong wristband
   - Wearing of more than one wristband
   - Partially missing information on the wristband
   - Erroneous information on the wristband
   - Illegible information on the wristband

   When the patient is unable to give his or her name, or when identification is attached to the bed or is missing, nursing personnel should be asked to identify the patient physically. Any variations in protocol should be noted on the test requisition. The CAP recommends that phlebotomists should refuse to collect blood from a patient when a wristband error is detected.
3. Test requisitions should be checked and the appropriate evacuate tubes assembled. All specimens should be properly labeled immediately after the specimen is drawn. Prelabeling is unacceptable.
4. The patient's name, unique identification number and room number or clinic, and date and time of collection are usually found on the label. In some cases, labels must include the time of collection of the specimen and the type of specimen. A properly completed request form should accompany all.

Capillary blood collection is performed with a sterile, disposable lancet. These lancets are individually wrapped and should be properly discarded in a puncture-proof container after a single use.

VENOUS BLOOD COLLECTION (PHLEBOTOMY)

Supplies and Equipment

1. Test requisition
2. Tourniquet and disposable gloves
3. Alcohol (70%) and gauze square or alcohol wipes
4. Sterile disposable needles (double-pointed or syringe type)
5. Evacuated blood tubes (appropriate to the test ordered) and a needle holder or a syringe (in special cases)
6. Any special equipment such as a stopwatch or warm water—refer to equipment required for special procedures
7. Spirits of ammonia breakable capsule (emergency use only)
8. Adhesive plastic strips or spots

Initiation of the Procedure

1. Identify the patient.
2. Assemble all necessary equipment at the patient's bedside.
3. Put on gloves.
4. If a needle and syringe are to be used, firmly secure the hub of the needle with its shield in place on the syringe. If an evacuated tube is to be used, screw the short end of the needle on the needle holder. The plastic shield is to remain on the needle until immediately before the venipuncture. The evacuated tube is placed into the holder and gently pushed until the top of the stopper reaches the guideline on the holder. Note: Do not push the tube all the way into the holder, or a loss of vacuum will result.

Selection of an Appropriate Site

Note: Venous blood should not be drawn near an intravenous (IV) infusion. It is preferable to draw the sample from the opposite arm, if possible, or from below the infusion site. If possible, the IV infusion should be shut off for 2 to 3 minutes before the sample is drawn. Whether the sample was drawn from below an IV site and the type of solution being administered should be noted on the test requisition. Obtaining a blood specimen from an IV line should be avoided because it increases the risk of mixing the fluid with the blood sample and producing incorrect test results.

1. Visually inspect both arms. Choose the arm that has not been repeatedly used for venipunctures and one that is free of bruises, abrasions, and sites of infection. In the arm, three veins are commonly used for venipuncture: the cephalic, basilic, and median cubital (Fig. 2.3).
2. Applying the tourniquet. Two general types of tourniquets are available. One type is a flat or rounded rubber tube,

(continued)

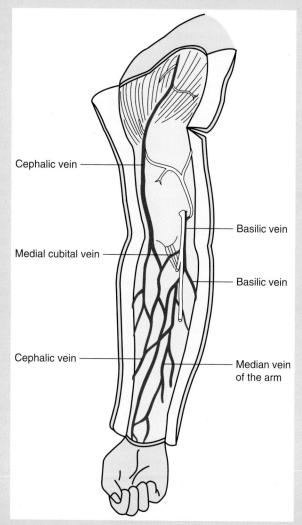

FIGURE 2.3 Anatomy of the veins of the arm. In the arm, three veins can be used for venipuncture: the cephalic, basilic, and median cubital.

and the other has Velcro ends for simple adjustment to the arm.

A. If a rubber tourniquet is used, slide the tourniquet under the arm a few inches above the expected venipuncture site. Evenly adjust both ends of the tourniquet (Fig. 2.4A).

B. Grasp both ends of the tourniquet a few inches above the patient's arm. Pull up on the ends to create tension in the tourniquet. Cross the right side of the tourniquet over the left side. With the index finger of the right hand, create a small loop in the right side of the tourniquet while continuing to hold tension in the tourniquet (Fig. 2.4B).

C. Slip this small loop under the left side of the tourniquet. The resulting application will allow for easy removal of the tourniquet with one hand, after the needle has been inserted into the vein (Fig. 2.4C). Note: Prolonged tourniquet application can elevate certain blood chemistry analytes. These are albumin, aspartate aminotransferase (AST), calcium, cholesterol, iron, lipids, total bilirubin, and total protein.

3. Ask the patient to make a fist (sometimes a roll of gauze is placed in the patient's hand). This usually makes the veins more prominent. With the index finger, palpate (feel) for an appropriate vein (Fig. 2.4D). Palpation is important for identifying the vein, which has a resilient feeling compared with the surrounding tissues. Large veins are not always a good choice because they have a tendency to roll as you attempt the venipuncture. Superficial and small veins should also be avoided. The ideal site is generally near or slightly below the bend in the arm. If no appropriate veins are found in one arm, examine the other arm by applying the tourniquet and palpating the arm. Do not leave the tourniquet on for more than 2 minutes. Veins in other areas such as the wrist, hands, and feet can be used as venipuncture sites; however, only experienced phlebotomists should use them.

Special Site Selection Situations

Five specific situations can create the potential for a difficult venipuncture or are potential sources of preanalytical (preexamination) error. These situations are

1. Edema of the extremities
2. IV lines
3. Scarring or burn patients
4. Dialysis patients
5. Postmastectomy patients

Edema

Edema is the abnormal accumulation of fluid in the intracellular spaces of the tissue. Venipuncture should not be performed in edematous areas because the extra fluid can make it difficult to palpate the veins, and the specimen may be contaminated with the fluid and produce erroneous test results.

IV Lines

Patients with fluid running in IV lines in their arms pose a common problem to phlebotomists. A limb with an IV running should not be used for venipuncture because of contamination to the specimen. The patient's other arm or an alternate site should be selected. If no alternate site can be found, the IV should be turned off by the physician and blood can be drawn from below the infusion site after a few minutes. The contents of the IV fluid should be documented on the requisition. After completing the venipuncture, the appropriate person should be notified to restart the infusion.

(continued)

BLOOD COLLECTION TECHNIQUES *(continued)*

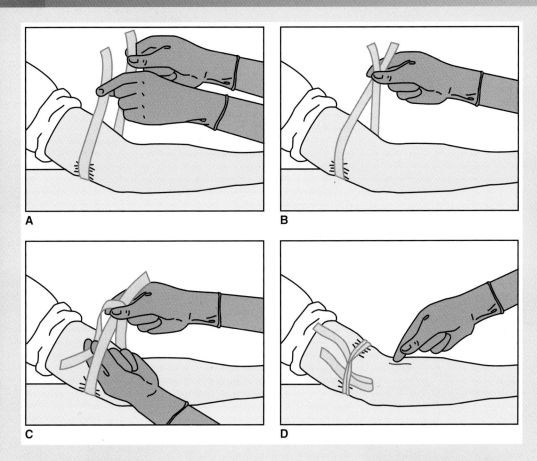

FIGURE 2.4 Selection of appropriate venipuncture site. **A:** Adjusting the tourniquet. Adjust both ends of the tourniquet evenly. **B, C:** Applying the tourniquet. Place tension on the tourniquet, cross one side over the other, and slip a small loop under one side of the tourniquet. A properly applied tourniquet can be removed with one hand by simply pulling on one end of it. **D:** Palpating the site. The index finger is used to feel for a suitable vein. This is the ideal site for venipuncture, usually near or slightly below the bend in the arm.

Scarring or Burn Patients

Veins are very difficult to palpate in areas where there is extensive scarring or burns. Burn areas also are more susceptible to infection because the protective barrier (the epidermis) has been disrupted. Venipunctures performed at these sites are unusually painful for the patient. Alternate sites or capillary blood collection should be used.

Dialysis Patients

Dialysis patients pose special problems when it comes to blood collection, frequency of testing and limited vein access. Blood should never be drawn from a vein in an arm with a cannula (temporary dialysis access device) or fistula (a permanent surgical fusion of a vein and an artery).

A trained staff member can draw blood from a cannula. Blood should never be drawn from a fistula or from a vein in an arm with a fistula. The preferred venipuncture site is a hand vein or a vein away from the fistula on the underside of the arm. In this case, a tourniquet may be used below the fistula but should be released as soon as the vein has been located.

In addition, special precautions should be taken to ensure that the dialysis patient does not bleed from the venipuncture site because most of these patients are medicated with heparin.

Postmastectomy Patients

If a mastectomy patient has had lymph nodes adjacent to the breast removed, lymphostasis (a lack of flow of lymphatic fluids in the affected area) results. Specimens drawn from the affected side of the body may not be representative. In addition, the patient is much more susceptible to infections. Therefore, venipuncture should not be performed on the same side as the mastectomy.

Preparation of the Venipuncture Site

1. After an appropriate site has been chosen, release the tourniquet.
2. Using a cotton ball saturated with 70% alcohol or an alcohol pad saturated with 70% alcohol, cleanse the skin in the area of the venipuncture site. Using a circular motion, clean the area from the center and move outward. Do not go back over an area once it has been cleansed.
3. Allow the site to dry.

Performing the Venipuncture (Fig. 2.5)

Note: It is preferable to avoid touching the cleansed venipuncture site. In unusual situations, it may be allowable to touch the area with an alcohol-wiped finger to reestablish the location of the vein.

(continued)

BLOOD COLLECTION TECHNIQUES *(continued)*

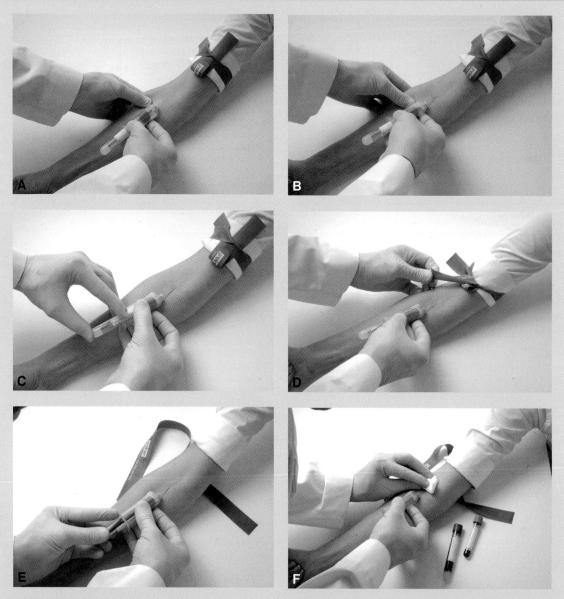

FIGURE 2.5 Phlebotomy procedure. After the site is prepared with an alcohol sterile wipe and gauze square, (**A**) anchor the skin from below by pulling the skin tight with the thumb of your free hand. **B**: The needle is gently inserted into the patient's vein. **C**: Apply the first tube. **D**: Release tourniquet. **E**: Remove and exchange tubes. **F**: After the appropriate evacuated tubes are filled, the procedure is terminated by covering the venipuncture site with a square of sterile gauze and applying pressure. A sterile adhesive bandage is then placed on the site. (Reprinted with permission from Ernst DJ. *Applied Phlebotomy*, Baltimore, MD: Lippincott Williams & Wilkins, 2005.)

1. Use one hand to hold the evacuated tube assembly or syringe. Use one or more fingers of the other hand to secure the skin area of the forearm below the intended venipuncture site. This will tighten the skin and secure the vein. Position the patient's arm in a slightly downward position.

2. Hold the needle with attached syringe or evacuated tube about 1 to 2 inches below and in a straight line with the intended venipuncture site. Position the blood draw-ing unit at an angle of about 20°. The bevel of the needle should be upward.

3. Gently insert the needle through the skin and into the vein. This insertion motion should be smooth. If an evacuated tube is used, one hand should steady the needle holder unit while the other hand pushes the tube to the end of the plastic holder. It is important to hold the needle still during the collection process to avoid interrupting the flow of blood.

(continued)

BLOOD COLLECTION TECHNIQUES *(continued)*

Multiple samples can be drawn by inserting each additional tube as soon as the tube attached to the needle holder has filled. The CLSI standards for the order of drawing multiple evacuated tubes areTo decrease the chance of bacterial contamination, blood cultures are always collected first. If a syringe is used, one hand should steady the barrel of the syringe while the other hand slowly pulls the plunger backward.

Termination of the Procedure

1. The tourniquet may be released as soon as the blood begins to flow into the evacuated tube or syringe or immediately before the final amount of blood is drawn.
2. Ask the patient to open the hand.
3. After the desired amount of blood has been drawn, place a gauze pad over the venipuncture site.
4. Withdraw the blood collecting unit with one hand and immediately press down on the gauze pad with the other hand (Fig. 2.5E).
5. If possible, have the patient elevate the entire arm and press on the gauze pad with the opposite hand. If the patient is unable to do this, apply pressure until bleeding ceases.
6. Place a nonallergenic adhesive spot or strip over the venipuncture site. Note: Failure to apply sufficient pressure to the venipuncture site could result in a hematoma (a collection of blood under the skin that produces a bruise).
7. Mix tubes with anticoagulant by inverting the tubes several times. If a syringe was used, carefully remove the needle before dispensing the blood into a test tube. Blood should never be forced back through the needle, and the syringe plunger should be slowly depressed. Discard the used needle into an appropriate safety container.
8. Label all test tubes as required by the laboratory.
9. Clean up supplies from the work area, remove gloves, and wash hands. Note: If the patient is an outpatient, wait a few minutes after the venipuncture is complete, and check to be sure that the patient does not feel dizzy or nauseated before discharge. Discard all contaminated supplies in a biohazard disposal bag.

Phlebotomy Problems

Occasionally, a venipuncture is unsuccessful. Do not attempt to perform the venipuncture more than two times. If two attempts are unsuccessful, notify the hematology supervisor. Problems encountered in phlebotomy can include the following:

1. Refusal by the patient to have blood drawn. The response to this problem is to politely excuse yourself from the patient's room, note the refusal on the requisition, and notify the hematology supervisor.
2. Difficulty in obtaining a specimen because the bore of the needle is against the wall of the vein. Slightly pulling back on the needle may solve this problem.

3. Movement of the vein. To guard against this problem, always have firm pressure on the arm below the intended venipuncture site. The needle can be moved to reach the vein, but excessive probing in the tissues must be avoided. Care must be exercised in moving the needle because a hematoma can form if both sides of the vessel wall are pierced.
4. An inadequate amount of blood in an evacuated tube. A "short draw," or lack of complete filling of an anticoagulated tube, can produce errors in test results. An excessive amount of EDTA will produce shrinkage of erythrocytes, and an insufficient amount of blood in a sodium citrate tube will introduce a dilutional problem if the specimen is tested for coagulation studies.
5. Improper anticoagulant. In most cases, anticoagulants cannot be substituted in a test. For example, blood smears cannot be prepared from a heparinized blood sample because with Wright stain the erythrocytes will stain too blue.
6. Sudden movement by the patient or phlebotomist that causes the needle to come out of the arm prematurely. Always anticipate this possibility. Quick action is needed! Immediately remove the tourniquet, place a gauze pad on the venipuncture site, and apply pressure until bleeding has stopped to prevent the formation of a hematoma. It is a good practice to have easy access to gauze pads whenever a venipuncture is being performed.
7. Blood clot formation in anticoagulated tubes. In the phlebotomy procedure, red-top (plain) evacuated tubes should be drawn first. Promptly after termination of the venipuncture procedure, any tubes containing an anticoagulant should be gently inverted several times to mix the specimen.
8. Fainting or illness subsequent to venipuncture. The first aid procedures of the laboratory should be practiced in this event. It is very important to prevent injury to the patient because of fainting or dizziness.

Ten Tips for Locating and Drawing from Difficult or Small Veins

It is not uncommon to have difficulty drawing a venous blood specimen. Tips for locating or drawing blood from difficult or small veins are

1. Adjust the position of the arm
2. Use a smaller gauge needle
3. Use a small syringe
4. Use a butterfly needle and multiple small syringes
5. Tighten the tourniquet
6. Loosen the tourniquet
7. Apply hot packs to the arm
8. Use a second tourniquet below the site
9. Use a hand or wrist vein or veins on the underside of the arm
10. Use a transilluminator device to identify the location of a vein

(continued)

BLOOD COLLECTION TECHNIQUES *(continued)*

Special Considerations for Pediatric and Geriatric Patients

Pediatric Patients

Phlebotomists should consider the limitations of their skills and self-confidence and consult with their immediate supervisor before attempting a difficult phlebotomy.

Procedure Box 2.1 lists some general tips in performing pediatric phlebotomy. Premature infants do not tolerate prolonged agitation or stimulation, so procedures should be done swiftly and efficiently. The amount of blood needed should be considered before selecting the site. It is also very important to examine all possible sites for venipuncture, if an obvious vein is not initially determined. Under no circumstances should a venipuncture be attempted on a child if the phlebotomist is uncertain of the vein or the feasibility of collecting all of the ordered tests in one needlestick.

Phlebotomists should always inspect the areas around a blood collection site for redness or bruising before collecting a sample. Also, excessive use of any area should be avoided and reported to the child's nurse. Warming a skin puncture site for a couple minutes increases the blood flow up to eight times and will preclude excessive squeezing and subsequent injury. Phlebotomists should report any difference in the condition of a site if immediately noted after blood collection.

Specimens from Children Younger than Age 1

Guidelines should be developed and revised as needed to reflect common practice for children younger than 1 year of age. Competency checklists should separate when a heelstick rather than venous blood can be used for an assay.

Some important points for phlebotomists who draw specimens from children younger than 1 year of age include:

1. Venipunctures should not be performed on children younger than 6 months of age unless there are specific testing requirements necessitating a venipuncture.

PROCEDURE Box 2.1
General Tips for Pediatric Phlebotomy

■ Work quickly on premature infants.
■ Warm blood collection site to increase the flow of blood.
■ Check potential blood collection sites for redness or bruising.
■ Do not attempt venipuncture unless obtaining enough blood collection for all ordered tests in one attempt is certain.
■ Report any changes in the condition of the site immediately after venipuncture.

---

2. Venipunctures on infants between 6 and 12 months of age should be done if the child is of at least average weight for age and the quantity of blood and/or the assays require a venipuncture.
3. Paternity testing on newborns, infants, and children requires from 1 to 3 mL of whole blood. Limiting the number of staff who are trained to perform paternity testing will assure proper procedure for "chain of custody."
4. Lead levels can be drawn via capillary puncture but preferably are obtained by venipuncture because of the potential for contamination and the subsequent need for recollection and/or confirmation.
5. If an extensive number of tests are ordered on a small child, an experienced phlebotomist should perform the procedure.

Geriatric Patients

Aging produces physiological conditions that accentuate naturally occurring changes in the skin and subcutaneously (e.g., slower healing time and more chance of infection). Because of increased susceptibility, venipuncture site preparation becomes even more important in the elderly than in other patients. In addition, arteries and veins change drastically with age. Blood vessels become less elastic and more fragile with aging and can be easily injured during a venipuncture attempt.

There are some important steps to consider when performing venipuncture on an elderly person. These include

1. Carefully identify the patient. Elderly patients may be confused and disoriented.
2. Take your time locating the "perfect" spot for the venipuncture. Look at both arms, the wrists, hands, and complete forearms.
3. Never slap the arm to dilate the vein because this could cause the patient to bruise.
4. Warm up the skin if the patient's limb feels cold and clammy.
5. Be very cautious when using tourniquets or bandages because the skin is fragile. Try placing the tourniquet over clothing, which will be more comfortable for the patient.
6. Remove the tourniquet just before inserting the needle to reduce the risk of rupturing the vein and causing a hematoma.
7. Consider using a smaller gauge needle (e.g., butterfly needles) to reduce trauma to the vein.
8. Use smaller pediatric vacuum tubes to reduce the vacuum draw back, if the vein is fragile and small.
9. Use one quick motion when inserting the needle; it is more effective and less painful.
10. Never probe for a vein.

(continued)

BLOOD COLLECTION TECHNIQUES *(continued)*

11. Veins must be well anchored by holding the skin alongside the vein instead of directly over the vein before a venipuncture attempt is made. This will prevent obstructing the vein and causing it to collapse.
12. Ask for assistance from another person to prevent a hematoma, if you anticipate that the patient will not hold still during the venipuncture or will not be able to apply pressure to the site after the procedure.
13. Pay special attention to the fragility of the skin. Bandages or tape can cause the skin to become raw and develop seeping areas. Elastic bandages will hold the gauze in place and not adhere to the skin.

Phlebotomy Complications

Patients can experience complications resulting from a phlebotomy procedure. These complications can be divided into six major categories: vascular (the most common), infection, cardiovascular, anemia, neurological, and dermatological.

Vascular Complications

Bleeding from the site of the venipuncture and hematoma formation are the most common vascular complications. The reasons for these mishaps include medications and existing medical conditions (e.g., coagulation disorders produced by a genetic defect or cancer). Bruises do not usually affect patient satisfaction. Uncommon vascular complications that are not usually related to the technique include pseudoaneurysm, thrombosis, reflex arteriospasm, and arteriovenous fistula formation (Procedure Table 2.1).

Infections

The second most common complication of venipuncture is infection. The most common infectious complications are cellulitis (inflammation of tissue) and phlebitis (inflammation of vessel or infection of vessel). Other infectious complications include sepsis (infection of the blood), septic arthritis (infection of the joint space), and osteomyelitis (infection of the bone). Infection of the joint space usually occurs in children in the femoral joint after an arterial puncture. Osteomyelitis is usually associated with capillary puncture because most skin preparation regimens remove the majority of microorganisms but not all of them. Deep puncturing of the skin allows microorganisms to enter and infect the deep tissues and bone.

Cardiovascular Complications

Cardiovascular complications include orthostatic hypotension, syncope, shock, and cardiac arrest.

Orthostatic hypotension results from changing from a sitting to a standing position or as the result of certain medica-

PROCEDURE Table 2.1
Vascular Complications of Phlebotomy

CONDITION	DESCRIPTION
Pseudoaneurysm	Fibrous capsule around encapsulated blood caused by a break in the blood vessel
Thrombosis	The patient usually has a coagulation disorder. Thrombosis in a vein produces edema and swelling. If thrombosis is in an arterial blood vessel, a decreased oxygen supply caused by impaired circulation can occur beyond the thrombosis.
Reflex arteriospasm	Occurs when a needle sticks an artery Prevents blood from moving through the vessel
Arteriovenous fistula	Abnormal connection between a vein and an artery can occur after repeated venipuncture.

tions. The lack of a compensatory blood pressure response produces hypotension that in turn produces syncope.

Syncope can be manifested as temporary loss of consciousness, fainting, light-headedness, dizziness, sweating, or nausea. The causes of syncope include vasovagal response, arrhythmia, orthostatic hypotension, volume depletion, shock, and cardiac arrest. A vasovagal response is a neurological response that can be triggered by emotion, stress, prolonged standing, warm temperature, fasting, pregnancy, or dehydration. The manifestations of this response are increased autonomic response, decreased heart rate and vasodilation, increased hypotension, and syncope. Treatment for syncope consists of having the patient lie down, loosening tight clothing, elevating the legs, ruling out chest pain and shortness of breath, and waiting for pressure and pulse to normalize.

Shock is manifested by the presence of cool, clammy, mottled skin; a weak and rapid pulse; and hypotension. The immediate treatment is to elevate the legs, use a warming blanket, and call a code.

Cardiac arrest manifests itself as chest pain, shortness of breath, arm or shoulder pain, nausea, and sweating. Treatment consists of immediately calling a code and beginning cardiopulmonary resuscitation (CPR) efforts.

(continued)

BLOOD COLLECTION TECHNIQUES *(continued)*

Anemia

Iatrogenic anemia is also known as nosocomial anemia, physician-induced anemia, or anemia resulting from blood loss for testing. Pediatric patients and adults in intensive care units and transplant patients are the most likely candidates to develop this iron-deficiency anemia. The medical consequences of iatrogenic anemia are fatigue, shortness of breath, and impaired performance of physical work. In severe cases, the treatment is blood transfusion.

Neurological Complications

Postphlebotomy patients can exhibit some neurological complications. These include diaphoresis, seizure, pain, and nerve damage. A physician should be consulted immediately.

Dermatological Complications

The most common dermatological consequence of phlebotomy is an allergic reaction to iodine in the case of blood donors. Other dermatological complications include necrosis, basal cell carcinoma (one case described), and scarring.

CAPILLARY BLOOD COLLECTION

Supplies and Equipment

1. Alcohol (70%) and gauze squares or alcohol wipes
2. Disposable gloves and sterile small gauze squares
3. Sterile disposable blood lancets
4. Equipment specific to the test ordered, such as glass slides for blood smears, micropipette and diluent for CBCs, or microhematocrit capillary tubes

Selection of an Appropriate Site

1. The fingertip (usually of the third or fourth finger), heel, and big toe are appropriate sites for the collection of small quantities of blood. The earlobe may be used as a site of last resort in adults. Do not puncture the skin through previous sites, which may be infected.

The plantar surface (sole) of the heel or big toe is an appropriate site in infants (Fig. 2.6A) or in special cases such as burn victims. Note: The ideal site in infants is the medial or lateral plantar surface of the heel, with a puncture no deeper than 2.0 mm beneath the plantar heel-skin surface and no more than half this distance at the posterior curve of the heel. CLSI recommendations are not to use fingers of infants. The back of the heel should never be used because of the danger of injuring the heel bone. The arch should never be punctured because tendons, cartilage, and nerves may be injured in this area.

2. The site of blood collection must be warm to ensure the free flow of blood; otherwise, the blood sample will not be truly representative of the blood in the vascular system. If necessary, massage the finger several times or place a warm cloth on the area for a few minutes to increase blood circulation to the site.

3. Osteomyelitis (infection of bone) is a potential complication in pediatric patients. This complication can be prevented by using good technique. It is important to avoid pushing too hard or too deeply with the lancet. Sites for the development of osteomyelitis are the heel, toes, or fingers. Treatment is long-term IV antibiotics.

Osteomyelitis can be prevented by warming an area to increase blood flow up to five times, selecting an appropriate site, cleansing the skin thoroughly, penetrating the skin no deeper than 2.4 mm, avoiding extra pressure, avoiding double cuts and previous puncture sites, and reducing the number of collections.

Preparation of the Site

1. Hold the area to be punctured with the thumb and index finger of a gloved hand.
2. Wipe the area with 70% alcohol and allow to air dry.
3. Wipe the area with a dry gauze square or cotton ball. If the area is not dry, the blood will not form a rounded drop and will be difficult to collect.

Puncturing the Skin

1. Use a disposable sterile lancet once and discard it properly in a puncture-proof container.
2. Securely hold the area and puncture once with a firm motion. The lancet should puncture across the creases of the fingerprint, not parallel with the grooves. If the finger is the chosen site, the area to be punctured should be in the portion of the finger that is rich in capillaries—not the fleshy part (Fig. 2.6B).
3. Wipe away the first drop of blood because it is not a true sample. The first drop of blood is mixed with lymphatic fluid and possibly alcohol.
4. Apply gentle pressure to the area to obtain subsequent drops. A good capillary puncture should require no forcing or hard squeezing of the site. If the site is squeezed too hard, lymphatic fluid will mix with the blood and produce inaccurate test results.

Collecting the Sample

1. If a blood smear is needed, follow the procedure in the next section of this chapter for the preparation of a push-wedge blood smear.
2. Allow micropipette or microhematocrit tubes to fill with free-flowing blood by capillary action. The tubes must be held horizontally to avoid introducing air bubbles or breaks in the column of blood.
3. If dilutions of the blood specimen are necessary, perform them promptly before the blood clots in the collecting tubes. Follow the specific methodology of the procedure

(continued)

BLOOD COLLECTION TECHNIQUES *(continued)*

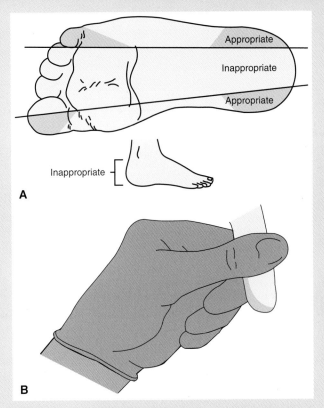

A

B

FIGURE 2.6 A: An infant heel. Shaded areas represent recommended safe areas for heel puncture. (Adapted with permission from McCall RE, Tankersley CM. *Phlebotomy Essentials*, 4th ed, Lippincott Williams & Wilkins, 2008, Fig 10.9, p. 371B.). **B:** Fingertip puncture. The shaded area is the preferred site for the collection of capillary blood from the finger.

to determine the quantities of diluent and whole blood that are needed.

4. Wipe the site frequently with a plain gauze square to prevent the accumulation of platelets, which will slow or stop the blood flow.

Termination of the Procedure

1. Wipe the area with alcohol.
2. Place a clean gauze square on the site and apply pressure. If the patient is unable to apply pressure to the site, hold the gauze square until the bleeding has stopped.
3. Label all specimens.
4. Place the used lancet into a puncture-proof container, remove gloves, and wash hands.

PREPARATION OF A BLOOD SMEAR

The preparation of a blood smear may be conducted at the patient's bedside or in the laboratory, if EDTA-anticoagulated blood is used. Two of the most basic procedures conducted by the hematology technologist or technician are the preparation and staining of blood smears. In this section, the

push-wedge and coverslip methods of blood smear preparation are presented.

THE PUSH-WEDGE METHOD

Specimen

Either EDTA-anticoagulated whole blood or free-flowing capillary blood can be used. If EDTA is used, smears must be prepared within 1 hour of collection. Before preparing the smear, store the blood at 18°C to 25°C. Adequate mixing is necessary before blood smear preparation.

Supplies and Equipment

Clean glass slides (plain or with one frosted end), a No. 2 lead pencil, and (optional) a specially designed pusher slide or a hemocytometer coverslip and pusher assembly.

Procedure

1. Place a small drop (0.05 mL) of well-mixed blood either directly from the freshly wiped fingertip puncture or with an applicator stick approximately 0.5 inch from one end of the slide. If frosted slides are used, place the blood near the frosted end of the slide.
2. Place the slide on a flat surface with the blood specimen to your right. Reverse this direction if you are left-handed.
3. Using a second pusher slide, place this slide slightly in front of the drop of blood. The angle of this pusher slide must be at approximately 45° (Fig. 2.7A).

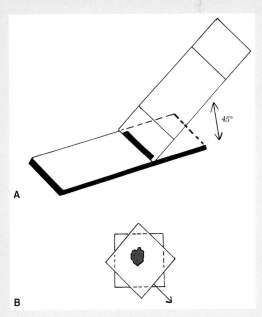

A

B

FIGURE 2.7 Push-wedge smear. **A:** Angle of slide. The proper angle of the pusher slide is approximately 45°. **B:** Coverslip preparation. Once a small drop of blood has spread by capillary action between the coverslips, they should be pulled apart smoothly in a horizontal plane.

(continued)

4. Draw the pusher slide back toward the drop of blood. Allow the drop of blood to spread about three fourths of the way across the bevel of the pusher slide. Do not allow the blood to spread to the edges. Quickly push this slide forward (away from the drop). This forward movement must be smooth and continue to the end of the slide.

5. Allow the smear to air dry before staining. The slides can be fanned in the air to dry them rapidly.

6. Label the slide using a No. 2 pencil. The labeling may be on the thick end (or frosted end) of the slide or on one edge of the slide.

Procedure Notes

1. A special pusher or spreader slide is commercially available to spread blood smears with margin-free edges. Some laboratories use a spreader device consisting of a straight artery clamp with the ends covered with rubber tubing. A rectangular (20 × 26 mm) hemocytometer coverslip is inserted between the ends of the clamp. The advantage of using a commercial spreader slide or the coverslip and pusher assembly is that the resulting smear has even slide margins that can be counted during the differential cell count.

2. The push-wedge method is recommended by CLSI as the reference method for differential leukocyte counting.

3. Normally, two smears are prepared. If free-flowing capillary blood is used, more than two smears may be desired.

Visual Evaluation of a Good Blood Smear

An ideal smear (Fig. 2.8) has the following characteristics.

1. It progresses from being thick at the point of origin to thin with a uniform edge at the termination point.

2. It does not touch the outer borders of the slide or run off the sides or ends of the slide.

3. It appears smooth, without waves or gaps.

4. It does not have any streaks, ridges, or troughs, which indicate an increased number of leukocytes carried to that area.

5. It is prepared with a proper amount of blood and spread to occupy approximately two thirds of the length of the glass slide.

Causes of a Poor Blood Smear

1. Prolonged storage of anticoagulated whole blood specimens. This can produce cellular distortion.

2. A delay in smear preparation. It is important to perform the blood smear immediately after placing the drop of blood on the slide. If this process is delayed, larger cells such as neutrophils and monocytes will be disproportionately located at the feathered edge when examined microscopically.

3. Dirty or poor-quality slides. Slides should be free of dust and grease spots.

4. Inappropriate size of blood droplet. Too large a drop of blood will produce a thick, long smear. Too small a drop of blood will produce a thin, short smear.

5. Improper angle of the pusher slide. The more the angle of the pusher slide is decreased, the longer the smear. The greater the angle, the thicker the smear.

6. Improper speed of the pushing movement. Slowly pushing the drop of blood will produce irregularities and affect the distribution of cells on the smear.

7. Improper pressure. The greater the pressure, the thinner the smear.

8. Humidity of the laboratory environment. High humidity can cause slides to dry too slowly. The prolonged drying of slides will produce erythrocyte distortion on microscopic examination.

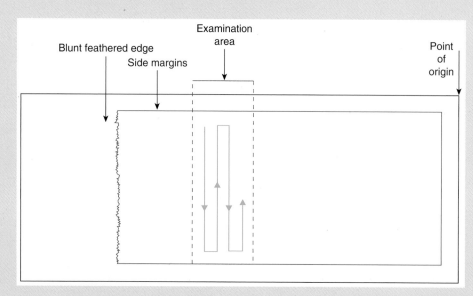

Blunt feathered edge
Side margins
Examination area
Point of origin

FIGURE 2.8 Ideal blood smear. An ideal peripheral blood smear should have side margins that do not touch the outer edges of the glass slide. The smear should become thinner from the point of origin to the termination in a blunt feathered edge. (Modified with permission from Koepke JA. Standardization of the manual differential leukocyte count, *Lab Med*, 11:371, 1980. ©1980 American Society for Clinical Pathology and ©1980 Laboratory Medicine.)

(continued)

COVERSLIP METHOD OF BLOOD FILM PREPARATION

Procedure

1. Hold two clean coverslips by their edges with the thumb and forefinger of each hand. Touch the center of one coverslip to a small drop of blood.
2. Immediately place the second coverslip on top of a very small drop of blood in a diagonal position.
3. Allow the blood to spread by capillary action. Just before the spreading action has almost stopped, evenly and smoothly pull the coverslips apart in the horizontal plane (see Fig. 2.6B).
4. Place the smears in an upright position and allow to air dry before staining.

Procedure Notes

1. The coverslip method produces a good distribution of leukocytes in all areas of the preparation.
2. Because of the smaller specimen amount, 50 leukocytes are counted per coverslip.
3. Owing to the small size of the coverslip, it is usually mounted (attached) to a conventional glass slide for staining.

Special Collection Procedures

In addition to the collection of venous or capillary blood specimens and the preparation of blood smears, some procedures are performed by the technologist or technician at the patient's bedside. This section describes basic procedures.

BONE MARROW PROCEDURE

Principle

Bone marrow examination is useful in the diagnosis of hematological disorders associated with cellular abnormalities. The diagnosis of disorders such as acute leukemia or multiple myeloma is usually confirmed by bone marrow examination. The management of patients undergoing treatment can also be monitored through the use of this procedure. Aspiration of bone marrow is performed only by a physician.

Sites of Aspiration

A specimen from a hematopoietically active area of the skeleton is needed (Fig. 2.9). Appropriate sites in an adult include the posterior iliac crest (preferred site), anterior iliac crest, and sternum. The tibia may be used in infants younger than 18 months of age.

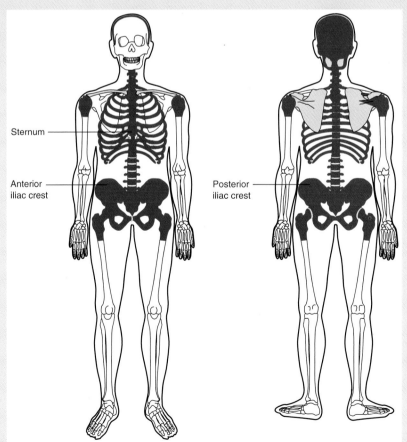

Sternum

Anterior iliac crest

Posterior iliac crest

FIGURE 2.9 Sites of bone marrow aspiration. The *red-shaded* areas indicate the sites in the skeletal system that contain productive marrow in adults. (Reprinted from Dzierzak E. Ontogenic emergence of definitive hematopoietic stem cells, *Curr Opin Hematol*, 10(3):230, 2003, with permission.)

(continued)

Supplies and Equipment

Bone marrow aspiration/biopsy equipment packs are frequently assembled and autoclaved in the central supply section of many hospitals, or they may be purchased in a kit form. If the laboratory is responsible for assembling the equipment, the following items are usually included:

1. Aspiration needles, biopsy needle, and various sizes of syringes and needles
2. Cotton balls and gauze, hemostat, 1% or 2% lidocaine, antiseptic solution, and surgical gloves
3. A bottle of Zenker solution or formalin fixative
4. A sterile container if microbiological cultures are requested
5. The laboratory may additionally supply liquid heparin, glass slides, a watch glass, and microbiological loop or capillary blood collection tubes with a small rubber bulb.

Procedure

After the physician has aspirated the specimen, the technician or technologist may be asked to prepare bone marrow films at the patient's bedside. Universal precautions must be observed throughout the procedure and during the clean-up phase.

1. Peripheral blood is usually mixed with the bone marrow aspirate in the syringe. A simple way of removing most of the unwanted peripheral blood is to place the entire contents of the syringe onto a watch glass and remove the small pieces of marrow with a microbiological loop or capillary pipette with a rubber bulb.
2. Depending on the established procedure, three different types of smears may be made: conventional push-wedge, coverslip, and squash techniques.
3. The previously described procedures for the push-wedge and coverslip techniques are followed. Squash preparations are prepared by placing the specimen in the middle of one slide and covering the specimen with a second slide. The slides are pressed together and then pulled apart longitudinally (see Fig. 2.9B).
4. The specimen remaining in the watch glass, and any additional specimens (e.g., from bone biopsy), are usually placed in fixative solution for histological processing.
5. All specimens must be labeled before leaving the patient's room. Properly dispose of contaminated supplies.

Routine Staining of Peripheral Blood Films

To examine cells on a blood smear in detail, it is necessary to stain the smear. The beginning student in hematology should become familiar with the principles and practice of routine staining of a blood smear before investigating specific characteristics of cells or performing other staining procedures. The most commonly used stain in the hematology laboratory is a Romanowsky-type stain.

STAINING PRINCIPLES

In 1891, Romanowsky and Malachowski first described the use of a stain that combined a polychrome (oxidized) methylene blue solution with eosin as a blood stain. Ten years later, this stain was refined by Leishman, who combined eosin with polychrome methylene blue, recovered the precipitate, and dissolved this precipitate in methyl alcohol. Today, Romanowsky-type stains are prepared by use of this modified technique.

A Romanowsky stain is defined as any stain containing methylene blue and/or its products of oxidation and a halogenated fluorescein dye, usually eosin B or Y. Romanowsky-based stains, such as Wright, Giemsa, or May-Grünwald stains, are alcoholic solutions with basic and acidic components. Stains of this type are referred to as polychrome stains because they can impart many colors and produce the Romanowsky effect. This effect imparts a typical color to certain cell components and reflects the combined action of the dyes contained in the stain at a pH of 6.4 to 7.0. The characteristic colors are purple in the cell nucleus, blue and pink in the cytoplasm, and various colors in specific granules.

Stain Preparation

The oxidation of methylene blue results in a solution containing primarily methylene blue; azures A, B, and C; methylene violet; and thionin symdimethylthionin. When eosin dye is added to this solution, the precipitate formed consists of eosinates of these products. Azure B eosinate appears to be the complex responsible for the characteristic Romanowsky effect. Stains with greater quantities of the azure B eosin will react rapidly and provide a better Romanowsky effect than those products containing a lesser amount of this salt. The content of azure B and eosin Y must be consistent and in correct proportions. Solutions of known composition and weights of azures can be prepared (e.g., Giemsa stain). A stock solution of the stain is dissolved in a mixture of glycerol and absolute methyl alcohol. The stock stain is then diluted with phosphate buffer pH 6.8 to permit ionization of the stains.

Staining Reactions

The specific stains in a Romanowsky-type stain and their associated reactions are as follows:

Methylene blue is a basic stain, which stains the nucleus and some cytoplasmic structures blue or purple color. These stained structures are thus basophilic (e.g., DNA or RNA).

Eosin is an acidic stain, which stains some cytoplasmic structures orange-red color. The orange-red staining structures are acidophilic (e.g., proteins with amino groups).

When both the basic and the acidic components of the mixture stain a cytoplasmic structure, a pink or lilac color develops. This is referred to as a neutrophilic reaction.

(continued)

STAINING PROCEDURE

Blood and other types of specimens can be stained using Romanowsky-based stains. These stains can be prepared in the laboratory or purchased in a ready-to-use form. Either manual or automated techniques can be used.

In some laboratories, blood smears are fixed separately in alcohol before the staining procedure is performed. This step enhances the retention of granules in blood cells. The usual fixative is methyl alcohol. Slides can be placed in anhydrous and acetone-free methanol for 1 minute or longer. Wright and other Romanowsky-based stains are dissolved in methyl alcohol; therefore, fixation normally takes place when the stain is applied to the blood smear.

Reagents and Equipment

1. Stains may be purchased in a ready-to-use form or may be prepared by diluting preweighed vials in methyl alcohol according to the manufacturer's directions.
2. A staining rack or Coplin staining jars are needed.

Procedure

1. Place a thoroughly dried and labeled slide on a level staining rack with the smear side facing up.
2. Place freshly filtered stain slowly on the slide until the smear is completely covered. Do not add excess stain. Staining times will vary. Commonly, 3 to 10 minutes may be needed for an acceptably stained blood smear.
3. At the end of the staining time, gently add buffer (pH 6.4) to the slide without removing the stain. The buffer should form a large bubble (convex shape) on the slide. Do not add excess buffer. Some technologists prefer to use ordinary tap water in place of the buffer.
4. Mix the stain and buffer by gently blowing on the slide. A well-mixed slide will have a metallic green sheen rise to the surface of the slide. The timing for this stage ranges from 2 to 5 minutes. If a Coplin jar is preferred for staining, the slides are dipped into the stain and buffer solutions.
5. Wash the stain and buffer off the slide with a gentle flow of tap water. Pick the slide up by its edges and wipe the back of the slide to remove any stain.
6. Allow the slide to air dry.

Sources of Error in Staining

Poor-quality staining can result from several factors:

1. Failure to filter the stain daily, or before use, can produce sediment on blood films. If the precipitated sediment is very heavy, it will be impossible to view the blood cell microscopically. Small amounts of sediment can be mistaken for platelets on microscopic examination.
2. Inaccurate buffer pH can produce too bright or too dark a staining reaction. The buffer solution must control the acid–base balance of the stain to produce the proper colors in the various components of the blood cells. An overly acidic buffer produces a blood smear that is too red on microscopic examination. If the buffer is too basic (alkaline), the blood smear will be too blue on microscopic examination.
3. Improper timing of staining or buffering can produce faded staining or altered colors of the blood smears. Too short a staining time produces a blood smear that is too red on microscopic examination. If the staining time is too long, the blood smear will be too dark on microscopic examination.
4. Deteriorated reagents or improper ratios of stain and buffer in the staining process can produce washed-out cellular colors.

CHAPTER HIGHLIGHTS

Quality in Phlebotomy

The role of the phlebotomist has never been more important. In the United States, it is estimated that more than 1 billion venipunctures are performed annually, and errors occurring within this process may cause serious harm to patients, either directly or indirectly.

Quality Assessment

The accuracy of laboratory testing begins with the quality of the specimen received by the laboratory. This quality depends on how a specimen was collected, transported, and processed. The term quality assessment or the older term, quality assurance, is used to describe management of the treatment of the whole patient. As it applies to phlebotomy, quality assessment includes preparation of a patient for any specimens to be collected, collection of valid samples, and proper specimen transport.

Patient Care Partnership

The delivery of healthcare involves a partnership between patients and physicians and other healthcare professionals. When collecting blood specimens, it is important that the phlebotomist considers the rights of the patient at all times.

The Phlebotomist as Laboratory Ambassador

A phlebotomist is frequently the only laboratory staff member that a patient sees. This means that the professional image of the laboratory is solely represented by the phlebotomist. The phlebotomist is expected to deliver unexcelled customer satisfaction.

Patients with Special Considerations

When working with children, it is important to be gentle and treat them with compassion, empathy, and kindness. Attempt to interact with the pediatric patient, realizing that both the patient and the parent (if present) may have anxiety about the procedure and be unfamiliar with the new settings. Acknowledge the parent and the child. Allow enough time for the procedure.

When obtaining a blood specimen from an adolescent, it is important to be relaxed and perceptive about any anxiety that he or she may have. General interaction techniques include allowing enough time for the procedure, establishing eye contact, and allowing the patient to maintain a sense of control.

It is extremely important to treat geriatric patients with dignity and respect. Do not demean the patient. It is best to address the patient with a more formal title such as Mrs., Ms., or Mr. rather than by his or her first name.

Blood Collection Supplies and Equipment

To make the phlebotomy procedure easier for the technician, the following suggestions should be remembered:

- Assemble supplies and have readily available.
- Use the minimal acceptable amount of blood for an individual assay or a group of assays.
- Collect the minimal acceptable amount of blood for each type of collection tube.
- Demonstrate a plan and an alternative plan each time a phlebotomy procedure is preformed.

A properly collected blood specimen is essential to a quality outcome in the laboratory.

Anticoagulants

Three types of anticoagulants are commonly used in the hematology laboratory:

1. K_2 EDTA
2. Sodium citrate
3. Heparin

Each of the anticoagulant types prevents the coagulation of whole blood in a specific manner.

Additives chosen for specific determinations must not alter the blood components or affect the laboratory tests to be done. If too little additive is used, partial clotting of whole blood will occur. This interferes with cell counts. By comparison, if too much liquid anticoagulant is used, it dilutes the blood sample and thus interferes with certain quantitative measurements.

Safe Blood Collection: Equipment and Supplies

An increased emphasis on safety has led to new product development by various companies. Newer designs of this equipment are reducing the incidence of post-phlebotomy needlesticks.

Evacuated tubes are the most widely used system for collecting venous blood samples. This system consists of a collection needle, a nonreusable needle holder, and a tube containing enough vacuum to draw a specific amount of blood. Evacuated tubes come in various (mL) sizes, including pediatric sizes, with color-coded stoppers. The stopper color denotes the type of anticoagulant or the presence of a gel separator.

Evacuated tubes are intended for one-time use. Use of evacuated tubes with double-pointed collection needles makes possible a closed sterile system for specimen collection. This preserves the quality of the specimen during transport before testing and protects the patient from infection. CLSI has set guidelines concerning the correct procedures for collecting and handling blood specimens. When collecting multiple tubes of blood, a specified "order of draw" protocol needs to be followed to diminish the possibility of cross-contamination between tubes caused by the presence of different additives. Errors in the order of draw can affect laboratory test results.

A variety of environment factors can impact the quality of evacuated tubes used to collect blood. Environmental factors affecting evacuated tubes include ambient temperature, altitude, humidity and sunlight.

Laser technology is the first radical change in phlebotomy in more than 100 years. The risk of an accidental needlestick injury haunts every phlebotomist. A laser device emits a pulse of light energy that lasts a minuscule fraction of a second. The laser concentrates on a very small portion of skin, literally vaporizing the tissue about 1 to 2 mm to the capillary bed. The device can draw a 100-μL blood sample, a sufficient amount for certain tests. The laser process is less painful and heals faster than when blood is drawn with traditional lancets. The patient feels a sensation similar to heat, as opposed to the prick of a sharp object.

REVIEW QUESTIONS

1. When the coagulation of fresh whole blood is prevented through the use of an anticoagulant, the straw-colored fluid that can be separated from the cellular elements is
   A. serum
   B. plasma
   C. whole blood
   D. platelets

2. Which characteristic is inaccurate with respect to the anticoagulant K_3 EDTA?
   A. Removes ionized calcium (Ca^{2+}) from fresh whole blood by the process of chelation
   B. Is used for most routine coagulation studies
   C. Is the most commonly used anticoagulant in hematology
   D. Is conventionally placed in lavender-stoppered evacuated tubes

3. Heparin inhibits the clotting of fresh whole blood by neutralizing the effect of
   A. platelets
   B. ionized calcium (Ca^{2+})
   C. fibrinogen
   D. thrombin

Questions 4 through 7: Match the conventional color-coded stopper with the appropriate anticoagulant.

4. _____ EDTA   A. Red
5. _____ Heparin   B. Lavender
6. _____ Sodium citrate   C. Blue
7. _____ No anticoagulant   D. Green

Questions 8 through 12: The following five procedural steps are significant activities in the performance of a venipuncture. Place these steps in the correct sequence.

8. _____   A. Select an appropriate site and prepare the site.
9. _____
10. _____   B. Identify the patient, check test requisitions, assemble equipment, wash hands, and put on latex gloves.
11. _____
12. _____   C. Remove tourniquet, remove needle, apply pressure to site, and label all tubes.
              D. Reapply the tourniquet and perform the venipuncture.
              E. Introduce yourself and briefly explain the procedure to the patient.

13. The appropriate veins for performing a routine venipuncture are the
    A. cephalic, basilic, and median cubital
    B. subclavian, iliac, and femoral
    C. brachiocephalic, jugular, and popliteal
    D. saphenous, suprarenal, and tibial

14. A blood sample is needed from a patient with IV fluids running in both arms. Which of the following is an acceptable procedure?
    A. Any obtainable vein is satisfactory.
    B. Obtain sample from above the IV site.
    C. Obtain sample from below the IV site with special restrictions.
    D. Disconnect the IV line.
    E. Do not draw a blood specimen.

15. The bevel of the needle should be held _____ in the performance of a venipuncture.
    A. sideways
    B. upward
    C. downward
    D. in any direction

16. A hematoma can form if
    A. improper pressure is applied to a site after the venipuncture
    B. the patient suddenly moves and the needle comes out of the vein
    C. the needle punctures both walls of the vein
    D. all of the above

17. Phlebotomy problems can include
    A. the use of improper anticoagulants
    B. misidentification of patients
    C. improper angle of the needle or having the needle up against the side of the vessel wall
    D. all of the above

18. Which of the following skin puncture areas is (are) acceptable for the collection of capillary blood from an infant?
    A. Previous puncture site
    B. Posterior curve of the heel
    C. The arch
    D. Medial or lateral plantar surface

19. The proper collection of capillary blood includes
    A. wiping away the first drop of blood
    B. occasionally wiping the site with a plain gauze pad to avoid the buildup of platelets
    C. avoiding the introduction of air bubbles into the column of blood in a capillary collection tube
    D. all of the above

20. A peripheral blood smear can be prepared from
    A. EDTA-anticoagulated blood within 1 hour of collection
    B. free-flowing capillary blood
    C. citrated whole blood
    D. both A and B

(continued)

REVIEW QUESTIONS (continued)

21. Identify the characteristic(s) of a good peripheral blood smear.
    A. It progresses from thick at the point of origin to thin.
    B. It has a blunt feathered termination.
    C. The outer margins do not touch the edges of the slide.
    D. All of the above.

22. Poor blood smears can be caused by
    A. a delay in preparing the smear once the drop of blood has been placed on the slide
    B. a drop of blood that is too large or too small
    C. holding the pusher slide at the wrong angle and poor drying conditions
    D. all of the above

23. If a blood smear is too long, the problem can be resolved by
    A. decreasing the angle of the pusher slide
    B. increasing the angle of the pusher slide
    C. using a larger drop of blood
    D. pushing the slide slower in smearing out the blood

24. The examination of bone marrow is useful in
    A. diagnosing a bleeding disorder
    B. diagnosing some disorders associated with erythrocytes and leukocytes
    C. diagnosing acute leukemias
    D. both B and C

25. Appropriate bone marrow aspiration sites in an adult are the
    A. anterior and posterior iliac crest
    B. sternum and posterior iliac crest
    C. tibia and sternum
    D. both A and B

Questions 26 through 28: Match the following type of staining effect with the color it imparts to blood cells.

26. _____ Basic stain   A. Orange-red color
27. _____ Acidic stain   B. Pink-lilac color
28. _____ Neutrophilic   C. Blue-purple color

Questions 29 through 32: Identify the following as Romanowsky-type or non–Romanowsky-type stains.

29. _____ Wright   A. Romanowsky-type
30. _____ May-Grünwald   B. Non–Romanowsky-type
31. _____ Giemsa
32. _____ Methylene blue

33. If a blood smear stains too red on microscopic examination of a Wright-stained preparation, possible causes include that
    A. the staining time was too long
    B. the stain was too basic
    C. the buffer was too acidic and the exposure time was too short
    D. the buffer was too basic and the exposure time was too long

REFERENCE

1. Lippi G, Fostini R, Guidi GC. Quality improvement in laboratory medicine: Extra-analytical issues, *Clin Lab Med*, 28(2):285–294, 2008.

BIBLIOGRAPHY

Adcock DM, et al. Effect of 3.2% vs. 3.8% sodium citrate concentration on routine coagulation testing, *Am J Clin Pathol*, 107:105–110, 1997.

American Hospital Association: Patient Care Partnership, www.aha.org (retrieved August 2005).

Avinoso D. Clot activator tubes, *Med Lab Obs*, 34(9):35, 2002.

BD Vacutainer Systems, *LabNotes*, 13(2):1–16, 2003.

BD Vacutainer Systems, *LabNotes*, 13(3): 2003.

Bush V. Why doesn't my heparinized plasma specimen remain anticoagulated? *LabNotes*, 13: 2003 (www.bd.com, retrieved July 2, 2003).

Bush V, Cohen R. The evolution of evacuated blood collection tubes, *LabNotes*, 19(1): 2009 retrieved August 20, 2009.

Clark K. Phlebotomy: Beyond the basics, *Adv Med Lab Prof*, 28(9):12–15, 1997.

CLSI. *Protection of Laboratory Workers from Infectious Disease Transmitted by Blood, Body Fluids and Tissue*, M29-A3. Wayne, PA: CLSI, 2005.

Dale JC. Phlebotomy Complications, Presented at Mayo Laboratory's Phlebotomy Conference, August 1996, Boston, MA.

Ernst D, Calam R. NCCLS simplifies the order of draw: A brief history, *Med Lab Obs*, 36(5):26, 2004.

Faber V. Phlebotomy and the aging patient, *Adv Med Lab Prof*, 29(1):24–25, 1998.

Foubister V. Quick on the draw—coagulation tube response, *CAP TODAY*, 16(10):38–42, 2002.

Gerberding JL. Occupational exposure to HIV in health care settings, *N Engl J Med*, 348(9):826–832, 2003.

Haraden L. Pediatric phlebotomy: Great expectations, *Adv Med Lab Prof*, 28(11):12–13, 1997.

Hurley TR. Considerations for the Pediatric and Geriatric Patient, Presented at Mayo Laboratory's Phlebotomy Conference, August 1996, Boston, MA.

Iverson LK. Changing Roles of Phlebotomist/Customer Satisfaction, Presented at Mayo Laboratory's Phlebotomy Conference, August 1996, Boston, MA.

Linke EG, Henry JB. Clinical pathology/laboratory medicine purposes and practice. In: Henry JB (ed.). *Clinical Diagnosis and Management by Laboratory Methods*, 18th ed, Philadelphia, PA: Saunders, 1991.

Reneke J, et al. Prolonged prothrombin time and activated partial thromboplastin time due to underfilled specimen tubes with 109 mmol/L (3.2%) citrate anticoagulant, *Am J Clin Pathol*, 109:754–757, 1998.

Sigma Diagnostics Summary Technical News and Notes, Vol. 1 and Vol. 2, St. Louis, MO: Sigma Diagnostics, 1985.

U.S. Department of Labor. Occupational Safety and Health Administration, US Department of Labor: Disposal of Contaminated Needles and Blood Tube Holders Used in Phlebotomy, Safety and Health Information Bulletin (www.osha.gov/dts/shib/ shib101503.html, retrieved May 2005).

U.S. Department of Labor Occupational Safety and Health Administration, US Department of Labor: Best Practice: OSHA's Position on the Reuse of Blood Collection Tube Holders, Safety and Health Information Bulletin (www.osha.gov/dts/shib/ shib101503.html, retrieved May 2005).

Ogden-Grable H, Gill GW. Preventing phlebotomy errors-potential for harming your patients, *Lab Med*, 36(7):430, 2005.

INTERNET SITES

http://www.bd.com/vacutainer/products.asp, BD Vacutainer Systems, BD Eclipse Blood Collection Needle Interactive Training Module, retrieved July 9, 2003.

http://www.cdc.gov/ncidod/sars/packingspecimens-sars.htm,retrieved October 10, 2003.

CHAPTER 3

Molecular Genetics and Cellular Morphology

Cellular ultrastructure and organization

- Describe the chemical composition and general function of cellular membranes.
- Explain the general membrane activities of passive and facilitated diffusion, active transport, osmosis, and endocytosis.
- Name and describe the structure and function of each of the cytoplasmic organelles found in a typical mammalian cell.
- Describe two cellular metabolites that are of importance to hematologists.
- Describe the features of the nucleus and define the terms heterochromatin and euchromatin.
- Relate the nuclear structures to the cellular activities that are associated with the nucleus.
- Describe the processes of mitosis and meiosis.
- Describe the process of apoptosis.

Molecular genetics in hematology

- Name at least three hematological abnormalities that can be detected by molecular methods.
- Explain the characteristics of the term minimal residual disease.
- Describe the polymerase chain reaction (PCR) amplification technique and variations.
- Describe the "gold standard" of genetic analysis.
- Compare the procedures and applications of dot blot, reverse dot blot, Southern blot, and Northern blot techniques.
- Define the acronym, FISH.
- Explain how microarrays are applied to hematological testing.
- Name four applications of molecular techniques as diagnostic tools in hematopathology.

CELLULAR ULTRASTRUCTURE AND ORGANIZATION

Cells, as the smallest organized units of living tissues, have the ability to individually perform all the functions essential for life processes. Although the range of morphological features varies widely, all cells conform to a basic model (Fig. 3.1A). Large cellular structures are observable on stained preparations with the light microscope. Smaller ultrastructures or organelles must be viewed with an electron microscope.

Cellular Membranes

Structure

Cellular membranes provide a semipermeable separation between the various cellular components, the organelles, and the surrounding environment. The cytoplasmic membrane, or outer membrane, defines the boundaries of the cell, while being resilient and elastic. Differences in membrane thickness reflect the various functional properties of specific cell types or organelles within the cell.

Chemically, membranes consist of proteins, phospholipids, cholesterol, and traces of polysaccharide. The most popular hypothesis to explain the arrangement of these molecular components is the **fluid mosaic model** (Fig. 3.1B). According to this model, the cell membrane is a dynamic fluid structure with globular proteins floating in lipids. The lipids, as phospholipids, are arranged in two layers. The polar (charged) phosphate ends of the phospholipids are oriented toward the inner and outer surfaces, while the nonpolar (fatty acid) ends point toward each other in the interior of the membrane. Protein molecules may be either integral (incorporated into the lipid bilayer) or peripheral (associated with either the outer or the inner surface of the membrane). Polysaccharides in the form of either glycoproteins or glycolipids can be found attached to the lipid and protein molecules of the membrane.

Membrane Functions

The lipid bilayer is directly responsible for the impermeability of the membrane to most water-soluble molecules. Proteins within the membrane act as transport molecules for the rapid penetration of polar and non–lipid-soluble substances. Additionally, protein molecules determine and protect the shape and structure of the membrane, often through attachment to underlying microtubules and microfilaments. In human red blood cells, the extrinsic protein, spectrin, in conjunction with the protein actin, forms a contractile network just under the cell membrane and provides the cell with the resistance necessary to withstand distorting forces during movement through the blood circulation. Membrane-bound carbohydrates act as surface **antigens**, which function in the process of cellular recognition and interaction between cells.

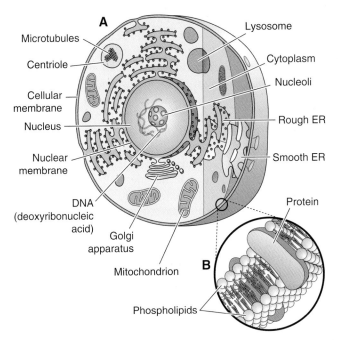

FIGURE 3.1 Cellular organization. Most of the organelles depicted in (**A**) are visible only with electron microscope examination. **A**: Cellular ultrastructures. **B**: Fluid mosaic model. The unique positioning of the phospholipids and free-floating proteins is characterized by the fluid mosaic model of the cellular membrane. ER, endoplasmic reticulum.

As a unit, the cytoplasmic membrane maintains cellular integrity of the interior of the cell by controlling and influencing the passage of materials in and out of the cell. This function is accomplished through the major membrane processes of osmosis, diffusion, active transport, and endocytosis.

The term **osmosis** is used to describe the net movement of water molecules through a semipermeable membrane (Fig. 3.2). Normally, water molecules move in and out of the cell membrane at an equal rate, producing no net movement. If a concentration gradient exists, the movement of water molecules will be greater from areas of low solute (e.g., sodium and chloride ions) concentration to areas of higher solute concentration. Osmosis is the basic principle underlying the previously popular erythrocyte, or red blood cell, fragility test that demonstrates changes in the erythrocytic

membrane. Alterations in the erythrocytic membrane, such as the loss of flexibility, can be observed by placing erythrocytes in solutions with varying solute concentrations.

Diffusion is an important process in overall cellular physiology, such as the physiological activities of the erythrocyte. This passive process through a semipermeable membrane may also be referred to as **dialysis**. Substances passively diffuse, or move down a concentration gradient from areas of high solute concentration to areas of low solute concentration, by dissolving in the lipid portion of the cellular membrane. Diffusion through the membrane is influenced by the solubility of molecules in lipids, temperature, and the concentration gradient. Lipid-soluble substances diffuse through the lipid layer at rates greater than through the protein portions of the membrane.

Small molecules, such as those of water or inorganic ions, are able to pass down the concentration gradient via **hydrophilic** regions. These hydrophilic regions are associated with the points where some of the membrane's protein molecules create a polar area, resulting in pore-like openings. However, movement of molecules through these regions is affected by electrical charges along the surface of the region, the size of the region, and the specific nature of the protein. Calcium ions affect the permeability of membranes. An increase in the concentration of calcium ions in the fluid surrounding the cell, or accumulation of calcium ions in the cytoplasm, can decrease the permeability of the membrane and has been demonstrated as a factor in the aging process of erythrocytes.

Active transport is another essential membrane function. Because the cellular membrane also functions as a metabolic regulator, enzyme molecules are incorporated into the membrane. One such enzyme, particularly important as a metabolic regulator, is sodium-potassium-adenosine triphosphatase (Na-K-ATPase). This enzyme provides the necessary energy to drive the sodium-potassium pump, a fundamental ion transport system. Sodium ions are pumped out of the cells into extracellular fluids, where the concentration of sodium is higher than it is inside the cell. This movement of molecules is referred to as moving against the concentration gradient. The energy-producing activities of the mitochondria are heavily dependent on this process (see "The Function of Mitochondria" in this chapter).

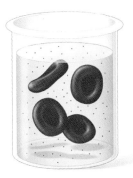
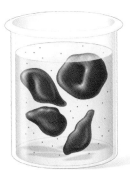
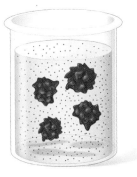

Normal (isotonic) solution

Hypotonic solution

Hypertonic solution

FIGURE 3.2 Effects of osmosis on red blood cells in different concentrations: isotonic, hypotonic, and hypertonic solutions. (Reprinted with permission from Braun CA. *Pathophysiology*, Baltimore, MD: Lippincott Williams and Wilkins, 2007).

Endocytosis (Fig. 3.3) is the process of engulfing particles or molecules, with the subsequent formation of membrane-bound vacuoles in the cytoplasm. Two processes, **pinocytosis** (the engulfment of fluids) and **phagocytosis** (the engulfment and destruction of particles), are forms of endocytosis. The vesicles formed by endocytosis either discharge their contents into the cellular cytoplasm or fuse with the organelles and the lysosomes. Phagocytosis is an important body defense mechanism and is discussed in more detail in Chapter 14.

Cell Volume Homeostasis

Maintenance of a constant volume despite extracellular and intracellular osmotic challenges is critical to the integrity of a cell. In most cases, cells respond by swelling or shrinking by activating specific metabolic or membrane-transport processes that return cell volume to its normal resting state. These processes are essential for the normal function and survival of cells.

Cells respond to volume changes by activating mechanisms that regulate their volume. The processes by which swollen and shrunken cells return to a normal volume are called regulatory volume decrease and regulatory volume increase, respectively. Cell volume can only be regulated by the gain or loss of osmotically active solutes, primarily inorganic ions such as sodium, potassium, and chloride or small organic molecules called organic osmolytes.

Regulatory loss and gain of electrolytes are mediated by membrane transport processes. In most animal cells, regulatory decreases in volume are accomplished by the loss of potassium chloride as a result of the activation of separate potassium and chloride channels or of the K^+/Cl^-

cotransporter. Regulatory increases in volume occur through the uptake of both potassium chloride and sodium chloride. Certain ion transport systems have multiple roles, participating in volume regulation, intracellular pH control, and transepithelial movement of salt and water.

Organic osmolytes are found in high concentrations in the cytosol of all organisms, from bacteria to humans. These solutes have key roles in cell volume homeostasis and may also function as general cytoprotectants. The accumulation of organic osmolytes is mediated either by energy-dependent transport from the external medium or by changes in the rates of osmolyte synthesis and degradation.

Volume accumulation induces a very rapid increase in the passive efflux of organic osmolytes. Generally, this process is slow. Cell swelling inhibits transportation of the genes coding for organic osmolyte transporters and the enzymes involved in osmolyte synthesis. As transcription decreases, levels of messenger RNA (mRNA) drop and the number of functional proteins declines over a period of many hours to days.

The sensing mechanism for cell size is not yet understood. A number of volume signals have been postulated, including swelling- and shrinkage-induced changes in membrane tension, cytoskeletal architecture, cellular ion concentrations, and the concentration of cytoplasmic macromolecules. No one signaling mechanism can account for the volume sensitivity of the various genes and membrane transport pathways that reactivate or are inactivated in response to perturbations in cell volume. Recent evidence suggests that cells can detect more than simple swelling or shrinkage. Disruption of cellular osmoregulatory mechanisms can give rise to a diverse group of disease states and their complications.

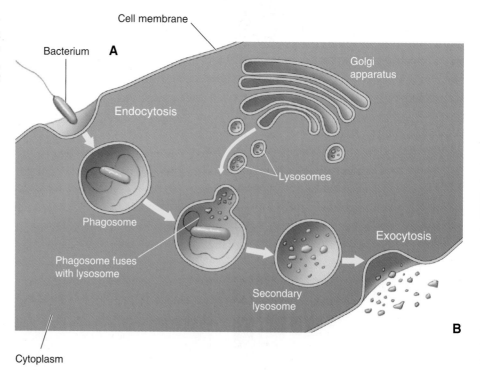

FIGURE 3.3 Vesicular transport. **A:** Endocytosis; **B:** Exocytosis. (Reprinted with permission from Premkumar K. *The Massage Connection Anatomy and Physiology*, Baltimore, MD: Lippincott Williams & Wilkins, 2004.)

Reactive and Neoplastic Growth Processes

The size and shape of particular cell types (Fig. 3.4) are constant. Individual cell features can vary because of infectious disease or malignancy, and groups of cells (tissues) can manifest a variety of changes as well. Terms that may be encountered in the study of hematological diseases include the following:

Anaplasia—highly pleomorphic and bizarre cytologic features associated with malignant tumors that are poorly differentiated.

Atrophy—decrease in the number or size of cells that can lead to a decrease in organ size or tissue mass.

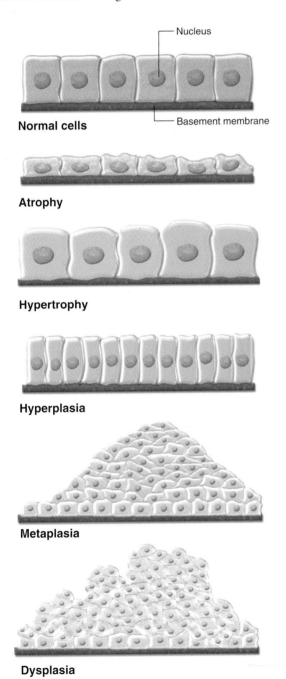

FIGURE 3.4 Adaptive cell changes. (Asset provided by Anatomical Chart Co.)

Dysplasia—abnormal cytologic features and tissue organization; often is a premalignant change.

Hyperplasia—increase in the number of cells in a tissue.

Hypertrophy—increase in the size of cells that can lead to an increase in organ size.

Metaplasia—change from one adult cell type to another (e.g., glandular to squamous metaplasia).

Cytoplasmic Organelles and Metabolites

Organelles (see Fig. 3.1A) are functional units of a cell. Most of the smaller organelles must be viewed with an electron microscope. Staining techniques are valuable in the identification of larger organelles and soluble substances in the cytoplasm.

Stains such as Wright stain (discussed in Chapter 2) aid in differentiating the features of cells found in the blood and bone marrow. The staining and morphological characteristics of blood cells are presented in the last section of this chapter. Specialized stains (discussed in Chapter 26) can be used to identify constituents such as lipids, glycogen, iron, enzymes, and nucleic acids in cells. In abnormal cells, the soluble substances in the cytoplasm can provide important clues to the cell's identity. A detailed discussion of representative cytochemical staining is included in Chapters 19, 21, and 26. The organelles and their respective functions are listed here.

Centrioles are two central spots inside of the centrosomes. These paired structures are cylindrical, and the long axes are always oriented at right angles to each other. Internally, each structure consists of nine (triplet) groups of microtubules. The centrioles divide and move to the opposite ends of the cell during cell division. They serve as points of insertion of the spindle fibers during cell division.

The **endoplasmic reticulum** (ER), an extensive lace-like network, is composed of membranes enclosing interconnecting cavities or cisterns. It is classified as either rough (granular) or smooth (agranular). The rough sections contain **ribosomes**. Rough ER is associated with protein production; smooth ER is thought to be the site of the synthesis of lipids such as cholesterol and also the site of the breakdown of fats into smaller molecules that can be used for energy.

The **Golgi apparatus** appears as a horseshoe-shaped or hook-shaped organelle with an associated stack of vesicles or sacs. In stained blood smears, the Golgi apparatus appears as the unstained area next to the nucleus. Functionally, the Golgi apparatus is the site for concentrating secretions of granules, packing, and segregating the carbohydrate components of certain secretions. Part of the Golgi apparatus and adjacent portions of the ER appear to form lysosomes. The Golgi-associated endoplasmic reticulum lysosome (GERL) concept focuses on the coordination of these cellular components. Products of the Golgi apparatus are usually exported from the cell when a vesicle of the Golgi apparatus fuses with the plasma membrane.

Lysosomes contain hydrolytic enzymes. Three types of lysosomes have been identified: primary, secondary, and tertiary. Lysosomes are responsible for the intracellular digestion of the products of **phagocytosis** or the disposal of worn-out or damaged cell components. In some instances, lysosomes fuse with vacuoles containing foreign substances engulfed by the cell. In this process, the lysosomes may rupture and these internal enzymes actually autolyze the entire cell.

Microbodies are small, intracytoplasmic organelles, limited by a single membrane that is thinner than the lysosome. Microbodies contain enzymes. These organelles are especially likely to contain oxidase enzymes that produce hydrogen peroxide. Their function, related to oxidative activity, is an important aspect of phagocytosis.

Microfilaments are solid structures, consisting of the protein **actin** and the larger **myosin** filaments. Microfilaments are the smallest components of the cytoskeleton. These structures are responsible for the amoeboid movement of cells, such as the phagocytic cells. In **cytokinesis**, the plasma membrane pinches in because of the contraction of a ring of microfilaments.

Microtubules are small, hollow fibers composed of polymerized, macromolecular protein subunits, **tubulin**. They are narrow and have an indefinite length. The formation of tubules occurs through rapid, reversible self-assembly of filaments. Microtubules may be concerned with cell shape (the cytoskeleton) and the intracellular movement of organelles and may have a passive role in intracellular diffusion. The mitotic spindle is composed of microtubules.

Mitochondria are composed of an outer smooth membrane and an inner folded membrane. Cells contain from hundreds to thousands of these rod-shaped organelles; however, mature erythrocytes lack mitochondria. The inner membrane functions as a permeable barrier. Each of the membranes has distinct functional differences. The cristae contain the enzymes and other molecules that carry out the energy-producing reactions of the cell. The granules of the matrix function as binding sites for calcium and contain some **deoxyribonucleic acid (DNA)** and some ribosomes that are similar to those found in microorganisms. The reaction located on the inner membrane of the mitochondria is enzyme-controlled, energy-producing, and electron transfer-oxidative.

Ribosomes, small dense granules, show a lack of membranes and are found both on the surface of the rough ER and free in the cytoplasm. They contain a significant proportion of **ribonucleic acid (RNA)** and are composed of unequally sized subunits. Ribosomes may exist singly, in groups, or in clusters. The presence of many ribosomes produces cytoplasmic basophilia (blue color) when a cell is stained with Wright stain. The complex of mRNA and ribosome serves as the site of protein synthesis. Numerous cytoplasmic ribosomes with few associated membranes suggest significant protein synthesis activity for internal use, such as in growing and dividing cells or in erythrocytic precursors in which hemoglobin is retained as it is synthesized. Cells, such as the plasma cell, that synthesize proteins for use outside of the cell tend to have greater amounts of rough ER except in the Golgi area.

Cellular Inclusions and Metabolites

Cells contain a variety of inclusions. Some of these structures are vacuoles with ingested fluids or particles, stored fats, and granules of glycogen and other substances. Numerous soluble cellular metabolites are present in the cytoplasm, but few have a clearly defined ultrastructural identity. Two metabolites of importance to hematologists are glycogen and ferritin.

Glycogen is a long-chain polysaccharide, a storage form of carbohydrate that is detectable with a special stain, the periodic acid-Schiff (PAS) stain (refer to Chapter 26). The size of these particles is about twice that of a ribosome. The beta form of glycogen is found in single particles in the neutrophilic leukocytes. Undoubtedly, increased glycogen concentrations in cells such as the neutrophilic leukocyte are related to the needs of the cells for a high energy reserve to carry out their body defense functions.

Ferritin is a common storage form of iron. Ferritin measures approximately 9 nm in diameter, which makes it substantially smaller than a ribosome. It is often found in iron-rich dense bodies referred to as **telolysosomes**. The term **siderosome** is used to refer to iron-saturated telolysosomes. Histologists refer to granular, iron-rich brown pigment as **hemosiderin**. Ferritin can be found in the macrophages of the spleen and bone marrow. The presence of ferritin in macrophages is indicative of the role these cells play in the recycling and storing of iron for hemoglobin synthesis (discussed in Chapter 5).

Nuclear Characteristics

Structure and Function

The overall average size of the nucleus is 10 to 15 μm. This structure, which is the largest organelle, functions as the control center of the cell and is essential for its long-term survival. The nucleus is surrounded by a nuclear envelope, which consists of an inner and an outer membrane with a gap between them of approximately 50 nm. The outer membrane is probably continuous at scattered points with the ER. Many large pores extend through this membrane envelope. The nuclear pores are usually bridged by a diaphragm that is more diffuse than a membrane and prevents materials from passing in and out freely.

Inside the nucleus, within the inner nucleoplasm, are the **nucleoli** (singular, nucleolus) and **chromatin**. Normally, the nucleus contains one or more small nucleoli that are not separated from the nucleoplasm by a specialized membrane. Morphologically, the nucleoli are irregularly shaped. Chemically, the nucleoli are composed mainly of RNA. Functionally, the nucleoli are the site of synthesis and processing of various species of ribosomal RNA. As the cell goes through various stages of growth and cellular division, the appearance of the nucleoli changes. These changes in the appearance are related to the rate of synthesis of ribosomal RNA.

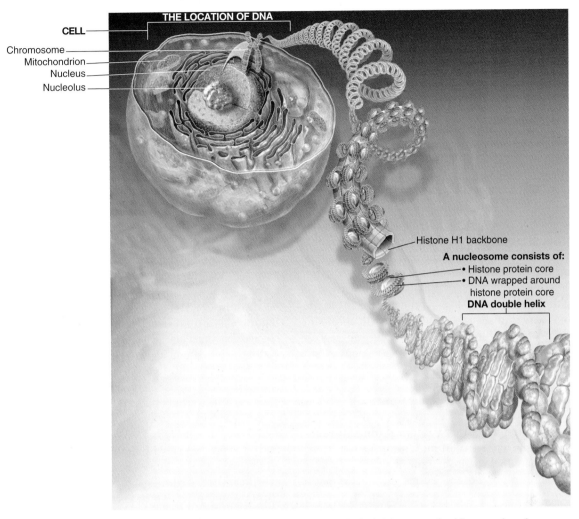

FIGURE 3.5 Understanding human DNA. The location of DNA (nucleolus); histone H1 backbone and nucleosome; DNA double helix. (Asset provided by Anatomical Chart Co.)

Chromatin Characteristics

The genetic material is composed of nucleic acids and protein (nucleoprotein), which is referred to as **chromatin** (Fig. 3.5). Despite the presence of protein in the chromatin, the DNA component stores genetic information. DNA has two functions:

1. To dictate the nature of proteins that can be synthesized, thereby controlling the function of the cell
2. To transmit information for cellular control from one generation to the next

Proteins associated with the nucleic acids are divided into basic, positively charged **histones** and less positively charged **nonhistones**. The histones are believed to be essential to the structural integrity of chromatin. Histones may be important in facilitating the conversion of the thin chromatin fibers seen during interphase into the highly condensed chromosomes seen in mitosis. The nonhistone proteins are thought to play other roles, including genetic regulation. A general model of the organization of DNA and histones (Fig. 3.6) depicts a regular spacing arrangement. The complete unit, the **nucleosome**, consists of a string of DNA wrapped around a histone core.

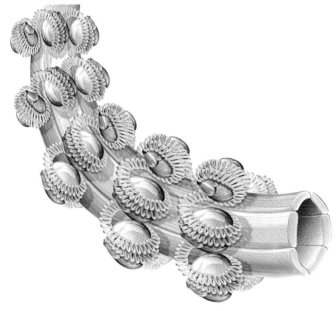

FIGURE 3.6 Understanding human DNA: DNA wrapped around histone protein. (Asset provided by Anatomical Chart Co.)

The chromatin arrangement within the nucleus demonstrates characteristic patterns when stained and viewed with a light microscope. These patterns are the most distinctive feature of a cell in terms of recognition of cell types and cell maturity. Chromatin is divided into two types: **euchromatin** (previously called parachromatin), the uncoiled, pale-staining areas, and, **heterochromatin** (previously called chromatin), the condensed, dark-staining areas.

Heterochromatin may be in patches or clumped toward the nuclear envelope in a thin rim. Small patches of heterochromatin may be associated with the nucleolus. **Chromatin in most primitive pluripotent stem cells, for example, embryonic stem cells, is in an open active state (euchromatin) and several genes are transcribed. During the cell differentiation process, the open type of euchromatin changes to the more condensed and genetically silent heterochromatin.** In general, the more restricted the function of a cell, the more predominant the heterochromatin. For example, in the maturation of an erythrocyte, the chromatin distribution is very diffuse in the young cells with abundant euchromatin. As the erythrocyte matures, dense aggregates of heterochromatin predominate before the nucleus is lost in the mature cell.

Several functional characteristics distinguish heterochromatin from euchromatin. Heterochromatin has a low expression level of chromatin-modifying factors, that is, epigenetic or chromatin plasticity. Heterochromatin replicates later during the S phase (described in the next section) of the cell cycle than does euchromatin. Labeled RNA shows that active transcription occurs within the euchromatin areas.

Chromosomes

The genetic material exists as diffuse elongated chromatin fibers during cellular interphase. However, during cellular division (mitosis), the individual strands condense into short visible structures, the **chromosomes.** The number of chromosomes in each cell is constant within each species. Humans have a complement of 46 chromosomes arranged into 23 pairs; one member of each pair is inherited from the father and the other from the mother. Each of the members of one chromosome pair is referred to as a chromosome homologue. Of the pairs, 22 are called autosomes; the remaining pair represents the sex chromosomes of which males have an X and a Y and females have two Xs.

The technique of staining cells to bring out the different parts more clearly was discovered around 1873. Basic dyes were used to stain the cells. The name chromosome was chosen because these structures showed the bright colors of the basic stain.

Chromosomes were first seen in human cells by Flemming in 1882; however, there were so many and they were so small that he could not accurately estimate the actual number. As a result of the squash technique developed in 1956, the entire chromosome complement of a cell can be spread out and flattened so that each chromosome can be seen clearly. Cells for chromosome studies can be taken from any area of the body including the bone marrow, circulating blood, and amniotic fluid. Most studies use leukocytes (white blood cells). Tissue culture technique allows these cells to be placed in a nutrient medium and stimulated to grow and divide very rapidly. Normally, mature blood cells do not divide, but the addition of a **mitogen**, such as colchicine, stimulates cell division in white blood cells of the lymphocyte type. Other cells such as red blood cells cannot divide. The cell selected for chromosome analysis is usually in the metaphase stage of cellular division.

In 1961, the Denver system of identifying human chromosomes was established. Chromosome pairs were numbered according to relative size and the position of their centromeres (the constricted area of a chromosome) and placed in groups according to letters. This arrangement of chromosome constitutes a **karyotype.** Differential staining of chromosomes (Fig. 3.7) using newer cytological techniques was introduced in the early 1970s. These methods, **chromosome banding techniques**, provide more information about the individual identity of chromosomes than previous methods. If chromosome preparations are denatured with heat and treated with Giemsa stain, a unique staining pattern emerges. The staining pattern with this technique is referred to as **C-banding.** Other banding techniques include fluorescent dyes that bind to nucleoprotein complexes. When chromosomes are treated with fluorochrome quinacrine mustard and viewed with a fluorescent microscope, precise patterns of differential brightness are seen. Each of the 23 human chromosome pairs can be distinguished by this technique; the bands produced are called **Q-bands.** Another technique that produces patterns similar to Q-bands involves the digestion of chromosomes with the enzyme trypsin, followed by Giemsa staining, that produces **G-bands** (Fig. 3.8). Chromosome analysis is being performed today by use of a laser technology (discussed in Chapter 27) that generates chromosome histograms.

The study of individual karyotypes and chromosome banding patterns is important to hematologists and geneticists. Supplementary information on hematological disorders, such as leukemias (discussed in Chapters 19 and 21), can aid in establishing a diagnosis and can provide information about the probable outcome (**prognosis**) in some cases.

Chromosomal Alterations

Chromosomes sometimes break, and a portion may be lost or attached to another chromosome. Deletion and translocation are the terms used to describe these conditions. **Deletion** is defined as the loss of a segment of chromosome. **Translocation** is the process in which a segment of one chromosome breaks away (is deleted) from its normal location. Translocation can happen frequently between homologous chromosomes while they are paired in meiosis (discussed in the next section). An abnormality or aberration can result when

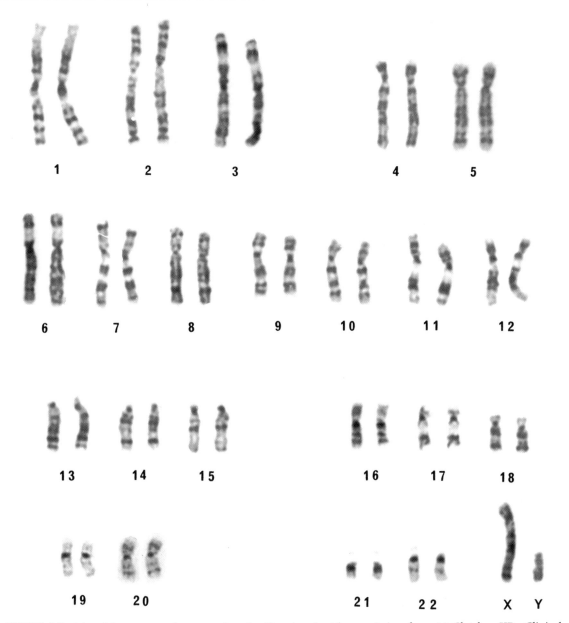

FIGURE 3.7 G-band karyotype of a normal male. (Reprinted with permission from McClatchey KD. *Clinical Laboratory Medicine*, 2nd ed, Philadelphia, PA: Lippincott Williams & Wilkins, 2002.)

the detached portion is lost or reattached. The Philadelphia chromosome, the first chromosomal abnormality discovered in a malignant disorder, is an example of a translocation from chromosome 22 to chromosome 9.

Trisomy is another abnormality of chromosomes that is of interest to hematologists. In trisomy, one of the homologous chromosomes fails to separate from its sister chromatid. This failure to separate leads to a set of three chromosomes in place of the normal pair. Trisomy is encountered in a variety of hematological malignancies.

Clinical Use of Cytogenetics

Clinical cytogenetics contributes to understanding inborn or acquired genetic problems by providing a low-power screening method for detecting isolated or missing chunks of chromosomes. The human genome consists of 3×10^9 base pairs (bp) of DNA distributed among 46 chromosomes. This genome contains at least 100,000 (and possibly as many as 1 million) genes, with gene sizes ranging from a few thousand to several hundred thousand base pairs. The resolution limit precludes microscopic recognition of genome regions smaller than 2 to 3 million bp, chromosome stretches sufficient to accommodate about 50 to 100 genes. In contrast, gene probing procedures are capable of discerning differences as small as 10 to 50 bp in fragments of individual cloned genes. The strength of cytogenetics is not in characterizing gene structure but in its utility in locating major rearrangements, which can then be characterized at the gene level by methods for DNA analysis.

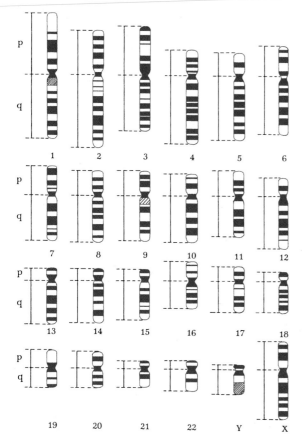

FIGURE 3.8 Chromosome banding. After the chromosomes are stained with Giemsa stain, the areas of the chromosomes referred to as G-bands can be seen. The p (*upper portion*) and q (*lower portion*) are easily visible.

Activities of the Nucleus

Mitosis

Mitosis (Fig. 3.9) is the process of replication in nucleated body cells (except ova and sperm cells). Cellular replication, or mitotic division, results in the formation of two identical daughter cells because the genes are duplicated and exactly segregated before each cell division. Originally, only two phases were recognized in mitosis: a resting phase or **interphase** (the period of time between mitoses) and **M phase** (the phase of actual cell division).

Mitosis, particularly the interphase period in bone marrow cells, is important to hematologists because special staining and flow cytometry techniques (discussed in Chapter 26) now make it possible to perform DNA cell cycle analysis in these cells. This type of analysis is useful in the treatment of various hematological disorders because the optimum time for the administration of chemotherapeutic drugs can be determined.

Interphase

Since the introduction of isotope techniques, it has been documented that in cells capable of reproduction, DNA is replicated or doubled during the interphase. Interphase is

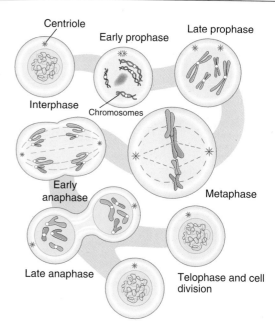

FIGURE 3.9 Cell mitosis. (*LifeART Super Anatomy Collection 2, CD-ROM*, Baltimore, MD: Lippincott Williams & Wilkins.). SA202029.

now divided into three subphases (see Fig. 3.9): G_1, first gap; S phase; and G_2, second gap. Under normal conditions, the amount of time that a cell spends in interphase is relatively constant for specific cell types.

1. The G_1 subphase lasts for approximately 6 to 8 hours. During this period, the nucleolus (nucleoli) becomes visible, and the chromosomes are extended and active metabolically. The cell synthesizes RNA and protein in preparation for cell division. As the G_1 period ends, cellular metabolic activity slows.

2. The S subphase lasts for approximately 6 hours. This is the time of DNA replication, during which both growth and metabolic activities are minimal. However, all metabolic activities do not stop because not all the DNA is replicated at the same time. The shorter chromosomes are replicated first, and the others follow according to their length. Some DNA strands complete replication and resume the output of their messages while others are still replicating. The protein portion of the chromosome is also duplicated, so that at the end of the S stage, each chromosome homologue has doubled but is held together by a single centromere (Box 3.1).

3. The G_2 phase is relatively short, lasting approximately 4 to 5 hours. This is the second period of growth, when the DNA can again function to its maximum in the synthesis of RNA and proteins in preparation for mitotic division. By the time a cell is ready to enter into mitotic division, proteins have been constructed in preparation for cell division, and both the DNA and the RNA are doubled. The centrioles have divided, forming a pair of new centrioles at right angles to each other.

BOX 3.1

Summary of DNA Structure and Activities

■ A single strand of DNA is composed of a chain of phosphorylated deoxyribose sugars, each attached to a purine (adenine or guanine) or pyrimidine (cytosine or thymine) base to form nucleotides. The sugars are bonded together between the OH (hydroxyl) group of the 3′ carbon at one end and the PO_4 group on the 5′ carbon of the next group. Every strand has a free 5′ phosphate on one end and a free 3′ hydroxyl on the other. This configuration results in a structural direction or polarity on each strand.

■ Each strand of DNA is arranged in a linear sequence consisting of any of the four nucleotide bases (adenine, thymine, cytosine, and guanine). These nucleotide bases come in close contact with the complementary nucleotide bases on the opposite strand of the two DNA strands, the double helix.

■ Hydrogen bonding produces interstrand pairing of complementary bases (adenine with thymine; cytosine with guanine). Two hydrogen bonds exist between adenine and thymine; three hydrogen bonds exist between cytosine and guanine.

■ The two strands of a DNA double helix run in opposite directions with the beginning 3′ carbon on one strand across from a free 5′ carbon on the opposing strand. This configuration is referred to as antiparallel.

■ DNA synthesis in vivo and in vitro is unidirectional, proceeding from the 5′ to 3′ end with growth of the new strand only at the 3′ end.

The Four Phases of Mitotic Division

The **M phase** is the period of actual cell division, which lasts from 30 to 60 minutes; however, not all human body cells duplicate at this rate. The rate is most rapid in the early embryo, with a progressive slowing throughout the rest of the fetal life and childhood. In adults, most cells undergo mitotic division only fast enough to replace cells, with the eventual loss in old age of many types of cells. Abnormal conditions (malignancies) can alter the rate of mitosis of particular cell lines during any stage of growth and development.

During mitosis, the replicated DNA and other cellular contents are equally distributed between the daughter cells. The four mitotic periods are prophase, metaphase, anaphase, and telophase (Box 3.2). Each state is visible in stained preparations by use of a conventional light microscope.

Prophase. In this stage of mitosis, the replicated strands of chromatin become tightly coiled, distinctive structures. The identical halves, referred to as **chromatids**, are joined at the centromere. The nucleolus and nuclear envelope disintegrate, with the fragments scattering in the

BOX 3.2

Characteristics of the Four Mitotic Periods

PROPHASE
The chromatin becomes tightly coiled.
Nucleolus and nuclear envelope disintegrate.
Centrioles move to opposite poles of the cell.

METAPHASE
Sister chromatids move to the equatorial plate.

ANAPHASE
Sister chromatids separate and move to opposite poles.

TELOPHASE
Chromosomes arrive at opposite poles.
Nucleolus and nuclear membrane reappear.
The chromatin pattern reappears.

cytoplasm. The centrioles, composed of microtubules, separate and migrate to the opposite poles of the cell. The microtubules aggregate to form the mitotic spindle that is attached to the centrioles.

Metaphase. During metaphase, the identical sister chromatids move to the center of the spindle (the equatorial plate). Each of the chromatid pairs is attached to a spindle fiber and aligned along the equator of the cell. The point of attachment is the centromere, a constriction that divides the chromatid into an upper and a lower portion.

Anaphase. This phase begins as soon as the chromatids are pulled apart and lasts until the newly formed chromosomes reach the opposite poles of the spindle. In this phase, the chromatid pairs are separated, with one half of each pair being pulled at their centromere by the spindle fibers toward each pole. Which half goes to which pole is random. Chromatids become chromosomes only after they have separated at the beginning of anaphase.

Telophase. The chromosomes arrive at opposite poles of the cell in early telophase. One of each kind of chromosome arrives at each of the poles of the cell. The nucleolus and nuclear membrane reappear and the spindle fibers disappear during this phase. Because the chromosomes uncoil and become longer and thinner, the chromosome structural formations disappear. The DNA and proteins (nucleoproteins) now assume their distinctive chromatin arrangement.

Following the stages that constitute nuclear division (**karyokinesis**), the cell undergoes cytokinesis. **Cytokinesis** is the division of cytoplasm. The cytoplasm around the two new nuclei becomes furrowed, and the cytoplasmic membrane pinches in. This pinching in is accomplished by the contraction of a ring of microfilaments that forms at the furrow. At the completion of cytokinesis, two new and identical daughter cells have been formed.

G$_0$ Phase

Following the M phase, some cells continue through the mitotic cycle repeatedly, but others lose their mitotic ability and enter a protracted state of mitotic inactivity, the G$_0$ phase. In some cases, cells will be stimulated by factors such as hormones (refer to Chapter 5 for a discussion of the hormone erythropoietin in the production of erythrocytes) to reenter the mitotic cycle. Abnormal proliferation of cells may result from overstimulation by extrinsic or intrinsic factors. Other nucleated cells, such as nerve cells, lose their ability to undergo mitosis and remain in the G$_0$ (zero growth) phase permanently.

Apoptosis

Apoptosis is referred to as programmed cell death. In multicellular organisms, homeostasis is maintained through a balance between cell proliferation (mitosis) and cell death (apoptosis).

During embryonic development, excess numbers of developing cells die; in hormone-responsive tissues (e.g., uterus), cyclical depletion of a particular hormone leads to death. In both of these situations, cell death occurs by the process of apoptosis.

Apoptosis can be influenced by a wide variety of regulatory stimuli. Cell survival appears to depend on the constant supply of survival signals provided by neighboring cells and the extracellular matrix. Inducers of apoptosis include the cytokines (e.g., tumor necrosis factor [TNF] family). A delicate balance between proapoptotic and antiapoptotic regulars of apoptosis pathways is at play on a continual basis, ensuring the survival of long-lived cells and the proper turnover of short-lived cells in various tissues, including the bone marrow, thymus and peripheral lymphoid tissues.

Apoptosis is caused by the activation of intracellular proteases, known as caspases. Two pathways of apoptosis exist: intrinsic and extrinisic. The intrinsic pathway focuses on mitochondria as initiators of cell death. In contrast, extrinsic apoptosis relies on TNF family death receptors for triggering apoptosis. In certain types of cells, these systems converge.

Cell death can be either physiologic or pathological Physiologic cell death in animals generally occurs through the mechanism of apoptosis. Apoptosis is characterized by chromatin condensation and fragmentation, cell shrinkage, and elimination of dead cells by phagocytosis. By comparison, necrotic cell death is a pathologic form of cell death resulting from acute cellular injury, which is characterized by rapid cell swelling and lysis.

Bcl-2 was the first antideath gene discovered. Since its discovery, multiple members of the human Bcl-2 family of apoptosis-regulating proteins have been identified. Bcl-2 family proteins regulate all major types of cell death, including apoptosis and necrosis.

Alterations in cell survival contribute to the pathogenesis of a number of human diseases (e.g., cancer). Certain diseases are associated with the inhibition of apoptosis; other diseases are associated with increased apoptosis. Programmed cell death plays a key role in controlling the size of the lymphocyte pool at many stages of lymphocyte maturation and activation. If lymphocytes never encounter an antigen after cellular maturation, they die by the process of apoptosis.

Meiosis

Meiosis (Fig. 3.10) is the process of cell division unique to **gametes** (ova and sperm). In contrast to mitosis, the process of meiosis produces four gametes with genetic variability. Gametes have *only* one of the homologues of each of the 23 pairs of chromosomes (the haploid [1n] number). Other nucleated human body cells contain 23 homologous pairs of chromosomes (the diploid [2n] number).

The phases of meiosis differ from mitosis in several important ways. During phase I of meiosis, the homologous sister chromatids in a tetrad formation undergo the process of **synapsis**, lining up end-to-end. Synapsis allows for the easy exchange of genetic material through **crossing over**. In phase II of meiosis, reduction division occurs, producing the haploid number in the resulting gametes.

The Foundations of Genetic Interactions

Genetics, the study of the transmission of inherited characteristics, is related to meiosis and is important in the study of inherited hematological disorders. During the past 30 years, a revolution has occurred in our understanding of genetic diseases. The identification of single-gene disorders is proceeding at an exponential rate. More than 200 human genes have been cloned, and the chromosomal map location is known for more than 140 of these genes. More than 100 genes are known to be associated with one or more diseases. The hemoglobinopathies and thalassemias (discussed in Chapter 13) have been extensively studied at the DNA level. Today, leukemias are being classified and treated at the molecular level. Information is also rapidly emerging about alterations in genes for factors VIII:C and IX of the coagulation system.

In 1953, Watson and Crick described the double-helix model of DNA in which genetic information is encoded into linear arrays in the form of the deoxyribonucleotide bases adenine (A), thymine (T), cytosine (C), and guanine (G). The two strands of DNA have antiparallel complementary sequences that pair by hydrogen bonding between the bases; thymine pairs with adenine, and cytosine with guanine. The genetic code, which stores hereditary information, is stored as triplets of nucleotides that encode for various amino acids. Genomes of different organisms are unique and distinguishable from one another. The human genome consists of double-stranded DNA (ds-DNA) molecules organized into chromosomes with cell nuclei. Most human DNA is in the right-handed beta configuration having 10.5 bp per helical turn.

A **gene** is a segment of DNA that is arranged along the chromosome at a specific position called a **locus**. Genes at a specific locus that differ in their nucleotide sequence are called **alleles**. Thus, in each somatic cell, one of the members of a set of alleles is maternally derived and the other paternally derived. Genes that lie close to each other in the linear array along the chromosomes have less opportunity for

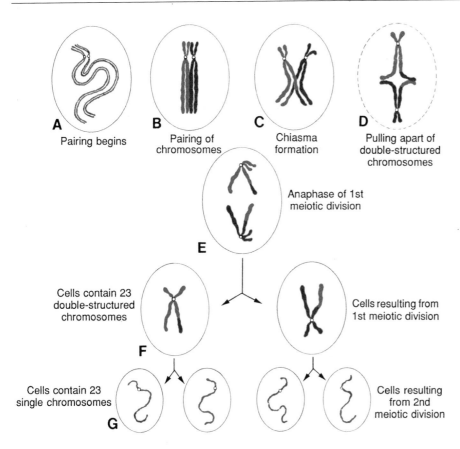

FIGURE 3.10 First and second meiotic divisions. **A:** Homologous chromosomes approach each other. **B:** Homologous chromosomes pair, and each member of the pair consists of two chromatids. **C:** Intimately paired homologous chromosomes interchange chromatid fragments (crossover). Note the chiasma. **D:** Double-structured chromosomes pull apart. **E:** Anaphase of the first meiotic division. **F, G:** During the second meiotic division, the double-structured chromosomes split at the centromere. At completion of division, chromosomes in each of the four daughter cells are different from each other. (Reprinted with permission from Sadler T. *Langman's Medical Embryology*, 9th ed, Baltimore, MD: Lippincott Williams & Wilkins, 2003.)

crossing over; genes that recombine once in every 100 meiotic opportunities are said to be 1 centimorgan (cM) apart. The relationship between the linear proximity of genetic loci and the recombinational frequency between them provides the basis for linkage mapping. However, this relationship is not always linear. Particular segments of DNA seem to be recombination hotspots and are predisposed to crossing over much more often than would be predicted from their DNA lengths.

Each gene has a unique sequence of nucleotides that is transcribed into mRNA. It is the sequence of nucleotides that determines gene function. In most cases, the coding sequences, or **exons**, are interrupted by intervening sequences, or **introns**. The entire gene, including both exons and introns, is transcribed in a pre-mRNA; however, the exon sequences are ultimately translated on the ribosomes into protein, but the intron sequences are spliced out as the pre-mRNA is processed into mature RNA. The sequences at the intron-exon junctions, called splices, are critical for mRNA processing and are important potential sites of mutation.

Genetic Alterations

A gene, as the functional unit of a chromosome, is responsible for determining the structure of a single protein or polypeptide. Normally, a gene is a very stable unit that undergoes thousands of replications, with perfect copies resulting each time. On rare occasions, a copy may be produced that varies slightly and leads to an alteration in transcription from

the long DNA molecule, with far-reaching consequences. A change in the gene is caused by **mutation** producing a change in the actual structure of DNA. A single-nucleotide change among the thousands of base pairs in a gene may have crucial consequences to the gene product. An example of such a gene alteration has been traced to Queen Victoria or one of her immediate ancestors; the alteration led to classic hemophilia (discussed in Chapter 24) that spread throughout the royal families of Europe.

Mutations usually affect a single base in the DNA. The sequence of nucleotide bases in the DNA is altered by the substitution of a single different base at one point along the DNA molecule. These mutations may act by affecting transcription of the gene, RNA processing to produce the mature mRNA, or translation of the mRNA into protein; or they may act by altering an important amino acid in the protein products.

The sickle cell mutation (Fig. 3.11) is the best known example of a single-nucleotide alteration. Human hemoglobin was one of the first proteins for which the genetic code was worked out and is a good example of the relationship between genes and proteins. The normal adult hemoglobin molecule (discussed in Chapter 5) consists in part of the protein globin. Globin is arranged into four chains in the form of two identical pairs. In each pair, the alpha chain consists of 141 amino acids and the beta chain contains 146 amino acids. The laboratory procedures of electrophoresis and chromatography allow determination of the exact sequence of amino acids on each of these two chains. In the case of sickle cell disease, hemoglobin S has a difference in one amino acid on

FIGURE 3.11 Sickle cell trait and anemia. When two persons with sickle cell trait (genotype: A/S) produce offspring, the expected genotypic ratio is 1:2:1, or a 25% chance of offspring with a normal hemoglobin (A/A), a 50% chance of offspring with sickle cell trait (A/S), and a 25% chance of offspring with sickle cell anemia (S/S). *Hgb*, hemoglobin.

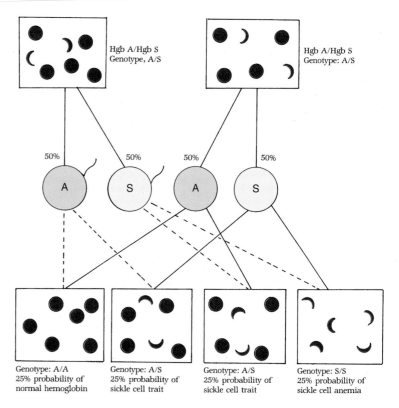

the beta chain (Fig. 3.12). On this chain, valine is substituted for glutamic acid at the sixth position on the chain because an A in the sixth codon is changed to a T; this changes the codon GAG (glutamic acid) to GTG (valine). In hemoglobin C disorder, a substitution of lysine for glutamic acid at the same position in the beta chain occurs.

Through meiosis, a parent with the trait may pass the mutation to another generation. In the case of sickle cell disease (anemia), an individual is *homozygous* for the trait. Because in the genetic expression of this disorder a lack of dominance exists, both genes of an allelic pair are partially and about equally expressed. Those individuals who are heterozygous for the trait are designated as suffering from sickle cell trait. The mode of inheritance of hemoglobin S is depicted in Figure 3.13. A further discussion of abnormal hemoglobins is presented in Chapter 13.

Linkage studies can be used for those families in which the precise mutation is unknown but the locus of the mutation is known, such as in the hemoglobinopathies. Linkage

analysis has proved highly useful as an indirect method of distinguishing between chromosomes carrying normal and mutant alleles. These polymorphisms represent so-called neutral mutations. Indirect analysis of this type has been used in the prenatal diagnosis of beta-thalassemia (see Chapter 13) and is available for hemophilia A. At the present time, prenatal diagnosis by DNA analysis is available for several hematological disorders including hemophilia A, hemophilia B, sickle cell disease, alpha-thalassemia, and beta-thalassemia.

Oncogenes

Cancer including leukemias and lymphomas is caused by alteration in oncogenes, tumor-suppressor genes, and microRNA genes. These alterations are usually somatic cell events but germ-line mutations can predispose a person to inherited or familial cancer. A single genetic change is rarely enough for the development of a malignancy. Most evidence suggests a multistep process of sequential alteration in several, often many, oncogenes, tumor-suppressor genes, or microRNA genes in the affected cells.

The first evidence that cancer arises from somatic genetic alterations came from studies of Burkitt lymphoma where one of three different translocations juxtaposes an oncogene, MYC, on chromosome 8q24 to one of the loci for immunoglobulin (Ig) genes. In chronic myelogenous leukemia (CML), which is initiated by a reciprocal to t(9;22) chromosomal translocation that fuses the ABL protooncogene to the BCR gene. The fusion gene encodes an oncogenic ABL fusion protein with enhanced tyrosine kinase activity. All leukemic cells in CML carry this chromosomal alteration.

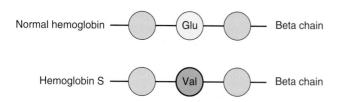

FIGURE 3.12 Hemoglobin S amino acid sequence. Hemoglobin S differs from hemoglobin A in one amino acid residue on the beta chain of the hemoglobin molecule. On this chain, valine (Val) is substituted for glutamic acid (Glu) at the sixth position of the chain.

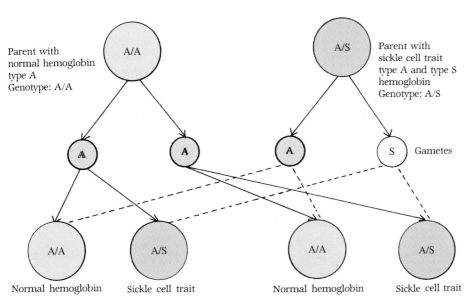

FIGURE 3.13 Inheritance of hemoglobin S.

Offspring probabilities are 50% normal hemoglobin A/A and 50% hemoglobin A and S (sickle cell trait)

Tumor protein, p53

p53, also known as protein 53 or tumor protein 53, is a transcription factor, encoded by the TP53 gene. p53 is described as the guardian of the genome because it conserves stability by preventing genome mutations.

p53 gene is important in regulation of the cell cycle and functions as a tumor suppressor. p53 can activate the repair of DNA when damaged, can hold the cell cycle at the G_1/S regulation point until DNA can be repaired and continue in the cell cycle, and can initiate apoptosis if DNA damage is beyond repair. Hematologic malignancies demonstrating a specific genetic alteration of p53 include acute myeloid leukemia, chronic lymphocytic leukemia, chronic myelogenous leukemia, myelodysplastic syndrome, and non-Hodgkin lymphoma.

Molecular Techniques in Hematology

The techniques of molecular biology are now being applied to hematology (Box 3.3). Since the inception of research on the Human Genome Project, molecular biology has a high profile in the field or medicine (see Box 3.4) with applications to the study of cancer and aging research. Single nucleotide polymorphisms (SNPs) comprise the most abundant source of genetic variation in the human genome. Since the decoding of the human genome and the resulting greater than 3 million SNPs, laboratory techniques have been able to associate disease states and pharmacological responses with individual SNPs.

Molecular genetic testing focuses on examination of nucleic acids (DNA or RNA) by special techniques to determine if a specific nucleotide base sequence is present. Applications of nucleic acid testing have expanded, despite higher costs associated with testing, in various areas of the clinical laboratory, including hematology (hematopathology) (see Box 3.5). The distinct advantages of molecular testing include greater accuracy in diagnosis, faster turnaround time, smaller required sample volumes, and increased specificity

and sensitivity in the detection of minimal residual disease after treatment for cancer.

Minimal Residual Disease

Minimal residual disease (MRD) is defined as the low level of disease, for example, leukemic cells, in a patient who appears to be in a state of clinical remission. In leukemia, the cells resistant to therapy remain in the bone marrow and/or peripheral blood. Following treatment, one million or more leukemic cells may persist, even when the residual leukemic cells are undetectable and the patient appears to

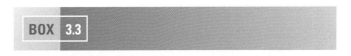

BOX 3.3

Common Molecular Techniques Used in the Clinical Laboratory

POLYMERASE CHAIN REACTION (PCR)
Reverse transcription PCR (RT-PCR)
Real-time PCR

LIGASE CHAIN REACTION NUCLEIC ACID AMPLIFICATION (LCR)

BRANCHED DNA (BDNA) AMPLIFICATION

PROBE-HYBRIDIZATION ASSAYS
Restriction fragment analysis with Southern blot hybridization
Liquid-phase hybridization (LPH)
In situ hybridization, including fluorescent ISH (FISH)

INTEGRATED PCR AND PROBE-HYBRIDIZATION ASSAYS

MICROARRAYS

2009 Nobel Prizes[a]

The 2009 Nobel Prize in medicine was awarded to Americans Elizabeth Blackburn, Carol Greider, and Jack Szostak. This trio of scientists has added a new dimension to understanding the cell, shedding light on disease mechanisms and stimulating the development of potential new therapies. They solved the mystery of how chromosomes can be copied in a complete way during cell divisions and how they are protected against degradation. The laureates have shown that the solution is to be found in the ends of the chromosomes—the telomeres—and in an enzyme that forms them. Telomeres are often compared to the plastic tips at the end of shoe laces that keep those laces from unraveling.

The 2009 Nobel Prize in chemistry belongs to Americans Venkatraman Ramakrishnan and Thomas Steitz and Israel's Ada Yonath—the first woman to receive it since 1964. This team of scientists created a detailed blueprints of ribosomes, the protein-making machinery within cells. This research is being used to develop new antibiotics.

[a]The Nobel Prize was established by Alfred Nobel, the Swedish scientist who invented dynamite.

be in complete molecular remission (CMR). CMR can be further defined as the failure to detect cancer cells by the most sensitive molecular methodology available and by being valid only when leukemic cells are undetectable in three sequential samples 1 month apart.

Molecular techniques, for example, PCR, real-time quantitative PCR (RQ-PCR), flow cytometry, and cytogenetic marker studies, are more sensitive to a low number of cells than morphologic appearance in the peripheral blood. PCR is able to detect one malignant cell in a population of 1 million cells.

Examples of Inherited Molecular Hematologic Disorders

HEMOGLOBINOPATHIES
Sickle cell anemia
Hemoglobin C, SC, E, or D disease
Thalassemias (α-thalassemia, β-thalassemia)

COAGULOPATHIES
Hemophilia (factor VIII, factor IX deficiencies)
Factor V Leiden

Molecular techniques permit early detection of leukemia relapse at subclinical levels, allow for early clinical intervention, perhaps before early progenitor cells, including CD34[+] cells, acquire genetic lesions that increase the aggressiveness of the clone.

In the past, molecular detection and monitoring of patients with chronic myeloid leukemia patients have been successful. Now, the current state of the art and development of molecular techniques in other leukemias, for example, childhood acute lymphoblastic leukemia (ALL), are of growing interest. Tumor load, type of leukemia, whether disease specific marker is identifiable, and technological limits will determine the optimum methodology for monitoring MRD.

Molecular Studies

PCR has been developed to detect and measure DNA sequences of interest. More recently, mRNA studies using reverse transcription PCR (RT-PCR) have become widespread.

Polymerase Chain Reaction

PCR is an in vitro method that amplifies low levels of specific DNA sequences in a sample to higher quantities suitable for further analysis. The three important applications of PCR are

1. Amplification of DNA
2. Identification of a target sequence
3. Synthesis of a labeled antisense probe

PCR is unrivaled as a means for direct cloning and gene sequence analysis. The first diagnostic application of PCR technology was in prenatal diagnosis of sickle cell anemia through amplification of beta globin sequences. PCR has become increasingly popular for detecting chromosomal breakpoints, fusion genes, and MRD after chemotherapy for leukemia and lymphoma.

To use this technology, the target sequence to be amplified must be known. Typically, a target sequence ranges from 100 to 1,000 base pairs in length. Two short DNA "primers" that are typically 16 to 20 base pairs in length are used. Namely, the oligonucleotides (small portions of a single DNA strand) act as a template for the new DNA. These primer sequences are complementary to the 3' ends of the sequence to be amplified. This enzymatic process is carried out in cycles (Figs. 3.14 and 3.15).

Each cycle theoretically doubles the amount of specific DNA sequence present and results in an exponential accumulation of the DNA fragment being amplified (amplicons) (Table 3.1). In general, this process is repeated approximately 30 times. At the end of 30 cycles, the reaction mixture should contain approximately 2^{30} molecules of the desired product. After cycling is completed, the amplification products can be examined in various ways. Typically, the contents of the reaction vessel are subjected to gel electrophoresis. This allows visualization of the amplified gene segments (e.g., PCR products, bands) and a determination of their specificity. Additional product analysis by probe hybridization or direct DNA sequencing is often performed to further verify the authenticity of the amplicon.

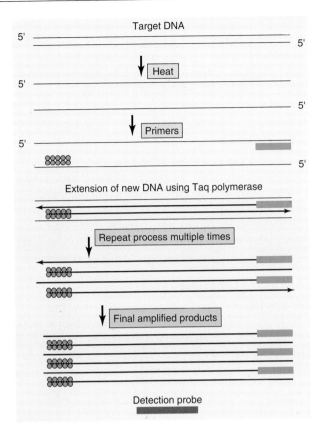

FIGURE 3.14 The PCR is depicted. The target DNA is first melted using heat (generally around 94°C) to separate the strands of DNA. Primers that recognize specific sequences within the target DNA are allowed to bind as the reaction cools. Using a unique, thermo-stable DNA polymerase called Taq and an abundance of deoxynucleoside triphosphates, new DNA strands are amplified from the point of the primer attachment. The process is repeated many times (called cycles) until millions of copies of DNA are produced, all of which have the same length defined by the distance (in base pairs) between the primer binding sites. These copies are then detected by electrophoresis and staining or through the use of labeled DNA probes that, similar to the primers, recognize a specific sequence located within the amplified section of DNA. (Reprinted with permission from Carrol Mattson Porlts, *Pathophysiology concepts of Altered Health States*, Seventh edition, Philadelphia: Lippincott Williams & Wilkins, 2005.)

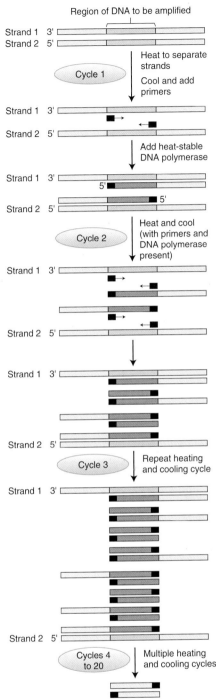

FIGURE 3.15 Polymerase chain reaction (PCR). (Reprinted with permission from Wilcox BR. *High-Yield Biochemistry*, Baltimore, MD: Lippincott Williams & Wilkins, 1999.)

Nested Primers

Adaptations of the PCR technique have been developed. One adaptation uses nested primers. This adaptation uses a two-step amplification process. In the first step, a broad region of the DNA surrounding the sequence of interest is amplified. This is followed by a second round of amplification to amplify the specific gene sequence to be studied. Another recent modification of the PCR technique has been used successfully to differentiate alleles of the same gene.

Real-Time PCR

Another method based on PCR is real-time PCR (RT-PCR). RT-PCR detects RNA from viable cells and thus targets genes expressed that are likely to have functional role, directly or indirectly, in cellular proliferation. The application of this technique is in the quantitation of specific DNA sequences of interest and for identification of point mutations.

This PCR variation uses fluorescence resonance energy transfer (FRET). This PCR variation is particularly appealing because the procedure is less susceptible to amplicon contamination and is more accurate in quantifying the initial copy number.

TABLE 3.1 PCR Amplification[a]	
Number of Cyclesh	**Number of DNA**
1	2
2	4
3	8
4	16
5	32
10	1024
20	>1,000,000

[a]The number of copies of a specific DNA sequence doubles with each amplification. PCR usually consists of a series of 20 to 40 repeated temperature changes called cycles; each cycle typically consists of 2 to 3 discrete temperature steps. Most commonly, PCR is carried out with cycles that have three temperature steps. The temperatures used and the length of time they are applied in each cycle depend on a variety of parameters. These include the enzyme used for DNA synthesis, the concentration of divalent ions and dNTPs in the reaction, and the melting temperature (Tm) of the primers. PCR may reach a plateau with no more copies produced because of reagent limitations, inhibitors, etc.

Real-time quantitative PCR (RQ-PCR or Q-PCR)

Quantification of specific sequences of DNA has been greatly simplified by real-time quantitative polymerase chain reaction (RQ-PCR or Q-PCR). In Q-PCR, the rate of accumulation of amplicons is proportional to the number of target transcripts in the starting material during the exponential phase of the PCR. This technique also offers increased specificity with the inclusion of the third reporter labeled oligonucleotide probe using hydrolysis-based technology, which anneals between forward and reverse primers. Hydrolysis is one of many methods now available for detection and quantification of target sequences.

A sensitivity of 1×10^{-5} is achievable by Q-PCR but contamination is a major concern and hence strict working practices must be adhered to; for example, RNA extraction, cDNA synthesis, and post PCR analysis must be geographically separated. Equally, false negatives due to a lack of mRNA or suboptimum integrity of mRNA and/or cDNA must be controlled for. This is achieved by concomitantly measuring one of the ubiquitously expressed housekeeping genes, for example, *ABL1*, *BCR*.

Consensus primer PCR and allele specific oligonucleotide PCR (ASO-PCR)

Consensus primer PCR and allele specific oligonucleotide PCR (ASO-PCR) are the two Ig PCR strategies for MRD studies. ASO-PCR utilizes primers designed to anneal to a unique patient-specific Ig sequence and subsequently is used to monitor sequential samples in follow-up studies. This qualitative method has a sensitivity of 1×10^{-2} to 1×10^{-4}.

ASO-PCR significantly improves the sensitivity of MRD studies, but ASO-PCR is time-consuming and expensive. Combination of ASO primers and consensus oligonucleotide probes make it accessible to Q-PCR, permitting precise quantification of MRD with a sensitivity of 1×10^{-4} to 1×10^{-5}.

Examples of Analysis of Amplification Products

DNA Sequencing

DNA sequencing is considered to be the "gold standard" method to which other molecular methods are compared. DNA sequencing displays the exact nucleotide or base sequence of a fragment of DNA that is targeted. The Sanger method, which uses a series of enzymatic reactions to produce segments of DNA complementary to the DNA being sequenced, is the most frequently used method for DNA sequencing.

Dot Blot and Reverse Dot Blot

These hybridization methods are used in the clinical laboratory for the detection of disorders in which the DNA sequence of the mutated region has been identified (e.g., sickle cell disease). These techniques are capable of distinguishing homozygous or heterozygous states for a mutation.

Dot Blot

Dot blot hybridization is a method used to detect single-base mutations using allele-specific oligonucleotides (ASOs). Unlike other assays, the dot blot does not require enzyme digestion or electrophoretic separation of DNA fragments. The procedure uses labeled oligonucleotide probes of approximately 15 to 19 bp. DNA is amplified in the region of a known mutation, denatured, and applied to separate areas of a membrane or filter. A probe designed to detect a normal DNA sequence is added to one area; a second probe for the detection of a sequence with the single-base mutation is applied to a second area. Ideally, only the labeled probe whose base sequences perfectly match those of the patient will hybridize.

Reverse Dot Blot

In this variation of the dot blot procedure, the ASO probes are bound to a filter, and denatured DNA from the patient is added to the immobilized ASO. Hybridization occurs only if the patient's DNA contains base sequences that are 100% complementary to those of the probe. A common variation of the reverse dot blot procedure is to bind oligonucleotide probes of a slightly longer length than in the reverse dot blot procedure to a 96-well microtiter plate. Biotin is used to label copies of the target sequence. The labeled copies are hybridized in the wells to the bound probes and detected using avidin conjugated to horseradish peroxidase. Subsequent addition of substrate produces a colored reaction that can be read photometrically.

Southern and Northern Blot Blotting Protocols

The Southern blot and Northern blot are used to detect DNA and RNA, respectively. These procedures share some common procedural steps: electrophoretic separation of the patient's nucleic acid, transfer of nucleic acid fragments to a solid support (e.g., nitrocellulose), hybridization with a labeled probe of known nucleic acid sequence, and autoradiographic or colorimetric detection of the bands created by the probe nucleic acid hybrid.

Southern Blot

Specimen DNA is denatured, treated with restriction enzymes to result in DNA fragments, and then the single-stranded DNA (ssDNA) fragments are separated by electrophoresis (Fig. 3.16). The electrophoretically separated fragments are then blotted to a nitrocellulose membrane, retaining their electrophoretic position and hybridized with radiolabeled ssDNA fragments with sequences complementary to those being sought. The resulting ds-DNA bearing the radiolabel is then, if present, detected by radiography.

The Southern blot procedure has clinical diagnostic applications for diseases or disorders associated with significant changes in DNA, a deletion or insertion of at least 50 to 100 bp (e.g., fragile X syndrome), or determination of clonality in lymphomas of T-cell or B-cell origin. If a single-base mutation changes an enzyme restriction site on the DNA resulting in an altered band or fragment size, the Southern blot procedure can be used to detect these changes in DNA sequences (referred to as restriction fragment length polymorphisms). Single-base mutations that can be determined by Southern blot include sickle cell disease and hemophilia A.

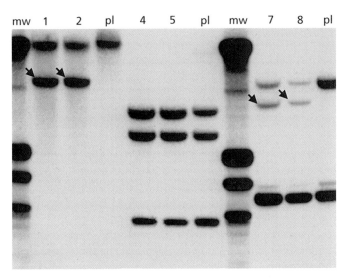

FIGURE 3.16 Southern blot detection of TCR gene rearrangement in a patient with peripheral T-cell lymphoma. Two separate lesions were investigated for evidence of a monoclonal T-cell population. Restriction digestion in the BamHI (1, 2) and EcoRI (7, 8) shows extra bands (*arrow*), which are not detected in the lane with DNA isolated from placenta (pl). Although HindIII digest (4, 5) shows no extra band, two rearranged bands detected by BamHI and EcoRI are sufficient to establish clonality. Because both lesions show similar banding pattern, these lesions are considered to be clonally identical. (Reprinted with permission from McClatchey KD. *Clinical Laboratory Medicine*, 2nd ed, Philadelphia, PA: Lippincott Williams & Wilkins, 2002.)

Northern Blot

This procedure is used for analysis of the proximal product of gene expression, mRNA. Cloned DNA probes can determine whether a given gene is expressed and, if so, how vigorously.

In Situ Hybridization

This is a tissue-based molecular diagnostic assay. Common in situ hybridization (ISH), including fluorescent in situ hybridization (FISH), probes are used in the diagnosis of hematological malignancies including CML, acute myelogenous leukemia (M3), Burkitt lymphoma, and other lymphomas (e.g., follicular lymphoma, mantle cell lymphoma, MALT lymphoma, and anaplastic large cell lymphoma).

Microarrays

Microarray (DNA chip) technologies are fast becoming routine tools for the high-throughput analysis of gene expression in a wide range of biological systems, including hematology.

Microarrays (Fig. 3.17) are basically the product of bonding or direct synthesis of numerous specific DNA probes on a stationary, often silicon-based, support. The chip may be tailored to particular disease processes. It is easily performed and readily automated.

Microarrays are miniature gene fragments attached to glass chips. These chips are used to examine gene activity of thousands or tens of thousands of gene fragments and to identify genetic mutations, using a hybridization reaction between the sequences on the microarray and a fluorescent sample. Following hybridization, the chips are scanned with high-speed fluorescent detectors and the intensity of each spot is quantitated. The identity and amount of each sequence are revealed by the location and intensity of fluorescence displayed by each spot. Computers are used to analyze the data. The applications of microarrays in clinical medicine include analysis of gene expression in malignancies (e.g., mutations in BRCA1), mutations of the tumor suppressor gene p53, genetic disease testing, and viral resistance mutation detection.

Hematopathology

The benefits of molecular techniques in hematopathology diagnosis and monitoring include:

■ Faster turnaround time
■ Smaller required sample volumes
■ Increased specificity and sensitivity

CML was the first human malignancy to be consistently associated with a chromosome abnormality (Table 3.2), the Philadelphia (Ph) chromosome. Today, molecular methods are used to identify changes ranging from a single chromosome disorder to alterations involving the interchange of DNA between chromosomes. Abnormalities of erythrocytes (sickle cell disease, and α- and β-thalassemias), leukocytes (acute myelogenous leukemia (AML), acute lymphoblastic

Microscope slide

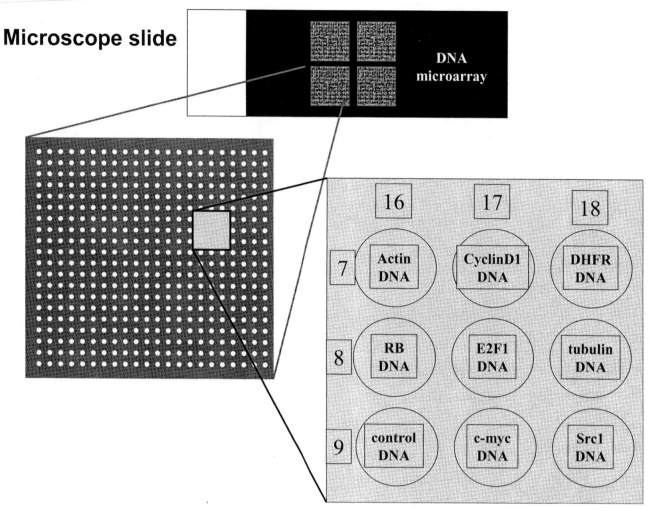

FIGURE 3.17 Gene expression profiling using microarray analysis. A solid surface (in this example, a glass micro-scope slide) contains thousands of spots. Each spot contains a large number of DNA fragments. For each spot, the DNA fragments are derived from one specific gene. (Courtesy of Ron Kerkhoven, Netherlands Cancer Institute, Amsterdam, The Netherlands.)

TABLE 3.2	Examples of Representative Chromosomal Translocations in Acute Leukemias

Type of Leukemia or Lymphoma	Translocation
Leukemias	
Acute myelogenous leukemia (M2)	t(8;21)
Acute myelogenous leukemia (M3)	t(15;17)
T-cell ALL	t(1;14) and variants
B-cell ALL	t(9;22)

leukemia (ALL), chronic myelogenous leukemia (CML), and lymphoma), and coagulation factors (hemophilia A, hemophilia B, and factor V Leiden defect) can be detected by molecular methods (Table 3.3).

Hematological malignancies were the first form of human cancer to be studied in depth at the molecular level. Investigation of the Philadelphia chromosome at the molecular level revealed a translocation-induced gene rearrangement involving the bcr and abl genes that results in activation of the abl cellular oncogene. FISH analysis is most commonly performed in the search for translocation (9;22) (bcr/abl), which is diagnostic of CML.

Cytogenetic, FISH, and other molecular genetic techniques can aid in establishing a diagnosis of a malignancy, for example, ALL, detecting blast transformation emerging from CML, or determining a patient's prognosis. In addition, molecular techniques provide a diagnostic tool for clinicians in order to

TABLE 3.3	Examples of Hematologic Disorders That are Detectable Using Molecular Diagnostics

Disorder

Hemoglobinopathies
  Sickle cell anemia
  β-Thalassemias
  α-Thalassemias
  α-Globin

Erythrocyte disorders
  Hereditary spherocytosis
  Hereditary elliptocytosis

Leukocyte disorders
  Chronic granulomatous disease
  Neutrophil NADPH oxidase

Lipid storage disorders
  Gaucher disease
  Niemann-Pick disease

Coagulopathies
  Factor V Leiden (inherited resistance to activated protein C [APC])

- Detect MRD in hematological malignancies
- Purge malignant cells (e.g., bcr-positive cells) from autologous bone marrow before infusion
- Monitor patients following bone marrow transplantation
- Discover an early relapse in patients treated for a hematological malignancy

Gene Rearrangement Studies

Gene rearrangement studies are important in diagnostic hematopathology as indicators of clonality and as aids in determining the cellular lineage of a particular malignant proliferation. Immunophenotyping categorizations are aided by the use of cluster designation (CD) for specific lineages of cells. CDs indicate a known cluster of monoclonal antibodies binding to a known antigen on the cell surface of hematopoietic cells.

Molecular diagnostic assays to detect heavy chain or kappa chain rearrangements are useful for establishing the diagnosis of B-cell neoplasms. T-cell receptor (TCR) beta, gamma, and delta rearrangements are useful in establishing the diagnosis of T-cell malignancies. The Ig and TCR gene rearrangements during normal B and T-lymphocyte development, respectively, generate unique fusions of variable, diversity, and joining (VDJ) segments, interspersed by random nucleotide (N) insertion and/or deletion. These B and T-clonal recombinations generate patient-specific DNA length and sequences which represent ideal molecular markers for detection and quantification of leukemic cells among normal lymphocytes in remission samples. Although it is sensitive, the technology is susceptible to false negatives due to clonal evolution during natural history of the disease; thus, some patients may relapse with a clone different to that observed at presentation.

CHAPTER HIGHLIGHTS

The Cell and Cellular Functions

Cells are the smallest organized units of a living organism. Cellular metabolism is responsible for the basic life processes within the human body. The cellular membrane has a variety of functions. These functions include cellular recognition and interaction between cells, osmosis, diffusion, active transport, and endocytosis. Endocytosis is important in defending the body against disease. The nucleus is a double-layered organelle containing both DNA in the form of chromatin and RNA in the nucleolus. The nucleus functions as the control center of the cell and is essential for its long-term survival. The RNA-containing nucleoli are contained within the nucleus. Both processes are important for the hematologist to understand because genetic errors can produce defective proteins, such as sickle cell hemoglobin.

Molecular Genetics in Hematology

Techniques in molecular genetics are beginning to be used extensively in hematology. A wide range of abnormalities can be detected with these techniques. PCR is an in vitro method that amplifies low levels of specific DNA sequences in a sample to higher quantities suitable for further analysis. PCR analysis can lead to the detection of gene mutations that signify the early development of cancer. Microarrays (DNA chips) are basically the product of bonding or direct synthesis of numerous specific DNA probes on a stationary, often silicon-based, support. Molecular biology provides new ways to establish a diagnosis, determine patient prognosis, and monitor disease.

REVIEW QUESTIONS

1. The smallest organized unit of living tissue is the
   A. nucleus
   B. cell
   C. organelle
   D. cytoplasm

2. The cell membrane's *major* components are
   A. carbohydrates and proteins
   B. proteins and lipids
   C. lipids and glycoproteins
   D. polysaccharides and lipids

3. Which of the following is a characteristic of osmosis?
   A. Requires energy (ATP)
   B. Movement of water molecules
   C. An unusual cellular activity
   D. Requires a carrier molecule

4. Which of the following is a characteristic of active transport?
   A. Requires energy (ATP)
   B. Movement of molecules up the concentration gradient
   C. Requires a carrier molecule
   D. All of the above

5. Phagocytosis is
   A. a type of endocytosis
   B. the engulfment of fluid molecules
   C. the engulfment of particulate matter
   D. Both A and C

Questions 6 through 9: Match the following organelles with their appropriate function.

6. _____ Centrioles
7. _____ Rough ER
8. _____ Smooth ER
9. _____ Golgi apparatus

A. Protein production
B. Concentration of secretory granules
C. Lipid synthesis
D. DNA synthesis
E. Points of attachment of the spindle fibers

Questions 10 through 13: Match the following organelles with their appropriate function.

10. _____ Lysosomes
11. _____ Microtubules
12. _____ Mitochondria
13. _____ Ribosomes

A. Energy production and heme synthesis
B. Protein synthesis
C. Cytoskeleton
D. Intracellular digestion
E. Carbohydrate synthesis

14. Glycogen is a
    A. protein
    B. lipid
    C. carbohydrate
    D. hormone

15. A cellular inclusion that represents a common storage form of iron is
    A. glycogen
    B. vacuoles
    C. Auer body
    D. ferritin

16. The nucleus of the cell contains
    A. chromatin, nucleoli, and nucleoplasm
    B. chromatin, nucleoli, and ribosomes
    C. DNA, RNA, and ribosomes
    D. DNA, RNA, and mitochondria

17. The overall function of DNA is
    A. protein and enzyme production
    B. control of cellular function and transmission of genetic information
    C. control of heterochromatin and euchromatin synthesis
    D. production of cellular energy and transmission of genetic information

18. Heterochromatin is
    A. genetically inactive
    B. found in patches or clumps
    C. genetically inactive and pale staining
    D. Both A and B

19. Chromosomal translocation is
    A. a frequent activity of homologous chromosomes in meiosis
    B. a rearrangement of genetic material
    C. the process in which a segment of one chromosome breaks away from its normal location
    D. All of the above

20. A chromosomal deletion is
    A. loss of a pair of chromosomes
    B. loss of a segment of chromosome
    C. attachment of a piece of a chromosome
    D. an exchange of genetic material

Questions 21 through 24: Match the following activities with the appropriate period of time. Use an answer only once.

21. _____ G_1
22. _____ S
23. _____ G_2
24. _____ G_0

A. DNA replication
B. Protracted state of mitotic inactivity
C. Immediately precedes actual mitotic division
D. Actual mitotic division
E. An active period of protein synthesis and cellular metabolism

(continued)

Questions 25 through 29: Match the following mitotic activities with the appropriate cellular activity. Use an answer only once.

25. _____ Prophase
26. _____ Metaphase
27. _____ Anaphase
28. _____ Telophase
29. _____ Cytokinesis

A. Chromosomes line up at the cell's equator
B. Two identical daughter cells form
C. Division of the cellular cytoplasm
D. Chromatids separate and move to opposite ends of the mitotic spindle
E. Chromosomes tightly coil and condense

30. In meiosis, the cells produced contain
  A. a 2n number of chromosomes
  B. 22 pairs of chromosomes
  C. 23 pairs of chromosomes
  D. 23 chromosomes
31. Hematologists are interested in inherited disorders. Which of the following are inherited disorders?
  A. Sickle cell trait
  B. Sickle cell anemia
  C. Hemophilia
  D. All of the above
32. Molecular techniques are being used to detect abnormalities of
  A. erythrocytes
  B. leukocytes
  C. some coagulation factors
  D. All of the above
33. The first inherited hematologic disorder to be diagnosed using molecular biologic assay was
  A. hemophilia A
  B. factor V Leiden
  C. sickle cell anemia
  D. CML
34. PCR testing is useful in
  A. forensic testing
  B. genetic testing
  C. disease diagnosis
  D. All of the above
35. The traditional PCR technique
  A. extends the length of the genomic DNA
  B. alters the original DNA nucleotide sequence
  C. amplifies low levels of specific DNA sequences
  D. amplifies the target region of RNA
36. PCR protocol
  A. doubles the specific amount of DNA with each cycle
  B. typically has three temperature steps
  C. repeats the number of cycles about 30
  D. all of the above
37. Variations of PCR include
  A. nested primers
  B. real-time PCR
  C. microarray analysis
  D. both A and B
38. The method considered to be the "gold standard" of molecular methods is
  A. DNA sequencing
  B. Southern blot
  C. Northern blot
  D. Dot blot
39. The Southern blot procedure has diagnostic applications for diseases or disorders associated with
  A. significant changes in DNA (e.g., deletion)
  B. determination of clonality in lymphomas of T- or B-cell origin
  C. detection of restriction fragment length polymorphisms
  D. all of the above
40. The Northern blot procedure can be used
  A. to mass-produce erythropoietin
  B. for analysis of the proximal product of gene expression
  C. for antenatal genetic counseling
  D. all of the above
41. All of the following are true of FISH except _____
  A. The acronym stands for fluorescent in situ hybridization.
  B. It is a tissue-based molecular diagnostic assay.
  C. It is a prenatal diagnosis of a genetic disorder.
  D. It is useful in the diagnosis of various anemias.
42. Microarrays are
  A. DNA probes bonded on glass chips
  B. tissue-based probes
  C. used to identify single-base mutations
  D. used to determine clonality in lymphomas
43. Molecular techniques provide a diagnostic tool to
  A. detect MRD in hematological malignances
  B. monitor patients following bone marrow transplantation
  C. detect an early relapse in a patient treated for a hematological malignancy
  D. all of the above

BIBLIOGRAPHY

Bao YP, et al. SN identification in unamplified human genomic DNA with gold nanoparticle probes, *Nucleic Acids Res,* 33(2):1–7, 2005.

Béné MC, Kaeda JS. How and why minimal residual disease studies are necessary in leukemia, *Haematologica,* 94(8):1135–1150, 2009.

Bruns DE, Ashwood ER, Burtis CA. *Fundamentals of Molecular Diagnostics,* St. Louis, MO: Elsevier, 2007.

Capetandes A. Polymerase chain reaction—the making of something big, *Med Lab Observer,* (31)2:26, 1999.

Croce CM. Oncogenes and cancers, *NEJM,* 358(5):502–510, 2008.

GEN-PROBE, New Directions in Molecular Diagnostic Testing, San Diego, CA: GEN-PROBE, 2000.

Glassman A, Hopwood VL, Schwartz DJ. Improving diagnosis of hematologic neoplasms. *ADV for Admin Lab,* 9(1):58–61, 2000.

Gocke CD. Molecular diagnostics of hematological malignancies, *Clin Lab Sci,* 19(1):32–38, 2006.

Gullans SR. Connecting the dots using gene-expression profiles, *NEJM,* 355(19):2042–2044, 2006.

Hanson CA. Clinical applications of molecular biology in diagnostic hematopathology, *Lab Med,* 24(9):562–572, 1993.

Kan YW. Development of DNA analysis for human diseases, *JAMA,* 267(11):1532–1536, 1992.

Kaufman HW, Strom CM. From peapods to laboratory medicine: molecular diagnostics of inheritable diseases, *Med Lab Observer,* 35(7):30–38, 2003.

Mifflin TE. Recent developments and uses of PCR in molecular diagnostics, *Adv Med Lab Prof,* 13(1):8–14, 2001.

Nadder TS. The new millennium laboratory: Molecular diagnostics goes clinical, *Clin Lab Sci,* 14(4):252–260, 2001.

Reed JC. Bcl-2-family proteins and hematologic malignancies: history and future prospects, *Blood,* 111:3322–3330, 2008.

Reed JC, Pellecchia M. Apoptosis-based therapies for hematologic malignancies, *Blood,* 106:408–416, 2005.

Saidman SL. Review of basic methods in molecular diagnostics, Current Concepts in Clinical Pathology Conference, June 2003, p. 94.

Schwartz M, Vissing J. Paternal inheritance of mitochondrial DNA, *N Engl J Med,* 347(8):576–579, 2002.

Turgeon ML. *Immunology and Serology in Laboratory Medicine,* 4th ed. St. Louis, MO: Mosby, 2009.

Uphoff TS. Basic concepts and innovations in molecular diagnosis, *Adv Med Lab Prof,* 14(18):13–15, 2002.

Vermes IL, et al. Impact of apoptosis (programmed cell death) for clinical laboratory sciences, American Association for Clinical Chemistry Annual Meeting Workshop, July 2000.

Walker J, Flower D, Rigley K. Microarrays in hematology, *Curr Opin Hematol,* 9(1):23–29, 2002.

Weiss RL. *ARUP's Guide to Molecular Diagnostics Clinical Laboratory Testing,* 2nd ed, Salt Lake City, UT: ARUP Laboratories, 2001.

Williams JL. Advances in understanding the molecular pathogenesis of neoplastic hematologic disorders, *Clin Lab Sci,* 17(4):221–222, 2004.

Wisecarver J. Amplification of DNA sequences, *Lab Med,* 28(3):191–196, 1997.

4 Hematopoiesis

- Explain the origin of blood cells and trace the sequential sites of cellular proliferation and development.
- Describe the development of hematopoietic progenitor cells.
- State the various functions of interleukins and hematopoietic growth factors.
- Name at least three growth factors.
- Name the cells in developmental order that will mature into erythrocytes, thrombocytes, plasma cells, and the five leukocyte types.

- Name and describe in detail the two overall features of a cell that are important in the identification of a cell and that may vary as a cell matures.
- Compare the nuclear characteristics of shape, chromatin pattern, and nucleoli in specific cell types and according to the age of the cell.
- Compare the cytoplasmic features of color, granulation, shape, quantity, vacuolization, and inclusions to cell maturity.
- Name and describe the average percentage and cellular characteristics of the six mature leukocytes found in normal peripheral blood.

HEMATOPOIESIS DEFINED

Hematopoiesis is the process of blood cell production, differentiation, and development. The hematopoietic system consists of the bone marrow, liver, spleen, lymph nodes, and thymus. Before investigating the general maturational characteristics of cells, knowledge of blood cell development is useful.

ORIGIN OF BLOOD CELLS

Hematopoietic stem cells (HSCs) are the foundation of the adult hematopoietic system. It is now widely accepted that the embryo produces the first adult repopulating HSCs.

Types of Human Stem Cells

Functionally, three types of human stem cells exist:

1. **Totipotential stem cells**. These cells are present in the first few hours after an ovum is fertilized. Totipotential stem cells, the most versatile type of stem cell, can develop into any human cell type, including development from embryo into fetus.
2. **Pluripotential stem cells**. These cells are present several days after fertilization. Pluripotent stem cells can develop into any cell type, except they cannot develop into a fetus.
3. **Multipotential stem cells**. These cells are derived from pluripotent stem cells. They can be found in adults, but they are limited to specific types of cells to form tissues. For example, bone marrow stem cells can produce all types of blood cells, bone cartilage, and adipose (fat) cells.

In tissues with a high cellular turnover, stem cell populations are essential for lifelong maintenance of organ function.

Somatic stem cells have been identified in several self-renewing organs, including the blood cell system. HSCs are ultimately responsible for the continuous daily production of all mature blood cell lineages. HSCs are historically the most thoroughly characterized type of adult stem cell. HSCs are functionally defined at the single-cell level by their dual capacity for self-renewal and multipotential differentiation. Signaling pathways are important control devices of HSC fate.

Stem cell therapy focuses on embryonic stem cell therapy, fetal stem cell therapy, cord stem cell therapy, and adult blood stem cell therapy.

Early Development of Blood Cells

Embryonic blood cells, excluding the lymphocyte type of white blood cell, originate from the mesenchymal tissue that arises from the embryonic germ layer, the mesoderm (Fig. 4.1). The mesodermally derived intraembryonic region —known as the aorta-gonad-mesonephros region or, at a slightly earlier developmental stage, the paraaortic splanchnopleure—produces, respectively, potent HSCs and multipotent progenitor cells before their appearance in the yolk sac. The mammalian embryo contains at least two spatially separated sources of hematopoietic cells.

The anatomical sites of blood cell development are as follows (see Fig. 4.2):

- Following gastrulation and mesoderm formation, the first hematopoietic cells are generated in the yolk sac. The first blood cells are primitive red blood cells (erythroblasts) formed during the first 2 to 8 weeks of life.
- The onset of circulation between the yolk sac and embryo proper confounds the precise determination of

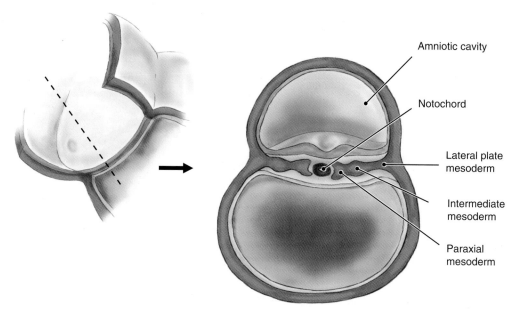

FIGURE 4.1 Cross-sectional view of the embryo at the time of mesoderm migration. The mesoderm cells coalesce into three distinct clumps, or colonies. The paraxial mesoderm tracks the path of the notochord. The intermediate mesoderm hovers just beside it for a short stretch of the embryo's length. The lateral plate mesoderm fills the rest of the space and forms an important contact with the ectoderm above (dorsally), the endoderm below (ventrally), and the extraembryonic shell to the outside. (Reprinted with permission from Hartwig W. *Fundamental Anatomy*, Baltimore, MD: Lippincott Williams & Wilkins, 2008.)

hematopoietic sources. Mesenchymal stem/progenitor cells and HSCs circulate together in the peripheral blood during the first trimester to the secondary ontogenic sites of hematopoiesis, the liver and bone marrow. Gradually, the **liver** becomes the site of blood cell development. By the second month of gestation, the liver becomes the major site of hematopoiesis, and granular types of leukocytes

have made their initial appearance. The liver predominates from about the second to fifth months of fetal life.

■ In the fourth month of gestation, the **bone marrow** begins to function in the production of blood cells. After the fifth fetal month, the bone marrow begins to assume its ultimate role as the primary site of hematopoiesis (medullary hematopoiesis).

FIGURE 4.2 Hemopoiesis in various organs before and after birth. (Reprinted with permission from Rubin E, Farber JL. *Pathology*, 3rd ed, Philadelphia, PA: Lippincott Williams & Wilkins, 1999.)

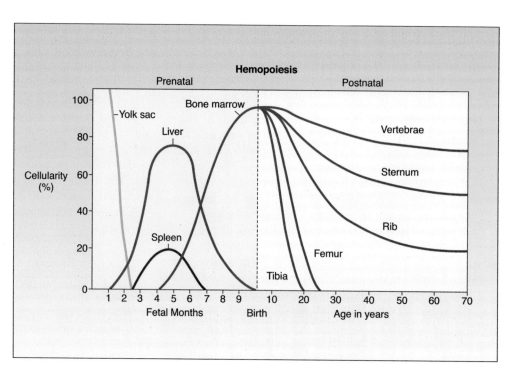

BONE MARROW SITES AND FUNCTION

Bone marrow is found within the cavities of all bones and may be present in two forms: yellow marrow, which is normally inactive and composed mostly of fat (adipose) tissue, and red marrow, which is normally active in the production of most types of leukocytes, erythrocytes, and thrombocytes (Figs. 4.3 to 4.5)

The bone marrow is one of the body's largest organs. It represents approximately 3.5% to 6% of total body weight and averages around 1,500 g in adults, with the hematopoietic marrow being organized around the bone vasculature (see Fig. 4.6). The bone marrow consists of hematopoietic cells (erythroid, myeloid, lymphoid, and megakaryocyte), fat (adipose) tissue, osteoblasts and osteoclasts, and stroma. Hematopoietic cell colonies are compartmentalized in the

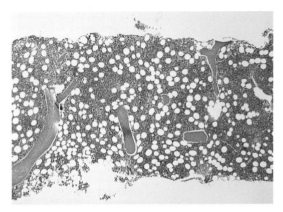

FIGURE 4.4 Bone marrow biopsy sections demonstrate normal cellularity. Approximately 40% to 50% cellularity in an otherwise healthy 60-year-old man. (Reprinted with permission from McClatchey KD. *Clinical Laboratory Medicine*, 2nd ed, Philadelphia, PA: Lippincott Williams & Wilkins, 2002.)

cords. Following maturation in the hematopoietic cords, hematopoietic cells cross the walls of the sinuses, specialized vascular spaces, and enter the circulating blood (Fig. 4.7).

During the first few years of life, the marrow of all bones is red and cellular. The red bone marrow is initially found in both the appendicular and the axial skeleton (Fig. 4.8A) in young persons but progressively becomes confined to the axial skeleton and proximal ends of the long bones in adults (Fig. 4.8B). By age 18, red marrow is found only in the vertebrae, ribs, sternum, skull bones, pelvis, and to some extent the proximal epiphyses of the femur and humerus.

In certain abnormal circumstances, the spleen, liver, and lymph nodes revert back to producing immature blood cells (**extramedullary hematopoiesis**). In these cases, enlargement of the spleen and liver is frequently noted on physical examination. This situation suggests that undifferentiated primitive blood cells are present in these areas and are able to proliferate if an appropriate stimulus is present. This situation occurs under the following conditions:

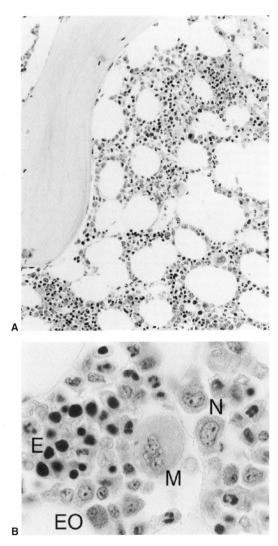

FIGURE 4.3 Normal bone marrow biopsy. Showing distribution of hematopoietic cells, fat, and trabecular bone: erythroid precursors (E), neutrophil precursors (N), eosinophil precursors (Eo), megakaryocyte (M). Giemsa; biopsies ×250 (**A**) and ×1000 (**B**). (Reprinted with permission from Handin RI, Lux SE, Stossel TP. *Blood: Principles and Practice of Hematology*, 2nd ed, Philadelphia, PA: Lippincott Williams and Wilkins, 2003.)

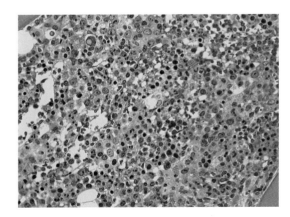

FIGURE 4.5 Bone marrow biopsy sections demonstrate normal cellularity. Virtually 100% cellular marrow from a newborn boy. (Reprinted with permission from McClatchey KD. *Clinical Laboratory Medicine*, 2nd ed. Philadelphia, PA: Lippincott Williams & Wilkins, 2002.)

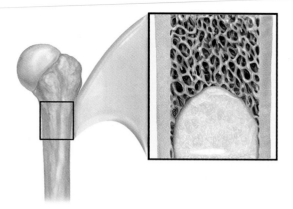

FIGURE 4.6 The development of blood cells: humerus bone, cortical bone, red bone marrow, and yellow bone marrow. (Asset provided by Anatomical Chart Co.)

1. When the bone marrow becomes dysfunctional in cases such as aplastic anemia, infiltration by malignant cells, or overproliferation of a cell line (e.g., leukemia).
2. When the bone marrow is unable to meet the demands placed on it, as in the hemolytic anemias (full discussions of the anemias are presented in Chapters 8 through 13).

CELLULAR ELEMENTS OF BONE MARROW

Progenitor Blood Cells

The pluripotent stem cell is the first in a sequence of steps of hematopoietic cell generation and maturation. The progenitor of all blood cells is called the **multipotential hematopoietic stem cell**. Stem cells carry out the ultimate burden of generating multilineage mature blood cells over the lifetime of the organism. During this span of time, the stem cell population may undergo quantitative and qualitative changes (Fig. 4.9).

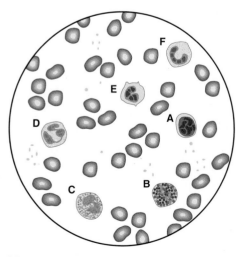

FIGURE 4.7 Normal peripheral blood cells. **A:** Lymphocytes. **B:** Basophils. **C:** Eosinophils. **D:** Segmented neutrophils. **E:** Monocytes. **F:** Band form neutrophil.

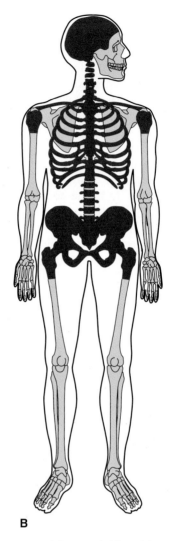

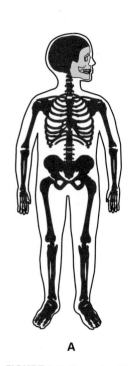

FIGURE 4.8 Sites of red bone marrow activity. **A:** Child: Red bone marrow (*red-shaded areas*) is located throughout the skeletal system in children. **B:** Adult: Yellow marrow replaces red marrow (*dark-shaded areas*) in the adult skeletal system. Red marrow activity occurs in the central portion of the skeleton. (Reprinted with permission from Dzierzak E. Ontogenic emergence of definitive hematopoietic stem cells, *Curr Opin Hematol*, 10(3):230, 2003.)

Stem cells have the capacity for self-renewal as well as proliferation and differentiation into progenitor cells. Recent research has demonstrated that blood, brain, and many other regions of the body have their own specialized stem cells that are capable of making replacement cells. Some of these stem cells are amazingly adaptable, a concept referred to as "stem cell plasticity," and are able to generate an assortment of seemingly unrelated types of cells. This research suggests that adults carry a reservoir of "master cells" inside their bone marrow that are capable of rebuilding almost any damaged tissue. These "master cells" are being called multipotent adult progenitor cells (MAPCs). MAPCs express an enzyme called telomerase that keeps cells from aging. In vitro, MAPCs can be coaxed into becoming muscle, cartilage, bone, liver, or different types of neurons and brain cells.

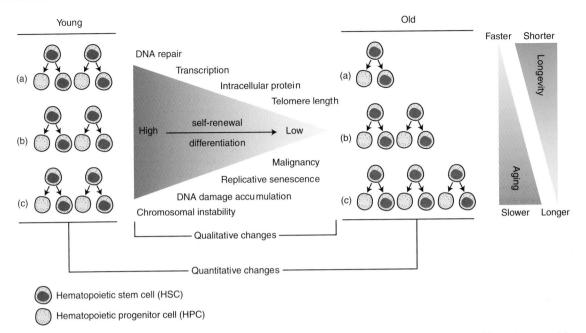

FIGURE 4.9 Over a lifetime, the size of the HSC population may decrease (a), remain the same (b), or increase (c). Examples of each can be found in individual inbred mouse strains and, by inference, may be found in individual humans. Irrespective of the quantitative changes, the quality of HSCs decreases during aging. Possible mechanisms include diminished capacity for DNA repair and transcription, decreased concentration of intracellular proteins, cross-linking of intracellular molecules, and shortened telomere length. The aggregate effects of accumulated DNA damage, increased chromosomal instability, and replicative senescence impair the self-renewal differentiation capabilities of aged HSCs and increase the probability of malignant transformation. Both qualitative and quantitative changes of HSCs are hypothesized to affect both the rate of aging and longevity of organisms. Fewer HSCs of diminished quality, according to the hypothesis, translate into faster progression of aging and shorter longevity. (Reprinted with permission from Liang W, Van Zant G. Genetic control of stem-cell properties and stem cells in aging, *Curr Opin Hematol*, 10(3):200, 2003.)

Hematopoietic cells can be divided into three phases according to cell maturity:

1. **Primitive, multipotential cells.** The most immature group capable of self-renewal and differentiation into all blood cell lines.
2. **Intermediate cells.** This group consists of committed progenitor cells destined to develop into distinct cell lines.
3. **Mature cells.** The most developed group with specific functions.

The multipotential stem cell is the progenitor of two major ancestral cell lines: lymphocytic and nonlymphocytic cells. The lymphoid stem cell is the precursor of either mature T cells or B cells/plasma cells. The nonlymphocytic (myeloid) stem cell progresses to the progenitor colony-forming unit, granulocyte-erythrocyte-monocyte-megakaryocyte (CFU-GEMM). The acronym CFU is used as a prefix to record the number of colony-forming units of different progenitor cells that are identified through in vitro clonal assays. The unit colony of CFU-GEMM leads to the development of distinct subsets of committed progenitor cells. The CFU-GEMM can lead to the formation of CFU-granulocyte macrophage/monocyte (CFU-GM), CFU-eosinophil (CFU-Eo), CFU-basophil (CFU-B), and CFU-megakaryocyte (CFU-Meg). In erythropoiesis, the CFU-GEMM differentiates into the burst-forming unit-erythroid

(BFU-E). Each of the CFUs in turn can produce a colony of one hematopoietic lineage under appropriate growth conditions.

The formation and development of mature blood cells from the bone marrow multipotential stem cell is controlled by growth factors and inhibitors as well as the microenvironment. The microenvironment or locale influences behavior and controls proliferation of multipotential cells. Bone seems to provide the microenvironment most appropriate for proliferation and maturation of cells.

Hematopoietic progenitor cells (HPCs) can be mobilized from the bone marrow to the blood by a wide variety of stimuli, including hematopoietic growth factors and chemokines (Fig. 4.10). Individual hematopoietic cytokines can be lineage specific or can regulate cells in multiple lineages, and for some cell types, e.g. stem cells, the simultaneous action of multiple cytokines is required for proliferative responses. HPCs in the bone marrow exist in a highly organized, three-dimensional microenvironment composed of a diverse population of stromal cells and an extracellular matrix rich in fibronectin, collagens, and various proteoglycans. Hematopoietic progenitor can be found in umbilical cord blood (UCB) as well. UCB hematopoietic cells have been employed successfully as a therapeutic source of autologous and allogeneic transplants for more than 20 years. Cryopreservation prolongs the storage time of UCB.

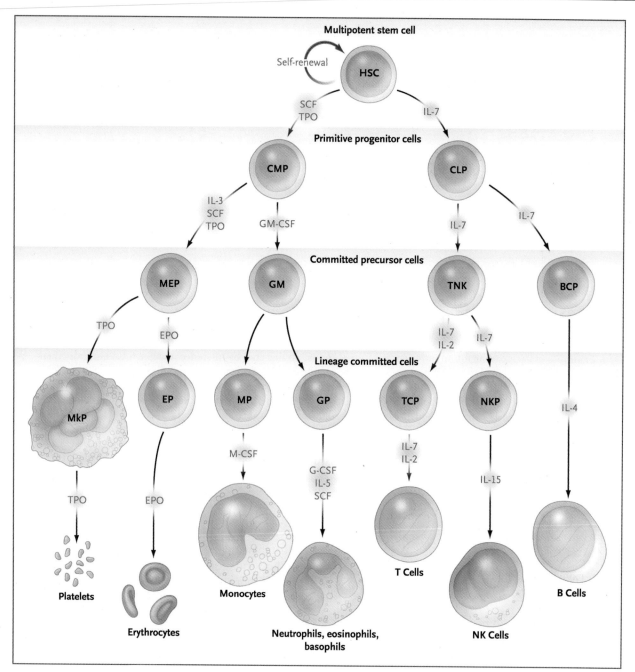

FIGURE 4.10 A General Model of Hematopoiesis. Blood cell development progresses from an HSC, which can undergo either self-renewal or differentiation into a multilineage committed progenitor cell: a common lymphoid progenitor (CLP) or a common myeloid progenitor (CMP). These cells then give rise to more differentiated progenitors, comprising those committed to two lineages that include T cells and natural killer cells (TNKs), granulocytes and macrophages (GMs), and megakaryocytes and erythroid cells (MEPs). Ultimately, these cells give rise to unilineage committed progenitors for B cells (BCPs), NK cells (NKPs), T cells (TCPs), granulocytes (GPs), monocytes (MPs), erythrocytes (EPs), and megakaryocytes (MkPs). Cytokines and growth factors that support the survival, proliferation, or differentiation of each type of cell are shown in *red*. For simplicity, the three types of granulocyte progenitor cells are not shown; in reality, distinct progenitors of neutrophils, eosinophils, and basophils or mast cells exist and are supported by distinct transcription factors and cytokines (e.g., IL-5 in the case of eosinophils, stem cell factor [SCF] in the case of basophils or mast cells, and G-CSF in the case of neutrophils). IL, interleukin; TPO, thrombopoietin; M-CSF, macrophage colony-stimulating factor; GM-CSF, granulocyte-macrophage CSF; EPO, erythropoietin. (Reprinted with permission from Kaushansky, K. Lineage-specific hematopoietic growth factors, *NEJM*, 354(19):2035, 2006, . Copyright © 2006 Massachusetts Medical Society. All rights reserved.)

Erythropoiesis

Erythropoiesis occurs in distinct anatomical sites called erythropoietic islands, specialized niches in which erythroid precursors proliferate, differentiate, and enucleate. Each island consists of a macrophage surrounded by a cluster of erythroblasts. Within erythroid niches, cell-cell and cell–extracellular matrix adhesion, positive and negative regulatory feedback, and central macrophage function occur. Erythroid cells account for 5% to 38% of nucleated cells in normal bone.

Granulopoiesis

Myeloid cells account for 23% to 85% of the nucleated cells in normal bone marrow. Granulopoiesis can be recognized as a maturational unit. Early cells are located in the cords and around the bone trabeculae. Neutrophils in the bone marrow reside in the proliferating pool and the maturation storage pool (see Chapter 14). Maturing cells spend an average of 3 to 6 days in the proliferating pool. If needed, cells from the storage pool can exit into the circulation rapidly and will have an average life span of 6 to 10 hours.

Lymphopoiesis

Unlike other cell lines, lymphocytes and plasma cells are produced in lymphoid follicles. Lymphocytes are randomly dispersed throughout the cords (see Chapter 16). Lymphoid follicles may also be observed, especially after the age of 50. Plasma cells are located along the vascular wall. Lymphoid cells typically account for 1% to 5% of the nucleated cells in the normal bone marrow.

Megakaryopoiesis

Megakaryopoiesis takes place adjacent to the sinus endothelium. Megakaryocytes protrude through the vascular wall as small cytoplasmic processes to deliver platelets into the sinusoidal blood. Megakaryocytes develop into platelets in approximately 5 days.

Other Cells Found in Bone Marrow

Marrow Stromal Cells

The meshwork of stromal cells is composed of reticulum cells, histiocytes, adipose cells, and endothelial cells. This structure is where the hematopoietic cells are suspended in a delicate semifluid state. Stromal cells produce an extracellular matrix composed of collagens and proteins (e.g., glycoproteins and proteoglycans). The extracellular matrix is critical for the maintenance of normal renewal and differentiation of bone marrow cells.

Mast Cells

Tissue mast cells, a connective tissue cell of mesenchymal origin, are normally observed in bone marrow. The abundant blue-purple granules that usually obscure the round or oval reticular nucleus contain heparin, histamine, serotonin, and proteolytic enzymes. Increased numbers of mast cells can be seen in a variety of abnormal conditions (e.g., chronic lymphoproliferative disorders or chronic infections).

Macrophages

Macrophages, also called reticulum cells or histiocytes, appear as large cells in the bone marrow. The appearance of the cytoplasms will vary, depending on what the cell has ingested (e.g., siderophages are macrophages containing iron-rich hemosiderin and ferritin). Gaucher cells are macrophages filled with uncatabolized glucocerebrosides.

Bone Cells

Osteoblasts are bone matrix–synthesizing cells that resemble plasma cells and are usually observed in groups. Although these cells are only occasionally seen in normal adult bone marrow aspirates, an increased number of cells is characteristically seen in aspirates from children and from patients who have metabolic disease. Osteoclasts resemble megakaryocytes. These are bone-remodeling cells.

INTERLEUKINS

In order to perform their specialized functions, highly differentiated blood cells are continuously produced by stem cells. More than a dozen growth and stromal factors drive cells to divide asymmetrically, undergo differentiation and carry out their end-cell function. Protein molecules that work in conjunction with hematopoietic growth factors to stimulate proliferation and differentiation of specific cell lines are the interleukins. Interleukins are cytokines that act independently or in conjunction with other interleukins to encourage hematopoietic growth. Interleukins are cell signaling molecules and a part of the cytokine super family of signaling molecules. The interleukins were first described as signals for communication between (inter—between) white blood cells (leuk—from leukocytes). Currently, it is well-known that these molecules are produced and used as signaling molecules in many cells of the body, in addition to immune cells.

Interleukins are basically the method of immune cross-talk and communication. Interleukins are the primary messengers and directors of the immune system. There are currently 35 well-known interleukins; however, there are many more to be found and characterized.

The interleukins are described in Table 4.1. This interacting network of inflammatory stimuli and cytokines suggests that these growth factors may have a limited role in hematopoietic homeostasis but a major role in host responses to infection or antigenic challenge. They can cause cellular proliferation, cell activation, inflammation, physiology changes such as fever and pain, and allergies as with histamine release and growth.

| TABLE | **4.1** | **Summary of Interleukins (ILs)** | |

Name	Source	Target Blood Cells	Function
IL-1	B cells, monocytes, dendritic cells. Appears to influence different progenitor cells indirectly in hematopoiesis. It may act in synergy with IL-3, M-CSF, G-CSF, and GM-CSF to stimulate cells.	T helper cells B cells NK cells Macrophages	Costimulation Maturation and proliferation Activation Inflammation
IL-2	Th1 cells	Activated T cells and B cells, NK cells, macrophages	Influences the proliferation and regulation of T cells, B cells, natural killer (NK) cells, and monocytes. It acts on activated B cells as a growth and differentiation factor.
IL-3	Activated Th3 cells, mast cells, NK cells, endothelium, eosinophils	Hematopoietic stem cells	Promotes the growth of early hematopoietic cell lines (e.g., proliferation of CFU-GEMM, CFU-M, CFU-Meg, CFU-Eo, and CFU-Bs colonies from bone marrow). IL-3 acts with M-CSF to stimulate proliferation of monocytes and macrophages. It also stimulates granulocyte, monocyte, eosinophil, and mast cell production.
		Mast cells	Growth and histamine release
IL-4	Th2 cells, just activated naive CD4+ cell, memory CD4+ cells, mast cells, macrophages Interacts with G-CSF to proliferate myeloid progenitor cells.	Activated B cells	Proliferation and differentiation, IgG1 and IgE synthesis
		T cells	Proliferation
IL-5	Th2 cells, mast cells, eosinophils	Eosinophils	Stimulates eosinophil colony production and interacts with GM-CSF and IL-3 in eosinophil induction.
		B cells	Differentiation, IgA production
IL-6	Macrophages, Th2 cells, B cells, astrocytes, endothelium	Activated B cells	Differentiation into plasma cells
		Plasma cells	Antibody secretion
		HSCs	Differentiation
		T cells, others	Induces acute phase reaction, hematopoiesis, differentiation, inflammation
IL-7	Bone marrow stromal cells and thymus stromal cells	Pre/pro-B cell, pre/pro-T cell, NK cells	Differentiation and proliferation of lymphoid progenitor cells, involved in B, T, and NK cell survival, development, and homeostasis, ↑ proinflammatory cytokines
IL-8	Macrophages, lymphocytes, epithelial cells, endothelial cells	Neutrophils, basophils, lymphocytes	An inflammatory cytokine that is chemotactic for both neutrophils and T cells. It is a potent stimulator of neutrophils, and it activates the respiratory burst and the release of both specific and azurophilic granular contents.
IL-9	Th2 cells, specifically by CD4+ helper cells	T cells, B cells	Acts as a potent CD4+ T lymphocyte growth factor. In addition, it has been demonstrated to support growth of BFU-E.

(continued)

Name	Source	Target Blood Cells	Function
IL-10	Monocytes, Th2 cells, CD8⁺ T cells, mast cells, macrophages, B cell subset	Macrophages B cells Mast cells Th1 cells Th2 cells	Cytokine production Activation inhibits Th1 cytokine production (IFN-γ, TNF-β, IL-2) Stimulation
IL-11	Bone marrow stroma	Bone marrow stroma	Multifunctional regulator of hematopoiesis
IL-12	Dendritic cells, B cells, T cells, macrophages	Activated T cells	Differentiation into cytotoxic T cells with IL-2, $\uparrow$ IFN-γ, TNF-α, $\downarrow$ IL-10
		NK cells	$\uparrow$ IFN-γ, TNF-α
IL-13	Activated Th2 cells, mast cells, NK cells	Th2 cells, B cells, macrophages	Stimulates growth and differentiation of B cells (IgE), inhibits Th1 cells and the production of macrophage inflammatory cytokines (e.g., IL-1, IL-6), $\downarrow$ IL-8, IL-10, IL-12.
IL-14	T cells and certain malignant B cells	Activated B cells	Induces growth and proliferation of B cells, inhibits Ig secretion
IL-15	Mononuclear phagocytes (and some other cells), especially macrophages following infection by virus(es)	T cells, activated B cells	Induces production of natural killer cells
IL-16	Lymphocytes, epithelial cells, eosinophils, CD8⁺ T cells	CD4⁺ T cells (Th cells)	CD4⁺ chemoattractant, increases the mobility of CD4⁺ T cells
IL-17	T helper 17 cells (Th17)	Epithelium, endothelium, other	$\uparrow$ Inflammatory cytokines
IL-18	Macrophages Acts as a synergist with IL-12 in some of its effects	Th1 cells, NK cells	Induces production of IFN-γ, $\uparrow$ NK cell activity
IL-19	—		Regulates the functions of macrophages, suppresses the activities of Th1 and Th2
IL-20	Biological activities similar to IL-10		Regulates proliferation and differentiation of keratinocytes
IL-21	Activated T helper cells, NKT cells	All lymphocytes, dendritic cells	Costimulates activation and proliferation of CD8⁺ T cells; augments NK cytotoxicity; augments CD40-driven B cell proliferation, differentiation, and isotype switching; promotes differentiation of Th17 cells
IL-22	Similar to IL-10 —		Activates STAT1 and STAT3 and increases production of acute phase proteins such as serum amyloid A, Alpha 1-antichymotrypsin and haptoglobin in hepatoma cell lines
IL-23	—		Increases angiogenesis but reduces CD8 T cell infiltration Acts as a stimulant on particular populations of memory T cells.
IL-24	—		Plays important roles in tumor suppression, wound healing, and psoriasis by influencing cell survival.
IL-25	—		Supports proliferation of cells in the lymphoid lineage. Induces the production of IL-4, IL-5, and IL-13, which stimulate eosinophil expansion

(continued)

Name	Source	Target Blood Cells	Function
IL-26	—		Enhances secretion of IL-10 and IL-8 and cell surface expression of CD54 on epithelial cells
IL-27	—		Regulates the activity of B lymphocytes and T lymphocytes
IL-28	—		Plays a role in immune defense against viruses
IL-29	—		Plays a role in host defenses against microbes
IL-30	—		Forms one chain of IL-27
IL-31	—		May play a role in inflammation of the skin
IL-32	—		Induces monocytes and macrophages to secrete TNF-α, IL-8, and CXCL2
IL-33	—		Induces helper T cells to produce type 2 cytokine
IL-35	Regulatory T cells		Suppression of T helper cell activation

CSF, macrophage colony-stimulating factor; G-CSF, granulocyte colony-stimulating factor; GM-CSF, granulocyte-macrophage colony-stimulating factor; CFU-GEMM, colony-forming unit-granulocyte, erythrocyte, monocyte, and megakaryocyte; CFU-M, colony-forming unit-macrophage; CFU-Meg, colony-forming unit-megakaryocyte; CFU-Eo, colony-forming unit-eosinophil; CFU-Bs, colony-forming unit-basophil; EBU, erythroid colony-forming unit.

HEMATOPOIETIC GROWTH FACTORS

Each hematopoietic growth factor is encoded by a single gene. The gene for erythropoietin is located on chromosome 7. For example, the genes for granulocyte-macrophage colony-stimulating factor (GM-CSF), interleukin-3 (IL-3), and monocyte colony-stimulating factor (M-CSF) are clustered on the long arm of chromosome 5. Chromosome 17 is the location of the granulocyte colony-stimulating factor (G-CSF)

gene. The cellular sources and other characteristics of growth factors are presented in Table 4.2.

The major role of hematopoietic growth factors appears to be regulating the proliferation and differentiation of HPCs as well as regulating the survival and function of mature blood cells. The biological effects of hematopoietic growth factors are mediated through specific binding to receptors on the surface of target cells.

TABLE 4.2	Characteristics of Human Hematopoietic Growth Factors

Growth Factor	Cellular Source	Progenitor Cell Target	Mature Cell Target
Erythropoietin	Peritubular cells of the kidney, Kupffer cells	CFU-E, late BFU-E, CFU-Meg	None
IL-3	Activated T lymphocytes	CFU-blast, CFU-GEMM, CFU-GM, CFU-G, CFU-M, CFU-Eo, CFU-Meg, CFU-Baso, BFU-E	Eosinophils, monocytes
G-CSF	Monocytes, fibroblasts, endothelial cells	CFU-G	Granulocytes
M-CSF	Monocytes, fibroblasts, endothelial cells	CFU-M	Monocytes
GM-CSF	T lymphocytes, monocytes, eosinophils, monocytes, fibroblasts, endothelial cells	CFU-blast, CFU-GEMM, CFU-GM, CFU-G, CFU-M, CFU-Eo, CFU-Meg, BFU-E	granulocytes

G-CSF, granulocyte colony-stimulating factor; M-CSF, macrophage colony-stimulating factor; GM-CSF, granulocyte-macrophage colony-stimulating factor; CFU-blast, colony-forming unit-blast; CFU-GEMM, colony-forming unit granulocyte, erythrocyte, monocyte, and megakaryocyte; CFU-GM, colony-forming unit-granulocyte and macrophage; CFU-EO, colony-forming unit-eosinophil; CFU-Meg, colony-forming unit-megakaryocyte; BFU-E, burst-forming unit-erythroid; CFU-G, colony-forming unit-granulocyte; CFU-M, colony-forming unit-macrophage; CFU-E, colony-forming unit-erythroid; CFU-Baso, colony-forming unit-basophil.

Hematopoietic growth factors are being used and tested in clinical trials for the treatment of a variety of hematological disorders. Erythropoietin, GM-CSF, G-CSF, M-CSF, and IL-3 are representative factors that have been identified, cloned, and produced through recombinant DNA technology. Specific factors are being used as adjunct therapy in a wide variety of diseases (e.g., to stimulate the production of granulocytes or lymphocytes).

Hematopoietic growth factors are capable of mobilizing HPCs. A striking feature of growth factors is the diversity of the target population. Examples of various factors and the target cells are

1. G-CSF and GM-CSF predominantly affect myeloid cells.
2. IL-7 stimulates T and B lymphocytes.
3. IL-12 targets natural killer cells.

The mobilization of HPCs from the bone marrow to the peripheral blood circulation is a complicated process regulated by multiple adhesive interactions between the HPCs and the bone marrow extracellular matrix. Mobilization of HPCs is by a wide variety of stimuli, including hematopoietic growth factors, chemotherapy, and chemokines. HPCs are selectively mobilized after the M phase of the cell cycle. Some of the molecules on HPCs that are important for mobilization are VLA-4 and VCAM-1, and possibly hyaluronan receptors. Hematopoietic growth factors interact with blood cells at different levels in the cascade of cell differentiation from the multipotential progenitor to the circulating mature cell. Once in the circulation, a preponderance of HPCs are in the G_0 or G_1 phase of the cell cycle.

EXAMINATION OF MATURING BLOOD CELLS

A comprehensive examination of bone marrow involves examination of both bone marrow smears and histological tissue sections. Traditional paraffin-reactive immunohistological reagents coupled with newer molecular techniques have improved the study of bone marrow biopsy specimens (see Chapter 26).

The examination of a stained peripheral blood smear is an important component of the **complete blood cell count** (CBC) procedure, which is routinely performed in the hematology laboratory. In this procedure (refer to the "Leukocyte Differential Count" in Chapter 26), white blood cells are examined, identified, and counted. Red blood cells and platelets are also carefully examined during this procedure.

To identify the normal cells (see Fig. 4.7) that appear on a blood smear and recognize immature cells that may appear in various disorders or in the bone marrow (refer to "Bone Marrow Examination" in Chapter 26), it is important to know the sequences of cellular development by name (Table 4.3) as well as the general maturational characteristics of blood cells. Specific cell-line maturational details and abnormalities that may be encountered in various types of cells are presented in relevant chapters in Parts 1, 2, and 3.

General Cellular Characteristics

The identification and stage of maturation of stained blood cells can be guided by a variety of systematic features (Table 4.4). Two important characteristics to observe initially in cell identification are

1. Overall cell size
2. Nuclear-cytoplasmic ratio

Overall Cell Size

The overall size of a blood cell is usually compared with the size of a mature erythrocyte. Except for the megakaryocytic maturational series, erythrocytes and leukocytes *decrease* in overall size as maturation progresses.

Nuclear-Cytoplasmic Ratio

The amount of space occupied by the nucleus in relationship to the space occupied by the cytoplasm is the **nuclear-cytoplasmic (N:C) ratio**. The size of the nucleus generally *decreases* as a cell matures. Consequently, the N:C ratio *decreases* in many cell types with maturation. Blast forms of erythrocytes, leukocytes, and megakaryocytes have a high (4:1) N:C ratio. As these cells mature, the ratio is reduced to 2:1 or 1:1 in most cells, except in thrombocytes, mature erythrocytes, and the lymphocyte type of leukocyte. Thrombocytes and erythrocytes lack a nucleus (**anuclear**), and mature lymphocytes frequently retain the original 4:1 to 3:1 N:C ratio.

Nuclear Characteristics

Nuclear characteristics play an important role in cell identification. Important features of the nucleus include

1. Chromatin pattern
2. Nuclear shape
3. Presence of nucleoli

Chromatin Patterns

The chromatin arrangement demonstrates characteristic patterns. These patterns are the most distinctive nuclear feature of a cell in terms of maturity and cell type recognition. In general, the overall pattern progresses from a loose-looking arrangement to a more clumped pattern as a cell matures. The terms used to describe various patterns include the following: smooth or homogeneous, fine, delicate, lacy or thready, smudged, clumped, or pyknotic (dense or compact). Examples of common chromatin features for each cell type are given here.

- **Lymphocytes** exhibit a smooth or homogeneous pattern of chromatin throughout development until the mature stage, when clumped heterochromatin is more obvious.
- **Granulocytes** progress from having a fine to a highly clumped pattern.
- **Monocytes** have a lacy pattern, which becomes finer as the cell matures.
- **Erythrocytes** continue to develop a more clumped pattern as maturation progresses, until the extremely dense (pyknotic) nucleus is lost (extruded) from the mature cell.

TABLE 4.3	Blood Cell Development Nomenclature of Normal Committed Cell Lines

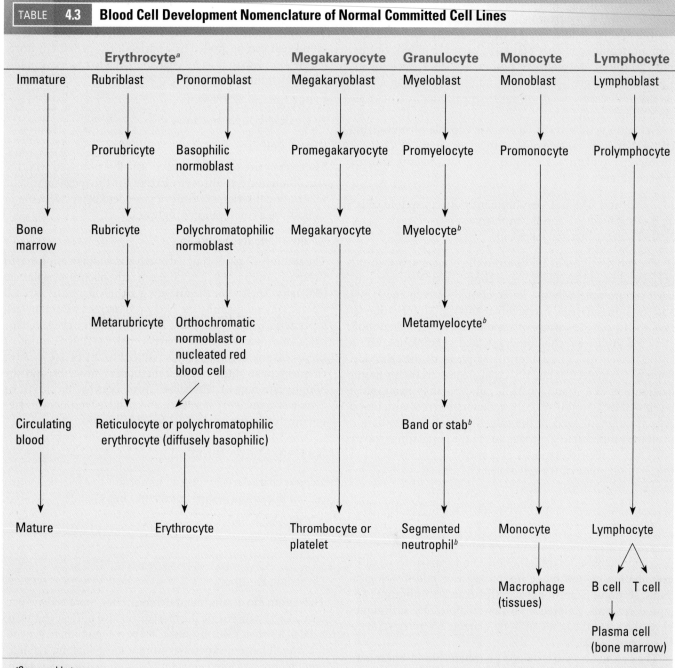

	Erythrocyte[a]		Megakaryocyte	Granulocyte	Monocyte	Lymphocyte
Immature	Rubriblast	Pronormoblast	Megakaryoblast	Myeloblast	Monoblast	Lymphoblast
	Prorubricyte	Basophilic normoblast	Promegakaryocyte	Promyelocyte	Promonocyte	Prolymphocyte
Bone marrow	Rubricyte	Polychromatophilic normoblast	Megakaryocyte	Myelocyte[b]		
	Metarubricyte	Orthochromatic normoblast or nucleated red blood cell		Metamyelocyte[b]		
Circulating blood	Reticulocyte or polychromatophilic erythrocyte (diffusely basophilic)			Band or stab[b]		
Mature	Erythrocyte		Thrombocyte or platelet	Segmented neutrophil[b]	Monocyte	Lymphocyte
					Macrophage (tissues)	B cell T cell
						Plasma cell (bone marrow)

[a]Comparable terms.
[b]These cell types may be neutrophilic, eosinophilic, or basophilic.

Nuclear Shape

The shape of the nucleus in young cells is either round or oval; however, monocytes may have a slightly folded nuclear shape. In the cells that retain their nucleus as they mature, nuclear shapes become very distinctive for particular cell types.

- **Lymphocytes** usually continue to have a round or oval nucleus. Some cells may have a small cleft in the nucleus.
- **Monocytes** have a kidney bean–shaped nucleus, but folded or horseshoe shapes are common.

- **Mature neutrophils**, **eosinophils**, and **basophils** have segmented nuclei attached to one another by fine filaments. The number of distinctive lobes ranges from two to five depending on the cell type.

Presence of Nucleoli

The presence or absence of nucleoli is important in the identification of cells. The three cell lines of erythrocytes, leukocytes, and megakaryocytes all have nucleoli in the earliest cell stages. As cells mature, nucleoli are usually not visible. These

TABLE 4.4	Summary of General Maturational Characteristics[a]
Morphological Feature	**Usual Development**
General cell size	Decreases with maturity
Nuclear-cytoplasmic ratio	Decreases with maturity
Nucleus	
Chromatin pattern	Becomes more condensed
Presence of nucleoli	Not visible in mature cells
Cytoplasmic characteristics	
Color	Progresses from darker blue to lighter blue, blue-gray, or pink
Granulation	Progresses from no granules to nonspecific to specific granules
Vacuoles	Increase with age

[a]The characteristics of specific cells vary.

changes in the appearance of the nucleoli are related to the rate of synthesis of ribosomal RNA.

The number of nucleoli varies depending on the cell type, as is shown in the following examples:

- **Lymphoblasts** have one or two nucleoli.
- **Myeloblasts** have one to five nucleoli.
- **Monoblasts** usually have one or two nucleoli but occasionally may have three or four.
- **Erythroblasts** may not have any nucleoli or may have up to two nucleoli that may stain darker than in other types of blast cells.
- **Megakaryoblasts** typically have one to five nucleoli.

Cytoplasmic Characteristics

A variety of cytoplasmic features aid in the microscopic identification of cell maturity and type. These features include

1. Staining color and intensity
2. Granulation
3. Shape
4. Quantity of cytoplasm
5. Vacuolization
6. Inclusion bodies

Staining Color and Intensity

The overall color and intensity of staining in a Wright-stained blood smear vary with cell maturity and type. In general, cytoplasmic color progresses from darker blue (indicating active protein synthesis) in younger cells to lighter blue or pink in mature cells. Most early cells have a medium-blue cytoplasm. Immature **erythrocytes** have a very distinctive dark-blue cytoplasm that becomes paler and gray looking as the cell synthesizes hemoglobin. As mature cells, **lymphocytes** are usually noted for their pale sky-blue cytoplasmic color. Variations in cytoplasmic color develop in many cells because of abnormalities or the presence of granules.

Granulation

The presence, size, and color of granules are important in cellular identification. In general, granulation progresses from *no* granules to *nonspecific* granulation to *specific* granulation.

The earliest, blast forms of leukocytes and megakaryocytes do not have granules, and erythrocytes never exhibit granulation throughout their life cycle. The granulocytic cell line of leukocytes is noted for distinctive granulation. The complete development of granules in leukocytes is discussed in Chapters 14 and 16.

Granules vary in several ways:

1. In size, ranging from very fine to coarse
2. In color, including red (**azurophilic**), blue (**basophilic**), and orange (**eosinophilic**)
3. In the amount of granulation per cell

Cytoplasmic Shape

The cytoplasmic outline or shape is useful in cellular identification. The most distinctive variation in cytoplasmic shape occurs in some **blast forms**, **monocytes**, and **megakaryocytes**. **Pseudopods** may be observed in mature monocytes and in some leukocyte blast forms. The megakaryocyte develops a more irregular outline as the cell matures.

Quantity of Cytoplasm

In some cell types, the actual quantity of cytoplasm increases with age. The megakaryocyte, in particular, develops extensive quantities of cytoplasm. Abnormalities of lymphocytes frequently demonstrate increased amounts of cytoplasm.

Vacuolization

Monocytes are frequently noted for having vacuoles throughout their life cycle and under normal conditions. Except for the monocyte, vacuolization of the cytoplasm is commonly seen in older cells and in abnormal conditions. Anticoagulants can also produce vacuoles as **artifacts** if the blood is stored for a longer-than-acceptable period. Severe bacterial infections, viral infections (e.g., infectious mononucleosis), and malignancies may produce a remarkable number of vacuoles in various leukocyte types.

TABLE 4.5	Normal Adult Values and Selected Characteristics of Mature Leukocytes in Peripheral Blood					
Type	Nuclear Shape Average	Chromatin	Cytoplasmic Color	Granules	Color of Granules	Percentage
Segmented neutrophil	Lobulated	Very clumped	Pink	Many	Pink, a few blue	56
Band form neutrophil	Curved	Moderately clumped	Blue/pink	Many	Pink	3
Lymphocyte	Round	Smooth	Light blue	Few or absent	Red	34
Monocyte	Indented or twisted	Lacy	Gray-blue	Many	Dusty blue	4
Eosinophil	Lobulated	Very clumped	Granulated	Many	Orange	2.7
Basophil	Lobulated	Very clumped	Granulated	Many	Dark blue	0.3

Inclusion Bodies

Cytoplasmic inclusions such as **Auer bodies** or **Auer rods** (discussed in Chapter 14) in **myelocytic** or **monocytic blast** forms or ingested particles are important to observe because they aid in the identification of cell types. Various **erythrocytic inclusions** (refer to Chapter 6) and **leukocytic inclusions** (refer to Chapters 15 and 17) are indicative of specific diseases. Some types of inclusions may be seen on a Wright-stained blood smear, but other inclusions (such as iron particles) require special staining techniques.

MATURE BLOOD CELLS IN PERIPHERAL BLOOD

Identification of blood cells by microscopic examination of a peripheral smear can be performed more systematically if the morphologist assesses the various maturational features as outlined in the preceding section. This process will simplify the identification of maturing and mature erythrocytes and leukocytes, including those that do not have all the classic features.

The normal average percentage of leukocytes in adults and selected characteristics of these cells found on a normal Wright-stained blood smear are presented in Table 4.5.

CHAPTER HIGHLIGHTS

Blood cells originate from the mesenchymal tissue that arises from the embryonic germ layer, the mesoderm. The process of blood cell development, hematopoiesis, follows a definite sequence of sites from embryonic life to fetal life to childhood to adult life. In abnormal situations, blood production may revert to a more primitive state, referred to as extramedullary hematopoiesis.

The stem cell is the first in a sequence of steps of hematopoietic cell generation and maturation. Hematopoietic cells can be divided into three phases according to cell maturity. The multipotential stem cell is the progenitor of the two major cell lines: lymphoid and nonlymphoid. Colony-forming units precede the blast stage of cell development.

Hematopoietic growth factors regulate the proliferation and differentiation of progenitor cells and the function of mature blood cells. These factors are being used to treat a variety of diseases and disorders.

Each cellular element has a name and associated characteristics for each stage of development. Certain maturational characteristics are shared by most hematopoietic cells. Characteristics such as overall size and N:C ratio are important in determining the stages of development. Nuclear characteristics, such as the presence of nucleoli and chromatin patterns, vary with cell type and cell maturity. Cytoplasmic features, such as color and the presence of granules, must be carefully observed in a peripheral blood examination. The presence of granules is indicative of specific cell types and is a feature of cellular age. Identification of blood cells can be performed more systematically if the morphologist assesses the various maturational features. This process simplifies the identification of many cells that do not have all the classic features associated with a particular cell line and is useful in determining the age of a cell.

REVIEW QUESTIONS

1. The normal sequence of blood cell development is
   A. yolk sac—red bone marrow—liver and spleen
   B. yolk sac—thymus—liver and spleen—red bone marrow
   C. yolk sac—liver and spleen—red bone marrow
   D. liver and spleen—yolk sac—red bone marrow

2. The maturational sequence of the thrombocyte (platelet) is
   A. megakaryoblast—promegakaryocyte—megakaryocyte—metamegakaryocyte—thrombocyte
   B. promegakaryocyte—megakaryocyte—metamegakaryocyte—thrombocyte
   C. megakaryoblast—promegakaryocyte—megakaryocyte—thrombocyte
   D. megakaryoblast—promegakaryocyte—metamegakaryocyte—thrombocyte

3. The maturational sequence(s) of the erythrocyte is (are)
   A. rubriblast—prorubricyte—rubricyte—metarubricyte—reticulocyte—mature erythrocyte
   B. prorubricyte—rubricyte—metarubricyte—reticulocyte—mature erythrocyte
   C. pronormoblast—basophilic normoblast—polychromatophilic normoblast—orthochromic normoblast—reticulocyte—mature erythrocyte
   D. both A and C

4. The cell maturation sequence of the segmented neutrophil is
   A. promyelocyte—myeloblast—myelocyte—metamyelocyte—band or stab—segmented neutrophil (PMN)
   B. myeloblast—promyelocyte—myelocyte—metamyelocyte—band or stab—segmented neutrophil (PMN)
   C. monoblast—promyelocyte—myelocyte—metamyelocyte—band or stab—segmented neutrophil (PMN)
   D. promyelocyte—myelocyte—metamyelocyte—band or stab—segmented neutrophil (PMN)

5. As a blood cell matures, the overall cell diameter in most cases
   A. increases
   B. decreases
   C. remains the same

6. As a blood cell matures, the ratio of nucleus to cytoplasm (N:C) in most cases
   A. increases
   B. decreases
   C. remains the same

7. The chromatin pattern, in most cells, as the cell matures
   A. becomes more clumped
   B. becomes less clumped
   C. remains the same

8. The presence of nucleoli is associated with
   A. immature cells
   B. all young cells, except myeloblasts
   C. only erythroblasts
   D. disintegrating cells

9. In the blast stage of development of leukocytes, the cytoplasm of the cell is
   A. dark blue and lacks vacuoles
   B. light blue and lacks granules
   C. light blue and has specific granules
   D. gray with many dark-blue granules

Questions 10 through 14: Match the cellular characteristics with the name of the appropriate mature leukocyte. Use an answer only once.

10. _____ Segmented neutrophil
11. _____ Monocyte
12. _____ Lymphocyte
13. _____ Band form neutrophil
14. _____ Eosinophil

A. Large orange granules
B. An elongated and curved nucleus
C. Light, sky-blue cytoplasm
D. Kidney bean–shaped nucleus
E. Averages approximately 56% of normal adult leukocytes in the peripheral blood

BIBLIOGRAPHY

Becerra SP, Amaral J. Erythropoietin—an endogenous retinal survival factor, *N Engl J Med*, 347(24):1968–1970, 2002.

Blank U, Karlsson G, Karlsson S. Signaling pathways governing stem-cell fate, *Blood*, 111(2):492–500, 2008.

Bunn HF. New agents that stimulate erythropoiesis, *Blood*, 109(3), 868–873, 2007.

Chasis JA, Mohandas N. Erythroblastic islands: niches for erythropoiesis. Blood, 112(3):470–476, 2008.

De la Fuente J, et al. Alpha₂beta₁ and Alpha₄beta₁ integrins mediate the homing of mesenchymal stem/progenitor cells during fetal life, *Hematol J*, 4(Suppl 2):13, 2003.

Durand C, Dzierzak E. Embryonic beginnings of adult hematopoietic stem cells. *Haematologica*, 90(1):100–108, 2005.

Dzierzak E. Ontogenic emergence of definite hematopoietic stem cells, *Curr Opin Hematol*, 10(3):229–234, 2003.

Fleming MD, Kutok JL, Skarin AT. Examination of the bone marrow. In: Handin RI, Lux SE, Stossel TP (eds.). *Blood*, 2nd ed, Philadelphia, PA: Lippincott Williams & Wilkins, 2003:59–79.

Golde DW. Hematopoietic growth factors, *Int J Cell Cloning*, 8(Suppl 1): 4–10, 1990.

Groopman JE, Molina J, Scadden DT. Hematopoietic growth factors, *N Engl J Med*, 321(21):1449–1459, 1989.

Hauke RJ. Hematopoietic growth factors, *Lab Med*, 31(11):613–615, 2000.

Kurec AS. A brave, new laboratory world. *Med Lab Observer*, 22–23, 2005.

Liang YG, Van Zant G. Genetic control of stem-cell properties and stem cells in aging, *Curr Opin Hematol*, 10(3):195–202, 2003.

Metcalf D. Hematopoietic cytokines. *Blood*, 111(2):485–491, 2008.

Nightingale SL. Hematopoietic growth factors workshop, *JAMA*, 262(10):1296, 1989.

Orazi A, O'Malley DP. Bone marrow immunohistochemistry, *Advance*, 22–24, 2003.

Thomas J, Liu F, Link DC. Mechanisms of mobilization of hematopoietic progenitors with granulocyte colony-stimulating factors, *Curr Opin Hematol*, 9(3):183–189, 2002.

Thompson CB. Apoptosis in the pathogenesis and treatment of disease, *Science*, 267:1456–1462, 1995.

Turgeon ML. *Immunology and Serology in Laboratory Medicine*, 4th ed, St. Louis, MO: Mosby, 2009.

Whichard ZL, et al, Hematopoiesis and its disorders: a systems biology approach, *Blood*, 115(12):2339–2347, 2010.

PART TWO

Erythrocytes

CHAPTER	5	Erythrocyte Maturation, Physiology, and Lifecycle

OBJECTIVES

Erythropoiesis

- Name the sites of erythropoiesis from the early embryonic stage of development until fully established in adults.
- Name the substances necessary for proper erythropoiesis.
- Describe the biochemical properties and sites of production of erythropoietin.
- Explain the normal condition that stimulates the production of erythropoietin and how it influences the production of erythrocytes.
- List the maturational times for the various erythrocyte developmental phases.
- Describe the major morphological features of each of the erythrocyte maturational stages.
- Explain the events that occur during reticulocyte maturation.
- Describe the normal distribution and replacement pattern of reticulocytes in the circulation.
- Define the terms **shift** or **stress** reticulocytes.
- Compare the morphological appearances of reticulocytes stained with Wright stain and a supravital stain, such as new methylene blue.
- Give the normal value of the uncorrected reticulocyte count.
- When given the necessary laboratory results, calculate the **corrected reticulocyte count** and the **reticulocyte production index**.

Disorders related to the erythrocyte maturation and production

- Describe the various types of conditions that can produce disorders of erythropoietin production.
- Compare the terms secondary polycythemia and relative polycythemia
- Compare the morphological characteristics of defective erythrocyte maturation and **megaloblastic maturation** with normal developmental features.

Characteristics and biosynthesis of hemoglobin

- Describe the chemical configuration of normal adult hemoglobin.
- Explain the physiological role of 2,3-diphosphoglycerate (2,3-DPG) in the oxygenation of the hemoglobin molecule.

- Relate the oxygen dissociation curve to the oxygen-binding activities of the hemoglobin molecule.
- Cite at least two examples of clinical conditions that can alter oxygen dissociation and explain what effect these conditions have on the oxygen dissociation curve.
- Describe the **Bohr effect** and other physical or chemical factors that affect the oxygen dissociation curve.
- Explain the elimination and transport of carbon dioxide.
- Briefly describe the overall synthesis of heme.
- Describe the sites and mechanism of transport and insertion of iron in the production of hemoglobin.
- Explain the factors that regulate the synthesis of globin in hemoglobin production.
- Specifically describe the outcomes of a deficiency in the production of globin.
- Name the embryonic hemoglobins and describe their chemical composition and site of formation.
- Explain the types of chains, developmental formation, and quantities of fetal hemoglobin.
- Identify the types of chains, site of formation, and quantities of adult hemoglobin A and A_2.
- Describe the formation and concentration of glycosylated hemoglobin in normal and hyperglycemic environments.
- Diagram and explain the inheritance patterns of normal hemoglobin and abnormal hemoglobin genotypes and phenotypes.
- Name at least four hemoglobin analysis methods and explain the purpose of each procedure.

Disorders related to hemoglobin biosynthesis

- Name one congenital and two acquired disorders that are related to defects in heme (porphyrin) synthesis.
- Describe the pathophysiology of sideroblastic anemia.
- Explain the remarkable laboratory characteristics of sideroblastic anemia.
- Compare the etiology and manifestation of hereditary hemochromatosis (HH).
- Compare various forms of globulin synthesis.

(continued)

Membrane characteristics and metabolic activities of erythrocytes

■ Describe the general characteristics, including the physical properties, of the erythrocyte membrane.

■ Explain the importance of enzymes in energy-yielding cellular reactions.

■ Describe the importance and physiology of the **Embden-Meyerhof** glycolytic pathway.

■ Explain the physiology of the **oxidative pathway** and the effects of a defect in this pathway.

■ Explain the importance of the **methemoglobin reductase** pathway to heme iron.

■ Describe the function of the **Luebering-Rapoport** pathway.

■ Detail the changes that take place at the end of the erythrocytic life span and describe the removal of cells from the circulation.

■ Explain the events of extravascular destruction of the erythrocyte.

■ Describe the details of intravascular destruction of the erythrocyte.

Measurement of erythrocytes

■ Name the procedures that assess the quantities of either erythrocytes or hemoglobin.

■ Cite the normal values of the erythrocyte count, hemoglobin, and packed cell volumes for various age groups.

■ Define each of the erythrocyte indices: mean corpuscular volume (MCV), mean corpuscular hemoglobin (MCH), and mean corpuscular hemoglobin concentration (MCHC).

■ Apply the appropriate formulas and calculate the MCV, MCH, and MCHC when given the erythrocyte values.

Case studies

■ Apply the laboratory data to the stated case studies and discuss the implications of these cases to the study of hematology.

ERYTHROPOIESIS

The mature erythrocyte is a biconcave disc with a central pallor that occupies the middle one-third of the cell. In the mature cell, the respiratory protein, hemoglobin, performs the function of oxygen–carbon dioxide transport. Throughout the life span of the mature cell, an average of 120 days, this soft and pliable cell moves with ease through the tissue capillaries and splenic circulation. As the cell ages, cytoplasmic enzymes are catabolized, leading to increased membrane rigidity (density), phagocytosis, and destruction.

The term used to describe the process of erythrocyte production is **erythropoiesis**. Erythropoiesis encompasses differentiation from the hematopoietic stem cell (HSC) through the mature erythrocyte. Erythropoiesis epitomizes highly specialized cellular differentiation and gene expression. As cells progress through the stages of erythropoiesis, their potential to differentiate into lymphoid or other hematopoietic cell types is restricted. They are increasingly committed to differentiate into erythrocytes.

To streamline their functional capacity, erythrocyte precursors shed most organelles and produce prodigious amounts of hemoglobin, which eventually comprises approximately 95% of the total cellular protein. Erythropoiesis is regulated partially by the combined actions of cytokine signaling pathways and transcription factors.

Molecular regulators of erythropoiesis can be categorized as those committing pluripotent precursors to an erythroid fate and those regulating the differentiation of erythroid progenitors into erythrocytes. Molecular chaperones, a diverse group of proteins, are important red cell maturation. Chaperones influence all aspects of normal cellular function including signaling, transcription, cell division, and apoptosis.

Hematopoiesis (see Chapter 4 for a complete discussion) begins with the development of primitive erythrocytes in the embryonic yolk sac, continues in extramedullary organs such as the liver in the developing fetus, and is ultimately located in the red bone marrow during late fetal development, childhood, and adult life.

Transport of oxygen to the tissues and transport of carbon dioxide from the tissues are accomplished by the **heme** pigment in hemoglobin, which is synthesized as the erythrocyte matures. The basic substances needed for normal erythrocyte and hemoglobin production are amino acids (proteins), iron, vitamin B_{12}, vitamin B_6, folic acid (a member of the vitamin B_2 complex), and the trace minerals cobalt and nickel. In adult humans, the daily production of more than 200 billion erythrocytes requires more than 20 mg of elemental iron. The vast majority of this iron comes from the recycling of senescent erythrocytes by macrophages of the mononuclear phagocytic system; only 1 to 2 mg of the daily iron supply derives from intestinal absorption, which at a steady state is sufficient only to replace iron lost by epithelial cell sloughing and functional and dysfunctional bleeding.

Abnormal erythropoiesis can result from deficiencies of any of these necessary substances. Defective erythropoiesis is frequently seen in underdeveloped countries where protein deficiencies are common. Other types of anemias (discussed in Chapters 10 and 11) can be caused by deficiencies in vitamin B_{12}, folic acid, or iron.

Erythropoietin

The substance **erythropoietin** is produced primarily by the kidneys. Peritubular cells are the probable site of synthesis in the kidneys. Extrarenal organs such as the liver also secrete this substance. Ten to fifteen percent of erythropoietin production occurs in the liver, which is the primary source of erythropoietin in the unborn. This glycoprotein hormone, with a molecular weight of 46,000, stimulates erythropoiesis and can cross the placental barrier between the mother and the fetus. Erythropoietin was the first human hematopoietic growth factor to be identified. The gene for erythropoietin is located on chromosome 7.

Blood levels of erythropoietin are inversely related to tissue oxygenation. The level can increase up to 20,000 mU/mL in response to anemia or arterial hypoxemia. Erythropoietin is detectable in the plasma (normal concentration up to 20 mU/mL). The red cell mass of the body is continuously adjusted to the optimal size for its function as an oxygen carrier, by messages transmitted to the bone marrow from the oxygen sensor in the kidney. Tissue hypoxia, a decrease in the oxygen content within the tissues, produces a dramatic increase in the production of erythropoietin. A heme protein is thought to be involved in the oxygen-sensing mechanism. The messages from the sensing mechanisms are mediated by erythropoietin, are modulated by cardiovascular and renal factors, and form a key link in the feedback loop that controls red cell production. Through the action of erythropoietin, the number of hemoglobin-containing erythrocytes increases, the oxygen-carrying capacity of the blood increases, and the normal level of oxygen in the tissues can be restored.

In 1985, the erythropoietin gene was cloned and expressed. This led the way to the development of recombinant (monoclonal) human erythropoietin, which reduces transfusion dependency and increases preoperative hemoglobin in patients whose bodies cannot respond to the need to produce erythropoietin. Recently, observations indicate that erythropoiesis-stimulating agents may be associated with serious adverse effects in patients with malignancy.

Erythropoietin has its predominant effect on the committed erythroid cells, colony-forming unit-erythroid (CFU-E), promoting their proliferation and differentiation into erythroblasts. It may also stimulate the differentiation of a more primitive erythroid progenitor, the burst-forming unit-erythroid (BFU-E), in association with so-called burst-promoting activity. Erythropoietin prevents erythroid cell apoptosis. Cell divisions accompanying terminal erythroid differentiation are finely controlled by cell cycle regulators. Disruption of these terminal divisions causes erythroid cell apoptosis. In reticulocyte maturation, regulated degradation of internal organelles involves a lipoxygenase, whereas survival requires the antiapoptotic protein Bcl-x.

In biochemical studies of the action of erythropoietin, it has been demonstrated that initially an increase in the production of several types of ribonucleic acid (RNA) takes place. This activity is followed by an increase in deoxyribonucleic acid (DNA) activity and protein synthesis. The number of cells at each stage before the polychromatophilic erythroblast stage is greater than at each preceding stage because of intervening cell divisions. After the polychromatophilic erythroblast stage, erythroid cells do not divide but undergo specialized maturation. Increased erythrocyte production and hemoglobin synthesis are ultimately the result.

Questions remain as to how many of the effects attributed to erythropoietin are direct. The androgen hormones and thyroid hormones can also stimulate erythropoiesis.

Erythropoietin also interacts with interleukin-3, granulocyte-macrophage colony-stimulating factor (GM-CSF), interleukin-1, and thrombocytopoiesis-stimulating factor to promote the production of megakaryocytes.

Recombinant human erythropoietin is produced from mammalian cells and was originally used in patients being treated with dialysis who had anemia due to chronic renal failure. In addition to possible uses in the treatment of various types of anemia, recombinant human erythropoietin is likely to be useful in a broad range of clinical applications.

General Characteristics of Maturation and Development

Erythrocytes are rapidly maturing cells. Once the stem cell differentiates into the erythroid cell line (Fig. 5.1), a cell matures through the nucleated cell stages in 4 or 5 days. Bone

Pronormoblast (Rubriblast)

Basophilic Normoblast (Prorubricyte)

Polychromatophilic Normoblast (Rubricyte)

Orthochromic Normoblast (Metarubricyte)

Polychromatophilic Erythrocyte (Reticulocyte)

Mature Red Blood Cell (Mature Erythrocyte)

FIGURE 5.1 Erythrocyte maturation. (Reprinted with permission from Anderson, SC. *Anderson's Atlas of Hematology*, Philadelphia, PA: Wolters Kluwer Health/Lippincott Williams & Wilkins, Copyright 2003.)

marrow reticulocytes have an average maturation period of 2.5 days. Once young reticulocytes enter the circulating blood, they remain in the reticulocyte stage for an average of 1 day and represent approximately 0.5% to 1.5% of the circulating erythrocytes.

Developmental Stages

Early Cells

All hematopoietic cell lines are derived from an original, common pool of ancestral pluripotent stem cells. Biologic systems function at the molecular, cellular, tissue, and organismismal levels. To perform their specialized functions, highly differentiated blood cells are continuously produced by stem cells. A combination of more than a dozen growth and stromal factors drive cells to divide asymmetrically, undergo differentiation, and carry out their end-cell functions. A simple erythrocyte, enucleated and without mitochondria, contains more than 750 proteins, ignoring posttranslational modifications. With at least a dozen types of highly specialized cells and platelets circulating a liquid phase consisting of 1,000 proteins, blood and its elements comprise a complex system.

When the pluripotent stem cell, the first in a sequence of steps of cell generation and maturation, differentiates into a nonlymphoid multipotential stem cell, it can become a colony-forming unit granulocyte-erythrocyte-monocyte-megakaryocyte (CFU-GEMM) depending on the presence of specific growth factors (see Fig. 4.10, Chapter 4).

In erythropoiesis, the CFU-GEMM differentiates into a BFU-E. The earliest cell in the erythrocyte series is the BFU-E. Like HSCs, BFU-Es are not actively proliferating. Most of these cells are in the G_0/G_1 phase of the cell cycle.

The next step in differentiation is the formation of colony-forming units (CFU-E). CFU-Es are actively proliferating. Most are in the S phase of the cell cycle. CFU-Es produce erythroid colonies of up to 100 cells. Under the influence of erythropoietin, the CFU-Es undergo a programmed series of cell divisions and cell maturation, culminating in the mature erythrocyte. As CFU-Es differentiate to late-stage erythroblasts, they cease to divide and accumulate in the G_0 phase before enucleation. Regulated cessation of cell division preceding erythroblast enucleation is crucial for normal erythrocyte production. If it is interrupted by drugs that interfere with DNA synthesis (e.g., methotrexate) or by deficiencies of vitamins required for DNA synthesis (e.g., folate and vitamin B_{12}), macrocytic anemia develops.

When cells differentiate into the erythroid line, the maturational changes are consistent with the overall nuclear and cytoplasmic changes seen in other cell lines (see Chapter 4). However, the erythrocyte becomes an **anuclear** mature cell (Table 5.1 and Fig. 5.2).

Rubriblast (Pronormoblast)

The **rubriblast** (Fig. 5.3) or **pronormoblast** (see Table 5.1) has an overall diameter of approximately 12 to 19 μm. The nuclear-to-cytoplasmic (N:C) ratio is 4:1. The large, round nucleus contains from zero to two nucleoli, is usually dark appearing, and has a fine chromatin pattern.

The cytoplasm stains a distinctive blue (**basophilic**) color with Wright stain and lacks granules. The distinctive blue color reflects the RNA activity needed to produce the protein required for hemoglobin synthesis. Studies with radioactive iron have demonstrated that most of the iron destined for hemoglobin synthesis is taken into the cell at this stage.

Prorubricyte (Basophilic Normoblast)

The second stage, the **prorubricyte** (Fig. 5.4) or basophilic normoblast, has an overall cell diameter of 12 to 17 μm and is only slightly smaller than the rubriblast. The N:C ratio remains high (4:1); however, this stage demonstrates morphological evidence of increasing maturity.

The nuclear chromatin becomes more clumped. Nucleoli are usually no longer apparent. The cytoplasm continues to appear basophilic with a Wright stain. This cell contains no evidence of the pink color that indicates hemoglobin development.

Rubricyte (Polychromatic Normoblast)

Hemoglobin appears for the first time in the third maturational stage, the **rubricyte** (Fig. 5.5) or **polychromatic normoblast**. At this stage, the overall cell size of 11 to 15 μm is slightly decreased from that of the prorubricyte stage. Further maturation is also demonstrated by the decreased N:C ratio of 1:1.

The chromatin continues to become increasingly clumped. The cytoplasm of cells in this stage shows variable amounts of pink coloration mixed with basophilia; this can give the cell a muddy, light gray appearance.

Metarubricyte (Orthochromic Normoblast)

The rubricyte matures into the metarubricyte (Fig. 5.6) or orthochromic normoblast. The overall cell is smaller (8 to 12 μm). The chromatin pattern is tightly condensed in this maturational stage and can be described as pyknotic (dense or compact). In the later period of this stage, the nucleus will be extruded from the cell. The metarubricyte is characterized by an acidophilic (reddish pink) cytoplasm. This coloration indicates the presence of large quantities of hemoglobin (Figs. 5.7 and 5.8). Three mitoses are believed to occur in the 2- to 3-day interval between the rubriblast and the end of the metarubricyte stage. Two thirds of these mitoses have been shown to occur in the rubricyte stage. After this stage, the cell is no longer able to undergo mitosis.

TABLE 5.1	Dual Nomenclature and Developmental Characteristics of Red Blood Cells		
Name	**Cellular Features**	**Name**	**Cellular Features**
1. Rubriblast or pronormoblast	Size: 12–19 μm in diameter	3. Rubricyte or polychromatic normoblast	Size: 11–15 μm in diameter
	N:C ratio 4:1		N:C ratio 1:1
	Nucleus		**Nucleus**
	Large, round nucleus		Increased clumping of the chromatin
	Chromatin has a fine pattern		**Cytoplasm**
	0–2 nucleoli		Color: variable, with pink staining mixed with basophilia
	Cytoplasm		
	Distinctive basophilic color		
	Without granules		
2. Prorubricyte or basophilic normoblast	Size: 12–17 μm in diameter	4. Metarubricyte or orthochromic normoblast or nucleated RBC (NRBC)	Size: 8–12 μm
	N:C ratio 4:1		**Nucleus**
	Nucleus		Chromatin pattern is tightly condensed
	Nuclear chromatin more clumped		**Cytoplasm**
	Nucleoli usually not apparent		Color: reddish-pink (acidophilic)
	Cytoplasm		
	Distinctive basophilic color		
		5. Reticulocyte (supravital stain) or polychromatic erythrocyte (Wright stain)	Size: 7–10 μm
			Cell is anuclear
			Diffuse reticulum
			Cytoplasm
			Overall blue appearance
		6. Erythrocyte	Average diameter: 6–8 μm

Reticulocyte

The **reticulocyte** stage is the next maturational stage. Part of this phase occurs in the bone marrow, and the later part of the stage takes place in the circulating blood (Fig. 5.9). Reticulocytes are discussed in greater detail in the following section.

This cell demonstrates a characteristic reticular appearance caused by remaining RNA if stained with a supravital stain, such as new methylene blue. In a Wright-stained blood smear, young reticulocytes with a high amount of RNA residual have a blue appearance, which is referred to as **polychromatophilia** (Fig. 5.10).

Rubriblast (pronormoblast)

Prorubricyte
(basophilic normoblast)

Rubricyte
(polychromatic normoblast)

Metarubricyte
(orthochromic normoblast)

Reticulocyte

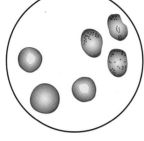

Reticulocyte appearance
with a supravital stain

Mature erythrocyte

FIGURE 5.2 Erythrocyte morphology. The morphological development of the erythrocyte is typical of blood cell maturation. The unique difference is that the erythrocyte loses its nucleus. If the erythrocyte is stained with a supravital stain, such as new methylene blue, reticulocytes, as depicted on the right, will be visible.

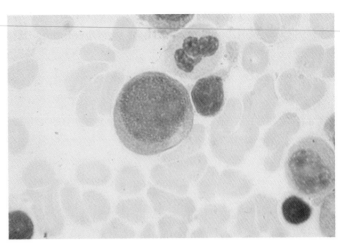

FIGURE 5.3 Pronormoblast (rubriblasts). (Reprinted with permission from Anderson, SC. *Anderson's Atlas of Hematology*, Philadelphia, PA: Wolters Kluwer Health/Lippincott Williams & Wilkins, Copyright 2003.)

the first day in the circulation, this immature erythrocyte is referred to as a **reticulocyte**.

Although the reticulocyte lacks a nucleus, it contains various organelles, such as mitochondria, and an extensive number of ribosomes. The formation of new ribosomes ceases with the loss of the nucleus in the late metarubricyte; however, while RNA is present, protein and heme synthesis continues. During reticulocyte maturation, the RNA is catabolized, and the ribosomes disintegrate. The loss of ribosomes and mitochondria, along with full hemoglobinization of the cell, marks the transition from the reticulocyte stage to full maturation of the erythrocyte.

Under normal conditions, the quantity of reticulocytes in the bone marrow is equal to that of the reticulocytes in the circulating blood. To maintain a stable reticulocyte pool in the circulation, the bone marrow replaces the num-

The overall cellular diameter ranges from 7 to 10 μm. This cell is anuclear.

Mature Erythrocyte

After the reticulocyte stage, the **mature erythrocyte** is formed. This cell has an average diameter of 6 to 8 μm. The survivability of erythrocytes can be determined by using radioactive chromium (^{51}Cr). A shortened life span can be observed in the hemolytic anemias (see Chapter 12).

Reticulocytes

As the erythrocyte develops, the nucleus becomes more and more condensed and is eventually lost. After the loss of the nucleus, an immature erythrocyte (reticulocyte) remains in the bone marrow for 2 to 3 days before entering the circulating blood. During this period in the bone marrow and during

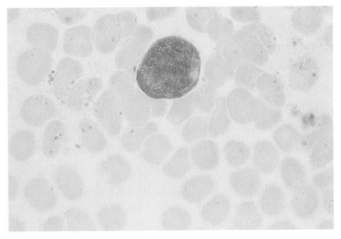

FIGURE 5.4 Basophilic normoblast (prorubricyte). (Reprinted with permission from Anderson, SC. *Anderson's Atlas of Hematology*, Philadelphia, PA: Wolters Kluwer Health/Lippincott Williams & Wilkins, Copyright 2003.)

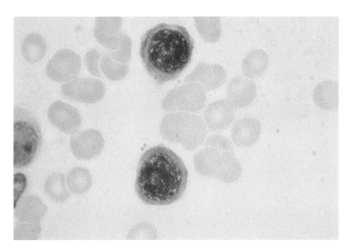

FIGURE 5.5 Polychromatophilic normoblast (rubricyte). (Reprinted with permission from Anderson, SC. *Anderson's Atlas of Hematology*, Philadelphia, PA: Wolters Kluwer Health/Lippincott Williams & Wilkins, Copyright 2003.)

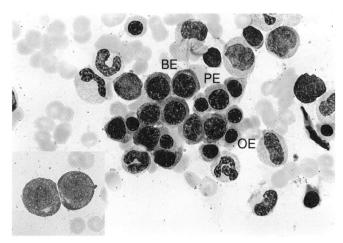

FIGURE 5.7 Erythroid maturation. (Reprinted with permission from Handin RI, Lux SE, Stossel TP. *Blood: Principles and Practice of Hematology*, 2 ed, Philadelphia, PA: Lippincott Williams & Wilkins, 2003.)

ber of erythrocytes that have reached their full life span. Because the normal life span or survival time is 120 days, 1/120th of the total number of erythrocytes is lost each day, and an equal number of reticulocytes is released into the circulation.

If, under the stimulus of erythropoietin, increased numbers of young reticulocytes are prematurely released from the bone marrow because of such conditions as acute bleeding, these reticulocytes are referred to as **stress** or **shift** reticulocytes. This situation is analogous to the appearance of immature leukocytes in the peripheral blood during the stress of infection.

The Reticulocyte Count

Peripheral smears of normal blood stained with Wright stain may demonstrate a slight blue tint in some erythrocytes. This morphological condition of erythrocytes, which is described in more detail in Chapter 6, is referred to as

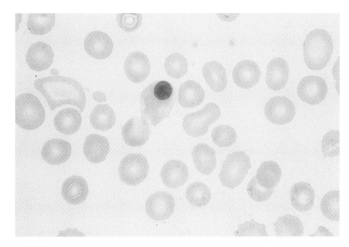

FIGURE 5.6 Orthochromatic normoblast (metarubricyte). (Reprinted with permission from Anderson, SC. *Anderson's Atlas of Hematology*, Philadelphia, PA: Wolters Kluwer Health/Lippincott Williams & Wilkins, Copyright 2003.)

polychromatophilia or **polychromasia**. However, a supravital stain, such as new methylene blue, precipitates the ribosomal RNA in these cells to form a deep-blue, meshlike network. Stress reticulocytes are recognizable on Wright-stained blood smears by their larger size and increased blue tint and may be accompanied by even younger erythrocytes, such as metarubricytes. When stained with a supravital stain, stress reticulocytes exhibit a much denser meshlike network.

The **reticulocyte count** procedure is frequently performed in the clinical laboratory as an indicator of the rate of erythrocyte production. Usually, the count is expressed as a percentage of total erythrocytes. The normal range is 0.5% to 2.0% in adults. In newborn infants, the range is 2.5% to 6.0%, but this value falls to the adult range by the end of the second week of life.

The reticulocyte count is of value as an indication of a shorter-than-normal erythrocyte survival, which is based on the deduction that the total red blood cell (RBC) mass in a steady state is equal to the number of new RBCs produced, multiplied by the 120-day life span of individual cells. When the RBC mass falls, it is the result of decreased RBC production or a shortened life span. Normal erythropoiesis corrects for a shorter life span by increasing the production rate, which the reticulocyte count measures. An elevated reticulocyte count accompanies a shortened RBC survival. **Reticulocytosis** indicates that the body is trying to maintain homeostasis.

Calculating and Expressing Reticulocyte Values

Traditionally, the reticulocyte count has been expressed as a percentage of the total number of circulating erythrocytes (e.g., 1%). However, this value may be erroneous because fluctuation in the percentage may be caused by a change in the total number of circulating erythrocytes rather than a true change in the number of circulating reticulocytes. To account for variations caused by erythrocyte

FIGURE 5.8 Erythroid maturation. RBC maturation/normoblasts. Pronormoblast (**A**); basophilic normoblasts (**B**); early (**C**) and late (**D**) polychromatophilic normoblasts; orthochromatic normoblast with stippling (**E**). Magnification, 1,000×; Wright stain. (Reprinted with permission from Greer JP (ed). *Wintrobe's Clinical Hematology*, 11 ed, Philadelphia, PA: Lippincott Williams & Wilkins, 2004.)

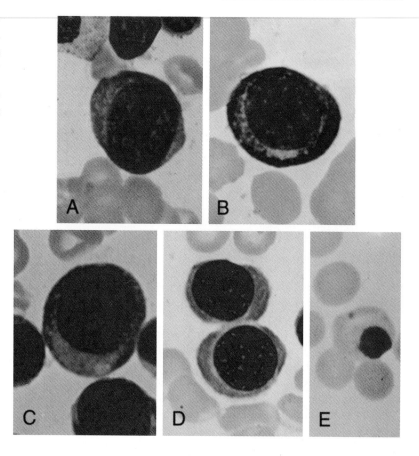

quantity, expression of reticulocytes in absolute rather than proportional terms is becoming the preferred method of reporting. The correction for anemia is helpful for clinical interpretation, and several different methods are used. The

CLSI proposes that the correction for anemia, the **corrected reticulocyte count**, be made mathematically by correcting the observed reticulocyte count to a normal packed RBC volume (hematocrit).

FIGURE 5.9 Changes in total body hemoglobin, blood hemoglobin concentration, reticulocyte count, and body weight in a representative premature infant. The vertical bars represent the infant's body weight. During the first 6 weeks of life, the blood hemoglobin concentration and total body hemoglobin fall as a result of decreased erythrocyte production, as evidenced by the low reticulocyte count. The more rapid decline in blood hemoglobin concentration from the third to the sixth week is the result of the increasing body size and dilution of the hemoglobin mass. After 6 weeks of age, hemoglobin production increases, as evidenced by the increased reticulocyte count and the rapid increase in total body hemoglobin. The blood hemoglobin concentration during that period may rise slightly, or not at all, because the total body size increases at approximately the same rate as the total hemoglobin mass. (Reprinted with permission from Mhairi G, et al. *Avery's Neonatology Pathophysiology and Management of the Newborn*, 6th ed, Philadelphia, PA: Lippincott Williams & Wilkins, 2005.)

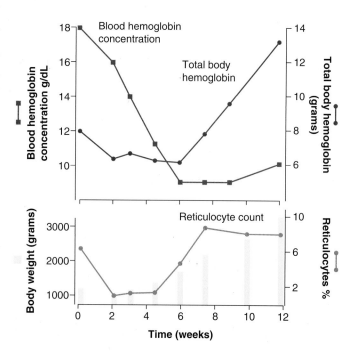

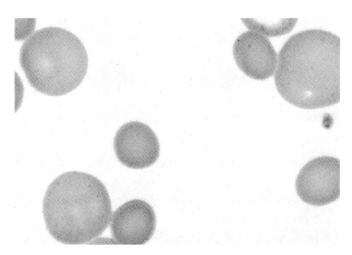

FIGURE 5.10 Polychromatophilia. (Reprinted with permission from Anderson, SC. *Anderson's Atlas of Hematology*, Philadelphia, PA: Wolters Kluwer Health/Lippincott Williams & Wilkins, Copyright 2003.)

Corrected Reticulocyte Count

Corrected reticulocyte count = reticulocyte count (%)

$$\times \frac{\text{patient's packed cell volume (hematocrit)}}{\text{normal hematocrit based on age and gender}} = \%$$

Example: If an adult male has a hematocrit of 30% (0.30 L/L) and a reticulocyte count of 3%, the corrected reticulocyte count would be

Corrected reticulocyte count

$$= 3\% \times \frac{0.30\,\text{L/L}}{0.45\,\text{L/L (adult male normal value)}}$$

$$= 0.3 \times \frac{0.30\,\text{L/L}}{0.45\,\text{L/L (adult male normal value)}} = 0.02 = 2.0\%$$

The normal value based on correction for anemia is the same as the previously stated normal reticulocyte values of 0.5% to 2.0%.

Reticulocyte Production Index

A simple percentage calculation of reticulocytes does not account for the fact that prematurely released reticulocytes require from 0.5 to 1.5 days longer in the circulating blood to mature and lose their netlike reticulum. Therefore, the reticulocyte count, even if corrected, will be elevated out of proportion to the actual increase in erythrocyte production because of the accumulation of these younger reticulocytes in the circulating blood. To correct for this situation, the use of the reticulocyte production index (RPI) was proposed.

The RPI measures erythropoietic activity when stress reticulocytes are present. The rationale for obtaining this value is that the life span of the circulating stress reticulocytes is 2 days instead of the normal 1 day. To compensate for

TABLE 5.2	Maturation Time Correction Factor
Hematocrit (%)	**Maturation Time (Days)**
45	1.0
35	1.5
25	2.0
15	2.5

the increased maturation time and consequent retention of residual RNA of the prematurely released reticulocytes, the corrected reticulocyte count is divided by a correction factor derived from the maturation timetable (Table 5.2).

Calculation of the Reticulocyte Production Index

$$\text{RPI} = \frac{\text{corrected reticulocyte count in \%}}{\text{maturation time in days}}$$

If the corrected reticulocyte count is 2.0% and the patient's hematocrit is 0.30 L/L, the RPI is

$$\text{RPI} = \frac{2.0}{1.75} = 1.14$$

Normal bone marrow activity produces an RPI index of 1. In hemolytic anemias, in which there is increased destruction of erythrocytes in the peripheral blood and a functionally normal marrow, this index may be from three to seven times higher than normal. In cases of bone marrow damage, erythropoietin suppression, or a deficiency of vitamin B_{12}, folic acid, or iron (hypoproliferative states), the index is 2 or less.

DISORDERS RELATED TO ERYTHROCYTE MATURATION AND PRODUCTION

Disorders of Erythropoietin

Polycythemia is the term used to refer to an increased concentration of erythrocytes (**erythrocytosis**) in the circulating blood that is above normal for gender and age. **Secondary,** or **absolute,** polycythemias reflect an increase in erythropoietin production and should *not* be confused with polycythemia vera (see Chapter 21) or relative polycythemias.

Secondary polycythemia produced by increased erythropoietin production results from tissue **hypoxia** caused by such diverse factors as defective high oxygen affinity type of hemoglobin, certain types of anemia, chronic lung disease, or inappropriate erythropoietin production. Smoking is a common cause of secondary erythrocytosis. Conditions of inappropriate erythropoietin production may result from

neoplasms, usually renal, or renal disorders that produce local hypoxia within the kidney. A more unusual cause of inappropriate erythropoiesis is **familial polycythemia,** an autosomal dominant trait that produces a defect in the regulation of erythropoietin. A reduction in erythropoietin production may also exist. In situations such as hypertransfusion, the quantity of erythropoietin is reduced.

Red Cell Increases

Increases in erythrocytes can result from conditions that are not related to increased erythropoietin production. These conditions include the **relative polycythemias**.

A relative polycythemia exists when an increase in the packed cell volume (hematocrit) or the total erythrocyte count is caused by decreased plasma volume. The total erythrocyte mass is not increased. Increases in the packed RBC volume or erythrocyte count reflect an increase in the volume or erythrocytes in proportion to the total blood volume. Loss of body fluids and plasma volume because of conditions producing dehydration, such as diarrhea or burns, can produce these increased results.

Defective Nuclear Maturation

A defect in maturation known as **megaloblastic maturation** (Fig. 5.11) can be seen in certain anemias, such as vitamin B_{12} or folate deficiencies (see Chapter 11). The most noticeable characteristic of this type of defect is that nuclear maturation lags behind cytoplasmic maturation. Because of an impaired ability of the cells to synthesize DNA, both the interphase and the phases of mitotic division are prolonged. This asynchronous pattern of maturation can be confusing because the nuclear development of the cell is much younger looking than the actual developmental age, which is expressed by the cytoplasmic development. Other important features of

megaloblastic maturation include an increased amount of erythrocytic cellular cytoplasm and increased overall erythrocyte size. The megaloblastic dysfunction also expresses itself in the maturation of leukocytes. Giant band-type leukocyte forms are frequently observed on blood smears.

CHARACTERISTICS AND BIOSYNTHESIS OF HEMOGLOBIN

In 1862, Felix Seyler identified the respiratory protein hemoglobin. He discovered the characteristic color spectrum of hemoglobin and proved that this was the true coloring matter of the blood. Following this discovery, research began on the reaction of hemoglobin with oxygen. Today, the activities of hemoglobin and oxygen are well-known and can be demonstrated by an oxygen dissociation curve.

Genetic Inheritance of Hemoglobin

Normal adult hemoglobin A is inherited in simple mendelian fashion. The genotype for this phenotype is A/A. Abnormalities of hemoglobin types may be seen in various hematological disorders; there are also approximately 350 variant types. Most defects in hemoglobin are related to either amino acid substitutions or diminished production of one of the polypeptide chains. Disorders referred to as hemoglobinopathies (discussed in detail in Chapter 13) represent disorders related to defective hemoglobin molecules.

Chemical Composition and Configuration of Hemoglobin

Normal adult hemoglobin (hemoglobin A) (Fig. 5.12) consists of four heme groups and four polypeptide chains with a total of 574 amino acids. The polypeptide chains are

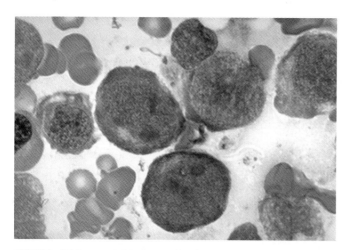

FIGURE 5.11 Megaloblastic anemia. A bone marrow aspirate from a patient with vitamin B_{12} deficiency (pernicious anemia) shows prominent megaloblastic erythroid precursors. (Reprinted with permission from Rubin E, Farber JL. *Pathology*, 3rd ed, Philadelphia, PA: Lippincott Williams & Wilkins, 1999.)

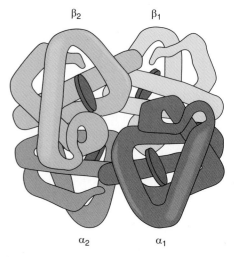

FIGURE 5.12 Structure of the hemoglobin. (Reprinted with permission from Porth CM. *Pathophysiology Concepts of Altered Health States*, 7th ed, Philadelphia, PA: Lippincott Williams & Wilkins, 2005.)

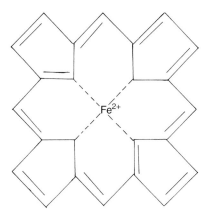

FIGURE 5.13 The heme portion of the hemoglobin molecule consists of one iron (Fe^{2+}) atom and four pyrrole rings that are joined to each other. A complete hemoglobin molecule consists of four heme molecules, each of which is attached to one molecule of the protein globin.

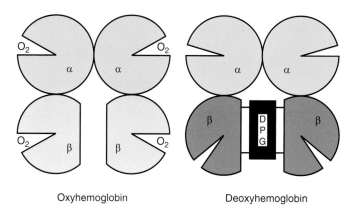

FIGURE 5.14 Hemoglobin molecular changes.

organized into two alpha chains and two beta chains. Each of the chains has an attached heme group (Fig. 5.13). Normal adult hemoglobin has 141 amino acids in each of the alpha chains and 146 amino acids in each of the beta chains. The specific sequence of these amino acids is known and is important in the identification of abnormal hemoglobins involving substitutions of specific amino acids.

In the native configuration of the hemoglobin molecule, the four hemes and four polypeptide chains are assembled in a very specific spatial configuration. Each of the four chains in the molecule coils into eight helices, forming an egg-shaped molecule with a central cavity. In the process of the binding of the first heme group to a molecule of oxygen, a change in the overall configuration of the hemoglobin molecule occurs. This altered configuration of the molecule favors the additional binding of oxygen to the remaining heme groups, if sufficient oxygen pressure is present. Metabolic processes within the erythrocyte ensure a suitable intracellular environment for hemoglobin that protects it from chemical changes that might result in the loss of its native structure or denaturation. If hemoglobin is denatured, it loses its ability to carry oxygen.

The Role of 2,3-Diphosphoglycerate

The major function of the hemoglobin molecule is the transport of oxygen to the tissues. The oxygen affinity of the hemoglobin molecule is associated with the spatial rearrangement of the molecule and is regulated by the concentration of phosphates, particularly 2,3-DPG in the erythrocyte. The manner in which 2,3-DPG binding to reduced hemoglobin (deoxyhemoglobin) affects oxygen affinity is complex. Basically, 2,3-DPG combines with the beta chains of deoxyhemoglobin and diminishes the molecule's affinity for oxygen (Fig. 5.14).

When the individual heme groups unload oxygen in the tissues, the beta chains are pulled apart. This permits the

entrance of 2,3-DPG and the establishment of salt bridges between the individual chains. These activities result in a progressively lower affinity of the molecule for oxygen. With oxygen uptake in the lungs, the salt bonds are sequentially broken; the beta chains are pulled together, expelling 2,3-DPG; and the affinity of the hemoglobin molecule for oxygen progressively increases.

In cases of tissue hypoxia, oxygen moves from hemoglobin into the tissues, and the amount of deoxyhemoglobin in the erythrocytes increases. This produces the binding of more 2,3-DPG, which further reduces the oxygen affinity of the hemoglobin molecule. If hypoxia persists, depletion of free 2,3-DPG leads to increased production of more 2,3-DPG and a persistently lowered affinity of the hemoglobin molecule for oxygen.

Oxygen Dissociation and Alterations

The structure of the hemoglobin molecule makes it capable of considerable molecular changes as it loads and unloads oxygen. Changes in oxygen affinity of the molecule are responsible for the ease with which hemoglobin can be loaded with oxygen in the lungs and unloaded in the tissues.

Oxygen Dissociation

The shape and position of the oxyhemoglobin dissociation curve (Fig. 5.15) graphically describe the relationship between oxygen content (percentage of saturation) and partial pressure of oxygen (PO_2). For comparative purposes, the position of the curve is usually explained by the P_{50} value. The P_{50} value is defined as the partial pressure of oxygen required to produce half saturation of hemoglobin, when the deoxyhemoglobin (reduced hemoglobin) concentration equals the oxyhemoglobin (oxygenated hemoglobin) concentration at a constant pH and temperature. In humans, the P_{50} value is 26.52 mm Hg for whole blood under accepted standard conditions of pH 7.4 and temperature of 37.5°C. An increase in oxygen affinity is demonstrated by a shift to the left in the curve, whereas a decrease in oxygen affinity is represented by a shift to the right.

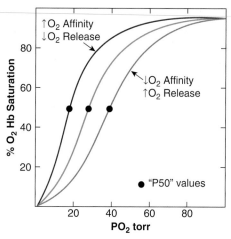

FIGURE 5.15 The oxygen dissociation curve of normal adult blood. The oxygen tension at 50% oxygen saturation (P50) is approximately 27 Torr. As the curve shifts to the right, the oxygen affinity of the hemoglobin decreases, and more oxygen is released at a given oxygen tension. With a shift to the left, the opposite effects are observed. A decrease in pH or an increase in temperature decreases the affinity of hemoglobin for oxygen. (Reprinted with permission from Mhairi G, et al. *Avery's Neonatology Pathophysiology and Management of the Newborn*, 6th ed, Philadelphia, PA: Lippincott Williams & Wilkins, 2005.)

In addition to the effect of 2,3-DPG, the oxygen-binding sites are also affected by their state of oxygenation. Oxygenation of one site on a hemoglobin molecule enhances affinity for oxygen at a different but chemically identical site. The sequence of molecular changes during oxygenation of hemoglobin probably occurs as follows. The first oxygen molecule binds to an alpha chain, causing a change in the three-dimensional structure of that chain. The addition of a second oxygen to the other alpha chain produces a change in the molecular structure, and the alignment of the chains to each other rapidly changes. The 2,3-DPG is expelled from the molecule, resulting in increased oxygen affinity, and oxygen is added to the remaining beta chain. These changes in molecular configuration are demonstrated by the sigmoid form of the hemoglobin oxygen dissociation curve.

Alterations

Fetal hemoglobin (hemoglobin F) has an increased affinity for oxygen. This increased affinity for oxygen is advantageous to the fetus because it results in increased placental oxygen transfer at low oxygen tension levels. The oxygen dissociation curve in the newborn is shifted to the left, owing to decreased levels of 2,3-DPG and the higher oxygen affinity of hemoglobin F. Hemoglobin variations caused by an amino acid substitution can alter the oxygen dissociation curve. These alterations in amino acids within the hemoglobin molecule are important in modifying oxygen transport. A variety of genetic hemoglobin abnormalities may distort the molecular structure or restrict the oxygenation. Other genetic abnormalities in the amino acid sequence of the hemoglobin molecule may affect oxygen transport by causing the oxidation of heme iron to methemoglobin.

Oxygen dissociation as represented by the sigmoid curve can be shifted to the right (decreased oxygen affinity) by a decrease in pH (Bohr effect), an increase in temperature, or hypoxic conditions such as altitude adaptation or anemia. An alteration in blood pH is responsible for the fact that the oxygen dissociation curve is shifted to the right in the acid microenvironment of hypoxic tissues. This causes an enhanced capacity to release oxygen where it is most needed. The reason for this shift in the oxygen affinity of hemoglobin is related to the acidity of the hemoglobin molecule. Oxyhemoglobin is a stronger acid than deoxyhemoglobin. Because deoxygenated hemoglobin is more alkaline than is oxygenated hemoglobin, and an alkaline pH stimulates glycolysis, 2,3-DPG production is thereby increased. This, in turn, decreases molecular affinity for oxygen. In summary, increased amounts of deoxyhemoglobin and increased amounts of 2,3-DPG produce decreased affinity for oxygen.

Carbon Dioxide Transport

The transport function of hemoglobin also includes support for carbon dioxide transport from the tissues to the lungs. Carbon dioxide can be carried to the lungs by three different mechanisms. These mechanisms are indirect and direct transport by erythrocytes, and transport in solution in plasma.

In the predominant indirect erythrocyte mechanism, which accounts for approximately three fourths of the activity for removing carbon dioxide, carbon dioxide diffuses into the erythrocytes, is catalyzed by the enzyme carbonic anhydrase, and is transformed into carbonic acid.

$$H_2O + CO_2 \rightarrow H_2CO_3$$

The hydrogen ion of carbonic acid is accepted by the alkaline deoxyhemoglobin, and the bicarbonate ion diffuses back into the plasma.

$$H_2CO_3 \rightarrow H^+ + HCO_3^-$$

Free bicarbonate diffuses out of erythrocytes into the plasma in exchange for plasma chloride (Cl^-) that diffuses into the cell. This process is called the **chloride shift**. Bicarbonate is carried back to the lungs by the plasma. In the pulmonary capillaries, bicarbonate is converted back into carbon dioxide and water and eliminated through respiration.

Approximately one fourth of the total carbon dioxide exchanged by erythrocytes in respiration is by a direct transport mechanism. In this mechanism, deoxyhemoglobin directly binds with carbon dioxide. This carbon dioxide reacts with uncharged amino groups of the four globin chains to form negatively charged carbamino hemoglobin. The carbamate groups form salt bridges with the positively charged deoxyhemoglobin molecule. This stabilizes the deoxy form and decreases oxygen affinity. Approximately 5% of carbon dioxide is carried in solution in plasma to the lungs.

Biosynthesis of Hemoglobin

Hemoglobin is synthesized during most of the erythrocytic maturation process. Approximately 65% of cytoplasmic hemoglobin is synthesized before the nucleus is extruded, and the remaining 35% is synthesized in the early reticulocyte. The major components of hemoglobin are heme and globin. Discussion of the synthesis of each of these components follows.

Formation of Heme From Porphyrin

Heme synthesis (Fig. 5.16) occurs in most body cells except for mature erythrocytes. Of all the body tissues, the red bone marrow and the liver are the most predominant heme (porphyrin) producers. Heme produced in the erythroid precursors is chemically identical to that in the cytochromes and myoglobin.

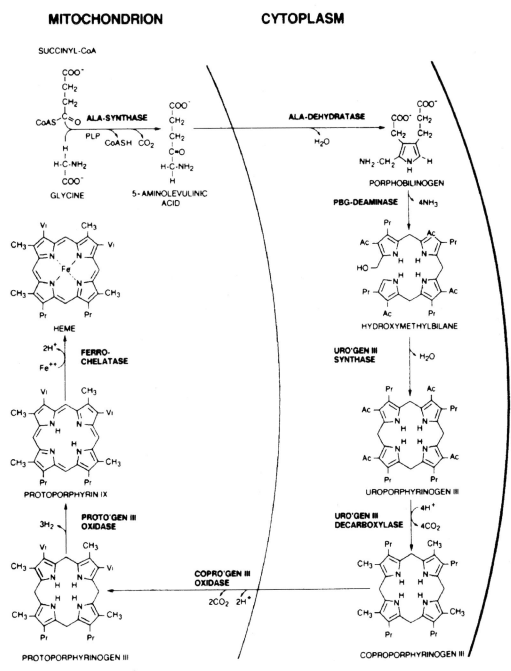

FIGURE 5.16 Heme biosynthetic pathway. Ac, acetate; ALA, σ-aminolevulinic acid; CoA, coenzyme A; CoAS, succinyl-CoA; CoASH, uncombined coenzyme A; COPRO'GEN, coproporphyrinogen; URO'GEN, uroporphyrinogen; Vi, vinyl. (Reprinted with permission from Greer JP [ed]. *Wintrobe's Clinical Hematology*, 12 ed, Philadelphia, PA: Lippincott Williams & Wilkins, 2009, p. 114.)

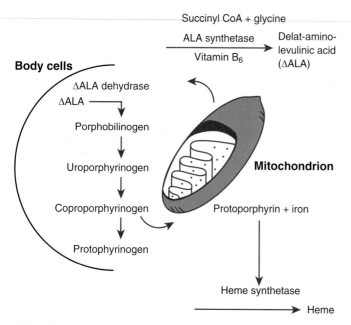

FIGURE 5.17 Sites of heme synthesis.

The synthesis of heme is a complex process that involves multiple enzymatic steps. The process begins in the mitochondrion (Fig. 5.17) with the condensation of succinyl-CoA and glycine to form 5-aminolevulinic acid. A series of steps in the cytoplasm produce coproporphyrinogen III, which reenters the mitochondrion. In the final enzymatic steps, iron is inserted into the ring structure of protoporphyrin IX to produce heme.

The preliminary activity in the synthesis of porphyrin, which precedes heme formation, begins when succinyl-coenzyme A (CoA) condenses with glycine. An unstable intermediate, adipic acid is formed from this condensation and is readily decarboxylated to delta-aminolevulinic acid (ALA). This initial condensation reaction occurs in the mitochondria and requires vitamin B_6. The most important limiting step in this reaction is the rate of conversion to delta-ALA, which is catalyzed by the enzyme ALA synthetase. The activity of this enzyme is influenced by both erythropoietin and by the presence of the cofactor pyridoxal phosphate (vitamin B_6).

Following the formation of delta-ALA in the mitochondria, the synthesis reaction continues in the cytoplasm. Two molecules of ALA condense to form the monopyrrole porphobilinogen (PBG). This reaction is catalyzed by the enzyme ALA dehydrase. Four molecules of PBG condense into a cyclic tetrapyrrole to form uroporphyrinogen I or III. The type III isomer is converted, by way of coproporphyrinogen III and protoporphyrinogen, to protoporphyrin.

The final steps, carried out in the mitochondria, involve the formation of protoporphyrin and the incorporation of iron to form heme. Four of the six ordinate positions of ferrous (Fe^{2+}) iron are chelated to protoporphyrin by the enzyme heme synthetase ferrochelatase. This step completes the formation of heme (Fig. 5.6), a colored compound consisting

of four pyrrole rings connected by methene bridges into a larger tetrapyrrole structure.

The Role of Iron in Hemoglobin Synthesis

Iron is the most abundant transition metal in the body. Iron uptake and release by the body are carefully controlled. Iron uptake is precisely controlled to maintain iron balance. In the duodenum (Fig. 5.18), dietary free iron is reduced to ferrous (+2) iron and taken up from the intestinal lumen into the enterocytes by the iron transport protein divalent metal transporter 1 (DMT1). DMT1 is instrumental in the uptake of iron by erythropoietic cells as well. Once absorbed, iron may be stored as ferritin in the enterocytes or exported into the circulation by another iron transport protein, ferroportin 1 (fpn1).

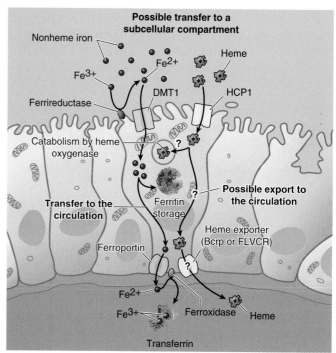

FIGURE 5.18 Intestinal absorption of iron. Mammalian iron absorption requires the transfer of iron across both the apical and basolateral membranes of duodenal enterocytes. Divalent metal transporter 1 (DMT1), located on the apical brush-border membrane, mediates the uptake of reduced, nonhemeiron (Fe^{2+}). A portion of this iron is retained within the cell for use or for storage in ferritin; the remainder is transferred to the circulation by ferroportin, a nonheme exporter. Released iron must be oxidized to bind to its plasma carrier protein, transferrin. A recent study suggests that the absorption of heme iron is mediated by HCP1, also expressed on the apical membrane. At least some heme is likely catabolized by heme oxygenase. This process may require the movement of heme into a membrane-bound subcellular compartment. Inorganic iron released from heme probably has the same fate as absorbed nonheme iron. The existence of two mammalian heme exporter proteins, Bcrp and FLVCR, raises the possibility that heme may transit the enterocyte intact and be exported into the serum. (Reprinted with permission from Andrews NC. Understanding heme transport, *NEJM*, 353:2508. Copyright © 2005 Massachusetts Medical Society. All rights reserved.)

Ferroportin is important as the last step in intestinal iron absorption and it allows macrophages to recycle iron by moving it out of macrophages in the liver, spleen, and bone marrow from damaged erythrocytes back into the circulation for reuse.

If there is insufficient hepcidin to control ferroportin, unregulated ferroportin activity causes hemochromatosis. This overloading of iron is due to mutations in ferroportin which has a dominant inheritance and a variable clinical phenotype.

In the plasma, ferric iron (+3) binds to transferrin which is delivered into cells by binding to transmembrane glycoprotein, transferrin receptors (TfR). It has been suggested that HFE protein interacts with TfRs to regulate cellular iron uptake.

In relation to the present discussion of hemoglobin synthesis, it is important to know that iron is delivered by a specific transport protein, **transferrin,** to the membrane of the immature cell. Iron in the ferric form (Fe^{3+}) is affixed to the cell membrane, and the transferrin is released back to the plasma. Most of the iron entering the cell is committed to hemoglobin synthesis and proceeds to the mitochondrion, where it is inserted into the protoporphyrin ring to form heme.

Hepcidin

Hepcidin, a liver-produced peptide hormone (Fig. 5.19), is the master regulatory hormone of systemic iron metabolism. The interaction of hepcidin with the plasma iron transporter, ferroportin, coordinates iron acquisition with iron utilization and storage.

The regulatory pathways that control hepcidin gene transcription are diverse but the role of hepcidin as a final common mediator of systemic and cellular iron transport and storage in response to iron stores, inflammation, erythropoiesis, and hypoxia is now well established. The production of hepcidin is controlled by the erythropoietic activity of the bone marrow, the amount of circulating and stored body iron, and inflammation. Hepcidin is the main regulator of intestinal iron absorption and macrophage iron release and ultimately influencing iron available for erythropoiesis.

Dietary iron absorption is regulated locally by hypoxia-inducible factor (HIF) signaling and iron-regulatory proteins (IRPs) in enterocytes and systematically by hepatic hepcidin. Hepcidin not only controls the rate of iron absorption but also determines iron mobilization from stores through

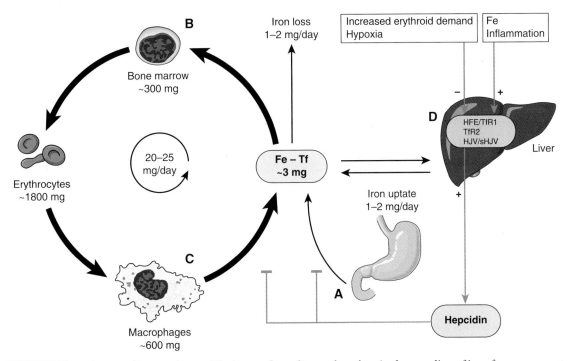

FIGURE 5.19 Pathways of iron exchange. The largest flux of iron takes place in the recycling of iron from senescent erythrocytes out of macrophages to incorporation in erythroid precursors. Note that values for the different tissues and fluxes are approximate. The liver and reticuloendothelial macrophages function as major iron stores. Only 1 to 2 mg of iron is absorbed and lost every day. Importantly, the total amount of iron in the body can be regulated by absorption only, whereas iron loss occurs only passively from sloughing of skin and mucosal cells as well as from blood loss. Hepcidin, a recently identified, antimicrobial, β-defensin–like peptide secreted by the liver, controls the plasma iron concentration by inhibiting iron export by ferroportin from duodenal enterocytes and reticuloendothelial macrophages. As a consequence, an increase in hepcidin production leads to a decrease in plasma iron concentrations. Hepcidin expression is regulated by iron concentration in hepatocytes, by inflammatory stimuli, by erythroid iron demand, and by hypoxia via pathways involving expression of the HFE, TRF2, and HJV genes. In HFE-, TfR2-, and HJV-related HH (hereditary hemochromatosis), hepcidin production is low despite increased liver iron, leading to inappropriately increased iron absorption. A, B, C, and D refer to sites with special functions in iron metabolism. (Reprinted with permission from Swinkels DW, et al. Hereditary hemochromatosis: genetic complexity and new diagnostic approaches, *Cl Chem,* 52(6):951, 2006; Figure 1.)

negatively modulating the function of ferroportin, the only identified cellular iron exporter to date. The regulation of hepatic hepcidin is accomplished by the coordinated activity of multiple proteins with different signaling pathways.

Hepcidin deficiency causes common iron overload syndromes but overexpression of hepcidin is responsible for microcytic anemia. In humans, genetic inactivation of hepcidin causes a rare form of juvenile hemochromatosis. In contrast, hepcidin overexpression in inflammation causes anemia of chronic disorders which has features of iron-restricted erythropoiesis. Cytokine-mediated increases in hepcidin appear to be an important causative factor in anemia of chronic disorders. Research is being conducted on pinpointing potent inhibitory factor for hepcidin expression and a negative feedback pathway for hepcidin regulation and how hepcidin expression can be limited to avoid iron deficiency.

Hepcidin transcription is activated by the bone morphogenetic protein (BMP) and the inflammatory JAK-STAT pathways but little is know about how hepcidin expression is inhibited. Iron excess or inflammatory cytokines stimulate hepcidin expression, which leads to reduced plasma iron levels as the result of iron retention in macrophages and reduced intestinal iron absorption. Hypoxia, high erythropoietic activity, and iron deficiency inhibit hepcidin expression by mostly unknown mechanisms to mobilize iron stores and increase iron absorption.

Hepcidin exerts its effection by binding to the iron efflux channel ferroportin, predominantly expressed on macrophages, intestinal enterocytes, and hepatocytes, causing ferroportin internalization and degradation. Hepcidin levels are inappropriately low in HH.

In inflammation, IL-6 triggers hepcidin activation binding to IL-6 and leads to activation and transcription that binds to a location (consensus sequence) in the hepcidin promoter. Constant induction of hepcidin by inflammatory cytokines is implicated in the pathogenesis of anemia of chronic inflammation/disorders.

Globin Structure and Synthesis

Both the structure and the production of globin in the hemoglobin molecule are under genetic control (Fig. 5.20). The specific sequences of amino acids are governed by the triplet code of DNA bases, which are genetically inherited. The rate of polypeptide synthesis is a function of the rate at which the DNA code is transcribed into messenger ribonucleic acid (mRNA).

Alpha Globin Locus

Each chromosome 16 has two alpha globin genes that are aligned one after the other on the chromosome. For practical purposes, the two alpha globin genes are identical. Each cell has two chromosomes 16; a total of four alpha globin genes exist in each cell. Each of the four genes produces about one quarter of the alpha globin chains needed for hemoglobin synthesis. The mechanism of this coordination is unknown. The transiently expressed embryonic genes that substitute for alpha very early in development, designated zeta, are also in the alpha globin locus.

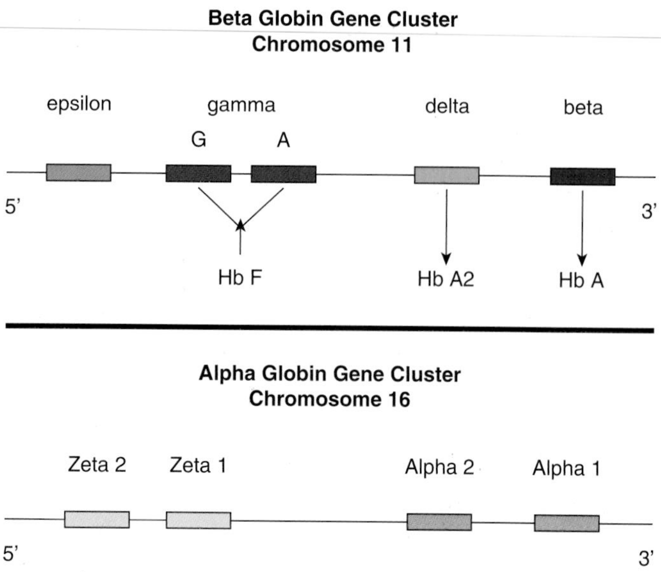

FIGURE 5.20 The globin gene loci. The upper figure represent the beta (β)globin locus on chromosome 11. The two gamma globin genes are active during fetal growth and produce hemoglobin F. The "adult" gene, β, becomes active after birth. The lower figure demonstrates the alpha (α)globin locus on chromosome 16. Each of the four α globin genes contribute to the synthesis of the α-globin protein.

Beta Globin Locus

The genes in the beta globin locus are arranged sequentially. The sequence of the genes is epsilon, gamma, delta, and beta. There are two copies of the gamma gene on each chromosome 11. The others are present in single copies. Each cell has two beta globin genes, one on each of the two chromosomes 11 in the cell. These two beta globin genes express their globin protein in a quantity that precisely matches that of the four alpha globin genes. The mechanism of this balanced expression is unknown.

The polypeptide chains of globin are produced, as are other body proteins, on the ribosomes. The alpha polypeptide chain unites with one of three other chains to form a dimer and ultimately a tetramer. In normal adult hemoglobin (hemoglobin A), these chains are two alpha and two beta chains.

DISORDERS RELATED TO HEMOGLOBIN BIOSYNTHESIS

Disorders of Heme (Porphyrin) Synthesis

Disorders in the synthesis of porphyrin (Fig. 5.21) or the heme moiety may be either inherited or acquired. Inherited defects include a rare autosomal recessive condition, congenital erythropoietic porphyria.

Acquired defects include lead poisoning, which inhibits heme synthesis at several points. In this defect, inhibition of several enzymes, including heme synthetase, impairs synthesis

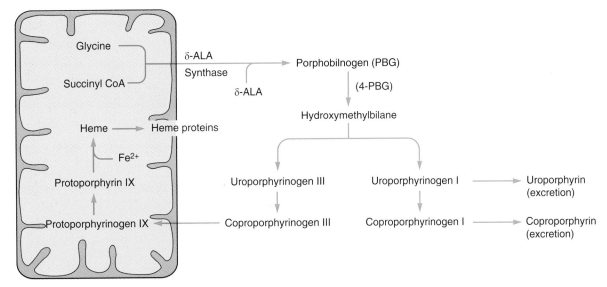

FIGURE 5.21 The heme biosynthetic pathway. Inherited defects of each of the heme biosynthetic enzymes except δ-aminolevulinic acid synthase have been described and lead to the clinical disorders known as the porphyrias. (Reprinted with permission from Mulholland MW, et al. *Greenfield's Surgery Scientific Principles and Practice*, 4th ed, Philadelphia, PA: Lippincott Williams & Wilkins, 2006.)

reactions at several points, including ALA to PBG and protoporphyrin to heme. Not only are there morphological abnormalities of the erythrocytes (discussed in Chapter 6), but the quantity of ALA that is normally excreted in small amounts in the urine is also increased in lead poisoning.

Porphyria is defined as a disease of heme metabolism in which a primary abnormality in porphyrin biosynthesis leads to excessive accumulation and excretion of porphyrins or their precursors by the biliary and/or renal route. Porphyrias can be classified based on various characteristics:

■ Clinical presentation (acute versus chronic)
■ Source of enzyme deficiency
■ Site of enzyme deficiency in the heme biosynthetic pathway

Clinically, patients with porphyria have either neurological complications or skin problems. Some patients have no symptoms. Distinct disease manifestation has led clinicians to divide porphyrias into two subgroups: acute neurologic and nonacute cutaneous based on the predominant clinical manifestation.

Porphyria is derived from the Greek word, *porphyra*, which means purple. The purple-red pigment (porphyrins) is responsible for the wine-red color characteristic of porphyric urine. PBG is normally excreted in small amounts in urine; however, it appears in significantly elevated amounts in acute intermittent porphyria, which may be detected by testing the urine with Ehrlich's aldehyde reagent. In addition to increased urinary PBG, mild anemia and neurological changes may be associated with porphyrias.

When porphyrin synthesis is impaired, the mitochondria become encrusted with iron, and some granules exist around the nucleus. These iron-containing granules in a nucleated

erythrocyte are visible if the cell is stained with a special stain, Prussian blue stain (Fig. 5.22). The cells are referred to as **sideroblasts**.

Disorders of Iron Metabolism

Genetic Defect of Iron

Genetic variations affect iron plasma concentrations in persons not affected by overt genetic disorders of iron metabolism. The SNP most strongly associated with lower serum

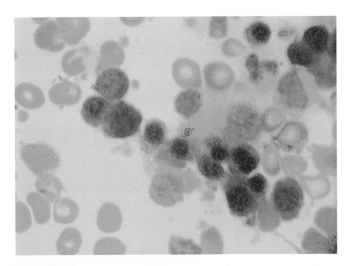

FIGURE 5.22 Iron stains of bone marrow bone marrow aspirate smear shows sideroblastic iron (note the small green granules present in the cytoplasm). (Reprinted with permission from McClatchey KD. *Clinical Laboratory Medicine*, 2nd ed, Philadelphia, PA: Lippincott Williams & Wilkins, 2002.)

iron concentration was rs4820268 ($p = 5.12 \times 10^{-9}$) located in exon13 of the transmembrane protease serine 6 (*TMPRSS6*) gene, an enzyme that promotes iron absorption and recycling by inhibiting hepcidin antimicrobial peptide transcription. The allele associated with lower iron concentrations was also associated with lower hemoglobin levels, smaller red cells, and high red blood cell distribution width (RDW). Therefore, an association of *TMPRSS6* variants with iron level has been established as **anemia**-related phenotypes.

Iron Overload

Conditions of iron overload can result from various causes. Too much iron accumulates in HH, porphyria cutanea tarda, and the iron-loading anemias, for example, hemolytic dyserythropoietic, myelodysplastic, and aplastic anemias.

In primary overload disorders, iron absorption from a normal diet is increased due to inherited alteration in factors that control iron uptake and retention. In comparison, secondary iron overload may arise in patients with chronic disorders or erythropoiesis or hemolytic anemias, for example, sideroblastic anemia as a consequence of iron therapy, due to excessive dietary or supplement ingestion of iron or from multiple RBC transfusions. In the United States, iron overload arises primarily from the genetic disorder, HH.

Sideroblastic Anemia

Excess iron accumulates as ferritin aggregates in the cytoplasm of immature erythrocytes. The amount of nonheme iron deposited depends on the ratio between the plasma iron level and the iron required by the cell. Sideroblastic anemia is associated with mitochondrial iron loading in marrow erythroid precursors (ringed sideroblasts) and ineffective erythropoiesis. Causes of sideroblastic anemia include

1. Congenital defect: hereditary sex linked (primarily males); autosomal
2. Acquired defect: primary (one of the myelodysplastic syndromes); may evolve into acute myelogenous leukemia
3. Association with malignant marrow disorders: acute myelogenous leukemia, polycythemia vera, myeloma, myelodysplastic syndromes
4. Secondary to drugs: isoniazid (INH), chloramphenicol; after chemotherapy
5. Toxins, including alcohol, and chronic lead poisoning

Diagnosis of sideroblastic anemia is based on variable red cell indices with a microcytic, hypochromic component of red cells on review of the peripheral smear; increased serum iron and serum ferritin (SF); and characteristic ringed sideroblasts on iron stain of bone marrow aspirate.

Treatment is pyridoxine trial in pharmacological doses. This approach is usually ineffective in acquired forms, but a significant number of patients with the sex-linked hereditary forms will respond. Other approaches include removing offending drugs or toxins and providing supportive care, such as blood product support and iron chelation as

indicated. Chemotherapy may also be used if the condition evolves into acute myelogenous leukemia.

Etiology

Sideroblastic anemias are associated with a variety of causes:

1. Drugs (e.g., isoniazid, chloramphenicol, alcohol, and cytotoxic drugs)
2. Diseases (e.g., hematological, neoplastic, and inflammatory)
3. Miscellaneous disorders (e.g., uremia, thyrotoxicosis, and porphyria)
4. Hereditary factors
5. Idiopathic origin

Hereditary and idiopathic types of sideroblastic anemia may be pyridoxine responsive or refractory.

Physiology

In this type of anemia, the body has adequate iron but is unable to incorporate it into hemoglobin synthesis. The iron enters the developing erythrocyte but then accumulates in the perinuclear mitochondria of metarubricytes (normoblasts). An established heme enzyme abnormality in sideroblastic anemia is a decrease in the activity of delta-aminolevulinic acid (delta-ALA) synthetase. Ringed sideroblasts are formed by mitochondria containing accumulated nonferritin iron that circles the normoblast (metarubricyte) nucleus. A Prussian blue stain reveals the iron as blue deposits circling the nucleus. Iron is normally deposited diffusely throughout the cytoplasm. Other forms of this anemia are associated with the administration of drugs or disease onset. If drugs are implicated, the drugs interfere with the activity of heme enzymes.

Laboratory Characteristics

Iron granules can be seen on bone marrow preparations stained for iron. Some of the granules may encircle the nucleus of erythrocytes, particularly of metarubricytes (normoblasts), to form ringed sideroblasts. There is increased erythropoietic activity in the bone marrow. Thus, the marrow is hypercellular, but the number of circulating reticulocytes is not elevated. The mature, nonnucleated erythrocytes are generally hypochromic with normocytic and/or microcytic erythrocytes.

Severe anemia is seen in hereditary types of sideroblastic anemia. The erythrocytes display significant hypochromia and microcytosis, target cells, basophilic stippling, and dimorphic RBC populations, although the leukocytes and platelets are usually normal. From 10% to 40% of the nucleated erythrocytes in the bone marrow are ringed sideroblasts. Megaloblastic changes in the marrow indicate complicating folate deficiency. In hereditary cases, transferrin saturation (TS) is high, and less than 50% of patients respond to pyridoxine therapy.

Idiopathic refractory types of sideroblastic anemia usually display moderate anemia. The peripheral blood is normocytic or macrocytic, with a small population of hypochromic erythrocytes. Some patients have significant stippling in the erythrocytes. The leukocytes and platelets are usually normal. The bone marrow demonstrates erythroid hyperplasia, with 45% to 95% of the nucleated erythrocytes being ringed sideroblasts. In 20% of patients, megaloblastic changes suggest a complicating folate deficiency. TS levels are increased (>90%) in approximately one third of patients, and SF levels are also increased with this form of anemia. Acute leukemia develops in approximately 10% of patients.

Hereditary Hemochromatosis

In contrast to iron overload caused by various conditions or disorders (e.g., multiple transfusions, alcohol abuse, or hepatocellular carcinoma), HH is a genetic error of metabolism that produces inappropriately increased (twofold to threefold greater than normal) GI absorption of iron. This autosomal recessive disorder, caused by a gene defect, was discovered in 1996. It causes a progressive iron overload and excessive accumulation in various organs because not only is there an excess of iron in the body but there is also an abnormal distribution of iron. The Centers for Disease Control and Prevention (CDC) estimate that more than 1 million Americans have hemochromatosis.

Classification and Characteristics

There are several distinct, inherited iron-loading disorders that have similar clinical presentations and are referred to as hemochromatosis:

1. **HFE-gene–related (Type 1).** A gene associated with HH was identified in 1996. The carrier frequency of HFE-associated hemochromatosis in the United States is approximately 1 in 8 to 1 in 10, and the homozygote frequency is approximately 1 in 200 to 1 in 250. This form of HH, a disorder described more than 100 years ago in western Europeans as "bronze diabetes," is prevalent in persons of northern European descent, particularly individuals of Celtic ancestry. It is the most common autosomal recessive genetic disease among whites, with a tight linkage to the HLA-A locus on chromosome 6. Estimates of prevalence are that 1 in 10 to 20 whites carry the disease gene and that 1 in 400 are homozygotes at risk for developing the clinical syndrome.

The gene identified at the HLA-A3 locus was named HFE. Two common mutations in the HFE gene, C282Y and H63D, are associated with HH. Its prevalence varies widely worldwide.

The disease pursues an insidious course and symptoms often do not occur until the fourth or fifth decade of life. Men are more frequently affected.

An interesting fact about HFE gene mutation is that individuals possessing mutations may have been favored by natural selection because they have enhanced uptake of iron from iron-poor diets, which minimizes their risk for iron deficiency and iron deficiency anemia (see Chapter 10).

2. **Juvenile hemochromatosis** (HJV). Patients with juvenile hemochromatosis caused by hemojuvelin (HJV) mutations (type 2A) share the same phenotype as that of patients with mutations that disrupt the hepcidin gene (HAMP, type 2B).

Hemojuvelin is a protein expressed in liver, skeletal muscle, and the heart. Membrane hemojuvelin positively modulates the iron regulator hepcidin. Type 2B is related to HAMP and the production of hepcidin. Mutation of the gene encoding for hemojuvelin causes juvenile hemochromatosis which is characterized by hepcidin deficiency and severe iron overload. No or very low hepcidin activation is the hallmark of juvenile hemochromatosis.

3. **Transferrin receptor 2 (TfR2) hemochromatosis is a different form of the disease that usually appears in midlife.** This form is associated with mutation in TFR2, the gene encoding transferrin receptor 2, found on human chromosome 7q22. It has not been established how the loss of transferrin 2 leads to iron overloading.

4. **Ferroportin disease related to the SLC40A1 gene that encodes for ferroportin.** Another type of hemochromatosis has been observed in two different families. This form of the disorder differs from the others in that it is inherited in an autosomal dominant pattern and is associated with increased iron in macrophages of mononuclear phagocytic system. This form also differs because it lacks linkage to the HLA locus.

Pathophysiology and Laboratory Characteristics

HH results from intestinal absorption of dietary iron in excess of bodily needs. The primary site for regulating iron absorption is in the cells of the duodenal mucosa. A patient destined to develop hemochromatosis begins early in life with a pattern of iron absorption that exceeds amounts appropriate to total body iron stores, and over the course of decades, excess iron accumulates in various tissues and damages them.

SF is generally viewed as an accurate reflection of body iron stores, but wide fluctuations in concentration are often seen. An elevated SF correlates with the degree of iron overload, if it is not confounded by coexisting liver disease, malignancy, or excessive alcohol intake. SF is an acute-phase reactant (protein) and is often elevated in various conditions other than HH.

Genetic testing can aid in diagnosis but cannot be used alone. The presence of abnormal TS and SF levels provides evidence of iron overload.

Although abnormally high amounts of iron are absorbed into the circulation in patients with hemochromatosis, the total amount of transferrin decreases because, at least in part, high iron levels cause a decrease in transcription of the transferrin gene. Furthermore, transferrin is synthesized in the liver, and levels of synthesis may decrease with the onset of liver disease. Thus, an increase in serum iron levels and a simultaneous decrease in transferrin levels combine to significantly increase TS levels. If saturation levels are consistently greater than 62% without any overt hepatic disease that would contribute to a decrease in transferrin synthesis,

TABLE 5.3	Comparative Chain Composition of Hemoglobin Types	
Hemoglobin Type	**Symbol**	**Polypeptide (Globin) Chains**
Embryonic		
Gower-1	$\delta_2\,\varepsilon_2$	2 zeta
		2 epsilon
Gower-2	$\alpha_2\,\varepsilon_2$	2 alpha
		2 epsilon
Portland-1	$\zeta_2\,\gamma_2$	2 zeta
		2 gamma
Hemoglobin F	$\alpha_2\,\gamma_2$	2 alpha
		2 gamma
Hemoglobin A	$\alpha_2\,\beta_2$	2 alpha
		2 beta
Hemoglobin A₂	$\alpha_2\,\beta_2$	2 alpha
		2 delta

the chances that the patient has HH are greater than 90%. A liver biopsy confirms the diagnosis.

Treatment

Treatment of iron load can be by therapeutic phlebotomy or iron chelation therapy. Removal of one unit (450 mL) of whole blood once or twice weekly is the safest and most effective way of removing iron from the body. Each unit of blood contains approximately 250 mg of iron. In patients with transfusion-dependent anemia, chelation is the only option for effective iron removal.

Disorders of Globulin Synthesis

Globin synthesis is highly coordinated with porphyrin synthesis. When globin synthesis is impaired, protoporphyrin synthesis is correspondingly reduced. Similarly, when porphyrin synthesis is impaired, excess globin is not produced.

However, there is no such fine regulation of iron uptake with impairment of either protoporphyrin or globin synthesis. When globin production is deficient, iron accumulates in the cytoplasm of cells as ferritin aggregates.

Defects of globulin synthesis are manifested in the thalassemias (see Chapter 13).

Ontogeny of Hemoglobin

In normal human development, several types of hemoglobin are produced. These hemoglobin types are hemoglobin A and a subfraction A_1, hemoglobin A_2, fetal hemoglobin, and embryonic hemoglobins. Each of these hemoglobin types has a distinctive composition of polypeptide chains (Table 5.3). Many other types of hemoglobin have been identified; however, these are referred to as variant or abnormal hemoglobins.

Embryonic Hemoglobins

Embryonic hemoglobins are primitive hemoglobins formed by immature erythrocytes in the yolk sac. These hemoglobins include Gower I, Gower II, and Portland types. They are found in the human embryo and persist until approximately 12 weeks of gestation (Fig. 5.23). In these hemoglobins, the zeta chain is analogous to the alpha chain of fetal and adult hemoglobin and may combine with epsilon or gamma chains to form various embryonic hemoglobin types. The epsilon chain is analogous to gamma, beta, and delta chains.

Fetal Hemoglobin

Fetal hemoglobin (hemoglobin F) is the predominant hemoglobin variety in the fetus and the newborn. This hemoglobin type has two alpha and two gamma chains. The gamma chains have 146 amino acids, as do beta chains. However, gamma chains differ from beta chains. Two types of gamma chains exist, differing in only one amino acid. Either an alanine or a glycine may be present at amino acid position 136.

Fetal hemoglobin appears by the fifth week of gestation and persists for several months after birth. This hemoglobin type is associated with hepatic erythropoiesis. Although bone marrow erythropoiesis begins at the fourth month of gestation, the bone marrow does not establish itself as the primary hematopoietic organ after 18 to 24 weeks of

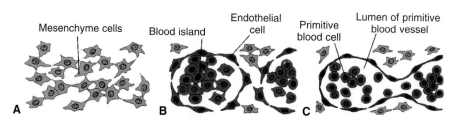

FIGURE 5.23 Successive stages of blood vessel formation. **A:** Undifferentiated mesenchyme cells. **B:** Blood island formation. **C:** Primitive capillary. Note the differentiation of mesenchymal cells into primitive blood cells and endothelial cells. (Reprinted with permission from Sadler T. *Langman's Medical Embryology*, 9th ed Image Bank, Baltimore, MD: Lippincott Williams & Wilkins, 2003.)

Mesenchyme cells | Blood island | Endothelial cell | Primitive blood cell | Lumen of primitive blood vessel | Primitive blood cell

gestation. Gradually, hemoglobin A replaces hemoglobin F in the circulating erythrocytes until the normal adult level of hemoglobin F (<2%) is attained. This process takes place until normal adult hemoglobin predominates, usually at about 6 months of age, although slight elevations may persist for 2 years. In abnormal cases, retention of hemoglobin F into adult life (15% to 30% of total hemoglobin) is referred to as hereditary persistence of fetal hemoglobin.

Glycosylated Hemoglobin (Hemoglobin A₁)

A subfraction of normal hemoglobin A is hemoglobin A_1. This subfraction can be termed **glycosylated hemoglobin** and includes the separate hemoglobin fractions A_{1a}, A_{1b}, and A_{1c}. This type of hemoglobin is formed during the maturation of the erythrocyte. Because proteins are vulnerable to modification after being synthesized by the ribosomes, this modification takes the form of glycosylation of hemoglobin in hyperglycemic persons. The formation of glycosylated hemoglobin is a slow, irreversible process that depends on the concentration of glucose in the body. Consequently, the concentration of glycosylated hemoglobin accurately reflects the patient's blood glucose level over the preceding weeks and has been recently used to monitor the control of diabetes.

Glycosylated hemoglobin is a stable hemoglobin and is structurally the same as hemoglobin A except for the *addition* of a carbohydrate group at the terminal valine of the beta chain. The concentration of hemoglobin A_1 is 3% to 6% in normal persons and 6% to 12% in both insulin-dependent and non–insulin-dependent diabetics.

Hemoglobin A

Although adult hemoglobin is predominantly of the A variety (95% to 97%), the A_2 type is also found in small quantities (2% to 3%). Hemoglobin A is composed of two alpha and two beta polypeptide chains. Hemoglobin A_2 is composed of two alpha and two delta chains. The delta chains differ from beta chains in eight of the 146 amino acids. Synthesis of delta chains begins during late fetal development, and the level of A_2 increases during the first year of life until the adult level is reached. The delta chains of hemoglobin A_2 are synthesized at only 1/40th the rate of beta chains. Therefore, the concentration of hemoglobin A_2 in a normal adult averages 2.5% of the total hemoglobin.

Variant Forms of Normal Hemoglobin

Carboxyhemoglobin, sulfhemoglobin, and methemoglobin are known as variant forms of normal hemoglobin. Unlike abnormal hemoglobins with permanent structural rearrangements of the hemoglobin molecule, these variants are typified by differing from normal hemoglobin only by the molecule that replaces oxygen.

Carboxyhemoglobin

Carbon monoxide poisoning is the most common type of accidental poisoning in the United States. Carbon monoxide, an insidious by-product of incomplete hydrocarbon combustion, is generated in toxic amounts from fossil fuels. Carbon monoxide is highly toxic in unventilated spaces. A stable gas at physiological temperatures, carbon monoxide diffuses rapidly across the alveolar capillary membrane and binds tightly to hemoglobin and other hemoproteins (e.g., myoglobin and cytochrome oxidase). Hemoglobin has the capacity to combine with carbon monoxide in the same proportion as with oxygen, but the affinity of the hemoglobin molecule for carbon monoxide is 210 times greater. This increased affinity results in the binding of carbon monoxide to hemoglobin to form carboxyhemoglobin even if the concentration of carbon monoxide is extremely low. The molecule forms an extremely stable compound, which renders the hemoglobin molecule useless for oxygen transport. Carboxyhemoglobin displaces oxygen and leads to tissue hypoxia.

A normal carboxyhemoglobin level is 1% to 3% as the result of endogenous carbon monoxide production by heme catabolism and low-level environmental carbon monoxide exposure. Slightly increased levels (an average of 5% per pack smoked per day) can be found in persons who smoke. Chronically increased levels can be associated with increased erythrocyte production. Levels of 20% to 30% carboxyhemoglobin saturation produce symptoms of dizziness, nausea, headache, and muscular weakness. Acute poisoning (beginning at levels of 15% to 20%) producing more than 40% saturation leads to sudden loss of consciousness and rapid death. Treatment of carbon monoxide poisoning is supplemental oxygen, which hastens the dissociation of carbon monoxide from hemoproteins in direct relation to the partial pressure of oxygen.

Sulfhemoglobin

This variant of hemoglobin contains sulfur. In vitro and in the presence of oxygen, hemoglobin reacts with hydrogen sulfide to form a greenish derivative called sulfhemoglobin. The formation of this variant produces an irreversible change in the polypeptide chains of the hemoglobin molecule due to oxidant stress, and further change can result in denaturation and the precipitation of hemoglobin as **Heinz bodies**. Sulfhemoglobin cannot transport oxygen, but it can combine with carbon monoxide to form carboxysulfhemoglobin. Sulfhemoglobin can be formed by the action of certain oxidizing drugs such as phenacetin and sulfonamides on hemoglobin in cases of bacteremia caused by *Clostridium welchii* and in enterogenous cyanosis. Concentrations of sulfhemoglobin in vivo are normally less than 1% and seldom exceed 10% of a patient's total hemoglobin. Elevated concentrations result in cyanosis but are usually otherwise asymptomatic.

Methemoglobin

This is a variant of hemoglobin, with iron in the ferric state, that is incapable of combining with oxygen. It can result from a metabolic defect (refer to "Methemoglobin Reductase Pathway" later in this chapter) or may occur because the structure of the hemoglobin molecule is abnormal because of the inheritance of an autosomal dominant trait. The genetically determined alteration in the amino acid composition of either alpha or beta globulin chains produces a hemoglobin molecule that has an enhanced tendency toward oxidation and a decreased susceptibility of the formed methemoglobin to reduce back to hemoglobin. Various forms of genetic alterations referred to as hemoglobin M disorders usually produce asymptomatic cyanosis.

Normally, 2% methemoglobin is formed each day. At this concentration, the abnormal hemoglobin is not harmful because the reduced ability of the erythrocytes to carry oxygen is insignificant. Higher concentrations of methemoglobin usually are avoided because of the presence of reducing systems. Cyanosis develops if methemoglobin levels exceed 10%; hypoxia develops if levels exceed 60%.

In addition to genetic reasons, increased methemoglobin production can result from environmental conditions such as exposure to certain drugs and oxidant chemicals. Once the offending agent is removed, methemoglobin disappears rapidly.

Infants are more susceptible to methemoglobin production because hemoglobin F is more easily converted to methemoglobin. In addition, the erythrocytes of infants are deficient in the required reducing enzymes. High nitrite quantities in food, water, or drugs can cause increased methemoglobin levels in infants.

Abnormal Hemoglobin Molecules

Abnormal hemoglobin molecules such as that seen in sickle cell anemia result from mutant, codominant genes (see Chapter 3). Persons with this mutant gene may be homozygous (S/S) or heterozygous (S/A) for the trait. The sickle gene may occur with hemoglobin C, E, or D, giving rise to SC, SE, or SD disease. In the case of hemoglobin S, the defective molecule of the normal glutamic acid amino acid residue at the sixth position of the beta globin chain is replaced by a valine amino acid residue. This amino acid substitution results in erythrocytes that are sickled when deoxygenated hemoglobin S polymerizes and forms intracellular aggregates that deform the cell and molecules of hemoglobin that are almost insoluble on deoxygenation. Altered solubility of the hemoglobin S molecule is owing to the substitution of a nonpolar amino acid residue for a polar residue near the surface of the chain. In abnormal hemoglobin C, the normal glutamic acid amino acid residue at the sixth position on the beta globin is replaced by a lysine amino acid residue. A comparison of the defective beta chains with the normal sequence of amino acids in hemoglobin A is presented in Figure 5.24.

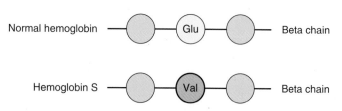

FIGURE 5.24 Comparison of normal and sickle hemoglobin molecules. Glu, glutamic acid; Val, valine.

Analysis of Hemoglobin

Since the first hemoglobinopathy was described in 1910, several techniques have been developed to study hemoglobin. They include hemoglobin electrophoresis with various media, such as paper, cellulose acetate, or agar; solubility testing; and denaturation of hemoglobin through the use of acid or alkaline solutions (see Chapter 17). A method for the preliminary identification of abnormal hemoglobin is **electrophoresis** (Fig. 5.25).

Alkaline Electrophoresis

This method of separating hemoglobin fractions is based on the principle that hemoglobin molecules in an alkaline solution have a net negative charge and move toward the anode in an electrophoretic system. This screening procedure can separate hemoglobins A, F, S, and C and other variant hemoglobins (Fig. 5.26). Those with a greater electrophoretic mobility than hemoglobin A at pH 8.6 are classified as the **fast hemoglobins**. Examples of fast hemoglobins are Bart hemoglobin and the two fastest variants, hemoglobin H and hemoglobin I. Hemoglobin C is the slowest common hemoglobin.

Various media, such as paper, cellulose acetate, or starch blocks, and different buffers may be used for electrophoresis. These alternative methods vary in their efficiency of separation. For example, cellulose acetate at alkaline pH is rapid and reproducible. This technique separates the hemoglobin fractions S, F, A, C, and A_2.

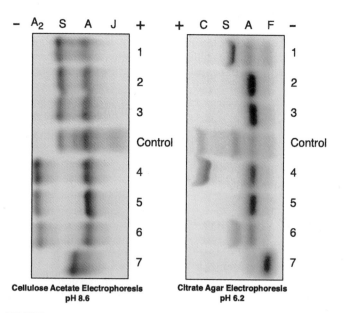

FIGURE 5.25 Examples of common hemoglobin variants on both cellulose acetate and citrate agar electrophoresis. 1, Hb S trait; 2, Hb G-Philadelphia trait; 3, Hb D-Punjab trait; 4, Hb C trait; 5, Hb E trait; 6, Hb O-Arab trait; 7, increased Hb F in a neonate. (Reprinted with permission from McClatchey KD. *Clinical Laboratory Medicine*, 2nd ed, Philadelphia, PA: Lippincott Williams & Wilkins, 2002.)

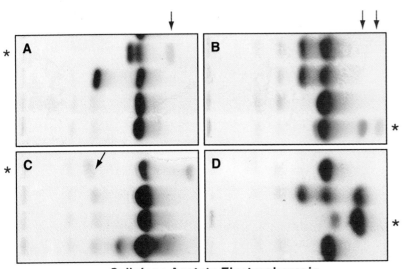

**Cellulose Acetate Electrophoresis
pH 8.6**

FIGURE 5.26 Cellulose acetate electrophoresis. **A:** Specimen from a neonate. Hb-Barts is present (*arrow*) indicating a thalassemia. **B:** Specimen from a 3-month-old. In addition to Hb-Barts, there is also a small amount of Hb H (*double arrow*). **C:** Hb H-Hb-Constant Spring. There is a fullness in the Hb A2 area indicating the presence of Hb-Constant Spring. **D:** Hb-Barts hydrops fetalis. There is no Hb A present. The majority of the hemoglobin is Hb-Barts, with a small amount of Hb-Portland. (Reprinted with permission from McClatchey KD. *Clinical Laboratory Medicine*, 2nd ed, Philadelphia, PA: Lippincott Williams & Wilkins, 2002.)

Citrate Agar Electrophoresis

This process takes place at an acid pH. In this method, hemoglobins are separated on the basis of a complex interaction between hemoglobin, agar, and citrate buffer ions. Citrate agar separates hemoglobin fractions that migrate together on cellulose acetate. These fractions are hemoglobins S, D, G, C, E, and O. All hemoglobin specimens that show an abnormal electrophoretic pattern in alkaline media should undergo electrophoresis on acid citrate agar. The combined information allows for a complete identification of many variant hemoglobins.

Denaturation Procedures

A procedure commonly used to determine the amount of fetal blood that has mixed with maternal blood following delivery is the **Kleihauer-Betke** (Fig. 5.27) procedure

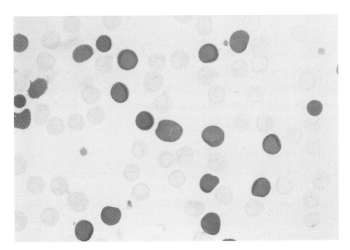

FIGURE 5.27 Kleihauer-Betke acid elution for fetal hemoglobin (Hb). Red blood cells containing HbF are deeply stained red; red cells containing HbA appear as pale pink ghosts. (Reprinted with permission from Greer JP (ed). *Wintrobe's Clinical Hematology*, 11 ed, Philadelphia, PA: Lippincott Williams & Wilkins, 2004.)

(see Chapter 26). This test involves acid denaturation of hemoglobin. Fetal hemoglobin resists denaturation, whereas adult hemoglobin does not. Occasionally, intermediate (partially denatured) cells may be seen that are almost surely fetal hemoglobin–containing cells. Elevated levels of hemoglobin F can be seen in beta-thalassemia, a form of anemia, and paroxysmal nocturnal hemoglobinuria (PNH).

Chromatography

Quantitation of hemoglobin A_1 can be accomplished by cation exchange minicolumn chromatography. However, the results of this technique can be affected by several types of hemoglobin in addition to hemoglobin A_1. Cellulose acetate and citrate agar electrophoresis should be used in conjunction with cation exchange chromatography to eliminate the possibility of interference by hemoglobin variants. Other assay methods for glycosylated hemoglobin include high-pressure liquid chromatography (HPLC) and colorimetric methods.

MEMBRANE CHARACTERISTICS AND METABOLIC ACTIVITIES OF ERYTHROCYTES

The mature erythrocyte has no nucleus or other organelles but is capable of existing in the blood circulation for an average of 120 days. An erythrocyte is more limited in metabolic activity than are other body cells. The cell has a limited ability to metabolize fatty acids and amino acids and lacks mitochondria for oxidative metabolism. Energy (Fig. 5.28) for metabolic processes is generated almost exclusively through the breakdown of glucose. The overall pathway of erythrocyte glycolysis may be subdivided into the major anaerobic Embden-Meyerhof glycolytic pathway and three supplementary pathways, which act in different ways to maintain the function of hemoglobin. The Embden-Meyerhof pathway uses glucose and generates adenosine

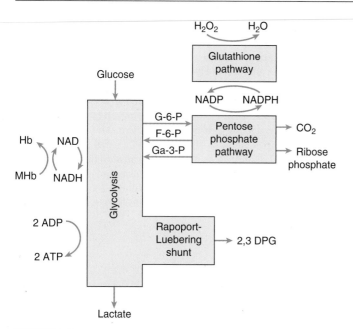

FIGURE 5.28 Energy metabolism in the erythrocyte. Main pathways are shown as boxes; major substrates and products of each are shown outside the boxes. More details of the pathways are given in Figure 5.29. ADP, adenosine diphosphate; ATP, adenosine triphosphate; 2,3-DPG, 2,3-diphosphoglycerate; F-6-P, fructose 6-phosphate; G-6-P, glucose 6-phosphate; Ga-3-P, glyceraldehydes 3-phosphate; Hg, hemoglobin; MHb, methemoglobin; NAD, NADH, nicotinamide adenine dinucleotide, NADP, NADPH, nicotinaamide adenine dinucleotide phosphate. (Adapted with permission from Greer JP (ed). *Wintrobes Clinical Hematology*, 12 ed, p. 150, Figure 7.28.)

triphosphate (ATP). This pathway also is essential in maintaining pyridine nucleotides in a reduced state to support the methemoglobin reductase pathway and 2,3-DPG synthesis, the Luebering-Rapoport pathway. In addition, the phosphogluconate pathway couples oxidative metabolism with pyridine nucleotide and glutathione reduction and protects erythrocytes from environmental oxidants. All these processes (Table 5.4) are essential for the erythrocyte to transport oxygen and to maintain the physical characteristics required for survival in the blood circulation.

Membrane Characteristics

Reticulocyte Membrane

Reticulocyte maturation is the final step of terminal erythroid differentiation. Erythroid differentiation occurs within erythroblastic islands surrounding a central macrophage. After nuclear extrusion, the immature reticulocytes continue to adhere to central macrophages before entry into the blood circulation. Various adhesion molecules, expressed on the surface of erythroblasts and immature reticulocytes mediate cell-cell and cell-extracellular matrix attachments within the erythroid niche. During steady-state erythropoiesis, reticulocytes remain and mature in the bone marrow for 24 to 48 hours and then circulate as recognizable reticulocytes for another 24 hours.

TABLE 5.4	Metabolic Pathways in the Erythrocyte
Metabolic Pathway	**Function**
Embden-Meyerhof pathway	Maintains cellular energy by generating ATP
Oxidative pathway or hexose-monophosphate shunt	Prevents denaturation of globin of the hemoglobin molecule by oxidation
Methemoglobin reductase pathway	Prevents oxidation of heme iron
Luebering-Rapaport pathway	Regulates oxygen affinity of hemoglobin

ATP, adenosine triphosphate.

During this time of maturation, changes in both protein content and membrane organization occur. It is known that membrane vesiculation leads to loss of membrane surface area. The membranes of young reticulocytes are mechanically much less stable than those of mature cells. Major reorganization of the membrane and structural components of a RBC accompany maturation of reticulocytes into discoid mature erythrocytes. Reticulocytes possess a significant amount of tubulin and actin in the membrane. These proteins are important during terminal erythroid differentiation in terms of cell division and cell motility. These proteins are not needed by mature erythrocytes and are lost during reticulocyte maturation.

The transition of a reticulocyte into a mature erythrocyte is accompanied by extensive changes in the structure and properties of the plasma membrane. These changes include

1. Increase in shear resistance
2. Loss of surface area (about 20%) due to loss of membrane lipid
3. Acquisition of a biconcave shape

Other changes to the cell include evolving from an immature reticulocyte with cytoplasmic organelles to an erythrocyte without organelles. In addition, immature reticulocytes undergo active endocytosis and exocytosis, a process which does not occur in mature erythrocytes.

Mature Red Blood Cell Membrane

The shape of the mature erythrocyte constantly changes as it moves through the circulation and performs extremely complex maneuvers. The cell is soft and pliable and can therefore move with ease through tissue capillaries and in the splenic microcirculation. The biconcave shape allows for maximum surface area and greatest flexibility.

The red cell membrane is a composite structure consisting of a membrane skeleton protein lattice and lipid bilayer to which the membrane skeleton is attached through interactions with transbilayer proteins.

The erythrocyte membrane has an important cytoskeleton. Different membrane-associated cytoskeletal protein networks are involved in the control of cell shape, attachments to other cells and to the substrate, and in organization of specialized membrane domains. The major components of the membrane skeleton are α- and β-spectrin, a fibrous polypeptide. The two isoforms of spectrin, alpha and beta, form a loosely wound helix. Spectrin tetramers are organized into a meshwork that is fixed to the membrane by the protein *ankyrin*. Ankyrin is itself connected to a transmembrane protein called "*band 3*" or *anion exchanger protein*. The purpose of *band 4.2* may be to stabilize the link between ankyrin and the anion exchanger. Spectrin is also linked to a transmembrane protein called *glycophorin C* by the protein known as *band 4.1*. The meshwork is anchored to the membrane at multiple sites. Band 4.1 R stabilizes the association of spectrin with *actin*. Phosphorylation of major proteins such as ankyrin and band 4.1 and 4.9 proteins can weaken the rigidity of the cytoskeleton. Disorders involving the cytoskeleton can produce altered shape and decreased deformability (see Chapter 6).

The membrane is approximately 40% by weight lipid, mostly phospholipids, and cholesterol between the phospholipids; carbohydrate approximately 8% by weight carbohydrate and linked to lipid or protein. Glycolipids are present on the outer leaflet in small concentrations and proteins that represent approximately 52% by weight, mostly glycoproteins.

More than 50 transmembrane proteins have been identified in the red cell, of which more than half carry blood group antigens. Antigens, such as those for type A or B and Rh type, are located on the outside or within the membrane. Antigens are chemically composed of oligosaccharides and glycoproteins. Some transmembrane components, for example, CD44, Lutheran blood antigens, and intercellular adhesion molecule-4 (ICAM-4), are adhesion proteins involved in interactions with other blood cells and endothelial cells.

Certain transmembrane proteins function as transporters or pumps. These include

1. Water transporter, aquaporin 1
2. Glucose transporters (GLOTI1 and GLUT4), sodium/hydrogen exchanger 1
3. Na-K-ATPase

The cell membrane is deformable and tolerant against mechanical stress and various pH and salt concentrations in vivo and in vitro. Cell shape changes reversibly depending on ATP level in the cell and intracellular calcium ion concentration. Two ideas explain the mechanism of shape regulation: the lipid bilayer coupled theory and the protein network scaffold theory.

Aging Red Blood Cell Membrane

Age-related changes in the RBC membrane occur. Plasma membrane Ca^{2+} (PMCA) and glycated hemoglobin, HbA1c, are reliable age markers for normal RBCs. An inverse correlation exists between PMCA strength and HbA1c content as an RBC ages. PMCA content declines with RBC age. This results in densification of the RBC membrane. At the end of the RBC lifecycle, a late reversal of membrane density caused by intracellular Ca^{2+} takes place in senescent RBCs.

Cytoplasmic Characteristics

In addition to hemoglobin, the cytoplasmic contents of the erythrocyte include potassium ions in excess of the concentration of sodium ions, glucose, the intermediate products of glycolysis, and enzymes. The Embden-Meyerhof pathway uses approximately 90% of the erythrocyte's total glucose. Efficient cellular metabolism depends on long-lived enzymes. The enzymes synthesized during early cell development have to be sufficient to provide the energy needed for these processes:

■ Maintaining hemoglobin iron in an active ferrous (Fe^{2+}) state
■ Driving the cation pump needed to maintain intracellular sodium ion (Na^+) and potassium ion (K^+) concentrations despite the presence of a concentration gradient
■ Maintaining the sulfhydryl groups of globins, enzymes, and membranes in an active reduced state
■ Preserving the integrity of the membrane

If metabolic pathways are blocked or inadequate, the life span of the erythrocyte is reduced and hemolysis results. Defects in metabolism can include

1. Failure to provide sufficient reduced glutathione, which protects other elements in the cell from oxidation
2. Insufficient energy-providing coenzymes such as reduced nicotinamide-adenine dinucleotide (NADH), nicotinamide-adenine dinucleotide phosphate hydrogenase (NADPH), and ATP

The most common erythrocytic enzyme deficiency, which involves the Embden-Meyerhof glycolytic pathway, is a deficiency of **pyruvate kinase**. In newborn infants, the activity of phosphofructokinase, the rate-controlling enzyme in glycolysis, demonstrates decreased activity. This contributes to a decrease in glucose consumption, which in turn contributes to shortened erythrocyte survival. A deficiency of glucose-6-phosphate dehydrogenase (G6PD) limits the regeneration of NADPH, which renders the cell vulnerable to the oxidative denaturation of hemoglobin.

Metabolic Activities

Embden-Meyerhof Pathway

This glycolytic pathway is the major source of the essential cellular energy. In the breakdown of a molecule of glucose to lactate, two ATPs are consumed during the hexose portion of the pathway but four ATPs are generated at the triose level. This net gain of two ATPs provides the high-energy phosphates needed for maintenance of the erythrocyte's shape and flexibility, for maintenance of membrane lipids, and for driving the sodium-potassium pump and calcium flux. The essential role of ATP in erythrocyte physiology is demonstrated in at least two conditions: premature cell death in vivo because of a deficiency in ATP due to inherited defects in glycolysis and the loss of viability that accompanies the depletion of ATP in vitro in stored blood for transfusion. The Embden-Meyerhof pathway also maintains pyridine nucleotides in a reduced state to permit their function in oxidation-reduction reactions within the cell.

Oxidative Pathway or Hexose Monophosphate Shunt

This energy system couples oxidative catabolism of glucose with reduction of NADP (nicotinamide-adenine dinucleotide phosphate) to NADPH (the reduced form of NADP), which is subsequently required to reduce glutathione. The pathway's activity is increased with the increased oxidation of glutathione. When the pathway is defective, the amount of reduced glutathione becomes insufficient to neutralize oxidants. This causes denaturation of globin, which precipitates as aggregates referred to as **Heinz bodies** (discussed in Chapter 6). Cells containing Heinz bodies are ultimately phagocytized and destroyed by the mononuclear phagocyte cells of the spleen. Although it is minimal, some activity in the aerobic pathway is essential for normal erythrocyte survival.

Methemoglobin Reductase Pathway

The methemoglobin reductase pathway is another important erythrocytic metabolic pathway that depends on the Embden-Meyerhof pathway for the reduced pyridine nucleotides that keep hemoglobin in a reduced state. Although the oxidative pathway, or hexose monophosphate shunt, is important in preventing denaturation of the globin of the hemoglobin molecule by oxidation, the function of the methemoglobin reductase pathway is to prevent the oxidation of heme iron. In the genetically inherited abnormalities in the amino acid sequence of the hemoglobin molecule, oxygen transport is affected by the oxidation of heme iron to methemoglobin.

Methemoglobin results from the oxidation of the reduced state (ferrous, Fe^{2+}) of heme to the trivalent (ferric, Fe^{3+}) form. In this form, hemoglobin can no longer combine reversibly with oxygen; therefore, the oxygen transport function of the molecule is lost. Maintenance of heme iron in a functional state ($Fe^{2}+$) requires the reducing action of NADH (the reduced form of nicotinamide-adenine dinucleotide), produced by the Embden-Meyerhof pathway, and the enzyme methemoglobin reductase. In the absence of this process, about 2% of the circulating hemoglobin is oxidized daily until 20% to 40% methemoglobin is present within the cell. Nonspecific reductants in the body are sufficient to keep the remaining hemoglobin reduced. A latent deficiency of methemoglobin reductase is compatible with the function of hemoglobin under normal conditions; however, high levels of methemoglobin can result when an afflicted person is challenged by an oxidant drug that denatures globin.

Methemoglobinemia—an increased concentration of hemiglobin, a derivative of hemoglobin in which iron is oxidized to the ferric state—results from either an increased production of hemiglobin or decreased NAD-reductase activity. The condition may be hereditary or acquired.

Luebering-Rapoport Pathway

This pathway is important in the oxygen-carrying capability of erythrocytes. Because of this pathway, the erythrocyte has a built-in mechanism that is low in energy expenditure and is capable of regulating oxygen transport during conditions of hypoxia and disorders of acid-base balance. The Luebering-Rapoport pathway permits the accumulation of 2,3-DPG. Erythrocytic DPG is essential for maintaining normal oxygen tension at a level necessary for oxygen transport, and it plays a regulator role in oxygen transport.

Regulation occurs in the following way. Whenever the oxygen supply to the peripheral tissues is reduced, the proportion of oxygen extracted from the blood in the systemic capillaries increases. An increase in deoxyhemoglobin (deoxygenated hemoglobin) within the erythrocyte results in increased binding of DPG and stimulates glycolysis. This may result from a pH change within the cell and the consequent increase in total erythrocytic DPG and ATP. An increase in DPG and ATP produces a shift to the right in the oxygen dissociation curve.

In **acidosis,** erythrocytic glycolysis is reduced, available oxygen is increased, and 2,3-DPG falls to a level just sufficient to normalize the oxygen tension. In conditions of **alkalosis,** the converse reaction takes place.

Catabolism of Erythrocytes

Exceptions to the normal erythrocytic life span occur in premature infants, whose erythrocytes have a mean life span of only 35 to 50 days, and in fetuses, in which case erythrocytes have an average life span of 60 to 70 days.

As an erythrocyte ages, the following processes occur:

1. The membrane becomes less flexible.
2. The concentration of cellular hemoglobin increases.
3. Enzyme activity, particularly glycolysis, diminishes.

When these changes have reached a critical point, the cell is no longer able to move through the microcirculation and is phagocytized. The spleen is the most active site for phagocytosis of aged cells because of its anatomy. Blood flow through the meshy splenic red cell pulp is slow, and the volume of plasma is reduced. This exposes aged or defective erythrocytes to phagocytosis. Intact erythrocytes return to the circulation via the small splenic venous sinusoids, where cell pliability is tested. The significant role of the spleen is demonstrated by the fact that erythrocytes with nuclear fragments (called **Howell-Jolly bodies**) and targeted erythrocytes (refer to Chapter 6) are seen after splenectomy.

Extravascular Catabolism

When an erythrocyte is phagocytized and digested by the macrophages of the reticuloendothelial system, the hemoglobin molecule is disassembled (Fig. 5.29). The resulting

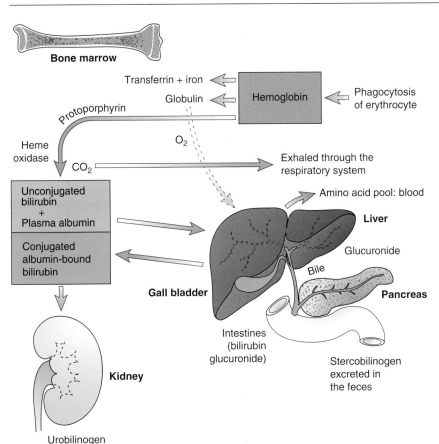

FIGURE 5.29 Extravascular catabolism of erythrocytes.

components are iron, protoporphyrin, and globin. Iron is transported in the plasma by transferrin to be recycled by the red bone marrow in the manufacture of new hemoglobin. Globin is catabolized in the liver into its constituent amino acids and enters the circulating amino acid pool. The porphyrin ring is broken at the alpha methene bridge by the heme oxidase enzyme. The alpha carbon leaves as carbon monoxide. The tetrapyrrole (bilirubin) resulting from the opened porphyrin ring is carried by plasma albumin to the liver, where it is conjugated to glucuronide and excreted in the bile. Both unconjugated (prehepatic) and conjugated (posthepatic) bilirubin are present in the plasma. Bilirubin glucuronide is excreted into the gut, converted by bacterial action, and excreted in the feces as stercobilinogen. A small amount of urobilinogen is reabsorbed into the blood circulation and excreted in the urine.

Intravascular Catabolism

Intravascular destruction is an alternate pathway for erythrocyte breakdown (Fig. 5.30). This process normally accounts for less than 10% of erythrocytic destruction. As the result of intravascular destruction, hemoglobin is released directly into the bloodstream and undergoes dissociation into alpha and beta dimers, which are quickly bound to the plasma globulin **haptoglobin**. The formation of this large molecular haptoglobin-hemoglobin complex prevents urinary excretion of plasma hemoglobin. This stable complex is removed from the circulation by the hepatocytes, where it is processed

by the cells in a manner similar to normal intact erythrocyte breakdown. Because haptoglobin is removed from the circulation as part of the haptoglobin-hemoglobin complex, the level of plasma haptoglobin decreases with hemolysis. Once plasma haptoglobin is depleted in the blood circulation, unbound hemoglobin alpha and beta dimers are rapidly filtered by the glomeruli in the kidneys, reabsorbed by the renal tubular cells, and converted to hemosiderin. The renal tubular uptake can process as much as 5 g/day of filtered hemoglobin. Once the capacity for renal tubular uptake has been exceeded, free hemoglobin and methemoglobin begin to appear in the urine. The renal processing of filtered hemoglobin can produce

1. Hemoglobin alone, if hemolysis is severe
2. Excretion of hemosiderin by itself
3. Excretion of both hemosiderin and hemoglobin; if desquamated tubular cells contain hemosiderin granules, this is evidence of a previous condition of hemoglobinemia

Hemoglobin that is neither bound by haptoglobin nor directly excreted in the urine is oxidized to methemoglobin. The heme groups in methemoglobin are released and taken up by another transport protein, **hemopexin**. Hemopexin is a plasma protein that binds heme with high affinity. Hemopexin-heme is cleared from the circulation by the low-density lipoprotein receptor–related protein (LRP/CD91, a multifunctional scavenger expressed in the brain, liver, macrophage/monocytes, and placenta). This

FIGURE 5.30 Intravascular catabolism of erythrocytes.

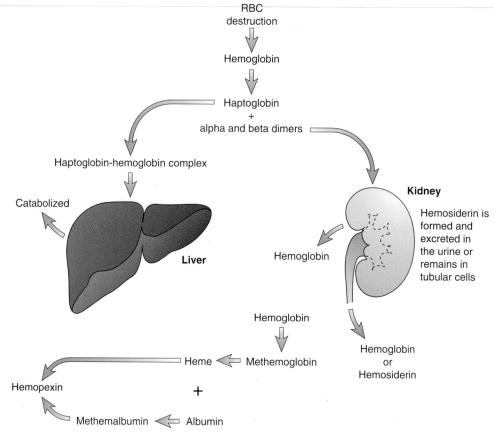

process is a biologically important pathway for eliminating potentially toxic-free heme.

Heme groups in excess of the hemopexin-binding capacity combine with albumin to form **methemalbumin** until more hemopexin is available. Once it is needed, hemopexin becomes available, and the complex is subsequently phagocytized by hepatocytes.

The combined depletion of haptoglobin and hemopexin and the presence of methemalbuminemia and hemosiderinuria can be seen in cases of intravascular hemolytic anemia and in intramarrow destruction of erythrocyte precursors. The presence of methemalbumin accompanied by hemopexin depletion *without* hemosiderinuria is associated with bleeding into the tissues (e.g., intra-abdominal bleeding in ectopic pregnancy.

MEASUREMENT OF ERYTHROCYTES

In evaluating erythrocytic disorders, it is necessary to have quantitative measurements of erythrocytes and evaluation of a peripheral blood smear as basic information. In this section, the erythrocyte indices of MCV, MCH, and MCHC are presented. The measurements of erythrocyte count, packed cell volume (hematocrit), and hemoglobin concentration may be performed manually (see Chapter 24). In Chapter 25, electronic methods of enumerating cells and additional measurements such as the RDW, including blood cell histograms,

are presented. Normal values for erythrocytes and related measurements appear in Table 5.5.

The erythrocyte indices are used to mathematically define cell size and the concentration of hemoglobin within the cell. They are

1. MCV
2. MCH
3. MCHC

Mean Corpuscular Volume

The MCV expresses the average volume of an erythrocyte. The formula is

$$MCV = \frac{\text{Patient's packed cell volume or hematocrit (L/L)}}{\text{Erythrocyte count} (\times 10^{12}/L)} = fL$$

Example: If the patient's hematocrit is 35%, or 0.35 L/L, and the erythrocyte count is $4.0 \times 10^{12}/L$, the MCV is determined thus:

$$MCV = \frac{0.35\,L/L}{4.0 \times 10^{12}} = 8.75 \times 10^{-15}\,L = 87.5\,fL^a$$

[a] One femtoliter (fL) = 10^{-15} L = 1 cubic micrometer (µm³)

TABLE 5.5	Values in the Measurement of Erythrocytes

| | Normal Adult Values | | | |
| | Men | | Women | |
	Conventional Units	SI	Conventional Units	SI
Hematocrit				
Packed cell volume	41.5–50.4%	0.415–0.504 L/L	36–45%	0.36–0.45 L/L
Erythrocyte count	$4.5–5.9 \times 10^6/\mu L$	$4.5–5.9 \times 10^{12}/L$	$4.5–5.1 \times 10^6/\mu L$	$4.5–5.1 \times 10^{12}/L$
Hemoglobin				
Concentration	14.0–18.0 g/dL	145–180 g/L	12.0–16.0 g/dL	120–160 g/L
Normal value of MCV	80–96	80–96 fL	80–96	80–96 fL
Normal value of MCH	27.5–33.2	27.5–33.2 pg	27.5–33.2	27.5–33.2 pg
Normal value of MCHC	33.4–35.6%	32–36 g/dL	33.4–35.6%	32–36 g/dL
Representative Average Pediatric Values				
At birth (cord blood)				
Packed cell volume	51%			
Erythrocyte count	$4.7 \times 10^{12}/L$			
Hemoglobin concentration	16.5 g/dL			
MCV	108 fL			
MCH	34 pg			
At 6–12 years of age				
Packed cell volume	40%			
Erythrocyte count	$4.6 \times 10^{12}/L$			
Hemoglobin concentration	13.5 g/dL			
MCV	86 fL			
MCH	29 pg			

SI = Systeme International d'Unites
Source: Perkins SL. Normal blood and bone marrow values in humans. In: Greer JP, et al. (eds.) *Wintrobes' Clinical Hematology,* 11th ed, Philadelphia, PA: Lippincott Williams & Wilkins, 2004, p. 2607; Handin RI, Lux SE, Stossel TP. *Blood,* 2nd ed, Philadelphia, PA: Lippincott Williams & Wilkins, 2003; Appendix 25 Red Blood Cell Values at Various Ages. p. 2216.
One femtoliter (fL) = 10^{15} L = 1 cubic micrometer; One picogram (pg) = 10^{12} g = 1 micromicrogram

Mean Corpuscular Hemoglobin

The MCH expresses the average weight (content) of hemoglobin in an average erythrocyte. It is directly proportional to the amount of hemoglobin and the size of the erythrocyte. The formula is

$$MCH = \frac{Hemoglobin\,(\times 10\,g/dL)}{Erythrocyte\,count\,(\times 10^{12}/L)} = pg$$

Example: If the patient's hemoglobin is 14 g/dL and the erythrocyte count is $4 \times 10^{12}/L$, the MCH would equal:

$$MCH = \frac{140\,g/dL}{4 \times 10^{12}/L} = 35 \times 10^{-12}\,g = 35\,pg^b$$

[b]One picogram (pg) = 10^{-12} g = 1 micromicrogram (μμg)

Mean Corpuscular Hemoglobin Concentration

The MCHC expresses the average concentration of hemoglobin per unit volume of erythrocytes. It is also defined as the ratio of the weight of hemoglobin to the volume of erythrocytes. The formula is

$$MCHC = \frac{Hemoglobin\,(g/dL)}{packed\,cell\,volume\,or\,hematocrit\,(L/L)} = g/dL$$

Example: If the patient's hemoglobin is 14 g/dL and the hematocrit is 45% or 0.45 L/L, the MCHC would equal:

$$MCHC = \frac{14\,g/dL}{0.45\,L/L} = 31\,g/dL$$

CHAPTER HIGHLIGHTS

Erythropoiesis

The mature erythrocyte contains the respiratory protein hemoglobin. Hemoglobin is vital to the erythrocyte's major function, transport of oxygen and carbon dioxide.

Erythropoiesis is the process of RBC production, which begins in the yolk sac of the embryo and ultimately continues throughout human life in the red bone marrow. Erythropoietin, a glycoprotein synthesized mainly by the kidneys, is produced in response to tissue hypoxia. The action of this substance is responsible for stimulating erythropoiesis and a subsequent increase in circulating erythrocytes.

Erythrocytes are rapidly maturing cells that undergo several mitotic divisions during the maturation process. After erythropoietin stimulation, the multipotential stem cell begins a series of maturational steps. The **rubriblast** is the first identifiable cell of this line, followed by the **prorubricyte, rubricyte, metarubricyte,** and **reticulocyte** stages in the bone marrow. Reticulocytes enter the circulating blood and fully mature into functional erythrocytes.

Disorders Related to Erythrocyte Maturation and Physiology

Disorders of erythrocyte maturation and physiology include

- Increased production of erythropoietin can produce a secondary polycythemia. But non–erythropoietin-related increases in erythrocytes can include the relative polycythemias or polycythemia vera.
- Defect in nuclear maturation can occur, for example, megaloblastic maturation.
- Disorders in the synthesis of porphyrin or the heme moiety can result in porphyrias.
- Conditions of iron overload, for example sideroblastic anemia.
- Genetic error of metabolism that produces inappropriately increased absorption of iron, for example, HH.
- Disorders of globulin synthesis, for example thalassemias.

Characteristics and Biosynthesis of Hemoglobin

Normal adult hemoglobin A, the predominant type of hemoglobin, is inherited in simple mendelian fashion. The genotype for this phenotype is A/A. It consists of four iron-containing heme groups and four polypeptide chains: two alpha and two beta chains. The oxygen affinity of the hemoglobin molecule is regulated by the concentration of phosphates, particularly 2,3-DPG, which diminishes the molecule's affinity for oxygen.

Abnormalities of hemoglobin types may be seen in various hematological disorders; there are also approximately 350 variant types. Most defects in hemoglobin are related to either amino acid substitutions or diminished production of one of the polypeptide chains. Iron uptake and release by the body are carefully controlled. Ferroportin is important as the last step in intestinal iron absorption, and it allows macrophages to recycle iron by moving it out of macrophages in the liver, spleen, and bone marrow from damaged erythrocytes back into the circulation for reuse. If there is insufficient hepcidin to control ferroportin, unregulated ferroportin activity causes hemochromatosis. It is important to know that iron is delivered by a specific transport protein, transferrin, to the membrane of the immature cell. Most of the iron entering the cell is committed to hemoglobin synthesis and proceeds to the mitochondrion, where it is inserted into the protoporphyrin ring to form heme.

Disorders referred to as hemoglobinopathies represent disorders related to defective hemoglobin molecules. Defects in either globin or porphyrin synthesis alter the synthesis of hemoglobin. A **sideroblast** is a nucleated erythrocyte in which iron deposits accumulate.

Several types of hemoglobin can be found during normal human growth and development: A, A_2, F, and embryonic forms. Genetic defects related either to amino acid substitutions or to diminished production of one of the polypeptide chains result in abnormal hemoglobin molecules. These conditions are referred to as **hemoglobinopathies**. One of the best-known hemoglobinopathies is sickle cell anemia.

Membrane Characteristics and Metabolic Activities of Erythrocytes

Although it lacks a nucleus and other organelles, the mature erythrocyte is capable of surviving and functioning in the circulation for an average of 120 days. Energy for metabolic processes is generated almost exclusively by glycolysis through the anaerobic Embden-Meyerhof and supplementary pathways, for example, the oxidative pathway, or hexose monophosphate shunt. If a defect exists in the oxidative pathway, this causes denaturation of globin, which precipitates as aggregates, Heinz bodies. The methemoglobin reductase pathway is essential to the prevention of oxidation of heme iron. The Luebering-Rapoport pathway is important to the oxygen-carrying capability of erythrocytes.

As the erythrocyte ages, the membrane becomes less flexible, with a loss of cell membrane; the concentration of cellular hemoglobin increases; and enzyme activity, particularly glycolysis, diminishes. When these changes reach a critical point, the erythrocyte is no longer able to move through the microcirculation and is phagocytized. When the erythrocyte is phagocytized and digested by the macrophages of the reticuloendothelial system, the hemoglobin molecule is disassembled. The resultant products are iron and globin. Iron is recycled back to the bone marrow by the plasma protein transferrin.

Globin is catabolized in the liver into its constituent amino acids and enters the amino acid pool. The porphyrin ring is broken down by the enzyme heme oxidase, and the alpha carbon is lost as carbon monoxide. The tetrapyrrole (bilirubin) resulting from the opened porphyrin ring is carried by plasma albumin to the liver, where it is conjugated to glucuronide and excreted as bile. Both unconjugated and conjugated bilirubin are present in the plasma. Bilirubin glucuronide is excreted in the feces after conversion to stercobilinogen. A small amount of urobilinogen is excreted in the urine.

An alternate pathway for erythrocyte breakdown is intravascular destruction. Normally, this accounts for less than 10% of erythrocyte breakdown. As the result of intravascular destruction, hemoglobin is released directly into the bloodstream and undergoes dissociation into its alpha and beta dimers, which are quickly bound to the plasma globulin **haptoglobin** or excreted directly. Hemoglobin, which is neither bound by haptoglobin nor directly

excreted in the urine, is oxidized to methemoglobin. In this oxidation process, heme groups are released and taken up by the transport protein **hemopexin**. If the hemopexin capacity is exceeded, heme groups combine with albumin to form methemalbumin, until more hemopexin becomes available.

Measurement of Erythrocytes

In the evaluation of erythrocytic disorders, it is necessary to have quantitative measurements of erythrocytes and a peripheral blood smear as basic information. Basic erythrocyte measurements include the erythrocyte count, packed cell volume (hematocrit), and hemoglobin concentrations. Several mathematically derived parameters based on these measurements are important to erythrocyte assessment. These parameters are the MCV, the MCH, and the MCHC. Together, they constitute the erythrocyte indices.

CASE STUDIES

CASE 5.1

The 6-month-old son of a 16-year-old mother was referred to the hospital laboratory by the well-baby clinic. The clinic's health officer noted that the baby was underweight and appeared pale. A complete blood cell (CBC) count was ordered.

■ Laboratory Data
The following determinations were obtained:

Hemoglobin 5.5 g/dL
Hematocrit 23%
RBC count 3.4×10^{12}/L
Total white blood cell (WBC) count 12×10^9/L

The differential leukocyte count revealed a normal distribution of leukocytes; however, the erythrocytes displayed a variety of morphological abnormalities.

■ Questions
1. What quantitative abnormalities were present in this baby's blood?
2. What are the MCV, MCH, and MCHC values, based on the data?
3. What type or types of abnormalities would be expected on the peripheral blood smear, on the basis of the erythrocyte indices?

■ Discussion
1. The baby's hemoglobin, hematocrit, and total erythrocyte count are all substantially below normal for a child of this age.
2. MCV, 67.6 fL; MCH, 16.2 pg; MCHC, 24 g/dL.
3. The indices demonstrate that the erythrocytes are smaller than normal and have a decreased amount of hemoglobin. These abnormalities should be very evident on the peripheral blood smear.

DIAGNOSIS: Microcytic hypochromic anemia

CASE 5.2

An Rh-negative woman, 25 years old, was admitted to the hospital's maternity ward. After a prolonged and difficult labor, she delivered a full-term infant daughter. A cord blood sample was submitted to the blood bank for Rh testing; this is a routine procedure if the mother is Rh negative.

■ Laboratory Data
The baby's cord blood sample revealed that the baby was Rh (D+) positive.

■ Follow-Up Testing
Because the mother had a long labor and there was evidence of greater-than-normal bleeding, her obstetrician ordered a Kleihauer-Betke test to determine whether one dose of immunoglobulin D would be sufficient to protect her from exposure to the baby's Rh-positive RBCs. A blood specimen was drawn from the mother. The figure shows a microscopic field of the Kleihauer-Betke results.

■ Questions
1. After examining the Kleihauer-Betke slide, which cells are the baby's?
2. What accounts for the appearance of the baby's erythrocytes?
3. What is the significance of increased fetal cells in the maternal circulation?

■ Discussion
1. The dense-appearing cells (A) are the erythrocytes containing fetal hemoglobin. The ghost cells (B) contain adult hemoglobin A.

(continued)

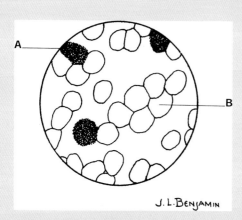

J. L. BENJAMIN

2. Cells containing hemoglobin F resist denaturation, but the cells containing adult hemoglobin are denatured. In all but rare cases in which hemoglobin F persists because of a hemoglobinopathy, increases in the number of fetal hemoglobin–containing cells are from the infant's blood and not from the mother's.
3. An increase in the number of fetal cells in the maternal circulation indicates that an increased amount of fetal blood crossed the placental barrier. If 2,000 erythrocytes are counted, the percentage of fetal cells is multiplied by 50 to estimate the amount of fetal whole blood present in the maternal circulation. For example, if 1.5% fetal cells are counted and multiplied by 50, 75 mL of fetal-maternal hemorrhage has occurred.

DIAGNOSIS: Increased fetal hemoglobin–containing erythrocytes in the maternal circulation

CASE 5.3

An 18-month-old Puerto Rican boy had recently been brought to upstate New York from a poor neighborhood in New York City. His mother reported that he had been very cranky lately. She attributed this condition to teething. He had a habit of chewing on his favorite painted wooden toys, which were family heirlooms. He was referred to the hospital laboratory from the well-baby clinic because he was lethargic and pale. A CBC was ordered.

■ **Laboratory Data**
The following determinations were obtained:

Hemoglobin 6.5 g/L
Hematocrit 22%
Total RBC count 3.0×10^{12}/L
Total WBC count 8.0×10^{9}/L
The peripheral blood smear revealed dense, dark-staining particles in some of the RBCs.

■ **Questions**
1. What are the erythrocyte indices in this patient?
2. Are any of the indices abnormal?

3. What are the dark-staining granules in the erythrocytes? What is their origin?

■ **Discussion**

1. MCV, 73 fL; MCH, 21.7 pg; MCHC, 29.5 g/dL.
2. Normal ranges: Yes. The MCV is low, the MCH is low, and the MCHC is low.
3. The dark-staining granules were determined to be basophilic stippling (see Chapter 6), a condition that represents a defect in heme synthesis. In this child, the blood lead level was increased.

DIAGNOSIS: Lead Poisoning; the Probable Etiology was the Leaded Paint on the Child's Toys

CASE 5.4

A 44-year-old white man consulted his primary care provider because of pain in his shoulder and fingers. The physical examination revealed no major abnormalities, but his liver was slightly enlarged and tender. CBC and blood chemistries were ordered.

■ **Laboratory Data**

Hemoglobin 13.5 g/dL
Hematocrit 40%
Serum iron 37 µg/dL N = 209 µg/dL
Serum transaminases slightly elevated
Serum ferritin 243.0 ug/L (extremely elevated)
Serum TS 95%

Follow-up laboratory data: A liver biopsy examination was performed. Tissue sections revealed fatty metamorphosis and an increase in fibrous tissue in portal areas consistent with early cirrhosis. Large amounts of parenchymal iron were noted with Prussian blue staining.

■ **Questions**
1. What is this patient's diagnosis based on the laboratory data?
2. What is the most common treatment for this disorder?
3. Which laboratory assays are of the greatest value in establishing this diagnosis?

■ **Discussion**
1. The patient's diagnosis is HH.
2. Therapeutic phlebotomy on a weekly basis is the usual treatment. In this case, the patient was phlebotomized weekly over a period of 10 months until his hematocrit reached 35% and iron saturation 15%. At that point, the therapeutic regimen was changed to phlebotomy every 2 to 3 months.
3. The single best screening test for a suspected case of hemochromatosis is serum TS. The normal level is less than 50% and is generally about 30%.

DIAGNOSIS: Hereditary hemochromatosis

REVIEW QUESTIONS

1. The progression of erythropoiesis from prenatal life to adulthood is
   A. yolk sac—red bone marrow—liver and spleen
   B. yolk sac—liver and spleen—red bone marrow
   C. red bone marrow—liver and spleen—yolk sac
   D. liver and spleen—yolk sac—red bone marrow

2. Which of the following is (are) characteristic(s) of erythropoietin?
   A. Glycoprotein
   B. Secreted by the liver
   C. Secreted by the kidneys
   D. All of the above

3. Which of the following is a characteristic of erythropoietin?
   A. Produced primarily in the liver of the unborn
   B. Gene for erythropoietin is found on chromosome 11
   C. Most erythropoietin is secreted by the liver in adults
   D. Cannot cross the placental barrier

4. Stimulation of erythropoietin is caused by
   A. tissue hypoxia
   B. hypervolemia
   C. inflammation
   D. infection

5. The maturational sequences of an erythrocyte are
   A. rubriblast—prorubricyte—metarubricyte—rubricyte-reticulocyte
   B. rubriblast—prorubricyte—rubricyte—metarubricyte-reticulocyte
   C. pronormoblast—basophilic normoblast—polychromatic normoblast—orthochromatic normoblast—reticulocyte
   D. both B and C

6. What is the immature erythrocyte found in the bone marrow with the following characteristics: 12 to 17 μm in diameter, N:C of 4:1, nucleoli not usually apparent, and basophilic cytoplasm?
   A. Rubriblast (pronormoblast)
   B. Reticulocyte
   C. Metarubricyte (orthochromatic normoblast)
   D. Prorubricyte (basophilic normoblast)

7. The nucleated erythrocyte with a reddish pink cytoplasm and condensed chromatin pattern is a
   A. rubricyte (polychromatic normoblast)
   B. basophilic normoblast (prorubricyte)
   C. metarubricyte (orthochromatic normoblast)
   D. either B or C

8. With a normal diet, an erythrocyte remains in the reticulocyte stage in the circulating blood for
   A. 1 day
   B. 2.5 days
   C. 3 days
   D. 120 days

9. In a Wright-stained peripheral blood film, the reticulocyte will have a blue appearance. This is referred to as
   A. megaloblastic maturation
   B. bluemia
   C. polychromatophilia
   D. erythroblastosis

10. In the reticulocyte stage of erythrocytic development,
    A. nuclear chromatin becomes more condensed
    B. RNA is catabolized and ribosomes disintegrate
    C. full hemoglobinization of the cell occurs
    D. both B and C

11. On a Wright-stained peripheral blood smear, *stress* or *shift* reticulocytes are
    A. smaller than normal reticulocytes
    B. about the same size as normal reticulocytes
    C. larger than normal reticulocytes
    D. noticeable because of a decreased blue tint

12. The normal range for reticulocytes in adults is
    A. 0% to 0.5%
    B. 0.5% to 1.0%
    C. 0.5% to 2.0%
    D. 1.5% to 2.5%

13. If a male patient has a reticulocyte count of 5.0% and a packed cell volume of 0.45 L/L, what is his *corrected* reticulocyte count?
    A. 2.5%
    B. 4.5%
    C. 5.0%
    D. 10%

14. If a male patient has a reticulocyte count of 6.0% and a packed cell volume of 45%, what is his RPI?
    A. 1.5
    B. 3.0
    C. 4.5
    D. 6.0

15. Normal adult hemoglobin has
    A. two alpha and two delta chains
    B. three alpha and one beta chains
    C. two alpha and two beta chains
    D. two beta and two epsilon chains

16. The number of heme groups in a hemoglobin molecule is
    A. 1
    B. 2
    C. 3
    D. 4

17. Increased amounts of 2,3-DPG _____ the oxygen affinity of the hemoglobin molecule.
    A. increases
    B. decreases
    C. does not alter

(continued)

18. After a molecule of hemoglobin gains the first two oxygen molecules, the molecule
    A. expels 2,3-DPG
    B. has decreased oxygen affinity
    C. becomes saturated with oxygen
    D. adds a molecule of oxygen to an alpha chain
19. If normal adult (A_1) and fetal hemoglobin F are compared, fetal hemoglobin has _____ affinity for oxygen.
    A. less
    B. the same
    C. a greater
20. Oxyhemoglobin is a _____ than deoxyhemoglobin.
    A. weaker acid
    B. stronger acid
21. Heme is synthesized predominantly in the
    A. liver
    B. red bone marrow
    C. mature erythrocytes
    D. both A and B

Questions 22 and 23: The initial condensation reaction in the synthesis of porphyrin preceding heme formation takes place in the (22) _____ and requires (23) _____.
22. _____
    A. liver
    B. spleen
    C. red bone marrow
    D. mitochondria
23. _____
    A. iron
    B. vitamin B_6
    C. vitamin B_{12}
    D. vitamin D
24. The final steps in heme synthesis, including the formation of protoporphyrin, take place in
    A. a cell's nucleus
    B. a cell's cytoplasm
    C. the spleen
    D. the mitochondria
25. An acquired disorder of heme synthesis is
    A. congenital erythropoietic porphyria
    B. lead poisoning
    C. hemolytic anemia
    D. hemoglobinopathy
26. The protein responsible for the transport of iron in hemoglobin synthesis is
    A. globin
    B. transferrin
    C. oxyhemoglobin
    D. ferritin

Questions 27 and 28: If globin synthesis is insufficient in a person, iron accumulates in the cell's (27) _____ as (28) _____ aggregates.
27. _____
    A. nucleus
    B. cytoplasm
    C. Golgi apparatus
    D. mitochondria
28. _____
    A. transferrin
    B. ferritin
    C. albumin
    D. iron
29. Increased erythropoietin production in secondary polycythemia can be caused by
    A. chronic lung disease
    B. smoking
    C. renal neoplasms
    D. all of the above
30. Relative polycythemia exists when
    A. increased erythropoietin is produced
    B. the total blood volume is expanded
    C. the plasma volume is increased
    D. the plasma volume is decreased
31. Which of the following is (are) characteristic(s) of megaloblastic maturation?
    A. Cells of some leukocytic cell lines are smaller than normal
    B. Nuclear maturation lags behind cytoplasmic maturation
    C. Cytoplasmic maturation lags behind nuclear maturation
    D. Erythrocytes are smaller than normal

Questions 32 and 33: When porphyrin synthesis is impaired, the (32) _____ become encrusted with (33) _____.
32. _____
    A. lysosomes
    B. nucleoli
    C. mitochondria
    D. vacuoles
33. _____
    A. protoporphyrin
    B. hemoglobin
    C. iron
    D. delta-aminolevulinic acid
34. Which of the following hemoglobin types is the major type present in a normal adult?
    A. A
    B. S
    C. A_2
    D. Bart

(continued)

35. The alkaline denaturation test detects the presence of hemoglobin
    A. A_{1C}
    B. F
    C. C
    D. S

Questions 36 through 39: Match the following hemoglobin types.

36. _____ A
37. _____ A_2
38. _____ F
39. _____ Embryonic
    A. Two alpha and two delta chains
    B. Zeta chains and either epsilon or gamma chains
    C. Two alpha and two beta chains
    D. Two alpha and two gamma chains

40. Fetal hemoglobin (hemoglobin F) persists until
    A. a few days after birth
    B. a few weeks after birth
    C. several months after birth
    D. adulthood

41. Cellulose acetate at pH 8.6 separates the hemoglobin fractions
    A. S
    B. H
    C. A
    D. both A and C

42. If an alkaline (pH 8.6) electrophoresis is performed, hemoglobin E has the same mobility as hemoglobin
    A. S
    B. F
    C. A
    D. C

43. The limited metabolic ability of erythrocytes is owing to
    A. the absence of RNA
    B. the absence of ribosomes
    C. no mitochondria for oxidative metabolism
    D. the absence of DNA

44. Which of the following statements is (are) true of the erythrocytic cytoplasmic contents?
    A. High in potassium ion
    B. High in sodium ion
    C. Contain glucose and enzymes necessary for glycolysis
    D. Both A and C

45. The Embden-Meyerhof glycolytic pathway uses _____ % of the erythrocyte's total glucose.
    A. 10
    B. 20
    C. 50
    D. 90

46. The Embden-Meyerhof pathway net gain of ATP provides high energy phosphates to
    A. maintain membrane lipids
    B. power the cation pump needed for the sodium-potassium concentration pump and calcium flux
    C. preserve the shape and flexibility of the cellular membrane
    D. all of the above

47. The end product of the Embden-Meyerhof pathway of glucose metabolism in the erythrocyte is
    A. pyruvate
    B. lactate
    C. glucose-6-phosphate
    D. the trioses

48. The net gain in ATPs in the Embden-Meyerhof glycolytic pathway is
    A. 1
    B. 2
    C. 4
    D. 6

49. The most common erythrocytic enzyme deficiency involving the Embden-Meyerhof glycolytic pathway is a deficiency of
    A. ATPase
    B. pyruvate kinase
    C. glucose-6-phosphate dehydrogenase
    D. lactic dehydrogenase

50. If a defect in the oxidative pathway (hexose monophosphate shunt) occurs, what will result?
    A. Insufficient amounts of reduced glutathione
    B. Denaturation of globin
    C. Precipitation of Heinz bodies
    D. All of the above

51. The function of the methemoglobin reductase pathway is to
    A. prevent oxidation of heme iron
    B. produce methemoglobinemia
    C. provide cellular energy
    D. control the rate of glycolysis

52. The Luebering-Rapoport pathway
    A. permits the accumulation of 2,3-DPG
    B. promotes glycolysis
    C. produces cellular energy
    D. produces acidosis

53. In conditions of acidosis,
    A. erythrocytic glycolysis is reduced
    B. available oxygen is increased
    C. DPG levels fall to a level sufficient to normalize oxygen tension
    D. all of the above

(continued)

54. As the erythrocyte ages,
- **A.** the membrane becomes less flexible with loss of cell membrane
- **B.** cellular hemoglobin increases
- **C.** enzyme activity, particularly glycolysis, decreases
- **D.** all of the above

55. Erythrocytic catabolism produces the disassembling of hemoglobin followed by
- **A.** iron transported in the plasma by transferrin
- **B.** globin catabolized in the liver to amino acids and then entering the amino acid pool
- **C.** bilirubin formed from opened porphyrin ring and carried by plasma albumin to the liver, conjugated, and excreted in bile
- **D.** all of the above

56. Which of the following statements are true of the intravascular destruction of erythrocytes?
- **A.** It accounts for less than 10% of normal erythrocyte breakdown.
- **B.** Hemoglobin is released directly into blood.
- **C.** Alpha and beta dimers are bound to haptoglobin.
- **D.** All of the above.

57. The upper limit of the reference range of hemoglobin in an adult male is

- **A.** 10.5 to 12.0 g/dL
- **B.** 12.5 to 14.0 g/dL
- **C.** 13.5 to 15.0 g/dL
- **D.** 14 to 18.0 g/dL

Questions 58 through 60: Match the specific erythrocytic indices with the appropriate formula.
58. _____ MCV
59. _____ MCH
60. _____ MCHC
- **A.** Packed cell volume or hematocrit (in L/L)/erythrocyte count ($\times 10^{12}$ /L) =fL
- **B.** Hemoglobin (in g/dL)/packed cell volume or hematocrit (in L/L) = g/dL
- **C.** Hemoglobin ($\times 10$ g/dL)/erythrocyte count ($\times 10^{12}$/L) = pg

Questions 61 through 63: Match the erythrocytic indices with the appropriate normal value.
61. _____ MCV
62. _____ MCH
63. _____ MCHC
- **A.** 32 to 36 g/dL
- **B.** 27 to 32 pg
- **C.** 80 to 96 fL

BIBLIOGRAPHY

Andrews NC. Forging a field: the golden age of iron biology, *Blood*, 112(2),:219–226, 2008.

Andrews NC. Understanding heme transport, *NEJM*, 353: 2508–2509, 2005.

Canmaschella C, Silvestri L. New and old players in the hepcidin pathway, *Haematologica*, 93(10):1441–1444, 2008.

Cazzola M, Della Porta MG, Malcovati L. Clinical relevance of anemia and transfion iron overload in myelodysplastic syndromes, *Hematology*, 166–173, 2008.

DeDomenico I, Lo E, Ward DM, Kaplan J. Human mutation D157G in ferroportin leads to hepcidin-independent binding of JAK2 and ferroportin down-regulation, *Blood*, 115(14):2956–2959, 2010.

Drakesmith H, et al. Ferroportin hemochromatosis: one molecule, two diseases, *The Hematologist*, 2(4):2–3, 2005.

Erwin JJM, et al. Hepcidin: from discovery to differential diagnosis, *Haematologica*, 93(1):90–97, 2008.

Fischer R, Harmatz PR. Non-invasive assessment of tissue iron overload, *Hematology*, Hematology Am Soc Hematol Educ Program. Vol. 1, Annual issue 215–221, 2009.

Fleming MD. The regulation of hepcidin and its effects on systemic and cellular iron metabolism, *Hematology*, 17:151–158, 2008.

Grim P. Why does this belly ache? *Discover*, 23:24–25, 2002.

Handin RI, Lux SE, Stossel TP (Ed). Iron overload. In: *Blood*, 2nd ed, Philadelphia, PA: Lippincott Williams & Wilkins, 2003:1418–1426.

Johnson GF. Understanding porphyrins and porphyria: An update, *Adv Med Lab Prof*, 28(11):14–17, 1997.

Kang JO. Chronic iron overload and toxicity: Clinical chemistry perspective, *Clin Lab Sci*, 14(3):202–219, 2001.

Kaushansky K. Leneage-specific hematopoietic growth factors, *NEJM*, 354:19:2034–2045, 2006.

Khumalo H, et al. Serum transferrin receptors are decreased in the presence of iron overload, *Clin Chem*, 44(1):40–44, 1998.

Kiechle FL. Molecular biology of porphyrias, *Lab Med*, 24(10): 648–653, 1993.

King D. Iron overload: Advances in hemochromatosis testing, *Adv Med Lab Prof*, 14(5):16–18, 2002.

Koepke JA. Reference values of reticulocytes, *Med Lab Observer*, 16:24, 1992.

Koepke JA. Reticulocyte count, *Med Lab Observer*, 27:12, 1995.

Laudicina RJ, Legrys VA. Hereditary hemochromatosis: A case study and review, *Clin Lab Sci*, 14(3):196–207, 2001.

Lew VL, et al. Effects of age-dependent membrane transport changes on the homeostasis of senescent human red blood cells, *Blood*, 110(4):1334–1342, 2007.

Liu J, et al. Membrane remodeling during reticulocyte maturaion, *Blood*, 115(10):2021–2027, 2010.

McLaren GD, Gordeuk VR. Hereditary hemochromastosis: insights from the Hemochromatosis and Iron Overload Screening (HEIRS) Study, *Hematology*, ASH 50th anniversary review edition, 195–206, 2009.

Melis MA. A mutation in the TMPRSS6 gene, encoding a transmembrane serine protease that suppresses hepcidin production, in familial iron deficiency anemia refractory to oral iron, *Haematologica*, 93(10):1473–1479, 2008.

Pagani A, et al. Hemojuvelin N-terminal mutants reach the plasma membrane but do not activate the hepcidin response, *Haematologica*, 93(10):1466–1472, 2008.

Parnas ML, Frank EL. Porphyrias, *Cl Lab News*, 36(4):8–10, 2010.

Piantadosi CA. Carbon monoxide poisoning, *N Engl J Med*, 347(14): 1054–1055, 2002.

Pietrangelo A. Clinical diagnosis and screening strategies for haemochromatosis, *Clin Lab Int*, 26(3):12–14, 2002.

Prouty HW. Correcting the reticulocyte count, *Lab Med*, 10(3): 161–163, 1979.

Romijn JA. Erythropoietin in anemia or renal failure in sickle cell disease, *N Engl J Med*, 325(16):1175, 1991.

Mleczko-Sanecka K, et al. SMAD7 controls iron metabolism as a potent inhibitor of hepcidin expression, *Blood*, 115(13):2657–2665, 2010.

Swinkels DW, et al. Hereditary hemochromatosis, *Cl Chem*, 52: 950–968, 2006.

Tanaka T. A genome-wide association analysis of serum iron concentrations. Blood First Edition Paper, prepublished online October 30, 2009 retrieved Nov. 1, 2009 (http://bloodjournal.hematologylibrary.org).

Unger EF, et al. Erythropoiesis-stimulating agents-time for reevaluation, *NEJM*, 362(3):189–192, 2010.

Waalen J, et al. Screening for hemochromatosis by measuring ferritin: a more effective approach, *Blood*, 111(7):3373–3382, 2008.

Weiss MJ, dos Santos CO. Chapteroning erythropoiesis, *Blood*, 113(10):2316–2142, 2009.

Weiss MJ. Handling heme, *Blood*, 106(7):2225–2226, 2005.

Zhang A, Enns CA. Molecular mechanisms of normal iron homeostasis, *Hematology*, ASH 50th anniversary review edition, 207–214, 2009.

CHAPTER 6

Erythrocyte Morphology and Inclusions

Erythrocytes: normal and abnormal

- Name and describe the variations in the size of a mature erythrocyte.
- Describe the chemical causes of variation in cell size.
- Correlate at least one clinical condition with each of the erythrocytic size variations: anisocytosis, macrocytosis, and microcytosis.
- Explain the terms used when a mature erythrocyte assumes an irregular shape.
- Explain the chemical or physical reasons for differences in cell shape.
- Correlate at least one clinical condition with each of these erythrocytic shape variations: acanthocytes, blister cells, burr cells, crenated red cells, elliptocytes, keratocytes, knizocytes, leptocytes, poikilocytosis, pyknocytes, schistocytes, sickle cells, spherocytes, stomatocytes, and teardrops.
- Compare the chemical basis for differences in erythrocyte color on a stained blood smear.
- Describe the alterations in color that can be seen in an erythrocyte.
- Correlate at least one clinical condition with the conditions of hypochromia and polychromatophilia.
- Name and describe the appearance of inclusions that may be seen in a variety of abnormal conditions.
- Explain the cellular or chemical basis of inclusions.
- Correlate at least one clinical condition with the following erythrocyte inclusions: basophilic stippling, Cabot rings, Heinz bodies, hemoglobin C crystals, Howell-Jolly bodies, Pappenheimer bodies, and siderotic granules.
- Define the alterations in erythrocyte distribution that may be encountered when examining a blood smear.
- Briefly describe the chemical reasons for alterations in erythrocyte distribution on a peripheral blood smear.
- Name the clinical conditions associated with alterations in erythrocyte distribution on a blood smear.
- Name and describe the morphology of malaria, Babesia, and leishmania parasites on a peripheral blood smear.

Case study

- Apply the laboratory data to the stated case study and discuss the implications of this case for the study of hematology.

ERYTHROCYTES: NORMAL AND ABNORMAL

Normal mature erythrocytes (discocytes) are biconcave and disc shaped and lack a nucleus. Some variations in size, shape, or color of erythrocytes may be seen on microscopic examination with a Wright or similar Romanowsky-type stain. In many disorders or disease states, erythrocytes may demonstrate variations in appearance or morphology as the result of pathological conditions.

The variations from normal can be classified as

1. Variation in size
2. Variation in shape
3. Alteration in color
4. Inclusions in the erythrocyte
5. Alterations in the erythrocyte distribution on a peripheral blood smear

Some differences in appearance may be misleading. Alterations in appearance may be caused by artifacts such as precipitated stain or proteins rather than an actual erythrocytic disorder. However, most erythrocyte deviations can be traced to specific chemical, physical, or cellular causes. This section discusses the appearance of erythrocytes on peripheral blood smears, the factors related to alterations in morphology, and the associated clinical disorders.

TYPES OF VARIATIONS IN ERYTHROCYTE SIZE

A normal erythrocyte (Fig 6.1) has an average diameter of 7.2 μm with a usual variation of 6.8 to 7.5 μm. The extreme size limits are generally considered to be 6.2 to 8.2 μm. This normal size is referred to as **normocytic.** Erythrocytes may be either larger than normal (**macrocytic**) or smaller than normal (**microcytic**) (Fig. 6.2). Macrocytic erythrocytes exceed the 8.2-μm diameter limit, whereas microcytic erythrocytes are smaller than the average 6.2-μm diameter.

The general term used in hematology to denote an increased variation in cell size is **anisocytosis** (Fig. 6.3). This term is nonspecific because it does not indicate the type of variation that is present. Anisocytosis is prominent in severe anemias.

The terms macrocytic, normocytic, and microcytic are the preferred terminology. Conditions in which a deviation from normal erythrocyte size occurs have a definite

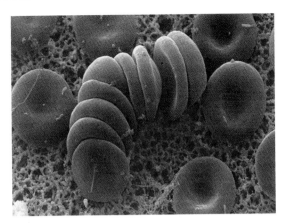

FIGURE 6.1 Scanning micrograph of normal RBCs shows their normal concave appearance. (Andrew Syred, Science Photo Lab, Science Source/Photo Researchers.)

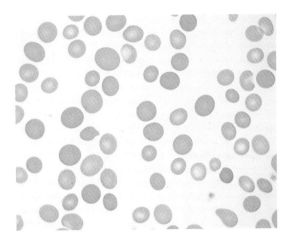

FIGURE 6.3 Anisocytosis: PB, 250×, Wright-Giemsa stain. (Reprinted with permission from McKenzie SB. *Textbook of Hematology*, 2nd ed, Baltimore, MD: Lippincott Williams & Wilkins, 1996.)

chemical or physiological basis. If more than one population of erythrocytes is present, such as following a transfusion of normocytic erythrocytes to a patient with many microcytic erythrocytes, more than one cell size may be present and the sizes of both populations should be recorded.

Macrocytosis is the result of a defect in either nuclear maturation or stimulated erythropoiesis. True macrocytes represent a nuclear maturation defect associated with a deficiency of either vitamin B_{12} or folate. These cells result from a disruption of the regular mitotic division in the bone marrow. Because of this defect, the cells appear as mature, enlarged erythrocytes in the circulating blood. The other type of macrocytosis is caused by increased erythropoietin stimulation, which increases the synthesis of hemoglobin in developing cells. This disorder causes a premature release of reticulocytes into the blood circulation. These cells not only will appear to be macrocytic but also may be basophilic and slightly hypochromic on a peripheral smear. **Microcytosis** is associated

with a decrease in hemoglobin synthesis. This decrease in hemoglobin content may be produced by a deficiency of iron, an impaired globulin synthesis, or a mitochondrial abnormality affecting the synthesis of the heme unit of the hemoglobin molecule. Disorders in which microcytosis may occur include malabsorption syndrome, iron deficiency anemia, and in the case of variant hemoglobin types, the hemoglobinopathies.

KINDS OF VARIATIONS IN ERYTHROCYTE SHAPE

The general term for mature erythrocytes that have a shape other than the normal round, biconcave appearance on a stained blood smear, or variations, is **poikilocytosis** (Fig. 6.4). Poikilocytes can assume many shapes (Fig. 6.5) but frequently resemble common objects such as eggs, pencils,

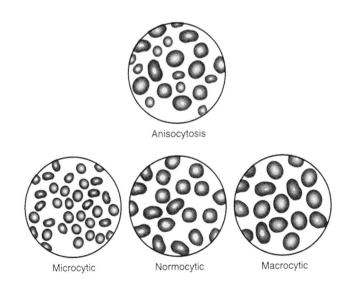

Anisocytosis

Microcytic   Normocytic   Macrocytic

FIGURE 6.2 Variations in erythrocyte size.

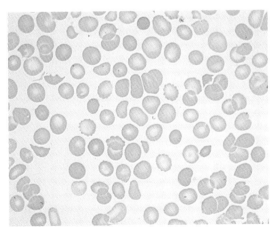

FIGURE 6.4 Hemolytic anemia: showing poikilocytosis and absence of platelets, but no signs of hemolysis. (Reprinted with permission from McKenzie SB. *Textbook of Hematology*, 2nd ed, Baltimore, MD: Lippincott Williams & Wilkins, 1996.)

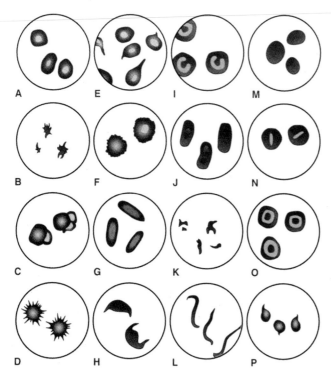

FIGURE 6.5 Variations in erythrocyte shape. A: normal RBCs (RBCs) (discocytes); B: acanthocytes; C: blister cells; D: burr cells; E: poikilocytes; F: crenated RBCs (echinocytes); G: elliptocytes; H: helmet cells (schizocytes); I: leptocytes; J: oval macrocytes (megalocytes); K: schistocytes (schizocytes); L: sickle cells (drepanocytes); M: spherocytes; N: stomatocytes; O: target cells (codocytes); P: teardrops (dacryocytes).

TABLE 6.1	Erythrocyte Nomenclature
Common Terms	**Synonyms (Greek Terminology)**
Acanthocyte	Acanthocyte
Blister cell	
Burr cell	Echinocyte
Crenated erythrocyte	Echinocyte
Elliptocyte	Elliptocyte
Helmet cell	Schizocyte
Normal erythrocyte	Discocyte
Oval macrocyte	Megalocyte
Ovalocyte	Elliptocyte
Pyknocyte	
Schistocyte	Schizocyte
Sickle cell	Drepanocyte, meniscocyte
Spiculated erythrocyte	
Spherocyte	Spherocyte
Stomatocyte	Stomatocyte
Target cell	Codocyte
Teardrop	Dacryocyte
Keratocyte	
Knizocyte	
Leptocyte	

and teardrops. Specific names have been given to many of these shapes. The names for specific kinds of poikilocytes include acanthocytes, blister cells, burr cells, crenated erythrocytes, echinocytes, elliptocytes, keratocytes, ovalocytes, pyknocytes, schistocytes, sickle cells, spiculated erythrocytes, spherocytes, stomatocytes, target cells, and teardrops. A newer nomenclature (Table 6.1) is preferred by many hematologists in place of the common names.

Deviation from the discoid shape of an erythrocyte represents a chemical or physical alteration of either the cellular membrane or the physical contents of the cell. In some cases, the exact mechanism is unknown. However, recent research in cell biology has contributed to an increased knowledge of many of these mechanisms. Each of the poikilocyte types has distinctive features and may be found in increased numbers in specific hematological and nonhematological disorders (Table 6.2). The following paragraphs give a brief description of each.

Acanthocytes (Fig. 6.6) have multiple thorny, spike-like projections that are irregularly distributed around the cellular membrane and may vary in size. Unlike echinocytes, acanthocytes have few spicules. Acanthocytes are prevalent in two very different disorders: **abetalipoproteinemia**, a rare hereditary disorder, and spur cell anemia.

In abetalipoproteinemia, acanthocytes represent an imbalance between erythrocyte and plasma lipids. The reason for this imbalance is that the patient does not absorb lipids in the small intestine. This results in decreased plasma lipids, which in turn produces a membrane defect. The loss of membrane integrity causes the cells to be more sensitive to external and internal forces. Acanthocytes are also found in cirrhosis of the liver with associated hemolytic anemia, following heparin administration; in hepatic hemangioma; in neonatal hepatitis, and postsplenectomy.

Blister cells (Fig. 6.7) are erythrocytes containing one or more vacuoles that resemble a blister on the skin. This cell has a significantly thinned area at the periphery or outer border of the cell membrane. The vacuoles may rupture. If rupturing does occur, distorted cells (**keratocytes** [Fig. 6.8]) and cell fragments (**schistocytes** [Fig. 6.9]) are produced. These cell alterations are found where there is damage to the membrane (e.g., severe burns). Blister cells result from the traumatic interaction of blood vessels and circulating blood such as fibrin deposits. Clinically, increased numbers can be seen as the result of pulmonary emboli in sickle cell anemia and microangiopathic hemolytic anemia.

Burr cells are erythrocytes having one or more spiny projections of cellular membrane. These cells are frequently

TABLE 6.2	Red Blood Cell Morphology and Related Conditions		
RBC Morphology	**Associated Clinical Conditions**	**RBC Morphology**	**Associated Clinical Conditions**
Variation in size		Pyknocytes	Acute, severe hemolytic anemias
Anisocytosis	Significant in severe anemias		G6PD deficiency
Macrocytes	Megaloblastic anemias and macrocytic anemias (pernicious anemia and folic acid deficiency)		Hereditary lipoprotein deficiency
			May be seen in small numbers during the first 2–3 months of life as infantile pyknocytes
Microcytes	Iron deficiency anemia	Schistocytes (schizocytes)	Hemolytic anemias related to burns or prosthetic implants
	Hemoglobinopathies		
Variation in shape			Renal transplant rejection
Acanthocytes	Abetalipoproteinemia	Sickle cells (drepanocytes)	Sickle cell anemia
	Cirrhosis of the liver with associated hemolytic anemia	Spherocytes	ABO hemolytic disease of the newborn
	Following heparin administration		Acquired hemolytic anemias
	Hepatic hemangioma		Blood transfusion reactions
	Neonatal hepatitis		Congenital spherocytosis
	Postsplenectomy		DIC
Blister cells	An indication of pulmonary emboli in sickle cell anemia		Storage phenomenon producing microspherocytes in the recipient
	Microangiopathic hemolytic anemia		
Burr cells (echinocytes)	A variety of anemias	Stomatocytes	Acute alcoholism
	Bleeding gastric ulcers		Alcoholic cirrhosis
	Gastric carcinoma		Glutathione deficiency
	Peptic ulcers		Hereditary spherocytosis
	Renal insufficiency		Infectious mononucleosis
	Pyruvate kinase deficiency		Lead poisoning
	Uremia		Malignancies
			Thalassemia minor
Crenated RBCs (echinocytes)	Diseases—none		Transiently accompanying a hemolytic anemia
	Result from osmotic imbalance		
Elliptocytes	Anemias associated with malignancy	Target cells (codocytes)	Hemoglobinopathies: Hb C disease, S-C, S-S, sickle cell thalassemia, thalassemia
	Hb C disease		
	Hemolytic anemias (occasionally)		Hemolytic anemias
	Hereditary elliptocytosis		Hepatic disease with or without jaundice

(continued)

RBC Morphology	Associated Clinical Conditions	RBC Morphology	Associated Clinical Conditions
	Iron deficiency anemia		
	Pernicious anemia		Iron deficiency anemia
	Sickle cell trait		Postsplenectomy
	Thalassemia		Artifact
Keratocytes	DIC	Teardrops (dacryocytes)	Homozygous beta-thalassemia
			Myeloproliferative syndromes
			Pernicious anemia
			Severe anemias
Knizocytes	Hemolytic anemia, including hereditary spherocytosis		
Leptocytes	Hepatic disorders	Alterations in color	
	Iron deficiency anemia	Hypochromia	Iron deficiency anemia
	Thalassemia	Polychromatophilia	Rapid blood regeneration
Poikilocytosis	Hemolytic anemias		
	Myelofibrosis		
	Pernicious anemia		
	Thalassemia		

RBC, red blood cell; G6PD, glucose-6-phosphate dehydrogenase; DIC, diffuse intravascular coagulation; Hb, hemoglobin.

elongated or assume irregular shapes such as a quarter moon. Burr cells are less spherical than acanthocytes. In vitro, burr cells can be produced as artifacts. Pointed projections on the outer edge are uniformly shaped. These erythrocytes have decreased deformability. The deformability depends on a variety of factors such as the relationship of the surface area of the cell to its volume, the type of hemoglobin present, or the lipid characteristics. This decreased deformability produces increased red cell

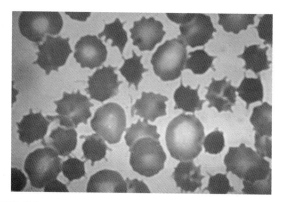

FIGURE 6.6 Acanthocytosis. In this smear of peripheral blood from a patient with abetalipoproteinemia, the erythrocytes display multiple irregular projections from the surface. (Reprinted from Rubin E, Farber JL. *Pathology*, 3rd ed, Philadelphia, PA: Lippincott Williams & Wilkins, 1999.)

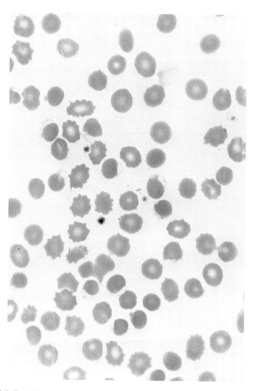

FIGURE 6.7 Blister cells are characteristic of Heinz body–mediated hemolysis. Blister cells appear to have a partially raised or blistered membrane. (Reprinted with permission from McClatchey KD. *Clinical Laboratory Medicine*, 2nd ed, Philadelphia, PA: Lippincott Williams & Wilkins, 2002.)

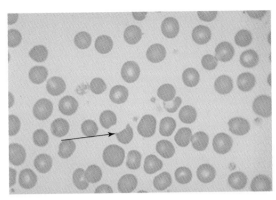

FIGURE 6.8 Keratocyte (horn). (Reprinted with permission from Anderson SC. *Anderson's Atlas of Hematology*, Philadelphia, PA: Wolters Kluwer Health/Lippincott Williams & Wilkins, Copyright 2003.)

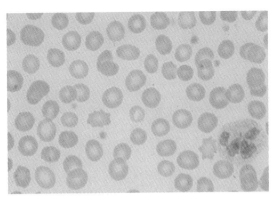

FIGURE 6.10 Echinocyte (burr). (Reprinted with permission from Anderson SC. *Anderson's Atlas of Hematology*, Philadelphia, PA: Wolters Kluwer Health/Lippincott Williams & Wilkins, Copyright 2003.)

rigidity and premature destruction. Clinically, burr cells are increased in a variety of anemias, bleeding gastric ulcers, gastric carcinoma, peptic ulcers, renal insufficiency, pyruvate kinase deficiency, and uremia. They may also occur as artifacts.

Echinocytes (crenated erythrocytes [Fig. 6.10]) have short, scalloped, or spike-like projections that are regularly distributed around the cell membrane. The projections can vary in number and appearance. Crenation can occur as the result of the physical loss of intracorpuscular water (see Chapter 3 for a discussion of osmosis). No disease states are related to crenation, but this cellular distortion results from an osmotic imbalance.

Elliptocytes (Fig. 6.11) are generally narrower and more elongated than megalocytes. These cells have a rod, cigar, or sausage shape. They represent a membrane defect in which the membrane is radically affected and suffers a loss of integrity. Associated clinical disorders include hereditary elliptocytosis, anemias associated with malignancy, hemoglobin (Hb) C disease, hemolytic anemias (occasionally), iron

deficiency anemia, pernicious anemia, sickle cell trait, and thalassemia.

Helmet cells (schizocytes) are usually the larger scooped out part of the cell (Fig. 6.12) that remains after the rupturing of a blister cell and are formed as a result of the physical process of fragmentation. These cell fragments are formed in the spleen and intravascular fibrin clots. (See the discussion of schistocytes below for a description of related clinical disorders.)

Keratocytes are erythrocytes that are partially deformed but not cut. The spicules, resembling two horns, result from a ruptured vacuole. Usually the cell appears like a half-moon or spindle. These cells are seen in conditions such as disseminated (diffuse) intravascular coagulation (DIC).

Knizocytes resemble a pinched bottle. This abnormality is associated with hemolytic anemias, including hereditary spherocytosis.

Leptocytes resemble target cells (codocytes) but the inner, central portion is not completely detached from the outer membrane. This variation of the target cell is clinically associated with hepatic disorders, iron deficiency anemia, and thalassemia.

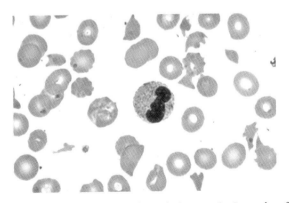

FIGURE 6.9 Microangiopathic hemolytic anemia. Irregular, fragmented erythrocytes (schistocytes) are seen in the blood smear of a patient with DIC. (Reprinted with permission from Rubin E, Farber JL. *Pathology*, 3rd ed, Philadelphia, PA: Lippincott Williams & Wilkins, 1999.)

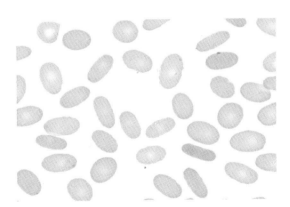

FIGURE 6.11 Hereditary elliptocytosis (HE). (Reprinted with permission from Anderson SC. *Anderson's Atlas of Hematology*, Philadelphia, PA: Wolters Kluwer Health/Lippincott Williams & Wilkins, Copyright 2003.)

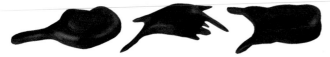

FIGURE 6.12 Poikilocytes, dacryocyte, drepanocyte, and keratocyte. RBCs of irregular shape: dacryocyte (tear drop) (*left*), drepanocyte (holly leaf) (*middle*), keratocyte (helmet cell) (*right*). (LifeART image copyright 2011 Lippincott Williams & Wilkins. All rights reserved.)

Oval macrocytes (megalocytes) have an oval or egg-like appearance (Fig. 6.13). Although these cells are similar in appearance to elliptocytes, megalocytes are macrocytic and have a fuller and rounder appearance. In contrast, elliptocytes tend to have a normal cell-size volume. Increases in this abnormality are seen in vitamin B$_{12}$ and folate deficiencies and may be observed in erythrocytes that are in the reticulocyte stage.

Pyknocytes (Fig. 6.14) are distorted, contracted erythrocytes that are similar to burr cells. These cells are seen in acute, severe hemolytic anemia; glucose-6-phosphate dehydrogenase (G6PD) deficiency; and hereditary lipoprotein deficiency and may be seen in small numbers during the first 2 to 3 months of life as infantile pyknocytes.

Schistocytes (schizocytes) (Fig. 6.15) are fragments of erythrocytes that are small and irregularly shaped. Because these cells are produced as the result of the breaking apart of an erythrocyte, the schistocyte is about half the size of a normal erythrocyte and may have a deeper red appearance. Increased numbers of schistocytes can be seen in hemolytic anemias related to burns and prosthetic implants as well as renal transplant rejections.

Sickle cells (drepanocytes) resemble a crescent (Fig. 6.16). At least one of the ends of the cell must be pointed. Generally, the membrane is smooth and the cell stains uniformly throughout. Sickle cells result from the gelation of polymerized deoxygenated Hb S. Polymerization of Hb S is influenced by both lowered oxygen levels and decreased blood pH. A variety of chemical factors contribute to membrane

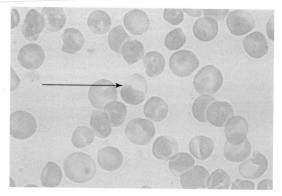

FIGURE 6.14 Pyknocyte (blister). (Reprinted with permission from Anderson SC. *Anderson's Atlas of Hematology*, Philadelphia, PA: Wolters Kluwer Health/Lippincott Williams & Wilkins, Copyright 2003.)

changes in these cells. The influx of sodium ions and other metabolic changes produce an extremely increased level of intracellular calcium ions. Alterations in the cellular contents produce cell membrane rigidity. The presence of sickle cells is associated with sickle cell anemia.

Spherocytes are erythrocytes that have lost their normal biconcave shape (Fig. 6.17). This type of cell has an extremely compact, round shape. It is usually smaller than 6 µm and has an intense orange-red color when stained. Spherocyte-like erythrocytes may appear as artifacts if a slide is examined at the thin end of a normal blood smear. Spherocytes occur as the ratio of surface area of the erythrocyte to the volume of the cell contents decreases because of the loss of cell membrane. This loss of cell membrane creates membrane instability. Membrane instability and the decreased deformability of the spherical cells lead to premature cell destruction. Spherocytes may be formed because of an inherited structural defect of the erythrocyte membrane or from direct physical trauma such as heat or chemical injury. Clinical disorders associated with spherocytes include acquired hemolytic anemia, blood transfusion reactions, congenital spherocytosis, and

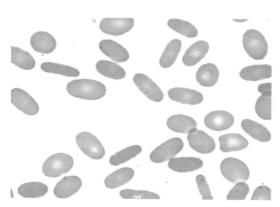

FIGURE 6.13 Ovalocyte (elliptocyte). (Reprinted with permission from Anderson SC. *Anderson Atlas of Hematology*, Philadelphia, PA: Wolters Kluwer Health/Lippincott Williams & Wilkins.)

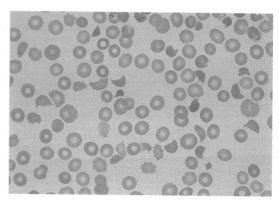

FIGURE 6.15 Peripheral blood smear contains schistocytes and increased reticulocytes in a patient with thrombotic thrombocytopenic purpura. (Reprinted with permission from Farhi D. *Pathology of Bone Marrow and Blood Cells*, 2nd ed, Philadelphia, PA: Lippincott Williams and Wilkins, 2009.)

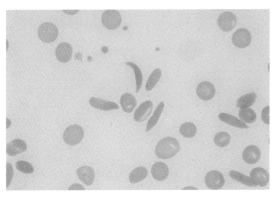

FIGURE 6.16 Drepanocyte (sickle). (Reprinted with permission from Anderson SC. *Anderson's Atlas of Hematology*, Philadelphia, PA: Wolters Kluwer Health/Lippincott Williams & Wilkins, Copyright 2003.)

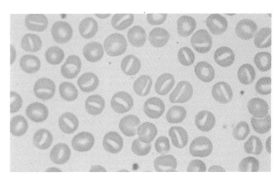

FIGURE 6.18 Stomatocyte. (Reprinted with permission from Anderson SC. *Anderson's Atlas of Hematology*, Philadelphia, PA: Wolters Kluwer Health/Lippincott Williams & Wilkins, Copyright 2003.)

DIC. Microspherocytes are associated with ABO hemolytic disease of the fetus and newborn and a storage phenomenon that produces microspherocytes in the recipient of a blood transfusion. Hereditary spherocytosis is a very heterogeneous form of hemolytic anemia.

Spiculated erythrocytes are irregularly contracted erythrocytes. Spiculated erythrocytes may also be referred to as burr cells, crenated cells, pyknocytes, spur cells, acanthocytes, and echinocytes. The terms **echinocyte** and **acanthocyte** are currently the preferred terms.

Stomatocytes (Fig. 6.18) have a slitlike opening that resembles a mouth. The slitlike opening is on one side of the cell. Stomatocytes result from increased sodium (Na^+) ion and decreased potassium (K^+) ion concentrations within the cytoplasm of the erythrocyte. Clinical conditions associated with an increase in stomatocytes include acute alcoholism, alcoholic cirrhosis, glutathione deficiency, hereditary spherocytosis, infectious mononucleosis, lead poisoning, malignancies, thalassemia minor, and transiently accompanying hemolytic anemia. These cells can also be seen in hereditary stomatocytosis and Rh null disease, which both lack the Rh antigen complex.

Target cells (codocytes) are erythrocytes that resemble a shooting target (Fig. 6.19). A central red bull's-eye is surrounded by a clear ring and then an outer red ring. The cells are thinner than normal, which may be because of an excessive ratio of membrane lipid to cell volume. Decreased intracellular volume in relationship to the membrane surface, as in thalassemia, may also account for thinner cells. In some instances, such as abnormal hemoglobins, the defect is related to a maldistribution of hemoglobin. In certain enzyme defects, cholesterol and phosphatidylcholine are abnormally increased within the erythrocyte and become incorporated into the membrane lipid. Clinically, target cells are seen in the hemoglobinopathies (Hb C disease, S-C and S-S disease, sickle cell thalassemia, and thalassemia), hemolytic anemias, hepatic disease with or without jaundice, and iron deficiency anemia as well as after a splenectomy. Laboratory-induced targeting can occur as an artifact.

Teardrop cells (dacryocytes) are usually smaller than normal erythrocytes (Fig. 6.20). As the term implies, teardrop

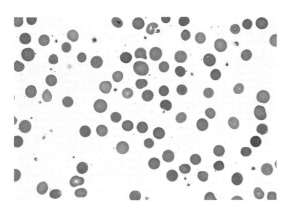

FIGURE 6.17 Hereditary spherocytosis, peripheral blood. Nearly all the red cells are microspherocytes or polychromatophilic cells. (Reprinted with permission from Farhi D. *Pathology of Bone Marrow and Blood Cells*, 2nd ed, Philadelphia, PA: Lippincott Williams & Wilkins, 2009.)

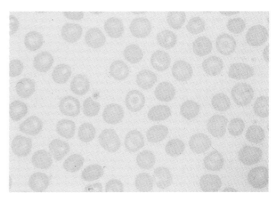

FIGURE 6.19 Codocyte (target). (Reprinted with permission from Anderson SC. *Anderson's Atlas of Hematology*, Philadelphia, PA: Wolters Kluwer Health/Lippincott Williams & Wilkins, Copyright 2003.)

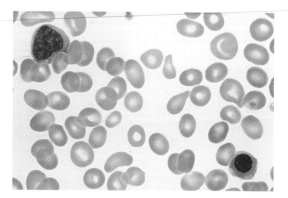

FIGURE 6.20 Typical peripheral blood smear of chronic idiopathic myelofibrosis with leukoerythroblastosis and teardrop RBCs. (Reprinted with permission from McClatchey KD. *Clinical Laboratory Medicine*, 2nd ed, Philadelphia, PA: Lippincott Williams & Wilkins, 2002.)

cells resemble tears. This cellular abnormality is associated with homozygous beta-thalassemia, myeloproliferative syndromes, pernicious anemia, and severe anemias.

ALTERATIONS IN ERYTHROCYTE COLOR

A normal erythrocyte has a moderately pinkish-red appearance with a lighter-colored center when stained with a conventional blood stain. The color reflects the amount of hemoglobin present in the cell. The lighter color in the middle, thinner portion of the cell does not normally exceed one third of the cell's diameter and is referred to as the central pallor. Under these conditions, the erythrocyte is referred to as **normochromic**. Normal and abnormal color variations reflect cytoplasmic chemical content.

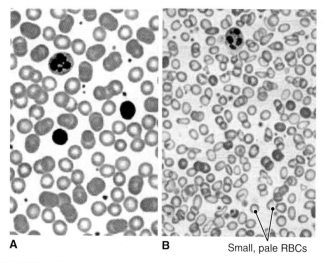

A   B   Small, pale RBCs

FIGURE 6.21 The blood in iron deficiency anemia. A: Normal blood smear. B: Blood smear in iron deficiency anemia. The red cells are small (microcytic) and pale (hypochromic). (Reprinted with permission from Thomas HM. *The Nature of Disease: Pathology for the Health Professions*, Philadelphia, PA: Lippincott Williams & Wilkins 2007.)

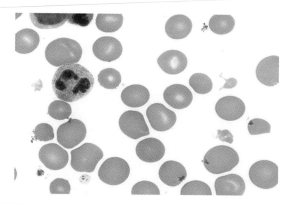

FIGURE 6.22 Erythropoietic porphyria. Polychromatophilia, nucleated RBCs in the peripheral blood, increased reticulocytes. (Reprinted with permission from Anderson SC. *Anderson's Atlas of Hematology*, Philadelphia, PA: Wolters Kluwer Health/Lippincott Williams & Wilkins, Copyright 2003.)

The general term for a variation in the normal coloration is **anisochromia**. A more specific term, **hypochromia**, is more commonly used when the central pallor exceeds one third of the cell's diameter (Fig. 6.21) or the cell has a pale overall appearance. In the case of hypochromia, inadequate iron stores result in a decrease in hemoglobin synthesis. Deficient hemoglobin content expresses itself as inadequate coloration or a lack of the typical red color associated with an erythrocyte on a peripheral smear. Hypochromia is clinically associated with iron deficiency anemia.

An alteration in the color of an erythrocyte may also reflect a state of cell immaturity. The term **polychromatophilia** is used if a nonnucleated erythrocyte has a faintly blue-orange color (Fig. 6.22) when stained with Wright stain. This cell lacks the full amount of hemoglobin, and the blue color is caused by diffusely distributed residual RNA in the cytoplasm.

Usually, the polychromatophilic erythrocyte is larger than a mature erythrocyte. If stained with a supravital stain, a polychromatophilic erythrocyte appears to have a thread-like netting within it and is called a **reticulocyte** (Fig. 6.23). Another term, **basophilic erythrocyte**, is used if the cell stained an intense

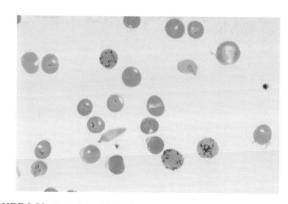

FIGURE 6.23 Peripheral blood smear with reticulocytes; staining is with new methylene blue dye. The blue granules represent precipitated, residual RNA. (Reprinted with permission from McClatchey KD. *Clinical Laboratory Medicine*, 2nd ed, Philadelphia, PA: Lippincott Williams & Wilkins, 2002.)

TABLE 6.3	Staining Characteristics of Erythrocytes and Inclusions		
		Stain	
Inclusion	**Feulgen**[a]	**Supravital**[b]	**Wright**
Basophilic stippling	Negative	Positive	Positive
Cabot rings	Negative	Negative	Positive
Howell-Jolly bodies	Positive	Positive	Positive
Polychromatophilia	Negative	Negative	Positive
Reticulocytes	Negative	Positive	Negative
Pappenheimer bodies	Negative	Positive	Positive
Heinz bodies[c]	Negative	Positive	Negative or positive

[a] Feulgen stain demonstrates the presence of DNA.
[b] Supravital stains (e.g., new methylene blue or brilliant cresyl blue) demonstrate the presence of RNA.
[c] Can be demonstrated with crystal violet stain.

blue or blue-gray color without a pink cast. Increased numbers of polychromatophilic erythrocytes are associated with rapid blood regeneration and increased bone marrow activity.

VARIETIES OF ERYTHROCYTE INCLUSIONS

Several types of inclusions can be seen in an erythrocyte stained with Wright stain. In addition to parasites such as malaria (discussed in the next section), substances that can be observed in peripheral blood smears include residual nucleic acids (DNA and RNA), aggregates of mitochondria, ribosomes, and iron particles. The nonparasitic inclusions include basophilic stippling (both a fine and coarse form), Cabot rings, Heinz bodies, Howell-Jolly bodies, Pappenheimer bodies, and siderotic granules.

Most inclusions are visible using Wright stain. However, some are only visible with other stains (Table 6.3). The inclusions are unique because they are composed of various biochemicals or organelles and are suggestive of specific abnormalities.

Basophilic stippling (fine) appears as tiny, round, solid-staining, dark-blue granules. The granules are usually evenly distributed throughout the cell and often require careful examination to detect them. Coarse basophilic stippling (Fig. 6.24) is sometimes referred to as **punctate stippling**. These granules are larger than in the fine form and are considered to be more serious in terms of pathological significance. Stippling represents granules composed of ribosomes and RNA that are precipitated during the process of staining of a blood smear. Stippling is associated clinically with disturbed erythropoiesis (defective or accelerated heme synthesis), lead poisoning, and severe anemias.

Cabot rings (Fig. 6.25) are ring-shaped, figure-eight, or loop-shaped structures. Occasionally, the inclusions may be formed of either double or multiple rings. These structures

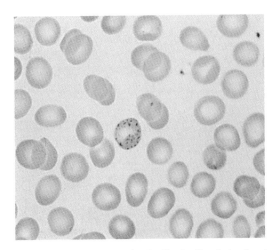

FIGURE 6.24 Hypochromia and red cell stippling in lead poisoning. (Reprinted with permission from Greer JP (ed.). *Wintrobe's Clinical Hematology*, 12th ed, Philadelphia, PA: Lippincott Williams & Wilkins, 2009.)

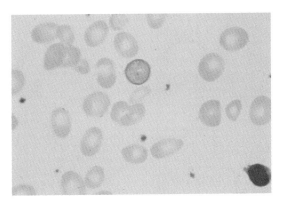

FIGURE 6.25 Cabot ring. (Reprinted with permission from Anderson SC. *Anderson's Atlas of Hematology*, Philadelphia, PA: Wolters Kluwer Health/Lippincott Williams & Wilkins, Copyright 2003.)

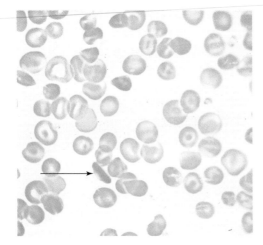

FIGURE 6.26 Hemoglobin C crystals. (Reprinted with permission from Anderson SC. *Anderson's Atlas of Hematology*, Philadelphia, PA: Wolters Kluwer Health/Lippincott Williams & Wilkins, Copyright 2003.)

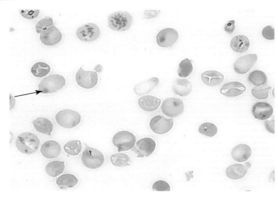

FIGURE 6.27 Heinz bodies. (Reprinted with permission from Anderson SC. *Anderson's Atlas of Hematology*, Philadelphia, PA: Wolters Kluwer Health/Lippincott Williams & Wilkins, Copyright 2003.)

stain a red or reddish purple color and have no internal structure. They may represent remnants of microtubules from the mitotic spindle. However, recent research suggests that these inclusions represent nuclear remnants or abnormal histone biosynthesis. Cabot rings can be seen in lead poisoning and pernicious anemia.

Crystals such as Hb C crystals appear as rodlike or angular opaque structures within some erythrocytes. These crystals are found in Hb C disease (Fig. 6.26). Hb H bodies may be seen with a brilliant cresyl blue stain and appear as blue globules, with many in each erythrocyte. These precipitated bodies represent polymers of the beta chains of HB A.

Heinz bodies (Fig. 6.27) are inclusions, 0.2 to 2.0 μm in size, that can be seen with a stain such as crystal violet or brilliant cresyl blue. They represent precipitated, denatured hemoglobin and are clinically associated with congenital hemolytic anemia, G6PD deficiency, hemolytic anemias secondary to drugs such as phenacetin, and some hemoglobinopathies.

Howell-Jolly bodies (Fig. 6.28) are round, solid-staining, dark-blue to purple inclusions, 1 to 2 μm in size. If present, cells contain only one or two Howell-Jolly bodies. Although these inclusions are most frequently seen in mature erythrocytes that lack a nucleus, they may be seen in immature, nucleated erythrocytes. Howell-Jolly bodies are not seen in normal erythrocytes. They are nuclear remnants predominantly composed of DNA. Howell-Jolly bodies are believed to develop in periods of accelerated or

FIGURE 6.28 Morphologic evidence of dyserythropoiesis in bone marrow smears from healthy volunteers. *A*: Intererythroblastic cytoplasmic bridge. *B*: Large Howell-Jolly body in an early polychromatic erythroblast. *C*: Two smaller Howell-Jolly bodies in a late polychromatic erythroblast. *D*: Karyorrhexis in a late polychromatic erythroblast. (Reprinted with permission from Stacey EM. *Histology For Pathologists*, 3rd ed, Philadelphia, PA: Lippincott Williams & Wilkins, 2007.)

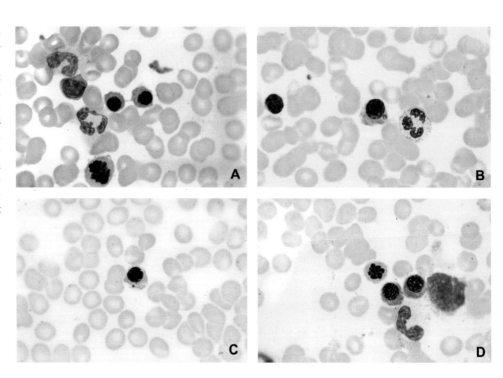

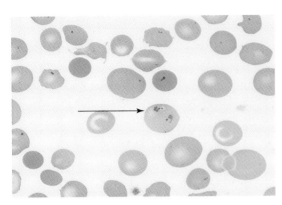

FIGURE 6.29 Pappenheimer bodies. (Reprinted with permission from Anderson SC. *Anderson's Atlas of Hematology*, Philadelphia, PA: Wolters Kluwer Health/Lippincott Williams & Wilkins, Copyright 2003.)

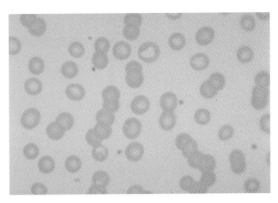

FIGURE 6.30 Rouleaux. (Reprinted with permission from Anderson SC. *Anderson's Atlas of Hematology*, Philadelphia, PA: Wolters Kluwer Health/Lippincott Williams & Wilkins, Copyright 2003.)

abnormal erythropoiesis, because the spleen cannot keep up with pitting these remnants from the cell. The presence of Howell-Jolly bodies is associated with hemolytic anemias, pernicious anemia, and particularly postsplenectomy, physiological atrophy of the spleen.

Pappenheimer bodies (siderotic granules) may be observed in Wright-stained smears as purple dots. These inclusions are infrequently seen in peripheral blood smears. Siderotic granules are dark-staining particles of iron in the erythrocyte that are visible with a special iron stain—Prussian blue. They appear as blue dots and represent ferric (Fe^{3+}) ions. Pappenheimer bodies (Fig. 6.29) and siderotic granules are probably identical structures. Pappenheimer bodies are aggregates of mitochondria, ribosomes, and iron particles. Clinically, they are associated with iron-loading anemias, hyposplenism, and hemolytic anemias.

ALTERATIONS IN ERYTHROCYTE DISTRIBUTION

Agglutination and rouleaux formation are two alterations in erythrocytic distribution that may be observed on a stained peripheral smear. **Agglutination,** or the clumping of erythrocytes, may be observed. **Rouleaux formation** (Fig. 6.30), the arrangement of erythrocytes in groups that resemble stacks of coins, is usually present in the thick portions of normal blood smears. If the rouleaux exist in thin areas of the blood smear where the erythrocytes should just touch each other or barely overlap, pathological rouleaux are present. True agglutination is caused by the presence of antibodies reacting with antigens on the erythrocyte. Thus, rouleaux formation is associated with the presence of cryoglobulins.

PARASITIC INCLUSIONS IN ERYTHROCYTES

Malaria

In its most severe form, malaria encompasses three major life-threatening manifestations: cerebral malaria, respiratory distress, and severe malarial anemia. Sever manifestations

are mostly restricted to young children, but it is also a major factor of morbidity in pregnancy-associated malaria. On a global basis, infection of red cells by protozoa is a common cause of hemolytic anemia. Malaria alone has a prevalence of 490 million cases, and in tropical Africa, the annual mortality attributable to malaria infection exceeds 2.3 million.

Etiology

The modern tendency is to refer to the various types of malaria by the name of their causative plasmodium agent: *Plasmodium vivax, P. falciparum, P. malariae,* and *P. ovale.* The life cycle of *Plasmodium* occurs in both humans and the mosquito.

The Disease Phase in the Mosquito

The disease cycle (Fig. 6.31) is initiated when the female mosquito of various species of anopheline mosquitoes bites an infected human. The infected blood of the person, which may contain male and female **gametocytes,** is drawn into the stomach of the mosquito. In the mosquito, the male or microgametocyte undergoes maturation and results in the production of **microgametes.** Concurrently, the female or macrogametocyte matures into a **macrogamete,** which may be fertilized by the microgamete to become a **zygote.** The active zygote is referred to as an **ookinete** and after constricting is referred to as an **oocyst.** The growth and development of the oocyte result in the production of a large number of thread-like **sporozoites,** which circulate throughout the body of the mosquito. The sporozoites that enter the salivary glands of the mosquito are ready to be inoculated into the next person bitten by the mosquito. The length of this cycle depends on factors such as the species of *Plasmodium* and the ambient temperature. It may range from as short as 8 days in *P. vivax* to as long as 35 days in *P. malariae*.

The Disease Phase in Humans

Sporozoites injected into the bloodstream of a human by an infected mosquito leave the circulatory system within 40 minutes and invade the liver cells of the human host. In the cells of the liver, all four species undergo an **asexual**

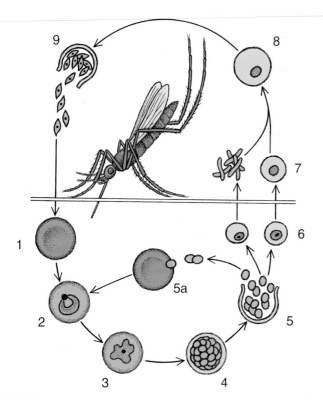

FIGURE 6.31 Malaria disease cycle plasmodium. Plasmodium: life cycle; (1) sporozoite invading RBC; (2) "ring" stage of development; (3) ameboid stage of development; (4) asexual division; (5) cell rupture with release of spore; (5a) reinfection of RBC by some spores; (6) development of other spores into sexual forms; (7) development into egg and sperm cells after mosquito sucks them in; (8) fertilized cell developing into cyst; (9) ruptured cyst releasing sporozoites. (Courtesy of Neil O. Hardy, Westpoint, CT.)

multiplication phase. This multiplication produces thousands of tiny **merozoites** in each infected cell. Subsequent rupture of the infected liver cells releases the merozoites into the circulation.

In the circulation, an **asexual cycle** takes place within the erythrocytes. This process, referred to as **schizogony**, results in the formation of 4 to 36 new parasites in each infected erythrocyte within 48 to 72 hours. At the end of this **schizogonic cycle**, the infected erythrocytes rupture, liberating merozoites, which in turn infect new erythrocytes. During the intraerythrocytic phase of the life cycle, malaria parasites hydrolyze host proteins. Hemoglobin is processed into individual amino acids, which are used for parasite protein synthesis. Erythrocyte cytoskeletal proteins are cleaved during erythrocyte invasion and rupture. A number of plasmodial protease enzymes (cysteine, aspartic, and metalloproteases and a neutral aminopeptidase) appear to be responsible for key cleavages of host proteins. Cysteine and aspartic proteases hydrolyze hemoglobin and cleave host cytoskeletal proteins. These and additional protease enzymes likely cleave the cytoskeleton to mediate erythrocyte rupture and invasion. Usually, after a patient has become clinically ill, gametocytes

appear in circulating erythrocytes. Gametocytes, derived from merozoites, grow but do not divide and finally form the male and female gametocytes. Gametocytes circulate in the blood for some time and if ingested by an appropriate species of mosquito undergo the **sexual cycle**, **gametogony**, which develops into **sporogony** in the mosquito.

Symptoms

There are usually no symptoms of malaria until several continuous life cycles have been completed. The simultaneous rupturing of erythrocytes liberates toxic products that characteristically produce chills followed by a fever in a few hours. A patient's temperature may rise to 104°F to 105°F. The symptoms last from 4 to 6 hours and recur at regular intervals, depending on the species of malaria.

Laboratory Data

The diagnosis of malaria is based on the demonstration of the parasite in the blood (refer to Chapter 3 for newer molecular tests and Chapter 26 for the manual procedure). Many of the general morphological features are shared by all of the malarial species but differences are usually sought to establish the species producing the illness (Table 6.4).

Molecular testing based on a hypervariable region with the 18s rRNA gene includes PCR kits (www.clonit.it), Milan, Italy, or differential diagnosis of a malaria infection by targeting the histidine-rich protein II (HRPII) antigen specific for *P. falciparum* and a pan-malaria antigen, common to all four malaria species capable of infecting humans (www. Inverness Medical).

Plasmodium vivax

Plasmodium vivax is the predominant species of malaria worldwide. It generally exhibits various stages in the asexual life cycle and many gametocytes in the blood (Figs. 6.32 and 6.33). The stages of the asexual cycle found in the blood depend on when the blood specimen is taken in relation to the febrile cycle. In the first few hours after symptoms begin, the majority of infected erythrocytes will contain very early forms of the parasite, **trophozoites**. Giemsa-stained smears will reveal minute blue discs with a red nucleus within the pink cytoplasm of the erythrocyte. Sometimes, the trophozoites are seen as crescent-shaped masses at the periphery of the erythrocyte (**accolé forms**). After this stage, an apparent vacuole forms in the blue cytoplasm of the parasite, which pushes the nuclear chromatin to the edge of the cell. At this point, the parasite resembles a signet ring. Two or more ring forms may be present in an erythrocyte and they are usually large. Very active trophozoites may assume irregular forms within the erythrocyte.

Between 6 and 24 hours after the beginning of the cycle, the trophozoites grow to approximately half the size of the infected cell and granules of brownish pigment appear. Infected erythrocytes are usually enlarged and pale staining. The cells may be irregularly shaped and may contain a number of fine red or pink granules known as **Schüffner dots** or **granules**. The nature of Schüffner dots is undeter-

TABLE 6.4	Red Blood Cell Morphological Features of Malarial Species			
Plasmodium sp.	Size	Inclusions	Cytoplasm	Merozoites
P. vivax	Enlarged	Schüffner dots	Blue discs with red nucleus	12–24
			Accolé forms	
			Signet-ring forms	
P. falciparum	Normal	Maurer dots	Minute rings	6–32
			Two chromatin dots	
			Accolé forms	
			Gametes crescent shaped	
P. malariae	Normal	Ziemann stippling	One ring with one dot	6–12
P. ovale	Enlarged	Schüffner dots	One ring form	6–14

mined. Although Schüffner dots may not always be seen, they can be seen in an erythrocyte infected from 15 to 20 hours or longer if the slide has been properly stained. If present, these inclusions are diagnostic of *P. vivax* or *P. ovale*. During the second 24 hours of the asexual cycle, the erythrocyte continues to increase in overall size and the parasite nearly fills the entire cell. The single nucleus divides repeatedly. During the stages of division, the parasite is known as a **schizont.** The cytoplasm finally segments to form separate small masses around each nucleus. The individual parasites thus produced are known as **merozoites**, and on rupture of the infected cell (at about 48 hours), they are released to infect new erythrocytes. There may be 12 to 24 merozoites present.

Fully mature gametocytes fill the cell almost completely and contain more pigment. Microgametocytes and macrogametocytes can be differentiated morphologically. The nucleus of the macrogametocyte is dense, whereas that of the microgametocyte forms a pale, loose network.

All the stages seen in thin films may also be found in thick-film preparations, but the parasites appear somewhat distorted. Young trophozoites may be seen but *cannot* be dis-tinguished from similar stages of *P. ovale* or *P. falciparum*. Gametocytes of *P. vivax*, *P. ovale*, and *P. malariae* are very similar in appearance. *P. malariae* is smaller and darker than the others and does *not* contain Schüffner dots.

Plasmodium falciparum

Plasmodium falciparum affects more than 500 million people each year. It is almost entirely confined to the tropics and subtropics. Fortunately, most cases of malarial anemia have a mild clinical outcome but more than 1 to 2 million fatalities occur each year. The current geographic distribution of group O individuals suggests a survival advantage if infected with *P. falciparum* to persons of group O in malaria-endemic regions.

Schizogony does not usually take place in peripheral blood. Young trophozoites and gametocytes are generally the only stages seen on the peripheral blood smear.

Young trophozoites are minute rings. Much more frequently than in other species, the ring may have two small chromatin dots. Multiple ring forms in a single erythrocyte are a common finding.

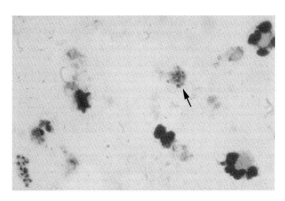

FIGURE 6.32 A thick blood film from a patient with *P. vivax* infection shows schizonts (*arrow*), trophozoites, and unlysed leukocytes.

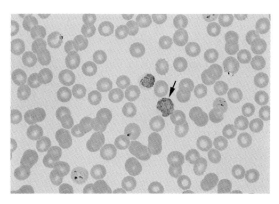

FIGURE 6.33 A blood film from a patient with *P. vivax* infection shows two microgametocytes and several ring forms. The microgametocytes have large nuclei with loose chromatin (*arrow*). Giemsa, ×3400.

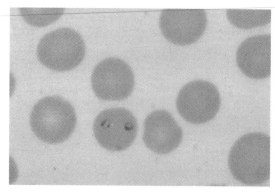

FIGURE 6.34 An erythrocyte (center) is infected with two delicate ring forms of *P. falciparum*, one of which has double chromatin.

The gametocyte in *P. falciparum* (Figs. 6.34 and 6.35) is characteristic. It appears as an elongated crescentic or sausage-shaped structure. The ends of the gametocytes may be pointed or bluntly rounded, and the remains of the erythrocyte may be seen in the concavity formed by the arched body of the parasite. Infected erythrocytes, which retain their original size, may develop a few irregular dark red- or pink-staining, rod- or wedge-shaped granules known as **Maurer dots.**

In thick blood smears, many early trophozoites can be seen. Because these cells are delicate, they frequently collapse and assume various shapes such as a comma or swallow. Gametocytes are easily recognizable by their shape, which is similar to that seen in the thin film.

Proteins exported from *P. falciparum* parasites into RBCs interact with the membrane skeleton and contribute to the pathogenesis of malaria. These proteins increase RBC membrane rigidity, decrease deformability, and increase adhesiveness, which produces intravascular sequestration of infected RBCs.

Plasmodium malariae

Plasmodium malariae occurs primarily in subtropical and temperate areas where other species of malaria are found but is seen less frequently than *P. vivax* or *P. falciparum*. All stages of development can be observed on a peripheral blood

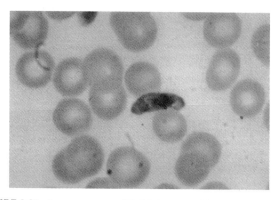

FIGURE 6.35 A gametocyte of *P. falciparum*. Giemsa, ×3700.

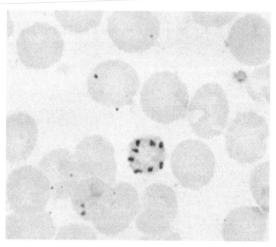

FIGURE 6.36 *Plasmodium malariae*: schizont with fewer than 13 segments in the erythrocyte.

smear (Fig. 6.36). The asexual cycle of *P. malariae* occupies 72 hours as compared with approximately 48 hours in other species. Ring forms of *P. malariae* are not easily distinguished from those of *P. vivax*. Only one ring form is usually found per erythrocyte and this form generally contains only one chromatin dot. Infected cells are not enlarged. As the parasite grows, it may almost fill the erythrocyte before schizogony.

The schizont stage contains 6 to 12 merozoites. Generally, abundant numbers of hematin granules are present and the cytoplasm of the erythrocyte may contain dust-fine, pale-pink dots, called **Ziemann stippling.** This stippling is seen only in heavily stained slides. Pigment is also produced in some quantity and is dark. The average number of merozoites is 8 and they may be arranged symmetrically in a rosette form around a central mass of pigment. Typically, they are irregularly displaced within the mature schizont.

Gametocytes are difficult to distinguish from growing trophozoites. When they are mature, they may be slightly larger than the mature trophozoites, tend to be oval, and contain proportionately more pigment than trophozoites at all stages. Thick smears do not assume the amoeboid shapes seen in other species but usually appear as small dots of nuclear material with rounded or slightly elongated masses of cytoplasm. Older trophozoites are compact and the predominant color may be that of the abundant pigment.

Plasmodium ovale

Plasmodium ovale is rather widely distributed in tropical Africa and replaces *P. vivax* in frequency on the West African coast. It has also been reported in South America and Asia. All stages of development may be present on the peripheral blood smear.

This form of *Plasmodium* is not as amoeboid as *P. vivax*. Infected erythrocytes may be enlarged and may be oval (Fig. 6.37). Only one ring form is present in each erythrocyte, and these ring forms contain only one chromatin dot.

There are 6 to 12 merozoites present in the schizont. The infected erythrocytes are enlarged and pale, and if properly

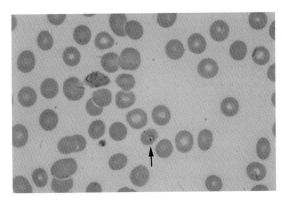

FIGURE 6.37 A blood film from a patient with *P. ovale* infection shows an immature schizont and a ring form. One of the infected erythrocytes shows the typical oval shape with fimbriated edges (*arrow*). Giemsa, ×3400.

stained, exhibit Schüffner dots in all stages. The margins of infected cells are often ragged and the erythrocytes are distinctly elongated, ovoid, or irregular in shape.

Thick films appear similar to those of *P. vivax*. Schizonts are larger than those in *P. malariae* but with no more than 12 merozoites. Schüffner dots can be observed.

Other Parasitic Inclusions

Several other types of parasites are associated with the blood. The family *Trypanosomatidae,* which includes the hemoflagellates, contains two genera that parasitize humans. These parasites may be seen in a variety of body locations including the circulating blood, the cardiac muscle, and the cerebrospinal fluid. *Leishmania* (Fig. 6.38) is found primarily in the cells of the mononuclear phagocytic system and may at times be seen in the circulating blood in large mononuclear cells.

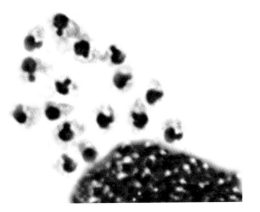

FIGURE 6.38 *Leishmania* sp. amastigotes bursting out of a macrophage, with characteristic nucleus and kinetoplast. (Reprinted with permission from Cagle PT. *Color Atlas and Text of Pulmonary Pathology*, Philadelphia, PA: Lippincott Williams & Wilkins, 2005.)

Babesiosis

Etiology

Babesiosis is a tickborne intraerythrocytic, protozoal parasite that can cause malaria-like symptoms and hemolytic anemia. It resembles *P. falciparum,* but babesiosis differs from malaria in that it is limited to erythrocytic propagation and that sexual reproduction is not evident.

Human infections in the United States have been attributed to *Babesia microti*, derived from rodents. There is increasing evidence to suggest that human babesiosis in North America may be caused by parasites that are antigenically and genotypically distinct from *Babesia microti.* Babesiosis may be transmitted via blood transfusions.

Epidemiology

Humans are opportunistic hosts for *Babesia* when bitten by nymph or adult ticks. Asplenic, elderly, and immunocompromised patients are at greatest risk for severe disease; however, babesiosis can be serious in immunologically normal persons. In the United States, the first case was reported from Nantucket, Massachusetts, in 1969. Babesiosis is emerging as a disease of public health significance in the United States with increased reports of clinical, even fatal, cases. Endemic areas in North America include the northeastern and northwestern United States, particularly Long Island, New York, and Nantucket and Martha's Vineyard, Massachusetts.

Signs and Symptoms

The clinical signs and symptoms of babesiosis are related to the parasitism of red blood cells (RBCs) by *Babesia* (Fig. 6.39). Fever, hemolytic anemia, and hemoglobinuria may result from *Babesia* infection. As with malaria, capillary blockage/microvascular stasis may occur as a result of RBC fragments, which explains liver, splenic, renal, and central nervous system involvement. With malaria, cells of the mononuclear phagocytic system in the spleen remove damaged RBC fragments from the circulation. RBC destruction results in hemolytic anemia. Babesiosis (Fig 6.3) elicits a B-lymphocyte response and a T-lymphocyte response.

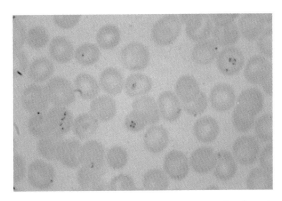

FIGURE 6.39 A thin blood film containing several infected erythrocytes. A typical tetrad form is in the center of the field. Giemsa, ×3400.

As with malaria, a T-cell–mediated cellular immunity is the primary immune response, and a secondary reactive polyclonal hypergammaglobulinemia occurs because of excessive B-lymphocyte reactivity.

Laboratory Findings

Hematology. The most important test to confirm the diagnosis of babesiosis in a patient with a malaria-like illness is a properly stained peripheral blood smear (see Fig. 6.3). Multiple peripheral-stained thin smears or stained buffy coat preparations may be necessary to detect low levels of *Babesia* parasitemia. Most patients with intact splenic function who are mildly to moderately ill with babesiosis have 10% or less of parasitemia in their peripheral blood. Patients with asplenia usually have greater degrees of parasitemia.

Wright or Giemsa stain on thin blood smears reveals the ring forms of babesiosis. Patients with *Babesia* infection, in addition to having intraerythrocytic ring forms, also may demonstrate merozoites arranged in a tetrad configuration that resembles a Maltese cross. Tetrad forms are pathognomonic of babesiosis. Babesiosis may be differentiated from malaria by the absence of pigment hemozoin, which is not present in babesiosis.

Other laboratory tests include a complete blood cell count (CBC) and erythrocyte sedimentation rate (ESR). A CBC should be obtained to look for Howell-Jolly bodies, leukopenia, lymphopenia, or thrombocytopenia. The ESR is typically elevated.

Chemistry. Serum protein electrophoresis results usually show a polyclonal gammopathy indicative of B-lymphocyte hyperreactivity in response to T-lymphocyte suppression by *Babesia*. Liver function tests should be obtained to look for elevated transaminase levels (SGPT/ALT), an elevated alkaline phosphatase level, hyperbilirubinemia, and a decreased haptoglobin level. These abnormalities may be present in patients with babesiosis.

A decreased haptoglobin level suggests a significant degree of intravascular hemolysis. A urine specimen should be obtained to check for hemoglobinuria. The frequency and degree of hemoglobinuria are related to the intensity of the *Babesia* infection.

Immunology/Serology. Immunoglobulin M (IgM) or IgG immune fluorescent assay (IFA) *B. microti* titers may be ordered in patients believed to have babesiosis who have negative findings on peripheral smears (e.g., low levels of parasitemia). A single IgM IFA titer of 1:64 or greater is diagnostic of babesiosis. Increased IgG IFA *Babesia* titers indicate past exposure rather than current infection. Polymerase chain reaction may be used to help diagnose recrudescent *Babesia* infection in patients who have previously had babesiosis or in those whose treatment is of questionable effectiveness.

CHAPTER HIGHLIGHTS

Normal, mature erythrocytes lack a nucleus, average 7.2 μm in diameter, and assume a discoid shape. However, in many hematological and nonhematological conditions, the red cell will deviate from its normal size, assume a variety of shapes, display color alterations, exhibit intracellular inclusions, or appear in an altered pattern of distribution. These characteristics are significant factors that can be observed during the examination of a peripheral blood film.

A variety of inclusions can be observed in abnormal erythrocytes when stained with Wright stain. These specific inclusions are termed basophilic stippling, Cabot rings, Howell-Jolly bodies, and Pappenheimer bodies (siderotic granules).

Alterations in erythrocyte morphology reflect chemical variances or physical abnormalities either of the red cell membrane itself or of its contents. Macrocytosis reflects either a nuclear maturational defect or stimulated erythropoiesis. Microcytosis is associated with a decrease in hemoglobin synthesis that can be produced by a deficiency of iron, impaired globulin synthesis, or a mitochondrial abnormality affecting the synthesis of heme.

Poikilocytosis may result from membrane defects caused by chemical alterations such as the decreased lipid in the cell membrane in acanthocytes. Examples of content abnormalities include sickle cells (drepanocytes), which are produced by the gelation of hemoglobin, and stomatocytes, which result from increased sodium ion and decreased potassium ion within the cellular contents.

Erythrocytic inclusions can represent parasitic infections such as malaria, DNA in Howell-Jolly bodies, RNA in basophilic stippling, aggregates of disintegrating ribosomes containing RNA in reticulocytes, nuclear remnants in Cabot rings, and aggregates of mitochondria, ribosomes, and iron particles in Pappenheimer bodies.

CASE STUDY

CASE 6.1

A 65-year-old retiree who spent his summer on Nantucket Island, MA, notes a small red bite on his leg about 6 weeks before going to see his family physician. He also noted that he had a fever and flu-like symptoms. He felt tired and was suffering from a loss of appetite. His physician ordered a CBC and reticulocyte count.

■ **Laboratory Data**
1. RBC 4.1×10^{12}/L
2. Hematocrit 39%

(continued)

CASE STUDY (continued)

3. Hemoglobin 13.3 g/dL
4. WBC 6.55 × 10⁹/L
5. Platelets 450 × 10⁹/L

■ Follow-Up

Because of the patient's symptoms and area of summer residence, his physician ordered a PCR and immunofluorescent assay titers to screen out babesiosis and ehrlichiosis.

■ Questions

1. What do the laboratory results suggest?
2. What evidence is there in the patient's history to suggest babesiosis?
3. Can babesiosis be fatal?

■ Discussion

1. The patient has a decreased hemoglobin, hematocrit, and RBC count. The follow-up PCR and immunofluorescent assay were positive for *B. microti*.
2. The small red bite on the patient's leg could have been from an infected tick. Nantucket Island is one of the areas in which tickborne diseases (e.g., Lyme disease, ehrlichiosis, and babesiosis) are endemic.
3. Yes. Babesiosis poses the greatest risk of fatality to individuals older than age 50, asplenic individuals, and immunocompromised individuals as a result of immunosuppressive drugs, malignancy, or human immunodeficiency virus infection.

DIAGNOSIS: Babesiosis

REVIEW QUESTIONS

1. The average diameter of a normal erythrocyte is _____ μm.
   A. 5.2
   B. 6.4
   C. 7.2
   D. 8.4

Questions 2 through 5: Match the following terms with the appropriate description.
2. _____ Macrocytic
3. _____ Microcytic
4. _____ Anisocytosis
5. _____ Poikilocytosis
   A. Variation in erythrocyte size
   B. Larger than normal
   C. Smaller than normal
   D. Variation in erythrocyte shape

Questions 6 through 9: Match the common terms for erythrocytes with the equivalent nomenclature.
6. _____ Normal erythrocyte
7. _____ Oval macrocyte
8. _____ Target cell
9. _____ Sickle cell
   A. Megalocyte
   B. Drepanocyte
   C. Codocyte
   D. Discocyte

Questions 10 through 13: Match the terms for erythrocytes with the appropriate morphological description.
10. _____ Echinocytes
11. _____ Helmet cells
12. _____ Schistocytes
13. _____ Spherocytes
   A. Short, scalloped, or spike-like projections that are regularly distributed around the cell
   B. Fragments of erythrocytes
   C. The scooped-out part of an erythrocyte that remains after a blister cell ruptures
   D. Compact round shape

Questions 14 through 17: Match the condition with the predominant erythrocyte type seen on a peripheral blood smear (use an answer only once).
14. _____ Associated with a defect in nuclear maturation
15. _____ Associated with a decrease in hemoglobin synthesis
16. _____ Represents an imbalance between erythrocytic and plasma lipids
17. _____ Results from the gelation of polymerized deoxygenated Hb S
   A. Microcytes
   B. Sickle cells
   C. Macrocytes
   D. Acanthocytes
18. Polychromatophilia is
   A. a blue-colored erythrocyte when stained with Wright stain
   B. caused by diffusely distributed RNA in the cytoplasm
   C. equivalent to a reticulocyte when stained with a supravital stain
   D. all of the above

(continued)

Questions 19 through 22: Match the following erythrocytic inclusions with the appropriate description.

19. _____ Basophilic stippling
20. _____ Howell-Jolly bodies
21. _____ Pappenheimer bodies
22. _____ Heinz bodies
   A. DNA
   B. Precipitated denatured hemoglobin
   C. Granules composed of ribosomes and RNA
   D. Aggregates of iron, mitochondria, and ribosomes

23. Which of the following is the term for erythrocytes resembling a stack of coins on thin sections of a peripheral blood smear?
   A. Anisocytosis
   B. Poikilocytosis
   C. Agglutination
   D. Rouleaux formation

Questions 24 through 27: Match the following erythrocyte morphology with the appropriate clinical condition or disorder.

24. _____ Macrocytes
25. _____ Microcytes
26. _____ Acanthocytes
27. _____ Echinocytes
   A. Iron deficiency anemia
   B. Abetalipoproteinemia
   C. Pernicious anemia
   D. No related disease state

Questions 28 through 31: Match the predominant erythrocyte morphology with the appropriate clinical condition or disorder.

28. _____ Leptocytes
29. _____ Microspherocytes
30. _____ Codocytes
31. _____ Dacryocytes
   A. Hepatic disorders
   B. Hemolytic disease of the fetus and newborn
   C. Hemoglobinopathies
   D. Pernicious anemia

Questions 32 through 35: Match the following erythrocyte inclusions with the appropriate clinical condition or disorder.

32. _____ Basophilic stippling
33. _____ Howell-Jolly bodies
34. _____ Heinz bodies
35. _____ Pappenheimer bodies
   A. Pernicious anemia
   B. G6PD deficiency
   C. Iron loading anemia
   D. Lead poisoning

Questions 36 through 39: Match the appropriate species of malaria with one of the following characteristics.

36. _____ *Plasmodium vivax*
37. _____ *Plasmodium falciparum*
38. _____ *Plasmodium malariae*
39. _____ *Plasmodium ovale*
   A. The schizont contains 6 to 12 merozoites; generally abundant in hematin granules; may contain Ziemann stippling.
   B. The most predominant species worldwide; 12 to 24 merozoites; may contain Schüffner dots or granules.
   C. Infected erythrocytes may be enlarged and oval shaped; may contain Schüffner dots; 6 to 14 merozoites in the schizont.
   D. Young trophozoites and gametocytes are generally the only stage seen in peripheral blood; gametocytes appear as crescent- or sausage-shaped structures in erythrocytes; Maurer dots may be present.

40. Nantucket Island is an endemic area for
   A. *P. vivax*
   B. *P. falciparum*
   C. Babesiosis
   D. all of the above

41. *Babesiosis* infection shares many of the same symptoms as
   A. *Plasmodium falciparum* malaria
   B. Lyme disease
   C. Ehrlichia
   D. None of the above

BIBLIOGRAPHY

Cserti CM, Dzik WH. The ABO blood group system and *Plasmodium falciparum* malaria, *Blood*, 110(7):2250–2258, 2007.

Cunha BA, Barnett B. Babesiosis, eMedicine (www.emedicine.com), retrieved October 9, 2003.

Glenister FK, et al. Functional alteration of red blood cells by a megadalton protein of *Plasmodium falciparum*, *Blood*, 113(4):919–928, 2009.

Haun DE, Leach A. Improving RBC morphology assessments, *Adv Med Lab Prof*, 13(24):21–23, 2001.

Kretchman DM, Rogers BS. Erythrocyte shape transformation associated with calcium accumulation, *Am J Med Technol*, 47(7):561–565, 1981.

Lehman D. Malaria and other bloodborne parasites, *Adv Med Lab Prof*, 28(10):19–21, 1997.

Mariani M, et al. Clinical and hematologic features of 300 patients affected by hereditary spherocytosis grouped according to the type of the membrane protein defect, *Haematologica* 93(9), 1310–1316, 2008.

Rosenthal PJ. Hydrolysis of erythrocyte proteins by protease of malaria parasites, *Curr Opin Hematol*, 9(2):140–145, 2002.

Winter G, Wahlgren M. Severe anemia in malaria: defense gone wrong?, *Blood* 106(10):3337–3338, 2005.

CHAPTER 7

Classification and Laboratory Assessment of Anemias

Causes of anemia

- Define the term **anemia**, based on a physiological description.
- Name the three causes of anemia.
- Explain some of the factors contributing to anemia.

Clinical signs and symptoms of anemia

- State what causes the clinical signs and symptoms of anemia.
- Briefly describe the usual complaints of an anemic patient.

Classification of anemias

- Describe the organization of anemias according to erythrocyte size and explain the limitation of such a system.

- Briefly explain the advantage of the categories of anemia using a pathophysiological basis.

Laboratory assessment of anemias

- List the three laboratory manifestations of anemia.
- Explain the grading system used to describe erythrocyte abnormalities on a peripheral blood film.
- Name the tests usually performed in the hematology laboratory to assist in the establishment of a specific anemia diagnosis.
- List the tests usually performed in other sections of the clinical laboratory that may be of assistance in establishing a specific anemia diagnosis.

CAUSES OF ANEMIA

Anemia is considered to be present if the hemoglobin concentration of the red blood cells (RBCs) or the packed cell volume of RBCs (hematocrit) is below the lower limit of the 95% reference interval for the individual's age, gender, and geographical location (see inside cover).

The causes of anemia fall into three major pathophysiological categories:

1. Blood loss
2. Impaired red cell production
3. Accelerated red cell destruction (hemolysis in excess of the ability of the marrow to replace these losses)

Anemia may be a sign of an underlying disorder. Dilutional anemia with normal or increased total red cell mass may occur with pregnancy, macroglobulinemia, and splenomegaly. Some anemias have more than one pathogenetic mechanism and go through more than one morphological state, such as blood loss anemia. In the case of accelerated red cell destruction, hemolysis in excess of the ability of the marrow to replace these losses occurs.

CLINICAL SIGNS AND SYMPTOMS OF ANEMIA

The clinical signs and symptoms of anemia can result from diminished delivery of oxygen to the tissues. Signs and symptoms of anemia are related to the lowered hemoglobin concentration. In addition, clinical signs reflect the rate of reduction

of hemoglobin and blood volume. If anemia develops slowly in a patient who is not otherwise severely ill, a hemoglobin concentration of as low as 6 g/dL may develop without producing any discomfort or physical signs if the patient is sedentary.

The usual complaints of an anemic patient are easy fatigability and dyspnea on exertion. Other general manifestations can include vertigo, faintness, headache, and heart palpitations. The most common physical expressions of anemia are pallor, low blood pressure, a slight fever, and some edema. In addition to these general signs and symptoms, particular clinical findings may be characteristically associated with a specific type of anemia.

CLASSIFICATION OF ANEMIAS

Many different types of anemias exist, with many causes and manifestations.

In an attempt to organize the anemias into understandable units, several classification schemes have been proposed. These classifications group anemias based on erythrocyte morphology, physiology, or probable etiology.

The method based on red cell morphology, which was originally proposed by Wintrobe, categorizes anemias by the size of the erythrocytes. Anemia also may be classified by red cell morphology as *macrocytic, normocytic,* or **microcytic** (see Fig. 6.2 and Fig. 7.1, and the section "Laboratory Assessment of Anemias" later in this chapter). The major limitation of such a classification is that it tells nothing about the etiology or reason for the anemia.

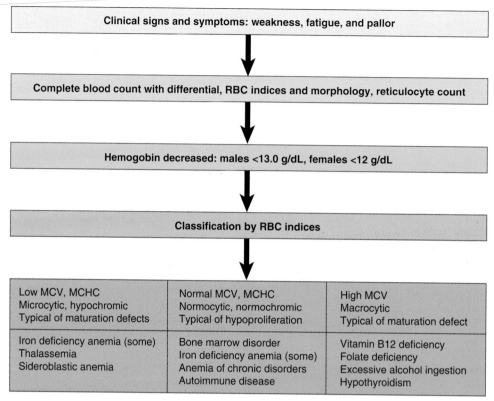

FIGURE 7.1 Algorithm for anemia testing classified by RBC size and other RBC indices.

Several schemes have been proposed to categorize anemias by etiology. None of these classifications are entirely satisfactory because within each classification the various subdivisions are not completely inclusive. However, the physiological system has merit because it describes the basic mechanism or probable mechanism responsible for the anemia.

Although many classification schemes exist, a classification system that divides the major pathophysiological characteristics into three major categories is easier to understand than other systems. The three major categories in this system are accelerated erythrocyte destruction, blood loss, and impaired RBC production. A modified organizational approach to this classification system is used in this chapter (Box 7.1) to discuss the more frequent types of anemias.

Although the incidence of certain anemias varies within different geographic areas of the world and among specific populations, some forms of anemia are generally more common than others. The most frequent forms of anemia result from either blood loss or iron deficiency conditions.

LABORATORY ASSESSMENT OF ANEMIAS

The laboratory investigation of anemias involves the quantitative and semiquantitative measurements of erythrocytes and supplementary testing of blood and body fluids. The results of these analyses provide the foundation for both the diagnosis and the treatment of anemia. In this section, the reader should become familiar with basic measurements associated with erythrocytes, various conditions and diseases that produce morphological alterations, and correlated testing that is necessary to categorize an anemia.

Categories of Anemia

BLOOD LOSS
Acute
Chronic

IMPAIRED PRODUCTION
Aplastic
Iron deficiency
Sideroblastic anemia
Anemia of chronic disease
Megaloblastic

HEMOLYTIC
Inherited defects
Acquired disorders

HEMOLYTIC-HEMOGLOBIN DISORDERS

Quantitative Measurements of Anemia

Anemia is physiologically defined as a condition in which the circulating blood lacks the ability to adequately oxygenate body tissues. The three major laboratory manifestations of anemia include

1. A decreased hemoglobin concentration
2. A reduced packed cell volume (microhematocrit) level
3. A decreased erythrocyte concentration

In addition to the direct measurement of hemoglobin, packed cell volume (microhematocrit), and erythrocyte count (see Chapter 26), a variety of other measurements or calculations can yield additional information. These assessments include

1. RBC indices (see Chapter 5)
2. The red cell histogram (see Chapter 27)
3. Red cell distribution width (RDW) or red cell morphology index (RCMI) (see Chapter 5)

Semiquantitative Grading of Erythrocyte Morphology

Direct observation of a peripheral blood smear (Fig. 7.2) for abnormalities in erythrocytic morphology or immature erythrocytes (described in Chapter 5) can yield additional information. In addition to the identification of erythrocyte abnormalities, erythrocyte morphology may be determined semiquantitatively to reflect the severity of the abnormalities. The best area on a blood smear for the examination of red cell morphology is where the red cells are barely touching each other but not overlapping. Additionally, under 10× (low power), it is possible to evaluate the relative number of white blood cells, with approximately 1 WBC for every 500 to 1,000 RBCs and 1 platelet for every 5 to 10 red cells.

Erythrocyte changes (Figs. 7.3 to 7.5) are commonly reported using either descriptive terms, such as **moderate** or **marked**, or grades on a numerical scale, such as 1+, 2+, 3+, or 4+. The characteristics of such a grading scale may vary

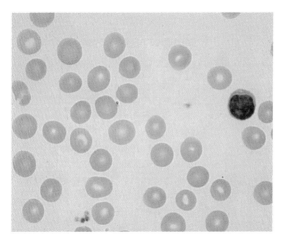

FIGURE 7.3 Peripheral blood smear showing morphologically normal RBCs, platelets, and a small lymphocyte. (Reprinted with permission from Topol EJ, et al. *Textbook of Cardiovascular Medicine*, 3rd ed, Philadelphia, PA: Lippincott Williams & Wilkins, 2006.)

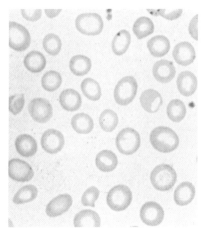

FIGURE 7.4 Nutritional anemia. Microcytosis and hypochromia in iron deficiency anemia. (Reprinted with permission from Lee G, Foerster J, Lukens J, et al. *Wintrobe's Clinical Hematology*, 10th ed, Philadelphia, PA: Lippincott Williams & Wilkins, 1998: 910.)

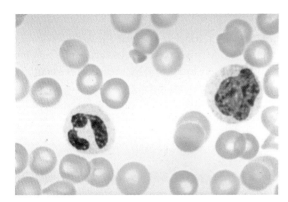

FIGURE 7.2 Normal peripheral blood smear. The mature erythrocytes are of normal size and show central pallor. A neutrophil and monocyte are also present. (Reprinted with permission from Rubin E, Farber JL. *Pathology*, 3rd ed, Philadelphia, PA: Lippincott Williams & Wilkins, 1999.)

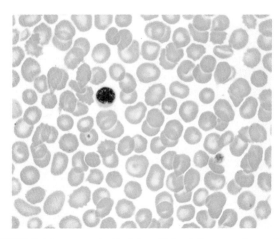

FIGURE 7.5 Macrocytosis. Peripheral blood from newborn; 250×, Wright-Giemsa stain.

TABLE 7.1	Grading of Erythrocyte Morphology
Numerical Scale	**Description**
0	Normal appearance or slight variation in erythrocytes.
1+	Only a small population of erythrocytes displays a particular abnormality; the terms **slightly increased** or **few** would be comparable.
2+	More than occasional numbers of abnormal erythrocytes can be seen in a microscopic field; an equivalent descriptive term is **moderately increased**.
3+	Severe increase in abnormal erythrocytes in each microscopic field; an equivalent descriptive term is **many**.
4+	The most severe state of erythrocytic abnormality, with the abnormality prevalent throughout each microscopic field; comparable terms are **marked** or **marked increase**.

Malarial smears
Platelet count
Reticulocyte count
Sickle cell testing
Glucose-6-phosphate dehydrogenase (G6PD) assay
Hemoglobin electrophoresis

Additional procedures may be of assistance in identifying specific types of anemias but are usually performed in other sections of the clinical laboratory. These procedures include

Antibody screening and identification tests
Direct antiglobulin (AHG) test
Measurements of bilirubin levels
Folic acid assay
Measurement of haptoglobin level
Lactic dehydrogenase (LDH) determination
Serum iron and total iron-binding capacity (TIBC)
Vitamin B_{12} assay
Occult blood testing
Urobilinogen screening

CHAPTER HIGHLIGHTS

Anemia is considered to be present if the hemoglobin concentration of the RBCs or the packed cell volume of RBCs (hematocrit) is below the lower limit of the 95% reference interval for the individual's age, gender, and geographical location. The causes of anemia fall into three major pathophysiological categories: blood loss, impaired red cell production, and accelerated red cell destruction. Anemia may be a sign of an underlying disorder.

The clinical signs and symptoms of anemia can result from diminished delivery of oxygen to the tissues. Signs and symptoms of anemia are related to the lowered hemoglobin concentration. The usual complaints of an anemic patient are easy fatigability and dyspnea on exertion. Many different types of anemias exist, with many causes and manifestations. Classifications group anemias based on erythrocyte morphology, physiology, or probable etiology. The method based on red cell morphology categorizes anemias by the size of the erythrocytes. Anemia also may be classified by red cell morphology as macrocytic, normocytic, or microcytic.

The laboratory investigation of anemias involves the quantitative and semiquantitative measurements of erythrocytes and supplementary testing of blood and body fluids. The results of these analyses provide the foundation for both the diagnosis and the treatment of anemia.

from one laboratory to another but will generally conform to the scale as presented in Table 7.1.

Supplementary Assessment of Anemias

Other procedures that support the diagnostic process of identifying an anemia may be needed. Some of these assays are performed in the hematology laboratory and others may be performed in another section of the clinical laboratory. A bone marrow examination (see Chapter 26) may be performed and may reveal an abnormal ratio of leukocytes to erythrocytes, the myeloid-erythroid (M:E) ratio. Other maturational irregularities or unusual cellular elements may be observed. The following procedures (see Chapter 26 for additional details) may provide supplementary information:
Fetal hemoglobin (Hb F) concentration

REVIEW QUESTIONS

1. The causes of anemia include
   A. blood loss
   B. impaired red cell production
   C. accelerated red cell destruction
   D. all of the above.

2. The clinical signs and symptoms of anemia can result from
   A. diminished delivery of oxygen to the tissues
   B. lowered hemoglobin concentration
   C. increased blood volume
   D. both A and B

(continued)

REVIEW QUESTIONS *(continued)*

3. Which of the following is a significant laboratory finding in anemia?
   A. Decreased hemoglobin
   B. Increased packed cell volume
   C. Increased erythrocyte count
   D. Normal erythrocyte indices

4. If you are grading changes in erythrocytic size or shape using a scale of 0 to 4+ and *many* erythrocytes deviate from normal per microscopic field, the typical score would be

   A. 1+
   B. 2+
   C. 3+
   D. 4+

5. Anemias can be categorized into
   A. hemolytic types
   B. blood loss types
   C. impaired production types
   D. all of the above

BIBLIOGRAPHY

Kahn F, et al. *Guide to Diagnostic Testing*, Philadelphia, PA: Lippincott Williams & Wilkins, 2002.

Pansky B. *Dynamic Anatomy and Physiology*, New York, NY: Macmillan, 1975.

Soloway HB, Peter JB. Interpretation of tests, *Diagn Med*, 8(4):10–11, 1985.

Wallach J. *Handbook of Interpretation of Diagnostic Tests,* 8th ed, Philadelphia, PA: Lippincott Williams & Wilkins, 2007.

Acute and Chronic Blood Loss Anemias

Acute blood loss anemia

■ Describe the etiology and physiology of acute blood loss.
■ Explain the significant hematological laboratory findings in acute blood loss.

Chronic blood loss anemia

■ Describe the etiology and physiology of chronic blood loss. Explain the significant hematological laboratory findings in chronic blood loss.

Case studies

■ Apply the laboratory data to the stated case studies and discuss the implications of these cases for the study of hematology.

ACUTE BLOOD LOSS ANEMIA

Etiology

The acute loss of blood is usually associated with traumatic conditions such as an accident or severe injury. Occasionally, acute blood loss may occur during or after surgery.

Physiology

An acute blood loss does not produce an immediate anemia. A severe hemorrhage or rapid blood loss amounting to more than 20% of the circulating blood volume reduces an individual's total blood volume and produces a condition of shock and related cardiovascular problems. Even if enough hemoglobin remains in the circulation, an oxygen impairment can exist because of circulatory failure. However, severe acute bleeding can be fatal as a result of the collapse of the circulatory system; immediate expansion of the blood volume is required (Table 8.1).

In acute blood loss, the body itself adjusts to the situation by expanding the circulatory volume, which produces the subsequent anemia. Fluid from the extravascular spaces enters the blood circulation and has a diluting effect on the remaining cells.

Laboratory Findings

Hematological findings are very different in the patient who has experienced an acute bleeding episode within the past 24 to 48 hours compared with a patient who has suffered from chronic bleeding for several months. Table 8.2 presents a profile of the typical findings in each case.

The earliest hematological change in acute blood loss is a transient fall in the platelet count, which may rise to elevated levels within 1 hour. The next change is the development of neutrophilic leukocytosis (from 10 to 35×10^9/L) with a shift to the left. The hemoglobin and hematocrit do not fall immediately but fall as tissue fluids move into the blood circulation. It can be 48 or 72 hours after the hemorrhage until the full extent of the red cell loss is apparent.

Assuming that the patient with acute bleeding was healthy before the episode, the peripheral blood film at 24 hours should be essentially normochromic and normocytic with normal red blood cell (RBC) indices (mean corpuscular volume [MCV], mean corpuscular hemoglobin [MCH], and mean corpuscular hemoglobin concentration [MCHC]). When an increased number of reticulocytes reach the circulating blood because of increased erythropoiesis, a transient macrocytosis develops. This phenomenon takes place beginning approximately 3 to 5 days after the blood loss and reaches a maximum approximately 10 days later.

It takes about 2 to 4 days after the blood loss for the total white blood cell (WBC) count to return to normal and about 2 weeks for the morphological changes to disappear. The return of the red cell profile to previous values takes longer.

CHRONIC BLOOD LOSS ANEMIA

Etiology

Chronic blood loss is frequently associated with disorders of the gastrointestinal (GI) tract, although chronic blood loss may be related to heavy menstruation in women or urinary tract abnormalities. In chronic anemias, blood loss of small amounts occurs over an extended period, usually months. The chronic and continual loss of small volumes of blood does not disrupt the blood volume.

TABLE 8.1	Clinical Features of Acute Hemorrhage in Healthy Young Adults	
Volume of Blood Loss (mL)	**Blood Volume (%)**	**Symptoms**
500–1,000	10–20	Few or none
1,000–1,500	20–30	At rest-(recumbent) asymptomatic
		Upright position-light-headedness, and hypotension, tachycardia
1,500–2,000	30–40	Symptomatic (recumbent)-thirst, shortness of breath, clouding or loss of consciousness; blood pressure, cardiac output, venous pressure decrease; pulse usually becomes rapid; extremities become cold, clammy, an pale.
2,000–2,500	40–50	Lactic acidosis, shock; irreversible shock, death

Source : Greer JP, et al. *Wintrobe's Clinical Hematology,* 11 ed, Philadelphia, PA: Lippincott Williams & Wilkins, 2004:975.

TABLE 8.2	Blood Loss Anemia	
	Acute (24 hours)	**Chronic (months)**
Etiology	Trauma	GI tract
		Menstruation
		Urinary tract
Blood volume disruption	Yes	No
Iron deficiency	No	Yes
Hematocrit (packed cell volume)	Usually normal	Decreased
WBC count	Increased	Normal
Platelets	Increased	Normal
Reticulocytes	Normal	Increased

If blood is lost in small amounts over an extended period, both the clinical and hematological features seen in acute bleeding are absent. Regeneration of RBCs occurs at a slower rate. The reticulocyte count may be normal or only slightly increased.

A noticeable anemia does not usually develop until after storage iron is depleted. At first, the anemia is normochromic and normocytic. Gradually, the chronic bleeding results in an iron deficiency, and the newly formed cells are morphologically hypochromic and microcytic. The WBC count is normal or slightly decreased. Platelets are commonly increased, and only later, in severe iron deficiency, are they likely to be decreased.

CHAPTER HIGHLIGHTS

Acute blood loss is usually associated with traumatic conditions during or after surgery. It does not produce an immediate anemia. A severe hemorrhage reduces an individual's total blood volume and can be fatal because of the collapse of the circulatory system.

In acute blood loss, the body attempts to adjust to the situation by expanding the circulatory volume, which produces the subsequent anemia. Fluid from the extravascular spaces enters the blood circulation and has a diluting effect on the remaining cells.

The earliest hematological change in acute blood loss is a transient fall in the platelet count, which may rise to elevated levels within 1 hour. The next change is the development of neutrophilic leukocytosis with a shift to the left. The hemoglobin and hematocrit do not fall immediately. It can be 48 or 72 hours after the hemorrhage until the full extent of the red cell loss is apparent.

Chronic blood loss lacks both the clinical and hematological features seen in acute bleeding. A noticeable anemia does not usually develop until after storage iron is depleted. In time, the peripheral blood smear becomes hypochromic and microcytic.

CASE STUDIES

CASE 8.1

A 38-year-old white woman was treated in the emergency department for severe lacerations and possible abdominal injuries sustained in an automobile accident. She was admitted to the hospital for observation and further evaluation. On admission, a complete blood

(continued)

count (CBC), urinalysis, and radiograph series were ordered.

■ **Laboratory Data**

Her CBC results were as follows:

Hemoglobin 10.5 g/dL
Hct 34%
RBC 3.8 × 10^{12}/L
WBC 12.0 × 10^9/L

The RBC indices were as follows:

MCV 89.6 fL
MCH 27.6 pg
MCHC 31 g/dL

The peripheral blood smear showed essentially normal RBC morphology and platelet distribution. Forty-eight hours after admission, a stat repeat CBC was ordered. The results were as follows:

Hemoglobin 8.0 g/dL
Hct 26%
RBC 2.9 × 10^{12}/L
WBC 15.5 × 10^9/L

The RBC indices were all within their normal ranges. A peripheral blood smear showed normal RBC morphology, although some polychromatophilia was noted. The distribution of platelets had increased. A follow-up platelet count was 0.60 × 10^{12}/L.

Subsequently, the patient was typed and cross-matched for 6 units of blood. Two units of whole blood cells were administered immediately. An emergency laparotomy revealed that the patient had injuries to both the liver and spleen.

■ **Questions**

1. Why was the patient's hemoglobin and hematocrit normal on admission but decreased after 48 hours?
2. What is the significance of this patient's increased leukocyte (WBC) and thrombocyte (platelet) count?
3. What is the reason for the polychromatophilia noted on the 48-hour peripheral blood film?

■ **Discussion**

1. The body adjusts to severe hemorrhaging by expanding the circulating volume at the expense of the extravascular fluid. This volume adjustment produces a delayed anemia. As the extravascular fluid enters the bloodstream, it dilutes the RBCs. The hemoglobin and hematocrit become decreased after 48 to 72 hours in such cases.
2. In acute blood loss, the platelets and circulating granulocytes increase within a few hours. Immature WBCs may also be seen. Increased leukocytes and platelets are a normal body response to stress. The body continually strives to maintain homeostasis.

3. Acute blood loss immediately begins to stimulate a healthy, normal bone marrow. Reticulocytosis becomes apparent within 24 hours and peaks at 7 to 10 days after severe blood loss. When erythrocyte restoration is completed, reticulocytosis ceases. Reticulocytes are seen as polychromasia or polychromatophilic RBCs when the RBCs are stained with Wright stain. A supervital stain such as new methylene blue needs to be used to visibly demonstrate reticulocytes in erythrocytes.

DIAGNOSIS: Acute Blood Loss

CASE 8.2

A 55-year-old white male college professor had been experiencing fatigue and shortness of breath when walking over the past several months. Getting more sleep at night did not help. He reported eating a balanced diet of fruits, vegetables, meat, and dairy products. Upon physical examination, he appeared slightly pale but had no other abnormalities. His primary care physician ordered a CBC, urinalysis, and fecal occult blood (×3) tests.

■ **Laboratory Data**

Laboratory findings were as follows:
Hemoglobin 12.5 g/dL
Hematocrit 32%
RBC 4.2 × 10^{12}/L
WBC count within normal limits
RBC indices:
MCV 42 fL
MCH 29.7 pg
Urinalysis: normal findings
Fecal occult blood (×3) positive

■ **Questions**

1. What is the most likely cause of this patient's anemia?
2. What type of red cell morphology would be expected on a peripheral blood smear?
3. What follow-up tests should be conducted?

■ **Discussion**

1. The most likely cause of this patient's anemia is chronic blood loss. The source of the bleeding could be the GI tract, in view of the fact that he had a positive test result for fecal blood.
2. Hypochromic, microcytic RBCs would be expected on his peripheral blood smear.
3. The source of the fecal blood needs to be located. In this case, the patient had a follow-up colonoscopy that revealed a number of nonmalignant, bleeding polyps.

DIAGNOSIS: Chronic Blood Loss

Questions 1 through 5: Match the following characteristics with either A or B.

1. _____ Disorders of the GI system or heavy menstruation
2. _____ Increased thrombocytes (platelets)
3. _____ Traumatic conditions
4. _____ Does not disrupt the blood volume
5. _____ Results in an iron deficiency and a hypochromic/microcytic erythrocyte morphology on a peripheral blood smear
   A. Acute blood loss
   B. Chronic blood loss

6. The erythrocyte morphology associated with anemia in an otherwise healthy individual caused by acute blood loss is usually
   A. microcytic
   B. megaloblastic
   C. normochromic
   D. hypochromic
7. Anemia caused by chronic blood loss is characterized by
   A. hypochromic, microcytic erythrocytes
   B. decreased packed cell volume
   C. increased platelets
   D. both A and B

BIBLIOGRAPHY

Greer JP, et al. *Wintrobe's Clinical Hematology*, 11 ed, Philadelphia, PA: Lippincott Williams & Wilkins, 2004.

Handin RI, Lux SE, Stossel TP. *Blood*, 2 ed, Philadelpha, PA: Lippincott Williams & Wilkins, 2003.

CHAPTER 9

Aplastic and Related Anemias

Acquired Aplastic anemia

- Describe the major characteristics of acquired aplastic anemia.
- Define the term **iatrogenic.**
- List at least three iatrogenic substances that can cause acquired aplastic anemia.
- Name at least four types of viral infection that have been associated with acquired aplastic anemia.
- Briefly describe how the immune process causes acquired aplastic anemia.
- Name the three phases of development of acquired aplastic anemia.
- Describe the clinical features of acquired aplastic anemia.
- Discuss the laboratory findings in acquired aplastic anemia.
- Explain how the laboratory findings in acquired aplastic anemia manifest themselves after acute radiation exposure.
- Discuss the role of bone marrow transplantation in the treatment of acquired aplastic anemia.

Congenital Red blood cell–related disorders

- Name three causes and examples of red cell aplasia.
- Identify the cause of pure red cell aplasia.

- Compare acquired pure red cell aplasia to chronic red cell aplasia.
- Describe the characteristics of Diamond-Blackfan syndrome, including the nature of the defect.
- Describe the mode of inheritance of Fanconi anemia.
- Explain the clinical signs and symptoms of Fanconi anemia.
- Name one treatment for Fanconi anemia.
- Compare the relationship between familial aplastic anemia and Fanconi anemia.
- Describe the laboratory features of familial aplastic anemia.
- Discuss the characteristics of transient erythroblastopenia of childhood.
- Name four types of congenital dyserythropoietic anemia.
- Describe the characteristics of congenital dyserythropoietic anemia.
- Explain the laboratory findings in congenital dyserythropoietic anemia.

Case studies

- Apply the laboratory data to the stated case studies and discuss the implications of these cases to the study of hematology.

APLASTIC ANEMIA

Aplastic anemia was first described by Paul Ehrlich in 1888 from an autopsy of a young pregnant woman. Aplastic anemia, an unusual hematologic disease, is either acquired or congenital in etiology. Aplastic anemia is one of a group of disorders, known as hypoproliferative disorders, that are characterized by reduced growth or production of blood cells. The other anemias in this category include those caused by deficiencies of erythropoietin (see Chapter 5), iron (see Chapter 10), and folic acid and vitamin B_{12} (see Chapter 11).

Etiology

Most cases of acquired aplastic anemia are the consequence of an immune-mediated destruction of hematopoiesis. Idiopathic aplastic anemia occurs in patients with no established history of chemical or drug exposure or viral infection. Other forms of aplastic anemia are iatrogenic and constitutional aplastic anemia. The term **constitutional aplastic anemia** designates a congenital or genetic predisposition to bone marrow

failure (see Diamond-Blackfan and Fanconi anemias later in this chapter).

Aplastic anemia are considered secondary to etiologic agents that are drug related (iatrogenic) and chemically related. Aplastic anemia is iatrogenic when the transient marrow failure follows cytotoxic chemotherapy or radiation therapy. Certain chemical or physical agents directly injure both proliferating and quiescent hematopoietic cells, leading to damage to DNA and ultimately to apoptosis. Drug-related and chemically related aplastic anemias account for 11% to 20% of all cases (Box 9.1). Ionizing radiation has been well documented as a cause of aplastic anemia. In addition, a variety of antigens—derived from chemicals, viruses, and perhaps altered self-antigens—have been inferred from clinical histories to initiate the immune process, but the precise nature of the antigenic stimulus has not been identified. Iatrogenic agents include

1. Benzene and benzene derivatives
2. Trinitrotoluene
3. Insecticides and weed killers

Etiologic Classification of Aplastic Anemia[a]

DIRECT TOXICITY
Iatrogenic causes
    Radiation
    Chemotherapy
Benzene
Intermediate metabolites of some common drugs

IMMUNE-MEDIATED CAUSES
Iatrogenic causes
    Transfusion-associated graft versus host disease
Eosinophilic fasciitis
Hepatitis-associated disease
Pregnancy
Intermediate metabolites of some common drugs
Idiopathic aplastic anemia

[a]Boldface type indicates relatively well-established mechanisms.

---

4. Inorganic arsenic
5. Antimetabolites (antifolate compounds and analogues of purines and pyrimidines)
6. Antibiotics

Benzene

Patients with community-acquired aplastic anemia rarely have a history of exposure to any substance that is toxic to the bone marrow, and even benzene is now infrequently associated with aplastic anemia in developed countries. However, exposure to burning oil wells in Kuwait during the Gulf War led to the development of aplastic anemia in at least one patient.

Burning gasoline aerosolizes many pollutants, one of which is benzene. Benzene can be metabolized in the liver to a series of phenolic and open-ring structures, including hydroquinones, which can inhibit the maturation and amplification of bone marrow stem and blast cells. In addition, the metabolites of benzene alter the function of stromal cells in the bone marrow so that they cannot adequately support the growth and differentiation of hematopoietic cells. The net result can be aplastic anemia, which does not typically develop until several years after exposure to benzene.

Drugs

Drugs have been associated with aplastic anemia. Unlike with anticancer agents and benzene, which, at sufficient doses, regularly result in marrow aplasia, idiosyncratic reactions to drugs are infrequent. The antibiotic chloramphenicol previously led the list of antibiotics that produced cases of aplastic anemia if not prescribed properly. Depending on the extent of damage, some cases of chemically induced aplastic anemia are reversible. Between 1988 and 1998, antibody-associated pure red cell aplasia was reported in three patients who had undergone treatment with recombinant human

erythropoietin (epoetin). Procedures for proper storage, handling, and administration of the drug reduced the incidence of aplastic anemia by more than 80%.

Other drugs that can produce aplastic anemia, depending on the dosage and duration of consumption, include tetracyclines, organic arsenicals, phenylbutazone, trimethadione, and methylphenylethylhydantoin.

Infections

Infections can also be responsible for acquired cases of aplastic anemia. Viral infections, particularly hepatitis B, hepatitis C, measles, Epstein-Barr virus, and cytomegalovirus, have been implicated. Type B19 human parvovirus (HPV) infects the erythroid replicating cells, causing aplastic crisis in patients with hemolytic anemia or in an immunocompromised host. The mechanism associated with the induction of aplastic anemia subsequent to viral infection includes the possibility of drug exposure during treatment, direct stem cell damage by the virus, depressed hematopoiesis by the viral genome, and virus-induced autoimmune damage. In addition, viral infections may be only secondary to bone marrow aplasia.

Hepatitis-associated aplastic anemia is a variant of aplastic anemia in which aplastic anemia follows an acute attack of hepatitis. Severe pancytopenia can occasionally occur 1 to 2 months after an episode of apparent viral hepatitis. The stereotypical syndrome of posthepatitis aplasia would seem to offer the opportunity to identify a specific infectious cause of aplastic anemia. In most patients, the hepatitis is non-A, non-B, non-C, and non-G. The hepatitis of the hepatitis-associated aplastic anemia does not appear to be caused by any of the known hepatitis viruses. Several features of the syndrome suggest that it is mediated by immunopathologic mechanisms. Although aplastic anemia is a rare sequela of hepatitis, there is a striking relationship between fulminant seronegative hepatitis and aplastic anemia.

Epidemiological studies suggest the involvement of an enteric microbial agent in the causation of aplastic anemia. Aplastic anemia not only is more common in the Far East (4% to 10% in the Far East compared with 2% to 5% of cases of aplastic anemia in the West), where hepatitis viruses are prevalent, but also is associated with poverty, rice farming, and past (but not recent) exposure to hepatitis A.

Hepatitis-associated aplastic anemia is often fatal if untreated. If a human leukocyte antigen (HLA)-matched related donor is not available for bone marrow transplantation, immunosuppressive treatment is given.

Pathophysiology

The pathophysiology is immune mediated in most cases, with activated type 1 cytotoxic T cells implicated. The molecular basis of the aberrant immune response and deficiencies in hematopoietic cells is now being defined genetically; examples are telomere repair gene mutations in the target cells and dysregulated T-cell activation pathways. Cellular immune suppression may occur transiently with certain viral infections such as parvovirus or as a result of drug action. Pure red cell aplasia is often associated with thymomas.

TABLE 9.1	**Phases of Aplastic Anemia**
Phase 1: Onset of Disease	After an initiating event (e.g., viral infection), the hematopoietic compartment is destroyed by the immune system.
	Small numbers of surviving stem cells support adequate hematopoiesis for some time, but eventually the circulating cell counts become very low and clinical symptoms appear.
Phase 2: Recovery	Either a partial response or a complete response can occur, at least initially, without increased numbers of stem cells.
	In a minority of patients, the primitive-cell compartment appears to repopulate over time by the process of self-renewal of stem cells.
Phase 3: Late Disease	Years after recovery, blood counts may fall as a relapse of pancytopenia occurs, or an abnormal clone of stem cells may emerge, leading to a new diagnosis of PNH, MDS, or AML.

Hematopoietic failure may occur at any level in the differentiation of bone marrow precursor cells. There may be insufficient or defective pluripotent stem cells (colony-forming unit, stem cells [CFU-S]) or committed stem cells (colony-forming unit, committed cells [CFU-C]). The microenvironment may be unable to provide for the normal development of hematopoietic cells. The appropriate humoral and cellular stimulators for hematopoiesis may be absent. In addition, bone marrow failure could result from excessive suppression of hematopoiesis by T lymphocytes or macrophages. Finally, stem cells could interact among themselves with one clone inhibiting the growth of another. In most cases of aplastic anemia, it is likely that damage to the hematopoietic stem cell by a known or unknown agent in some way alters the ability of the cell to proliferate or differentiate.

In most patients with acquired aplastic anemia, bone marrow failure results from immunologically mediated, tissue-specific organ destruction. The course of the disease can be separated into distinct phases (Table 9.1). The bone marrow is unlikely to recover spontaneously, and most patients die of infection or bleeding complications within a few years.

A model for the interaction between the immune system and hematopoietic cells in patients with aplastic anemia has been developed from laboratory observations (Fig. 9.1). An early experiment showed that mononuclear cells from the blood and marrow of patients with aplastic anemia suppressed hematopoietic colony formation by normal marrow

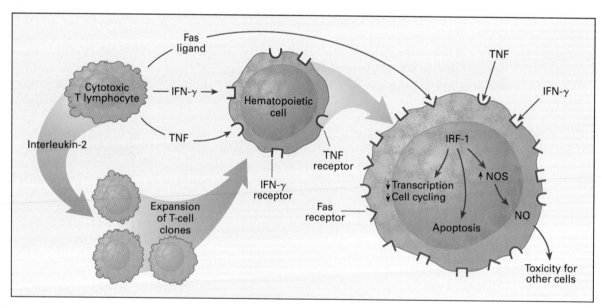

FIGURE 9.1   Immune destruction of blood cell production. Hematopoietic cell targets are affected by many factors. Activated cytotoxic T lymphocytes play a major role in tissue damage, partially through secreted cytokines such as IFN-γ and TNF. Increased production of interleukin-2 (IL-2) leads to polyclonal expansion of T cells. However, activation of the Fas receptor leads to apoptosis in target cells. Some effects of IFN-γ are mediated through interferon regulatory factor 1 (IRF-1), which inhibits the transcription of cellular genes and entry into the cell cycle. IFN-γ is a potent inducer of many cellular genes, including inducible nitric oxide synthase (NOS), and production of the toxic gas nitric oxide (NO) may further diffuse toxic effect. In addition, direct cell–cell interactions between lymphocytes and targets probably occur. (Adapted with permission from Young NS, Maciejewski J. The pathophysiology of acquired aplastic anemia, *N Engl J Med*, 336(19):1368, 1997.)

cells; the removal of T cells from patients' samples sometimes improved in vitro colony formation by the affected marrow. Blood and marrow from patients also contained increased numbers of activated cytotoxic lymphocytes, and the activity and numbers of these cells decreased with successful antithymocyte globulin (ATG) therapy. INF-α and TNF suppress the proliferation of early and late hematopoietic progenitor cells and stem cells. This suppression is greater when the INF-α and TNF are secreted into the marrow microenvironment than when they are added to cultured cells.

The immunological events that precede the destruction of hematopoietic cells are not as clear as the mechanism of suppression of proliferation (Fig. 9.2). Involvement of lymphocytes of the CD4 or helper class has been inferred from overrepresentation of the class II histocompatibility antigen HLA-DR2 in white patients, and a more specific haplotype has been linked to the disorder in Japanese patients. Nevertheless, both the dysregulatory events that lead to loss of tolerance and to autoimmune destruction of hematopoietic cells and the initial antigen exposure that triggers immune system activation are unknown.

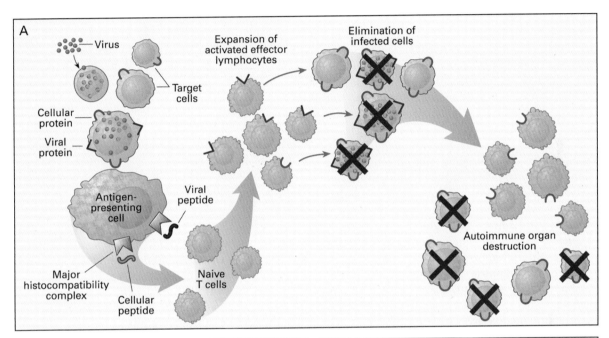

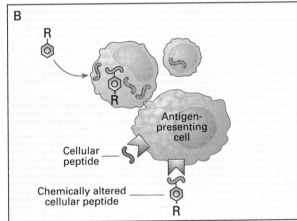

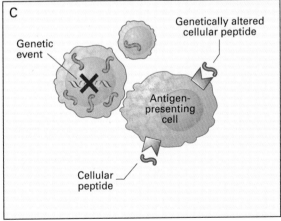

FIGURE 9.2 Destruction of bone marrow initiated by antigenic stimulation. **A:** Viral infection of hematopoietic cells with subsequent immune response results in the destruction of infected cells. This process is initiated with the production of viral proteins and the excessive or aberrant production of normal cellular proteins, which are released and are taken up by antigen-presenting cells. The proteins are processed into peptides in the antigen-presenting cells and then form complexes with major histocompatibility complex molecules that are then presented to naive T cells. Infected cells are subsequently destroyed. Rarely, the lymphocyte response persists and affects normal cells, resulting in autoimmune organ destruction. **B:** Drug-induced aplastic anemia may occur in a process similar to viral infection of hematopoietic cells after reactive drug metabolites, formed in marrow cells, bind to cellular proteins. This leads the immune system to recognize the complex as foreign, and the destructive sequence is initiated. **C:** A product of a chromosomal translocation or an oncogene may also initiate a T-cell response that expands to include nonmalignant cells, which leads to marrow hypocellularity in MDS by a sequence similar to viral and drug-induced processes. (Adapted with permission from Young NS, Maciejewski J. The pathophysiology of acquired aplastic anemia, *N Engl J Med*, 336(19):1369, 1997.)

Laboratory studies of patients' lymphocytes and their products support the concept of pathophysiological roles for lymphocytes and lymphokines in the destruction of hematopoietic cells. Alpha-INF expression is prevalent in acquired aplastic anemia and may be a specific marker of this disease. Local production of this inhibitory lymphokine in the target organ, the bone marrow, may be important in mediating aplastic anemia. Measurement of this lymphokine's message may be useful in distinguishing acquired aplastic anemia from other forms of bone marrow failure.

Clinical Features

Acquired aplastic anemia is characterized by total bone marrow failure with a reduction in circulating levels of red blood cells, white blood cells, and platelets. It is not a common disease. The clinical course may be acute and fulminating, with profound pancytopenia and a rapid progression to death, or the disorder may have an insidious onset and a chronic course. The signs and symptoms depend on the degree of the deficiencies and include bleeding from thrombocytopenia, infection from neutropenia, and signs and symptoms of anemia. Splenomegaly and lymphadenopathy are absent.

Recent studies have shown that long-term survivors of acquired aplastic anemia may be at high risk for subsequent malignant diseases or late clonal hematologic diseases, often years after successful immunosuppressive therapy. Paroxysmal nocturnal hemoglobinuria (PNH) occurs in approximately 9% of patients, and myelodysplasia (MDS) and acute myelogenous leukemia (AML) occur at a cumulative incidence rate of approximately 16% 10 years after treatment. The incidence of solid tumors is similarly increased after immunosuppression and after bone marrow transplantation. One hypothesis has postulated that aplastic anemia is primarily a preleukemic condition.

Laboratory Findings

Aplastic anemia is caused by damage or destruction of the hemopoietic tissue of the bone marrow that results in deficient production of blood cells (Fig. 9.3). If all the cell lines (erythrocytic, leukocytic, and thrombocytic) are affected, the disorder is referred to as **pancytopenia**. However, if only one cell line is involved, it is usually the erythrocytic cells.

A diagnosis of severe aplastic anemia is made when at least two of the three peripheral blood values fall below critical levels: granulocytes less than 0.5×10^9/L, platelets less than 20×10^9/L, or reticulocytes less than 1.0% in the presence of anemia. The bone marrow is either significantly or moderately hypocellular, with less than 30% of residual hematopoietic cells. Most severely affected patients have neutrophil counts less than 2.0×10^9/L, platelet counts less than 20×10^9/L, or reticulocyte counts less than 0.6%.

Red blood cells usually are normochromic and normocytic. In some cases, there may be varying degrees of anisocytosis and poikilocytosis or macrocytosis. The red cell distribution

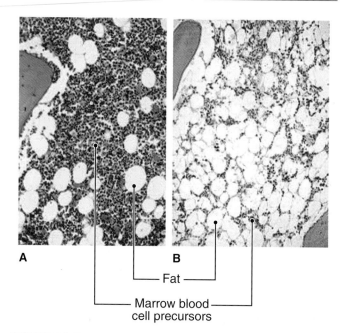

FIGURE 9.3 Bone marrow in aplastic anemia. **A:** Normal bone marrow. **B:** Bone marrow in aplastic anemia. Few bone marrow cells are present. Most of the tissue shown is fat. (Reprinted with permission from McConnell TH. *The Nature of Disease Pathology for the Health Professions*, Philadelphia, PA: Lippincott Williams & Wilkins, 2007.)

width (RDW) is normal in nontransfused patients. Leukopenia with a significant decrease in granulocytes and a relative lymphocytosis are noticeable. Thrombocytopenia is typically present. Serum iron usually is increased; this is a valuable early sign of erythroid hypoplasia and reflects the decreased plasma iron turnover. In addition, the erythrocyte use of iron is decreased. Both effective and total erythropoiesis are decreased in aplastic anemia.

The bone marrow reveals very few early erythroid and myeloid cells at any stage of differentiation, and megakaryocytes are scanty if present at all. Primitive progenitor and stem cells, which normally constitute approximately 1% of marrow cells, cannot be identified by their appearance.

If acute exposure to radiation is the inciting agent, the production of new red blood cells (reticulocyte count) falls, but the red blood cells decline slowly because of their long survival. Within the first few hours, there is a neutrophilic leukocytosis caused by a shift from the marginal and probably the marrow storage pools as well. A decrease in lymphocytes occurs after the 1st day and is responsible for early leukopenia. After approximately 5 days, granulocytes begin to decrease. The platelets decrease later. Platelets are often the last to return to normal in the recovery phase.

Treatment

Aplastic anemia responds to immunosuppressive therapy, but success in treating this disease appears to be related to the degree of organ destruction, the capacity for tissue regeneration, and, perhaps most importantly, a drug regimen that can control a misdirected and extraordinarily potent immune response.

Almost universally fatal just a few decades ago, aplastic anemia can now be cured or ameliorated by stem cell transplantation or immunosuppressive drug therapy. Treatment strategies depend on the age of the patient and the availability of an identical familial donor. Allogenic bone marrow transplantation is indicated in patients younger than 40 years of age, if a suitable donor is available. Bone marrow transplantation is recommended in younger patients who have an identical twin donor or an HLA-matched donor. Two-year survival rates are 60% to 70%, with 5% to 15% of patients not surviving the transplant procedure.

In the absence of a donor and in older patients, the treatment of choice is immunosuppression. Combined immunosuppressive therapy protocols including several treatment steps such as antilymphocyte globulin (ALG), cyclosporine-A (Cy-A), splenectomy, and lymphocytapheresis have been developed. Immunosuppression with ATGs and cyclosporine is effective at restoring blood-cell production in the majority of patients, but relapse and especially evolution of clonal hematologic diseases remain problematic.

CONGENITAL RED BLOOD CELL–RELATED DISORDERS

Many patients with inherited bone marrow failure syndromes (IBMFS) initially exhibit aplastic anemia. The IBMFS include:

■ Fanconi anemia,
■ congenital amegakaryocytic thrombocytopenia, and rarely,
■ Diamond-Blackfan anemia.

It is important to distinguish between IBMFS and acquired aplastic anemia. The prevalence of IBMFS is poorly defined and previously underestimated. Acquired aplastic anemia, MDS, or AML may present with the manifestation of an IBMFS.

Telomeres

Impaired erythrocyte production can be caused by a variety of factors. Recently, heterozygous mutations in TERC, telomerase RNA component, the gene for the RNA component of telomerase, have been found to cause short telomeres in congenital aplastic anemia and in some cases of apparently acquired hematopoietic failure. Mutations in TERT may be a risk factor for marrow failure.

In humans, telomere are hexameric repetetive DNA sequences (TTAGGG in the leading strand and CCCTAA in the lagging strand) capped by specific proteins at the extremities of linear chromosomes. Telomere shorten with every cell cycle, and telomere reduction has been suggested to be fundamental to normal senescence of cells, tissues

and organism. Telomeres cannot be fully duplicated during cell division. This insufficiency, the "end-replication problem" causes telomere shortening after every cell division. Telomeres are additionally shortened by post-replicative DNA processing or by direct damage. When critically short, telomeres signal cell proliferation arrest, senescence, and apoptosis by p53, p21, and PMS2. If a cell bypasses these inhibitory pathways and continues to proliferate, extremely short telomeres lose their function of chromosomal protection and promote chromosomal instability. To counter telomere shortening, highly proliferative cells, for example, stem cells and lymphocytes, express the enzyme, telomerase. Most mature cells do not express telomerase and cannot elongate their telomeres.

In stem and progenitor cells, telomerase expression is tightly regulated and these cells contain very low levels of telomerase. As a result of this low level of telomerase enzyme expression in adult stem and progenitor cells, telomeres eventually shorten with age. In peripheral blood leukocytes, telomeres are long at birth but display rapid erosion in the first two decades of life, continuing to shorten with age at a slower rates. Telomeres also are relatively shorter in lymphocytes than granulocytes.

Molecular mechanisms have evolved to maintain the length and protective function of telomeres. These mechanisms include:

■ telomerase (TERT), a reverse transcriptase enzyme, that uses an RNA molecule (TERC) as the template to elongate the 3′ ends of telomeres and
■ Shelterin, a collection of DNA-binding proteins, that cover and protect telomeres.

Mutations in genes that function to repair telomeres in hematopoietic tissue result in defects in telomere repair and protection. The hematologic disorders of aplastic anemia and AML are associated with inherited mutations in telomere repair or protection genes. Telomeres were first measured to be short in approximately one-third of patients with acquired aplastic anemia more than a decade ago. Patients with the shortest telomeres appear to be more likely to develop late malignant clonal complications. Granulocytes were subsequently found to be affected by telomere erosion in acquired marrow failure. Telomere shortening also is common in congenital aplastic anemias. Patients with Fanconi anemia have some degree of telomere attrition mainly in granulocytes.

Originally, telomere shortening was thought to be the result of a "stressed" hematopoietic stem cell, which overproliferates in response to marrow destruction. Mutation in a gene, DKC1, and similar genes was discovered. Mutations in the telomerase complex genes or in the telomere-protecting complex (shelterin) cause telomere erosion and disease.

Adequate telomere length maintenance is pivotal for hematopoiesis, and excessive telomere loss permeates the pathogenesis of bone marrow failure and malignancy. Short telomeres inhibit cell proliferation and predispose to chromosomal instability.

Techniques to measure telomeres include:

1. Southern blot analysis,
2. quantitative PCR (qPCR) and
3. flow-FISH (a combination of flow cytometry and fluorescence in situ hybridization).

The most accurate and reliable seems to be flow-FISH in which telomere lengths in different cell types can be distinguished.

Laboratory Findings in Bone Marrow Failure Syndromes

Hematology

Peripheral cytopenias range from absent to severe. Unexplained red cell macrocytosis, especially if a family history of marrow failure exists. In many cases, red cell macrocytosis is the only hematologic abnormality. Macrocytosis may be masked, if a concurrent iron deficiency or thalassemia trait is present. Elevated levels of hemoglobin F are common. Cells in the bone marrow may exhibit dysplastic changes, for example, micromegakaryocytes with only a single or double nuclei, pseudo-Pelger Huët anomalies, mild megaloblastic features with nuclear:cytoplasmic dyssynchrony or multinucleated erythroid precursors.

A minority of patients with aplastic anemia has heterozygous mutations in genes encoding the telomerase components TERT or TERC (5% to 10% of cases; mutation in shelterin components are rarely found). Patients with aplastic anemia carrying telomerase mutations have an increased risk of developing cancer, particularly AML. Telomerase mutation correlated with chromosomal abnormalities, especially trisomy 8 and inv(16).

Hypoproliferation of the erythroid elements, without corresponding decreases in other cell lines, is characteristic of pure red cell aplasia. Pure red cell aplasia exists in three forms but a number of variant and intermediate forms have been recognized. Examples of red cell aplasia are

■ Congenital—Diamond-Blackfan syndrome
■ Acquired chronic—idiopathic, associated with thymoma and lymphoma
■ Acute (transient)—parvovirus, other infections, drugs, riboflavin deficiency

Pure Red Cell Aplasia

This is a disorder primarily involving disturbed erythropoiesis. Immune suppression of erythropoiesis is believed to play a role in this form of red cell aplasia. An immune system etiology is supported by the fact that some patients respond to steroid treatment. Patients with pure red cell aplasia have antibodies against erythroid precursor cells and lymphocytes capable of inhibiting erythropoiesis.

Erythroid precursors are absent from the bone marrow, and evidence of hemolysis or hemorrhage is not present in red cell aplasia. The level of serum erythropoietin is usually increased. An aplastic crisis can develop in some patients with hemolytic anemia and concomitant infection. Other causes of acquired red cell aplasia include malnutrition and neoplasia. Thymoma (tumor of the thymus gland) is a frequent finding.

Acquired pure red cell aplasia characterized by selective failure of red blood cell production rarely occurs in middle-aged adults. Reticulocytopenia and a cellular marrow devoid of all but the most primitive erythroid precursors are characteristic. Leukocyte and platelet production are normal. Approximately half of reported cases have been associated with thymoma, usually a noninvasive spindle cell type. Only 5% to 10% of patients with thymoma have anemia. Remission of anemia occurs in approximately one fourth of cases after surgical removal of thymoma.

Chronic acquired red cell aplasia has been associated with other conditions, such as drugs, collagen vascular disorders, and lymphoproliferative disorders. Most of these anemias appear to be part of a spectrum of autoimmune cytopenias in which the target cells are either erythroid stem cells or normoblasts. Antibodies that react with these cells have been identified in some patients. Corticosteroids and immunosuppressive drugs have been used as therapy, but less than 50% of patients achieve satisfactory remission.

Diamond-Blackfan Anemia

Diamond-Blackfan anemia (DBA), first reported in 1936, is one of a heterogeneous group of disorders characterized by proapoptotic hematopoiesis, bone marrow failure, low stature, birth defects, and cancer predisposition known as the inherited bone marrow failure syndromes. DBA was later categorized by Diamond and Blackfan as a congenital hypoplastic anemia. In 2010, there were 595 patients registered in the Diamond-Blackfan Anemia Registry of North America. DBA is the preferred name for this disorder, but other names for DBA include

■ Blackfan-Diamond syndrome
■ Congenital pure red cell aplasia
■ Congenital hypoplastic anemia

Classically, DBA has been included within the inherited bone marrow failure syndromes and shares many aspects with other syndromes that may present erythroblastopenia (e.g., Fanconi anemia).

Pathophysiology

DBA was the first recognized inherited bone marrow failure syndrome (IBMFS) in which a ribosomal disorder was identified. Congenital mutations in the gene, RPS19,and other genes encoding ribosomal proteins causes Diamond-Blackfan anemia. The list of genes responsible for DBA (see Table 9.2) is rapidly growing. RPS19 was the first ribosomal gene implicated in human disease and is the most frequently mutated gene in DBA with a total of 77 mutations described. The majority ore whole gene deletions, translocations, or truncating mutation universally present in only a single allele.

TABLE 9.2	Genetic Tests for Inherited Bone Marrow Failure Syndromes	
Syndrome	Inheritance Pattern	Gene
Fanconi anemia	Autosomal recessive	FANCA, FANCC, FANCD1, FANCD2, FANCE, FANCF, FANCG, FANCI, FANCJ, FANCL, FANCM, FANCN
Fanconi anemia	X-linked recessive	FANCB
Diamond-Blackfan anemia	Autosomal dominant	RPS19, RPS17, RPS24, PRL35A, RPS5, RPL11, RPS7, RPL36, RPS15, RPS27A

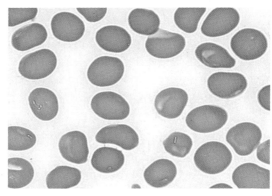

FIGURE 9.4 Congenital Pure Red Cell Aplasia (Diamond-Blackfan Anemia) Peripheral smear. Anemia resulting from marrow failure. Aplastic anemia is characterized by a bone marrow cellularity of less than 20% (**A**). The aplastic process is selective to the erythroid lineage in pure red cell aplasia (**B**). Both aplastic anemia and pure red cell aplasia may result from a parvovirus infection that produces characteristic changes in the bone marrow, including vacuolated erythroid precursors (**C**). (Armitage JO. *Atlas of Clinical Hematology*, Philadelphia, PA: Lippincott Williams & Wilkins, 225.) (Reprinted with permission from Anderson SC. *Anderson's Atlas of Hematology*. Wolters Kluwer Health/Lippincott Williams & Wilkins, 2003.)

To date, all DBA genes encode protein components of either the small 40S or large 60S ribosomal subunits which associated to form the translationally active 80S ribosome. In eukaryotic cells, assembly of rRNA and ribosomal proteins, along with associated proteins and small nucleolar RNAs, occurs in the nucleolus. This leads to the production of pre-60S and pre-40S preribosomal particles. These particles are exported to the cytoplasm where the final steps in assembly and maturation of ribosomes occur.

Mutations in genes encoding ribosomal proteins and the resulting defects in ribosome biogenesis or function appear to be capable of causing anemia and other hematologic abnormalities. The central hematopoietic defects in DBA are thought to be the hypoproliferation of erythroid cells and the enhanced sensitivity of hematopoietic progenitors to apoptosis. In addition, another potential mechanisms is that defective maturation of ribosomal subunits could delay translation of globin genes. This delay would result in a relative excess of free heme, which would also lead to erythroid-specific apoptosis and anemia.

Laboratory Manifestations

The majority of patients are diagnosed in the first year of life, with pallor and lethargy being the most common presenting symptoms. The classic diagnostic criteria for DBA (Fig. 9.4) are

- Anemia appearing prior to the 1st birthday
- Normal or slightly decreased neutrophil count
- Variable platelet counts, often increased
- Macrocytosis
- Normal bone marrow cellularity with few red cell precursors

It is now evident that nonclassical cases of DBA occur. In patients beyond 1 year old, those with mild or no ane-mia and consistent congenital anomalies may be suffering from DBA. DBA may be present more commonly than previously thought, but other causes of red cell failure are more common.

The disorder is characterized by a slowly progressive and refractory anemia, with no concurrent leukopenia or thrombocytopenia. The severe anemia is normochromic and slightly macrocytic; reticulocyte level is low; leukocytes are normal or slightly decreased; platelets are normal or increased; the marrow usually shows a reduction in all developing erythroid cells but normal granulocytic and megakaryocytic cell lines. In a small number of cases, residual erythroid precursors are detected. These precursors are mostly pronormoblasts.

Fetal hemoglobin is elevated (5% to 25%) and the fetal membrane "i" antigen is present. A notable characteristic of DBA is an elevated red blood cell adenosine deaminase level.

Treatment

Approximately 75% of patients respond at least partially to steroids. The overall long-term survival rate is approximately 65%, although many patients require long-term steroid treatment.

Fanconi Anemia

Fanconi anemia is the best described congenital form of aplastic anemia. There are at least 13 different Fanconi anemia subtypes. Although aplastic anemia is rare during childhood, Fanconi anemia occurs most frequently (accounting for approximately 25% to 30% of cases of childhood aplastic anemia).

Fanconi anemia is inherited through an autosomal recessive mode with the exception of the FA-B subtype which is

X-linked (see Table 9.2). The Fanconi genes have been localized to chromosomes 9q and 20q. Chromosomal analysis usually reveals frequent chromatid breaks, gaps, rearrangements, reduplications, and exchanges.

Fanconi anemia is twice as common in males as in females and can be confused with pure red cell aplasia and thrombocytopenia-absent radius syndrome.

Clinical Signs and Symptoms

Clinical signs and symptoms of Fanconi anemia commonly include low birth weight (<2,500 g), skin hyperpigmentation (café au lait spots), and short stature. Other manifestations can include skeletal disorders (aplasia or hypoplasia of the thumb), renal malformations, microcephaly, hypogonadism, mental retardation, and strabismus.

Laboratory Findings

Among patients with congenital malformations, only 28% are diagnosed before the onset of hematologic manifestations. Progressive pancytopenia (see Fig. 9.5) usually becomes apparent by 5 years of age. If moderate to severe pancytopenia is present, the hemoglobin concentration is between 5 and 6 g/dL at diagnosis. In addition, there is a predisposition to neoplasia and nonhematopoietic developmental anomalies. Susceptibility to an immune cytokine may be a marker of the genetic defect.

The current gold standard for diagnosing patients with Fanconi anemia is the demonstration of increased chromosomal breakage following exposure to clastogenes, for example, mitocytic C (MMC) and diepoxybutane (DEB). This response distinguishes Fanconi anemia from most of the other chromosomal breakage syndromes., both prenatally and postnatally. Prenatal HLA typing has made it possible to ascertain whether a fetus is HLA identical to an affected sibling.

Therapy

Traditional therapy includes bone marrow transplantation to ward off hemorrhage and infection as well as administration of steroids and androgens. Bone marrow transplantation has been the treatment of choice for patients with an HLA-identical unaffected sibling. Transplantation from other donors has produced poor results.

Cryopreserved umbilical cord blood transplantation from a sibling shown by prenatal testing to be unaffected by the disorder, to have a normal karyotype, and to be HLA identical to the patient is considered a viable alternative. Cord blood contains a high percentage of CD34$^+$ cells that are known as the stem cell marker by cluster designation (CD) terminology. Human hematopoietic stem cells are thought to reside in a small fraction (1% to 4%) of bone marrow cells. Stem cells that are as CD34$^+$/CD38$^-$ represent a more primitive cell that is capable of greater proliferation in culture. It is estimated that this primitive cell population accounts for 4% of the stem cell fraction in cord blood compared with only 1% in bone marrow. A pretransplantation conditioning procedure developed specifically for the treatment of such patients makes use of the hypersensitivity of abnormal cells to alkylating agents that cross-link DNA and to irradiation.

Another recent treatment strategy is the use of recombinant granulocyte colony-stimulating factor (CSF). This treatment has been successful in reducing neutropenia but is ineffective in stimulating erythrocyte or thrombocytic cell lines. Patients who respond to this treatment suffer from fewer and less severe infections.

Familial aplastic anemia is a subset of Fanconi anemia with a low incidence of congenital abnormalities. Some patients may have a relative with classic Fanconi anemia. The age of diagnosis varies from younger than 1 year to 77 years of age. A few children present with bleeding manifestations secondary to a thrombocytopenia. As their disease progresses, they develop pancytopenia and hypocellular bone marrow. Patients may have pancytopenia and hypocellular marrow without major developmental anomalies. In some cases, there may be skin hyperpigmentation or stunted growth.

Transient Erythroblastopenia of Childhood

The more common diagnosis for a child with pure red cell aplasia is acquired transient erythroblastopenia of childhood (TEC). TEC occurs in previously healthy children, usually younger than 8 years of age, with most cases occurring between the ages of 1 and 3 years. A history of a viral infection within the past 3 months is frequent. It is usually self-limited, with recovery occurring within 1 or 2 months without therapy. The pathogenesis appears to involve humoral inhibition of erythropoiesis or decreased stem cells in many of the patients who have been studied, but parvovirus is not a cause. Erythroid marrow recovery is usually 1 to 2 weeks after onset.

TEC is characterized by a moderate to severe normocytic anemia and severe reticulocytopenia. The bone marrow generally is normocellular and shows virtual absence of erythroid precursors, except for a few early forms.

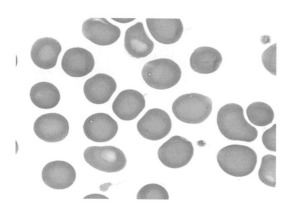

FIGURE 9.5 Fanconi Anemia Peripheral Smear. (Reprinted with permission from Anderson SC. *Anderson's Atlas of Hematology.* Wolters Kluwer Health/Lippincott Williams & Wilkins, 2003.)

Congenital Dyserythropoietic Anemia

Four types of congenital dyserythropoietic anemia (CDA) have been identified. They are characterized by indirect hyperbilirubinemia, ineffective erythropoiesis, and peculiarly shaped multinuclear erythroblasts. Type 1 CDA demonstrates a mildly macrocytic anemia with prominent anisocytosis and poikilocytosis. This form is apparent at birth and is not a threat to life. Type 2 (the most common type of CDA) CDA patients have a positive acidified serum test. Their erythrocytes are similar to those of patients with PNH because the red cells in both abnormalities are susceptible to hemolysis in acidified normal serum. However, type 2 CDA red cells differ from PNH red cells because they react strongly with both anti-i and anti-I. Type 3 CDA is similar to type 1 CDA because patients frequently demonstrate giant multinucleated erythroblasts. Megaloblastic changes are not prominent, and the red cells are not susceptible to lysis by acidified normal serum. A proposed type 4 classification exists. It is similar to type 2 but differs, in part, because of the lack of serological abnormalities.

Physiology

The pathogenesis of bone marrow failure is not entirely certain. One hypothesis states that a foreign agent, such as a drug or virus, may enter the body and attach itself to the pluripotent hemopoietic stem cells. This attachment may then provoke the body into defending itself against what is perceived as a foreign body. The patient's own body defense mechanism may destroy the stem cells. In addition, cellular and humoral abnormalities in hematopoietic regulation and an altered marrow microenvironment have been implicated as possible factors in aplastic anemia.

Laboratory Findings

If all cell lines are involved, the patient will have a decreased hemoglobin, hematocrit (Hct or packed cell volume), and red cell count with decreased leukocyte and platelet counts. If only the red cell line is affected, only the hemoglobin, Hct, and red cell count will be affected. If a bone marrow examination is performed, the erythroid cell line and perhaps the leukocyte and thrombocyte cell lines will all demonstrate a lack of maturational activity.

CHAPTER HIGHLIGHTS

Aplastic anemia is one of a group of disorders, known as hypoproliferative disorders, that are characterized by reduced growth or production of blood cells. The other anemias in this category include those caused by deficiencies of erythropoietin, iron, and folic acid and vitamin B_{12}.

The sudden appearance of aplastic anemia or pure red cell aplasia is often caused by an immune process, either antibodies directed against the stem cell or a cellular immune mechanism (T lymphocytes) that suppresses stem cell proliferation. Cellular immune suppression may occur transiently with certain viral infections such as parvovirus or as a result of drug action. Hematopoietic failure may occur at any level in the differentiation of bone marrow precursor cells. In most patients with acquired aplastic anemia, bone marrow failure results from immunologically mediated, tissue-specific organ destruction.

Aplastic anemia is characterized by total bone marrow failure with a reduction in circulating levels of red blood cells, white blood cells, and platelets. It is not a common disease. If all the cell lines (erythrocytic, leukocytic, and thrombocytic) are affected, the disorder is referred to as **pancytopenia**. If only one cell line is involved, it is usually the erythrocytic cells. A diagnosis of severe aplastic anemia is made when at least two of the three peripheral blood values fall below critical values: granulocytes less than 0.5×10^9/L, platelets less than 20×10^9/L, and reticulocytes less than 0.6%.

Aplastic anemia responds to immunosuppressive therapy and, in some cases, bone marrow transplantation..

Fanconi anemia is the best-described congenital form of aplastic anemia. Progressive pancytopenia usually becomes apparent by the age of 5 years. If moderate to severe pancytopenia is present, the hemoglobin concentration is between 5 and 6 g/dL at diagnosis. In addition, there is a predisposition to neoplasia and nonhematopoietic developmental anomalies, including acute leukemia, in patients with Fanconi anemia. Most patients die by their mid-to-late teens.

Related disorders include hypoproliferation of the erythroid elements, for example, pure red cell aplasia. Pure red cell aplasia exists in three forms. Intermediate forms include Diamond-Blackfan syndrome, acquired chronic, and acute transient forms. Pure red cell aplasia is a disorder primarily involving disturbed erythropoiesis.

CASE STUDIES

CASE 9.1

A 22-year-old white woman was admitted to the hospital because of severe menstrual bleeding. She had numerous petechiae and some purpura. The patient was a religious missionary who had recently returned from a 2-year assignment in Haiti. Six months ago, she developed a severe respiratory infection. She was treated by a local Haitian physician at that time but was not hospitalized because of the lack of medical facilities on the island. She had refused to return home for further treatment at that time.

Initially, she received a cephalosporin-type antibiotic but later received chloramphenicol because her symptoms persisted. At the time of admission, she showed no evidence of a respiratory disorder. However, she had recently

(continued)

discontinued the chloramphenicol that she had taken continuously for 5 months.

On admission, the following tests were ordered: CBC, platelet count, cold agglutinin antibody screen, urinalysis, and chest radiograph.

■ **Laboratory Data**

The results of the tests were as follows:

Hemoglobin 5.5 g/dL
Hct 18%
RBC 1.85×10^{12}/L

The RBC indices were as follows:

MCV 97.2 fL
MCH 29.7 pg
MCHC 31 g/dL

Her WBC count was 2.1×10^9/L. On the peripheral blood smear, the RBCs had a normochromic, normocytic appearance. Platelets were severely diminished on the blood film. Her platelet count was 6.5×10^9/L. The result of the screening test for cold agglutinins was negative. Urinalysis results were normal.

Thirty-six hours after admission the patient died of a massive cerebral hemorrhage. Tests performed on specimens obtained at autopsy revealed that the patient's bone marrow showed an almost total absence of hematopoiesis. A blood culture was positive for the Gram-negative rod *Proteus vulgaris*.

QUESTIONS

1. What is the most likely cause of this patient's pancytopenia?
2. How do certain drugs affect the body's cellular elements?
3. What caused the patient's death?

DISCUSSION

1. This patient's reduced erythrocytes, leukocytes, and thrombocytes (pancytopenia) had probably been induced by the drug chloramphenicol. Certain drugs depress bone marrow activity at a critical dosage level. Chloramphenicol is most notorious for its depression of hematopoiesis. The patient's prolonged use of this drug with its known high tissue toxicity index undoubtedly produced this bone marrow failure.
2. Various types of antibiotics function in different ways in the human body. Penicillin, for example, inhibits the cell wall synthesis of peptidoglycans, which constitute the major cell wall chemical in Gram-positive microorganisms. Many antibiotics interfere with protein synthesis. In the case of chloramphenicol, the specific in vivo action is unclear. However, in vitro studies have demon-

strated that chloramphenicol inhibits protein synthesis and mitochondrial synthetic activity.
3. This patient died of bacteremia (septicemia) caused by the Gram-negative microorganism *P. vulgaris*. Because the patient's body defenses had been severely compromised because of the effects of chloramphenicol, she was unable to effectively ward off a massive bacterial infection.

DIAGNOSIS: **Drug-induced Aplastic Anemia**

CASE 9.2

A 6-year-old African boy who had recently immigrated to the United States from Liberia was taken to the emergency department because of a high fever. Physical examination showed bilateral syndactyly and contractures of the fingers. His temperature was 100°F. A CBC was ordered.

LABORATORY DATA

RBC 2.1×10^{12}/L
Hematocrit 18%
Hemoglobin 6.0 g/dL
WBC 1.31×10^9/L
Platelets 45×10^9/L

QUESTIONS

1. What do the laboratory results suggest?
2. Is the boy's physical appearance suggestive of a hematologic abnormality?
3. What is the cause of Fanconi anemia?
4. What innovative treatments are available to patients with Fanconi anemia?

DISCUSSION

1. Decreased red blood cells, white blood cells, and platelets are indicative of a deficiency of all bone marrow elements. This condition is called pancytopenia.
2. Yes. The developmental defects of thumb and radius are suggestive of Fanconi anemia. The childhood onset of pancytopenic anemia further supports the diagnosis.
3. Fanconi anemia is a rare autosomal recessive genetic disorder. Fanconi anemia is one of the well-known chromosome instability syndromes. Hypersensitivity to alkylating or DNA cross-linking agents (e.g., mitomycin C) is used as a standard laboratory assay to confirm the diagnosis.
4. Most patients with Fanconi anemia have a short life expectancy. Recently, a child with Fanconi anemia made news by being the recipient of an umbilical cord blood stem cell transplant from her genetically screened and selected newborn brother.

DIAGNOSIS: **Fanconi Anemia**

REVIEW QUESTIONS

1. Acquired aplastic anemia may be caused by
   A. benzene or benzene derivatives
   B. ionizing radiation and vitamin B_{12}
   C. purine or pyrimidine analogues
   D. all of the above

2. The sudden appearance of aplastic anemia or pure red cell aplasia is often caused by
   A. a hemolytic process
   B. an immune process
   C. acute leukemias
   D. chronic leukemias

3. Aplastic anemia can occur years before a diagnosis of _____ is made.
   A. paroxysmal nocturnal hemoglobinuria
   B. myelodysplasia
   C. acute myelogenous leukemia
   D. all of the above

4. If a patient with aplastic anemia is referred to as exhibiting pancytopenia, which cell lines are affected?
   A. Erythrocytes
   B. Leukocytes
   C. Thrombocytes
   D. All of the above

Questions 5 to 8: Match the following. (Use an answer only once)

5. _____ Fanconi anemia
6. _____ Familial aplastic anemia
7. _____ Pure red cell anemia
8. _____ Diamond-Blackfan syndrome
   A. A subset of Fanconi anemia
   B. A rare congenital form of red cell aplasia
   C. Is characterized by selective failure of red blood cell production
   D. The best-described congenital form of aplastic anemia

9. Hematopoietic cell targets in aplastic anemia are affected by
   A. activated cytotoxic T lymphocytes
   B. activation of the Fas receptor
   C. direct cell–cell interactions between lymphocytes and target cells
   D. all of the above

10. Fanconi anemia is associated with abnormal genes located on chromosomes __q___, __q___.
   A. 9, 20
   B. 5, 22
   C. 9, 12
   D. 8, 23

BIBLIOGRAPHY

Ayari AS, et al. Prevalence, severity and outcome of 20 children and adolescents with Fanconi anemia, *J Hematol*, 4(Suppl 2):48, 2003.

Bennett CL, et al. Pure red cell aplasia and epoetin therapy. *NEJM*, 351(14):1403–1408, 2004.

Calado RT. Telomeres and marrow failure. *Am Soc Hematol, Educational program*, Vol. 1, Annual issue, 338–342, 2009.

Choesmel V, et al. Impaired ribosome biogenesis in Diamond-Blackfan anemia, *Blood*, 109(3):1275–1292, 2007.

D'Andrea AD. Susceptibility pathways in Fanconi's anemia and breast cancer, *NEJM*, 362(20):1909–1919, 2010.

Dianzani I, Loreni F. Daimond-Blackfan anemia: a ribosomal puzzle, *Haematologica*, 93(11):1601–1604, 2008.

Gan SS, et al. Mycophenolate mofetil and aplastic anemia, *J Hematol*, 4(Suppl 2):47, 2003.

Keohane EM. Acquired aplastic anemia. *Cl Lab Sci*, 17(3):165–170, 2004.

Lipton JM. Diamond-Blackfan anemia: novel mechansims-ribosomes and the erythrron. *Blood*, 109(3):850, 2007.

Mikhailova EA, et al. Program of combined immunosuppressive therapy, *J Hematol*, 4(Suppl 2):46, 2003.

Miniero R, et al. Treatment of severe aplastic anemia (SAA) with mycophenolate mofetil: a case report, *J Hematol*, 4(Suppl 2):47, 2003.

Montanaro M, et al. Pure red cell aplasia, thrombotic thrombocytopenic purpura and rapidly fulminating myocarditis in a patient presenting acute B19 human parvovirus infection: a case report, *J Hematol*, 4(Suppl 2):47, 2003.

Narla A, Ebert BL. Ribosomopathies: human disorders of ribosome function, *Blood*, 115(16):3196–3205, 2010.

Petrov L, et al. Immunosuppressive therapy in severe and very severe aplastic anemia, *J Hematol*, 4(Suppl 2):45–46, 2003.

Ray MA, et al. Enhanced alternative splicing of the FLVCR1 gene in Diamond Blackfan anemia disrupts FLVCR1 expression and function that are critical for enythropoiesis. *Haematologica*, 93(11):1617–1626, 2008.

Seiwerth RS, et al. Transplantation of CD 34-enriched peripheral blood stem cells from a haploidentical donor in a patient with severe anemia, *J Hematol*, 4(Suppl 2):47, 2003.

Shimamura A. Clinical approach to marrow failure. *Am Soc Hematol, Educational program*, Vol. 1, Annual issue, 329–336, 2009.

Stern MA, Eckman J, Offermann MK. Aplastic anemia after exposure to burning oil, *N Engl J Med*, 331(1):58, 1994.

Tulpule A, et al. Knockdown of Fanconi anemia genes in human embryonic stem cells reveals early developmental defects in the hematopoietic lineage, *Blood*, 115(17):3453–3462, 2010.

Yamaguchi H, et al. Mutations in TERT, the Gene for Telomerase Reverse Transcriptase in Aplastic Anemia, *NEJM*, 352(14):1413–1424, 2005.

Young NS, Maciejewski J. The pathophysiology of acquired aplastic anemia, *N Engl J Med*, 336(19):1365–1372, 1997.

10

Iron Deficiency Anemia and Anemia of Chronic Inflammation

Iron deficiency anemia

- Name conditions that can contribute to iron deficiency anemia (IDA).
- Name three of the most common groups vulnerable to IDA.
- Describe the physiology of iron metabolism, including the iron needs of children and normal dietary sources.
- Characterize the signs and symptoms of IDA.
- Explain the value of soluble transferrin receptors.

Anemia of inflammation or anemia of chronic disorders

- Describe the etiological basis of anemia of chronic inflammation or chronic disorders.

- Explain the cause of anemia of chronic inflammation or anemia of chronic disorders.
- Discuss the laboratory characteristics of anemia of chronic inflammation or chronic disorders.

Case studies

- Apply knowledge of etiology, pathophysiology, and laboratory findings to case studies of IDA and anemia of chronic inflammation or anemia of chronic diseases.

SCOPE OF THE PROBLEM

A common false assumption is that IDA due to inadequate nutrition is confined to developing or underdeveloped countries. It is not. Worldwide, more than 40% of children have an IDA that is frequently associated with infections. Cellular immune insufficiency occurs during iron deficiency because of a reduction in the proliferative capacity of T lymphocytes in infants with IDA. Challenged immunity resulting from the IDA and impaired development have significant public health implications.

Older, anemic adults are more likely to experience physical decline and disability and to have higher rates of hospitalization than those without anemia. Even adults with mild anemia have an increased risk of functional impairment and morbidity and mortality. About one third of all cases of anemia in the elderly are related to blood loss, nutritional deficiencies of folate or vitamin B_{12}, or a combination of both. Another one third of cases are due to chronic kidney disease, chronic inflammation, or both, and the final one third of cases are unexplained.

IRON DEFICIENCY ANEMIA

Iron is an essential element in the synthesis of hemoglobin. Iron deficiency is a common form of anemia. Although iron deficiency is a well-defined category of anemia, confusing this type of anemia with other forms of anemia does occur. Diagnosing and treating an iron-deficient patient correctly are especially important in high-risk populations. The failure to do so can produce a significant public health problem.

Early Diagnosis

Early diagnosis of iron deficiency is essential in nonanemic infants and toddlers (under 2 years of age). Prevention of cognitive and psychomotor skills decline in young children relies on detection of iron deficiency before full manifestation of anemia is present in the circulating blood. In addition, a correct diagnosis is essential for proper treatment. Confusing iron deficiency with other forms of anemia impacts proper treatment. Early diagnosis of iron deficiency is equally important in pregnant women to reduce maternal-fetal morbidity.

Etiology

Although an individual's need for dietary iron is small and will only manifest itself after iron storage sites in the body have been depleted, IDA is one of the most frequently encountered types of anemias. Four pathophysiological categories can contribute to the development of IDA (see Fig. 10.1).

IDA may result from various categories with multiple conditions in each category (Box 10.1). The major categories that result in IDA are

1. Decreased iron intake. A deficiency of this type results when not enough iron is consumed to meet the normal, daily required amount of iron (e.g., fad diets and an imbalanced vegetarian diet).
2. Increased iron utilization. An increased demand for iron that is not met, such as during pregnancy, the growth years, or periods of increased blood regeneration.

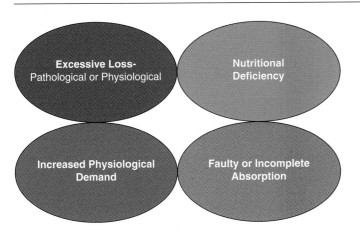

FIGURE 10.1 Factors in iron deficiency.

3. Excessive loss of iron (physiological or pathological iron deficiency). An excessive loss of iron can result from acute or chronic hemorrhage or heavy menstruation.
4. Faulty or incomplete iron absorption (physiological iron deficiency). Conditions of faulty or incomplete iron absorption can be caused by achlorhydria in certain disorders or following gastric resection; or chronic diarrhea. If a gastroenterologic evaluation fails to disclose a likely cause of IDA, or in patients refractory to oral iron treatment, screening for celiac disease, autoimmune gastritis, and *Helicobacter pylori* is recommended. Twenty to twenty-seven percent of patients with unexplained IDA

BOX 10.1

Examples of Causes of Iron Deficiency Anemia

DECREASED IRON INTAKE
Iron deficient diets

INCREASED IRON UTILIZATION
Postnatal growth spurt
Adolescent growth spurt

IRON LOSS (PHYSIOLOGICAL)
Menstruation
Pregnancy

FAULTY OR INCOMPLETE IRON ABSORPTION
Autoimmune gastritis
Celiac disease
H. pylori infection

IRON LOSS (PATHOLOGICAL)
GI bleeding
Urogenital bleeding
Pulmonary hemosiderosis
Intravascular hemolysis
Malignancy (e.g., colon cancer)

---

have autoimmune gastritis, 50% have evidence of active *H. pylori* infection, and 4% to 6% have celiac disease.
5. Pathological iron loss in adult males and postmenopausal females with iron deficiency. An evaluation of abnormal occult bleeding, especially gastrointestinal (GI) bleeding, is needed.

Iron deficiency may result from several other less commonly occurring conditions including a disorder of iron utilization, sideroblastic anemia; selected hemoglobinopathies; anemia related to chronic disorders; chronic inflammation; parasitic infections such as hookworm; and a deficiency of the plasma iron transporting protein, transferrin.

Epidemiology

Although a high prevalence of iron deficiency existed in the 1960s in the American population, intensified efforts to combat iron deficiency in this country appear to have successfully reduced anemia in some vulnerable age subgroups, such as infants. In the most recent survey in the United States, iron deficiency continues to be common in toddlers, adolescent girls, and women of childbearing age (Table 10.1). In adults, the prevalence of anemia rises rapidly after age 50. The Third National Health and Nutrition Examination Survey (NHANES III)

TABLE 10.1 Prevalence of Iron Deficiency (1999–2000)

Gender and Age	Iron Deficiency (%)
Both sexes	
1–2	7
3–5	5
6–11	4
Females[a]	
12–15	9
16–19	16
20–49	12
White, non-Hispanic	10
Black, non-Hispanic	19
Mexican American	22
50–69	9
70 and older	6
Males	
12–15	5
16–69	2
70 and older	3

[a]Nonpregnant only. (Adapted from Centers for Disease Control and Prevention; Iron Deficiency—United States, 1999–2000, *MMWR*, 51(40):897–899, 2002.)

statistics reveal that roughly 11% of adults 65 years and older, and more than 20% of those 85 and older, are anemic.

Various racial and ethnic groups exhibit lower average hemoglobin levels. Up to 30% of African Americans carry the deletion in the alpha thalassemia gene. In the heterozygous state, that is, silent carrier, a low normal or slightly decreased hemoglobin level and mean corpuscular volume (MCV) can be observed. Patients who are homozygotes, that is, alpha thalassemia trait, typically exhibit a slight microcytic anemia. Even when factors such as alpha thalassemia gene deletion, iron deficiency, sickle cell trait, and renal insufficiency were removed from an observed group, African Americans still had significantly lower hemoglobin levels compared to a corresponding white population. Further studies are needed to describe average hemoglobin levels based on precise race, ethnicity, and age.

Physiology

Humans have 35 to 50 mg of iron per kilogram of body weight. The average adult has 3.5 to 5.0 g of total iron. Normal iron loss is very small, amounting to less than 1 mg/day. Iron is lost from the body through exfoliation of intestinal epithelial and skin cells, the bile, and urinary excretion. To compensate for this loss, the adult male has a replacement iron need of 1 mg/day. However, additional iron is needed during the growth years, pregnancy, and lactation. Some women require supplementary iron because of heavy menstrual blood loss.

Operational iron consists of iron used for oxygen binding and biochemical reactions. In humans, most operational iron is found in the heme portion of hemoglobin or myoglobin. Most operational iron is incorporated into the hemoglobin molecules of erythrocytes and is recycled. In normal adults, hemoglobin contains two thirds of the iron present in the body.

Iron Needs in Infants and Children

In the normal infant at term, iron stores are adequate to maintain iron sufficiency for approximately 4 months of postnatal growth. In the premature infant, total body iron is lower than in the full-term newborn, although the proportion of iron to body weight is similar. Premature infants have a faster rate of postnatal growth than infants born at term, so unless the diet is supplemented with iron, they become iron depleted more rapidly than full-term infants. Iron deficiency can develop by 2 to 3 months of age in premature infants. Iron intake must supplement the approximately 75 mg of iron per kilogram of body weight that is present at birth. Iron losses from the body are small and relatively constant except during episodes of diarrhea or during the feeding of whole cow's milk, when iron losses may be increased. Approximately two thirds of iron losses in infancy occur when cells are extruded from the intestinal mucosa and the remainder when cells are shed from the skin and urinary tract. In the normal infant, these losses average approximately 20 μg/kg/day. Infants aged 7 to 12 months need 11 mg of iron a day. Babies younger than 1 year should be given iron-fortified cereal in addition to breast milk or an infant formula supplemented with iron.

Breast milk and cow's milk both contain about 0.5 to 1.0 mg of iron per liter, but its bioavailability differs significantly. The absorption of iron from breast milk is uniquely high, about 50% on average, and tends to compensate for its low concentration. In contrast, only about 10% of iron in whole cow's milk is absorbed. About 4% of iron is absorbed from iron-fortified cow's milk formulas that contain 12 mg of iron per liter. Reasons for high bioavailability of iron in breast milk are unknown.

Dietary Iron

There are two broad types of dietary iron. Approximately 90% of iron from food is in the form of iron salts and is referred to as nonheme iron. The extent to which this type of iron is absorbed is highly variable and depends both on the person's iron status and on the other components of the diet. The other 10% of dietary iron is in the form of heme iron, which is derived primarily from the hemoglobin and myoglobin of meat. Heme iron is well absorbed, and its absorption is less strongly influenced by the person's iron stores or the other constituents of the diet. There is little meat in the diet of most infants; therefore, most of their dietary iron is nonheme, and their intake is highly influenced by other dietary factors. Ascorbic acid enhances the absorption of nonheme iron, as do meat, fish, and poultry. Inhibitors of absorption include bran, polyphenols, oxalates, phytates, vegetable fiber, the tannin in tea, and phosphates. Heme iron itself promotes the absorption of nonheme iron. For example, adults absorb approximately four times as much nonheme iron from a mixed meal when the principal protein source is meat, fish, or chicken than when it is milk, cheese, other dairy products, or eggs. The beverage is also important. Orange juice doubles the absorption of nonheme iron from the entire meal, whereas tea decreases it by 75%.

Following the oral intake of iron (Fig. 10.2) in the ferric (Fe^{3+}) state, stomach secretions reduce the iron to the ferrous (Fe^{2+}) state. These stomach secretions, referred to as reducing agents, include glutathione, ascorbic acid, and sulfhydryl groups of proteins and digestion products. Gastric juice plays an important but poorly understood role in promoting absorption. The low pH of gastric juice makes iron available from hemoglobin-containing meat in the diet and other sources. However, very little iron is absorbed by the stomach.

Most of the iron passes from the stomach to the duodenum and upper jejunum, where it can be absorbed readily. Absorption by the GI epithelial cells is finely tuned to admit just enough iron to cover losses, without permitting either excess or deficiency of body iron to develop. Absorption normally admits approximately 5% to 10% of a total dietary intake of 10 to 20 mg/day.

Most absorbed iron becomes attached to the plasma protein transferrin, which is formed in the liver. Transferrin, a beta globulin, is a glycoprotein. Transferrin chelates iron within the intestinal lumen and shuttles it into the mucosal cells of the small intestine.

The internal iron transport of most mammals consists of transferrin transport of iron between donating tissues and

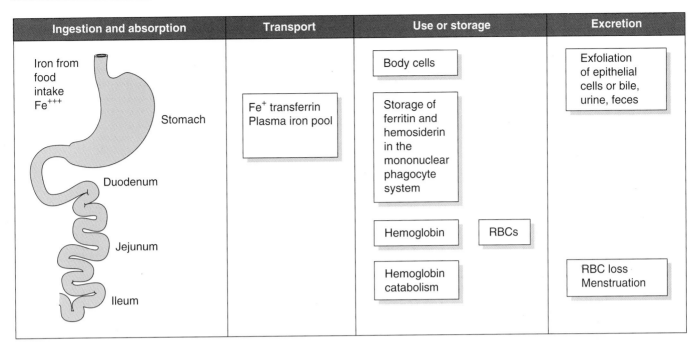

Ingestion and absorption	Transport	Use or storage	Excretion

FIGURE 10.2 Iron physiology.

transmembrane transferrin receptors, designed to procure iron for the cell. The cellular uptake of iron begins with the binding of the transferrin-iron complex to a specific receptor. Under normal circumstances, the iron required for cellular metabolism is acquired via transferrin receptors. Cells of different organ systems show considerable differences in the concentration of cellular transferrin receptors, the highest concentrations being found in cells of organs with the highest requirements, such as the hemoglobin synthesizing erythroid bone marrow cells and placental trophoblasts. The concentration of cell surface transferrin receptors is carefully regulated by transferrin receptor mRNA according to the internal iron content of the cell and its individual iron requirements. Iron-deficient cells contain increased numbers of receptors, whereas receptor numbers are downregulated in iron-replete cells.

Circulating transferrin receptor concentrations do not differ between healthy males and females, although concentrations are slightly higher in blacks than in nonblacks. Concentrations vary in populations living at different altitudes, with higher concentrations occurring at higher altitudes.

Circulating transferrin receptor concentrations increase in tissue iron deficiency, reflecting the degree of iron deficiency in the erythroid precursors of the marrow. When iron stores decline, serum ferritin concentrations drop until iron stores are depleted, at which time the ferritin concentration falls below the lower limit of the reference interval. With further iron loss, and as iron-deficient erythropoiesis begins, circulating transferrin receptor concentrations begin to increase and continue to do so as the severity of iron-deficient erythropoiesis increases, reflecting the increasing number of receptors on the erythroid cells of the bone marrow. The ratio of transferrin receptor to ferritin displays an inverse linear relationship to iron status, covering the spectrum from usual iron stores in health to substantial functional iron deficiency. The measurement of transferrin receptors is especially valuable in physiological conditions in which iron stores are depleted, making it difficult to clearly distinguish iron-deficient erythropoiesis from depleted iron stores. Such situations are commonly encountered in childhood and adolescence and during pregnancy, when iron stores are uniformly low to absent but iron-deficient erythropoiesis is not necessarily present.

Intracellular migration of transferrin-iron complexes produces an invagination of the cell membrane that results in a vacuole. Iron is subsequently released, and the transferrin is returned to the plasma to resume iron transport once again.

Any remaining iron is retained in the cells, where it combines with the protein apoferritin to form ferritin. Storage iron is the second largest iron compartment in the body. Most storage iron is found in hepatocytes and macrophages, where it is sequestered in ferritin. If the amount of apoferritin is insufficient, the remaining iron will be deposited and stored in tissues as hemosiderin. Iron is taken from these storage deposits and transported back to erythroid precursors by transferrin.

The first line of iron supply is the mononuclear phagocyte system. In iron deficiency, any increase in iron supply must come from the GI tract, because body tissues are already depleted of storage iron. At the time that iron has been depleted from these iron stores, an iron deficiency will manifest itself.

Pathophysiology

An IDA does not develop rapidly in most cases. Three sequential phases evolve until the manifestation of clinical signs and symptoms become apparent. Each phase is associated with specific characteristics (see Table 10.2). The phases are

TABLE 10.2 Sequential Phases of Iron Deficiency[a]			
	Stage 1 (Prelatent) Decrease in Storage Iron	Stage 2 (Latent) Decrease in Iron Available for Erythropoiesis	Stage 3 (Anemia) Decrease in Circulating Red Blood Cell Parameters and Decrease in Oxygen Delivery to Peripheral Tissues
Bone marrow iron stores	Decreased	Absent	Absent
Serum ferritin level	Decreased	<12 µg/L	<12 µg/L
Transferrin saturation	Normal	<16%	<16%
Free erythrocyte protoporphyrin, zinc protoporphyrin	Normal	Increased	Increased
Serum transferrin receptor	Normal	Increased	Increased
Reticulocyte hemoglobin content	Normal	Decreased	Decreased
Hemoglobin	Normal	Normal	Decreased
MCV	Normal	Normal	Decreased
Clinical signs and symptoms			Present

[a]The changes in laboratory measurements are progressive.
MCV, mean corpuscular volume.
Source: Greer JP, et al. *Wintrobe's Clinical Hematology*, 11th ed. (Table 28.2 Stages in the Development of Iron Deficiency), 2004:989.

■ Stage 1: Prelatent—decrease in storage iron
■ Stage 2: Latent—decrease in iron available for erythropoiesis
■ Stage 3: Anemia—decrease in circulating red blood cell parameters and decrease in oxygen delivery to peripheral tissues

Clinical Signs and Symptoms

The history and physical presentation are the typical initial observations in the diagnostic workup of a patient with symptoms of paleness, fatigue, and/or weakness.

Papilledema may be caused by IDA. The mechanism may be related to abnormal hemodynamics, as in other states of increased blood flow to the brain. Anemia may lead to reversible bulging of the fontanelles in infants with iron deficiency rather than papilledema. Patients with IDA and headache should undergo a careful examination of the optic fundi to rule out papilledema because this can lead to visual loss if left untreated.

IDA in children is associated with psychomotor and mental impairment in the first 2 years of life. Currently, more than one third of children in the United States demonstrate evidence of iron insufficiency, 7% have iron deficiency without anemia, and 10% have IDA.

Pica, the compulsive ingestion of nonnutritive substances (e.g., ice, wooden toothpicks, chalk, or dirt) has a well-documented association with iron deficiency. It may be a habit that induces iron deficiency by replacing dietary iron sources or inhibiting the absorption or iron. However, considerable evidence suggests that iron deficiency is usually the primary event and pica a consequence. Pica may occur in as many as half of iron-deficient patients.

Laboratory Characteristics

Hematology Studies

The first step in laboratory evaluation is a complete blood count including observation of the peripheral blood smear and a platelet count. The red blood cell parameters of hemoglobin, microhematocrit and red blood cell count, are the cornerstones for calculation of the red blood cell indices (MCV, mean corpuscular hemoglobin [MCH], and mean corpuscular hemoglobin concentration [MCHC]). The platelet count and white blood cell count should be noted. The MCV can separate macrocytic, normocytic, and microcytic red blood cell presentations. When searching for an IDA, normochromic, normocytic as well as microcytic, and hypochromic presentations can be encountered. Approximately, one third of patients with iron deficiency will present with normal red blood cell morphology because they are in an early phase of iron depletion. Another evaluation of mature erythrocyte indices as a new marker of iron status is the percentage of hypochromic red blood cells (% HYPO). This marker has been demonstrated to be the most sensitive and specific parameter of functional iron deficiency.

A reticulocyte count is additionally helpful. A reticulocyte count equal to or greater than 2.5% demonstrates increased erythropoiesis. Common categories of disorders associated with anemia in the presence of erythropoiesis are acute bleeding (after at least 24 hours), hemoglobinopathies, or hemolytic anemias.

In the presence of a reticulocyte count less than 2.5%, the red blood cell indices can form the algorithmic basis for separating anemias into categories. Reticulocyte hemoglobin content (CHr) is an effective early indicator of iron deficiency. This early alert is particularly important in infants and toddlers, who can suffer cognitive and psychomotor developmental problems as a result of inadequate iron in the synthesis of hemoglobin.

Measurement of hemoglobin content in reticulocytes is available on the Sysmex XE2100 (Ret He and RBC He) and the Bayer ADVIA 2120 (CHr and CH) analyzers. With a Ret He cutoff level of 27.2 pg, iron deficiency can be diagnosed with a sensitivity of 93.3% and a specificity of 83.2%. These assays are considered to be a reliable marker of cellular hemoglobin content and can be used to identify the existence of iron deficiency states early in erythrocyte hemoglobinization.

A typical IDA (Fig. 10.3) profile includes a decreased hemoglobin and hematocrit (perhaps a normal erythrocyte count). The red cell indices demonstrate a decreased MCV, MCH, and MCHC. Although this anemia may initially be normochromic or normocytic, or may only have some anisocytosis and hypochromia, a full manifestation of the anemia will exhibit both the hypochromic and the microcytic red cell patterns (Table 10.3; Fig. 10.4).

Other hematological findings related to the anemia include the following: platelets are usually normal but may be increased following acute blood loss; the leukocyte count is usually normal; the reticulocyte count is decreased or normal. A bone marrow examination reveals a marked decrease in stainable iron and erythroid hyperplasia.

Clinical Chemistry Studies

Iron studies (Table 10.4) are used to establish a differential diagnosis of microcytic, hypochromic anemia. These studies are of value at this stage of investigation because a microcytic, hypochromic red blood cell appearance can be associated with not only iron deficiency but thalassemias or sideroblastic anemias as well. Interpretation of the assays is dependent on the stage of iron deficiency in an IDA patient.

Iron-Deficient Pronormoblast (Iron-Deficient Rubriblast)

Iron-Deficient Basophilic Normoblast (Iron-Deficient Prorubricyte)

Iron-Deficient Polychromatophilic Normoblast (Iron-Deficient Rubricyte)

Iron-Deficient Orthochromic Normoblast (Iron-Deficient Metarubricyte)

Iron-Deficient Polychromatophilic Erythrocyte

Iron-Deficient Erythrocyte (Hypochromic/Microcytic)

FIGURE 10.3 Iron deficiency maturation drawing. (Reprinted with permission from Anderson SC, Poulsen KBV. *Anderson's Atlas of Hematology*, Philadelphia, PA: Wolters Kluwer Health/Lippincott Williams & Wilkins, Copyright 2003.)

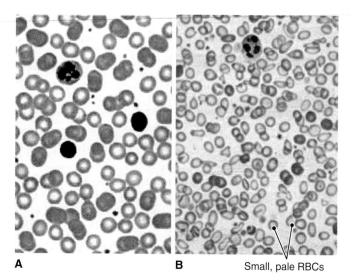

A   **B**   Small, pale RBCs

FIGURE 10.4. The blood in iron deficiency anemia. **A:** Normal blood smear. **B:** Blood smear in iron deficiency anemia. The red cells are small (microcytic) and pale (hypochromic). (Reprinted with permission from McConnell TH. *The Nature of Disease: Pathology for the Health Professions*, Philadelphia, PA: Lippincott Williams & Wilkins, 2007.)

When total body iron is low, transferrin levels increase, but the relative and absolute amounts of serum iron decline. Low serum iron levels, some down to 10 to 15 g/dL, characterize iron deficiency. The percent saturation is extremely low because more transferrin is available for less iron. Iron turnover and the percentage of serum iron used in red cell production increase as a way of getting the most possible mileage out of the little iron that is available. Transferrin saturation alone can be very misleading.

Serum ferritin is a currently accepted laboratory assay for diagnosing iron deficiency. A ferritin value of 12 µg/L or less is a highly specific indicator of iron deficiency. Ferritin is an acute-phase reactant. Because of this, diagnosis of iron

deficiency in hospitalized or ill patients can be difficult when these patients have normal or increased ferritin values even when iron deficient. Conditions associated with increased serum ferritin include infection, malignancy, iron overload, inflammation, and liver disease. The low sensitivity of ferritin for iron deficiency in these patients may require a bone marrow biopsy or a trial of iron therapy to differentiate iron deficiency from other causes of anemia.

A newer test is **soluble transferrin receptor (sTfR)**. The complete transferrin receptor is a membrane-bound protein that captures transferrin with its two iron atoms from extracellular fluid. A fragment of TfR finds its way into serum and appears to reflect production of TfR in the body. As the supply of transferrin-bound iron declines, hungry cells produce more TfR, which results in a higher serum concentration of the fragment. An apparent, and potentially major, advantage is the ability of sTfR to provide differentiation of IDA from anemia of chronic inflammation disorders (ACDs). The use of sTfR, in conjunction with ferritin and reticulocyte index, could reduce the need for bone marrow examinations to confirm iron deficiency or differentiate it from ACD.

Soluble transferrin receptor, a truncated form of the membrane-associated transferrin receptor, has been reported to be an indicator of erythropoietic activity and the diagnosis of iron deficiency and is not an acute-phase reactant. Therefore, it has been proposed as a laboratory test to identify iron deficiency in hospitalized and chronically ill patients. This could reduce the need for a bone marrow biopsy or trial of iron therapy. An additional application of sTfR with the MCH is in predicting maternal thyroid status.

Ferritin detects deficient iron stores; sTfR detects increased erythropoiesis. sTfR is not superior to ferritin for the routine clinical evaluation of patients with suspected iron deficiency.

The main value of the sTfR assay is in the differential diagnosis of microcytic anemias. Assay of transferrin receptor with calculation of the transferrin receptor:ferritin ratio is a useful addition to this evaluation. Because circulating

TABLE 10.3	Red Blood Cell Characteristics in Children and Adults		
Age	Lowest Normal Hemoglobin (g/dL)	Normal RBC MCV	Fetal Hemoglobin (%)
Birth	14.0	100–130	55–90
3–6 months	10.5	75–90	5–25
1–4 years	11.0	70–85	<2
4 years to puberty	11.5	75–90	<2
Adult (female)	12.0	80–95	<2
Adult (male)	14.0	80–95	<2

Source: Greer JP, et al. *Wintrobe's Clinical Hematology*, 11th ed., [(Table 27.1 Red Blood Cell Characteristics in Childhood]), 2004:948.

TABLE 10.4 Iron Studies			
Classic Iron Studies	Fe Def Without anemia	Fe Def With mild anemia	Fe Def With severe anemia
Marrow RE iron stores	+	0	0
Serum iron level	N/↓	N/↓	↓
Fe binding capacity	N or ↑	N or ↑	↑
Hemoglobin	N	Slight ↓	↓
Microcytic hypochromic	N	2+	4+
Ferritin	↓	↓	↓
Free RBC protoporphrin level (FEP)	N or ↑	↓	↓

transferrin receptors do not increase in anemia secondary to inflammatory disorders, they are helpful for distinguishing ACD from IDA. In situations in which IDA coexists with ACD, transferrin receptor concentrations increase secondary to the underlying iron deficiency. With serum ferritin concentrations greater than 30 μg/L in patients with frank inflammatory disease, measurement of circulating transferrin receptor is warranted to exclude concurrent iron deficiency. Transferrin receptor concentrations are also increased in other causes of microcytic anemia, including sideroblastic anemia and the thalassemias; however, these diseases can be distinguished from IDA by ferritin concentrations being within the reference interval or greater.

ANEMIA OF INFLAMMATION OR ANEMIA OF CHRONIC DISORDERS

Etiology

Anemia of inflammation (AOI) or anemia chronic diseases or disorder (ACD) is the second most prevalent anemia after IDA. This form of anemia is a common complication in patients with disorders as diverse as inflammation, infection, malignancy, or various systemic diseases. Approximately half of AOI/ACD cases are caused by subacute or chronic infections, such as tuberculosis, lung abscess, and bacterial endocarditis. Other cases may be caused by neoplasms, rheumatoid arthritis, rheumatic fever, systemic lupus erythematosus (SLE), uremia, or chronic liver disease. A hematologic abnormality is often minor and underlies pathology elsewhere in the body.

Pathophysiology

AOI/ACD is a hypoproliferative anemia resulting from underproduction of red cells. Although the life span of erythrocytes is mildly shortened in this disorder (in some patients,

the average erythrocyte survival time is 90 days), decreased erythrocyte survival is not an isolated or major factor in the development of anemia.

Multiple mechanisms contribute to anemia associated with inflammation or malignancy (Table 10.5). The principal pathogenesis of ACD is believed to be related to a recently described molecule, hepcidin. Body iron metabolism is regulated by several molecules. Hepcidin, a small 25-amino acid polypeptide hormone, is a key molecule in controlling iron absorption and recycling. In the liver, hepcidin gene expression is regulated by at least two pathways:

1. A pathway dependent on iron availability and involves signaling from the surface of the hepatocyte through the BMP receptor complex.
2. A pathway that regulates hepcidin gene expression by the IL-6–mediated inflammatory signaling pathway.

Hepcidin is released by the liver and circulates to interact with its cellular receptor, the iron export channel ferroportin, to block release of iron from cells, for example, tissue

TABLE 10.5 Mechanisms Associated with Anemia of Inflammation/Malignancy
1. Increased hepcidin production
2. Alterations in production of proinflammatory cytokines; interleukins (IL-1), (IL-6); tumor necrosis factor alpha (TNFα); interferons
3. Hemolysis (drug induced, microangiopathic, autoimmune)
4. Effects of chemotherpay
5. Nutritional deficiencies
6. Blood loss

macrophages and jejunal enterocytes. Hepcidin is also produced in human monocytes.

Hepcidin is able to induce iron sequestration and hypoferremia. Hepcidin blocks cellular efflux by binding to and inducing the degradation via internalization of ferroportin at the level of both enterocytes and macrophages of the mononuclear phagocytic system (MPS). Excessive production of hepcidin results in MPS iron blockage and a defective iron supply for erythropoiesis, and defective endogenous erythropoietin production, which results in anemia.

Characteristics of AOI associated with malignancy can be

- Inadequate production of erythropoietin (Epo) in response to the anemia
- Inadequate response of the erythroid marrow to endogenous Epo
- Impaired release of iron due to increased hepcidin production producing a functional iron deficiency
- Alterations in production of several proinflammatory cytokines
- Decreased erythrocyte production because of direct bone marrow infiltration by malignant tumor cells or by primary marrow cell malignancies
- Increased erythrocyte destruction present in immune or microangiopathic hemolytic anemia
- Acute or chronic blood loss
- Toxic effects of invasive therapy (e.g., chemotherapy or radiation therapy)
- Indirect multiple causes such as anemia associated with malignant disease, anemia associated with major organ failure, and various hemolytic anemias

The systemic diseases that produce AOI are accompanied by the release of acute-phase reactants in the blood (e.g., elevated C-reactive protein [CRP], fibrinogen, haptoglobin, and ceruloplasmin). This response becomes unified in a common pathway of metabolic events initiated by interleukin-1β (IL-1-β) from activated macrophages. IL-1-β then initiates a cascade of events mediated by the cytokines released from macrophages, lymphocytes, and other numerous cells within the body. IL-1-β is specifically responsible for production of fever, neutrophilia, leukocytosis, acute-phase protein synthesis, stimulation of production of lymphokines, and the release of lactoferrin from granulocytes.

Anemia associated with renal disease is usually caused by decreased production of erythropoietin by damaged kidneys. In chronic liver disease, anemia can result from many conditions, including AOI. If alcoholism is the cause of liver disease, ethanol is known to have direct toxic effects on bone marrow hematopoietic precursor cells, marrow cellularity, and red cell morphology.

Laboratory Characteristics

Laboratory assays that suggest inflammation or infection include elevated platelet counts, elevated total leukocyte counts, and evidence of acute-phase reactants. CRP is

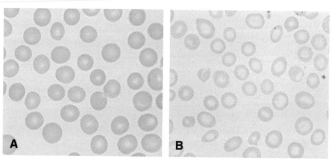

FIGURE 10.5. A blood smear showing normal erythrocytes (**A**) compared with a blood smear revealing microcytic, hypochromic erythrocytes in a patient with iron deficiency anemia (**B**). (Reprinted with permission from Willis MC. *Medical Terminology: A Programmed Learning Approach to the Language of Health Care*, Baltimore, MD: Lippincott Williams & Wilkins, 2002.)

frequently a surrogate marker that may or may not correlate with hepdicin levels.

Hematology Studies

This form of anemia is usually a mild hypoprolific anemia with a hematocrit usually fixed in the 28% to 32% range, but in some cases (e.g., uremia), the hemoglobin may be as low as 5 g/dL. The peripheral blood smears (Fig. 10.5) usually show normochromic and normocytic erythrocytes, but one fourth to one third of patients display hypochromic and microcytic erythrocytes. In patients with abnormal red cell morphology, it is less significant than in IDA. An ACD patient with normochromic, normocytic red blood cells may be suffering from conditions such as an autoimmune disorder or chronic renal disease. A compensatory erythroid hyperplasia of the bone marrow or reticulocytosis is not present. Normal or increased bone marrow iron stores are observed within macrophages (Fig. 10.6).

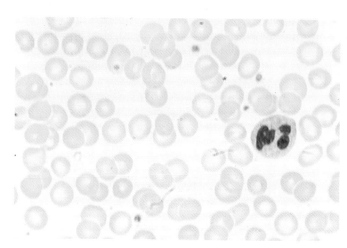

FIGURE 10.6. Anemia of chronic diseases. (Reprinted with permission from Armitage JO. *Atlas of Clinical Hematology*, Philadelphia, PA: Lippincott Williams & Wilkins, 2004.)

In patients with AOI caused by malignancy, a variety of abnormalities can be observed on a peripheral blood smear. Leukoerythroblastosis, the presence of both immature erythrocytes and leukocytes, can be seen. In addition, abnormal erythrocyte morphology can include teardrop red blood cells, schistocytes, helmet cells, fibrosis, and hypochromia.

The total leukocyte count is consistent with the type and degree of infection present in the patient; the platelets are normal in quantity. In the bone marrow, hemosiderin is increased or normal; sideroblasts are decreased. The reticulocyte count is usually less than 2%.

Clinical Chemistry Studies

Abnormalities in iron metabolism are associated with this disorder. Serum iron levels and transferrin (iron-binding capacity) are decreased. Serum iron is low because recycling of iron from macrophages is impaired. The total iron-binding capacity (TIBC) and transferrin saturation levels are decreased or normal. It is confusing to rely on the percentage of saturation of the iron-binding capacity to distinguish between iron deficiency and inflammation. The percentage of saturation may be very low in inflammation with abundant iron in the marrow. Total serum iron-binding capacity is superior to the percentage of saturation as an indicator of iron deficiency. If the TIBC is increased, IDA must be ruled out. Serum ferritin levels are variable. sTfR is low because its synthesis is impaired by proinflammatory cytokines. The combination of low serum iron and iron-binding capacity combined with stainable iron in the bone marrow is virtually diagnostic of ACD (Table 10.6).

It is not uncommon for AOI to coexist with IDA, particularly in women of childbearing age. In these cases, characteristics of both IDA and ACD coexist.

Treatment

Treatment of the underlying cause of anemia is the most direct. If anemia is severe, blood transfusion may be considered. Iron therapy is inappropriate because patients lack iron availability, not iron concentration. Recombinant human erythropoietin, rHu-EPO (Procrit, epoetin alfa), is a newer treatment alternative. Although AOI is not entirely caused by erythropoietin deficiency, high concentrations of this hormone have been able to counteract the suppressive effects of cytokines (e.g., IL-1). Clinical studies have demonstrated that the administration of rHu-EPO ameliorates anemia in infants with infections.

CHAPTER HIGHLIGHTS

Iron Deficiency Anemia

Although an individual's need for dietary iron is small and will only manifest itself after iron storage sites in the body have been depleted, IDA is one of the most frequently encountered types of anemias.

IDA may result from nutritional deficiency, faulty or incomplete iron absorption, increased demand for iron that is not met, or excessive loss of iron. Iron deficiency may result from several other less commonly occurring conditions including a disorder of iron utilization, **sideroblastic anemia**; selected hemoglobinopathies; anemia related to chronic

TABLE 10.6	Comparison of Classic Iron deficiency Anemia Versus Anemia of Inflammation/Chronic Disorders	
	IDA	**ACD**
Serum iron	Significant decrease	Decreased
TIBC	Increased	Decreased
Serum ferritin	Decreased	Normal to increased
Transferrin	Increased	Decreased or normal
Soluble transferrin		
Receptor (serum sTfR)	Increased	Normal
Transferrin		
Saturation	Decreased	Decreased
Peripheral blood	Microcytic	Normochromic
RBC morphology	Hypochromic	Normocytic or microcytic, hypochromic

IDA, iron deficiency anemia, ACD, anemia of chronic diseases or disorders; TIBC, total iron-binding capacity.

disorders; chronic inflammation; parasitic infections such as hookworm; and a deficiency of the plasma iron transporting protein **transferrin**.

Humans have 35 to 50 mg of iron per kilogram of body weight. The average adult has 3.5 to 5.0 g of total iron. Normal iron loss is very small, amounting to less than 1 mg/day. Iron is lost from the body through exfoliation of intestinal epithelial and skin cells, the bile, and urinary excretion. To compensate for this loss, the adult male has a replacement iron need of 1 mg/day. However, additional iron is needed during the growth years, pregnancy, and lactation. Some women require supplementary iron because of heavy menstrual blood loss. Seventy percent of iron is functional or essential, and 30% is stored or nonessential iron. Most functional iron is incorporated into the hemoglobin molecules of erythrocytes and is recycled.

In the normal infant at term, iron stores are adequate to maintain iron sufficiency for approximately 4 months of postnatal growth. In the premature infant, total body iron is lower than in the full-term newborn, although the proportion of iron to body weight is similar. Iron deficiency can develop by 2 to 3 months of age in premature infants. Iron intake must supplement the approximately 75 mg of iron per kilogram of body weight that is present at birth.

There are two broad types of dietary iron. Approximately 90% of iron from food is in the form of iron salts and is referred to as nonheme iron. The other 10% of dietary iron is in the form of heme iron, which is derived primarily from the hemoglobin and myoglobin of meat.

IDA in children is associated with psychomotor and mental impairment in the first 2 years of life. Pica, the compulsive ingestion of nonnutritive substances, has a well-documented association with iron deficiency.

A typical IDA will exhibit the following laboratory characteristics: the hemoglobin and Hct are both decreased, whereas the red cell count may be normal initially but will decrease as the iron deficiency state continues, and the red cell indices demonstrate decreased MCV, MCH, and MCHC.

Examination of the blood film in this anemia characteristically reveals a hypochromic, microcytic pattern. Although this anemia may initially be normochromic or normocytic, or may only have some anisocytosis and hypochromia, a full manifestation of the anemia will exhibit both the hypochromic and the microcytic red cell patterns.

Serum ferritin is currently the accepted laboratory test for diagnosing iron deficiency, and a ferritin value of 12 µg/L or less is a highly specific indicator of iron deficiency. A newer test is sTfR. Ferritin detects deficient iron stores; sTfR detects increased erythropoiesis. sTfR is not superior to ferritin for the routine clinical evaluation of patients with suspected iron deficiency.

Anemia of Chronic Inflammation or Anemia of Chronic Diseases

Anemia of chronic inflammation or chronic disorders (AOI/ACD) results from long- or short-term inflammation. AOI/ACD is the term that is used to describe the anemia associated with inflammation, chronic infection, malignancy, or various systemic diseases.

AOI/ACD is not related to any nutritional deficiency. AOI/ACD is associated with and is caused by one or more of the many biochemical changes that occur during inflammation. The life span of erythrocytes is mildly shortened in this disorder, but this mechanism is not a major factor in the development of anemia. The main defect is related to hepcidin.

CASE STUDIES

CASE 10.1

A 10-month-old Central American child was referred to the laboratory for testing after being seen by a pediatrician. The phlebotomist noted that the child was very pale and listless. The following tests were ordered: complete blood count (CBC), platelet count, reticulocyte count, total serum bilirubin, total serum iron and TIBC, and a stool examination for occult blood, ova, and parasites. The results were as follows:

■ **Laboratory Data**
Hemoglobin 5.6 g/dL
Hct 24%
RBC 3.5 × 10^{12}/L
WBC 10.5 × 10^9/L

The RBC indices were as follows:

MCV 68.6 fL
MCH 16 pg
MCHC 23 g/dL

The peripheral blood smear revealed significant anisocytosis, microcytosis, hypochromia, and poikilocytosis. A normal distribution of platelets was present. Additional laboratory findings were as follows:

Platelet count 200 × 10^9/L
Reticulocyte count 0.5%
Total serum bilirubin 0.9 mg/dL
Serum iron 40 µg/dL
TIBC 465 µg/dL
Percent saturation of transferrin 8.6%

(continued)

CASE STUDIES (continued)

A stool examination was negative for occult blood, ova, and parasites.

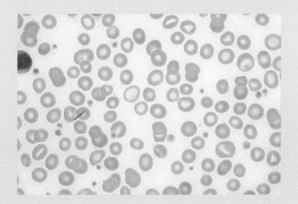

(Reprinted with permission from Anderson SC, *Anderson's. Atlas of Hematology*, Philadephia, PA: Wolters Kluwer Health/Lippincott Williams & Wilkins, Copyright 2003.)

■ Questions

1. What category of anemia is suggested by the morphology of the RBCs on the peripheral blood smear?
2. What laboratory assays would be of additional value in establishing the diagnosis?
3. What is the most probable cause of the patient's anemia?

■ Discussion

1. The demonstration of hypochromic, microcytic erythrocytes in a peripheral blood film suggests IDA.
2. The RBC indices reveal both a decreased MCV and MCH. These findings support the RBC morphology observations of microcytosis and hypochromia. Several follow-up laboratory assays were valuable in establishing the etiology of this patient's anemia. These tests were the serum iron, TIBC, and percent saturation. A decreased serum iron and percent saturation were present, along with an increased TIBC. The serum bilirubin and reticulocyte count were normal. No evidence of bleeding or parasitic infections was detected.
3. The most probable cause of this patient's anemia is iron deficiency. The laboratory findings demonstrate an iron deficit with no evidence of either hemolysis or blood loss. Small children are among the most frequent victims of inadequate dietary iron. The newborn begins life with 350 to 500 mg of iron. A daily intake of 1 mg/kg (2.2 lb) of body weight is needed during infancy to keep pace with growth. Some iron-poor foods, such as milk, never become useful sources for the absorption of iron. Children in underdeveloped countries frequently suffer from a combination of poor diet and parasitic infections. IDA is a frequent by-product of a diet consisting largely of milk and unsupplemented by fortified food products during the early years of development.

DIAGNOSIS: Iron Deficiency Anemia

CASE 10.2

A 75-year-old woman started feeling a bit weak. The patient reported limited red meat intake. A cholecystectomy was performed at age 60 and some bowel was removed. The patient has occasional diarrhea but considers this a minor inconvenience. The patient has experienced some bilateral loss of sensation in the feet and a tingling that was getting worse and more frequent over the past few months. She takes over-the-counter medications and her husband's pills for indigestion. The patient complained of arthritis; she has been taking nonsteroidal anti-inflammatory drugs for 5 years, and she has started low-dose methotrexate for arthritis flare-ups.

The physician is certain that she is anemic and requests a CBC and differential, iron, TIBC, and % Sat/ferritin.

No malignancies or GI bleeding is noted. Blood loss from the GI tract has been ruled out. Profound atrophic gastritis with patches of inflammation is noted, as is *H. pylori* at stomach biopsy study.

■ Laboratory Data

Hemoglobin 10 g/dL (reference value, 12 g/dL)
Hematocrit 33% (reference value, 36% to 45%)
MCV 83 fL (reference value, 81 to 98 fL)
RDW 17.5 % (reference value, 11.5% to 14.5%)
Iron 25 µg/dL (reference value, 50 to 170 dL)
TIBC 250 µg/dL (reference value, 250 to 450 µg/dL)
% Sat 10% (reference value, 15% to 50%)
Ferritin 45 µg/L (reference value, 12 to 120 µg/L)
Serum folate 4 ng/mL (reference value, 3 to 16 ng/mL)
RBC folate 100 ng/mL (reference value, 130 to 628 ng/mL)
Vitamin B$_{12}$ 100 pg/mL (reference value, 200 to 900 pg/mL)

■ Questions

1. Is ferritin a reliable laboratory indicator of iron stores?

■ Discussion

1. Ferritin is an iron-storage molecule. The amount in serum reflects iron storage: every 1 µg/L indicates (very roughly) 10 mg of body stores. Concern about the use of this indicator in the elderly arises because a range of inflammatory diseases increase ferritin; therefore, its concentration no longer reflects iron stores. Ferritin acts as an acute-phase reactant. In this case, the increased ferritin was caused by the inflammation of rheumatoid arthritis, illustrating the diagnostic pitfall of placing too much faith in ferritin.

Atrophic gastritis is common in the elderly and is almost certainly caused, to some extent, by *H. pylori.*

(continued)

Follow-up

The patient was given the usual course of intramuscular vitamin B_{12} and oral folate, 1 mg/day. The following were the laboratory results at her 3-month follow-up:

Hemoglobin 11 g/dL
MCV 75 fL
TIBC 500 μg/dL
RDW 15
Ferritin 8 μg/L
Iron 35 μg/dL
% Sat 7%
Bone marrow ordered for refractory anemia

Diagnostic Problems

This case presented some challenging diagnostic problems. The patient had an extremely elevated red blood cell distribution width index (RDW), which suggested a mixed red cell population.

A mixed vitamin B_{12}/iron deficiency is well recognized in the literature but seldom considered in practice. Note the normal MCV that became microcytic when the vitamin B_{12} deficiency was corrected.

A microbiological component to nutritional deficiency, *H. pylori,* is very common in the elderly and, ulcers or no ulcers, requires consideration. Biopsy is not necessary for reasonably reliable identification of affected persons; serologic tests are available. However, after the gastric damage has been done, nutritional support may be necessary.

Nonresponse to a particular form of oral iron supplement could involve gastric pH, bowel loss or disease, malabsorption secondary to vitamin B_{12} deficiency, or other components of her diet which reduce iron absorption.

DIAGNOSIS: Iron Deficiency and Vitamin B_{12} Deficiency Anemia

CASE 10.3

A 35-year-old woman with type I diabetes was admitted to the hospital with severe anemia, vomiting, and fever. She had not felt well for the past several months. She had lost more than 25 lb without dieting.

Physical examination revealed a pale and slightly obese female with a distended abdomen. She was the mother of two young children, ages 3 and 5. Her menstrual periods were regular.

A CBC, blood glucose, urinalysis, and pregnancy test were ordered.

Laboratory Data

Hemoglobin 11.40 g/dL
RBC 4.06×10^{12}/L
Hematocrit 35.5%
MCV 87 fL
MCH 28.1
MCHC 32 g/dL
RDW 16%
WBC 22.1×10^9/L

Her peripheral blood smear showed abnormal erythrocyte morphology, anisocytosis, poikilocytosis, and some teardrop (dacryocytes) cells. Her serum blood glucose was elevated. Her urinalysis was normal, except for an elevated blood glucose. The result of her pregnancy test was negative.

A follow-up ultrasound of the abdomen revealed a 20-cm extrauterine mass. Subsequent surgical excision of the mass revealed a malignant epithelial tumor of the left ovary with metastases to the pelvic lymph nodes, opposite ovary, and right lung.

Questions

1. Does this patient have AOI?
2. Which hematopoietic cells are involved in an inflammatory response?
3. What are the characteristic iron and iron storage results in anemia of chronic inflammation?

Discussion

1. This patient has AOI subsequent to a malignancy. In cases of malignancy, it has been shown that anemia may develop when the neoplasm persists for even a few weeks.
2. Cellular reactions to injury involving inflammation are macrophages, lymphocytes, and neutrophils.
3. Typically, patients with anemia of chronic inflammation demonstrate low serum iron and decreased TIBC with increased iron stores in macrophages.

DIAGNOSIS: Anemia of Inflammation Secondary to Metastatic Carcinoma Originating in the Ovary

1. The etiology of IDA is
   A. nutritional deficiency
   B. faulty iron absorption
   C. excessive loss of iron
   D. all of the above
2. Iron deficiency is still common in
   A. toddlers
   B. adolescent girls
   C. women of childbearing age
   D. all of the above

Questions 3 through 7: Match the following categories with an appropriate example. (Use an answer only once)
3. _____ Decreased iron intake
4. _____ Faulty iron absorption
5. _____ Pathological iron loss
6. _____ Physiological iron loss
7. _____ Increased iron utilization
   A. Sprue
   B. Colon cancer
   C. Adolescent growth spurt
   D. Menstruation
   E. Meat-poor diet
8. The average adult has _____ g of total iron.
   A. 0.2 to 1.4
   B. 1.5 to 3.4
   C. 3.5 to 5.0
   D. 5.1 to 10.0
9. Most functional iron in humans is found in
   A. the bone marrow
   B. the liver
   C. hemoglobin molecules of erythrocytes (RBCs)
   D. the free hemoglobin in the circulation

Questions 10 and 11: Approximately (10) _____% of iron from food is in the form of (11) _____ iron.
10.
   A. 25
   B. 50
   C. 70
   D. 90
11.
   A. Nonheme
   B. Heme
12. Most ingested iron is readily absorbed into the body in the
   A. stomach and duodenum
   B. duodenum and upper jejunum
   C. ileum and duodenum
   D. upper jejunum and ileum
13. Transferrin represents a
   A. storage form of iron
   B. beta globulin that moves iron
   C. glycoprotein that moves iron
   D. both B and C

14. In IDA, the erythrocytic indices are typically
   A. MCV increased, MCH decreased, and MCHC decreased
   B. MCV decreased, MCH decreased, and MCHC decreased
   C. MCV decreased, MCH increased, and MCHC decreased
   D. MCV decreased, MCH decreased, and MCHC normal
15. The peripheral blood smear demonstrates _____ red blood cells in IDA.
   A. microcytic, hypochromic
   B. macrocytic, hypochromic
   C. macrocytic and spherocytic
   D. either A or B
16. In IDA, the
   A. serum iron is severely decreased and the TIBC is increased
   B. serum iron is decreased and the TIBC is normal
   C. serum iron is normal and the TIBC is normal
   D. serum iron is increased and the TIBC is normal
17. Anemias of inflammation/chronic diseases can be caused by
   A. inflammation
   B. infection
   C. malignancy
   D. all of the above
18. AOI can result from
   A. inappropriately decreased erythropoietin
   B. suppression of erythropoiesis by cytokines from activated macrophages and lymphocytes
   C. impaired iron metabolism
   D. all of the above
19. The typical peripheral blood film of a patient with AOI typically reveals _____ erythrocytes.
   A. microcytic, hypochromic
   B. macrocytic, hypochromic
   C. normocytic, normochromic
   D. many spherocytes
20. Leukoerythroblastosis can appear as _____ on a peripheral blood smear.
   A. immature leukocytes
   B. immature erythrocytes
   C. immature thrombocytes
   D. both A and B
21. What is the most appropriate treatment for AOI?
   A. Red blood cell transfusion
   B. Iron therapy
   C. Erythropoietin injections
   D. Treatment of the inflammatory condition
22. Sideroblastic anemia can be caused by
   A. congenital (chromosomal) defect
   B. drugs (e.g., chloramphenicol)

(continued)

C. association with malignant disorders (e.g., acute myelogenous leukemia)
D. all of the above

23. A common feature of sideroblastic anemia is
A. ringed sideroblasts
B. decreased serum iron
C. decreased serum ferritin
D. macrocytic red blood cells

24. The greatest portion of operational body iron is normally contained in what compound?
A. Hemoglobin
B. Ferritin

C. Cytochromes
D. Myoglobin

25. Storage iron in the human body is
A. found in hepatocytes
B. found in macrophages
C. sequestered as ferritin
D. all of the above

26. The most sensitive assay for the diagnosis of hereditary hemochromatosis (HH) is
A. serum iron
B. serum iron–binding capacity
C. transferrin
D. transferrin saturation

BIBLIOGRAPHY

Andrews NC. Forging a field: the golden age of iron biology, *Blood*, 112(2):219–230, 2008.

Adamson JW. The anemia of inflammation/malignancy: mechanisms and management, *Am Soc of Hematol: ASH Education Book*, 159–164, 2008.

Bamberg R. Occurrence and detection of iron-deficiency anemia in infants and toddlers, *Clin Lab Sci*, 21(4):225–231, 2008.

Bergamaschi G, et al. Anemia of chronic disease and defective erythropoietin production in patients with celiac disease, *Haematologica*, 93(12):1785–1790, 2008.

Beutler E, Waalen J. The definition of anemia: what is the lower limit of normal of the blood hemoglobin concentration? *Blood*, 107 (5):1747–1750, 2006.

Beutler E, West C. Hematologic differences between African-Americans and whites: the roles of iron deficiency and (alpha) thalassemia on hemoglobin levels and MCV, *Blood*, 106(2):740–745, 2005.

Beutler E, Studenski S. Toward a better understanding of anemia in older adults, *The Hematologists*, ASH News and Reports, 2(4):7, 2005.

Bovy C. Mature erythrocytes indices: new markers of iron availability, *Hematologia*, 90(4):549–551, 2005.

Brandão M, et al. The soluble transferrin receptor as a marker of iron homeostasis in normal subjects and in HFE-related hemochromatosis, *Haematologica*, 90(1): 31–37, 2005.

Brugnara C, et al. Reticulocyte hemoglobin content to diagnose iron deficiency in children, *JAMA*, 281(23):2225–2230, 1999.

Culleton BF, et al. Impact of anemia on hospitalization and mortality in older adults, *Blood*, 107(10):3841–3846, 2006.

Ekiz C, et al. the effect of iron deficiency anemia on the function of the immune system. *Hematol J*, 5:579–583, 2005.

Greendyke RM, et al. Serum levels of erythropoietin and selected other cytokines in patients with anemia of chronic disease, *Am J Clin Pathol*, 101:338, 1994.

Hedenus M, et al. Darbepoetin alfa significantly increases hemoglobin and reduces transfusions in patients with lymphoproliferative malignancies: Results of a randomized double-blind, placebo-controlled study, *Hematol J*, 4(Suppl 2):253, 2003.

Hershko C, et al. Mechanism of iron regulation and of iron deficiency, *Eur Hemtol Assoc*, 1(1):1–8, 2007.

Jolobe O. Reticulocyte hemoglobin content vs. soluble transferrin receptor and feritn index in iron deficiency anemia accompanied with inflammation, *Int J Lab Hem*, 30:175–176, 2008.

Laudicina RJ. Anemia in an aging population, *Clin Lab Sci*, 21(4): 232–239, 2008.

Looker AC, et al. Prevalence of iron deficiency in the United States, *JAMA*, 277(12):973–976, 1997.

Lux SE. Hematologic aspects of systemic disease. In: Handin RI, Lux SE, Stossel TP (eds.). *Blood*, 2nd ed, Philadelphia, PA: Lippincott Williams & Wilkins, 2003:1977–2009.

Malope BI, et al. The ratio of serum transferrin receptor and serum ferritin in the diagnosis of iron status, *Br J Haematol*, 115:84–89, 2001.

Patel KV, Guralnik JM. Prognostic implications of anemia in older adults, *Haematologica*, 94(1):1–2, 2009.

Patel KV. Variability and heritability of hemoglobin concentration: an opportunity to improve understanding of anemia in older adults, *Hematologica*, 93(9):1281–1283, 2008.

Price EA, Schrier SL. Anemia in the older adult. www.UpToDate.com. Retrieved April 6, 2010.

Skikne BS. Circulating transferrin receptor assay: Coming of age, *Clin Chem*, 44(1):7–9, 1998.

Tsang CW, et al. Hematologic indices in an older population sample: Derivation of healthy reference values, *Clin Chem*, 44(1):96–101, 1998.

Turgeon ML. Anemia: is it iron deficiency? Presented at MEDLAB 2009 Arab Health Conference, Dubai, UAE, Jan 29, 2009.

Weiss G, Goodnough LT. Anemia of chromic disease, *NEJM*, 352(10):1011–1023, 2005.

Weiss G. Pathophysiology, diagnosis and treatment of the anemia of chronic disease, *Eur Hemtol Assoc*, 1(1):9–16, 2007.

CHAPTER 11

Megaloblastic Anemias

Megaloblastic anemias
- List four causes of vitamin B$_{12}$ deficiency.
- List three causes of folic acid deficiency.
- Briefly describe the epidemiology of pernicious anemia.
- Explain the physiology, including the immune nature, of pernicious anemia.
- Describe the clinical signs and symptoms of pernicious anemia.
- Delineate the laboratory findings in pernicious anemia.

- Explain the usual management of and therapy for pernicious anemia.
- Compare megaloblastic anemia caused by folic acid deficiency with pernicious anemia.

Case study
- Apply knowledge of etiology, epidemiology, physiology, clinical signs and symptoms, laboratory findings, and management therapy to the case studies.

MEGALOBLASTIC ANEMIAS

Megaloblastic anemias can be classified into two major categories based on etiology. The major divisions are vitamin B$_{12}$ (cobalamin, Cbl) deficiency and folic acid deficiency.

The term **megaloblastic** refers to the abnormal marrow erythrocyte precursor seen in processes, such as pernicious anemia, associated with altered DNA synthesis. Macrocytes can occur in the absence of a megaloblastic process. For example, an increased mean corpuscular volume (MCV) can result simply from an increase in the number of circulating reticulocytes, which are larger than mature erythrocytes.

The most common causes of megaloblastic anemia are acquired, although congenital forms exist. Deficiencies in cobalamin, folate, or both account for the majority of cases. The most common disorder of cobalamin deficiency is pernicious anemia. Less common manifestations can occur as the result of a gastrectomy, inflammatory disorders of the terminal ileum, or infestation with fish tapeworm *Diphyllobothrium latum*. Folic acid deficiency is usually caused by inadequate dietary intake.

Red blood cells in megaloblastic anemias (Fig. 11.1) have an abnormal nuclear maturation and imbalance between nuclear and cytoplasmic maturation. The absence of vitamin B$_{12}$ or folates impairs DNA synthesis, which slows nuclear replication and delays each step of maturation. The premitotic interval is prolonged. This results in a large nucleus, increased cytoplasmic RNA, and early synthesis of hemoglobin. Many cells never undergo mitosis and breakdown in the bone marrow, producing extremely increased levels of serum lactic dehydrogenase (LDH). This deficiency can impair maturation in myelogenous white blood cells and megakaryocytes, producing leukopenia with neutrophilic hypersegmentation and thrombocytopenia. Megakaryocyte fragments and giant platelets may be seen on peripheral blood smears. Megaloblastic anemias such as pernicious anemia are also characterized by active intramedullary hemolysis.

In addition to hematological manifestations, neuropsychiatric disturbances, such as peripheral neuropathy or depression, are also common with cobalamin or folate deficiency and may occur in the absence of significant hematological manifestations. These neuropsychiatric conditions are reversible if treated promptly by cobalamin or folate replenishment.

Usually, the measurement of serum cobalamin or folate levels is sufficient to make the diagnosis. Inherited enzyme deficiencies are rare causes of megaloblastic anemia.

Etiology

Megaloblastic anemia caused by vitamin B$_{12}$ deficiency is associated with

1. Increased utilization of vitamin B$_{12}$ because of parasitic infections such as *D. latum* (tapeworm) and pathogenic bacteria in disorders such as diverticulitis and small bowel stricture.
2. Malabsorption syndrome caused by gastric resection, gastric carcinoma, and some forms of celiac disease or sprue.
3. Nutritional deficiency or diminished supply of vitamin B$_{12}$. Cobalamin is synthesized by bacteria and is found in soil and in contaminated water. Foods of animal origin (e.g., meat, eggs, and milk) are the primary dietary sources. The amount of cobalamin in the average Western diet (5 to 15 µg/day) is more than sufficient to meet normal requirements. The body can store large amounts of cobalamin. Because of this, it can take 2 to 5 years for a

Promegaloblast (Megaloblastic Rubriblast)

Basophilic Megaloblast (Megaloblastic Prorubricyte)

Polychromatophilic Megaloblast (Megaloblastic Rubricyte)

Orthochromic Megaloblast (Megaloblastic Metarubricyte)

Polychromatophilic Megalocyte (Megaloblastic Reticulocyte)

Megalocyte (Oval Macrocyte)

FIGURE 11.1 Megalocyte maturation drawing. (Reprinted with permission from Anderson S, Poulsen K. *Anderson's Atlas of Hematology*, Philadelphia, PA: Lippincott Williams & Wilkins, 2003.)

deficiency to develop even in the presence of severe malabsorption.
4. Pernicious anemia, the condition associated with chronic atrophic gastritis.

Megaloblastic anemia caused by folic acid deficiency is associated with

1. Abnormal absorption caused by celiac disease or sprue
2. Increased utilization caused by pregnancy or some acute leukemias
3. Treatment with antimetabolites that act as folic acid antagonists

Epidemiology

Research studies have recently documented that 1.9% of persons older than 60 years have undiagnosed pernicious anemia. Earlier studies suggested that pernicious anemia is restricted to Northern Europeans; however, newer studies report the disease in both blacks and Latin Americans. The median age at diagnosis is 60 years. Slightly more women than men are affected.

Although the disease is silent for a span of 20 to 30 years until the end stage, the underlying gastric lesion can be predicted many years before anemia develops. The underlying gastritis that causes pernicious anemia is immunologically related to an autoantibody to intrinsic factor (IF), a serum inhibitor of IF, and autoantibodies to parietal cells.

A genetic predisposition to pernicious anemia is suggested by the clustering of the disease and of gastric autoantibodies in families, and by the association of the disease and gastric autoantibodies with the autoimmune endocrinopathies. Approximately 20% of the relatives of patients with pernicious anemia have pernicious anemia. These relatives, especially first-degree female relatives, also have a higher frequency of gastric autoantibodies than normal subjects. In contrast to some other autoimmune diseases, there is little evidence of an association between pernicious anemia and particular molecules of the major histocompatibility complex (MHC).

Pernicious anemia may be associated with autoimmune endocrinopathies and antireceptor autoimmune disease. These diseases include chronic autoimmune thyroiditis (Hashimoto thyroiditis), insulin-dependent diabetes mellitus, Addison disease, primary ovarian failure, primary hypoparathyroidism, Graves disease, and myasthenia gravis.

Physiology

Normal red cell maturation is dependent on many hematological factors, two of which are the vitamin B_{12} coenzymes (also called cobalamin) and folates. Megaloblastic dyspoiesis occurs when one of these factors is absent.

Vitamin B_{12} and a variety of structurally similar compounds, known as cobalamin analogues, that lack the functional coenzyme activity of the vitamin occur in nature as a product of certain microorganisms. It becomes available to humans through the food chain. About one third of the body's average total of 5,000 µg is stored in the liver. The average loss of vitamin B_{12} is approximately 5 µg/day. An adult requires about 5 µg of vitamin B_{12} per day to balance this loss, with a greater need during unusual periods such as pregnancy. A normal diet contains 5 to 30 µg.

Folates are abundant in yeast, many leafy vegetables, and organ meats such as liver and kidneys. An ample amount of folate is present in most well-balanced diets containing vegetables, fruits, dairy products, and cereals. The human body stores little folic acid. Storage amounts would last about 3 to 4 months if a complete absence of dietary folates existed. However, a chronically inadequate diet can produce folic acid deficiency anemia. In addition to a poor diet, alcohol is the most common pharmacological cause of folic acid deficiency. However, folic acid antagonists, such as certain drugs used to treat leukemias and oral contraceptives, appear to reduce the absorption of folic acid.

Vitamin B_{12} (Cobalamin) Transport

Cobalamin transport is mediated by three different binding proteins that are capable of binding the vitamin at its required physiological concentrations:

1. intrinsic factor (IF),
2. transcobalamin II (TC II), and
3. R proteins.

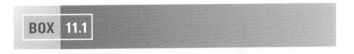

FIGURE 11.2 Vitamin B$_{12}$ physiology.

IF, a glycoprotein, is synthesized and secreted by the parietal cells of the mucosa in the fundus region of the stomach in several mammalian species, including humans. In health, the amounts of IF secreted by the stomach greatly exceed the quantities required to bind ingested cobalamin in its coenzyme forms. At a very acidic pH, cobalamin splits from dietary protein and combines with IF to form a vitamin-IF complex (Fig. 11.2). Binding by IF is extraordinarily specific and is lost with even slight changes in the cobalamin molecule. This complex is stable and remains unabsorbed until it reaches the ileum. In the ileum, the vitamin-IF complex attaches to specific receptor sites present only on the outer surface of microvillus membranes of ileal enterocytes.

The release of this complex from the mucosal cells with subsequent transport to the tissues depends on TC II. TC II is a plasma polypeptide synthesized by the liver and probably several other tissues. Like IF, TC II, which turns over very rapidly in the plasma, acts as the acceptor and principal carrier of the vitamin to the liver and other tissues. Receptors for TC II are observed on the plasma membranes of a wide variety of cells. TC II is also capable of binding a few unusual cobalamin analogues, and it stimulates cobalamin uptake by reticulocytes.

The R proteins comprise an antigenically cross-reactive group of cobalamin-binding glycoproteins. The R proteins bind cobalamin and various cobalamin analogues. Their function is unknown, but they appear to serve as storage sites and as a means of eliminating excess cobalamin and unwanted analogues from the blood circulation through receptor sites on liver cells. R proteins are produced by leukocytes and perhaps other tissues. They are present in plasma as TC I and TC III as well as in saliva, milk, and other body fluids. TC I probably serves only as a backup transport system for endogenous cobalamin. Endogenous vitamin is synthesized in the human gastrointestinal tract by bacterial action, but none is adsorbed.

Vitamin B$_{12}$ (Cobalamin) and Folic Acid Deficiencies

In addition to dietary and other causes of deficiencies of cobalamin (Box 11.1), a deficiency of TC II can produce a vitamin deficiency. Folic acid deficiencies (Box 11.2) appear to be less related to transport but are typically associated with

BOX 11.1

Examples of Conditions Contributing to Cobalamin (Vitamin B$_{12}$) Deficiency

DIETARY
Malnutrition

MEDICATIONS (INHIBITORS)
H2 receptor antagonists
Proton-pump inhibitor drugs

MALABSORPTION
Achlorhydria
Gastric resection

INTESTINAL
Overgrowth of intestinal organisms, e.g., short bowel syndrome)
Sprue
Diphyllobothrium latum infestation

IMPAIRED UTILIZATION
Transcobalamin II deficiency or abnormality

INCREASED DEMAND
Pregnancy
Inhibitors: Achlorhydria

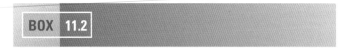

Potential Causes of Folate Deficiency

Inadequate intake
Increased demands, e.g., pregnancy, infancy
Malabsorption disorders, e.g., sprue
Biologic competition for dietary folate, e.g., bacterial overgrowth in the intestine
Medications (inhibitors), e.g., anticonvulsants, chemotherapy agents, methotrexate
Alcohol

conditions of either dietary inadequacy, medications acting as inhibitors, or malabsorption syndromes.

In pernicious anemia, the deficiency is caused by reduced IF secondary to gastric atrophy. In the majority of cases of pernicious anemia, anti-IFs or antibodies to parietal cells (large cells on the margin of the peptic glands of the stomach)

have been reported. Most authorities consider the demonstration of these antibodies to support the theory that pernicious anemia is an autoimmune disorder. The presence of IF-blocking antibodies is diagnostic of pernicious anemia.

Pathophysiology

Pernicious anemia applies only to the condition associated with chronic atrophic gastritis.

Gastric Pathological Findings

There are three regions of the stomach: the fundus and the body, both of which contain acid-secreting gastric parietal cells and pepsinogen-secreting zymogenic cells, and the antrum, which contains gastrin-producing cells. Autoimmune gastritis, associated with pernicious anemia, involves the fundus and the body of the stomach only. The pathological process associated with autoimmune gastritis appears to be directed toward the gastric parietal cells (Fig. 11.3). Autoantibodies to parietal cells bind to both the α and β subunits of gastric H^+/K^+-ATPase, the antigen recognized by parietal cell autoantibodies (Fig. 11.4).

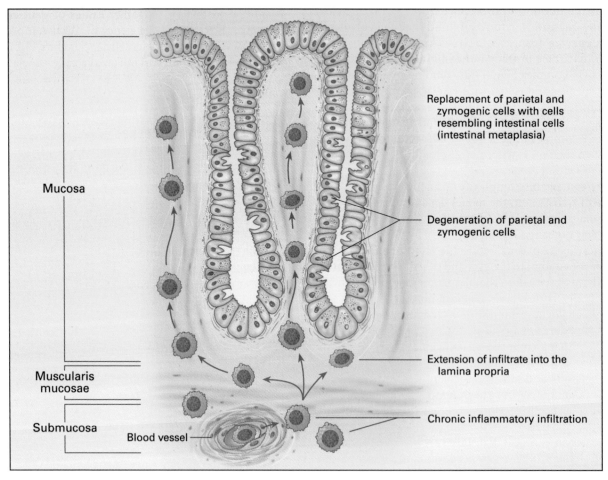

FIGURE 11.3 The gastric lesion of pernicious anemia. The early lesion is characterized by chronic infiltration of the gastric submucosa with inflammatory cells. Extension of the chronic inflammatory infiltrate into the lamina propria is associated with degeneration of gastric parietal and zymogenic cells. The advanced lesion is characterized by loss of parietal and zymogenic cells and replacement cells resembling those of the intestinal mucosa (intestinal metaplasia). (Reprinted with permission from Toh B-H, et al. Pernicious anemia, *N Engl J Med*, 337(20):1442, 1997. Copyright©1997 Massachusetts Medical Society. All rights reserved.)

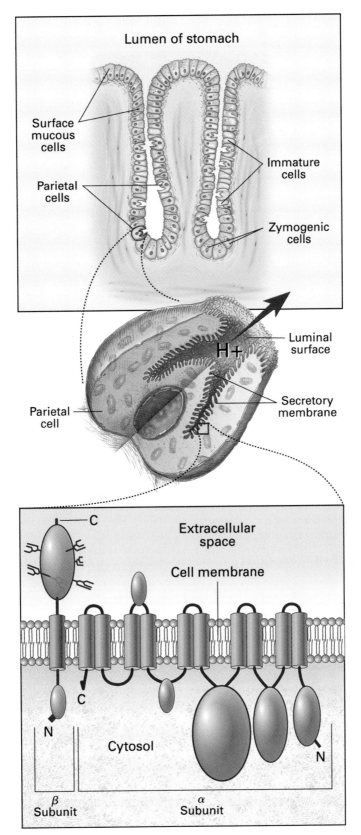

FIGURE 11.4 Gastric parietal cell H⁺/K⁺-ATPase as the molecular target in autoimmune gastritis with pernicious anemia. The top panel represents a gastric gland, showing the location of parietal cells in relation to zymogenic cells, immature cells, and surface mucous cells. The middle figure represents a stimulated gastric parietal cell, showing the lining membrane of the secretory canaliculus on which gastric H⁺/K⁺-ATPase is located. The bottom panel represents the catalytic α and glycoprotein β subunits of gastric H⁺/K⁺-ATPase, showing their orientation in the lining membrane of the secretory canaliculus of the parietal cell. N, N-terminal of protein; C, C-terminal of protein. (Reprinted with permission from Toh B-H, et al. Pernicious anemia, *N Engl J Med*, 337(20):1443, 1997. Copyright ©1997 Massachusetts Medical Society. All rights reserved.)

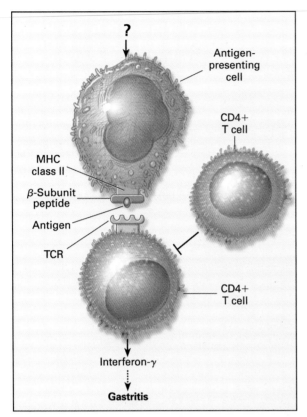

FIGURE 11.5 The development of autoimmune gastritis. CD4 Th1 T cells are activated by binding of their T-cell antigen receptors (TCR) with a complex of a peptide of the β subunit of the gastric H⁺/K⁺-ATPase and a MHC class II molecule on antigen-presenting cells. The mechanism of activation of the antigen-presenting cells and the pathway by which pathogenic T cells mediate gastritis are not known. Other CD4 cells may prevent expansion of pathogenic CD4 T cells. (Reprinted with permission from Toh B-H, et al. Pernicious anemia, *N Engl J Med*, 337(20):1445, 1997. Copyright ©1997 Massachusetts Medical Society. All rights reserved.)

Autoimmune type A gastritis exhibits autoantibodies to gastric parietal cells and to IF, achlorhydria, low serum pepsinogen concentrations, and high serum gastrin concentrations. Most patients with pernicious anemia exhibit anti-IF and/or antiparietal antibodies. The demonstration of these antibodies supports the theory that pernicious anemia is an autoimmune disorder (Fig. 11.5).

Clinical Signs and Symptoms

Pernicious anemia is frequently seen in those of Northern European ancestry, with clinical presentation during the fourth or fifth decade of life.

Acquired megaloblastic anemias tend to have a very insidious onset, with symptoms that may have been present for years before the diagnosis is made. Because of the pivotal role of cobalamin in metabolism, multiple organ systems can be affected in pernicious anemia.

Patients may note changes in their skin color to a lemon-yellow appearance. The nail beds, skin creases, and periorbital areas may become hyperpigmented owing to melanin deposition. Angular cheilitis (cracking at the corners of the mouth), dyspepsia, and diarrhea can occur. Glossitis and a painful tongue are frequently observed.

Early graying of the hair can be seen. Patients may complain of tiredness, dyspnea on exertion, vertigo, or tinnitus secondary to anemia. Congestive heart failure, angina, or palpitations may be noted. Neurological and cognitive abnormalities may be seen in cobalamin deficiency. Paresthesias, loss of balance, visual changes, paraplegia, memory loss, dementia, and other psychiatric disturbances have been described. The degree to which these symptoms are present may not be correlated with the degree of anemia. If the disease is severe, infection, bleeding, or bruising may occur owing to granulocytopenia.

Vitamin B_{12} deficiency in infants can cause neurological symptoms. If untreated, permanent neurological damage can result. Two reported cases of B_{12}-deficient infants occurred in exclusively breast-fed infants whose mothers had undiagnosed pernicious anemia.

Laboratory Findings

Pernicious anemia, the most common megaloblastic anemia, is a prototype of the entire group. The hematological picture is the same whether the cause is vitamin B_{12} or folic acid deficiency. However, supporting laboratory assays will differ for the various megaloblastic anemias.

The hemoglobin and red cell counts are usually extremely low in this anemia. However, the **microhematocrit** (packed cell volume) may not reflect the actual decrease in erythrocytes because of the enlarged size of the red cells. This increase in red cell size is typically reflected in the **mean corpuscular volume** (MCV), which may be as high as 130 fL. The **mean corpuscular hemoglobin** (MCH) varies but is usually increased in 90% of cases. Concurrent conditions that decrease the MCV, such as thalassemia or iron deficiency, may cause the MCV to be normal. The **mean corpuscular hemoglobin concentration** (MCHC) is usually normal. In this anemia, platelet counts are usually moderately decreased. The total white blood cell count will classically demonstrate a leukopenia, particularly a neutropenia.

Examination of a peripheral blood smear reveals a moderate to significant anisocytosis and poikilocytosis with many macrocytic, ovalocytic red cells (Figs. 11.6 and 11.7). Erythroid precursors, notably metarubricytes, may also be observed. Red cell inclusions such as basophilic stippling, Howell-Jolly bodies, and Cabot rings may be observed. Abnormalities in leukocytes may include hypersegmented (more than four lobes) neutrophils and an increase in the percentage of eosinophils (eosinophilia). Platelets are also typically decreased in number.

The reticulocyte count is less than 1% in untreated pernicious anemia and is low for the degree of anemia. However, subsequent to vitamin B_{12} treatment, assuming that the patient does not have antibodies against IF, the reticulocyte count can increase up to 25% in 5 to 8 days.

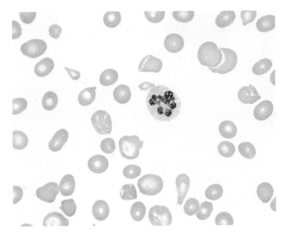

FIGURE 11.6 Pernicious anemia: peripheral blood smear showing oval macrocytes and hypersegmented neutrophil nucleus.

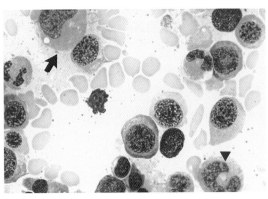

FIGURE 11.8 Bone marrow aspirate smear in megaloblastic anemia demonstrates numerous large erythroblasts having a fenestrated nuclear chromatin. The nuclear appearance has been likened to that of a piece of salami. Nuclear changes are also evident in the developing neutrophils: giant metamyelocytes (*arrow*) and giant bands (*arrowhead*). (Reprinted with permission from McClatchey KD. *Clinical Laboratory Medicine*, 2nd ed, Philadelphia, PA: Lippincott Williams & Wilkins, 2002.)

Pancytopenia may be seen in advanced cases. In severe anemia with a hematocrit of less than 20%, promegaloblasts and nucleated erythrocytes may be seen, caused by extramedullary hematopoiesis in the spleen and very early marrow release. A dimorphic population of red cells may be present with concurrent iron deficiency. The red cell distribution width is high.

The bone marrow (see Fig. 11.8) is usually hypercellular with megaloblastic changes in either the erythroid line or all lines, but it can be hypocellular and mimic aplastic anemia. Erythrocyte precursors are enlarged with a decreased nuclear-cytoplasmic ratio. Nuclear-cytoplasmic asynchrony, with relative immaturity of the nucleoplasm, is typical. Changes give red cells a dysplastic appearance, and a mistaken diagnosis of myelodysplastic syndrome can be made. Granulocytic precursors may also display nuclear-cytoplasmic dissociation and enlargement. Characteristically, giant metamyelocytes with large, incompletely segmented nuclei are seen. The number of mitoses are increased and the myeloid-erythroid ratio (M:E ratio) is diminished to 1:1 or less. Iron stores are increased, unless iron deficiency is coincidentally present.

Clinical chemistry analyses and immuno assays are valuable in the diagnosis of pernicious anemia (see Table 11.1). Folic acid deficiency anemias present the same erythrocytic picture as pernicious anemia but have a different chemical and immunologic profile. Assays of importance in megaloblastic anemia testing include serum vitamin B_{12}, serum folate, serum methylmalonic acid, total homocysteine, intrinsic factor blocking antibody (IF-antibody), parietal cell antibody (IgG), and gastrin levels. Ancilllary findings include increase LDH and bilirubin levels.

The now obsolete Schilling test was done to establish the cause of vitamin B_{12} deficiency in a patient with undetectable IF antibody and no clear history of gastric or ileal disease or surgery. Assays for anti-IF measure antibodies to IF. Antibodies are evident in approximately 60% of patients with pernicious anemia. Most patients with pernicious anemia (80%) have parietal cell antibodies. In the presence of parietal cell antibodies, gastric biopsy almost always demonstrates gastritis. Low-antibody titers to parietal cells are often found with no clinical evidence of pernicious anemia or atrophic gastritis and are sometimes seen in older adult patients.

Achlorhydria, the absence of hydrochloric acid (HCl) in the stomach, is an important finding in pernicious anemia. An absence of free HCl in gastric fluid is a universal feature of this form of megaloblastic anemia. Achlorhydria results from atrophy of the parietal cells of the stomach. The LDH is significantly increased owing to the increased intramedullary destruction of megaloblastic bone marrow cells.

If cobalamin deficiency is suspected, it becomes important to determine the source of the deficiency. Conditions that can contribute to cobalamin (vitamin B_{12}) or folate deficiency and the resulting impaired production of erythrocytes are presented in Table 11.2.

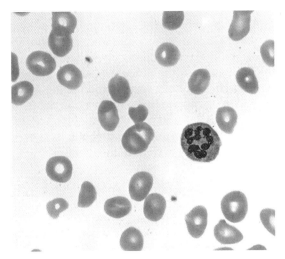

FIGURE 11.7 Megaloblastic anemia is characterized by hypersegmented neutrophils and the presence of well-hemoglobinized macrocytes and macroovalocytes. (Reprinted with permission from McClatchey KD. *Clinical Laboratory Medicine*, 2nd ed, Philadelphia, PA: Lippincott Williams & Wilkins, 2002.)

TABLE 11.1	Megaloblastic Anemia Testing[a]			
Basic Testing	Level	Follow Up Testing	Level	Interpretation
Vitamin B$_{12}$	>400 pg/mL			Not PA
	>400 pg/mL if neurologic symptoms	Serum Methylmalonic acid (MMA) and homocysteine		May confirm B$_{12}$ deficiency
	100–400 pg/mL	Serum methylmalonic acid (MMA)	<0.4 µmol/L	Not PA
			≥0.4 µmol/L Optional testing IF blocking antibody, parietal cell antibody, IgG, gastrin levels	PA
	<100 pg/mL		Optional testing IF blocking antibody, parietal cell antibody, IgG, gastrin levels	PA
Folate	Low			Folate deficiency
	Low or Normal	RBC folate		

[a]Presence of macrocytic red blood cells.
PA, pernicious anemia.

Treatment and Monitoring Therapy

The standard treatment for vitamin B$_{12}$ deficiency is regular monthly intramuscular injections of at least 100 µg of vitamin B$_{12}$ to correct the vitamin deficiency. This regimen corrects the anemia and may correct the neurological complications if administered soon after the onset of symptoms. A further suggestion is that elderly patients with gastric atrophy should take tablets containing 25 µg to 1 mg of vitamin B$_{12}$ daily to prevent vitamin B$_{12}$ deficiency. This recommendation supposes that approximately 1% of vitamin B$_{12}$ is absorbed by mass action in the absence of IF.

A successful response to treatment with cobalamin (**vitamin B$_{12}$**) or folate begins within 8 to 12 hours in the bone marrow, with resolution of megaloblastic hematopoiesis. The reticulocyte count begins to increase 2 to 3 days after treatment and peaks in 5 to 8 days; higher and later peaks occur in more severe anemia. The hematocrit begins to increase in approximately 1 week and will normalize within 4 to 8 weeks. The MCV typically increases for the first 3 to 4 days, presumably because of reticulocytosis, and then begins to decrease. The normal reference range is expected to be reached in 25 to 78 days. Resolution of neurological abnormalities is dependent on the duration of loss. Most neurological symptoms will show maximal improvement within 6 months of initiation of therapy. Serum iron levels will begin to fall within 24 hours of successful treatment, but the patient must be observed over the next 2 to 3 weeks.

CHAPTER HIGHLIGHTS

Megaloblastic anemias can be classified into vitamin B$_{12}$ deficiencies and folic acid deficiencies.

Earlier studies suggested that pernicious anemia was restricted to Northern Europeans; however, newer studies report the disease in both blacks and Latin Americans. The median age at diagnosis is 60 years. Slightly more women than men are affected.

The term **megaloblastic** refers to the abnormal marrow erythrocyte precursor seen in processes, such as pernicious anemia, associated with altered DNA synthesis. Macrocytosis can occur in the absence of a megaloblastic process. For example, an increased MCV can result simply from an increase in the number of circulating reticulocytes, which are larger than mature erythrocytes. The most common disorder of cobalamin deficiency is pernicious anemia.

Pernicious anemia is immunologically related to an autoantibody to IF, a serum inhibitor of IF, and autoantibodies to parietal cells. A genetic predisposition to pernicious anemia is suggested by the clustering of the disease and of gastric autoantibodies in families, and by the association of the disease and gastric autoantibodies with autoimmune endocrinopathies.

Normal red cell maturation is dependent on many hematological factors, two of which are the vitamin B$_{12}$ coenzymes (also called cobalamin) and folates. Macrocytic anemias and megaloblastic dyspoiesis occur when one of these factors is absent.

Red blood cells in megaloblastic anemia have an abnormal nuclear maturation and imbalance between nuclear and cytoplasmic maturation. The absence of vitamin B$_{12}$ or folates impairs DNA synthesis, which slows nuclear replication and delays each step of maturation. The premitotic interval is prolonged. This results in a large nucleus, increased cytoplasmic RNA, and early synthesis of hemoglobin. Many cells never undergo mitosis and breakdown in the bone marrow, producing extremely increased levels of serum LDH.

In addition to dietary and other causes of deficiencies of cobalamin, a deficiency of TC II can produce a vitamin deficiency. Folic acid deficiencies appear to be less related to transport but are typically associated with conditions of either dietary inadequacy or malabsorption syndromes.

TABLE 11.2	Comparison of Selected Laboratory Findings in Various Types of Anemia	
Disorder	**Test**	**Result**
Aplastic anemia (Chapter 9)	Hemoglobin	Severely decreased
	PCV	Severely decreased
	Erythrocyte count	Severely decreased
	WBC count	Severely decreased
	Platelet count	Severely decreased
	MCV	Normal
	Serum iron	N/A
	TIBC	N/A
	Percent saturation	N/A
	Serum ferritin	N/A
Iron deficiency anemia (Chapter 10)	Hemoglobin	Decreased
	PCV	Decreased
	Erythrocyte count	Decreased
	WBC count	Normal
	Platelet count	Normal
	MCV	Decreased
	Serum iron	Severely decreased
	TIBC	Increased
	Percent saturation	Severely decreased
	Serum ferritin	Decreased
Anemia of chronic diseases (Chapter 10)	Hemoglobin	Decreased
	WBC count	Variable
	MCV	Usually normal
	MCH	Usually normal
	Platelet count	Normal
	Serum iron	Decreased
	TIBC	Decreased or normal
	Percent saturation	Decreased or normal
	Serum ferritin	Variable
Megaloblastic anemia (Chapter 11)	Hemoglobin	Severely decreased
	PCV	Severely decreased
	Erythrocyte count	Decreased
	WBC count	Slightly decreased
	Platelet count	Slightly decreased or normal
	MCV	
	Serum iron	Increased
	TIBC	Increased
	Percent saturation	Normal or decreased
	Serum ferritin	Increased

PCV, packed cell volume; WBC, white blood cell (leukocyte) count; MCH, mean corpuscular hemoglobin; MCV, mean corpuscular volume; TIBC, total iron–binding capacity; N/A, not applicable.

In pernicious anemia, the deficiency is caused by reduced IF secondary to gastric atrophy. In the majority of cases of pernicious anemia, anti-IFs or antibodies to parietal cells (large cells on the margin of the peptic glands of the stomach) have been reported. Most authorities consider the demonstration of these antibodies to support the theory that pernicious anemia is an autoimmune disorder. The presence of IF-blocking antibodies is diagnostic of pernicious anemia.

Pernicious anemia is frequently seen in those of Northern European ancestry, with clinical presentation during the fourth or fifth decade of life.

Pernicious anemia, the most common megaloblastic anemia, is a prototype of the entire group. The hematological picture is the same whether the cause is vitamin B_{12} or folic acid deficiency. However, supporting laboratory assays will differ for the various megaloblastic anemias.

CASE STUDY

CASE 11.1

A 50-year-old white woman had seen her physician and reported having no energy and feeling tired all the time. She also reported experiencing mild pain in the abdominal region. The physician ordered a routine CBC.

■ **Laboratory Data**

The results of the blood count were as follows:

Hemoglobin 6.2 g/dL
Hct 22%
RBC 1.7×10^{12}/L
WBC 4.0×10^9/L
Her RBC indices were as follows:
MCV 129.4 fL
MCH 36.5 pg
MCHC 28 g/dL

The peripheral blood smear demonstrated abnormalities of erythrocytes and leukocytes. On receipt of the laboratory data, the physician ordered the following additional tests: vitamin B_{12} and folate assays, reticulocyte count, serum iron and TIBC, serum bilirubin, and serum LDH. A fecal examination for occult blood was additionally ordered. The results of the tests were as follows:

Vitamin B_{12}: 121 pmol/L (decreased)
Serum folate level: normal
Reticulocyte count: 0.4%
Serum iron and TIBC: normal
Serum bilirubin: 1.8 mg/dL (slightly increased)
Serum LDH: >3,000 units (significantly increased)

The test result for occult blood was negative.

■ **Questions**

1. What category of anemia is suggested by the hematological findings in this case?

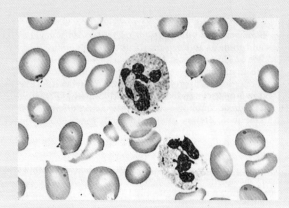

(Reprinted with permission from Rubin E, Farber JL. *Pathology*, 3rd ed, Philadephia, PA: Lippincott-Raven, 1999:1076.)

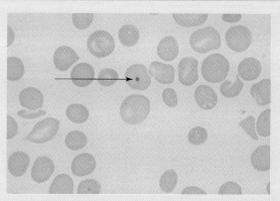

(Reprinted with permission from Anderson SC, *Anderson's Atlas of Hematology*, Philadephia, PA: Wolters Kluwer Health/ Lippincott Williams & Wilkins, Copyright 2003.)

2. What specific kind of anemia can be diagnosed based on the laboratory findings?
3. What is the etiology and physiological process in this anemia?

■ **Discussion**

1. The increased RBC size as seen on the peripheral blood (macrocytes) and the increased MCV indicate a macrocytic-megaloblastic–type anemia.
2. The two most common megaloblastic anemias are pernicious anemia and folic acid deficiency. Supporting laboratory assays can differentiate between these two types of anemias. In this case, a decreased vitamin B_{12} level, normal folic acid level, significantly increased LDH level, and absence of hydrochloric acid in the stomach support the diagnosis of pernicious anemia.
3. Many drugs can cause megaloblastic anemia by interfering with DNA synthesis, functioning as folic acid antagonists, or inhibiting purine and pyrimidine synthesis. Classic pernicious anemia is a chronic disease with a familial incidence, although no clear pattern of genetic transmission exists. Pernicious anemia usually becomes apparent in midlife or later. The macrocytosis in pernicious anemia is the result of a defect in nuclear maturation or DNA impairment. Because RNA synthesis is normal, the normal nuclear-cytoplasmic ratio is maturationally asynchronous. The disease complex includes atrophy of the gastric mucosa and changes caused by the deficiency of vitamin B_{12}. Atrophic gastric mucosa secretes neither IF nor hydrochloric acid. A few patients have antibodies to IF in their gastric juice and serum. This antibody condition causes a failure in the absorption of vitamin B_{12} even if it is available.

DIAGNOSIS: **Megaloblastic Anemia (Pernicious Anemia)**

REVIEW QUESTIONS

1. Megaloblastic anemias can be caused by
   - A. tapeworm infestation
   - B. gastric resection
   - C. nutritional deficiency
   - D. all of the above

2. Megaloblastic anemia related to folic acid deficiency is associated with
   - A. abnormal absorption
   - B. increased utilization
   - C. nutritional deficiency
   - D. all of the above

3. The underlying type A gastritis that causes pernicious anemia is immunologically related to
   - A. autoantibody to IF
   - B. low serum gastrin
   - C. autoantibody to parietal cells
   - D. both A and C

4. Cobalamin transport is mediated by
   - A. IF
   - B. TC II
   - C. R proteins
   - D. all of the above

5. In megaloblastic anemia, the typical erythrocytic indices are
   - A. MCV increased, MCH increased, and MCHC normal
   - B. MCV increased, MCH variable, and MCHC normal
   - C. MCV increased, MCH decreased, and MCHC normal
   - D. MCV normal, MCH increased, and MCHC normal

6. The peripheral erythrocyte morphology in folate deficiency is similar to pernicious anemia, and the RBCs are
   - A. small
   - B. normal size
   - C. large

7. In a case of classic pernicious anemia, the patient has
   - A. leukopenia
   - B. hypersegmented neutrophils
   - C. anemia
   - D. all of the above

8. The reticulocyte count in a patient with untreated pernicious anemia is characteristically
   - A. 0%
   - B. 0.3%
   - C. <1.0%
   - D. approximately 1.8%

Questions 9 through 15: Match the following clinical chemistry assays with their expected value in pernicious anemia: (An answer can be used more than once.)

9. _____ Serum haptoglobin–binding capacity
10. _____ Serum B_{12}
11. _____ Folate
12. _____ Serum iron
13. _____ Percent transferrin
14. _____ Serum LDH
15. _____ Unconjugated bilirubin
   - A. Decreased
   - B. Normal
   - C. Increased
   - D. Significantly increased

BIBLIOGRAPHY

Andres E, Boichot B, Schlienger J. Food cobalamin malabsorption: A usual cause of vitamin B_{12} deficiency, *Arch Intern Med*, 160:2061, 2000.

Carson-DeWitt RS. Pernicious anemia. In: Olendorf D, Jeryan C, Boyden K (eds), *Gale Encyclopedia of Medicine*, 1st ed, Farmington Hills, MI: The Thomson Corp., 1999:2224.

El-Newihi HM, et al. Gastric cancer and pernicious anemia appearing as pseudoachalasia, *SMJ*, September 1996 (retrieved from www.sma.org/ smj/96sept13.htm on February 21, 2003).

Emery E, Homans AC, Colletti RB. Vitamin B_{12} deficiency: a cause of abnormal movements in infants, *Pediatrics*, 99(2):255, 1997.

Harriman GR, et al. Vitamin B_{12} malabsorption in patients with acquired immunodeficiency syndrome, *Arch Intern Med*, 149:2039–2041, 1989.

Hillman RS, Finch CA. *Red Cell Manual*, 7th ed, Philadelphia, PA: FA Davis, 1996.

Kapadia C, Donaldson RM. Disorders of cobalamin (vitamin B_{12}) absorption and transport. *Ann Rev Med*, 36:93–110, 1985.

Moridani M, Ben-Poorat S. Laboratory investigation of vitamin B12 deficiency, *Labmedicine*, 37(3):166–174, 2006.

Snow CF. Laboratory diagnosis of vitamin B_{12} and folate deficiency, *Arch Intern Med*, 159:1289–1298, 1999.

Toh B-H, et al. Pernicious anemia. *N Engl J Med*, 337(20):1441–1448, 1997.

Turgeon ML. *Immunology and Serology in Laboratory Medicine*, 4 ed, St. Louis, MO: Elsevier, 2009.

CHAPTER 12

Hemolytic Anemias

OBJECTIVES

Hemolytic anemias

- Define the term **hemolytic anemia.**
- Name two categories of inherited hemolytic disorders.
- Explain the basis of structural membrane defects.
- Name and discuss five types or varieties of membrane defects.
- Explain the consequences of erythrocytic enzyme deficiency in two defects.
- Name and briefly explain three categories of acquired hemolytic anemia.
- Name three types of autoimmune hemolytic anemia (AIHA).
- Cite an example of isoimmune hemolytic anemia.
- Name four mechanisms of drug-induced hemolytic anemia.

- Describe the physiology and typical laboratory findings in hemolytic anemia.

Paroxysmal nocturnal hemoglobinuria (PNH)

- Characterize the etiology of PNH.
- Explain the physiology of PNH.
- Describe the clinical signs and symptoms, laboratory findings, and treatment protocol of PNH.

Case studies

- Apply knowledge of characteristics, physiology, clinical signs and symptoms, laboratory findings, and treatment to the case studies presented.

HEMOLYTIC ANEMIAS

The common denominator in hemolytic anemia is an increase in erythrocyte destruction initiated primarily by trapping of cells in sinuses of the spleen or liver and producing a decrease in the normal average life span of the erythrocyte. Increased bone marrow activity may compensate temporarily for this reduction. When the bone marrow fails to increase the production of erythrocytes to offset the loss of cells caused by hemolysis, anemia develops. Most anemias have a hemolytic component, and even in the anemias of marrow failure, the erythrocyte is somewhat defective. This is particularly evident in the case of dyserythropoietic syndromes, megaloblastic anemias, and thalassemias.

Hemolytic disruption of the erythrocyte involves an alteration in the erythrocytic membrane. The causes of this membrane alteration can be divided into

- Inherited hemolytic disorders (**intrinsic hemolytic anemia**)
- Acquired hemolytic disorders in which a factor outside the erythrocyte acts on it (**extrinsic hemolytic anemia**)

Further subdivisions within each classification are based on the causative mechanism. The terms **intravascular** and **extravascular hemolysis** refer to the site of destruction of the red blood cell, within the circulating blood or outside it, respectively (Table 12.1).

Inherited Hemolytic Anemia

Etiology

Inherited hemolytic disorders may affect the basic membrane structure, the erythrocytic enzymes, or the hemoglobin molecules within the red cell. Box 12.1 outlines selected examples of the genetically based hemolytic anemias.

Structural Membrane Defects

Primary defects of the red cell membrane head the list as a matter of taxonomy, not of prevalence. The cell membrane allows the erythrocyte with the flexibility and resilience to undergo numerous passages through the spleen during its 120-day life span. The ability of erythrocytes to deform and subsequently return to their original biconcave disc shape is determined by

1. Flexibility of the membrane, which relies on the structural and functional integrity of the membrane skeleton
2. Cytoplasmic viscosity determined primarily by hemoglobin
3. Cell surface-area-to-volume ratio

Some aspects of the erythrocyte membrane proteins (see Fig. 3-1B) are important in the pathophysiology of hemolytic anemia. Structural proteins, forming the erythrocyte skeleton, are α and β spectrin, actin, and protein 4.1. Red cell band 3 is the major integral membrane protein that regulates exchange and facilitates the transfer of CO_2 from tissues to lungs. Ankyrin is the major connecting protein that links the

TABLE 12.1	Comparison of Intravascular and Extravascular Hemolysis	
	Intravascular	**Extravascular**
Site of destruction of erythrocytes	Within blood vessels	Spleen or liver
Mechanism	Activation of complement IgM or IgG	Cell-mediated phagocytosis of IgM- or IgG-coated cells
Laboratory findings	Hemoglobinuria direct antiglobulin test Hemosiderinuria	Positive direct antiglobulin test Erythrocytes

membrane skeleton to the membrane bilayer. Mutations in any of the genes coding for the major membrane proteins can

- Alter the amount or function of the expressed proteins
- Compromise the integrity of the membrane
- Contribute to abnormal erythrocyte morphology

Most membrane defects result from genetic aberrations of cytoskeletal components, some represent rare disorders of cation permeability, and others arise from abnormalities of the lipid bilayer or integral membrane proteins. Genetic aberrations of nearly half of these skeletal and integral proteins are associated with hereditary hemolytic anemias. Inherited abnormalities in the skeletal protein network of the erythrocyte membrane can produce decreased membrane stability, decreased cell flexibility, and deviations from the normal discoid shape. Loss of membrane is another related disturbance. Membrane defects are commonly related to structural or quantitative defects in the skeletal protein, spectrin, or to abnormalities in the membrane's association with the other skeletal proteins. Cell membrane instability and decreased flexibility cause red cells to be removed from the circulation by the spleen. If the rate of hemolysis exceeds the erythropoietic compensatory mechanism of the bone marrow, anemia can result.

Examples of disorders in which skeletal protein defects have been described include hereditary spherocytosis and a variant, hereditary pyropoikilocytosis (HPP); hereditary elliptocytosis; and hereditary stomatocytosis. Another disorder in this grouping is hereditary xerocytosis.

Hereditary spherocytosis

Hereditary spherocytosis (HS) (Fig. 12.1) is a very heterogeneous form of hemolytic anemia transmitted in the majority of cases as an autosomal dominant trait; it is the most common prevalent hereditary hemolytic anemia among people of Northern European descent. It is not restricted to any single race. Manifestations of the disorder range from almost-normal carriers of the trait to cases of severe hemolytic anemia. Anemia may manifest itself anytime, from early infancy to later life.

BOX 12.1	

Examples of Inherited Hemolytic Anemias

STRUCTURAL MEMBRANE DEFECTS
Acanthocytosis
Hereditary spherocytosis
Hereditary elliptocytosis
Hereditary stomatocytosis
Hereditary xerocytosis
Rh_{null} disease

ERYTHROCYTIC ENZYME DEFECTS
G6PD deficiency
Glutathione reductase
Hexokinase
Pyruvate kinase

DEFECTS OF THE HEMOGLOBIN MOLECULE
Hb C disorder
Hb S-C disorder
Hb S-S disorder (sickle cell anemia)
Thalassemia

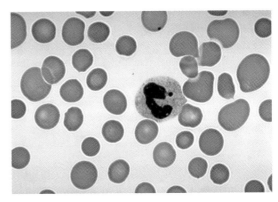

FIGURE 12.1 Hereditary spherocytosis. The peripheral blood smear shows many erythrocytes with decreased diameter, intense staining, and no central pallor (spherocytes). (Reprinted with permission from Rubin E, Farber JL. *Pathology*, 3rd ed, Philadelphia, PA: Lippincott Williams & Wilkins, 1999.)

HS results from the loss of erythrocytic membrane surface, as vesicles, due to membrane protein defects. The underlying abnormality is a defect in the interaction between the cell membrane skeleton and the bilayer. The defect mainly involves decreased proteins linked to spectrin-ankyrin-band 3 associations and weak contacts between spectrin and the negatively charged lipids of the inner half of the membrane bilayer. The identification of the red cell membrane defect has no major clinical implications but may be useful for a differential diagnosis from other hematologic disorders that mimic this form of hemolytic anemia.

Hemolysis is extravascular, occurring only in the presence of the spleen. In HS, secondary to membrane loss, the cell has a decreased surface-area-to-volume ratio, which changes the shape of the cell from discoid to spherocyte. Spherocytes have reduced cellular flexibility. The underlying mechanism of hemolysis is probably caused by physical fragmentation of the membrane; however, contraction of the membrane surface by another mechanism is a possibility. A deficiency of spectrin and defective binding of spectrin to band 4.1 or some other cytoskeletal abnormality may be present. Spherocytic cells demonstrate an abnormal permeability to sodium ion (Na^+), causing an influx of sodium at 10 times the normal rate.

Clinical severity is heterogeneous, depending on the protein lesion, but in the majority of cases, diagnosis is based on clinical and laboratory data. Some patients have compensated hemolytic disease, no anemia, little or no jaundice, and slight splenomegaly. Other patients may be severely anemic. Hemoglobin concentration can range from normal to decreased. Peripheral blood smears demonstrate the characteristic spherocytes. The mean corpuscular volume (MCV) is normal or slightly decreased. The mean corpuscular hemoglobin (MCH) is normal, but the mean corpuscular hemoglobin concentration (MCHC) is generally greater than 36%. Spherocytes are responsible for an increased MCHC. The osmotic fragility test is sensitive in 99% of cases. In some cases, diagnosis is not so straightforward in mild cases of HS or in the presence of associated diseases or can be falsely positive as in AIHA. A new screening method, a flow cytometric method, has been developed. Preliminary results of this assay indicate that this rapid and simple screening method is quite specific for HS.

Splenectomy corrects the anemia and hemolysis in severely afflicted patients. Spectrin-deficient patients show increased reticulocyte numbers and levels of unconjugated bilirubin postsplenectomy. Spherocytes can still be found. Some asplenic persons are at increased risk for life-threatening and fatal bacterial infections. Splenectomy carries a substantial risk for sepsis in children and adults (2.2% mortality rate).

Hereditary elliptocytosis

Figure 12.2 represents a comparatively common heterogeneous group of inborn disorders characterized by an overabundance of red blood cells and, in some individuals, by a hemolytic process.

Hereditary elliptocytosis (HE) and a closely related subtype of HE, HPP, are caused by defects in the membrane skeleton.

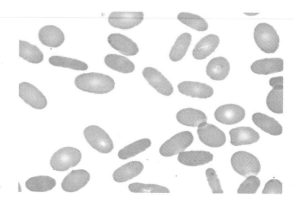

FIGURE 12.2 Ovalocyte (elliptocyte). (Reprinted with permission from Anderson SC. *Anderson's Atlas of Hematology*, Philadelphia, PA: Wolters Kluwer Health/Lippincott Williams & Wilkins.)

The majority of HE-associated defects occur in spectrin, the principal structural component of the red cell membrane skeleton. The pathogenesis and consequent morphological phenotype result from defects in horizontal interactions between components of the membrane skeleton, which include spectrin dimer self-association and spectrin-actin-protein 4.1 complex formation. HE is usually transmitted by a single (dominant) autosomal gene. In its homozygous form, it may produce a severe hemolytic anemia in infancy. The heterozygous form may show hemolysis.

Nine clinical variants of HE have been delineated, but these have been consolidated into three major categories based on the grounds of clinical severity and red cell morphology: common HE, spherocytic elliptocytosis, and stomatocytic elliptocytosis.

Spherocytic HE is a unique subset of elliptocytosis caused by dual inheritance of two nonallelic genes: one for mild HE and one for mild HS. This phenotypic hybrid is responsible for approximately 15% to 20% of HE cases in white families of European origin. The clinical course mimics that of conventional HS.

Stomatocytic HE is a unique variant peculiar to Melanesia and neighboring island groups. The red cells are only moderately oblong, and many of them display a transverse bridge of hemoglobin that connects with the opposite rim to create two central areas of pallor. Hemolysis is mild or absent.

The most prominent peripheral blood smear finding in HE is an increase in oval and elongated red cells (elliptocytes) to greater than 25% of the red blood cell population. A defect of the membrane cytoskeleton causes the elliptical red cell form, and it is acquired in the circulation. In addition, the membrane may fragment under the stresses of circulation. Moderate weakening causes elliptocytosis, but severe weakening causes membrane fragmentation and elliptocytosis.

Several different membrane molecular defects are suspected as causes. Of the known mutations, the most common is a functional defect of tetramer assembly of varying degrees due to decreased association of spectrin dimers and tetramers, caused by defective spectrin chains. Other abnormalities may include a deficiency in band 4.1, which binds spectrin to actin, and various abnormal interactions among several membrane proteins, including defective binding of ankyrin of integral protein.

Cells have a nearly normal life span. A very small proportion (10%) of patients with common HE have significant chronic hemolytic anemia. If membrane fragmentation exists, the life span is shortened. In addition, red cells are abnormally permeable to sodium ion (Na^+).

Most patients show little or no hemolysis. No anemia exists if the hemolysis is compensated for by erythropoiesis. However, a variant in black infants is associated with moderately severe anemia at birth and neonatal jaundice.

In symptomatic patients, splenectomy may be indicated. This will prevent hemolysis and protect the patient from chronic hemolysis, but the elliptocytes will remain.

Hereditary pyropoikilocytosis

HPP is a rare autosomal recessive disorder, representing a subset of common hereditary elliptocytosis HE, seen primarily in blacks. It is manifested in infancy or early childhood as a severe hemolytic anemia with significant poikilocytosis. As the name of the disorder implies, bizarre red cell shapes are evident when a peripheral blood smear is examined. MCV values range from 55 to 74 fL because of the prevalence of microspherocytes and red blood cell fragments. This multiformity of the poikilocytosis is unmatched in any other hemolytic disease.

Hereditary stomatocytosis

Hereditary stomatocytosis (Fig. 12.3) can be seen in the genetic hemoglobin defect, thalassemia, and in lead poisoning, HS, and alcoholic cirrhosis. The cellular appearance stems from a cation abnormality, because the erythrocytes contain increased sodium (Na^+) and decreased potassium (K^+). The specific membrane abnormality has not been identified, but abnormal membrane permeability has been implicated in the pathogenesis of hereditary stomatocytosis. Because the intracellular osmolality is exceeded and the intracellular concentration of cations increases, water enters the cell and overhydrated erythrocytes take on the appearance of stomatocytes or erythrocytes with a mouth-like opening. The cells are uniconcave. The MCHC is usually decreased and the MCV may be increased.

Anemia is usually mild to moderate. Bilirubin is increased and reticulocytosis is moderate. Peripheral blood smears have 10% to 50% stomatocytes. Osmotic fragility and autohemolysis are increased. Autohemolysis is partially corrected with glucose and adenosine triphosphate (ATP). Splenectomy yields variable responses.

In addition, Rh_{null} disease is also associated with the presence of stomatocytes. The lack of the Rh complex and stomatocytic membrane abnormality have not been explained.

Hereditary Xerocytosis

Hereditary xerocytosis is a permeability disorder. In vitro, the thermal instability of spectrin suggests a defect in qualitative spectrin abnormality. The net loss of intracellular K^+ exceeds the passive Na^+ influx, yielding a net Na^+ gain. This causes the red cell to dehydrate. The MCHC increases and the red cell appears contracted and spiculated. When the MCHC increases beyond 37%, cytoplasmic viscosity increases and cellular deformability decreases. Rigid red cells are trapped in the spleen and removed from the circulation.

Peripheral blood smears demonstrate budding, fragments, microspherocytes, and bizarre red cell fragments. The osmotic fragility test is abnormal, especially after incubation. Autohemolysis is increased and the hemolysis is not corrected with glucose.

Rh_{null} Disease

Rh_{null} disease, or Rh deficiency syndrome, is a rare hereditary disorder causing mild, compensated chronic hemolytic anemia. This disorder is associated with stomatocytosis, spherocytosis, and the deletion of all Rh-Hr determinants including the Landsteiner-Weiner (LW) antigen from the red blood cells. Rh_{null} cells are abnormally permeable to K^+ and partly compensate for this leakiness and the resultant cation deficiency by reinforcing the number and activity of Na-K-ATPase pumps. The abnormal red cell morphology may be related to the increased K^+ leak rate. The resulting anemia is mild but variable. Typically, the hemoglobin concentration is between 11 and 13 g/dL and reticulocytes are moderately increased. Many of the red blood cells are spheroidal or stomatocytic. Hemoglobin F levels are often elevated.

Acanthocytosis

Acanthocytes (Fig 12.4) are dense contracted or spheroidal red blood cells with multiple thorny projections or spicules. Acanthocytes are prevalent in two very different constitutional disorders: abetalipoproteinemia and spur cell anemia. Abetalipoproteinemia is a rare derangement of lipid metabolism resulting from a genetic inability to synthesize apolipoprotein B (apoB), the protein that coats chylomicrons. Most red cell membrane lipids are in exchange equilibrium with the corresponding plasma lipoprotein lipids. Acanthocytes are a manifestation of the profound disturbances in plasma lipoprotein levels found in this disorder.

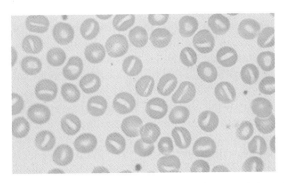

FIGURE 12.3 Stomatocyte. (Reprinted with permission from Anderson SC. *Anderson's Atlas of Hematology*, Philadelphia, PA: Wolters Kluwer Health/Lippincott Williams & Wilkins, Copyright 2003.)

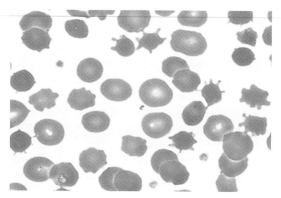

FIGURE 12.4 Hereditary acanthocytosis. (Reprinted with permission from Anderson SC. *Anderson's Atlas of Hematology*, Philadelphia, PA: Wolters Kluwer Health/Lippincott Williams & Wilkins, Copyright 2003.)

Moderate anemia may develop in young children, but adults suffer from only mild anemia. MCV, MCH, MCHC, and osmotic fragility are normal.

Spur Cell Hemolytic Anemia

This form of acanthocyte-associated hemolytic anemia is seen in patients with established alcoholic cirrhosis. A fatal hemolytic process will develop in approximately 5% to 10% of patients. Hemolysis usually becomes severe and may necessitate maintenance transfusions. In most patients, the hemoglobin concentrations level off at 5 to 7 g/dL. Reticulocyte counts fluctuate between 10% and 20%, and ^{51}Cr-labeled red cell half-life survival may be as short as 5 to 6 days. Maintenance blood transfusions are common.

Other causes of acanthocytosis can include neonatal hepatitis, infantile pyknocytosis, the McLeod blood group, and severe malnutrition (e.g., anorexia nervosa).

Neuroacanthocytosis

Neuroacanthocytosis (NA) is a heterogeneous group of neurodegenerative disorders associated with acanthocytosis in peripheral blood. Clinically, NA is characterized by a combination of neurobehavioral changes. The cause of the disorder is unknown, but recent evidence is increasing that the erythrocytic membrane is defective, with major integral membrane protein band 3 being reported in a few cases. Two cases of NA have expressed an alteration of erythrocyte membrane protein 4.1R. It is hypothesized that brain protein 4.1R could play a role in the neurodegenerative disorder.

Erythrocytic Enzyme Defects

Like the structural membrane defects, erythrocytic enzyme defects are inherited. The anemias in this group are caused by deficiencies of

1. Glucose-6-phosphate dehydrogenase (G6PD)
2. Pyruvate kinase (PK)
3. Methemoglobin reductase

The clinical effects of these enzymopathies vary widely. Some individuals manifest no hematological abnormalities, but the erythrocytes share the abnormality that produces a malfunction in other tissues. Certain inborn or genetic errors may produce hematological disorders other than hemolytic anemia. In a number of erythrocytic enzyme defects, such as deficiencies in hexokinase, glucose-phosphate isomerase, and PK, the sole clinical manifestation is hemolytic anemia. Many genetic enzyme errors cause multisystem disease with a hemolytic syndrome as one component.

Glucose-6-Phosphate Dehydrogenase

Glucose-6-phosphate dehydrogenase (G6PD Deficiency), the most common aerobic erythrocyte enzyme deficiency, is related to oxidant stress induced by several drugs, infection or fava beans, in afflicted individuals. Drugs such as primaquine can induce a hemolytic episode in approximately 10% of American black males, whereas the drugs chloramphenicol, quinine, and quinidine and the legume fava beans can precipitate a hemolytic incident in nonblacks.

The X-linked enzymopathy, G6PD deficiency, affects 400 million people worldwide. Some areas of the Middle East have an extremely high prevalence of G6PD deficiency, for example, 62% of male Kurdish Jews and 24% of male Bahrainis.

More than 400 variants of this enzyme have been identified by their biochemical properties. To date, more than 60 G6PD-deficient class I mutations have been identified. A Mediterranean variant, a missense genetic mutation, has been detected at the molecular level throughout the coding region of G6PD gene. G6PD is inherited as an incomplete dominant trait. Full expression of the trait is seen in homozygous males. In females, full expression of the disorder occurs when two mutant genes are inherited. If only one mutant gene is inherited by a female (heterozygous), two populations of red blood cells exist. One population of red blood cells has a normal enzyme content; the other red blood cells are G6PD deficient.

The erythrocyte, unlike other body cells, cannot compensate for an unstable enzyme. The absence of organelles to carry out oxidative phosphorylation on a compensatory basis creates unique problems for the red cells. The enzyme G6PD catalyzes this reaction:

$$\text{Glucose-6-phosphate} + \text{NADP} \xrightarrow{\text{G6PD}} 6\text{-phosphogluconate} + \text{NADPH}$$

This is the first step in the pentose-phosphate pathway (aerobic-glycolytic pathway). Nicotinamide-adenine dinucleotide phosphate (NADPH) produced by this reaction is an important intracellular reducing agent. An excess intermediate product, oxidized glutathione, accumulates in the red cell because of the absence of NADPH and forms insoluble complexes with hemoglobin that result in Heinz body formation.

Laboratory findings (see Fig. 12.5) in this disorder include a quantitatively decreased level of G6PD, a positive autohemolysis test result, and the presence of Heinz bodies on peripheral blood smears prepared for Heinz body screening. Heinz bodies are not visible on routinely stained, Wright-stain preparations.

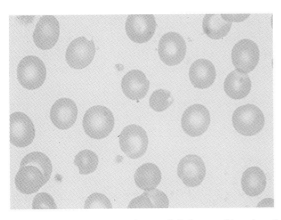

FIGURE 12.5 Glucose-6-phosphtase deficiency. (Reprinted with permission from Anderson SC. *Anderson's Atlas of Hematology*, Philadelphia, PA: Wolters Kluwer Health/Lippincott Williams & Wilkins, Copyright 2003.)

Pyruvate Kinase

The second most common inherited erythrocyte enzyme deficiency is in PK. PK is an autosomal recessive trait. The Pennsylvania Amish have a high frequency of PK deficiency, but it exists worldwide. The heterozygote allele frequencies range between 1% and 3.6% in North America, Europe, and parts of Asia. A study in African Americans suggested that the frequency of the heterozygote allele was 2.4 times more common in Africans than in whites.

The human PK-LR gene codes for red cell PK. PK is essential in the Embden-Meyerhof pathway of anaerobic glycolysis. Mature erythrocytes lack mitochondria and are exclusively dependent on anaerobic glycolysis for the generation of ATP. A deficiency of PK and subsequent deficiency in generating ATP produces loss of water and results in cell shrinkage, distortion of the shape of the cell, and increased membrane rigidity. These changes subsequently lead to premature destruction of erythrocytes in the spleen and liver as well as hemolytic anemia.

PK-deficient erythrocytes have been shown to be resistant to malaria, perhaps due to ATP depletion, which impairs parasite invasion in vitro. Low ATP concentration also increases 2,3-diphosphoglycerate (DPG), which disrupts spectrin, actin, and protein 4.1 interactions and causes membrane instability and impacts intracellular parasite survival. It also inhibits G6PD leading to increased oxidative stress. In vivo, other factors such as splenic clearance, early phagocytosis, and decreased cyto-adherence of parasitized red cells occur in PK deficiency.

Peripheral blood smears of patients with PK deficiency usually appear as normochromic, normocytic erythrocytes with varying degrees of polychromatophilia (reticulocytosis). Patients with this disorder have elevated 2,3-DPG because of the abnormal enzyme block.

Diagnosis of the disorder is based on a specific assay for the PK enzyme. The fluorescent screening test is based on the following coupled enzyme assay:

$$PEP + ADP + Mg^{2+} \xrightarrow{\text{PK enzyme}} Pyruvate + ATP$$

$$\underset{\text{(UV Fluorescence)}}{Pyruvate} + NADH + H^+ \xrightarrow{\text{LDH enzyme}} \underset{\text{(No Fluorescence)}}{Lactate + NAD^+}$$

This assay reflects the fact that NADH fluoresces when it is illuminated with long-wave ultraviolet (UV) light, but NAD does not fluoresce.

Methemoglobin Reductase Deficiency

Hemoglobin that is oxidized from the ferrous to the ferric valency state is called methemoglobin. Approximately 1% of circulating hemoglobin in normal individuals is methemoglobin. Hereditary deficiency of the enzyme NADH-methemoglobin reductase results in increased levels of methemoglobin. A deficiency in the enzyme, also called NADH diaphorase, can result from inheritance of an autosomal recessive trait or in conjunction with hemoglobin M disease, or as a result of exposure to toxic substances or various drugs. The predominant clinical manifestation of methemoglobin reductase deficiency is cyanosis because the methemoglobin cannot carry oxygen to the tissues (see Chapter 13 for an additional discussion of this disorder).

Acquired Hemolytic Anemia

Etiology

Acquired hemolytic anemias can be classified according to the agent or condition responsible for inducing the hemolysis. Selected examples of agents and conditions associated with acquired hemolytic anemias are presented in Box 12.2.

A major distinction exists between acute hemolysis of red cells, which results from damage done directly to the cell membrane, and hemolytic anemias caused by immunologic responses.

Drugs, Chemicals, and Venoms

Intravascular hemolysis can result from exposure to environmental agents and conditions. Fortunately, the destruction of erythrocytes usually ceases when the conditions no longer exist. This is in contrast to congenital membrane defects, which are continuous. Lead from gasoline, paint, or other industrial products directly interferes with ATP production and inhibits heme synthesis.

Quinine sensitivity is a new, unusual cause of hemolytic uremic syndrome. Adult hemolytic uremic syndrome of acute onset with accompanying microangiopathic hemolytic anemia, thrombocytopenia, renal failure, neutropenia, and low-grade disseminated intravascular coagulation (DIC) has been observed. Quinine, in one case in tonic water, was implicated by the finding of quinine-dependent antibodies reactive with platelets, granulocytes, and erythrocytes in patient serum.

This recently described syndrome can occur with or without associated DIC or granulocytopenia. Only a small percentage of patients taking quinidine and quinine have this sensitivity (quinine and quinidine appear to do so more often than other

Examples of Agents and Conditions Associated With Acquired Hemolytic Anemias

CHEMICALS, DRUGS, VENOMS
Aniline
Copper (Wilson disease)
Lead from gasoline or paint
Naphthalene (found in moth balls)
Nitrobenzene
Phenacetin
Phenol derivatives
Resorcinol
Sulfonamides

INFECTIOUS MICROORGANISMS
Bacteria: *Clostridium* sp., cholera, *E. coli O157:H7*, typhoid fever
Protozoa: *Leishmania*, malaria (*Plasmodium* sp.), toxoplasmosis

IMMUNE MECHANISMS (ANTIBODIES)
Autoimmune anemia due to cold-reactive antibodies
Cold hemagglutinin disease
Idiopathic or secondary
Paroxysmal cold hemoglobinuria
Autoimmune anemia due to warm-reactive antibodies
Drug induced
Idiopathic
Secondary
Lymphoproliferative disorders (CLL, malignancies, systemic lupus erythematosus, viruses)
Hemolytic disease of the fetus and newborn (HDFN)
Incompatible blood transfusion
Paroxysmal nocturnal hemoglobinuria

PHYSICAL AGENTS
Severe burns

TRAUMATIC AND MICROANGIOPATHIC HEMOLYTIC ANEMIAS
Disseminated intravascular coagulation
E. coli O157:H7
Hemolytic uremic syndrome
Prosthetic cardiac valves
Thrombotic thrombocytopenic purpura

agents). Platelets are the preferred target for drug-induced antibodies, but granulocytes, erythrocytes, and probably other tissues are sometimes affected. Patients usually recover spontaneously when the provoking drug is withdrawn. The mechanism by which drugs promote selective binding of these immunoglobulins to target glycoproteins is not fully understood, but evidence suggests that the inciting medications bind reversibly to specific protein domains to form complexes

or to induce conformational changes (neoantigens) for which the antibodies are specific. Deposition of fibrin in glomeruli and renal failure are characteristic features of the hemolytic uremic syndrome. Plasminogen-activator inhibitor type 1 (PAI-1) is believed to be the circulating inhibitor of fibrinolysis in the hemolytic uremic syndrome.

Venoms from some types of snakes contain hemolysins that can produce intravascular hemolysis and also initiate DIC.

Infectious Microorganisms

Several mechanisms of infectious organisms (Table 12.2) cause destruction of erythrocytes. The intraerythrocytic protozoa (e.g., malaria) rupture red cells. Malarial anemia is the major cause of morbidity and mortality of millions of individuals living in endemic areas who are infected by the malarial species, *Plasmodium falciparum*.

In some cases, such as with *Clostridium perfringens*, hemolytic toxin is released from bacteria. In other cases, extravascular hemolysis can be caused by infectious agents such as *Bartonella*.

A significant infectious cause of hemolytic uremic syndrome was discovered a decade ago. *Escherichia coli O157:H7* has emerged as a major cause of both sporadic cases and outbreaks of diarrhea in North America. The first report was associated with consumption of undercooked ground beef from a chain of fast-food restaurants. Little was known about the pathophysiology, epidemiology, or clinical sequelae of infection with *E. coli O157:H7*. Several studies have shown that infection with *E. coli O157:H7* is responsible for most cases of the hemolytic uremic syndrome, which is a major cause of acute renal failure in children. This microorganism is estimated to cause more than 20,000 infections and as many as 250 deaths each year. Shiga toxins 1, 2, or both cause microangiopathic hemolytic anemia as a result of endothelial cell injury.

Immune Mechanisms (Antibodies)

A wide variety of disorders of acquired hemolytic anemia result from immune mechanisms. In these disorders, the survival of erythrocytes is reduced because of the deposition of immunoglobulin or complement, or both, on the cell membrane. The immune hemolytic anemias can be grouped according to the presence of autoantibodies, isoantibodies, or drug-related antibodies (Box 12.3).

Autoimmune anemias can be due to cold-reactive or warm-reactive antibodies. Other types of disorders in this category include hemolytic disease of the fetus and newborn (HDFN) and fetus, incompatible blood transfusion, and PNH.

Autoimmune Hemolytic Anemias

AIHAs are caused by an altered immune response resulting in production of antibody against the patient's own erythrocytes, with subsequent hemolysis. The definitive cause of autoantibody production is unknown.

Development of AIHA in patients with lymphoproliferative or autoimmune disorders may be related to some abnormality with B cells, T cells, macrophages, or the interaction between these cells. Some unusual aspects of the epidemiology of AIHA are association with

| TABLE 12.2 | Representative Microorganisms Associated With Hemolytic Anemia |

Bacteria	Parasites	Viruses
Bartonella bacilliformis	Babesia microti	Cytomegalovirus
Borrelia recurrentis	B. divergens	Epstein-Barr
Clostridium perfringens	Leishmania sp.	
Escherichia coli O157	Plasmodium falciparum	
Haemophilus influenzae	Trypanosoma brucei gambiense	
Mycobacterium tuberculosis	T. brucei rhodesiense	
Mycoplasma pneumoniae		
Neisseria meningitides		
Salmonella typhi		
Streptococcus species		
Vibrio cholerae		

- Blood transfusion
- Pregnancy
- Immune hemolysis with allogeneic hematopoietic cell transplantation
- Immune hemolysis with orthotopic solid-organ transplantation

Warm-Type Autoimmune Hemolytic Anemia

In warm-type AIHA (Table 12.3), there is immunoglobulin G (IgG) coating of erythrocytes with or without complement fixation. The predominant type of reported cases of AIHA are of the warm type. Autoantibodies are usually directed at Rh antigens but also can be anti-U, anti-LW, anti-Kell, and Jk^a or Fy^a.

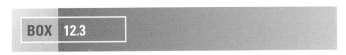

BOX 12.3

Classification of Immune Hemolytic Anemia

AUTOIMMUNE HEMOLYTIC ANEMIAS
Associated with warm-type antibodies
Associated with cold-type antibodies
Associated with both warm- and cold-type antibodies

ISOIMMUNE HEMOLYTIC ANEMIAS
Hemolytic disease of the fetus and newborn (HDFN)
Rh incompatibility
ABO incompatibility

DRUG-INDUCED HEMOLYTIC ANEMIA
Adsorption of immune complexes to red cell membrane
Adsorption of drug to red cell membrane
Induction of autoantibody to drugs
Nonimmunological adsorption of immunoglobulin to red blood cell membrane

Clearance of the erythrocyte occurs mostly in the spleen. In the absence of complement fixation, it appears that the Fc portion of the immunoglobulin molecule bound to the red blood cell interacts with the Fc receptor present on the membrane of splenic macrophages. Therefore, sensitized red blood cells are retained, phagocytosed, or fragmented by splenic macrophages during their passage through the spleen.

Moderate to severe anemia can result. Peripheral blood smears frequently exhibit spherocytosis, schistocytes, polychromasia, and nucleated erythrocytes. The percentage of reticulocytes is high in approximately half of affected patients.

The clinical course of patients with warm-type AIHA is characterized by periods of remission and relapse. In secondary AIHA, the course and prognosis are related to the nature of the underlying disease. In idiopathic AIHA, the complications can be severe and fatal.

Cold-Type Autoimmune Hemolytic Anemia

In AIHA associated with cold-type autoantibody (e.g., cold hemagglutinin disease), the erythrocytes are usually coated with IgM. The antibody is usually anti-I. Complement fixation occurs frequently. If the entire complement system is activated, intravascular hemolysis can occur. Extravascular hemolysis can occur if complement activation is incomplete and no lysis of the red blood cells occurs.

IgG can be a cause of paroxysmal cold hemoglobinuria.

Warm- and Cold-Type Autoimmune Hemolytic Anemias

AIHA associated with both warm and cold autoantibodies is mediated by IgG warm antibodies and complement as well as IgM cold hemagglutinins. A high percentage of patients also have systemic lupus erythematosus. Autoimmune hemolysis in pregnancy from a combination of warm and cold antibodies has an estimated incidence of 1 in 50,000 pregnancies. Pregnancy outcomes are usually favorable, if the autoantibody is idiopathic or pregnancy-associated.

TABLE 12.3 Comparison of Warm and Cold Autoimmune Hemolytic Anemia		
	Warm AIHA	**Cold AIHA**
Optimal temperature of reactivity	37°C	4°C
Immunoglobulin class	IgG	IgM
Complement activation	±	+
Site of hemolysis	Extravascular	Intravascular

Isoimmune Hemolytic Anemia

This form of anemia usually occurs in newborn infants because of transplacental passage of maternal antibodies directed toward antigens of the baby's cells. Isoimmune hemolytic anemia is most commonly the result of ABO incompatibility between the mother and the baby (e.g., the mother is group O, whereas the baby is group A).

Drug-Induced Immune Hemolytic Anemia

Drugs causing drug-induced immune hemolytic anemia (DIIHA) are most commonly cefotetan, ceftriaxone, and peperacillin. DIIHA is rare with an incidence estimated at about 1 in 1 million of the population. AIHA is about 10 times more likely to occur than DIIHA. Immune hemolytic anemia may occur following the administration of drugs (e.g., insulin), antihistamines, and sulfonamides.

Two types of drug-related antibodies exist:

1. drug-independent antibodies, for example, antibodies that can be detected in vitro without adding any drug. In vivo and in vitro characteristics are identical to red blood cell antibodies.
2. drug-dependent antibodies, for example, antibodies that will only react in vitro in the presence of drug bound to RBCs or added to the patient's serum in a test system to detect drug antibodies.

With drug-dependent mechanisms, one mechanism is universally accepted. Some drugs bind covalently to proteins on the RBC membrane. This does no harm to the RBCs. If the patient produces an IgG antibody to the drug the antibody will bind to the drug on the RBCs, macrophages will phagocytize, and extravascular RBC destruction occurs. Occasionally, complement may be involved. The prototype drug demonstrating this type of reaction is penicillin but cefotetan can react by this mechanism.

Most drugs that cause acute and severe intravascular hemolysis potentially leading to death usually involve drug-dependent antibodies that activate complement.

Other mechanisms of interaction of a drug-induced antibody with the red cell membrane are currently being investigated.

Physical Agents

Hemolysis occurs within 24 hours of suffering severe burns. Because the red cells become fragile after exposure to heat, they form fragments and microspheres. These structures are removed by the spleen, with a subsequent rapid drop in the circulating red cell volume.

Microangiopathic red cell destruction

DIC is one example of a microangiopathic hemolytic anemia. DIC is a consumptive coagulopathy that involves depositions of microthrombi in the blood vessels. These depositions form surfaces that damage circulating red cells. Traumatic injury caused by repeated impact of the capillary bed produces red cell damage in **march anemia**, a condition diagnosed in soldiers after intense marches. Damage to capillary beds can also be seen in long-distance runners and individuals who play high-impact sports.

Other examples of microangiopathies include

- Thrombotic thrombocytopenic purpura (TTP)
- Hemolytic uremia syndrome (HUS)
- HELLP syndrome (Hemolysis, Elevated Liver enzyme levels, Low Platelet count)

Medical Conditions

Various lymphoproliferative disorders and disseminated malignancy can be the cause of red cell hemolysis. One example of such a condition is chronic lymphocytic leukemia (CLL).

Pathophysiology

The normal erythrocyte has an average life span of 120 days. As the red cell becomes older, membrane changes occur and the cell is phagocytized. Most red cell destruction (80% to 90%) is presumed to be extravascular, within macrophages of the mononuclear phagocyte system of the liver and spleen. The red cell membrane and hemoglobin become separated. The red cell membrane remnants are phagocytized and eventually leave the body.

Hemoglobin is then further reduced into its two major components: heme and globin. The globin portion is further reduced to its constituent amino acids. Although some of the amino acids are further catabolized, most of the amino acids become part of the circulating amino acid pool and are reused in the synthesis of new proteins. The heme portion is broken down into iron, carbon monoxide, and biliverdin. Most of the iron will be recycled into new molecules of hemoglobin. Biliverdin will be converted to bilirubin. After entering into the plasma portion of the circulating blood as unconjugated bilirubin, being bound to albumin, and being transported to the liver where it is converted to conjugated bilirubin, it is finally excreted into the biliary system.

When red blood cell destruction is increased, the formation of unconjugated bilirubin exceeds the ability of the liver to conjugate it. This condition produces elevated levels of unconjugated bilirubin in the blood plasma, and jaundice may result.

Some normal erythrocyte catabolism occurs intravascularly. In this situation, free hemoglobin is released into the blood plasma and is rapidly bound to the glycoprotein haptoglobin. This large molecular complex of hemoglobin and haptoglobin cannot pass through the renal glomeruli. Most of the molecular complex is taken up by the liver, whereas some is taken by the bone marrow.

If the amount of intravascular hemoglobin increases, all the available haptoglobin will become saturated. Remaining free hemoglobin continues to circulate in the plasma and may dissociate into smaller components capable of passing through the glomeruli. If these smaller hemoglobin components are not reabsorbed by the proximal tubular cells of the kidney, the hemoglobin will be excreted in the urine (hemoglobinuria).

Diagnostic Tests

Hemolysis is characterized by increased erythrocyte destruction and increased hematopoietic activity in normal bone marrow.

The patient with hemolytic anemia is expected to have decreased hemoglobin, Hct, and red blood cell count. Blood smear examination will typically reveal the presence of many spherocytic erythrocytes (see Fig. 12.6), a hallmark abnormality in hemolytic anemia. Other red cell abnormalities include acanthocytes, schistocytes, stomatocytes, polychromatophilia, target cells, and early erythroid forms such as rubricytes (see Fig 12.7).

The reticulocyte count (see Chapters 5 and 26) is usually increased unless hematopoiesis is suppressed. An osmotic fragility test will exhibit increased fragility as a result of the presence of spherocytes.

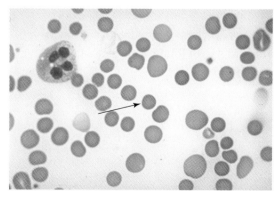

FIGURE 12.6 Spherocyte. (Reprinted with permission from Anderson SC. *Anderson's Atlas of Hematology*, Philadelphia, PA: Wolters Kluwer Health/Lippincott Williams & Wilkins, Copyright 2003.)

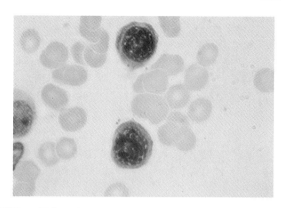

FIGURE 12.7 Polychromatophilic normoblast (rubricyte). (Reprinted with permission from Anderson SC. *Anderson's Atlas of Hematology*, Philadelphia, PA: Wolters Kluwer Health/Lippincott Williams & Wilkins, Copyright 2003.)

Clinical chemistry assays used to reflect increased erythrocyte destruction are unconjugated (indirect bilirubin) and serum haptoglobin. Bilirubin levels, a manifestation of the catabolism of heme derived from erythrocyte phagocytized by the mononuclear phagocytic system (MPS), rarely exceed 3 to 4 mg/dL. Serum haptoglobin, an indicator of intravascular and extravascular hemolysis, is decreased in the presence of erythrocyte destruction. Haptoglobin levels reflect clearance by the MPS of a complex formed in the pathway between liberated hemoglobin and circulatory haptoglobin. Rapid clearance is reflected in decreased haptoglobin levels. Falsely elevated levels of haptoglobin arise in inflammatory conditions or malignancies; falsely decreased levels can result from a genetically controlled deficiency of haptoglobin in black populations or because of decreased synthesis of this protein by the liver caused by hepatocellular disease. Supporting laboratory tests can include

Antiglobulin (AHG) (direct and indirect) test
Occult blood screening (to rule out bleeding)
Chromium 51 red cell survival studies
Bone marrow studies
Determinations of G6PD values
Heinz body preparation (see Fig. 12.8)

Prussian blue iron stain of urinary sediment to detect the hemosiderin- and ferritin-containing renal tubular cells sloughed off several days after a hemolytic episode.

Table 12.4 and Box 12.4 give, respectively, the typical laboratory findings in a hemolytic anemia and the supplementary tests that may be needed to establish a differential diagnosis.

PAROXYSMAL NOCTURNAL HEMOGLOBINURIA

Etiology

PNH is commonly regarded as a type of hemolytic anemia. It is actually a rare, acquired, clonal blood disorder caused by a nonmalignant clonal expansion of one or

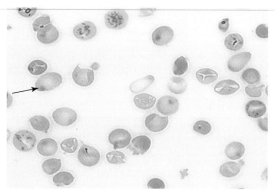

FIGURE 12.8 Heinz bodies. (Reprinted with permission from Anderson SC. *Anderson's Atlas of Hematology*, Philadelphia, PA: Wolters Kluwer Health/Lippincott Williams & Wilkins, Copyright 2003.)

more hematopoietic stem cells that have acquired somatic mutation of the X-chromosome gene, PIGA. PNH results in a deficiency of cell-surface glycosyl phosphatidylinositol anchored proteins (GPI-APs) that are normal expressed on hematopoetic cells. This red cell membrane defect renders one population of red cells significantly sensitive to complement. Chronic intravascular hemolysis of PNH is mediated by the alternative pathway of complement.

PNH expresses itself with hemolytic anemia, bone marrow failure, and thrombosis. Intravascular hemolysis in this disorder is characterized by intermittent (paroxysmal) sleep-associated (nocturnal) blood in the urine (hemoglobinuria). Some patients with PNH suffer from chronic hemolysis that is not associated with sleep and manifest no obvious hemoglobinuria.

Epidemiology

Twenty-five percent of cases will evolve into or from aplastic anemia. Approximately 5% to 10% of patients will have terminal acute myelogenous leukemia.

The median age of patients at diagnosis is 42 years (range, 16 to 75 years). Median survival after diagnosis is 10 years. Spontaneous long-term remission can occur.

Pathophysiology

Mutations occur in a gene termed PIG-A and result in the failure to present a large class of proteins on the hematopoietic cell surface. These proteins share a unique linkage to the surface membrane through a glycolipid structure called the GPI anchor. Absence of a GPI-anchored receptor prevents several proteins from binding to the red cell membrane. These include the complement-regulatory proteins, CD55 and CD59, whose absence results in enhanced complement-mediated lysis. This explains the characteristic intravascular hemolysis in the syndrome.

The biochemical basis of marrow failure in patients with PNH is unknown. Some observers have suggested that clones emerge because they are favored by certain extrinsic conditions. Patients may harbor clones with different PIG-A gene mutations, a finding consistent with the independent proliferation of genetically altered hematopoietic stem cells under some selective pressure.

Clinical Signs and Symptoms

PNH begins insidiously in patients between the age of 30 and 60 years. Irregular episodes of hemoglobinuria associated with sleep are a startling manifestation of this disorder. Many

TABLE 12.4	Typical Profile of Quantitative Laboratory Findings in Hemolytic Anemias
Test	**Result**
Hemoglobin, hematocrit, RBC count	Decreased
Serum haptoglobin	Decreased
Red blood cell survival (^{51}Cr)	Decreased
Lactic dehydrogenase (LDH) isoenzymes (LD_1 and LD_2)	Increased
Bilirubin (total)	Usually increased
Antiglobulin test	Positive or negative

of the clinical manifestations of the disease result from complement-mediated intravascular hemolysis. Clinical manifestations include chronic hemolysis, thrombosis, recurrent infections, and a tendency toward bone marrow aplasia.

The leading cause of death in PNH is thrombosis, but related late-developing bacterial and fungal infections can also be life-threatening events. PNH is a chronic disease. Patients have an average life expectancy of more than 10 years.

Laboratory Findings

Most patients have severe anemia with hemoglobin concentrations less than 6 g/dL. Peripheral blood smears may reveal hypochromic, microcytic red cells if an iron deficiency state has developed owing to cell lysis. The sucrose hemolysis (sugar-water) test is a diagnostic procedure (see thepoint. lww.com/Turgeon5e). Flow cytometry is becoming more commonly used because it is more specific and sensitive than the sucrose lysis test. Hemosiderinuria, the excretion of an iron-containing pigment derived from hemoglobin on disintegration of red cells, is a classic manifestation of chronic intravascular hemolysis. The use of flow cytometry for immunophenotyping erythrocytes for the diagnosis of PNH is increasing.

Treatment

Treatment includes blood transfusion therapy, antibiotics, and anticoagulants. Allogeneic bone marrow transplantation is the only curative therapy. Eculizumab, a monoclonal antibody that blocks terminal complement activation, is highly effective in reducing hemolysis, improving quality of life, and reducing the risk for thrombosis in PNH patients.

PAROXYSMAL COLD HEMOGLOBINURIA

Paroxysmal cold hemoglobinuria is the least common type of AIHA. It is transient and self-limiting but can produce serious hemolysis of erythrocytes. It occurs almost exclusively in children in association with viral disorders. Erythrocyte destruction is the result of a cold-reacting, IgG autoantibody termed autohemolysin. This autoagglutinin, the Donath-Landsteiner antibody with anti-P specificity, only attaches to erythrocytes at cooler temperatures and then activates complement in warmer temperatures. This type of antibody activity is called biphasic hemolysis.

CHAPTER HIGHLIGHTS

The common denominator in hemolytic anemia is an increase in red cell destruction and a decrease in the normal average life span of the erythrocyte. Increased bone marrow activity may compensate temporarily for this reduction. However, when the bone marrow fails to increase the production of erythrocytes to offset the loss of cells caused by hemolysis, anemia develops.

Hemolytic disruption of the red cell always involves an alteration in the erythrocytic membrane. The causes of this membrane alteration can be divided into inherited hemolytic disorders (**intrinsic hemolytic anemia**) and acquired hemolytic disorders in which a factor outside the red blood cell acts on it (**extrinsic hemolytic anemia**). Further subdivisions within each classification are based on the causative mechanism. The terms **intravascular** and **extravascular hemolysis** refer to the site of destruction of the red blood cell, within the circulating blood or outside it, respectively.

Inherited hemolytic disorders may affect the basic membrane structure, the erythrocytic enzymes, or the hemoglobin molecules within the red cell. A variety of membrane defects are inherited. These are **hereditary spherocytosis, hereditary elliptocytosis, hereditary stomatocytosis, hereditary pyropoikilocytosis**, and **hereditary xerocytosis.**

Like the structural membrane defects, erythrocytic enzyme defects are inherited. The clinical effects of these enzymopathies vary widely. In a number of erythrocytic enzyme defects, such as deficiencies in hexokinase, glucose-phosphate isomerase, and PK, the sole clinical manifestation is hemolytic anemia.

The acquired hemolytic anemias can be classified according to the agent or condition responsible for inducing the hemolysis. These categories include chemicals, drugs, and venoms; infectious organisms; immune or antibody causes; physical agents; and trauma.

Autoimmune anemias can be caused by cold-reactive or warm-reactive antibodies. Other types of disorders in this category include HDFN and fetus and fetus, incompatible blood transfusion, and PNH.

Patients with hemolytic anemia will have decreased hemoglobin, Hct, and red blood cell count. Blood smear examination will typically reveal the presence of many spherocytic erythrocytes. Other red cell abnormalities may include acanthocytes, schistocytes, stomatocytes, polychromatophilia, target cells, and early erythroid forms such as metarubricytes.

PNH is an acquired intravascular hemolytic disorder characterized by intermittent (paroxysmal) sleep-associated (nocturnal) blood in the urine (hemoglobinuria). PNH is a very complex disease that is more common than originally thought. This disorder is sometimes classified as a chronic myeloproliferative syndrome because of its potential to transform into acute leukemia or one of the myelodysplastic syndromes. Clinically, the disorder manifests itself and is sometimes classified as chronic hemolytic anemia.

Most patients have severe anemia with hemoglobin concentrations less than 6 g/dL. Peripheral blood smears may reveal hypochromic, microcytic red cells if an iron deficiency state has developed owing to cell lysis. Autohemolysis is increased after 48 hours, and hemolysis may increase with the addition of glucose to the test. Both the sucrose hemolysis (sugar-water) test and Ham test (acid-serum lysis) are useful diagnostic procedures.

CASE 12.1

5-year-old white boy was admitted with a fractured tibia following a playground accident. A CBC was ordered on admission.

■ **Laboratory Data**

The results of the admission CBC were as follows:

Hemoglobin 10.2 g/dL
Hct 27%
RBC 3.6×10^{12}/L
WBC 12.5×10^9/L
The RBC indices were as follows:

MCV 96.4 fL
MCH 28.3 pg
MCHC 38 g/dL

The peripheral blood smear revealed anisocytosis, some spherocytosis, and polychromatophilia. Platelet distribution was normal on the smear. Following receipt of the CBC results, the boy's physician ordered a serum biliruulocyte count, and an osmotic fragility test. The findings of these tests were as follows:

Total serum bilirubin 2.4 mg/dL
Reticulocyte count 2.0%
Negative findings on direct and indirect AHG test
Increased osmotic fragility

■ **Questions**

1. What category of anemia is suggested by the laboratory findings?
2. What is the most probable etiology of this patient's anemia?
3. Describe the mechanism responsible for the increased bilirubin result.

■ **Discussion**

1. When the spherocytes in the peripheral blood film are coupled with the laboratory results of an increased

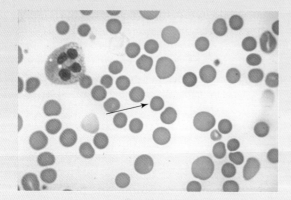

(Reprinted with permission from Anderson SC, *Anderson's Atlas of Hematology*, Philadephia, PA: Wolters Kluwer Health/ Lippincott Williams & Wilkins, Copyright 2003.)

reticulocyte count, increased bilirubin, decreased haptoglobin, and a negative direct AHG test, a diagnosis of chronic hemolytic anemia is suggested. The increased osmotic fragility further demonstrates that the RBCs have a decreased surface-area-to-volume ratio or spherocytic shape. These findings are reflective of most cases of chronic hemolytic anemia; however, spherocytes are not evident in approximately 20% to 25% of patients.

2. The laboratory findings of anemia and spherocytosis, and the inability to demonstrate antibodies either in the circulating blood or adhering to the RBCs in vivo, coupled with the associated clinical findings of jaundice, splenomegaly, and skeletal changes in this child, suggest a congenital membrane defect. In this case, the diagnosis of HS, which occurs at a frequency of 1 in 5,000, was made.

3. This disorder is usually an autosomal dominant trait with a variable hemolytic process. Although the condition is usually corrected by splenectomy, the spherocytosis remains. Physiologically, a decrease in the lipid content of the RBC membrane has been described as the source of the spherocytes. A membrane lipid alteration affects the permeability of the cell membrane to sodium ion (Na^+). As a result of the lack of permeability, the sodium increases within the cell and, in turn, demands greater glycolytic enzyme adenosine triphosphatase (ATPase) activity. ATP is needed to help maintain the normal, discoid erythrocytic shape. If ATP depletion occurs, the stability of the membrane will be altered and result in the formation of spherocytes. The spleen adversely affects RBCs. The erythrocytes must pass through the splenic cords, where the Hct is increased and blood flow is slow. The amount of available glucose diminishes, and blood pH is lowered. These conditions place a metabolic stress on the RBC, which depletes ATP. In stressed cells, such as in HS, the membrane becomes more unstable and is lost more readily than normally.

DIAGNOSIS: **Hereditary Spherocytosis**

CASE 12.2

A 44-year-old white woman was seen in the emergency department. She complained of fatigue and weakness. Over the past 2 weeks, she had noted that the whites of her eyes and her skin were becoming yellowish looking. On physical examination, the spleen was palpable. The emergency department physician ordered a CBC, serum bilirubin, and urinalysis.

■ **Laboratory Data**

The test findings were as follows:

Hemoglobin 8.5 g/dL
Hct 27% SI

(continued)

RBC 3.0×10^{12}/L
MCV 90 fL
MCH 28.3 pg
MCHC 32 g/dL

The WBC count was 9.0×10^9/L. The peripheral blood smear was essentially normochromic and normocytic; however, moderate polychromatophilia, spherocytes, rare basophilic stippling, 2 metarubricytes/100 WBC, and rouleaux formation were noted. The distribution of platelets on the peripheral smear was normal. The total serum bilirubin was 4.2 mg/dL, and the patient's urine was pinkish red.
The patient was admitted to the hospital. The following tests were ordered by her attending physician: reticulocyte count, direct and indirect AHG, and serum haptoglobin. These test results were as follows:

Reticulocyte count 13%
Direct AHG 3+
Indirect AHG 2+
Serum haptoglobin decreased

The blood bank subsequently identified the serum antibody as a cold agglutinin. An elution (removal of antibodies from the RBCs that they are coating) demonstrated that the same cold agglutinin was responsible for the positive direct AHG test result.

■ **Questions**
1. Which category and specific type of anemia are present in this case?
2. What is the etiology of this anemia?
3. What mechanism produced this patient's spherocytosis?

■ **Discussion**
1. The laboratory findings of a decreased hemoglobin, Hct, RBC count, and spherocytes on the peripheral blood smear coupled with an increased reticulocyte count, decreased haptoglobin, elevated bilirubin, and hemoglobinuria are typical findings in a patient who is suffering from increased RBC destruction. Supplementary laboratory testing in this case assisted in establishing a differential diagnosis. The positive direct and indirect AHG test results demonstrated that the hemolytic process was being caused by a circulating antibody. Further, blood bank results established that the antibody was a cold-type antibody rather than a warm-type antibody or a complement-related problem. This information is needed to differentiate this type of spherocytic-hemolytic anemia from other, similar anemias. In addition to the test data, the patient's medical history indicated no history of a recent blood transfusion to account for the presence of these circulating antibodies. Therefore, the diagnosis of AIHA was established.
2. The annual incidence of AIHA is approximately 1 per 80,000 in the United States. Of these cases, 70% are of the

warm antibody type, and 16% are cold-reacting antibodies. The antibodies of the cold type are usually IgM. Patients who have this disorder suffer either acute life-threatening hemolysis or a chronic hemolytic anemia. Half of cases of AIHA of either the warm or the cold variety are secondary to an underlying disease such as a lymphoproliferative disorder or viral infection. The remaining cases have an unknown etiology and are classified as idiopathic.
3. Spherocytes are often formed in AIHA as the cell membrane of antibody-coated RBCs is lost following interaction of the RBCs with splenic macrophages. RBCs coated with IgG or complement are partially phagocytized and bind to the macrophages. The macrophage subsequently removes portions of the RBC membrane and releases the RBC in its spherocytic form with a typically decreased surface-area-to-volume ratio. In AIHA, the slow flow of blood through the spleen provides an ample opportunity for the macrophages to come in contact with coated RBCs. This loss of membrane decreases the ability of RBCs to pass through the sinuses. Thus, the cells become trapped within the splenic cords. These events produce a cell that is highly vulnerable to hemolysis.

DIAGNOSIS: **Autoimmune Hemolytic Anemia due to Cold Antibody**

CASE 12.3
A newborn girl, who was well hydrated, began developing jaundice at 24 hours of age. The mother's prenatal information sheet noted that she was O-negative and had received immunoglobulin (IgG) after the delivery of each of her prior two children. This was her third child. No irregular antibodies were present during her initial prenatal blood screening during the first trimester of pregnancy. The neonatologist ordered the following tests on the neonate: CBC, serum bilirubin, blood type and Rh, and direct antihuman globulin test.

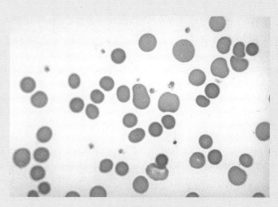

(Reprinted with permission from Anderson SC, *Anderson's Atlas of Hematology*, Philadephia, PA: Wolters Kluwer Health/ Lippincott Williams & Wilkins, Copyright 2003.)

(continued)

■ **Laboratory Data**

The results of the tests were as follows:

Hemoglobin 15.6 g/dL
Hct 50% SI
RBC 4.71 × 10^{12}/L
MCV 106.2 fL
MCH 33.1 pg
MCHC 31 g/dL

The peripheral smear revealed anisocytosis, macrocytosis, slight spherocytosis, 3+ polychromatophilia, and 3 metarubricytes/100 WBCs. The total serum bilirubin was 10.5 mg/dL. The infant was type O-positive. The result of the AHG test was positive (2+).

Following receipt of these laboratory findings, the physician ordered blood type and Rh determinations for both the mother and the baby, a direct AHG test on the routinely collected cord blood sample, and an irregular antibody screen on the mother. These tests revealed that the mother was type O-negative.

Her irregular antibody screening was positive. The antibody was identified as anti-c̄. A further antibody elution study of the neonate's cells revealed the presence of anti-c̄. The mother's full genotype was determined as being D-negative, C-positive, c̄-negative, E-positive, and e-positive. The neonate's genotype was D-positive, C-negative, c̄-positive, E-positive, and e-positive.

■ **Questions**

1. Is this an inherited or acquired anemia?
2. Which category of anemias does this case represent?
3. What is the cause of the baby's increased red cell destruction?

■ **Discussion**

1. The neonate's decreased hemoglobin, Hct, and RBC count; elevated bilirubin; and positive direct AHG on both the cord blood specimen and the blood sample suggest an acquired anemia. The presence of the antibody anti-c in the mother's serum postpartum and the identification of the antibody adhering to the baby's RBCs as anti-c confirmed that the baby has an acquired anemia. This type of acquired, hemolytic anemia in the newborn is referred to as HDFN, originally called erythroblastosis fetalis.

2. An increased bilirubin and decreased RBC count with both spherocytes and immature RBCs (metarubricytes) indicate that a hemolytic process is taking place. The identification of antibody in the mother's serum and on the neonate's cells confirmed that this hemolytic anemia was acquired.

3. Although an incompatibility in the ABO blood group system between the mother and the neonate is the most frequent type of HDFN, in this case, both the mother and the baby were type O. In ABO incompatibility, the most frequent cases occur when the mother is type O

and the baby is type A. The neonate's direct AHG test result in ABO incompatibility is frequently negative or only slightly positive. In this case, no atypical or irregular antibodies had been detected during prenatal testing during the first trimester of the mother's pregnancy. However, the antibody did exist postpartum. Although the mother was Rh-negative, she did not exhibit the presence of anti-D. The mother's medical history indicated that she had delivered two Rh-positive babies in the past but had been given an IgD substance postpartum as a preventive measure. However, she had apparently been sensitized to the c antigen during a previous pregnancy. When pregnant with this child, she built c antibodies that crossed the placental barrier and attached themselves to the c antigen on the baby's RBCs. The anti-c antibody is a warm-reacting, IgG-type antibody that is small enough to pass through the placental barrier and cause hemolytic disease. The antibody attaches itself if the specific c antigen is present on the fetal cells. This coating of fetal cells with antibody makes the RBC membrane vulnerable to hemolysis, which subsequently leads to increased erythrocyte destruction. In this case, it was important to identify the disorder not only for the newborn's sake but for the mother's sake as well. Because the mother did not demonstrate anti-D in her circulation and met the other necessary criteria, she was again eligible to receive IgD to protect any further babies against HDFN caused by the anti-D antibody.

DIAGNOSIS: Hemolytic disease of the fetus and newborn (HDFN)

CASE 12.4

A 30-year-old white man saw his family physician because of increasing fatigue over the previous few months. Physical examination revealed a pale but otherwise normal-appearing adult, although the liver and spleen appeared to be very slightly enlarged. The patient reported that his first urine of the morning was occasionally dark brown. His physician ordered a CBC, urinalysis, and liver and spleen scan.

■ **Laboratory Data**

The following determinations were obtained:

Hemoglobin 8.5 g/dL
Hematocrit 25%
RBC count 2.6 × 10^{12}/L
Total WBC count 4.4 × 10^9/L

The differential leukocyte count revealed an increase in lymphocytes (60%), but the percentages of other leukocytes were within the normal range. The urine demonstrated the presence of hemosiderin. Serum iron level and reticulocyte count were additionally requested. The total serum iron level was decreased, and the reticulocyte count was increased to 13%.

(continued)

CASE STUDIES *(continued)*

■ Questions
1. What is this patient's corrected reticulocyte count?
2. What is the RPI?
3. From what type of defect is this patient suffering?

■ Discussion
1. The corrected reticulocyte count is as follows:

$$\text{Reticulocyte count (\%)} \times \frac{\text{patient's hematocrit}}{\substack{\text{normal hematocrit based} \\ \text{on age and gender}}} = \%$$

$$0.13 \times \frac{0.25 \text{L/L}}{0.45 \text{L/L}} = 7.2\%$$

2. The RPI is as follows:

$$\frac{\text{Corrected reticulocyte count in \%}}{\text{Normal maturation time of 2 days}} = \frac{7.2}{2} = 3.5\%$$

3. The occasional presence of brown urine on early morning voiding is suggestive of hemolysis. Because these episodes were described as intermittent by the patient, a diagnosis of PNH would be suspected. That condition is a rare, acquired chronic hemolytic anemia. The episodes of intravascular hemolysis typically occur while the patient is asleep. During sleep, the blood pH decreases, making it easier for RBCs to lyse because of a membrane defect. This disorder represents an acquired erythrocytic membrane defect that renders one population of RBCs sensitive to lysis by normal plasma complement components. Hemosiderinuria is an important diagnostic feature of this disorder. Demonstration of PNH in vitro depends on the lysis of PNH erythrocytes by complement. A leukocyte alkaline phosphatase cytochemical stain may also be valuable because PNH is one of two disorders that show a decreased score. The other disorder is chronic myelogenous leukemia (discussed in Chapter 21).

DIAGNOSIS: Paroxysmal Nocturnal Hemoglobinuria

REVIEW QUESTIONS

1. Hemolytic disruption of the erythrocyte involves
   A. an alteration in the erythrocyte membrane
   B. a defect of the hemoglobin molecule
   C. an antibody coating the erythrocyte
   D. physical trauma

Questions 2 and 3: Match the following.
2. _____ Intravascular hemolysis
3. _____ Extravascular hemolysis
   A. Destruction of RBCs outside the circulatory blood
   B. Destruction of RBCs within the circulatory blood
4. Which of the following tests is not useful in determining increased erythrocyte destruction?
   A. Reticulocyte count
   B. Total leukocyte count
   C. Serum haptoglobin
   D. Unconjugated bilirubin

Questions 5 through 8: Match the following disorders with the appropriate category of defect (an answer may be used more than once):
5. _____ G6PD deficiency
6. _____ Hereditary spherocytosis
7. _____ Thalassemia
8. _____ Pyruvate kinase (PK) deficiency
   A. Structural membrane defect
   B. Erythrocytic enzyme defect
   C. Defect of the hemoglobin molecule

Questions 9 through 13: Match the following (use an answer only once):
9. _____ Hereditary spherocytosis
10. _____ Hereditary elliptocytosis
11. _____ Hereditary pyropoikilocytosis (HPP)
12. _____ Hereditary stomatocytosis
13. _____ Hereditary xerocytosis
   A. An overabundance of oval-shaped red cells
   B. A permeability disorder
   C. The most common prevalent hereditary hemolytic anemia among people of Northern European descent
   D. Can be seen in the genetic hemoglobin defect, thalassemia
   E. A subgroup of common hereditary elliptocytosis
14. Heinz bodies are associated with the congenital hemolytic anemia
   A. G6PD deficiency
   B. abetalipoproteinemia
   C. hereditary spherocytosis
   D. hemolytic anemias
15. A hemolytic crisis may be precipitated in 10% of American black males suffering from G6PD deficiency by
   A. fava beans
   B. primaquine
   C. quinine
   D. quinidine

(continued)

REVIEW QUESTIONS (continued)

16. What is the most common glycolytic enzyme deficiency associated with the aerobic pathway of erythrocyte metabolism?
    A. Glucose-6-phosphate dehydrogenase (G6PD)
    B. Pyruvate kinase (PK)
    C. Methemoglobin reductase deficiency
    D. Hexokinase deficiency

17. What is the most common glycolytic enzyme deficiency associated with the anaerobic pathway of erythrocyte metabolism?
    A. Glucose-6-phosphate dehydrogenase (G6PD)
    B. Pyruvate kinase (PK)
    C. Methemoglobin reductase deficiency
    D. Hexokinase deficiency

18. What laboratory assay would specifically indicate a deficiency of G6PD enzyme?
    A. Heinz bodies on peripheral blood smears
    B. Reticulocyte count
    C. Hemoglobin and hematocrit
    D. Osmotic fragility test

19. What enzyme deficiency causes methemoglobinemia?
    A. Glucose-6-phosphate dehydrogenase (G6PD)
    B. Pyruvate kinase (PK)
    C. NADH-methemoglobin reductase
    D. Hexokinase deficiency

20. Acquired hemolytic anemia can be caused by
    A. chemicals or drugs
    B. infectious organisms
    C. antibody reactions
    D. all of the above

21. The infectious microorganism directly associated with hemolytic uremic syndrome is
    A. *Pasteurella tularensis*
    B. *E. coli O157-H7*
    C. *Staphylococcus aureus*
    D. *Clostridia botulinum*

Questions 22 through 24: Match the following immune-mediated acquired hemolytic anemias with their respective answer (use an answer only once).

22. _____ Warm-type autoimmune hemolytic anemia (AIHA)

23. _____ Cold-type AIHA
24. _____ Isoimmune hemolytic anemia
    A. IgM, usually anti-I
    B. Rh antibodies are the most frequent cause
    C. Usually occurs in newborn infants

25. The erythrocyte alteration characteristically associated with hemolytic anemias is
    A. hypochromia
    B. macrocytosis
    C. spherocytosis
    D. burr cells

26. What laboratory procedures would reflect a typical hemolytic anemia?
    A. Increased osmotic fragility
    B. Increased total serum bilirubin
    C. Increased reticulocyte count, unless hematopoiesis is suppressed
    D. All of the above

27. Which of the following is not associated with hemolytic anemia?
    A. Decreased hemoglobin and packed cell volume
    B. Increased reticulocyte count
    C. Increased serum haptoglobins
    D. Decreased erythrocyte survival

28. Paroxysmal nocturnal hemoglobinuria exhibits sensitivity of one population of red blood cells to
    A. warm antibodies
    B. cold antibodies
    C. complement
    D. either A or B

29. Paroxysmal nocturnal hemoglobinuria episodes are usually associated with
    A. cold temperatures
    B. hot temperatures
    C. sleep
    D. certain foods or drugs

30. The defect in PNH probably is a (an) _____ associated defect of the red cell membrane.
    A. structural protein
    B. hemoglobin
    C. antibody
    D. enzyme

BIBLIOGRAPHY

Aster RH. Quinine sensitivity: A new cause of the hemolytic uremic syndrome, *Ann Intern Med*, 119(3):243–244, 1993.

Au WU, et al. Late onset glucose 6-phosphate dehydrogenase deficiency in Chinese women, *J Hematol*, 4(Suppl 2):50, 2003.

Bell BP, et al. A multistate outbreak of *Escherichia coli O157:H7*-associated bloody diarrhea and hemolytic uremic syndrome from hamburgers, *JAMA*, 272(17):1349–1353, 1994.

Bergstein JM, Riley M, Bang NU. Role of plasminogen-activator inhibitor type 1 in the pathogenesis and outcome of the hemolytic uremic syndrome, *N Engl J Med*, 327(11):755–759, 1992.

Bianchi P, et al. A lethal variant of pyruvate kinase deficiency associated with a missense mutation (G409) and a large deletion in the PR-PK gene, *Hematol J*, 4(Suppl 2):57, 2003.

Bick RL. Paroxysmal nocturnal hemoglobinuria, *Lab Med*, 25(3): 148–151, 1994.

Bissell M, Domen R (eds.). Quantifying fetomaternal hemorrhage by fluorescence microscopy, *CAP TODAY*, 16(10):80, 2002.

Boyce T, Swerdlow DL, Griffin PM. *Escherichia coli O157:H7* and the hemolytic-uremic syndrome, *N Engl J Med*, 333(6):362–363, 1995.

Caprari P, et al. Erythrocyte membrane protein 4.1R defect in patients affected by neuroacanthocytosis, *Hematol J*, 4(Suppl 2):60, 2003.

Costa FF, et al. Linkage of dominant hereditary spherocytosis to the gene for the erythrocyte membrane-skeleton protein ankyrin, *N Engl J Med*, 323(15):1046, 1990.

Durand PM, Coetzer TL. Pyruvate kinase deficiency protects against malaria in humans, *Haematologica*, 93(6):939–940, 2008.

Fernandes LMR, et al. Diagnosis of hereditary spherocytosis by flow cytometry-preliminary results, *Hematol J*, 4(Suppl 2):62, 2003.

Gaetani M, et al. Structural and functional effects of hereditary hemolytic anemia-associated point mutations in the alpha spectrin tetramer site, *Blood*, 111(12):5712–5720, 2008.

Hillmen P, et al. Natural history of paroxysmal nocturnal hemoglobinuria, *N Engl J Med*, 333(19):1253–1258, 1995.

Kostova GK, et al. Serum EPO and transferring receptors are useful in evaluation of the pathophysiology of anemia in malignancy, *Hematol J*, 4(Suppl 2):56, 2003.

Leach AP, Gaumer HR. Diagnosis and detection of PNH using GPI anchored proteins, *Clin Lab Sci*, 9(4):191–197, 1996.

Lindorfer MA, et al. A novel approach to preventing the hemolysis of paroxysmal nocturnal hemoglobinuria: both complement-mediated cytolysis and C3 deposition are blocked by a monoclonal antibody specific for the alternative pathway of complement, *Blood*, 115(11):2283–2291, 2010.

Luban NLC. Hemolytic disease of the newborn and fetus: progenitor cells and late effects, *N Engl J Med*, 338(12):830–831, 1998.

Mariani M, et al. Clinical and hematologic features of 300 patients affected by hereditary spherocytosis grouped according to the type of the membrane protein defect, *Haematologica*, 93(9):1310–1316, 2008.

Martin JTN, et al. Paroxysmal nocturnal haemoglobinuria clones in patients with aplastic aneaemia, myelodysplastic syndrome and paroxysmal nocturnal haemoglobinuria, *Hematol J*, 4(Suppl 2):58, 2003.

Mortazavi Y, et al. Molecular characterization of G6PD deficiency in south east Iran, *J Hematol*, 4(Suppl 2):55, 2003.

Ong MG, Hawthorne LM. Autoimmune hemolytic anemia in pregnancy, *Lab Medicine*, 41(5):264–266, 2010.

Pavlov AD, Fedina NV, Skobin VB. The use of RHU-EPO in anemic infants with infections, *Hematol J*, 4(Suppl 2):53, 2003.

Scamurra D, Davey FR. Anemias associated with spherocytic erythrocytes, *Lab Med*, 16(2):83–88, 1985.

Schilling RF. Estimating the risk for sepsis after splenectomy in hereditary spherocytosis, *Ann Intern Med*, 122(3):187–188, 1995.

Smith LJ. Paroxysmal noctural hemoglobinuira, *Clin Lab Sci*, 17(3):172–175, 2004.

Steensma DP, Hoyer JD, Fairbanks VF. Hereditary red blood cell disorders in Middle Eastern patients, *Mayo Clin Proc*, 76:285–293, 2001.

Tarr PI, et al. Hemolytic-uremic syndrome in a six-year-old girl after a urinary tract infection with shiga-toxin-producing *Escherichia coli* O103:H2, *N Engl J Med*, 335(9):635–638, 1996.

Hemoglobinopathies and Thalassemias

Hemoglobin defects

- Describe the common denominator in hemoglobinopathies.
- Name the three major categories of classification of hemoglobin defects.
- List the components and percentage of normal adult hemoglobin.
- Compare the disease state and trait condition of a hemoglobinopathy.

Sickle cell disease

- Describe the etiology of sickle cell disease (SCD).
- Explain the epidemiology of SCD.
- Describe the clinical signs and symptoms of SCD.
- Briefly explain the symptoms of SCD in children.
- Describe the symptoms of SCD associated with pregnancy.
- Discuss the clinical manifestations of SCD in adults.
- Characterize the general signs and symptoms in the categories of pain, pulmonary complications, and stroke associated with SCD.
- Outline laboratory findings that are typical of SCD.
- Briefly describe the value of the techniques of hemoglobin electrophoresis and deoxyribonucleic acid (DNA) analysis.

- Explain the process of prenatal diagnosis of SCD.
- Delineate the general management of SCD.

Sickle cell syndromes

- Describe the conditions of sickle β-thalassemia, sickle-C (SC), and sickle cell trait.

Thalassemia

- Compare the conditions of α- and β-thalassemia.
- Outline the laboratory findings in thalassemia.

Other hemoglobinopathies

- Describe the general characteristics of hemoglobin (Hb) C disease, Hb SC disease, Hb D disease, Hb E disease, Hb H disease, methemoglobinemia, and unstable hemoglobins.

Case studies

- Apply knowledge of etiology, epidemiology, pathophysiology, clinical signs and symptoms, laboratory findings, and treatment to the case studies presented.

HEMOGLOBIN DEFECTS

The hemoglobinopathies encompass a heterogeneous group of disorders associated with genetic mutations in both the alpha-globin and beta-globin genes.

Demographics

Sickle cell disease (SCD) and β-thalassemias are the most common monogenic diseases of man. They are found in the "malaria belt" that extends from the Mediterranean (see Box 13.1) and sub-Saharan Africa through Southeast Asia and southern China. These hemoglobin mutations occur at high incidences in these regions because heterozygotes have a selective advantage against infection with *Plasmodium falciparum*.

The sickle mutant has the highest frequency of occurrence in Central Africa. Thalassemia major can be traced back to the Mediterranean. Thalassemias are uncommon in North America but are a worldwide public health issue, particularly in many developing countries. The Middle East, South Asia, and the Orient have α-thalassemia as a prevalent hemoglobinopathy.

Sickle cell anemia is particularly common among people whose ancestors come from Sub-Saharan Africa, South

America, Cuba, Central America, Saudi Arabia, India, and Mediterranean countries such as Turkey, Greece, and Italy. In the Uniteds States, it affects around 72,000 people, most of whose ancestors come from Africa. The disease occurs in about 1 in every 500 African American births and 1 in every 1,000 to 1,400 Hispanic American births. About 2 million Americans, or 1 in 12 African Americans, carry the sickle cell allele.

Because of rapid growth in the Asian and Hispanic segments of the U.S. population, the geographic distribution of hemoglobinopathies is expected to become significantly different in the future.

These epidemiologic changes in the prevalence of nonsickling hemoglobin disorders will produce challenges for public health programs, including newborn screening.

Etiology

Hemoglobinopathies, for example, SCD, are inherited single-gene disorders that affect the amino acid residual sequence or production of normal hemoglobin. It is estimated that around 7% of the world population carries a globin-gene mutation, and in the majority of cases, it is inherited as an autosomal recessive trait. However, some of these disorders

Percentage of Eastern Mediterranean Region with an Abnormal Hemoglobin[a]

PROPORTION OF POPULATION	COUNTRY
>10%	Cyprus (17%), Bahrain (13%)
6%–10%	Iraq, Morocco, Oman, Qatar, Saudi Arabia, Sudan, Syria, Yemen.
4%–6%	Iran, Kuwait, Lebanon, Libya, Pakistan, Tunisia, United Arab Emirates.
<4%	Afghanistan, Ethiopia, Egypt, Jordan

[a]Thalassemias and hemoglobinopathies are considered but not enzymopathies, e.g. G6PD, or red cell membrane defects. Data derived from Angastiniotis and Modell.

Examples of Selected Hemoglobinopathies

ABNORMAL MOLECULAR STRUCTURE
Hb SS (sickle cell anemia)
Hb SA (sickle cell trait)
Hb C disease or trait

RATE OF SYNTHESIS
β-Thalassemia
α-Thalassemia

COMBINATION OF TWO MOLECULAR ALTERATIONS OR A MOLECULAR ABNORMALITY AND SYNTHESIS DEFECT
Hb S–Hb C
Hb S–β-thalassemia

are caused by the inheritance of an autosomal dominant gene that will produce hemolytic disease in its heterozygous state. Disorders associated with autosomal recessive genes need to be in the homozygous state to produce the disease.

Hemoglobinopathies may have a hemolytic manifestation. Approximately 25% of all hemoglobinopathies demonstrate the decreased red cell survival due to red cell membrane deformity that characterizes hemolytic disease. Although hemoglobinopathies and thalassemias are two genetically distinct disease groups, the clinical manifestations of both include anemia of variable severity and variable pathophysiology.

Disease Versus Trait

In the genetic manifestation of the hemoglobinopathies, the distinction between the disease state and the trait condition is made. A disease is defined as either the homozygous occurrence of the gene for the abnormality or the possession of a heterozygous, dominant gene that produces a hemolytic condition. In the case of sickle cell anemia, the trait must be inherited from both parents. A trait is described as the heterozygous and normally asymptomatic state. A review of inheritance and the synthesis of hemoglobin can be found in Chapter 5.

Abnormal Hemoglobin Molecules

Abnormal hemoglobins including hemoglobinopathies and thalassemias can be classified into three major categories:

1. Abnormal molecular structure of one or more of the polypeptide chains of globulin in the hemoglobin molecule, for example, sickle cell anemia.
2. A defect in the rate of synthesis of one or more particular polypeptide chains of globulin in the hemoglobin molecule, for example, the thalassemias.

3. Disorders that are a combination of abnormal molecular structure with a synthesis defect, for example, Hb E–β-thalassemia.

More than 700 abnormal hemoglobins have been described in the literature. The majority of hemoglobinopathies (hemoglobin variants) result from β-chain abnormalities.

At the molecular level, a single-base DNA substitution in the corresponding triplet codon produces one amino acid change and a defect in the chemical structure of the hemoglobin molecule. Selected examples of hemoglobinopathies within each of the three major categories are listed in Box 13.2.

Normal adult hemoglobin contains the following components: Hb A (95% to 98%), Hb A_2 (2% to 3%), Hb A_1 (3% to 6%), and fetal hemoglobin (Hb F) (<1%). The major fraction is Hb A. Typically, the individual with a hemoglobinopathy will demonstrate an alteration in this pattern.

SICKLE CELL DISEASE

SCD is a general term for abnormalities of hemoglobin structure, for example, hemoglobinopathies, in which the sickle gene is inherited from at least one parent. These genetic disorders are characterized by the production of Hb S, anemia, and acute and chronic tissue damage secondary to the blockage of blood flow produced by abnormally shaped red blood cells.

Sickle cell anemia (Hb SS), the most common form of hemoglobinopathy, is an expression of the inheritance of a sickle gene from both parents (see Chapter 3). Other sickle cell disorders result from the coinheritance of the sickle gene. Common variants include Hb SC disease and β-thalassemia.

Patients with this disease are living longer, new treatments are becoming available for adults as well as children, and early detection does matter. Almost every state in the United States screens the blood of all newborns for SCD.

Etiology

The sickle cell gene must be inherited from both parents. Hb S is different from Hb A because of a single nucleotide change (GAT to GTT) that results in the substitution of valine for glutamic acid at the sixth position on the β chain of the hemoglobin molecule (see Chapter 3). This results in abnormalities in polymerization (or gelation), with deoxygenation that leads to sickling. The end result of the polymerization is a permanently altered membrane protein. Two thirds of the red blood cells (RBCs) are removed by extravascular mechanisms.

Epidemiology

SCD is found most commonly in persons of African ancestry, but it also affects persons of Mediterranean, Caribbean, South and Central American, Arab, and East Indian ancestry. The sickle cell carrier state confers a selective advantage to *Plasmodium falciparum* malaria, because of preferential sickling of only the parasitized cells. The prevalence of the disease in some regions reflects this selective advantage or protective mechanism.

Hb SC disease affects an estimated 1 in 835 African American births, and SC β-thalassemia (S β-thalassemia) affects 1 in 1,667 African American live births. As a result, it is one of the most common genetic diseases in the United States.

Sickle cell anemia, the homozygous form of SCD, is the most common inherited hematological disease affecting humans. More than 50,000 Americans have sickle cell anemia.

The life expectancy of patients with SCD has improved considerably since 1960. The median age at death for individuals with sickle cell anemia is 42 years for men and 48 years for women, considerably younger than the general African American population. For Hb SC disease, the median age at death is 60 years for men and 68 years for women.

Pathophysiology

Sickling

When Hb S is deoxygenated, it becomes polymerized and produces sickling (Fig. 13.1). Subsequent hemolysis is probably a result of the extent of the red cell's capacity to sickle. The erythrocytic membrane in sickle cell anemia possesses significant membrane abnormalities, with an excessive increase in ionized calcium in the cell playing a role in the produced abnormality. Ionized calcium in the Hb SS cell is twice normal, with the most dense cells having four times the normal amount of ionized calcium.

Polymerization of Hb S occurs under conditions of extremely reduced oxygen and increased acidity in the

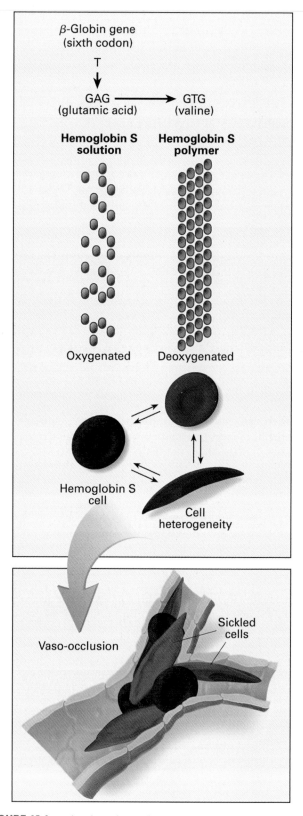

FIGURE 13.1 Pathophysiology of SCD. In Hb S, a substitution of T for A in the sixth codon of the β-globin gene leads to the replacement of a glutamic acid residue by a valine residue. On deoxygenation, Hb S polymers form, causing cell sickling and damage to the membrane. Some sickle cells adhere to endothelial cells, leading to vasoocclusion. (Reprinted with permission from Steinberg MH. Management of sickle cell disease, *N Engl J Med*, 340(13):1022, 1999. Copyright © 1999 Massachusetts Medical Society. All rights reserved.)

blood. Sickling is promoted by low oxygen tension, low pH, increased 2,3-diphosphoglycerate, high cellular concentration of hemoglobins, loss of cell water, Hb C, and Hb O–Arab. Sickling is retarded by Hb A, Hb F (at least 30%), Hb J, and α-thalassemia.

When sickling occurs, it subsequently leads to an increased mean corpuscular hemoglobin concentration (MCHC) in proportion to the number of molecules in the deoxygenated state. Deoxyhemoglobin S is less soluble than deoxyhemoglobin A or oxyhemoglobin S.

Recently, the understanding of the molecular basis of SCD has progressed rapidly. It is now possible to describe the structure of the gel of polymerized deoxyhemoglobin S and to begin to understand the mechanism of the formation of this gelatinous hemoglobin solution in red cells. It is believed that with deoxygenation, a continuum of cellular changes begins.

The first stage progresses from the formation of small amounts of polymer to larger amounts of highly ordered polymer as the result of severe and prolonged deoxygenation. This polymerization produces the resultant sickling. The red cell flexibility, which is governed by the amount and alignment of this intracellular polymer, is the principal determinant of the flow of sickled red cells.

Because cells that have large amounts of ordered polymer may be caught in the capillaries and venules, some cells at relatively high oxygen saturation with polymer but no deformability may have difficulty traversing the constriction of the precapillary arterioles. When the sickled cells attempt to travel through these small vessels, they become stuck and the vessels become obstructed. This initiates a pattern of blood not flowing properly to the tissue and creating a lack of oxygen. The lack of oxygen causes more sickling and more deprivation of oxygen to the tissues. This process can cause intense pain.

When sickled cells receive oxygen, they return to their normal shape. Repeated cycles of sickling and unsickling lead to the RBCs becoming permanently damaged. This process ends in hemolysis, which leads to anemia. In addition, repeated episodes of this type lead to the necrosis of body tissues.

Vasoocclusion

The adherence of sickled erythrocytes to the vascular endothelium may contribute to painful vasoocclusion. Sickle cell adherence involves several receptor-mediated processes and may be triggered by the appearance of adhesion molecules on activated endothelial cells. Thrombin has been demonstrated to increase the adhesiveness of endothelial cells for sickled erythrocytes, which results in vasoocclusion and painful crises.

Clinical Signs and Symptoms

Acute crises are caused by recurrent obstruction of the microcirculation by intravascular sickling. Aside from the painful crisis, sickling takes its toll on the body in other ways.

TABLE 13.1	Causes of Death Among Children With SCD	
Cause	**Percentage of Total Deaths**	
Infection	44	
Splenic sequestration	16	
Sudden, unexpected death	14	
Cerebrovascular accident	12	
Congestive heart failure	7	
Miscellaneous	7	

Through the years, the cumulative damage from vascular occlusion can lead to organ and tissue failure. Other complications may include an enlarged heart, progressive loss of pulmonary or renal function, stroke, arthritis, liver damage, and other complications. There is significant activation of coagulation with consequent increase in fibrinolysis during both the sickle cell crisis and in the steady state.

There is variation in the severity of SCD. Many patients are reasonably well and have relatively few complications. However, 5% to 10% of patients account for 40% to 50% of hospital visits.

Symptoms in Children

In sickle cell anemia, splenic dysfunction is a potentially life-threatening complication that develops during infancy. The red blood cells become trapped in the spleen, leaving the infant vulnerable to shock and infection from encapsulated bacteria, particularly members of the *Streptococcus pneumoniae* and *Haemophilus influenzae* species. Infectious crises are the most frequent cause of death in patients younger than 5 years (Table 13.1).

Symptoms are not present unless the patient is older than 6 months. Vasoocclusive disease develops between the ages of 12 months and 6 years. Chronic manifestations in children include a progressive lag in growth and development after the first decade of life and chronic destruction of bone and joints, with ischemia and infarction of the spongiosa.

Symptoms Associated with Pregnancy

In pregnancy, there is no increase in disease manifestation but there is an increase in maternal mortality of 20% and fetal mortality of 20%.

Clinical Manifestations in Adults

SS homozygotes have a severe hemolytic anemia, with hematocrit values ranging between 15% and 30%. Red cells with relatively low Hb F levels are likely to become sickled cells and, therefore, have short life spans. In cases in which erythropoiesis is also suppressed, anemia becomes increasingly severe. The two main causes of erythropoietic suppression are aplastic crises and megaloblastic erythropoiesis. Aplastic crises result from infection, particularly with parvovirus, whereas megaloblastic erythropoiesis occasionally occurs owing to the induction of folic acid deficiency by the increased requirements of the hyperplastic marrow. The hematocrit can plummet rapidly as a result of combined impairment in red cell production and ongoing hemolysis.

Acute chest syndrome is a significant cause of death in patients of all ages who have sickle cell anemia. Higher blood viscosity leads to several complications, including complications in the shoulders and hips, multiorgan dysfunction, and possibly some of the pain associated with the disease. There is an increased incidence of pigmented gallstones in 30% to 60% of adults, with symptoms in 10% to 15%. Renal manifestations include papillary necrosis. Leg ulcers may occur.

Fifty percent of patients with sickle cell anemia survive beyond the fifth decade. A large proportion of those who die have had no overt chronic organ failure but die during an acute episode of pain, chest syndrome, or stroke.

Patients with more symptomatic disease are at higher risk of early death. Risk of early death is inversely associated with the level of Hb F. Patients with sickle cell anemia who had hemoglobin values less than 7.1 g/dL and elevated white blood counts (>15.0 × 10⁹/L) have a slightly higher risk.

General Signs and Symptoms

Pain

Painful sickle cell crisis is the hallmark of sickle cell anemia and is the most common complaint of patients with this disease. Acute painful episodes, often called vasoocclusive crises, are the most frequent complication of SCD and are a common reason for visits to the emergency department and admission to the hospital. High-dose methylprednisolone decreases the duration of pain in children and adolescents with SCD, but they have more rebound attacks after therapy is discontinued.

Pulmonary Complications

Thoracic bone infarction is common in patients with SCD who are hospitalized with acute chest pain. Incentive spirometry can prevent the pulmonary complications (atelectasis and infiltrates) associated with the acute chest syndrome in patients with SCDs who are hospitalized with chest or back pain above the diaphragm. The cause of acute chest syndrome is uncertain.

Stroke

Twenty-four percent of SCD patients have a stroke by the age of 45 years. Because Hb S tends to form intracellular polymers that distort the red cell, the disease is characterized clinically by chronic hemolytic anemia, recurrent bouts of pain, and organ infarction, including stroke.

Cerebral infarction in SCD is associated with an occlusive vasculopathy involving the distal intracranial segments of the internal carotid artery as well as the proximal middle and anterior cerebral arteries. Transcranial ultrasonography can identify children with SCD who are at highest risk for cerebral infarction. Blood transfusions decrease stroke risk in patients deemed high risk by transcranial Doppler. However, transcranial Doppler has poor specificity, and transfusions are limited by alloimmunization and iron overload. Transfusion withdrawal may be associated with an increased rebound stroke risk. Periodic ultrasound examinations and the selective use of transfusion therapy could make the primary prevention of stroke an achievable goal. Recent genome-wide association studies may provide methods for modulating Hb F production enough to attenuate stroke risk and other complications.

Laboratory Testing

In addition to decreased hemoglobin (5 to 9.5 g/dL), hematocrit, and red blood cell count, a persistent increase in the white blood cell (WBC) count of 12,000 to 15,000 × 10⁹/L is common. The red cell morphology on peripheral blood smear can include moderate to significant anisocytosis, poikilocytosis, and hypochromia. Red cell abnormalities may include target cells, microcytes, polychromatophilia, and basophilic stippling. Howell-Jolly bodies may be present if hyposplenism is present. If the patient is in an acute crisis state, sickled red cells (drepanocytes) may be seen on peripheral smears (Fig. 13.2 and Box 13.3).

Laboratory features of this chronic hemolytic state include reticulocytosis (8% to 12%), which may increase the mean corpuscular volume (MCV) to levels up to 100 fL; elevated serum; unconjugated bilirubin and methemalbumin; decreased serum haptoglobin and hemopexin; increased serum lactate dehydrogenase (LDH); mildly increased aspartate transaminase (AST); and increased urine urobilinogen.

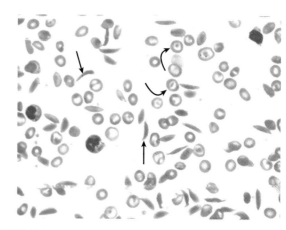

FIGURE 13.2 Sickle cell anemia. Sickled cells (*straight arrows*) and target cells (*curved arrows*) are evident. (Reprinted with permission from Raphael R, Strayer DS. *Rubin's Pathology: Clinicopathologic Foundations of Medicine*, 5th ed, Philadelphia, PA: Lippincott Williams & Wilkins, 2008.)

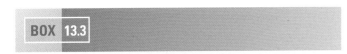

Common Laboratory Signs of Hemolysis in SCD

Reticulocytosis (polychromasia)
Unconjugated hyperbilirubinemia
Increased fecal and urine urobilinogen
Decreased serum haptoglobin
Decreased serum hemopexin
Increased serum methemalbumin
Elevated LDH
Mild elevation in AST

Special Laboratory Testing

Other diagnostic laboratory tests include thin-layer isoelectric focusing (IEF) or high performance liquid chromatography (HPLC). Hemoglobin electrophoresis, IEF, and HPLC are all acceptable, reliable, and accurate methods of testing. Globin DNA analysis is also advocated as an alternative method, although the procedure is costly and limited in the number of genotypes it can identify.

Definitive diagnosis includes reassessment of the hemoglobin phenotype, measurement of hemoglobin concentration and red cell indices, inspection of red cell morphology, and correlation with the clinical history.

Hemoglobin Electrophoresis

As early as 1949, Linus Pauling ascribed the altered electrophoretic mobility of the hemoglobin in patients with sickle cell anemia to a change in the hemoglobin (Fig. 13.3). This cemented the fact that there was a direct link between defective hemoglobin molecules and their pathological consequences, setting the groundwork for the concept of molecular disease.

In SCD, hemoglobin electrophoresis shows 80% to 95% Hb S, 0% to 20% Hb F, and a normal amount of Hb A_2.

High-Pressure Liquid Chromatography

Electrophoresis at acid and alkaline pH has been in use for many years but cation-exchange HPLC is emerging as the method of choice for quantification of Hb A_2 and Hb F and identification of hemoglobin variants. This method streamlines the preliminary and follow-up tests for the identification of both hemoglobinopathies and thalassemias in most cases.

DNA Analysis

With the discovery of reverse transcriptase and the cloning of the human globin genes, it became possible to probe specifically for the globin genes in the human genome. The hemoglobin disorders represent the first groups of disease to which DNA analysis was applied.

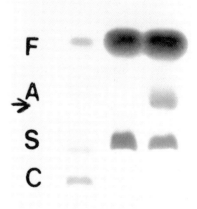

FIGURE 13.3 Hemoglobin electrophoresis in agar using a citric acid–citrate buffer at pH 6.2. **Left lane:** A control mixture of Hb C, Hb S, and Hb F. **Middle lane:** Cord blood from a neonate with sickle cell anemia shows Hb S and Hb F, but not Hb A (a similar pattern would be seen in Hb S–β-thalassemia and Hb S HBFH). **Right lane:** Cord blood from a neonate with sickle cell trait shows Hb S, Hb F, and Hb A. (Reprinted with permissoin from McClatchey KD. *Clinical Laboratory Medicine*, 2nd ed, Philadelphia, PA: Lippincott Williams & Wilkins, 2002.)

This analysis has led to better understanding of the basic mechanism of diseases, clinical application, and in some countries, control of the diseases. Virtually all cases of SCD and most cases of thalassemia can be diagnosed by direct DNA analysis with polymerase chain reaction (PCR).

Prenatal Diagnosis

Prenatal diagnosis of abnormal hemoglobin is important because of the high frequency of SCD. As DNA from the fetus is available in the amniocytes, fetal diagnosis can be made by amniocentesis at about the 14th week of gestation. The current widespread use of chorionic villus biopsy allows DNA diagnosis to be performed at the 7th to 10th week of gestation.

Screening of Newborns for Sickle Cell Anemia and Carriers

The principal hemoglobin in the newborn is Hb F. The distribution is 80% Hb F and 20% Hb A in a normal term infant. Hb F is composed of two α- and two γ-globulins. During the last trimester, there is a progressive increase in β-globin synthesis and a decrease in γ-chain synthesis. In a normal term infant, approximately 80% of the non-α globulin is γ-globin and 20% is β-globin.

Screening for SCD in newborns at birth is mandated in all 50 states and the District of Columbia. Sickle cell anemia (Hb SS) affects 1 in 375 African American newborns born in the United States and smaller proportions of children in other ethnic groups. Without prompt diagnosis and the initiation of prophylactic antibiotics and pneumococcal conjugate vaccination by 2 months of age, children with sickle cell anemia are vulnerable to life-threatening pneumococcal infections. Early detection of sickle cell anemia followed by prophylactic oral penicillin substantially reduces the risk of serious infections during the first few years of life. Additional benefits result from pneumococcal conjugate vaccination and parental education about early warning signs of infection.

Screening tests will identify approximately 50 sickle cell carriers for every infant diagnosed with SCD. An infant with sickle cell trait has both a normal β gene and a β S gene, and the infant will have a predominance of Hb F and both Hb A and Hb S. There always will be more Hb A than Hb S in these infants because α chains preferentially pair with normal β chains.

Screening of newborn infants is an important step in disease control. Although universal newborn screening can reliably identify all infants with sickle cell hemoglobinopathies, the initial screening result must not be considered the definitive diagnosis. Confirmatory testing should occur no later than 2 months of age.

Blood collection on the first day of life poses no problem for hemoglobin screening, provided the infant has not received a blood transfusion. A cord blood sample can be used, but it has the potential of being contaminated with blood from the mother. Blood collected from a heelstick is the method of choice because it is easy to obtain and it is the same method used for other newborn screening (e.g., phenylketonuria, hypothyroiditis, and galactosemia). Samples collected onto a filter paper from a heelstick remain stable for at least 1 week at room temperature. Specimens must be drawn prior to any blood transfusion due to the potential for a false negative result as a result of the transfusion. Extremely premature infants may have false positive results when adult hemoglobin is undetectable.

In the United States, most state-based screening programs use either thin-layer IEF or HPLC as the initial screening techniques performed on capillary blood collected from a heelstick and absorbed onto a filter paper. The sensitivity and specificity of each of these tests approach 100% for sickle cell anemia. Thin-layer IEF provides resolution of Hb A, S, and C from Hb F and detection of other abnormal hemoglobins. Metabisulfite sickle cell preparations and solubility testing are not acceptable screening methods for newborns or Hb S confirmation in early infancy.

Management of Sickle Cell Disease

The management of SCD consists of the following:

1. Monitoring the severity of the anemia and transfusing blood only when necessary
2. Treating acute and chronic pain according to a rational guideline
3. Diagnosing organ failure and administering appropriate therapy; over time, recurrent vasoocclusion and its associated vasculopathy result in significant progressive organ failure

Treatment

Bone marrow transplant offers the only potential cure for sickle cell anemia. However, finding a donor is difficult and the procedure has serious risks associated with it, including death.

Conventional management of sickle cell anemia is primarily supportive. It is important to detect infections early and treat them with antibiotics, as these infections may trigger painful and aplastic crises. General supportive care includes daily oral folate supplementation, antibiotic prophylaxis in childhood, Pneumovax, *Haemophilus influenzae* vaccine, meningococcal vaccine, a yearly flu shot, a yearly eye examination, prompt treatment of infections, and avoidance of dehydration. Treatment of pain crises includes hydration, adequate analgesia, and adequate oxygenation. Exchange transfusions may play a limited role in treatment, but possible reasons for their use include prevention of stroke recurrence, acute chest syndrome, in preparation for elective surgery, refractory priapism, refractory pain crises, and splenic sequestration crises.

Experimental treatment approaches include

- Gene therapy. Gene therapy involves inserting a normal gene into the bone marrow of patients with sickle cell anemia to produce normal hemoglobin. Another approach is to attempt to turn off the defective gene while reactivating another gene responsible for the production of Hb F.
- Butyric acid. Butyric acid is normally used as a food additive but it may increase the amount of Hb F in the blood.
- Clotrimazole. This over-the-counter antifungal medication helps prevent a loss of water from red blood cells, which may reduce the number of sickle cells that form.
- Nitric oxide. Abnormal function of the cells lining blood vessels may contribute to the complications of SCD. Disruption in the synthesis of nitric oxide, an important regulator of blood vessel relaxation, contributes to these abnormalities. Treatment with nitric oxide may prevent sickle cells from clumping together.
- Nicosan. This is an herbal treatment in early trials in the United States. Nicosan has been used to prevent sickle crises in Nigeria, West Africa.

Infectious Diseases

The primary treatment is prevention of infectious diseases. Vaccination including pneumococcal, influenza A, and *H. influenzae* immunizations are indicated. In addition, splenectomy is recommended for children who survive the initial splenic sequestration crisis.

Blood Transfusion

Blood transfusion and exchange transfusion are means of treatment of anemia. The major indications for blood transfusion in SCD are

- To improve oxygen-carrying capacity and transport
- To dilute circulating sickle red blood cells to improve microvascular perfusion

Transfusion should be considered in a patient with

1. Hemoglobin less than 5.0 g/dL and significant signs and symptoms of anemia associated with erythroid aplasia or hypoplasia (aplastic crisis)
2. Angina or high output failure
3. Acute hemorrhage
4. Acute central nervous system complications
5. Acute chest syndrome with hypoxia
6. Sequestration crisis
7. Preoperative preparation (general anesthesia)

Exchange transfusion may be considered in patients with cerebrovascular accident, fat embolism, acute chest syndrome, eye surgery, unresponsive acute priapism, leg ulcers, and before injection of contrast material. Prolonged hypertransfusion or an exchange transfusion regimen will result in iron overload and the consequent need for iron chelation therapy.

Drug Therapy

Drug therapy consists of hydroxyurea, a cytostatic agent. Hydroxyurea, a ribonucleotide reductase inhibitor, stimulates the production of Hb F but suppresses bone marrow production. Fetal hemoglobin is a potent inhibitor of the polymerization of deoxyhemoglobin S. The exact mechanism of action of hydroxyurea remains uncertain. Hydroxyurea therapy can ameliorate the clinical course of sickle cell anemia in some adults with three or more painful crises per year (Fig. 13.4). In addition to moderating acute painful episodes, hydroxyurea has been demonstrated to reduce the frequency of hospitalizations and the need for blood.

The beneficial effects of hydroxyurea do not become manifest for several months, and its use must be monitored carefully. Because of the effect of bone marrow suppression, patients must be monitored every 2 weeks to ensure that a life-threatening decrease in the number of hematopoietic cells, especially granulocytes and platelets, does not occur. In addition, the long-term safety of hydroxyurea in patients with sickle cell anemia is uncertain.

Hydroxyurea alone can reduce symptoms of anemia that require some patients to undergo frequent transfusions. However, by combining hydroxyurea and human recombinant erythropoietin, and adding iron supplements to the treatment, patients reportedly manifest increased

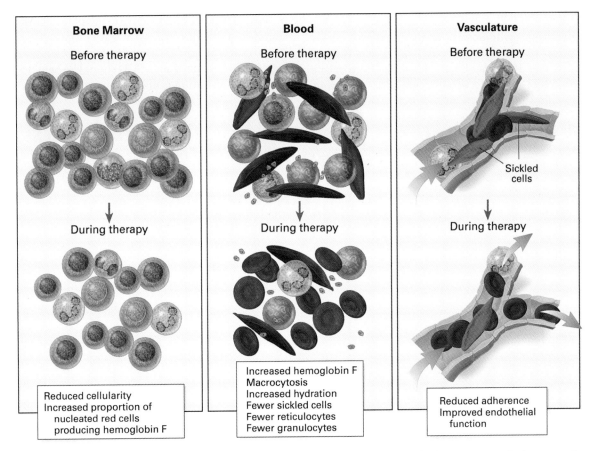

FIGURE 13.4 Mechanisms of action of hydroxyurea in SCD. By selectively killing cells in the bone marrow, hydroxyurea increases the number of erythroblasts that produce Hb F. It has no known direct effects on gene expression. Bone marrow cellularity may also be diminished. Higher concentrations of Hb F reduce the polymerization of Hb S and the numbers of deformed, dense, and damaged erythrocytes. Cells with a high Hb F content survive longer attenuating hemolysis and leading to a reduction in reticulocyte counts. The numbers of circulating granulocytes, monocytes, and platelets are diminished. The likelihood of vasoocclusion is reduced by the reduction in the number of dense, poorly deformable erythrocytes that can adhere to and perturb the endothelium. (Reprinted with permission from Steinberg MH. Management of sickle cell disease, *N Engl J Med*, 340(13):1026, 1999.)

levels of the Hb F protein in their blood. By increasing the production of red blood cells containing the protein, the effect of the drug is to interfere with the process that makes hemoglobin abnormal in those who suffer from the disease.

Novel Pharmaceutical Therapies

Currently, hydroxyurea is the only FDA approved drug for treating SCD. Significant progress in developmental research of novel drugs for the treatment of SCD has been made recently. Novel therapies can:

■ increase the production of fetal hemoglobin,
■ improve red blood cell hydration,
■ increase the availability of nitric oxide and
■ possess anti-inflammatory effects.

Novel therapies include nitric oxide, anti-inflammatory agents, for example, statins, and anticoagulants and anti-platelet agents. Because of the complex pathophysiology of SCD, it is unlikely that a single new agent will prevent or treat all of the sequelae of SCD. It is most likely that patients will benefit the most from a treatment strategy that combines agents with different mechanisms of action.

Bone Marrow Transplant

Bone marrow transplantation as a treatment for sickle cell anemia was first used in Europe. Children and adolescents younger than 16 years of age who suffer from severe complications (e.g., stroke, recurrent acute chest syndrome, or refractory pain) and have an HLA-matched donor available are the best candidates for transplantation. Approximately 1% of patients meet these criteria. A significant problem is development of regimen-related mortality due to infection and graft-versus-host disease.

Hematopoietic stem cell

Hematopoietic stem cell (HSC)-targeted gene transfer is an attractive approach for the treatment of some of the hematopoietic disorders caused by single gene defects, e.g. SCD, β thalassemia.

Prevention

Genetic counseling may be useful in the prevention of sickle cell anemia. When the parents are both hemoglobin SA (carriers), antenatal diagnosis can be performed during

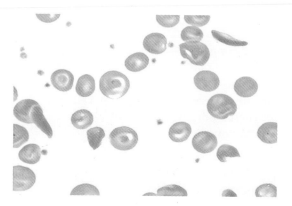

FIGURE 13.5 Hb S/β-thalassemia. (Reprinted with permission from Anderson SC. *Anderson's Atlas of Hematology*, Philadelphia, PA: Wolters Kluwer Health/Lippincott Williams & Wilkins, Copyright 2003.)

the 18th to 20th weeks of pregnancy by analyzing DNA from amniotic fluid.

Experimental therapy includes induction of Hb F by short-chain fatty acids and membrane-active drugs. Short-chain fatty acids appear to modulate gene expression directly by interacting with transcriptionally active elements of the genes. Membrane-active drugs block cation-transport channels in erythrocyte membranes and can shift cellular cation content and cell density toward normal values. Reversing cellular dehydration in SCD should be beneficial, because Hb S polymerization is highly concentration dependent.

SICKLE CELL SYNDROMES: PATHOGENESIS AND NEW APPROACHES

Sickle cell anemia was the first molecular disease to be recognized. The severity of illness in SCD differs with the quantity of Hb S in the erythrocytes. The various states associated with the presence of Hb S are listed in Table 13.2 in the order of clinical severity.

Sickle β-Thalassemia

The inheritance of the sickle gene from one parent and a β-thalassemia gene from the other results in the compound heterozygous state: sickle β-thalassemia (Fig. 13.5). This

TABLE 13.2	Various Clinical States Associated with the Presence of Hb S			
Genotype	Percentage Hb S	Percentage Non-S Hb	Clinical Severity (Scale 0–4)	Other Clinical Features
SS	80–98	2–15 (fetal)	3–4	10%–20% reticulocytosis; rare splenomegaly
S β-thalassemia	60–90	10–30	1–3	Splenomegaly; microcytosis; 4+ target cells
SC	50	50 (hgb C)	1–3	Splenomegaly, 4+ target cells
AS sickle trait	30–40	60–70 (hgb A)	0	Normal morphology; no splenomegaly

disorder is variable in its clinical manifestations but tends to be milder in blacks than in Mediterranean persons. Patients have moderately severe hemolytic anemia. Splenomegaly occurs in 70% of cases.

Patients who are unable to produce any Hb A (S β⁰-thalassemia) have disease as severe as that of SS patients. Those with S β+ thalassemia can make a small amount of Hb A and have less extensive hemolysis and vasoocclusive phenomena.

S β-thalassemia can be diagnosed by examining the blood film and through hemoglobin electrophoresis. The blood film reveals hypochromic, microcytic red cells with polychromatophilia, target cells, stippling, and, rarely, sickled cells. Hemoglobin electrophoresis reveals that 60% to 90% of the hemoglobin is S and 10% to 30% is fetal (F). The therapy is the same as for SS disease. Splenectomy may be beneficial if the spleen is sequestering red cells in significant amounts. Hb S/β-thalassemia is less severe than SCD. The spleen remains functional, but retinopathy is more common.

Sickle-C Disease

In Hb SC disease, the patients have only Hb S and C, with an absence of Hb A and normal or increased levels of Hb F. The complications associated with this disorder are less severe than SCD with three exceptions: proliferative retinopathy,

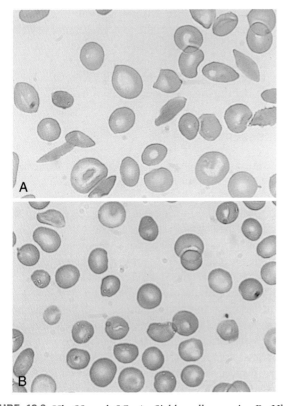

FIGURE 13.6 Hb SS and SC. A. Sickle cell anemia. B. Hb SC disease. (Reprinted with permission from Greer JP, et al. *Wintrobe's Clinical Hematology*, 11th ed, Philadelphia, PA: Lippincott Williams & Wilkins, 2004.)

aseptic necrosis of femoral heads, and acute chest syndrome secondary to fat emboli in the final months of pregnancy. Mild anemia occurs in 10% of patients with the hemoglobin being less than 10 g/dL. Sickle cells are rarely seen on a peripheral blood smear, but approximately 50% of red blood cells on a peripheral blood smear are target cells. The spleen remains functional.

The compound heterozygous state SC (Fig. 13.6) disease is almost as common among adults as SS disease, although the gene frequency for Hb C is 25% that for Hb S. The clinical manifestations in SC disease are highly variable. There are two reasons why SC is a disease whereas AS (i.e., sickle cell trait) is benign. First, in SC red cells, the intracellular hemoglobin concentration is significantly elevated because of the presence of Hb C. Second, SC red cells have at least a 10% higher level of Hb S than SA red cells. Patients with SC disease experience a mild to moderate hemolytic anemia and usually have splenomegaly. Target cell and occasional plump sickle forms are noted in the blood film. Complications commonly include retinopathy, hematuria from medullary infarcts, and aseptic necrosis of the femoral head (Box 13.4).

Sickle Cell Trait

Approximately 8% of black Americans are heterozygous for Hb S. Thus, their red cells contain Hb S and A. Sickle cell trait provides a survival advantage over individuals with normal hemoglobin in regions where malaria, *P. falciparum*, is endemic. Sickle hemoglobin impairs malaria growth. Sickle cell trait does not provide absolute protection, but individuals are more likely to survive the acute illness. Life expectancy and morbidity of individuals with sickle trait (AS) resemble those of a comparable group with Hb A. AS red

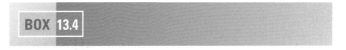

BOX 13.4

Abnormalities Reported with Sickle Cell Trait

ASSOCIATIONS WITH SICKLE CELL TRAIT VERY LIKELY
Splenic infarction at high altitude
Hyposthenuria
Hematuria
Bacteriuria and pyelonephritis in pregnancy

ASSOCIATION WITH SICKLE CELL TRAIT POSSIBLE
Pulmonary embolism
Complications induced by prolonged use of tourniquet
Renal papillary necrosis
Proliferative retinopathy
Avascular necrosis of bone
Intravascular sickling with strenuous exertion (especially in uninformed or noncompliant patients)

cells sickle far less readily than SS red cells. Accordingly, AS heterozygotes develop sickling crises rarely and only when severely hypoxic.

There are no manifestations of anemia, red blood cell abnormalities, increased risk of infection, or increased mortality associated with sickle cell trait. Electrophoresis of whole blood reveals that 35% to 45% of hemoglobin in patients with sickle cell trait is Hb S. Clinical signs and symptoms associated with sickle cell trait include hematuria, splenic infarction at high altitude (over 10,000), hyposthenuria, bacteriuria, and pyelonephritis in pregnancy.

THALASSEMIA

Demographics

Thalassemia is a growing global public health problem, with an estimated 900,000 births of clinically significant thalassemia disorders expected to occur in the next 20 years. An increase will occur in disorders previously uncommon in many parts of the world. In particular, Hb E–β-thalassemia and Hb H disease account for much of the projected increases in thalassemia. Worldwide, Hb E–β-thalassemia is one of the most frequent hemoglobinopathies. The incidence of Hb E approaches 60% of the populations in many regions of Southeast Asia. In coastal regions of North America, its prevalence is rapidly growing. α-thalassemia diseases, often considered benign, are now recognized to be more severe than originally reported. Hb H, Hb H–constant spring (CS), and homozygous α-thalassemia affect at least a million people worldwide. California considers Hb H disease a public health problem and has initiated a neonatal screening program for Hb H and particularly Hb H–CS. Homozygous α-thalassemia, usually fatal, is also being more commonly detected.

Etiology

Thalassemias are caused by an abnormality in the rate of synthesis of the globin chains. This is in contrast to the true hemoglobinopathies (e.g., Hb S and Hb C) that result from an inherited structural defect in one of the globin chains that produces hemoglobin with abnormal physical or functional characteristics.

Inheritance of thalassemia is autosomal; whether it is autosomal dominant or recessive is questionable because heterozygotes are not always symptomatic. Globin structural genes are found on chromosomes 11 and 16. The α chain and its embryonic counterpart, the ζ chain, are located on chromosome 16. Two genes on each homologous chromosome, four per diploid cell, specify the α-globin sequence. Only one gene per chromosome, two per diploid cell, specifies most of the non-α chain on chromosome 11. The γ chain is also represented by two sites per chromosome. In terms of the genetic basis of α- and β-thalassemia, this represents an important difference.

All thalassemia genes that have been studied to date have been found to contain mutations that directly alter gene structure and subsequently gene function. One of five processes is now believed to be responsible for the genetic defect in thalassemia. These processes are

1. A nonsense mutation leading to early termination of the globin chain synthesis
2. A mutation in one of the noncoding intervening sequences of the original globin chain gene, which causes inefficient splicing to mRNA
3. A mutation in the promoter area that decreases the rate of gene expression
4. A mutation at the termination of the gene that leads to lengthening of the globin chain with additional amino acids; the mRNA becomes unstable and causes a reduction in globin synthesis
5. A total or partial depletion of a globin gene, probably as the result of unequal chromosomes crossing over

Pathophysiology

Thalassemias are characterized by the absence or decrease in the synthesis of one of the two constituent globin subunits of a normal hemoglobin molecule. In α-thalassemia, decreased synthesis of α-globulin results in accelerated red cell destruction because of the formation of insoluble Hb H inclusion in the mature erythrocyte. The more severe β-thalassemia reflects the extreme insolubility of α-globin, which is present in excess in the red cell because of decreased β-globin synthesis. Studies of RNA metabolism in erythroid cells have suggested that many patients with β-thalassemia have a defect in RNA processing. This defect affects efficient RNA splicing during protein globin synthesis.

β-Thalassemia

β-thalassemia is one of the most common single-gene disorders. Most mutations that cause β-thalassemia are point mutations, and rarely by deletions, in functionally important regions of the β-globin gene. More than 200 point mutations in or around the β-globin gene are known to cause decreased production of β-globin, which in turn leads to the excess accumulation of unstable γ-globin chains, ineffective erythropoiesis, and shortened red cell survival. It is still not known how accumulation of excess unmatched α-globulin in β-thalassemia and β-globulin in α-thalassemia leads to erythrocyte hemolysis in the peripheral blood and, particularly in β-thalassemia, premature destruction of erythroid precursors in marrow (ineffective erythropoiesis). Ineffective erythropoiesis now appears to be caused by accelerated apoptosis.

Any combination of normal β genes and β-thalassemia genes is possible, producing a wide variety of phenotypes. In the production of normal hemoglobin, equal quantities of α and β chains are synthesized, which results in a 1:1 α:β chain

TABLE 13.3 β-Thalassemia Types	
Phenotype	**Clinical Descriptions**
Thalassemia minor (Thalassemia trait)	Mild anemia, microcytosis, abnormal erythrocyte morphology, splenomegaly
Thalassemia intermedia	Moderate anemia and ineffective erythropoiesis, microcytosis, abnormal erythrocyte morphology, splenomegaly, iron overload, not transfusion-dependent
Thalassemia major (Cooley anemia)	Severe anemia caused by ineffective erythropoiesis, transfusion-dependent, organ damage (heart, liver, etc.) secondary to iron overload, extramedullary erythropoiesis, hepatosplenomegaly

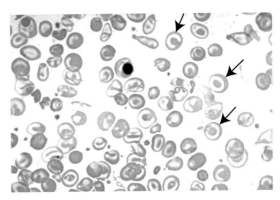

FIGURE 13.7 Thalassemia. The peripheral blood erythrocytes are hypochromic and microcytic and show anisocytosis, poikilocytosis, and target cells (*arrows*). (Reprinted with permission from Raphael R, Strayer DS. *Rubin's Pathology: Clinicopathologic Foundations of Medicine*, 5th ed, Philadelphia, PA: Lippincott Williams & Wilkins, 2008.)

ratio. In β-thalassemia, synthesis of β chains is decreased or absent; therefore, an excess of α chains results.

This underproduction of β chains contributes to a decrease in the total erythrocyte hemoglobin production, ineffective erythropoiesis, and a chronic hemolytic process. The excess free α chains are unstable and precipitate within the cell, causing membrane damage. Marrow macrophages destroy precipitate-filled erythrocytes in the bone marrow, which results in ineffective erythropoiesis. Precipitate-filled circulating erythrocytes are destroyed prematurely in the spleen. This also contributes to the anemia of thalassemia.

β-thalassemia has two main variants (Table 13.3). These descriptions usually reflect the clinical severity of the hemoglobinopathy. In homozygous β-thalassemia, symptoms are usually manifested in early life after hemoglobin synthesis switches from γ-chain to β-chain synthesis several months after birth. Infants fail to grow, and splenomegaly is common. Severe anemia is the most outstanding feature of the disorder and is responsible for many related problems.

Although the clinical severity of β-thalassemia varies considerably, most patients who are homozygous for β-thalassemia become dependent on transfusions and develop transfusion-related complications of iron overload, alloimmunization, and potential viral infection. Patients who have undergone splenectomy and who undergo transfusion therapy infrequently can suffer from thromboembolic phenomena, both venous and arterial. Abnormalities in the levels of coagulation factors and their inhibitors have been reported to result in what is defined as chronic hypercoagulable state. Abnormalities of the red cell membrane contribute to this hypercoagulability.

Laboratory Findings

In β-thalassemia, hematological findings include decreased hemoglobin, hematocrit, and red cell count. The hemoglobin concentration can be as low as 2 or 3 g/dL in homozygous patients. Peripheral blood smears reveal anisocytosis, poikilocytosis, hypochromia, target cells, polychromatophilia, and few to many nucleated red cells (Fig. 13.7). Erythrocytes are significantly microcytic and hypochromic. The red cell indices (MCV, MCH, MCHC) are significantly reduced. In addition, the red cell distribution width (RDW) is increased because of the anisocytosis. Other laboratory findings include increased reticulocyte formation (5% to 10%), decreased osmotic fragility, moderately increased bilirubin, increased serum iron, and saturated total iron-binding capacity (TIBC). Serum ferritin is a sensitive, accurate marker in determination of iron status. Soluble transferring receptor index is useful and is more specific than soluble transferring receptor because serum ferritin may be increased because of other pathology.

Hemoglobin electrophoresis reveals increased Hb F and decreased Hb A. A variable form of homozygous β-thalassemia demonstrates no Hb A, increased Hb A₂, and decreased Hb F. The absence of Hb A is owing to the absence of β-chain synthesis.

Heterozygous β-thalassemia could be mistaken for a mild iron deficiency anemia on a peripheral blood smear. Other laboratory findings include decreased MCV, increased Hb A₂ on electrophoresis, and decreased osmotic fragility. Table 13.4 summarizes the significant test results in SCD, sickle cell trait, and thalassemia.

Prenatal Diagnosis

Prenatal diagnosis of β-thalassemia ideally is conducted in the first trimester of pregnancy using chorionic villus tissue for DNA analysis by PCR to detect point mutations or deletions. Later, second trimester fetal blood analysis is done to estimate relative rates of synthesis of globin chains of hemoglobin. This is performed to estimate relative rates of synthesis of globin in mid-trimester fetuses and base the diagnosis on the beta-to-alpha (β/α) biosynthetic ratio.

TABLE 13.4	Summary of Selected Laboratory Findings in Hemoglobinopathies	
Disorder	**Test**	**Result**
SCD	Hemoglobin	Decreased
	PCV	Decreased
	Erythrocyte count	Decreased
	Hb S	Significantly increased
	Hb A	Decreased
	Hb F	Increased
Sickle cell trait	Hemoglobin	Normal
	PCV	Normal
	Erythrocyte count	Normal
	Hb S	Increased
	Hb A	Slightly decreased
	Hb F	Normal or slightly increased
Homozygous β-thalassemia	Hemoglobin	Decreased
	PCV	Decreased
	Erythrocyte count	Decreased
	Hb S	Negative
	Hb A	Significantly decreased
	Hb F	Increased

PCV, packed cell volume.

Beginning in the early 1990s, methods were developed to perform diagnostic testing before implantation in high-risk patients. Preimplantation genetic diagnosis (PGD) involves performing conventional in vitro fertilization, followed by extracting one or two cells from the resulting blastomeres on day 3. PCR can then be used to detect thalassemia mutations within the cells. Unaffected blastomeres may then be selected for implantation. PGD has now been extended to HLA typing of embryonic biopsies. This allows for the selection of an embryo that is not affected by thalassemia and that may also serve as a stem-cell donor for a previously affected child in the same family. Some of these are ethically controversial or even illegal in some countries.

Newborn Screening

Historically, newborn screening programs have focused on identifying infants with classic β thalassemia major. In the U.S., clinically significant forms of α-thalassemic disorders, HbH including HbH Constant Spring and HbE disorders are becoming increasingly recognized.

Testing for hemoglobinopathies is incorporated into existing programs because of the increasing prevalence of hemoglobinopathies in the United States.

Initial screening methods differ between states, but most newborn screening programs employ HPLC or IET as the preferred first-line technique to make a presumptive diagnosis of a clinically significant hemoglobinopathy. In HbH disorders, accurate quantification of the percentage of Hb Bart's can be used to identify newborns whose levels exceed a specified threshold and require follow-up testing. Prematurity or a previous blood transfusion can create screening problems.

If an abnormal is identified, ethnicity information and parental studies are helpful in guiding the sequence of diagnostic tests for specific hemoglobinopathies. Second-tier testing includes molecular diagnostic testing to distinguish β thalassemia major from Hereditary Persistence of Fetal Hemoglobin (HPFH), HbEβ thalassemia from HbEE, and HbH disease from α thalassemia trait. Genomic microarrays have recently been advocated as a potential diagnostic tool for newborn screening.

Treatment

Medical therapy of thalassemia is one of the most spectacular medical successes of the last two decades. Thalassemia has been transformed from a lethal disease of infancy into a chronic disease of adulthood with a dramatic increase in both survival and life expectancy. In cases of severe anemia, regular blood transfusions are required to prevent death but accumulation of iron from the transfused blood is a problem. To overcome this problem, iron chelation treatment is used. Three iron chelators are available in different parts of the world:

- deferiprone (unlicensed in North America but widely available elsewhere),
- deferoxamine, and
- deferasirox (the newest iron chelator).

The combined use of deferiprone and deferoxaminehas proven to be effective in improving cardiac function and a patient's quality of life.

Bone marrow transplantation from HLA-identical related donors is an accepted treatment for patients with homozygous β-thalassemia. Hematopoietic stem-cell transplantation is the only available curative approach for thalassemia but it is limited by high cost and the scarcity of HLA-matched, related donors. Cost is a particular challenge for patients in developing countries.

Scientists are working to develop a gene therapy that may offer a cure for thalassemia. Such a treatment might involve inserting a normal β-globin gene (the gene that is abnormal in this disease) into the patient's stem cells, the immature bone marrow cells that are the precursors of all other cells in the blood.

Another form of gene therapy could involve using drugs or other methods to reactivate the patient's genes that produce Hb F—the form of hemoglobin found in fetuses and newborns. Scientists hope that spurring production of Hb F will compensate for the patient's deficiency of adult hemoglobin.

In contrast to treatment in developed countries, less developed countries offer entirely different treatment. Safe transfusion and iron chelation therapy are not universally available. Unfortunately, many patients with thalassemia in underdeveloped countries die in childhood or adolescence.

Prevention

Careful counseling and prenatal diagnosis in Sardinia reduced the incidence of homozygous β-thalassemia by more than 90%.

α-Thalassemia

In contrast to β-thalassemia, with most cases caused by point mutations, the major cause of α-thalassemia is deletions that remove one or both α-globulin genes from the affected chromosome 16. α-thalassemias can be classified into four types on the basis of genotype and the total number of abnormal genes that result:

1. Silent carrier state (one inactive α gene)
2. α-thalassemia trait (two inactive α genes)
3. Hb H disease (three inactive α genes)
4. Hydrops fetalis with Hb Bart (four inactive α genes)

In silent carrier state, a patient is missing only one functioning α gene. The three remaining α genes direct the synthesis of an adequate number of α chains for normal hemoglobin synthesis; therefore, patients have no clinical manifestation of hemoglobinopathy. Hemoglobin electrophoresis, red blood cell measurements, and peripheral blood smears are essentially normal.

Hemoglobin constant spring, an unusual form of the silent carrier state, has one deletion and represents an mRNA termination defect. It is a hemoglobin formed from the combination of two structurally abnormal α chains, each elongated by 31 amino acids at the carboxy-terminal end, and two normal β chains. The homozygous state is phenotypically similar to mild α-thalassemia.

Patients with α-thalassemia trait (α-thalassemia-1) have two missing α genes. The imbalance of α- and β-chain synthesis creates an excess in β chains.

Three deletions are present in patients with Hb H disease. Hb H, formed from tetrads of β chains, is unstable and has a high affinity for molecular oxygen (10 × the affinity of Hb A). Erythrocytes containing Hb H produce precipitated Hb H when incubated with brilliant cresyl blue (Fig. 13.8). These erythrocytes have a decreased life span because of the damage to the cell membrane by the precipitated Hb H and the poor handling of inclusions by the normal pitting function of the spleen. Hb H disease is a chronic, moderately severe hemolytic anemia that occurs most frequently in individuals from Southeast Asia. A slight variation in the degree of anemia exists. Conditions such as pregnancy, infection, or the consumption of oxidant drugs worsen the condition. Hemoglobin levels usually range from 8 to 10 g/dL. Red cell indices (MCV, MCH, MCHC) are decreased. The reticulocyte count is increased from 5% to 10%. Hemoglobin electrophoresis demonstrates Hb H (4% to 30%), small amounts of Hb Bart, and a normal or decreased amount of Hb A_2.

Two distinct α-thalassemia syndromes are caused by acquired mutations of the α-globin genes: Hb H disease associated with myeloproliferative or myelodysplastic disorders, and Hb H disease associated with mental retardation. Other variations include Hb H constant spring and homozygous constant spring.

Hydrops fetalis with Hb Bart (see Fig. 13.9) represents a state of four deletions. This lack of α-chain production is incompatible with life. Affected fetuses die either in utero or shortly after birth.

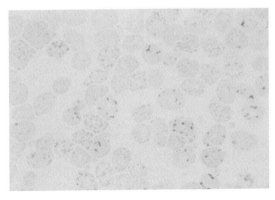

FIGURE 13.8 α-Thalassemia (three-gene deletion) Hb H disease. (Reprinted with permission from Anderson SC. *Anderson's Atlas of Hematology*, Philadelphia, PA: Wolters Kluwer Health/Lippincott Williams & Wilkins, Copyright 2003.)

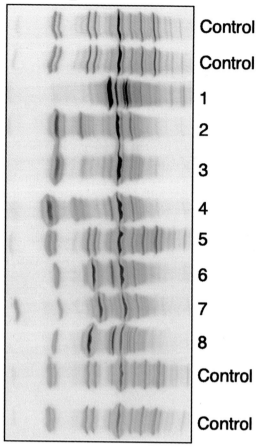

CM877749-13

FIGURE 13.9 IEF gel with examples of common hemoglobin variants. *1*, increased Hb F in a neonate. There is also Hb Bart present, indicating α-thalassemia; *2*, Hb O–Arab trait; *3*, Hb E trait; *4*, Hb C trait; *5*, control consisting of Hbs C-S-G, J, and N; *6*, Hb D–Punjab trait; *7*, Hb G–Philadelphia trait; *8*, Hb S trait. Most specimens also show the aging bands owing to glycerated hemoglobin and methemoglobin. (Reprinted with permission from McClatchey KD. *Clinical Laboratory Medicine*, 2nd ed, Philadelphia, PA: Lippincott Williams & Wilkins, 2002.)

OTHER HEMOGLOBINOPATHIES

Hemoglobin C Disease

This hemoglobinopathy is prevalent in the same geographic area as Hb S (sickle cell) disease. Hb C differs from Hb A by the substitution of a single amino acid residual, lysine, for glutamic acid in the sixth position from the amino (NH_2) terminal end of the β chain. This is the exact point of substitution of Hb S; however, the amino acid is different.

Deoxyhemoglobin C has decreased solubility and forms intracellular crystals Figure 13.10. Erythrocyte morphology is usually normochromic and normocytic, with more than 50% target cells on peripheral blood smear examination. Clinical manifestations include mild, chronic hemolytic anemia

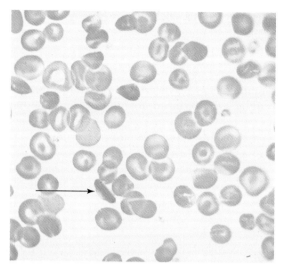

FIGURE 13.10 Hb C crystals. Cell type: Mature red blood cells. Description: Hexagonal, rod-shaped inclusions with blunt ends that stain very dark; formed within the cell membrane; remainder of cell has a clear area. Clinical conditions: Hb CC disease. (Reprinted with permission from Anderson SC. *Anderson's Atlas of Hematology*, Philadelphia, PA: Wolters Kluwer Health/Lippincott Williams & Wilkins, Copyright 2003.)

with associated splenomegaly. Hb C trait is symptomless. Laboratory findings include target cells and possibly mild hypochromia.

Hemoglobin SC Disease

This disorder results from the inheritance of one gene for Hb S from one parent and one gene for Hb C from the other parent. The course of this disease is generally milder than SCD, although Hb C tends to aggregate and potentiate the sickling of Hb S.

Clinical signs and symptoms are similar to mild sickle cell anemia. Laboratory examination of a peripheral blood smear usually reveals target cells, folded erythrocytes, and occasionally, intracellular crystals (see Fig. 13.6).

Hemoglobin D Disease

Hb D has several variants. Patients who are homozygous or heterozygous are asymptomatic. Some target cells may be seen on examination of a peripheral blood smear. Hb D migrates to the same position as Hb S and Hb G at an alkaline pH but migrates with Hb A at an acid pH.

Hemoglobin E Disease

This hemoglobinopathy occurs with the greatest frequency in Southeast Asia. Hb E/β-thalassemia is now a worldwide clinical problem. In some areas of Thailand, the frequency of the Hb E trait is almost 50%. Hb E syndromes appear in both homozygous (E/E) and heterozygous forms (A/E) and as compound heterozygotes in combination with α-, β-thalassemias, and other structural variants. Hb E results from the substitution of lysine for glutamic acid in the β chain of hemoglobin.

Clinical presentation is diverse. It can range from entirely asymptomatic (A/E) to mildly anemic (E/E) to severely anemic (E/β).

In the homozygous state, patients suffer from a mild microcytic anemia with decreased erythrocyte survival. Target cells are visible on peripheral blood smears. In addition to assays to differentiate Hb E anemia from iron deficiency anemia, electrophoresis (cellulose acetate, basic pH) is the procedure used to characterize the hemoglobin pattern. In the United States, most cases of Hb E and its syndromes are discovered through prenatal and newborn screening programs in high-risk populations (e.g., Southeast Asians).

Hemoglobin H Disease

Hb H disease is a mild to severe chronic hemolytic anemia. The disease most frequently results from an absence of three of the four α-globin genes (see α-thalassemia).

This hemoglobin variant primarily affects individuals throughout Southeast Asia, the Mediterranean islands, and parts of the Middle East. Because of the large influx of immigrants from Southeast Asia in the past 20 to 30 years, the prevalence of Hb H disease in the United States has increased significantly.

Hb H migrates at a fast rate at an alkaline pH during hemoglobin electrophoresis. The complete blood count may give important clues to the presence of Hb H disease. All patients exhibit significantly abnormal findings. The results are similar to those in iron deficiency anemia, except that in Hb H disease, the red blood cell count and RDW are usually greater and the MCV is usually lower. A peripheral blood smear exhibits more target cells, anisocytosis, poikilocytosis, and polychromasia than in patients with iron deficiency. The reticulocyte count is generally between 5% and 10% but may be within the normal range. Serum ferritin can be normal or elevated.

Methemoglobinemia

Methemoglobinemia is a disorder associated with elevated methemoglobin levels in the circulating blood. Causes of methemoglobinemia include acquired toxic substances, Hb M variants, and NADH-methemoglobin reductase (also called diaphorase) deficiency.

Hb M has five variant forms. It displays a dominant inheritance resulting from a single substitution of an amino acid in the globin chain that stabilizes iron in the ferric form. NADH-diaphorase is the enzyme that reduces cytochrome b5, which converts naturally occurring ferric iron back to the ferrous state.

Patients with congenital methemoglobinemia tolerate baseline methemoglobin levels of up to 40% without symptoms other than cyanosis. Patients with acquired

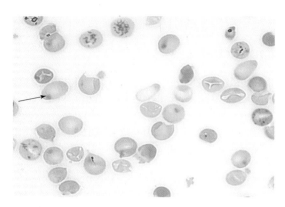

FIGURE 13.11 Heinz bodies. Crystal violet stain. (Reprinted with permission from Anderson SC. *Anderson's Atlas of Hematology*, Philadelphia, PA: Wolters Kluwer Health/Lippincott Williams & Wilkins, Copyright 2003.)

methemoglobinemia caused by foreign oxidants begin to develop symptoms of hypoxia at methemoglobin levels of 20% to 40%. The symptoms produced by methemoglobinemia do not respond to oxygen therapy. Initial therapy consists of removal of any toxin that may be causing the accelerated hemoglobin oxidation. Except in cases of Hb M disease and in patients with glucose-6-phosphate dehydrogenase (G6PD) deficiency, methylene blue effectively treats methemoglobinemia by quickly reducing the ferric heme iron to its useful ferrous state. If life-threatening levels of methemoglobin are present, exchange transfusion may be the therapy of choice.

Unstable Hemoglobins

Unstable hemoglobins are hemoglobin variants in which amino acid substitutions or deletions weaken the binding forces that maintain the internal portion of the globin chains of the hemoglobin molecule. Most unstable hemoglobins are inherited as autosomal dominant disorders.

Instability may cause abnormal hemoglobin to denature and precipitate in erythrocytes such as Heinz bodies. As a result, red blood cells become rigid, membrane damage occurs, and hemolysis results. Hemolysis is usually associated with a change in the normal environment such as the presence of an oxidizing drug or an infection. Heinz bodies (Fig. 13.11) are associated with α- or β-chain abnormalities. Tetramers of normal chains, such as Hb Bart and Hb H, appear in thalassemias.

HEREDITARY PERSISTANCE OF FETAL HEMOGLOBIN

Retention of Hb F (fetal hemoglobin) into adult life is abnormal. The level of expression is 15% to 30% of total hemoglobin. This abnormality is referred to as hereditary persistence of Hb F.

CHAPTER HIGHLIGHTS

Hemoglobin Defects

Hemolytic anemias are characterized by decreased red cell survival caused by inherited or acquired mechanisms. Hemoglobinopathies may have a hemolytic manifestation. Approximately 25% of all hemoglobinopathies demonstrate the decreased red cell survival that characterizes hemolytic disease.

The common denominator in the hemoglobinopathies is that all represent an inherited or genetic defect related to hemoglobin. This defect may result in an abnormal structure of the hemoglobin molecule or a deficiency in the synthesis of normal adult hemoglobin. Hemoglobinopathies can be classified into abnormal molecular structure of one or more of the polypeptide chains of globulin in the hemoglobin molecule; a defect in the rate of synthesis of one or more of the polypeptide chains of globulin in the hemoglobin molecule; and a combination of abnormal molecular structure with a synthesis defect.

Normal adult hemoglobin contains the following components: Hb A (95% to 98%), Hb A_2 (2% to 3%), Hb A_1 (3% to 6%), and Hb F (<1%). The major fraction is Hb A. Typically, the individual with a hemoglobinopathy will demonstrate an alteration in this pattern.

The hemoglobinopathies are inherited diseases. Some of these disorders are caused by the inheritance of an autosomal dominant gene that will produce hemolytic disease in its heterozygous state. Others are autosomal recessive genes and need to be in the homozygous state to produce the disease.

In the hemoglobinopathies, the distinction between the disease state and the trait condition is made. A disease is defined as either the homozygous occurrence of the gene for the abnormality or the possession of a heterozygous, dominant gene that produces a hemolytic condition. A trait is described as the heterozygous and normally asymptomatic state.

Sickle Cell Disease

SCD is a general term for abnormalities of hemoglobin structure and function, hemoglobinopathies, in which the sickle gene is inherited from at least one parent. These genetic disorders are characterized by the production of Hb S, anemia, and acute and chronic tissue damage secondary to the blockage of blood flow produced by abnormally shaped red blood cells.

Sickle cell anemia (Hb SS), the most common form of hemoglobinopathy, is an expression of the inheritance of a sickle gene from both parents. Other sickle cell disorders result from the coinheritance of the sickle gene. Common variants include Hb SC disease and β-thalassemia (S β-thalassemia).

SCD is found most commonly in persons of African ancestry, but it also affects persons of Mediterranean, Caribbean, South and Central American, Arab, and East Indian ancestry. The high prevalence in some regions is owing to a selective advantage of the carrier state to malaria infection.

In the United States, an estimated 8% of the African American population carries the trait, and approximately 1 in 375 African American newborns is born with sickle cell anemia.

Hb SC affects an estimated 1 in 835 African American births, and sickle cell β-thalassemia (S β-thalassemia) affects 1 in 1,667 African American live births. As a result, it is one of the most common genetic diseases in the United States.

When Hb S is deoxygenated, it becomes polymerized and produces sickling. Subsequent hemolysis is probably a result of the extent of the red cell's capacity to sickle. Acute crises are caused by recurrent obstruction of the microcirculation by intravascular sickling. Aside from the painful crisis, sickling takes its toll on the body in other ways. Through the years, the cumulative damage from vascular occlusion can lead to organ and tissue failure. Other complications may include an enlarged heart, progressive loss of pulmonary or renal function, stroke, arthritis, and liver damage.

In addition to decreased hemoglobin, hematocrit, and red blood cell count, a persistent increase in the WBC count is common. The red cell morphology on peripheral blood smear can include moderate to significant anisocytosis, poikilocytosis, and hypochromia. Red cell abnormalities may include target cells, microcytes, polychromatophilia, and basophilic stippling. Howell-Jolly bodies may be present if hyposplenism is present. If the patient is in an acute crisis state, sickled red cells (drepanocytes) may be seen on peripheral smears.

Other diagnostic laboratory tests can include sickle cell screening tests, hemoglobin electrophoresis, the alkali denaturation test, an acid elution test, and determination of the osmotic fragility of erythrocytes.

Conventional management of sickle cell anemia is primarily supportive. It is important to detect infections early and treat them with antibiotics, as these infections may trigger painful and aplastic crises. Drug therapy consisting of erythropoietin injections with the drug, hydroxyurea, is a treatment protocol.

Genetic counseling may be useful in the prevention of sickle cell anemia when the parents are both SA heterozygotes.

Sickle cell anemia was the first molecular disease to be recognized. The severity of illness in SCD differs with the quantity of Hb S in the erythrocytes. The various states associated with the presence of Hb S are S β-thalassemia and SC disease.

Thalassemia

The thalassemia syndromes are among the most common genetic diseases in humans. These syndromes are caused by an abnormality in the rate of synthesis of the globin chains. This is in contrast to the true hemoglobinopathies (e.g., Hb S and Hb C) that result from an inherited molecular defect in one of the globin chains that produces hemoglobin with abnormal physical or functional characteristics.

One of five processes is now believed to be responsible for the genetic defect in thalassemia. These processes are mutations of various types leading to early termination of globin chain synthesis, inefficient splicing of mRNA, a decrease in the rate of gene expression, a reduction in globin synthesis, or a total or partial depletion of a globin.

Classical thalassemia has two main variants: major and minor. These descriptions, however, usually reflect the clinical severity of the hemoglobinopathy. Thalassemia major, also known as Mediterranean or Cooley anemia, is usually equivalent to β-thalassemia in a homozygous form. A third type of thalassemia, Δ-thalassemia, occurs rarely but it is not clinically significant because the Δ chain is a component of the minor hemoglobin, Hb A$_2$.

In β-thalassemia, hematological findings include decreased hemoglobin, hematocrit, and red cell count. The hemoglobin concentration can be as low as 2 or 3 g/dL in homozygous patients. In contrast, heterozygous β-thalassemia could be mistaken for a mild iron deficiency anemia on a peripheral blood smear. Other laboratory findings include decreased MCV, increased Hb A$_2$ on electrophoresis, and decreased osmotic fragility.

β-thalassemia is one of the most common single-gene disorders. More than 100 mutations in or around the β-globin gene are known to cause decreased production of β-globin, which in turn leads to the excess accumulation of unstable γ-globin chains, ineffective erythropoiesis, and shortened red cell survival.

α-thalassemia is a group of disorders characterized by decreased synthesis of α chains. α-Thalassemias can be classified into four types on the basis of genotype and the total number of abnormal genes that result.

Other Hemoglobinopathies

Hb C disease is prevalent in the same geographic area as Hb S (sickle cell) disease. Hb C differs from Hb A by the substitution of a single amino acid residual, lysine, for glutamic acid in the sixth position from the amino (NH$_2$) terminal end of the β chain. This is the exact point of substitution of Hb S; however, the amino acid is different.

Hb E disease occurs with the greatest frequency in Southeast Asia. In some areas of Thailand, the frequency of the Hb E trait is almost 50%. Hb E results from the substitution of lysine for glutamic acid in the β chain of hemoglobin.

Hb H disease is a mild to severe chronic hemolytic anemia. The disease most frequently results from an absence of three of the four α-globin genes.

Methemoglobinemia is a disorder associated with elevated methemoglobin levels in the circulating blood. Causes of methemoglobinemia include acquired toxic substances, Hb M variants, and NADH-diaphorase (NADH-methemoglobin reductase) deficiency.

Unstable hemoglobins are hemoglobin variants in which amino acid substitutions or deletions weaken the binding forces that maintain the internal portion of the globin chains of the hemoglobin molecule. Most unstable hemoglobins are inherited as autosomal dominant disorders.

Hereditary persistence of Hb F is a group of conditions characterized by the abnormal persistence of total hemoglobin synthesis in adult life.

CASE STUDIES

CASE 13.1

An 18-year-old black woman was admitted to the hospital for elective surgery. She had a routine preoperative CBC and urinalysis.

■ **Laboratory Data**
The results of these tests were as follows:

Hemoglobin 13.0 g/dL
Hct 40%
RBC 4.35 × 10^{12}/L
WBC 7.3 × 10^9/L

The RBC indices were as follows:

MCV 92 fL
MCH 29.9 pg
MCHC 33 g/dL

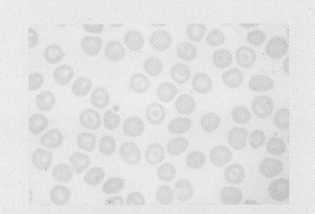

(Reprinted with permission from Anderson SC, *Anderson's Atlas of Hematology*, Philadephia, PA: Wolters Kluwer Health/Lippincott Williams & Wilkins, Copyright 2003.)

(continued)

The patient's peripheral blood smear revealed a normochromic, normocytic pattern; however, a moderate number of target cells (codocytes) were noted throughout the smear. A repeat blood smear obtained from fingertip blood again had a moderate number of codocytes present. The urinalysis revealed no abnormalities. A hematology technician notified the surgeon and anesthetist of the abnormal RBC morphology.

On receipt of these results, the anesthetist postponed surgery and ordered a sickle cell preparation, sickle cell screening test, and hemoglobin electrophoresis. The results were

Sickle cell preparation positive
Hb S screening test positive
Hb electrophoresis: Hb A 63%, Hb F 3%, and Hb S 34%

■ **Questions**

1. Why was it important to establish a diagnosis in this patient's asymptomatic state?
2. What kind of disorder does this patient have?
3. What is the etiology of this patient's condition?

■ **Discussion**

1. This patient has sickle cell trait, which, under ordinary conditions, is usually asymptomatic except for the presence of codocytes on a peripheral blood smear. However, the fact that the patient was to undergo elective surgery made it important for the anesthetist to be aware of the patient's condition to carefully monitor the patient to prevent hypoxia.
2. The presence of a great number of true codocytes on a peripheral film is highly suggestive of hemoglobinopathy. Because the codocytes (target cells) persisted on repeated smears, the possibility that the target appearance was an artifact was eliminated. Supplementary laboratory assays provided the differential information needed to establish the diagnosis of sickle cell trait. The profile of this patient is typical of sickle cell trait. She is a heterozygous Hb A–Hb S. Both the sickle cell preparation, which exposed the cells to reduced oxygen levels, and the Hb S screening test confirmed the electrophoresis findings of the presence of the abnormal type S hemoglobin.
3. This patient has hemoglobinopathy, which is a genetically inherited trait. In her case, she received only one gene for S-type hemoglobin and was fortunate to have received a normal gene for A-type hemoglobin. Approximately 10% of American blacks possess the sickle cell trait. Identifying its existence in an individual is important for two reasons. Exposure to reduced oxygen levels will cause some of the cells of the individual to sickle, and the genetic consequences to future offspring are an impor-

tant aspect of prenatal counseling in both men and women who possess the trait.

DIAGNOSIS: Sickle Cell Trait

CASE 13.2

The 5-year-old son of a Liberian exchange student was hospitalized because of severe diarrhea, abdominal distention, and splenomegaly. The child had been previously diagnosed in Europe as suffering from sickle cell anemia and had experienced several episodes of sickle cell crisis. On admission, the following tests were ordered: CBC, platelet count, bilirubin determination, hemoglobin electrophoresis, Hb S screening test, electrolyte studies, urinalysis, and stool culture.

■ **Laboratory Data**

The results of the tests were as follows:

Hemoglobin 5.8 g/dL
Hct 19%
RBC $2.0 \times 10^{12}/L$

The RBC indices were as follows:

MCV 96 fL
MCH 29 pg
MCHC 31 g/dL

The total WBC count was $8.7 \times 10^9/L$. The peripheral blood smear revealed moderate anisocytosis, macrocytosis, microcytosis, poikilocytosis, polychromatophilia, occasional Howell-Jolly bodies, moderate basophilic stippling, many sickled RBCs (drepanocytes), and 12 (nucleated RBCs) metarubricytes/100 WBCs. The distribution of platelets was normal on the blood smear, and the total platelet count was $0.42 \times 10^{12}/L$.

The patient's total serum bilirubin was 6.0 mg/dL. Hemoglobin electrophoresis demonstrated Hb S 78% and Hb F 22%. The Hb S screening test result was positive. A routine urinalysis was positive for occult blood, and the stool culture was normal. The patient had severely abnormal electrolytes.

■ **Questions**

1. What is the cause of this patient's condition?
2. What is the clinical course of this disease?
3. Explain the presence of the drepanocytes on the peripheral blood film.

■ **Discussion**

1. This patient had been previously diagnosed as having sickle cell anemia. However, the current crisis was undoubtedly precipitated by the dehydration caused by severe diarrhea. Although the exact trigger mechanism is not really known, events such as dehydration, fatigue, and emotional stress can trigger a crisis episode in patients with sickle cell anemia.

(continued)

CASE STUDIES (continued)

2. Sickle cell anemia takes a chronic clinical course. The course of the disease is characterized by hemolytic episodes, severe organ damage, and painful, acute episodes involving both bones and muscles. Painful crises are a feature of this disease. The crises correspond to obstruction of the microcirculation by the sickled cells, followed by ischemia, which produces the associated pain and sometimes consequent necrosis of tissues.

3. Congestion in the microcirculation, tissue hypoxia, and the lowering of blood pH are all factors that promote the gelation of Hb S. With this gelation, the sickle cell assumes its characteristic shape. Many of these cells will assume a discoid shape following reoxygenation; however, dense sickle cells are irreversibly sickled. These cells have a distinctive boat shape and will not resume the normal discoid shape after reoxygenation.

DIAGNOSIS: Sickle Cell Anemia

CASE 13.3

A 21-year-old white female college student of Greek ethnicity visited her gynecologist in San Francisco. She appeared to be healthy and was 3 months pregnant. She was concerned about her future child because she had been diagnosed as a child as having heterozygous β-thalassemia. However, she had never had any "blood problems" but knew that her disorder had been inherited. The following tests were ordered: CBC, urinalysis, and hemoglobin electrophoresis.

■ Laboratory Data

The results of these tests were as follows:

Hemoglobin 11.1 g/dL
Hct 29%
RBC 4.2×10^{12}/L

Her WBC count was 5.8×10^9/L. The peripheral blood smear revealed the presence of significant microcytosis, 2+ hypochromia, and some codocytes (target cells). Her RBC indices were as follows:

MCV 69 fL
MCH 26.4 pg
MCHC 37 g/dL

The distribution of platelets was normal on the peripheral smear. The hemoglobin electrophoresis revealed a slight increase in the Hb A_2 fraction (patient, 3.5%; normal, 2% to 3%) and the F fraction (patient, 2%; normal, <1%). The urinalysis was normal.

On receipt of these results the physician referred the patient to a research laboratory for prenatal testing and counseling.

■ Questions

1. Explain the asymptomatic state and peripheral blood findings in this patient.
2. What kind of advanced prenatal testing can be performed?
3. Is there an option for carriers who do not want to risk having a child with thalassemia?

■ Discussion

1. Patients with heterozygous b-thalassemia are frequently asymptomatic. The expression of this disorder can range from an asymptomatic state, as in this patient, to a fairly severe anemia. Her peripheral blood film is typical of the heterozygous patient with microcytosis, hypochromia, and codocytes. This condition can be confused with iron deficiency anemia until further laboratory studies are conducted, such as serum iron and TIBC and hemoglobin electrophoresis.

2. Modern prenatal testing for hematological disease began in 1974. Before that time, chromosomal studies were performed on amniotic fluid in older women with a high risk of Down syndrome or to determine fetal sex if the patient was at risk for a sex-linked disorder. Methods for obtaining fetal blood in utero were established in 1974, and this led to the development of prenatal diagnosis of any blood disorder that expressed itself in utero. The first disorders to be studied were the hemoglobinopathies, specifically thalassemia. Recently, a third technique that uses amniotic fluid was developed for use with DNA probes. Sampling of fetal blood remains the method of choice for the detection of hematological diseases for which DNA probes are not available.

During the midtrimester, blood is aspirated from the placenta. To determine the proportion of fetal blood in the sample, RBC size (MCV) is performed immediately on the specimen. Fetal erythrocytes have an average MCV of 140 fL, compared with adult or maternal RBCs, which have an average MCV of 100 fL. The sample is then labeled with a radioactive substance and incubated to label newly synthesized globin chains. Mutant β-globins are detected with this technique because they separate from normal β-globin on chromatographic analysis. The diagnosis of α- or β-thalassemia can be made based on either the absence of or the substantially reduced amount of globin in the sample. By this method, 25% of the samples lead to a diagnosis of thalassemia in cases in which the fetus is at risk. This frequency is proportional to the expected frequency for autosomal recessive disorders. If amniocentesis studies are done, the fluid is obtained at 16 to 20 weeks of gestation. The sample must contain enough fetal cells to provide DNA for studies of the globin genes. Earlier studies may now be done using chorionic villi specimens. All these procedures are aimed at the early diagnosis of hematological diseases of genetic origin.

(continued)

3. Assisted reproductive therapy is an option for carriers who do not want to risk having a child with thalassemia. A new technique, PGD, used in conjunction with in vitro fertilization, may enable parents with thalassemia or thalassemia trait to give birth to healthy babies. Embryos created in vitro are tested for the thalassemia gene before being implanted into the mother, allowing only healthy embryos to be selected.

DIAGNOSIS: Prenatal Patient with Thalassemia Minor (Heterozygous β-thalassemia)

CASE 13.4

A 23-year-old Italian woman is noted to be suffering from mild anemia in a preemployment physical examination. The patient denied any significant illness in the past. She has no history of joint or abdominal pain and she was not sickly as a child. She had been told on several occasions that she has anemia and was given medications containing iron. She has not noted any unusual bleeding. Her menstrual periods are regular at monthly intervals and they last for about 3 days. She has never been pregnant. She has no history of excessive alcohol intake.

Physical examination revealed an enlarged spleen. She has no icterus, purpura, or lymphadenopathy. Her liver is not enlarged.

■ Laboratory Data

Hemoglobin 11.0 g/dL
Hematocrit 35%
RBC 5.0×10^{12}/L
WBC 9.5×10^9/L

The peripheral blood smear shows target cells, an occasional sickle-shaped cell, microcytes, and slight hypochromia. The reticulocyte count is 7.2%.

■ Questions
1. What is the differential diagnosis?
2. What test will aid in the differential diagnosis?
3. What is the probable diagnosis?
4. How do you account for this patient's benign course?
5. Why does the patient have disease, compared to AS individuals who are asymptomatic?
6. What complications might arise in the future?

■ Discussion
1. Striking target cells are seen in liver disease and hemoglobinopathies. The fact that hemolysis is present and this patient lacks clinical evidence of liver disease both favor the latter alternative.
2. The following will aid in the differential diagnosis: hemoglobin electrophoresis, serum Fe/TIBC to rule out

iron deficiency, liver function tests, and solubility test for the presence of hemoglobin S. This patient's liver function was normal. The hemoglobin electrophoresis on acrylamide gel was abnormal.
3. Sickle β+ thalassemia
4. The extent of polymer formation is less in S β+ thalassemia, owing primarily to lower MCHC and less crowding of hemoglobin molecules in the red cell. The ability to synthesize some Hb A also reduces intracellular polymer formation.
5. Cells contain much more Hb S and therefore will form more polymer.
6. Proliferative retinopathy and avascular necrosis of hip; these complications are particularly common in sickle β+ thalassemia and in SC disease for unclear reasons.

DIAGNOSIS: Sickle β-thalassemia

CASE 13.5

A 50-year-old white woman wanted to realize a lifelong dream of trekking in Nepal. One year before her expected date of departure, she began a vigorous exercise program to build up her strength and endurance for this trip. She was in excellent health at the beginning of her training and at her departure from the East Coast of the United States for Katmandu, Nepal.

After a few days on the trail, as the group was approaching the base camp at 6,500 ft, the patient began to experience shortness of breath, abdominal pain in her left upper quadrant, and blood in her urine. She was rushed to the nearest emergency station and then transported by air lift to Katmandu.

In Katmandu, the patient was examined and found to have a very slightly enlarged spleen with slight tenderness. A CBC and urinalysis were ordered.

■ Laboratory Data

RBC 3.82×10^{12}/L
Hematocrit 29%
Hemoglobin 9.5 g/dL
WBC 15.1×10^9/L
Platelets 455×10^9/L
MCV 74 fL
MCH 25 pg
MCHC 33 g/dL

■ Leukocyte Differential

1% band neutrophils
68% segmented neutrophils
5% eosinophils
1% monocytes
25% lymphocytes

(continued)

The peripheral blood smear revealed 2+ polychromatophilia, 2+ anisocytosis, and 2+ target cells.

Urinalysis showed 3+ blood.

■ **Questions**

1. What is the significance of the laboratory findings?
2. Do any of the other findings suggest a hemoglobinopathy?
3. What other tests would be valuable?
4. What precipitated the incident?
5. This woman is not of African ancestry. How can she be a sickle cell carrier?

■ **Discussion**

1. The targeted red cells could be caused by an artifact, and a repeat blood smear should be made. However, the presence of polychromatophilia, targeted red blood cells, and a slight anemia are suggestive of hemoglobinopathy.
2. Yes. The presence of an enlarged spleen indicates that a hematological condition might exist. Painless hematuria that is otherwise unexplained can occur in sickle cell trait.
3. A reticulocyte count and hemoglobin electrophoresis were ordered for this patient. In this case, the results revealed an increased reticulocyte count (3.5%), and the hemoglobin electrophoresis revealed the presence of Hb A and Hb S.
4. In the United States, the heterozygous state (sickle cell trait [AS]) is usually considered to be a benign condition in about 9% of Americans of African descent. However, at moderately high altitudes (5,400 to 9,600 ft above sea level), sickle cell carriers can express clinical symptoms (e.g., splenic infarction causing abdominal pain). Increased fragility of RBCs seen in sickle cell trait can lead to hematuria. Other conditions that can precipitate a sickle cell crisis in carriers include anesthesia, unpressurized aircraft, congestive heart failure, and lower respiratory tract problems.
5. In addition to being found in persons of African ancestry, sickle cell anemia and trait occur in Mediterranean countries (e.g., Sicily), the Arabian peninsula, and India. Isolated cases have been found in other countries.

DIAGNOSIS: Sickle Cell Trait

CASE 13.6

A 30-year-old pregnant Thai woman was referred to a hematologist because of anemia. The hematologist ordered a hemoglobin, hematocrit, and RBC indices; serum iron; percent saturation; and urinalysis.

■ **Laboratory Data**

Hematocrit 27%
Hemoglobin 8.1 g/dL
MCV 65 fL
MCH 20 pg
MCHC 30 g/dL

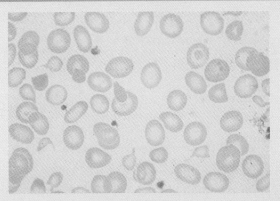

(Reprinted with permission from Anderson SC. *Anderson's Atlas of Hematology*, Philadephia, PA: Wolters Kluwer Health/ Lippincott Williams & Wilkins, Copyright 2003.)

Serum iron and percent saturation were within normal limits. Urinalysis results were also normal.

■ **Questions**

1. What is the cause of this patient's low hemoglobin and hematocrit?
2. What follow-up laboratory assays should be ordered?
3. What confirmatory laboratory assay should be performed?
4. What is the etiology of her hemoglobinopathy?

■ **Discussion**

1. During pregnancy many women suffer from iron deficiency anemia, which is characterized by a decreased hemoglobin and hematocrit and decreased red blood cell indices. However, this patient was not iron deficient according to her serum iron and percent saturation values.
2. Because of the patient's Asian ancestry and the exclusion of iron deficiency anemia as a diagnosis, a hemoglobin electrophoresis was ordered. The results of the procedure demonstrated an abnormal hemoglobin band whose migration pattern was suggestive of Hb H.
3. Hb H is an unstable hemoglobin. Demonstration of Heinz bodies, inclusions formed by precipitated unstable hemoglobin in red blood cells that are oxidatively denatured and stained with brilliant cresyl blue stain, confirms the presence of the unstable hemoglobin.
4. The genetic defect responsible for the presence of Hb H is a gene deletion. α-Thalassemias are most frequently caused by deletion mutations that affect globin chain synthesis. Anemia associated with thalassemia is caused by diminished production of functional hemoglobin and increased destruction of red blood cells compromised by intracellular inclusions.

DIAGNOSIS: α-Thalassemia

REVIEW QUESTIONS

1. The common denominator in the hemoglobinopathies is that all are
   A. structural defects in the erythrocyte membrane
   B. metabolic defects in the erythrocytic physiology
   C. inherited or genetic defects related to hemoglobin
   D. acquired defects related to hemoglobin

2. Hemoglobinopathies can be classified as
   A. abnormal hemoglobin globulin structure
   B. a defect of hemoglobin globulin synthesis
   C. a combination of defects of both structure and synthesis
   D. all of the above

3. Normal adult hemoglobin contains the following components: Hb A (95% to 98%), Hb A_2 (2% to 3%), Hb A_1 (3% to 6%), and Hb F (<1%).
   A. True
   B. False

4. In the hemoglobinopathies, a trait is described as
   A. heterozygous and asymptomatic
   B. heterozygous and symptomatic
   C. homozygous and asymptomatic
   D. homozygous and symptomatic

5. In sickle cell anemia the cause is
   A. a change of a single nucleotide (GAT to GTT)
   B. the substitution of valine for glutamic acid at the sixth position on the beta chain of the hemoglobin molecule
   C. not genetic
   D. both A and B

6. In sickle cell disease the abnormality is related to
   A. the rate of synthesis of hemoglobin
   B. an abnormal molecular structure of hemoglobin
   C. an acquired defect
   D. a membrane dysfunction

7. One of the two most common monogenetic diseases of man is
   A. sickle cell trait
   B. sickle cell anemia
   C. α-thalassemia
   D. Hb SC disease

8. If a patient with sickle cell anemia is in an acute crisis state, peripheral blood smears may exhibit
   A. leptocytes
   B. drepanocytes
   C. ovalocytes
   D. stomatocytes

9. What estimated percentage of black Americans are heterozygous for Hb S?
   A. 4%
   B. 8%
   C. 12%
   D. More than 25%

10. What factors contribute to the sickling of erythrocytes in sickle cell anemia crisis?
    A. Increase in blood pH and increase in oxygen
    B. Extremely hot weather
    C. Extremely reduced oxygen and increased acidity in the blood
    D. Sickling is spontaneous

11. The most common complaint associated with sickle cell anemia?
    A. Acute pain
    B. Organ or tissue failure
    C. Stroke
    D. All of the above

12. Thalassemias are characterized by
    A. abnormal amino acid sequence of the hemoglobin molecules
    B. defective iron synthesis
    C. absence or decrease in synthesis of one or more globlin subunits
    D. skeletal membrane defects

13. Homozygous β-thalassemia patients have
    A. no manifestations of anemia
    B. only mild anemia
    C. moderate anemia
    D. severe transfusion-dependent anemia

14. In α-type thalassemia, with three inactive α genes, which of the following is characteristic?
    A. Hb A_2
    B. Hb A
    C. Hb H
    D. Hb F and A_2

15. What is the primary risk to thalassemia major patients who receive frequent and multiple blood transfusions?
    A. Iron overload
    B. Citrate toxicity
    C. Polycythemia
    D. Hyperviscosity

16. The peripheral blood smear in silent state patients with α-thalassemia typically appears as
    A. normochromic, normocytic
    B. microcytic, hypochromic
    C. macrocytic, normocytic
    D. macrocytic, hypochromic

17. The characteristic hemoglobin concentration in a patient's silent state with heterozygous β-thalassemia is
    A. Hb A level normal
    B. Hb A_2 increased
    C. Hb A_2 level decreased
    D. Hb F level increased

(continued)

REVIEW QUESTIONS *(continued)*

18. Deoxyhemoglobin C has
    A. decreased solubility
    B. increased solubility
    C. the ability to form intracellular crystals
    D. both A and C
19. The incidence of Hb E hemoglobinopathy is highest in
    A. Southeast Asia
    B. China
    C. Vietnam
    D. Native Americans
20. Most unstable hemoglobins
    A. are inherited autosomal dominant disorders
    B. result from amino acid substitutions or deletions
    C. are hemoglobin variants
    D. all of the above

BIBLIOGRAPHY

Abou-Diwan C, Young AN, Molinaro RJ. Hemoglobinopathies and clinical laboratory testing, *Med Lab Observ*, 41(8):10–16, 2009.

Abdulrahman, J. Hemoglobinopathies in the United Arab Emirates: current screening and diagnostic techniques. Unpublished Master's Thesis: Northeastern University, Boston, 2006.

Ahmed S, et al. Screening extended families for genetic hemoglobin disorders in Pakistan, *N Engl J Med*, 347(15):1162–1168, 2002.

Alymara V, et al. Evaluation of pulmonary function in patients with β-thalassemia Major, *J Hematol*, 20(4 Suppl 2):61, 2003.

Angelucci E, Baronciani D. Allogenic stem cell transplantation for thalassemia major, *Hematologia*, 93(12):1780, 2008.

Ataga KI. Novel therapies in sickle cell disease, *Am Soc Hematol*, , 54–60, 2009 (50th Anniversary Issue).

Camberlein E, et al. Anemia in β-thalassemia patients targets hepatic hepcidin transcript leels independently of iron metabolism genes controlling hepcidin expression, *Haematologica*, 93(1):111–115, 2008.

Cao A, Galanello R. Effect of consanguinity on screening for thalassemia, *N Engl J Med*, 347(15):1200–1202, 2002.

Chen FE, et al. Genetic and clinical features of hemoglobin H disease in Chinese patients, *N Engl J Med*, 343(8): 544–550, 2000

Chui D. Thal for Thal, *Blood*, 110(8):2788–2789, 2007.

Cohen AR. Iron chelation therapy: you gotta have heart, *Blood*, 115(12), 2333–2334, 2010.

Colombatti R, et al. Hospitalization of children with sickle cell disease in a region with increasing immigration rates, *Haematologica*, 93(3):463–464, 2008.

Farmaki KF. Combined chelation therapy in patients with thalassaemia major: Research protocol or routine therapy, *J Hematol*, 4(Suppl 2):64, 2003.

Hoppe CC. Newborn screening for non-sickling hemoglobinopathies, *Am Soc Hematol*, 19–40, 2009 (50th Anniversary Issue).

Khoury MJ, et al. Population screening in the age of genomic medicine, *N Engl J Med*, 348(1):50–58, 2003.

Matsui NM. P-selectin mediates the adhesion of sickle erythrocytes to the endothelium, *Blood*, 98(6):1955–1962, 2001.

Mayo Clinic Staff. www.MayoClinic/sickle cell anemia.com. Retrieved 16 December 2009.

Persons DA. Hematopoietic stem cell gene transfer for the treatment of hemoglobin disorders, *Am Soc Hematol*, 690–697, 2009 (50th Anniversary Issue).

Platt OS, Guinan EC. Bone marrow transplantation in sickle cell anemia—the dilemma of choice, *N Engl J Med*, 335(6):426–427, 1996.

Rund D, Rachmilewitz E. β-Thalassemia, *NEJM*, 353:11, 2005.

Steensma DP, Hoyer JD, Fairbanks VF. Hereditary red blood cell disorders in middle eastern patients, *Mayo Clinic Proc*, 76:285–293, 2001.

Steinberg MH. Management of sickle cell disease, *N Engl J Med*, 340(13):1021–1030, 1999.

Thien SL. Genetic modifiers of β-thalassemia. *Haematologica*, 90(5):649–660, 2005.

Turgeon ML. *Clinical Hematology*, 4th ed, Philadelphia, PA: Lippincott Williams & Wilkins, 2003.

U.S. Department of Health and Human Services. Guideline: laboratory screening for sickle cell disease, *Lab Med*, 24(8):515–522, 1993.

Verduzco LA, Nathan DG. Sickle cell disease and stroke, *Blood*, 114(25):5117–5125, 2009.

Vichinsky VP. *Changing Patterns of Thalassemia Worldwide, Annals of the New York Academy of Sciences-Cooley's Anemia: Eighth Symposium*, 1054:18–24, 2006.

Voon HPJ, Vadolas J. Controlling α-globin: a review of α-globin expression and its impact on β-thalassemia, *Haematologica*, 93:1868–1876, 2008.

Voskaridou E, et al. The effect of prolonged administration of hydroxyurea on morbidity and mortality in adult patients with sickle cell syndromes: results of a 17-year, single-center trial (LaSHS), *Blood*, 115(12):2354–2363, 2010.

Wadia MR, et al. Usefulness of automated chromatography for rapid fetal blood analysis for second trimester prenatal diagnosis of β-thalassemia, *Prenat Diagn*, 22:153–157, 2002.

Ware RE, Aygun B. Advances in the use of hydroxyurea, *Am Soc Hematol*, 62–68, 2009 (50th Anniversary Issue).

Zago MA, et al. Hydroxyurea treatment reduces the exposure of phosphatidylserine on erythrocytes and platelets in sickle cell anemia, *J Hematol*, 4(Suppl 2):60, 2003.

CHAPTER **14**

Leukocytes: The Granulocytic and Monocytic Series

OBJECTIVES

The granulocytic series

- Briefly explain the factors related to the development of multipotential progenitor cells into specific leukocyte cell lines.
- List each type of immature neutrophil found in the proliferative compartment of the bone marrow along with the percentage of each and the approximate time spent in each developmental stage.
- List each type of neutrophil found in the maturation-storage compartment of the bone marrow along with the percentage of each and the approximate time spent in this phase.
- Describe the chemical factors and cellular characteristics that permit neutrophils to leave the bone marrow and enter the peripheral circulation.
- Define the terms **marginating** and **circulating pools** and discuss the length of time the neutrophils, eosinophils, and basophils spend in each pool.
- Describe the nuclear and cytoplasmic characteristics of the neutrophils, eosinophils, and basophils throughout the maturation process.
- Explain the appearance and etiology of the various morphological abnormalities encountered in mature granulocytes.
- Describe the abnormalities associated with mature granulocytes in body fluids.

The monocytic-macrophage series

- Discuss the differentiation of monocytes and macrophages from the multipotential stem cell.

- Compare the bone marrow maturation of the monocyte with that of the neutrophil.
- Describe the nuclear and cytoplasmic characteristics of the monocyte as it develops.

Normal values and functional properties of granulocytes and macrophages

- List the normal values for neutrophils, eosinophils, basophils, and monocytes in normal peripheral blood.
- Explain the activities of the acute inflammatory response.
- Describe the characteristics of sepsis syndrome.
- Describe the general characteristics and specific details of phagocytosis.
- Discuss the specialized functions of eosinophils, basophils, and monocytes.

Assessment methods

- Describe the rationale for each of the methods used in the assessment of inflammatory conditions.

Case study

- Apply laboratory data to the stated case study and discuss the implication of this case to the study of hematology.

INTRODUCTION

The cellular elements of the blood are produced from a common, multipotential hematopoietic cell. This cell, the progenitor cell, undergoes mitotic division. Subsequent maturation of progenitor cells produces the major categories of the cellular elements of the circulating blood: the erythrocytes, leukocytes, and thrombocytes.

On the basis of function, leukocytes can be divided into the granulocytic, monocytic, and lymphoid series. This chapter discusses the granulocytic leukocytes, which can be further subdivided on the basis of morphology into neutrophils,

eosinophils, basophils, and the monocytic-macrophage series.

THE GRANULOCYTIC SERIES

Production of Neutrophils, Eosinophils, and Basophils

Factors that regulate the commitment of a human hematopoietic progenitor cell to a specific cell line, such as the granulocytic cell type, and their function are influenced by the hematopoietic growth factors, the interleukins, and the microenvironment (see Chapter 4).

Cells that are committed to differentiation as granulocytes have been cloned in vitro and have produced a mixture of granulocytes and macrophage cells. Further growth of these cells is dependent on **colony-stimulating factor** (CSF) and interleukins. The presence of different CSFs favors interleukins, and the microenvironment of the progenitor cell favors differential development of either the granulocytic (**myeloid**) series or the macrophage-monocytic series. In addition to the differentiation of granulocytes and monocytes, different CSFs stimulate specific differentiation, such as the development of eosinophils.

Sites of Development and Maturation

The development, distribution, and destruction of neutrophils, eosinophils, and basophils are collectively referred to as **granulocytic kinetics**. The neutrophil, basophil, and eosinophil each begin as a multipotential cell in the bone marrow. Throughout the normal processes of differentiation, multiplication, and maturation, these cells remain in the bone marrow. After developing into either band or segmented forms, mature cells enter into the blood circulation.

Development and Proliferation of Neutrophils, Eosinophils, and Basophils

When the colony-forming-unit-granulocyte-erythrocyte-megakaryocyte (CFU-GEMM) progenitor cell differentiates into the colony-forming-unit-granulocyte-macrophage (CFU-GM) progenitor cell, the cell line becomes committed to developing into a myeloblast; the maturational development from the myeloblast through the myelocyte stage and mitotic division take place in what is referred to as the bone marrow's **proliferative compartment** (Fig. 14.1A). This is also called the **mitotic pool** and includes cells capable of DNA synthesis.

The **myeloblast** is the first identifiable cell in the granulocytic series. Myeloblasts constitute approximately 1% of the total nucleated bone marrow cells. This stage lasts approximately 15 hours. The next stage, the **promyelocyte**,

constitutes approximately 3% of the nucleated bone marrow cells. This stage lasts about 24 hours. The **myelocyte** is the next maturational stage, with approximately 12% of the proliferative cells existing in this stage. The stage from myelocyte to **metamyelocyte** lasts an average of 4.3 days. Once the metamyelocyte stage has been reached, cells have undergone four or five cell divisions and the **proliferative phase** comes to an end.

Following the proliferative stage, granulocytes enter a **maturation-storage compartment** (Fig. 14.1B). The metamyelocytes and band forms mature into segmented granulocytes in this compartment of the bone marrow. The relative proportions of these cells are approximately 45%, 35%, and 20%, respectively. The segmented neutrophils in the maturation-storage compartment are frequently referred to as the **marrow reserve**. This reserve constitutes a 4- to 8-day supply of neutrophils. It is estimated that neutrophilic granulocytes normally remain in the maturation-storage phase for 7 to 10 days. Eosinophils remain for about 2.5 days, and basophils remain in this phase for the shortest period, approximately 12 hours.

Distribution of Neutrophils, Eosinophils, and Basophils

The release of neutrophils from the bone marrow into the circulatory system is a complex process. Certain characteristics (Fig. 14.2) and physiological regulators promote movement of the granulocytes through the sinusoid wall of the bone marrow, which is normally an anatomical barrier. Some of the factors that influence cellular release include

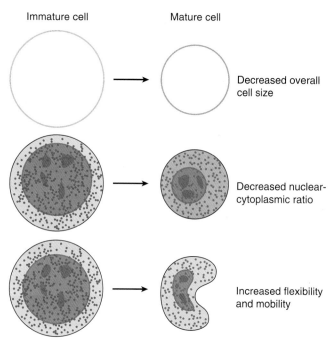

FIGURE 14.2 Comparative maturational characteristics. As cells mature, they are able to move through the sinusoids of the bone marrow because of a decreased overall cell size, a decreased nuclear-cytoplasmic ratio, and increased flexibility and mobility.

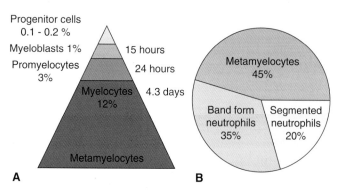

FIGURE 14.1 Bone marrow compartments. **A:** Proliferative. **B:** Maturation-storage.

the interleukins. Cellular characteristics include an overall reduction in cell size and a smaller nuclear-cytoplasmic ratio. The greater flexibility and mobility of mature cells enhance the migration of cells through the marrow sinusoids into the peripheral blood pool.

The peripheral blood circulation is subsequently divided into two pools of equal size: the **circulating** and the **marginating** pools. The marginating granulocytes adhere to the endothelium of the blood vessels. Some granulocytes are additionally found in the spleen. Mature granulocytes in the peripheral blood are only in transit to their potential sites of action in the tissues. The movement of granulocytes from the circulating pool to the peripheral tissues occurs by a process called **diapedesis**. Once in the peripheral tissues, granulocytes, particularly the neutrophils, are able to carry out their function of **phagocytosis**.

The average life span of a segmented neutrophilic granulocyte in the circulating blood is approximately 7 to 10 hours. Once mature cells have migrated into the tissues, their life span is considered to be several days, unless the cells encounter antigens, toxins, or microorganisms. Eosinophils are in the peripheral blood for a few hours and are believed to reside in the tissues for several days. Basophils have an average circulation time of about 8.5 hours. If excessive numbers of eosinophils are present because of a disease state, damaged or degenerated eosinophils give rise to **Charcot-Leyden crystals** found in body secretions, such as the sputum and stool. If cells are not prematurely destroyed while defending the body, they are sloughed off with various body secretions, such as the urine, saliva, or gastrointestinal secretions. An alternative route for the removal of granulocytes from the circulation is phagocytosis by the mononuclear phagocyte cells of the spleen.

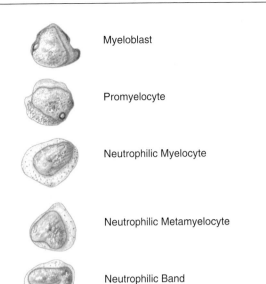

Myeloblast

Promyelocyte

Neutrophilic Myelocyte

Neutrophilic Metamyelocyte

Neutrophilic Band

Segmented Neutrophil
(Polymorphonuclear Neutrophil)

FIGURE 14.3 Neutrophilic series. (Reprinted with permission from Anderson SA, Poulsen KB. *Anderson's Atlas of Hematology*, Philadelphia, PA: Lippincott Williams & Wilkins, 2003.)

Normal Maturational Characteristics of Neutrophils, Eosinophils, and Basophils

Myeloblast

In the maturational sequence (Fig. 14.3; Table 14.1), the earliest morphologically identifiable granulocytic precursor

TABLE 14.1	**Maturational Characteristics of Neutrophilic Granulocytes**					
	Myeloblast	**Promyelocyte**	**Myelocyte**	**Metamyelocyte**	**Band**	**Segmented**
Size (µm)	10–18	14–20	12–18	10–18	10–16	10–16
N:C ratio	4:1	3:1	2:1–1:1	1:1	1:1	1:1
Nucleus						
Shape	Oval or round	Oval or round	Oval or indented	Indented	Elongated, curved	Distinct lobes (2–5)
Nucleoli	1–5	1–5	Variable	None	None	None
Chromatin	Reticular	Smooth	Slightly clumped	Clumped	Very clumped	Densely packed
Cytoplasm						
Inclusions	Auer rods	None	None	None	None	None
Granules	None	Heavy	Fine	Fine	Fine	Fine
		Nonspecific	Specific	Specific	Specific	Specific
Amount	Scanty	Slightly increased	Moderate	Moderate	Abundant	Abundant
Color	Medium blue	Moderate blue	Blue-pink	Pink	Pink	Pink

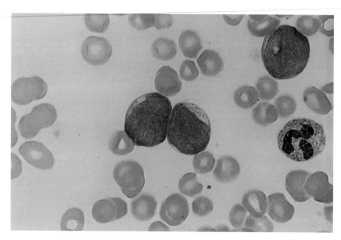

FIGURE 14.4 Type I (**left cell**) and II (**right cell**) myeloblasts. (Reprinted with permission from McClatchey KD. *Clinical Laboratory Medicine*, 2nd ed, Philadelphia, PA: Lippincott Williams & Wilkins, 2002.)

is the **myeloblast** (Fig. 14.4). This cell has an average overall diameter of 10 to 18 μm. The nuclear chromatin is finely reticular, with one to five light-staining nucleoli. The cytoplasm appears as a small rim of basophilic cytoplasm that lacks granules. **Auer rods** (Fig. 14.5), which are aggregates of fused lysosomes, may appear as red, needle-like crystalline cytoplasmic inclusions. These inclusions may appear alone or in groups. Auer rods are pathological, not normal, inclusions.

Promyelocyte

The **promyelocyte** (Fig. 14.6) represents the second maturational stage seen in granulocytes. The outstanding feature of this cell is the presence of prominent granulation that may actually obscure the other morphological features of the cell. These granules are primarily **azurophilic** granules and are rich in the enzymes myeloperoxidase and chloroacetate esterase.

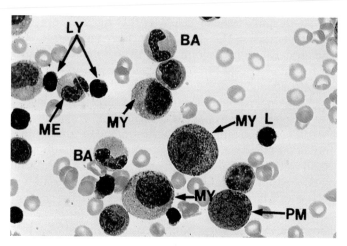

FIGURE 14.6 Photomicrograph of a bone marrow aspirate smear shows erythroid and granulocytic maturation. MB, myeloblast; PM, promyelocyte; MY, myelocyte; ME, metamyelocyte; MO, monocyte; PN, pronormoblast; BN, basophilic normoblast; PCN, polychromatophilic normoblast; ON, orthochromatic normoblast; PC, plasma cell. (Reprinted with permission from McClatchey KD. *Clinical Laboratory Medicine*, 2nd ed, Philadelphia, PA: Lippincott Williams & Wilkins, 2002.)

The promyelocyte is larger than the blast stage, with an average diameter of 14 to 20 μm. The N:C ratio is lower in the promyelocyte than in the myeloblast. The nuclear chromatin is more condensed than in the blast, and nucleoli are present. The cytoplasm is a pale grayish blue.

Myelocyte

The **myelocyte** (Fig. 14.7) is the third maturational stage. This cell is characterized by the recognizable appearance of secondary or specific cytoplasmic granulation. The separate cell types—neutrophils, eosinophils, and basophils—become visibly recognizable at this stage. Neutrophilic granules are fine and stain a blue-pink color with Wright stain. Eosinophilic granules are larger than neutrophilic granules. These round or oval-shaped granules are orange and have a glassy or semiopaque texture. Basophilic granules have a dark blue-black color and a dense appearance. The myelocyte has an average diameter of 12 to 18 μm. The

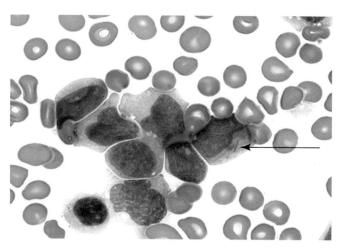

FIGURE 14.5 Auer rods. (Reprinted with permission from Anderson S, Poulsen K. *Anderson's Atlas of Hematology*, Philadelphia, PA: Lippincott Williams & Wilkins, 2003.)

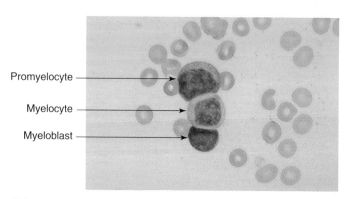

FIGURE 14.7 Myeloblast, myelocyte, promyelocyte. (Reprinted with permission from Anderson S, Poulsen K. *Anderson's Atlas of Hematology*, Philadelphia, PA: Lippincott Williams & Wilkins, 2003.)

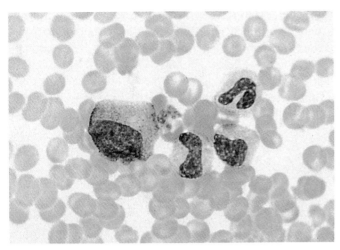

FIGURE 14.8 Two neutrophil myelocytes (one large and one small), a neutrophil metamyelocyte, and a juvenile neutrophil (stab form) from a normal marrow smear. (Reprinted with permission from Mills SE. *Histology For Pathologists*, 3rd ed, Philadelphia, PA: Lippincott Williams & Wilkins, 2007.)

N:C ratio continues to decrease. The nucleus has a more oval appearance than in previous stages, nucleoli are no longer visible, and the chromatin is much more clumped than in previous stages.

Metamyelocyte

The **metamyelocyte** (Fig. 14.8) is the fourth maturational stage. Its most characteristic feature is that the nucleus begins to assume an indented or kidney bean shape, which will continue to elongate as the cell matures through this phase. The chromatin continues to become more condensed or clumped. The color of the specific granulation continues to become a major distinguishing feature.

Mature Forms

Two stages of granulocytes are observed in the circulating blood: the **band form** and the **segmented form** (Fig. 14.9). The band form has a typical elongated nucleus.

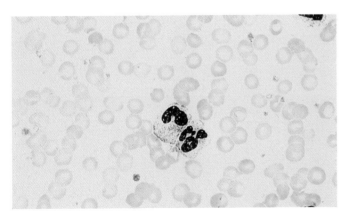

FIGURE 14.9 Peripheral blood smear from a normal individual. Segmented neutrophil. (Reprinted with permission from McClatchey KD. *Clinical Laboratory Medicine*, 2nd ed, Philadelphia, PA: Lippincott Williams & Wilkins, 2002.)

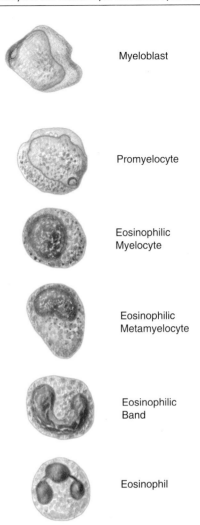

Myeloblast

Promyelocyte

Eosinophilic Myelocyte

Eosinophilic Metamyelocyte

Eosinophilic Band

Eosinophil

FIGURE 14.10 Eosinophilic series. (Reprinted with permission from Anderson SA, Poulsen KB. *Anderson's Atlas of Hematology*, Philadelphia, PA: Lippincott Williams & Wilkins, 2003.)

A mature, segmented neutrophil has a characteristic multilobed nucleus. The separate lobes are attached to each other by a fine thread-like filament. The filament, between separate lobes may be hidden. The nucleus of the basophil can be difficult to see because it is usually obscured by dark, large granules.

The band form of neutrophils, eosinophils, and basophils and, in the final stage of maturation, the segmented neutrophils, eosinophils (Fig. 14.10), and basophils (Fig. 14.11) are the cell forms normally found in the circulating blood.

Mast cells (tissue basophils) are not observed in the blood of healthy persons. These cells have an appearance similar to that of the blood basophil. Mast cells have a round or oval nucleus. The granules of the mast cell do not overlie the nucleus as they do in basophils.

Granulation in Mature Forms

Although all granules are commonly produced by the rough endoplasmic reticulum and transported to the Golgi apparatus for packaging, the granules of each cell type stain

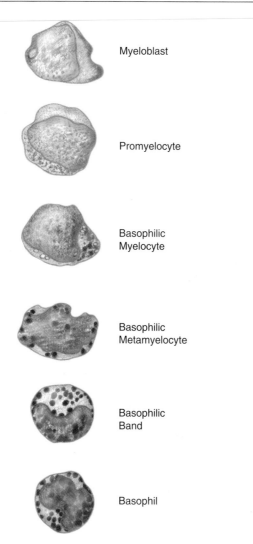

- Myeloblast
- Promyelocyte
- Basophilic Myelocyte
- Basophilic Metamyelocyte
- Basophilic Band
- Basophil

FIGURE 14.11 Basophilic series. (Reprinted with permission from Anderson SA, Poulsen KB. *Anderson's Atlas of Hematology*, Philadelphia, PA: Lippincott Williams & Wilkins, 2003.)

differently because their contents vary. The characteristics of these granules are as follows.

The granules of **segmented neutrophils** are rich in various antibacterial substances, including lysosomal hydrolases, lysozyme, and myeloperoxidase. Some of these granules are typical lysosomes.

Eosinophilic granules differ from neutrophilic granules in that they lack lysozyme. These granules are of two types:

1. Smaller round granules, which have been identified as not containing crystalloids. These granules exist in small quantities in the mature eosinophil and are rich in acid phosphatase.
2. Larger crystalline granules, which are more numerous. These crystalline granules are elliptical, are larger than the granules of the neutrophil, and have an amorphous matrix surrounding an internal crystalline structure. The crystals are thought to represent the enzyme peroxidase (*not* the same as the myeloperoxidase found in neutrophils), and the matrix contains acid phosphatase.

Basophilic granules contain heparin and histamine. **Mast cells** have granules that have an enzyme content similar to those of the blood basophil.

THE MONOCYTIC-MACROPHAGE SERIES

Cells of the mononuclear phagocyte system include the monocytes and macrophages. Macrophages (Fig. 14.12) have a variety of names, including **histiocytes** in the loose connective tissues, **Kupffer cells** in the sinusoids of the liver, **osteoclasts** in bone, and **microglial cells** in the nervous system. The name of the cell changes with the location of the cell; however, mature macrophages are distributed throughout the body. These cells, along with the reticular cells of the spleen, thymus, and lymphoid tissues, are collectively referred to as the **mononuclear phagocyte** (Fig. 14.13). The predominant phagocytic cell, the segmented neutrophil, is confined to the circulating blood unless it is recruited into the tissues.

Production and Development of Monocytes and Macrophages

Cells of the macrophage system are formed from the progenitor cells in the bone marrow. These cells are derived from the CFU-GM, which can differentiate into either the megakaryocyte-colony-forming- unit (CFU-M) and develop into a monocyte or macrophage or the granulocyte-colony-forming-unit (CFU-G) and develop into a segmented neutrophil. A monocyte is influenced by hematopoietic growth factors to transform into a macrophage in the tissues. Functionally, monocytes and macrophages have phagocytosis as their major role, although they also have regulatory and secretory functions.

In contrast to the granulocytic leukocytes, the promonocyte will undergo two or three mitotic divisions in approximately 2 to 2.5 days. Monocytes are released into the circulating blood within 12 to 24 hours after their precursors

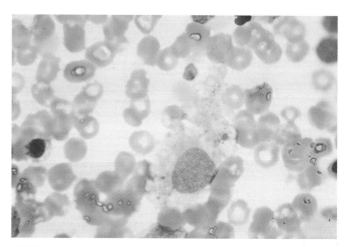

FIGURE 14.12 Macrophage. (Reprinted with permission from Anderson SA, Poulsen KB. *Anderson's Atlas of Hematology*, 2003.)

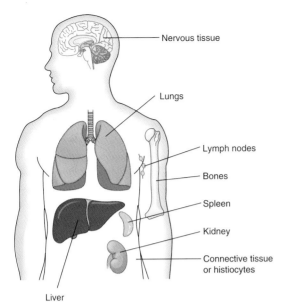

FIGURE 14.13 Mononuclear phagocyte system. Phagocytic cells are located in many body organs. Promonocyte precursors in the bone marrow develop into circulating monocytes in the peripheral blood. Monocytes ultimately become distributed throughout the body as macrophages. Neutrophils are located in the circulating blood, except when they enter the tissues during acute inflammation. (Adapted with permission from Cohen BJ, Wood DL. *Memmler's The Human Body in Health and Disease*, 11th ed, Philadelphia, PA: Lippincott Williams & Wilkins, 2009.)

have completed their last mitotic division. Monocytes have no large reserve of cells in a maturation-storage pool as do the granulocytes. Once the monocytes have entered the

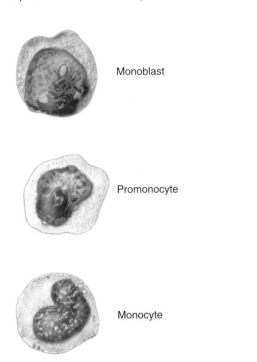

FIGURE 14.14 Monocyte maturation series. (Reprinted with permission from Anderson SA, Poulsen KB. *Anderson's Atlas of Hematology*, 2003.)

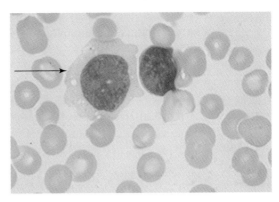

FIGURE 14.15 Monoblast. (Reprinted with permission from Anderson S, Poulsen K. *Anderson's Atlas of Hematology*, Philadelphia, PA: Lippincott Williams & Wilkins, 2003.)

circulation, cells may be located in a **circulating** or **marginating pool**. The ratio of circulating to marginating cells is 1:3.5. Monocytes are estimated to have a circulatory half-life of approximately 8.5 hours. The life span of tissue monocytes is variable. However, cells in noninflammatory areas have been demonstrated to live for months to years.

Morphological Characteristics

Morphological identification of the monocyte (Fig. 14.14) is more difficult than that of the neutrophilic, eosinophilic, or basophilic granulocytes. Monoblasts (Fig. 14.15), promonocytes (young monocytes), and monocytes vary greatly in their morphological appearance (Table 14.2). The monocytic series does have a characteristic nuclear chromatin pattern. The chromatin is clumped, although the clumps are smaller and more elongated than in neutrophils. This pattern can be described as lace-like. The shape of the nucleus of the monocyte may be round or oval, but it is frequently convoluted or twisted.

Mature monocytes (Fig. 14.16) are the largest mature cells seen in peripheral blood. They may exhibit an irregular cytoplasmic outline. These cytoplasmic irregularities can include pseudopods. Vacuoles are also commonly observed. Classically, the cytoplasm is blue-gray in color, with fine granulation resembling ground glass.

REFERENCE RANGES OF GRANULOCYTES AND MONOCYTES

Healthy adults and children have a relatively consistent number of each of the granulocytic and monocytic types of leukocytes. Normal variations occur along with daily rhythmic fluctuations; racial differences also occur.

The major function of the granulocytic leukocytes is **phagocytosis**, a body defense mechanism. Neutrophilic granulocytes are the major phagocytic cell of the circulating blood. Eosinophils and basophils are less effective as phagocytes but have additional specialized functions associated with body defense.

TABLE 14.2 Characteristics of Monocytes			
	Monoblast	**Promonocyte**	**Mature Monocyte**
Size (μm)	12–20	12–20	12–18
N:C ratio	4:1	3:1–2:1	2:1–1:1
Nucleus			
Shape	Oval, folded	Elongated, folded	Horseshoe shaped, folded
Nucleoli	1–2 or more	0–2	None
Chromatin	Fine	Lace like	Lace like
Cytoplasm			
Inclusions	Vacuoles variable	Vacuoles variable	Vacuoles common
Granules	None	None or fine	Fine, dispersed
Amount	Moderate	Abundant	Abundant
Color	Blue	Blue-gray	Blue-gray
Shape	Monocytes frequently demonstrate irregular cytoplasmic shape with pseudopods		

Each type of granulocyte and the monocytes have an established normal range (Table 14.3) and an average percentage on a stained blood smear (refer to Chapter 3). Significant differences in the total leukocyte count do occur between black and white persons. Blacks have a lower total leukocyte count compared with whites, owing to a decreased number of neutrophils. Individual variations in the total leukocyte count occur, with a daily fluctuation of as much as 20%. Peak levels occur in the middle of the night and the early morning.

Variations may also occur with specific cells. For example, smoking causes a mild elevation of neutrophils. Monocytes have periodic oscillations of 0.2×10^9/L every 3 to 6 days.

Eosinophils have a well-documented daily fluctuation, with a diurnal (time-related) variation in the number of circulating cells. The quantity of circulating eosinophils tends to be highest late at night during sleep, decreases during the morning, and begins to rise at midafternoon. This rhythmic variation in a person's eosinophil count is related to the fluctuation of the hormone adrenal glucocorticosteroid.

In women, the menstrual cycle affects the eosinophil count, with the number of circulating eosinophils dropping at the time of ovulation and rising during menstruation. The summer season may produce higher counts in a person without allergies. Exercise produces a brief rise in eosinophils, whereas stress can lower eosinophil counts.

FUNCTIONAL PROPERTIES OF GRANULOCYTES AND MONOCYTES

One of the major functional properties of granulocytes and monocytes is **phagocytosis**. Defense against infectious disease is the responsibility of both the phagocytic and the immune

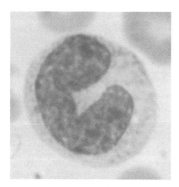

FIGURE 14.16 Blood cell, monocyte. (Reprinted with permission from Cohen BJ, Wood DL. *Memmler's The Human Body in Health and Disease*, 11th ed, Philadelphia, PA: Lippincott Williams & Wilkins, 2009.)

TABLE 14.3 Reference Leukocyte Values for a Normal Adult Population	
WBC Cell Type	**Reference Range (%)**
Neutrophils-Bands	0–3
Neutrophils-Segmented	40–74
Eosinophils	1–4
Basophils	0.5–1
Lymphocytes	34
Monocytes	2–6

Source: Adapted from Handin, RI, Lux SE, Stossel TP. *Blood*, 2nd ed, philadelphia, PA: Lippincott williams & Wilkins, 2003, Appendix 6, p. 2194.

systems in humans. The activities of these two systems are somewhat coordinated and interdependent.

Phagocytosis is the process that enables particular cells to engulf and disable particles, such as bacteria. Defects in phagocytosis (e.g., chronic granulomatous disease, in which there is defective killing of phagocytosed microorganisms) can be fatal.

Body defense systems include phagocytic cells (neutrophils, monocyte, and macrophages), cells that release inflammatory mediators (basophils, mast cells, and eosinophils), and natural killer cells. The molecular components of body defenses include complement, acute-phase proteins, and cytokines (e.g., interferons).

Upon initiation of inflammation, local inflammatory signals, for example, chemokines, cytokines, and adhesion molecules, initiate an orchestrated process of actively recruiting neutrophils into the tissue. Neutrophils act quickly in body defense by recognizing pathogen-associated molecular patterns (PAMPs) through encoded toll-like receptors (TLRs). Human neutrophils express the majority of TLRs. Furthermore, they act in concert with other components of the immune system, by expressing receptors for antibody (fraction crystallizable receptors [FcRs]) and complement (complement receptors [CRs]). Recently, interleukin-17A (IL-17A) and IL-17F, two cytokines produced by a subset of T helper cells have been found to indirectly induce the recruitment of neutrophils in inflammation.

Human peripheral blood monocytes are a heterogeneous population of leukocytes, distinguishable by the expression of CD14 and CD16 membrane markers. Monocyte subset phenotypes include inflammatory and resident monocytes. These subsets differentially express cell adhesion molecules and chemokine receptors that implies alternate recruitment mechanisms to a site of inflammation. Monocytes are not just phenotypically different but subsets use alternate sets of cell adhesion molecules and chemokine receptors that contribute to different functions and are recruited at different time points after initiation of inflammation. Classical monocytes with CD14$^+$CD16$^-$ membrane markers produce lower amounts of proinflammatory cytokines but contribute more effectively to bacterial clearance by phagocytosis compared with nonclassical monocytes. Nonclassical CD14^{lo}CD16$^+$ monocytes are more potent in presenting antigens in the immune response.

General Characteristics

Although the major cells associated with phagocytosis are the neutrophilic leukocytes (neutrophils) and the monocytes-macrophages, the neutrophils are the principal leukocytes involved in a localized inflammatory response. The inflammatory exudate (pus), which develops rapidly in an inflammatory response, is primarily composed of neutrophils and monocytes.

Neutrophils are steadily lost to the respiratory system, the gastrointestinal system, and the urinary system, where they participate in generalized phagocytic activities. Although the eosinophils and basophils are capable of participating

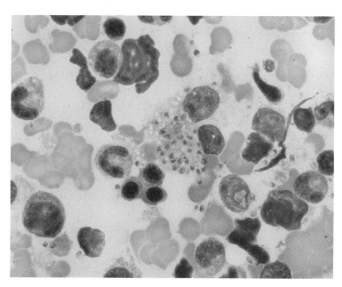

FIGURE 14.17 Bone marrow aspirate from a patient with AIDS and progressive disseminated histoplasmosis. Highly characteristic image shows macrophage filled with 1- to 2-μm yeast cells (Wright stain, original magnification ×400). (Reprinted with permission from Crapo JD, et al. *Baum's Textbook of Pulmonary Diseases*, 7th ed, Philadelphia, PA: Lippincott Williams & Wilkins, 2004.)

in phagocytosis, they possess less phagocytic activity. Their ineffectiveness is owing to both the small number of these cells in the circulating blood and the lack of powerful lytic enzymes. Eosinophils and basophils are functionally important in body defense in other ways.

The Role of Macrophages

Macrophages (Fig. 14.17) participate in the phagocytic process and are particularly important in the processing of antigens as part of the immune response. Macrophages exist as either **fixed** or **wandering cells**. Fixed macrophages line the endothelium of capillaries and the sinuses, the bone marrow and organs, spleen, and lymph nodes. Specialized macrophages, such as the **pulmonary alveolar macrophages**, are the dust phagocytes of the lung and function as the first line of defense against inhaled foreign particles and bacteria. Macrophages and their known precursor, monocytes, migrate freely into the tissues from the blood to replenish and reinforce the macrophage population. When there is tissue damage and inflammation, cellular activity increases with the release of substances that attract macrophages.

Acute Inflammatory Response

Acute inflammation is of short duration and is characterized by vascular and cellular changes. In an acute inflammatory response, cells and molecules of the immune system move into the affected site (Figs. 14.18 and 14.19). The process of movement of fluids, proteins, and leukocytes (primarily neutrophils) into the interstitial tissue is called exudation.

Activation of complement generates C3b, which coats the surface of the pathogen. The neutrophil chemoattractant and

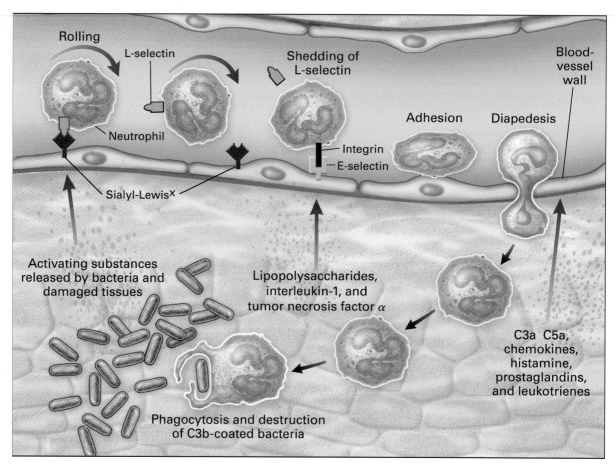

FIGURE 14.18 Acute inflammatory disease. (Reprinted with permission from Delves PJ, Roitt IM. The Immune System, Part I, *N Engl J Med*, 343(1):37–49, 2000. Copyright © 2000 Massachusetts Medical Society. All rights reserved.)

activator C5a is also produced and, together with C3a and C4a, triggers the release of histamine by degranulating mast cells. This in turn causes the contraction of smooth muscles and a rapid increase in vascular permeability.

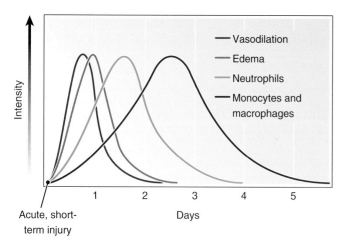

FIGURE 14.19 Timing of acute inflammatory events. The graph shows both intensity and duration for vasodilation, edema, neutrophils, and monocytes and macrophages. (Reprinted with permission from McConnell TH. *The Nature Of Disease Pathology for the Health Professions*, Philadelphia, PA: Lippincott Williams & Wilkins, 2007.)

Substances released from a pathogen and from damaged tissues upregulate the expression of adhesion molecules on the vascular endothelium, alerting passing cells to the presence of infection. The cell surface molecule L selectin on neutrophils recognizes carbohydrate structures, for example, sialyl-Lewis, on the vascular adhesion molecules. The neutrophil rolling along the vessel wall is arrested in its course by these interactions. As the neutrophil becomes activated, it rapidly sheds L selectin from its surface and replaces it with other cell surface adhesion molecules (e.g., integrins). These integrins bind the molecule E selectin, which appears on the blood vessel wall under the influence of inflammatory mediators (e g., bacterial lipopolysaccharide and the cytokines, interleukin-1 and tumor necrosis factor-α). Complement components and other inflammatory mediators all contribute to the recruitment of inflammatory cells as does an important group of chemoattractant cytokines called chemokines.

Activated neutrophils pass through the vessel walls, moving up the chemotactic gradient to accumulate at the site of infection, where they are positioned to phagocytize any C3b-coated microbes. Mutations in the genes for a number of different adhesion molecules have been described in patients with leukocyte-adhesion deficiencies, some of which are associated with life-threatening infections.

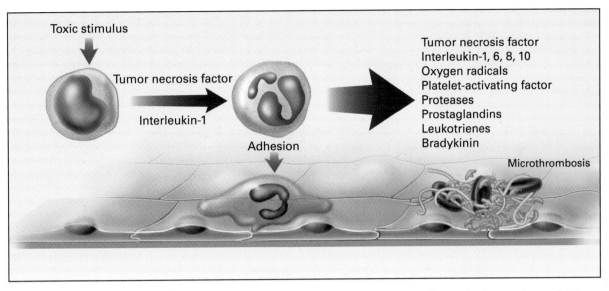

FIGURE 14.20 Early biomechanical events in sepsis. (Reprinted with permission from Wheeler AP, Bernard GR. Treating patients with severe sepsis, *N Engl J Med*, 340(3):208, 1999. Copyright © 2005 Massachusetts Medical Society. All rights reserved.)

Sepsis

Neutrophils have been regarded as a help and a hindrance. Although neutrophils were believed to be essential for the killing of pathogens, excessive release of oxidants and proteases by neutrophils is also believed to be responsible for injury to organs.

Sepsis is an infection-induced syndrome defined as the presence of two or more of the following features of systemic inflammation:

Fever or hypothermia
Leukocytosis or leukopenia
Tachycardia and tachypnea
Supranormal minute ventilation

Early biochemical events in sepsis (Fig. 14.20) include the key element, cytokines. The most widely investigated cytokines are tumor necrosis factor, interleukin-1 and interleukin-8, which are generally proinflammatory, and interleukin-6 and interleukin-10, which tend to be anti-inflammatory. A trigger (e.g., microbial toxin) stimulates the production of tumor necrosis factor and interleukin-1, which in turn promote endothelial cell–leukocyte adhesion, release of proteases and arachidonate metabolites, and activation of clotting. Interleukin-8, a neutrophil chemotaxis, may have an especially important role in promoting tissue inflammation (Fig. 14.21).

Steps in Phagocytosis

Phagocytosis can be divided into three stages (Fig. 14.22). These stages are **movement of cells, engulfment,** and **digestion**. If microorganisms are not effectively immobilized, stage 4, subsequent phagocytic activity may take place.

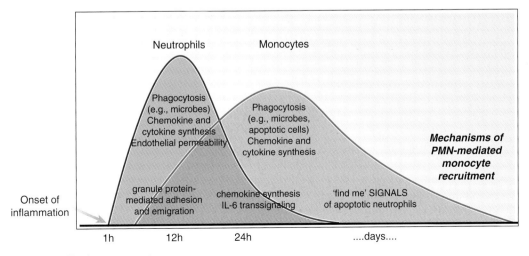

FIGURE 14.21 Summary of leukocyte recruitment pattern.

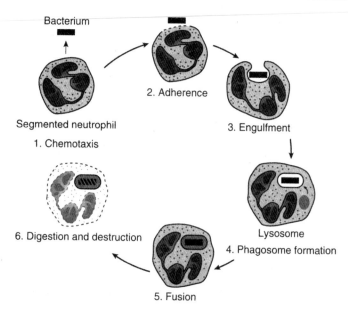

1. Chemotaxis
Segmented neutrophil
Bacterium
2. Adherence
3. Engulfment
Lysosome
4. Phagosome formation
5. Fusion
6. Digestion and destruction

FIGURE 14.22 Phagocytosis. Step 1 depicts the movement of a segmented neutrophil toward the site of bacterial invasion, chemotaxis. Step 2 depicts the initiating event in engulfment, the adherence of the phagocytic membrane to the bacterial cell wall. This process can be enhanced by opsonization. If the surface tensions of the membranes are conducive to engulfment, the phagocytic cell membrane invaginates and engulfs the bacterium (step 3), and a phagosome is formed (step 4). The phagosome fuses with one or more lysosomal granules (step 5). Digestion of the bacterium occurs (step 6) and normally results in autolysis of the phagocyte.

Stage 1: Movement of Cells

Various phagocytic cells continually circulate throughout the blood, lymph, gastrointestinal system, and respiratory tract. The physical occurrence of damage to tissues and inflammation due to trauma or microbial multiplication releases substances that attract phagocytic cells.

Cells are guided to the site of injury by the concentration gradient of chemotactic substances. This event is termed **chemotaxis.** Chemotactic factors polarize and orient attached neutrophils for locomotion. Cells acquire a characteristic asymmetric shape with the formation of pseudopodia. The movement of neutrophils is a process called **extravasation**. Extravasation of polymorphonuclear leukocytes (PMNs) to the site of inflammation precedes a second wave of emigrating monocytes. Monocyte subsets are affected differently by signals generated from PMNs. PMN granule proteins induce adhesion as well as emigration of inflammatory monocytes to the site of inflammation involving β_2-integrins and formyl-peptide receptors. PMNs create an environment, including rapidly undergoing apoptosis, that is favorable for extravasation and accumulation of inflammatory monocytes at the site of inflammation.

Actively motile segmented neutrophils are able to gather at the site of inflammation quickly, but monocytes are slower to arrive. Segmented neutrophils can be found in the beginning exudate in less than 1 hour.

Large numbers of intracapillary neutrophils are retained in the narrow capillaries of the pulmonary circulation without impeding regional alveolar blood flow, thus accommodating the marginated pool. The marginating pool of neutrophils, adhering to the endothelial lining of capillaries, migrates through the vessel wall to the intestinal tissues. This amoeboid movement is called **diapedesis**.

Stage 2: Engulfment

After the phagocytic cells have arrived at the site of injury, the invading microorganisms or particles can be engulfed through active membrane invagination. Leukocyte-specific CD18 integrins mediate neutrophil adhesion during migration and function as phagocytic receptors for bacterial uptake and killing.

It is important to realize that phagocytosis is an active process that requires a large expenditure of energy by the cells. The required energy is primarily provided by anaerobic **glycolysis**.

The principal factor in determining whether phagocytosis can occur is the physical nature of the surfaces of both the foreign particle and the phagocytic cell. Bacteria must be more hydrophobic than the phagocyte. Some bacteria, such as *Streptococcus pneumoniae*, possess a hydrophilic capsule and are not normally phagocytized. Most nonpathogenic bacteria are easily phagocytized because they are very hydrophobic.

Certain soluble factors, including complement (a plasma protein), coupled with antibodies, and substances such as acetylcholine, enhance the phagocytic process. Enhancement of phagocytosis through the process of **opsonization,** the coating of a particle with immunoglobulin and/or complement, speeds up the ingestion of particles. If the surface tensions are conducive to engulfment, the phagocytic cell membrane invaginates, a process that leads to the formation of an isolated vacuole, a **phagosome,** within the cell.

Stage 3: Digestion

Digestion follows ingestion of particles, the required energy being provided primarily by anaerobic glycolysis. The vacuole formed during the engulfment process fuses with one or more lysosomal granules that contain various lytic enzymes. The granules of neutrophils contain various antibacterial substances such as lysosomal hydrolases, lysozyme, and myeloperoxidase. The action of the oxygen-dependent myeloperoxidase-mediated system, hydrogen peroxide, and an oxidizable cofactor serve as major factors in the actual killing of bacteria within the vacuole. Other oxygen-independent systems, such as alterations in pH, lysozymes, lactoferrin, and the granular cationic proteins, also participate in the bactericidal process.

An energy-dependent respiratory burst accompanies phagocytosis. The respiratory burst generates oxidizing compounds through the hexose-monophosphate shunt. Oxidizing compounds produced from partial oxygen reduction are important in bacteriocidal activity. Utilization of reduced nicotinamide adenine dinucleotide phosphate (NADPH) or reduced nicotinamide adenine dinucleotide (NADH) as an electron donor subsequent to the activation of a membrane-bound oxidase produces superoxide (O_2^-) from oxygen. Hydrogen peroxide (H_2O_2) is either generated from superoxide spontaneously or catalyzed by superoxide dismutase.

$$2 O_2 + NADPH \rightarrow 2 O_2^- + NADP^+ + H^+$$

$$2 O_2^- + 2 H^+ \rightarrow H_2O_2 + O_2$$

The killing effect of H_2O_2 is potentiated by the formation of peroxide-halide. This reaction requires the enzyme myeloperoxidase, found in the primary granules of neutrophilic granulocytes.

$$H_2O_2 + Cl^- \xrightarrow{\text{myeloperoxidase}} HOCl + H_2O$$

Monocytes are particularly effective as phagocytic cells because of the large amounts of lipase in their cytoplasm. Although monocytes accumulate at a site of acute inflammation more slowly, they persist longer. Their metabolic burst is less extreme than neutrophils, but their capacity to kill many microbes is more diverse compared with that of neutrophils. Lipase digests the lipid-rich cell wall of bacteria such as *Mycobacterium tuberculosis*. Monocytes are further able to bind and destroy cells coated with complement-fixing antibodies because of the presence of membrane receptors for specific components or types of immunoglobulin.

As a result of the release of lytic enzymes, the cytoplasmic membrane of the phagocytic cell is usually ruptured, and the engulfing cell itself is phagocytized by macrophages. Macrophage digestion proceeds without risk to the cell unless the ingested material is toxic. However, if the ingested material damages the lysosomal membrane, the macrophage will also be destroyed because of the release of lysosomal enzymes.

Stage 4: Subsequent Phagocytic Activity

If invading microorganisms are not phagocytized at entry into the body, they may establish themselves in secondary sites, such as the lymph nodes or various body organs. Undigested bacteria produce a secondary inflammation, where neutrophils and macrophages again congregate. If bacteria escape from secondary tissue sites, **bacteremia** will develop. In patients whose conditions are unresponsive to antibiotic intervention, this situation can be fatal.

In cases of **acquired immunodeficiency syndrome (AIDS)**, researchers at the National Cancer Institute have found evidence of the virus in mononuclear phagocytes. Infected phagocytes were found in brain and lung tissue specimens from AIDS patients, indicating that the brain infection might have been caused by the phagocytes.

Phagocytes harboring AIDS virus were found to be more powerfully infective than T lymphocytes (discussed in Chapter 16). The infected phagocytes may be responsible for passing the virus back to the rest of the immune system, with other infected cells passing the virus back to healthy phagocytes.

Protozoan organisms, such as *Leishmania donovani* (popularly referred to as **kala-azar**), are cleared by the mononuclear phagocyte cells of the liver, spleen, and bone marrow. The **Leishman-Donovan bodies,** which are oblong or round,

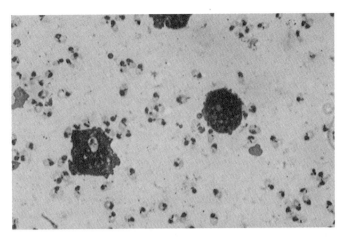

FIGURE 14.23 A spleen imprint shows many Leishman-Donovan (L-D) bodies, which are composed of a round nucleus and a rod-shaped kinetoplast. Giemsa, ×3300.

multiply in the phagocytic cells. Repeated multiplication produces extensive numbers of parasitized macrophages and monocytes (Fig. 14.23). Infection with the pathogenic fungus *Histoplasma capsulatum,* which also infiltrates the mononuclear phagocytic system and appears within macrophages of the bone marrow, can mimic kala-azar.

Specialized Functions of Granulocytes

Eosinophils

The eosinophil is considered to be a homeostatic regulator of inflammation that leaves the circulating blood when adrenal cortical hormone increases. Functionally, this means that the eosinophil attempts to suppress inflammatory tissue reactions to prevent the excessive spread of inflammation.

Eosinophils proliferate in response to antigenic stimulation and contain substances that inactivate factors released by mast cells and basophils. The primary function of eosinophils appears to be their reactions with products from mast cells, lymphocytes, and other soluble substances in the blood, such as the coagulation factors, complement, and hormones.

Although eosinophils are ineffective in protecting the body against invading foreign particles, they do play a role in the body defense mechanism. Eosinophils regulated allergic diseases and granulomatous and fibrotic disorders, and eosinophil recruitment in response to helminthic parasite infection has been well documented. Eosinophils have the ability to interact with the larval stages of some helminthic parasites and to damage them by means of oxidative mechanisms. Certain proteins released from eosinophilic granules are known to damage antibody-coated *Schistosoma* parasites.

Basophils

Basophils and mast cells (in tissues) share significant phenotypic and functional properties. Both cell lines possess metachromatic granules containing histamine and proteoglycans and express the high-affinity immunoglobulin E (IgE) receptor through which they can be activated to degranulate and synthesize inflammatory mediators. Histamine plays an important role in acute, systemic allergic reactions. Degranulation (loss of granules) occurs when an antigen, such as pollen, binds to two adjacent immunoglobulin E (IgE)-type antibody molecules located on the surface of basophils. The release of the contents of these basophilic granules results in increased vascular permeability, smooth muscle spasm, and vasodilation. If this reaction is severe, it can result in **anaphylactic shock**.

A class of compounds, the **leukotrienes**, mediates the inflammatory functions of leukocytes. The observed systemic reactions that are related to these compounds were previously attributed to the slow-reacting substance of anaphylaxis (SRS-A).

Monocytes

In addition to phagocytosis, monocytes are able to synthesize various biologically important compounds, including transferrin, complement, interferon, and certain growth factors. In cellular immunity, monocytes assume a killer role. In this role, they are activated by sensitized lymphocytes to phagocytize offending cells or antigen particles. This is important in fields such as tumor immunology.

ASSESSMENT METHODS

Inflammation almost always follows acute tissue damage. Diagnostic categories of acute inflammation can include bacterial causes and nonbacterial causes such as trauma, chronic inflammation, and viral disease. Among the many laboratory tests that have been advocated for the diagnosis of inflammation, the total leukocyte count, the percentage of band and segmented neutrophils determined by a differential leukocyte count, the absolute neutrophil cell count, and the erythrocyte sedimentation rate (ESR) are the most common. Other tests include direct cell counts of eosinophils or basophils, the leukocyte alkaline phosphatase (LAP) cytochemical stain, and neutrophilic function tests.

Total Leukocyte Count

The total leukocyte count can be elevated above 10×10^9/L in conditions such as pregnancy or strenuous exercise. The total count may be depressed because of overwhelming bacterial infection (sepsis) or immunosuppressive agents. A diagnosis of acute inflammation is generally based on a total leukocyte count greater than 10.5×10^9/L in combination with other factors.

Differential Blood Smear Evaluation

Some authorities advocate doing away with the identification of band forms on the leukocyte differential procedure (see Chapter 26) because of individual variability in cell identification and limited usefulness. Patients with stress conditions can demonstrate an increase in the number of band forms in the presence of a normal total leukocyte count. The normal average for band

neutrophils is considered to be 3% in adults; newborn infants have a somewhat higher normal average. A neutrophilic band count greater than 11% is considered to be consistent with an inflammatory condition. When the percentage of band forms and other immature neutrophils such as metamyelocytes and myelocytes increases, the condition is sometimes referred to as a shift to the left. The normal average for segmented neutrophils is 56% and approximately 4% for monocytes.

Absolute Cell Counts

The absolute number of segmented neutrophils and bands is considered to be a less specific index of inflammation than other tests because the total leukocyte count drops in many patients with overwhelming infection. This condition results from the movement of circulating granulocytes into the tissue sites of infection. However, the absolute count may be valuable in other cases of inflammation. An example of the method of calculating an absolute cell count is presented in Box 14.1.

Erythrocyte Sedimentation Rate

The ESR, or sed rate, is a nonspecific indicator of disease with increased sedimentation of erythrocytes in acute and chronic inflammation and malignancies. Although this procedure is nonspecific, it is one of the most commonly performed laboratory tests.

Very few tests have as long a history as the ESR. A Swedish physician, Fahraeus, is credited with the discovery of this test in 1915. However, the sedimentation of blood was one of the principles on which ancient Greek medicine was based. The Greek philosophy of the four humors (fluids) in the human

BOX 14.1

Absolute Cell Counts

Absolute count[a] = absolute cell value = total leukocyte count × percentage of cell type

PATIENT DATA
Total leukocyte count: 15.0×10^9/L
Differential blood smear results: bands 12%, segmented neutrophils 80%, lymphocytes 8%

SAMPLE CALCULATION
Absolute segmented neutrophil value = total leukocyte count × % of segmented neutrophils
Absolute value = 15.0×10^9/L $\times 0.80 = 12.0 \times 10^9$/L segmented neutrophils

[a]This formula can be used to determine the absolute value of any cell appearing on a leukocyte differential blood smear.

Normal absolute values include segmented neutrophils 1.4–6.5 × 10⁹/L, bands 0–0.7 × 10⁹/L, lymphocytes 1.2–3.4 × 10⁹/L.

body was established in the 5th century B.C. and further developed by Aristotle. This belief proposed that these fluids formed the body. On the basis of this philosophy, each person had a predisposition for a particular disease depending on the predominance of one of the four fluids: blood, phlegm, yellow bile, or black bile.

In 1836, Nasse recognized that a property of plasma, later identified as increased proteins, produced an increased sinking speed of erythrocytes in whole blood. The work of Nasse went unnoticed for nearly a century because medicine was undergoing a radical reform, moving away from the humoral philosophy of the Greeks toward the cellular pathology theories of Virchow (see Chapter 18). With the reestablishment by Fahraeus of the significance of the empirical basis of Greek medicine, Alf Westergren began working concurrently on refining the technique.

Except for some refinements, the ESR procedure continues to be an established parameter of inflammation in the modern clinical laboratory. The Westergren method (see Chapter 24) has been selected by the CLSI as the standard method of choice.

Assessment of Eosinophils and Basophils

Examination of a peripheral blood smear normally demonstrates an average of approximately 4% eosinophils. Because this method of estimation is only semiquantitative, an absolute eosinophil count, either by manual chamber counting (see Chapter 24) or by the use of automated equipment, is preferred. This procedure is required only if an extreme increase in eosinophils is demonstrated on a peripheral blood smear or if clinical symptoms suggest an increase.

The basophil is the least numerous of the granulocytes. Normally, differential smears of normal blood have only one basophil, if any. An increase in basophils is very significant and is seen in conditions such as chronic myelogenous leukemia and polycythemia vera.

Leukocyte Alkaline Phosphatase Test

This procedure is discussed in detail in Chapters 21 and 26. The value of this cytochemical stain is in differentiating malignant disorders from leukemoid reactions.

Neutrophilic Function

A number of diseases are associated with leukocyte dysfunctions related to locomotion, chemotaxis, adhesion, or the ability of cells to destroy infectious organisms. In vitro assays of the rate of cell movement and the directional orientation of the movement as well as the ability of granulocytes to destroy organisms have been in existence for more than 20 years. A defect in cell adhesiveness, for example, leukocyte adhesion defect (LAD), can lead to decreased cell locomotion.

A test that assesses the killing ability of granulocytes is the nitroblue tetrazolium (NBT) test. In the routine clinical laboratory, this procedure is infrequently performed.

Functional abnormalities expressed by patients with congenital neutropenia include defective migration, bacterial killing, or increased apoptosis.

Neutrophilic Hypersegmentation Index

Mature segmented neutrophils have from two to five nuclear lobes (segments). Counting the number of lobes can be performed to determine the neutrophilic hypersegmentation index (NHI). A right shift or increase in the number of lobes to five or more occurs in various conditions, for example, sepsis, chronic nephritis. The NHI is clinically useful in vitamin B_{12} deficiency (pernicious anemia) and folic acid diagnosis.

Three methods exist for calculating the NHI:

1. Lobe average. This is determined by counting the number of lobes in a number of neutrophils, for example, 200, and dividing by the total number of neutrophils for the average number of lobes. The reference value is 2.5 to 3.3.
2. Percentage of neutrophils with five or more lobes. Count the number of lobes in randomly selected segmented neutrophils, for example, 200. Add up the total number of lobes for each segmented neutrophil counted and divide by the total number of cells counted. The reference range is greater than 3%.
3. Hypersegmentation index. To calculate this index, use a minimum of 200 segmented cells.

$$\frac{Number\ of\ neutrophils\ with\ 5\ or\ more\ lobes \times 100}{Number\ of\ neutrophils\ with\ 4\ lobes}$$

Values greater than 16.9 are considered to indicate hypersegmentation. This method is considered to be the most sensitive method.

CHAPTER HIGHLIGHTS

The following types of leukocytes are found in peripheral blood, in order of frequency: neutrophils, lymphocytes, monocytes, eosinophils, and basophils. The function of the entire leukocytic system is to defend the body against disease, with each type of leukocyte having a unique function.

The Granulocytic Series

The cellular elements of the blood are derived from a single, multipotential stem cell. This stem cell undergoes differentiation, multiplication, and maturation within the bone marrow. After a progenitor cell becomes committed to a specific cell line, mitosis and early development take place in the proliferative compartment of the bone marrow. A neutrophilic granulocyte matures in the following sequence: stem cell, myeloblast, promyelocyte, myelocyte, and metamyelocyte. Once the metamyelocyte stage has been reached, the proliferative phase comes to an end. In the next phase of bone marrow development, the maturation-storage compartment, metamyelocytes, and most band-type neutrophils mature into segmented granulocytes or polymorphonuclear neutrophils.

Release of granulocytes from the bone marrow is influenced by a variety of factors. These factors are chemical and physical. Chemical factors include neutrophil-releasing factor and leukocytosis-inducing factor. Physical factors include greater flexibility and mobility of cells, allowing the cells to pass through the sinusoid barrier of the bone marrow.

The earliest identifiable neutrophil-eosinophil-basophil precursor in the bone marrow is the myeloblast. This cell has a high N:C ratio and frequently contains Auer rods in the cytoplasm. The second stage of development is the promyelocyte, a heavily granulated cell, which may retain visible nucleoli in the nucleus. Following the promyelocyte, the myelocyte is the third stage. In this stage, granules that distinguish neutrophils, eosinophils, and basophils begin to become apparent. Myelocytes mature into metamyelocytes. The nucleus of the myelocyte progresses from an indented structure to an elongated structure as it matures. The last two maturational stages are the band and segmented forms. Band forms have a condensed chromatin pattern in the nucleus and a thin, elongated, curved nuclear shape. The segmented neutrophil is typified by the multiple segments of the nucleus that are attached to one another by fine filaments.

The Monocytic-Macrophage Series

Cells of the mononuclear phagocyte system include the monocytes and their bone marrow precursors, the macrophages. Macrophages have a variety of names, depending on their tissue location. Collectively, they are referred to as the mononuclear phagocyte system.

Morphological identification of monocytes is more difficult than granulocyte identification. A convoluted nuclear shape is typical of monocytes. The promonocyte, or young monocyte, has a greater N:C ratio than the mature monocyte. The cytoplasm is gray-blue, with fine granules that resemble ground glass. Vacuoles can frequently be observed.

Normal Values and Functional Properties of Granulocytes and Monocytes

Defense against infectious disease is the responsibility of both the phagocytic and the immune (antigen-antibody)

system. The neutrophils defend the body against infectious agents and local noninfectious challenges. Macrophages participate in the phagocytic process and are important in the processing of antigens as part of the immune system. Macrophages may be of either fixed or wandering type. Fixed types are located in the mononuclear phagocyte system.

Infection with a pathogen triggers an acute inflammatory response involving cells and molecules of the immune system. Sepsis is an infection-induced syndrome with classic features. Tumor necrosis factor and certain interleukins act as proinflammatory or anti-inflammatory factors in the activation of clotting, or tissue inflammation.

Physical trauma initiates the events of phagocytosis. The attraction of phagocytic cells to the site of injury is termed **chemotaxis**. The neutrophils are the most abundant of the cells participating in phagocytosis and arrive at the site rapidly. Monocytes are slower in arriving. Engulfment of foreign particles, such as bacteria, is the next step. Digestion of bacteria follows engulfment. Antibacterial enzymes contained in granules, and alterations within the cell such as a change in pH, destroy the engulfed bacteria. Lytic enzymes disrupt the cellular membrane of the phagocytic cells, which are in turn phagocytized by macrophages. Macrophage digestion proceeds without risk to the cell unless the ingested material is toxic. If bacteria are not phagocytized or destroyed at entry, they may establish themselves at secondary sites, and bacteremia develops.

Both the eosinophils and basophils can participate in the phagocytic process, but they are relatively ineffective, for a variety of reasons. However, eosinophils and basophils have separate important and specialized functions. Eosinophils prevent the excessive spread of inflammation. Histamine found in basophils is important in acute allergic reactions, the most important being anaphylactic shock.

Assessment Methods

Several laboratory tests can be used to assess the inflammatory response. Two important indicators are the total leukocyte count and the differential count of leukocytes on a peripheral blood smear. Other assessments include the absolute cell count, ESR, absolute counts of eosinophils and basophils, the LAP test, and neutrophilic function tests.

CASE STUDY

CASE 14.1

An 18-year-old woman came to the emergency department because of severe abdominal pain. She had no fever or nausea. Her periods had been regular.

■ **Laboratory Data**
a. Hemoglobin 13.5g/dL
b. Hematocrit 40%

c. Total RBC 4.0×10^{12}/L
d. Total WBC 28.5×10^9/L

A peripheral blood smear examination revealed the following:

e. Segmented PMNs 26%
f. Band neutrophils 42%
g. Lymphocytes 32%

(continued)

A few nucleated red blood cells were observed per 100 WBCs on the peripheral blood smear.

■ **Questions**

1. What abnormalities appeared in the patient's laboratory values?
2. What could cause this type of abnormality?
3. How could leukemia be differentiated from a leukemia-like, leukemoid, reaction or lymphoma?

■ **Discussion**

1. A leukoerythroblastic reaction is evident because of the presence of both immature granulocytes and nucleated erythrocytes.
2. This type of reaction could be associated with malignant diseases (e.g., leukemias or lymphomas) or exogenous stress from a variety of nonmalignant disorders (e.g., severe infection or inflammation, ovarian cysts, or inflammatory bowel disease).
3. To distinguish between a leukemic condition and a leukemoid reaction, the LAP test could be used. An increased score is associated with a leukemoid reaction or a variety of malignancies (e.g., lymphoma, multiple myeloma, polycythemia vera). Decreased scores are associated with chronic myelogenous leukemia and some other conditions.

DIAGNOSIS: Leukemoid Reaction Subsequent to Ovarian Cysts

REVIEW QUESTIONS

1. The granulocyte cells that are believed to descend from a common multipotential stem cell in the bone marrow are
   A. neutrophils and eosinophils
   B. basophils and lymphocytes
   C. lymphocytes and monocytes
   D. Both A and B

2. The types of granulocytic leukocytes found in the proliferative compartment of the bone marrow are
   A. myeloblasts, myelocytes, and metamyelocytes
   B. myeloblasts, promyelocytes, and myelocytes
   C. myeloblasts, promyelocytes, myelocytes, and metamyelocytes
   D. myeloblasts, promyelocytes, myelocytes, metamyelocytes, and band neutrophils

3. The types of granulocytic leukocytes found in the maturation-storage compartment of the bone marrow are
   A. metamyelocytes, band form neutrophils, segmented neutrophils, mature eosinophils, and mature basophils
   B. only band form neutrophils, segmented neutrophils, mature eosinophils, and mature basophils
   C. metamyelocytes, band form neutrophils, segmented neutrophils, mature eosinophils, and mature basophils
   D. segmented neutrophils, immature and mature monocytes, and mature lymphocytes

4. Release of neutrophils from the bone marrow is believed to be influenced by
   A. CSF
   B. interleukins
   C. interferon
   D. all of the above

5. The stages of neutrophilic granulocyte development are
   A. promyelocyte, myeloblast, myelocyte, metamyelocyte, and band and segmented neutrophils
   B. myeloblast, promyelocyte, myelocyte, metamyelocyte, and band and segmented neutrophils
   C. myelocyte, myeloblast, promyelocyte, metamyelocyte, and band and segmented neutrophils
   D. myeloblast, promyelocyte, metamyelocyte, myelocyte, and band and segmented neutrophils

6. Marginating granulocytes in the peripheral blood can be found
   A. in the circulating pool
   B. in the tissues
   C. adhering to the vascular endothelium
   D. all of the above

7. The major function of neutrophilic granulocytes is
   A. antibody production
   B. destruction of parasites
   C. phagocytosis
   D. suppression of inflammation

8. The half-life of circulating granulocytes in normal blood is estimated to be
   A. 2.5 to 5 hours
   B. 7 to 10 hours
   C. 24 hours
   D. 2 days

9. Identify the cell with these characteristics: prominent primary granules that are rich in myeloperoxidase and chloroacetate esterase and has a diameter of 14 to 20 μm.
   A. myeloblast
   B. promyelocyte
   C. myelocyte
   D. promonocyte

(continued)

10. The earliest granulocytic maturational stage in which secondary or specific granules appear is
    A. myeloblast
    B. monoblast
    C. promyelocyte
    D. myelocyte

11. The mature granulocytes seen in the peripheral blood of healthy persons include
    A. band form and segmented neutrophils
    B. eosinophils and basophils
    C. lymphocytes and monocytes
    D. Both A and B

12. The granules of segmented neutrophils contain
    A. lysosomal hydrolases
    B. lysozymes
    C. myeloperoxidase
    D. all of the above

13. Which of the following are contents of basophilic granules?
    A. Heparin
    B. Histamine
    C. Myeloperoxidase
    D. Both A and B

14. The tissue basophil can be referred to as a/an
    A. mast cell
    B. macrophage
    C. mononuclear cell
    D. antibody-producing cell

15. A leukocyte with the morphological characteristics of being the largest normal mature leukocyte in the peripheral blood and having a convoluted or twisted nucleus is the
    A. myelocyte
    B. metamyelocyte
    C. promonocyte
    D. monocyte

16. The reference range of PMN neutrophil count in adults is
    A. 20 – 40%
    B. 40 – 60%
    C. 60 – 80%
    D. 80 – 100%

17. The principal leukocyte type involved in phagocytosis is the
    A. monocyte
    B. neutrophil
    C. eosinophil
    D. basophil

18. The mononuclear phagocyte system consists of reticular cells. These cells can be found in the
    A. connective tissue
    B. spleen
    C. lymph nodes
    D. all of the above

19. The immediate precursor of the macrophage is the
    A. myeloblast
    B. monoblast
    C. promonocyte
    D. monocyte

20. The correct sequence(s) of events in successful phagocytosis is (are)
    A. chemotaxis, opsonization, phagosome formation, and the action of antibacterial substances
    B. opsonization, chemotaxis, phagosome formation, and the action of antibacterial substances
    C. engulfment, opsonization, digestion, and destruction of bacteria or particulate matter
    D. Both A and C

21. The major function of eosinophils is
    A. suppression of inflammatory reactions
    B. destruction of protozoa
    C. participation in anaphylaxis
    D. phagocytosis

22. Monocytes are capable of
    A. phagocytosis
    B. synthesis of biologically important compounds
    C. assuming a killer role
    D. All of the above

23. The hematology tests that are useful in the early diagnosis of acute inflammation are the
    A. total leukocyte count and total erythrocyte count
    B. total leukocyte count and white blood cell differential count
    C. ESR and absolute neutrophil cell count
    D. Both B and C

24. The total leukocyte count can be increased in certain states. Select the conditions when this is not true.
    A. Strenuous exercise
    B. Overwhelming bacterial infection
    C. Sepsis
    D. Use of immunosuppressive agents

25. Acute inflammation is based on
    A. total leukocyte count >10.5×10^9/L
    B. neutrophilic band count <2%
    C. symptoms of long duration
    D. an increase in lymphocytes

26. On the basis of the following data, calculate the absolute value of the segmented neutrophils. Total leukocyte count = 12×10^9/L; percentage of segmented neutrophils on the differential count = 80%. The absolute segmented neutrophil value is
    A. 2.5×10^9/L
    B. 4.5×10^9/L
    C. 6.5×10^9/L
    D. 9.6×10^9/L

(continued)

27. An increase in metamyelocytes, myelocytes, and promyelocytes can be referred to as
    A. leukocytopenia
    B. a shift to the right
    C. a shift to the left
    D. Pelger-Huet anomaly

28. What is the normal range of the segmented neutrophil absolute value?
    A. 1.4 to 6×10^9/L
    B. 2.5 to 6.5×10^9/L
    C. 3.5 to 8×10^9/L
    D. 5.5 to 10×10^9/L

29. The absolute value of segmented neutrophils can be an unreliable indicator of overwhelming infection because
    A. it drops in many patients because the circulating granulocytes are mobilized into the tissue site of infection
    B. the bone marrow reserve becomes exhausted
    C. the infection suppresses granulocytic production
    D. All of the above

30. The CLSI-recommended method for the ESR is the
    A. Wintrobe method
    B. Westergren method
    C. Duke
    D. Ivy

BIBLIOGRAPHY

Akin, C. What does a basophil do? *Blood,* 110(3):790, 2007.

Baer DM (ed.). Absolute neutrophil critical values, *Med Lab Observ,* 34(9):34, 2002.

Bunting M, et al. Leukocyte adhesion deficiency syndromes: Adhesion and tethering defects involving β_2 integrins and selectin ligands, *Curr Opin Hematol,* 9(1):30–35, 2002.

Dale DC, Boxer L, Liles WC. The phagocytes: neutrophils and monocytes, *Am Soc Hematol,* ASH 50th Anniversary Review, 121–128, 2008.

Delves PJ, Roitt IM. The immune system, *N Engl J Med,* 343(1):37–50, 2000.

Dinarello CA. The role of the interleukin-1-receptor antagonists in blocking inflammation mediated by interleukin-1, *N Engl J Med,* 343(10): 732–734, 2000.

Etzioni A. Integrins: The molecular glue of life, *Hosp Pract,* (www.hosppract.com/issues/2000/03/etzioni.htm). Retrieved November 14, 2002.

Gerard C. Complement C5a in the sepsis syndrome—Too much of a good thing, *N Engl J Med,* 348(2):167–169, 2003.

Hotchkiss RS, Karl IE. The pathophysiology and treatment of sepsis, *N Engl J Med,* 348(2):138–150, 2003.

Klein C. Congenital neutropenia, *Am Soc Hematol,* 344–348, 2009; 50th Anniversary edition 2009.

Koepke JA, Bull BS, Simson E, van Assendelft, OW. *Reference and Selected Procedure for the Human Erythrocyte Sedimentation Rate (ESR) test. H2-T2. Approved Standard,* 4th ed, Villanova, PA: NCCLS, 1977.

Markell EK, et al. *Medical Parasitology,* Philadelphia, PA: Saunders, 1986:314.

McCabe BH. A brief history of the erythrocyte sedimentation rate, *Lab Med,* 16(3):177–178, 1985.

Mueller H, et al. Tyrosine kinase Btk regulates E-selectin-mediated integrin activation and neutrophil recruitment by controlling phospholipase C (PLC)γ2 and PI3Kγ pathways, *Blood,* 15(15): 3118–3127, 2010.

Nimrichter L, et al. E-selectin receptors on human leukocytes, *Blood,* 112(9):3744–3752, 2008.

Pelletier M, et al. Evidence for a cross-talk between human neutrophils and Th17 cells, *Blood,* 115(2):335–343, 2010.

Peters-Golden M, Henderson WR Jr. Leukotrienes, *NEJM,* 357: 1841–1854, 2007.

Phipps S, et al. Eosinophils contribute to innate antiviral immunity and promote clearance of respiratory syncytial virus, *Blood,* 110(5):1578–1586, 2007.

Ridker PM, et al. C-Reactive protein and other markers of inflammation in the prediction of cardiovascular disease in women, *N Engl J Med,* 342 (12):836–837, 2000.

Saffar AS, Gounni AS. Neutrophils in health and disease. *MedLab Mag,* 1(1):18–19, 2009.

Statland BE (ed.). Normal values for bands, *Med Lab Observ,* 17(4):12, 1985.

Soehnlein O, Lindbom L, Weber C. Mechanisms underlying neutrophil-mediated monocyte recruitment, *Blood,* 114(21):4613–4621, 2009.

Van Ziffle JA, Lowell CA. Neutrophil-specific deletion of Syk kinase results in reduced host defense to bacterial infection, *Blood,* 114(23):4871–4882, 2009.

Wheeler AP, Bernard GR. Treating patients with severe sepsis, *N Engl J Med,* 340(3):207–214, 1999.

Wilson JM, Ziemba SE. Neutrophils fight infectious disease but may promote other human pathologies, *Lab Med,* 30(2):123–128, 1999.

Nonmalignant Disorders of Granulocytes and Monocytes

OBJECTIVES

Quantitative disorders

- Define the terms leukocytosis and leukocytopenia.
- List examples of common conditions that can cause leukocytosis or leukocytopenia.
- List at least one representative condition in which an increase or decrease in neutrophils, eosinophils, basophils, or monocytes can be found.

Morphological abnormalities of mature granulocytes

- Describe the appearance of cells when the following abnormalities are present: toxic granulation, Döhle bodies, hypersegmentation, Pelger-Huët anomaly, May-Hegglin anomaly, Chédiak-Higashi syndrome, Alder-Reilly inclusions, *Ehrlichia*, and abnormalities of mature granulocytes in body fluids.
- Briefly describe the conditions associated with the previously listed abnormalities of mature granulocytes.

Qualitative disorders

- Describe the consequences of defective locomotion and chemotaxis.
- Explain two defects in microbicidal activity.
- List and describe other functional anomalies of neutrophils.

Monocyte-macrophage disorders

- Compare defects found in monocyte-macrophage disorders, Gaucher disease, and Niemann-Pick disease.

Case studies

- Apply laboratory data to the stated case studies and discuss the implications of these cases to the study of hematology.

The diagnosis of nonmalignant disorders of granulocytes and monocytes is dependent on laboratory assays along with a patient's history and physical examination. Nonmalignant disorders of granulocytes range from general increases or decreases in the total leukocyte count to qualitative disorders, such as a defect in the killing ability of the leukocytes. A variety of laboratory tests are used to assess disorders related to granulocytes and monocytes.

QUANTITATIVE DISORDERS

Quantitative disorders of leukocytes may reflect either a general increase (**leukocytosis**) or decrease (**leukocytopenia**) in the total leukocyte count, or a specific disorder (Table 15.1). Increases in neutrophils, eosinophils, and basophils are referred to as **neutrophilia**, **eosinophilia**, and **basophilia**, respectively. An increase in monocytes is called **monocytosis**. Decreases in these cellular elements are referred to as **neutropenia**, **eosinopenia**, **basopenia**, and **monocytopenia**, respectively.

Leukocytosis

Leukocytosis is an increase in the concentration or percentage of any of the leukocytes in the peripheral blood: neutrophils, eosinophils, basophils, monocytes, or lymphocytes.

Although an increase in the total leukocyte count may be caused by an increase in lymphocytes (see Chapter 16), an increase in neutrophils is the most frequent cause of nonmalignant increases in the total leukocyte count because of their proportionally higher concentrations in circulating blood.

Nonmalignant leukocytosis can be caused by various conditions in several general categories. These categories include

1. Increased movement of immature cells out of the bone marrow's proliferative compartment
2. Increased mobilization of cells from the maturation-storage compartment of the bone marrow to the peripheral blood
3. Increased movement of mature cells from the marginating pool to the circulating pool
4. Decreased movement of mature cells from the circulation into the tissues

Neutrophilia

An increase in the number of neutrophils can be present in some forms of leukemia and nonmalignant conditions, such as inflammatory conditions or infection. Neutrophilia can also be caused by physical stimuli such as heat and cold, surgery, burns, stressful activities such as vigorous exercise, nausea, and vomiting. In addition, some drugs and hormones may produce neutrophilia.

TABLE 15.1	Leukocytic Increases or Decreases and Examples of Related Disorders
Neutrophilia	Neutrophilia Inflammatory conditions Infection Physical stimuli (e.g., heat or cold) Surgery Burns Stress Some drugs and hormones Some types of leukemia
Eosinophilia	Active allergic disorders (e.g., asthma and hay fever) Dermatoses Nonparasitic infections Some forms of leukemia Parasitic infections (nonprotozoan)
Basophilia	Ulcerative colitis Hyperlipidemia Smallpox and chickenpox Chronic sinusitis Chronic myelogenous leukemia Polycythemia vera
Monocytosis	Infections (e.g., tuberculosis and bacterial endocarditis) Fever of unknown origin Inflammatory bowel disease Rheumatoid arthritis Hematological disorders (e.g., hemolytic anemia)
Neutropenia	Bone marrow injury or infiltration Starvation Anorexia nervosa Cyclic neutropenia Increased destruction or utilization Entrapment in the spleen
Eosinopenia	Glucocorticosteroid hormones Acute bacterial or viral inflammation
Basopenia	Hormones (e.g., corticotropin and progesterone) During ovulation Thyrotoxicosis
Monocytopenia	No known conditions

Eosinophilia

Persistently and significantly increased numbers of eosinophils are most frequently observed in active allergic disorders, such as asthma and hay fever. Other causes of eosinophilia include dermatoses, nonparasitic infections, some forms of leukemia, and parasitic infections. Patients with significant eosinophilia usually demonstrate some abnormal morphology. Vacuolization and degranulation can be observed. Charcot-Leyden crystals can be found in the tissues, exudates, sputum, and stool of patients with active eosinophilic inflammation.

Eosinophilia is an index of host reaction to parasites and varies considerably from one patient to another. It is *not* characteristic of any of the protozoan infections. In general, tissue parasites provoke a higher eosinophilia than do parasites that live only in the lumen of the bowel. Significant eosinophilia (20% to 70% or higher) is most frequently seen in trichinosis, strongyloidiasis, hookworm infection, filariasis, schistosomiasis, and fasciolopsiasis. Moderate eosinophilia (6% to 20%) is related to trichuriasis, ascariasis, paragonimiasis, taeniasis, and eosinophilic meningitis.

Basophilia

The number of circulating basophils is not remarkably affected by factors such as time of day, age, and physical activity. Basophilia is considered to exist when the number of basophils exceeds 0.075×10^9/L. Hormones can cause an increase in basophils, and basophils can be seen in many disorders, including ulcerative colitis, hyperlipidemia, smallpox, chickenpox, chronic sinusitis, chronic myelogenous leukemia, and polycythemia vera.

Monocytosis

Because the normal value of circulating monocytes is not precisely defined, the association of monocytosis with disease may not be entirely accurate. Monocytosis is a significant absolute increase in circulating monocytes, which can represent a reactive monocytosis to many diseases. Some of the disorders commonly associated with monocytosis include infections (e.g., tuberculosis and bacterial endocarditis), fever of unknown origin, inflammatory bowel disease, rheumatoid arthritis, and various hematological disorders (e.g., hemolytic anemia). An increase in tissue macrophages may reflect a response to foreign antigens.

Leukocytopenia

The major leukocyte type associated with leukocytopenia or granulocytopenia is the segmented neutrophil.

Neutropenia

A reduction in the number of circulating neutrophils is referred to as **neutropenia**. Causes of neutropenia include underproduction of cells caused by bone marrow injury or infiltration of the marrow by malignant cells as well as nutritional deficiencies (such as those caused by starvation or anorexia nervosa). Other causes include cyclic neutropenia, a hereditary disorder; increased destruction or utilization of neutrophils; and entrapment in the spleen.

Most transient neutropenias in children are acquired disorders, and viral infections are a common cause. Congenital neutropenia can be caused by a variety of conditions. A rare congenital disorder of young children is congenital agranulocytosis of the Kostmann type. Another uncommon congenital disorder is **myelokathexis**, the inability to release mature granulocytes into the blood. Other rare causes of congenital neutropenia include reticular dysgenesis, type IB glycogen storage disease, and transcobalamin-II deficiency.

Eosinopenia

This is a rare, stress-related condition that may be caused by several factors. Eosinopenia is frequently related to the action of glucocorticosteroid hormones or occurs as an aftermath of acute bacterial or viral inflammation.

Basopenia

This condition may be caused by hormones, such as corticotropin and progesterone, or it may occur at the time of ovulation. Patients with thyrotoxicosis may also have basopenia.

Monocytopenia

No conditions are known to be related to a decrease in monocytes.

MORPHOLOGICAL ABNORMALITIES OF MATURE GRANULOCYTES

Abnormalities of mature granulocytes, particularly neutrophils, can be observed in stained smears of peripheral blood. These conditions include the more frequently observed disorders of toxic granulation, Döhle bodies, and hypersegmentation as well as rarely observed disorders such as Pelger-Huët anomaly, May-Hegglin anomaly, Chédiak-Higashi syndrome, and Alder-Reilly inclusions.

Toxic Granulation

This is a condition in which prominent dark granulation, either fine or heavy, can be observed in band and segmented neutrophils or monocytes (Fig. 15.1) Toxic granules are azurophilic (primary) granules that are peroxidase-positive. The granulation may represent the precipitation of ribosomal protein (RNA) caused by metabolic toxicity within the cells.

The extent of toxic granulation is usually graded on a scale of 1+ to 4+, with 4+ being the most severe. Grading of the granulation is dependent on the coarseness and amount of granulation within the cellular cytoplasm. This condition is most frequently associated with infectious states. It may be seen in conditions such as burns and malignant disorders or as the result of drug therapy.

Döhle Bodies

These inclusion bodies are seen as single or multiple, light-blue–staining inclusions on Wright-stained blood smears (Fig. 15.2). They are usually seen near the periphery of the cytoplasm. These inclusions are predominantly seen in neutrophils, although they may be seen in monocytes or lymphocytes. Döhle bodies represent aggregates of rough

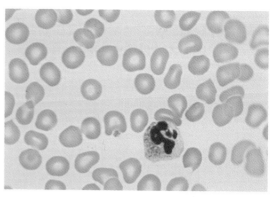

FIGURE 15.1 Toxic granulation. (Reprinted with permission from Anderson SC. *Anderson's Atlas of Hematology*, Wolters Kluwer Health/Lippincott Williams & Wilkins, 2003.)

endoplasmic reticulum (RNA) and may be associated with a variety of conditions such as viral infections, burns, or certain drugs. Döhle body–like inclusions may be seen in **May-Hegglin anomaly.**

Hypersegmentation

Hypersegmentation is most frequently seen in segmented neutrophils with more than five lobes or nuclear segments (Fig. 15.3). This condition is frequently associated with deficiencies of vitamin B_{12} or folic acid and exists along with abnormally enlarged, oval-shaped erythrocytes. Pseudohypersegmentation may be seen in old segmented neutrophils.

Pelger-Huët Anomaly

This genetically acquired, autosomal dominant disorder produces **hyposegmentation** of many of the mature neutrophils (Fig. 15.4). The nuclear shape may resemble a dumbbell or a pair of eyeglasses. Although the segments fail to lobulate normally, other characteristics, such as chromatin clumping and cytoplasmic maturation, are normal. Heavy chromatin

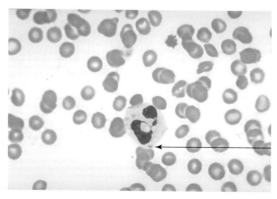

FIGURE 15.2 Döhle Body. (Reprinted with permission from Anderson SC. *Anderson's Atlas of Hematology*, Wolters Kluwer Health/Lippincott Williams & Wilkins, 2003.)

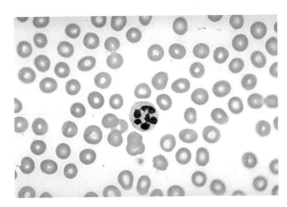

FIGURE 15.3 Hypersegmentation. (Reprinted with permission from Anderson SC. *Anderson's Atlas of Hematology*, Wolters Kluwer Health/Lippincott Williams & Wilkins, 2003.)

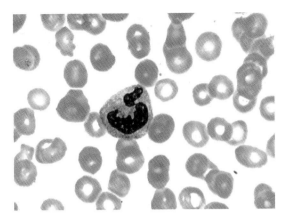

FIGURE 15.5 May-Hegglin anomaly shows large platelets and prominent Dohle bodies in the cytoplasm. (Reprinted with permission from McClatchey KD. *Clinical Laboratory Medicine*, 2nd ed. Philadelphia, PA: Lippincott Williams & Wilkins, 2002.)

clumping distinguishes Pelger-Huët anomaly from the left shift of infection. Abnormal nuclear maturation is presumed to be a reflection of abnormal nucleic acid metabolism, although the specific abnormality is unknown. A pseudoanomaly may be drug induced or may occur in a maturational arrest associated with some acute infections. The function of the cell is considered to be normal despite the morphological abnormality. Therefore, it is considered to be a benign anomaly.

May-Hegglin Anomaly

This genetic condition is characterized by the presence of Döhle body–like inclusions in neutrophils, eosinophils, and monocytes (Fig. 15.5). Abnormally large and poorly granulated platelets and thrombocytopenia (a decreased number of platelets) frequently coexist in this condition.

Although approximately 50% of patients do not have symptoms; others have manifested abnormal bleeding tendencies. The cause of the hemostatic defect is unclear, but it is proportionate to the degree of thrombocytopenia.

Chédiak-Higashi Syndrome

This rare disorder is a hereditary disease (autosomal recessive trait). It is primarily seen in children and young adults and is characterized by very large granules (Fig. 15.6). These gigantic, peroxidase-positive deposits represent abnormal lysosomal development in neutrophils and other leukocytes, such as monocytes and lymphocytes. Neutrophils display impaired chemotaxis and delayed killing of ingested bacteria. Patients with this disorder suffer from frequent infections, which suggests that neutrophils with this defect are not efficient bacteriocidal cells.

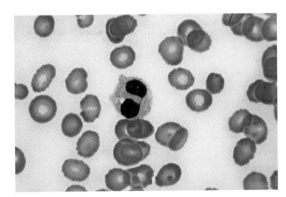

FIGURE 15.4 Pelger-Huet anomaly showing abnormal, bilobed segmentation of mature neutrophils. (Reprinted with permission from McClatchey KD. *Clinical Laboratory Medicine*, 2nd ed. Philadelphia, PA: Lippincott Williams & Wilkins, 2002.)

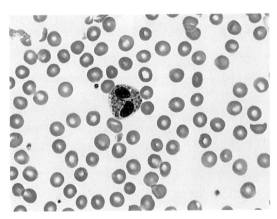

FIGURE 15.6 Chediak-Higashi syndrome shows neutrophil. (Reprinted with permission from McClatchey KD. *Clinical Laboratory Medicine*, 2nd ed. Philadelphia, PA: Lippincott Williams & Wilkins, 2002.)

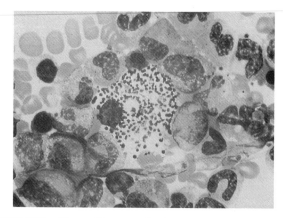

FIGURE 15.7 Alder-Reilly anomaly shows prominent cytoplasmic inclusions surrounded by a clear halo. Macrophage. (Reprinted with permission from McClatchey KD. *Clinical Laboratory Medicine*, 2nd ed. Philadelphia, PA: Lippincott Williams & Wilkins, 2002.)

Alder-Reilly Inclusions

These purple-red particles are precipitated mucopolysaccharides seen primarily in neutrophils, eosinophils, and basophils (Fig. 15.7). Occasionally, they are seen in monocytes and lymphocytes. These inclusions can resemble very coarse toxic granulation. Alder-Reilly granules are most commonly seen in patients with Hurler, Hunter, and Maroteaux-Lamy types of genetic mucopolysaccharidosis. Most of these disorders are transmitted as autosomal recessive genes.

Ehrlichia

In the United States, human diseases caused by *Ehrlichia* species have been recognized since the mid-1980s. The ehrlichioses represent a group of clinically similar diseases caused by *Ehrlichia chaffeensis*, *E. ewingii*, and a bacterium extremely similar or identical to *E. phagocytophila*.

Human ehrlichiosis caused by *E. chaffeensis* was first described in 1987. The disease occurs primarily in the southeastern and south central regions of the United States and is primarily transmitted by the lone star tick, *Amblyomma americanum*. Human granulocytic ehrlichiosis (HGE) represents the second recognized ehrlichial infection of humans in the United States and was first described in 1994. HGE is transmitted by the black-legged tick (*Ixodes scapularis*) and the western black-legged tick (*I. pacificus*) in the United States.

E. ewingii is the most recently recognized human pathogen. Disease caused by *E. ewingii* has been limited to a few patients in Missouri, Oklahoma, and Tennessee, most of whom have had underlying immunosuppression. The full extent of the geographic range of this species, its vectors, and its role in human disease is currently under investigation.

Ehrlichia are small, Gram-negative bacteria that primarily invade leukocytes. Ehrlichia typically appear as minute, round bacteria (cocci), ranging from 1 to 3 μm in diameter. In the leukocytes, ehrlichia divide to form vacuole-bound colonies known as morulae, the Latin word for mulberry, referring to the mulberry-like clustering of the dividing organisms. The formation of morulae is a defining characteristic of this group of bacterial pathogens (Fig. 15.8).

Abnormalities of Mature Granulocytes in Body Fluids

Certain abnormal inclusions can be seen in granulocytes obtained from body fluids. Examples of such inclusions are bacteria and *Histoplasma capsulatum*.

In Wright-stained sediments of body fluids, such as cerebrospinal fluid (refer to Chapter 25 for a complete discussion of the examination of body fluids) and pus from an abscess, engulfed bacteria can be observed as the result of phagocytosis. When this staining method is used, most bacteria appear as dark-blue, round, or elongated structures in the cytoplasm.

H. capsulatum is a fungus. This organism lives intracellularly in cells of the mononuclear phagocyte system, cells of the bone marrow, or cells from sputum or effusion specimens. The fungus appears as a tiny oval body with a clear halo surrounding a small nucleus.

QUALITATIVE DISORDERS

Defective Locomotion and Chemotaxis

Defective locomotion and defects in chemotaxis represent qualitative defects. Leukocyte mobility may be impaired in diseases such as rheumatoid arthritis, cirrhosis of the liver, and chronic granulomatous disease (CGD). Defective locomotion or leukocyte immobility can be seen in patients receiving corticosteroids and in lazy leukocyte syndrome. A significant defect in the cellular response to chemotaxis is seen in patients who have diabetes mellitus, Chédiak-Higashi

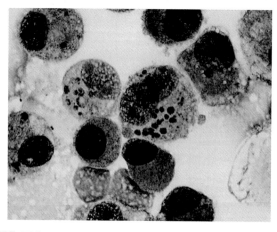

FIGURE 15.8 *Ehrlichia chaffeensis* cultivated in vitro in a macrophage cell line (canine DH82 cells). Note the multiple, large, round intracytoplasmic aggregates of bacteria. Romanowsky stain, original magnification 1,000×. (Reprinted with permission from McClatchey KD. *Clinical Laboratory Medicine*, 2nd ed. Philadelphia, PA: Lippincott Williams & Wilkins, 2002.)

anomaly, and sepsis as well as in patients with high levels of antibody IgE, such as those with Job syndrome.

Defects in Microbicidal Activity

Neutrophils and monocytes possess oxidase systems capable of killing ingested microorganisms in the process of phagocytosis (see Chapter 14). These disorders include CGD, myeloperoxidase (MPO) deficiency, and other functional anomalies of neutrophils.

Chronic Granulomatous Disease

CGD is the most serious disorder related to a defect in microbicidal activity. It consists of a group of genetic disorders in which neutrophils and monocytes ingest, but cannot kill, catalase-positive microorganisms such as *Staphylococcus aureus*, Gram-positive enteric bacteria, and various fungi, especially *Aspergillus*. CGD is a rare disorder; the inability to kill microorganisms leads to recurrent life-threatening infections by catalase-positive organisms during the 1st year of life. In CGD, stimulated phagocytes do not generate O_2^-, produce H_2O_2, or consume O_2 at an accelerated rate via the hexose monophosphate (HMP) shunt; the respiratory burst is not activated, and free radical forms of reduced O_2 are not produced.

In many patients with CGD, the disease is X-linked, but in about one fourth of families, the disease is transmitted by autosomal recessive genes. In most of these cases, both parents have had normal neutrophil functions and their cytochrome *b* concentrations are normal, unlike the X-linked cases. Abnormal oxidase activity is detectable by negative nitroblue tetrazolium (NBT) screening test, an indirect test for respiratory burst power. In addition to the two main categories of CGD, X-linked and the autosomal recessive forms, some cases do not conform to either classification. These cases are believed to be caused by point mutations. Rare causes of CGD include severe deficiency or instability of leukocyte glucose-6-phosphate dehydrogenase (G6PD).

Myeloperoxidase Deficiency

MPO deficiency (Alius-Grignaschi anomaly) is a benign inherited disorder that is usually transmitted by autosomal recessive genes. This disorder is manifested by the absence of MPO enzyme from neutrophils and monocytes, but not eosinophils. A lack of MPO, which mediates oxidative destruction of microbes by H_2O_2, creates a microbicidal defect in phagocytes. The functional abnormality is not severe. Infections are not usually serious.

A partial deficiency of MPO has been observed in patients with acute and chronic leukemias, myelodysplastic syndromes, Hodgkin disease, and carcinoma.

Other Functional Anomalies of Neutrophils

At least 15 hereditary defects and 30 additional disorders of neutrophil function have been described. A functional anomaly of neutrophils includes lactoferrin deficiency.

Lactoferrin deficiency is a rare disorder. In this disorder, specific granules are reduced in quantity and almost devoid of the specific granule protein, lactoferrin. This deficiency causes several dysfunctions including unresponsiveness to chemotactic signals and diminished adhesiveness to surfaces of particles. This deficiency leads to pyogenic infections, particularly deep-seated skin abscesses.

MONOCYTE-MACROPHAGE DISORDERS

Qualitative disorders of monocytes-macrophages are manifested as lipid storage diseases, including several rare autosomal recessive disorders. The macrophages are particularly prone to accumulate undegraded lipid products, which subsequently leads to an expansion of the reticuloendothelial tissue. Monocytic disorders include Gaucher disease and Niemann-Pick disease.

Gaucher Disease

This inherited disease is caused by a disturbance in cellular lipid metabolism. Gaucher disease is most frequently discovered in children, and the prognosis varies from patient to patient. If the disease is mild, the patient may live a relatively normal life; if it is severe, the patient may die prematurely.

The disorder represents a deficiency of β-glucocerebrosidase, the enzyme that normally splits glucose from its parent sphingolipid, glucosylceramide. As the result of this enzyme deficiency, cerebroside accumulates in (macrophages) histiocytes (Fig. 15.9). Gaucher cells are rarely found in the circulating blood. The typical Gaucher cell is large, with one to three eccentric nuclei and a characteristically wrinkled cytoplasm. These cells are found in the bone marrow, spleen, and other organs of the reticuloendothelial system. The production of erythrocytes and leukocytes decreases as these abnormal cells infiltrate into the bone marrow.

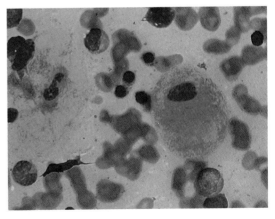

FIGURE 15.9 Gaucher disease. Bone marrow aspirate shows macrophage with prominent blue cytoplasmic fibrils. (Reprinted with permission from McClatchey KD. *Clinical Laboratory Medicine*, 2nd ed. Philadelphia, PA: Lippincott Williams & Wilkins, 2002.)

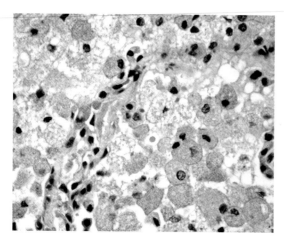

FIGURE 15.10 Higher power shows foamy macrophages with uniform-appearing lipid droplets in Niemann-Pick disease. (Reprinted with permission from Cagle PT. *Color Atlas and Text of Pulmonary Pathology*, Philadelphia, PA: Lippincott Williams & Wilkins, 2005.)

Niemann-Pick Disease

This disease is similar to Gaucher disease because it is also an inherited abnormality of lipid metabolism. Niemann-Pick disease afflicts infants and children; the patient's average age at death is 5 years.

This disorder represents a deficiency of the enzyme that normally cleaves phosphoryl choline from its parent sphingolipid, sphingomyelin. Sphingomyelin accumulates in the tissue macrophages (Fig. 15.10). The characteristic cell in this disorder, Pick cell, is similar in appearance to the Gaucher cell; however, the cytoplasm of the cell is foamy in appearance.

CHAPTER HIGHLIGHTS

Quantitative Disorders

Disorders of the quantitative type involve either an increase in leukocytes (leukocytosis) or a decrease in leukocytes (leukocytopenia). Any of the leukocyte types can be affected. A nonmalignant increase in specific granulocytes is referred to as neutrophilia, eosinophilia, or basophilia. An increase in monocytes is monocytosis. Neutrophils can be associated with physical stress, infection, inflammation, and drugs and hormones. Eosinophilia can be related to bronchial asthma, parasitic infections, and pulmonary and gastrointestinal disorders. Basophilia can be associated with asthma, smallpox, chickenpox, and drug therapy. Monocytosis is not a precisely defined state; however, tuberculosis, fever of unknown origin, and inflammatory bowel disease are a few of the disorders associated with an increase in circulating monocytes.

Decreases in leukocytes are caused primarily by either decreased production of normal granulocytes or increased destruction of circulating granulocytes. Neutropenia may be caused by bone marrow injury or nutritional deficiencies. Eosinopenia is rare and can be stress related. Basopenia can be induced by the action of hormones, such as cortisone.

Qualitative Disorders

Qualitative abnormalities include defective locomotion and defective bacterial killing. Qualitative disorders of monocytes-macrophages include Gaucher disease and Niemann-Pick disease. Both these disorders represent enzyme deficiencies that result in the accumulation of undegraded lipid products in macrophages.

CASE STUDIES

CASE 15.1

The 18-month-old son of a Nigerian exchange student was taken to his family doctor because he was losing weight and had been experiencing frequent fevers. The child had no history of disease or allergies. Physical examination revealed a well-nourished male infant. His rectal temperature was 101.8°F. The pediatrician ordered a complete blood count.

■ Laboratory Data

The patient had a slightly decreased hemoglobin and hematocrit. His total leukocyte count was $11.0 \times 10^9/L$. The total leukocyte differential count was as follows:

Neutrophilic bands 4%
Segmented neutrophils 35%
Lymphocytes 19%
Monocytes 2%
Eosinophils 40%

Allergy testing revealed no remarkable results. A stool examination was negative for ova and parasites.

■ Questions

1. What is the most probable cause of this child's eosinophilia?
2. Could pinworms (*Enterobius vermicularis*) be suspected?
3. What is the most probable source of this infection?

■ Discussion

1. In the absence of physical signs or symptoms such as asthma or other respiratory distress and with no history of allergies, the etiology of the eosinophilia must be considered to be systemic, that is, a condition throughout the body such as an invasive parasitic condition.
2. Children frequently suffer from pinworm infections. This parasitic infection is easily transmitted. However, the degree of eosinophilia is not usually as pronounced as in this case. In this case, a Scotch tape examination was subsequently performed and was negative for *E. vermicularis*.

(continued)

3. A subsequent muscle biopsy revealed trichinosis. Trichinosis is contracted by eating pork that is infected with the parasite and is improperly cooked. Because of laws that prohibit the marketing of hogs that have been fed garbage in the United States, trichinosis is uncommon today. However, in underdeveloped countries, improper swine management and improper food preparation can result in the transmission of this disease to humans.

DIAGNOSIS: Eosinophilia caused by trichinosis

CASE 15.2

An 18-year-old female college freshman complaining of severe abdominal pain was brought to the emergency department by the college nurse. She had no history of prior illness but had begun having pain immediately after eating dinner. Physical examination revealed tenderness in the lower right quadrant.

No abdominal masses were noted. The patient had a temperature of 100°F (37.8°C). A complete blood count and urinalysis were ordered.

■ **Laboratory Data**

The hemoglobin and hematocrit values were within normal range. The total leukocyte count was 20×10^9/L. The leukocyte differential smear revealed the following:

Segmented neutrophils 72%
Band form neutrophils 16%
Lymphocytes 2%
Monocytes 6%
Eosinophils 4%

The result of urinalysis was essentially normal except for the presence of ketone bodies.

■ **Questions**

1. From what general type of disorder is this patient suffering?
2. What is the absolute segmented neutrophil value? Is it normal?
3. What is the probable diagnosis?

■ **Discussion**

1. The patient has symptoms and laboratory findings that support the classification of an acute inflammatory disorder.
2. The absolute value of segmented neutrophils is 20×10^9/L $\times 0.72 = 14.4 \times 10^9$/L. The patient's absolute segmented neutrophil value is above normal. The normal range for segmented neutrophils is 1.5 to 6.0×10^9/L.
3. The initial symptom of pain in the lower right quadrant progressively became more severe, and the patient developed the classic rebound phenomenon found in acute appendicitis. The increased total leukocyte count and

increased band form neutrophils supported the physical findings. Additionally, the presence of ketone bodies was consistent with acute appendicitis, although they may also be found in other disorders such as starvation and diabetic ketosis.

DIAGNOSIS: Acute Inflammation of the Appendix (Appendicitis)

CASE 15.3

A 45-year-old woman with a known diagnosis of diabetes mellitus visited her physician because of difficulty and pain on urination. Physical examination revealed that the patient had a slightly elevated temperature but no other abnormalities. A complete blood count, urinalysis, and urine culture were ordered.

■ **Laboratory Data**

The patient's hemoglobin and hematocrit were normal. However, the total leukocyte count was 28.5×10^9/L, with the following leukocyte differential results:

Segmented neutrophils 79%
Neutrophilic bands 10%
Eosinophils 2%
Lymphocytes 9%

Most of the segmented neutrophils displayed dark, coarse granulation. Many of the neutrophils were also vacuolated.

The patient's urine had an elevated concentration of protein, increased numbers of leukocytes, and many bacteria. The urine culture had a heavy growth of a Gram-negative rod, *Pseudomonas* species.

■ **Questions**

1. What is the dark, coarse granulation in the neutrophils?
2. Does this condition alter the phagocytic effectiveness of the leukocytes?
3. What is the most probable explanation of the patient's elevated leukocyte count?

■ **Discussion**

1. The granulation observed is toxic granulation. This disorder is commonly seen in the hematology laboratory. However, care must be taken not to overlook the rarer finding of Chédiak-Higashi syndrome. The inclusion granules in this disorder are gigantic.
2. No. Toxic granulation is believed to represent the precipitation of ribosomal RNA due to metabolic toxicity occurring in the cell. This metabolic toxicity may shorten the life span of the cell, but the cell can remain fully functional until it dies.
3. Toxic granulation can be observed in granulocytes in a variety of conditions, including severe infections, burns, and drug therapy.

(continued)

In this case, the combination of an elevated total leukocyte count, toxic granulation, and a positive urine culture with a Gram-negative rod suggests that both the toxic granulation and the elevated leukocyte count were caused by a severe urinary tract infection. Although the patient also had diabetes, that would not have directly affected the total leukocyte count. However, patients with diabetes tend to be more susceptible to bacterial infections than nondiabetic persons owing to their circulatory problems and defective chemotaxis.

DIAGNOSIS: Toxic granulation caused by bacterial infection

CASE 15.4

A 6-month-old black child was admitted to the hospital for repair of an inguinal hernia. Routine preoperative laboratory testing was ordered.

■ **Laboratory Data**

Hemoglobin and hematocrit were normal, and the total leukocyte count was 7.5×10^9/L. The differential results revealed the following:

Band-type neutrophils 25%
Segmented neutrophils 10%
Lymphocytes 62%
Monocytes 2%
Eosinophils 1%

■ **Questions**

1. What is the condition most probably being observed in the neutrophils?
2. What is the etiology of this disorder?
3. Is it clinically significant?

■ **Discussion**

1. Further observation of the band-type neutrophils revealed that the nuclear chromatin was very coarsely clumped. The degree of clumping was much more than would normally be seen in bands and more consistent with the degree of chromatin clumping observed in segmented neutrophils. The cells classified as segmented neutrophils usually had only two lobes as compared with the multiple lobes seen in normal segmented neutrophils. Hypolobulation of neutrophils presents a peripheral blood picture that mimics an increase in neutrophilic bands. Because the total leukocyte count was within normal range, one would have expected the percentage of bands to be normal also. However, major discrepancies between these two measurements should alert the hematology technologist that an error has occurred. Repeated review of the peripheral smear confirmed that

the band-type neutrophils were actually hypolobulated neutrophils. The condition was Pelger-Huët anomaly.

2. Pelger-Huët anomaly exists as a congenital disorder. This trait is inherited in an autosomal dominant manner. In persons who are heterozygous for this trait, more than three fourths of the mature neutrophils may be hypolobulated. Homozygous states for this trait are rare. A condition of pseudo–Pelger-Huët anomaly may be observed in leukemias, such as chronic granulocytic leukemia, or it may be induced by drugs such as the sulfa drugs or those used in chemotherapy.

3. Congenital Pelger-Huët anomaly has not been associated with any specific clinical disease. The abnormal nuclear maturation is presumed to be a reflection of abnormal nucleic acid metabolism, although the specific abnormality is unknown. Functionally, these leukocytes do not show any abnormality.

DIAGNOSIS: Congenital Pelger-Huët anomaly

CASE 15.5

A 31-year-old white man was admitted to the burn unit of a local hospital following an accident at a local foundry. Several STAT laboratory blood tests were ordered, including a complete blood count.

■ **Laboratory Data**

The hemoglobin, hematocrit, and red blood cell (RBC) count were all slightly elevated. The total leukocyte count was 15.8×10^9/L. The differential count was as follows:

Band neutrophils 12%
Segmented neutrophils 65%
Lymphocytes 23%

Light blue-gray inclusions were observed in the cytoplasm of many of the bands and segmented neutrophils.

■ **Questions**

1. What is the etiology of the abnormal quantitative findings in this patient's complete blood count?
2. What are the blue-gray vacuoles in the cytoplasm of the leukocytes?
3. Is this abnormality diagnostically significant?

■ **Discussion**

1. The concentration of the RBCs that produced the slightly elevated hemoglobin, hematocrit, and RBC count was undoubtedly caused by the loss of fluids as the result of the serious burns. Elevation of the total leukocyte count is frequently seen as a response to stress, as in this type of trauma.

2. The blue-gray inclusions in the cytoplasm are Döhle bodies. However, care must be taken to distinguish these

(continued)

more common inclusions from May-Hegglin anomaly. The absence of unusual platelets and the admitting diagnosis would be helpful in not mistaking the more frequently encountered Döhle bodies from the May-Hegglin anomaly.

3. Döhle bodies are frequently seen in traumatic or toxic conditions such as severe burns. These leukocytic inclusions may also be seen in severe infections, during pregnancy, and as the result of cancer chemotherapy. Patients with viral infections, such as measles or hepatitis, may also have Döhle bodies. Although they are indicative of a metabolic abnormality, they are not specific for a particular disorder. However, it is diagnostically significant as a sign of abnormal stress on the bone marrow.

DIAGNOSIS: Döhle inclusion bodies caused by extensive burns

CASE 15.6

A 4-year-old white girl was taken to her pediatrician because of increasing fatigue when playing and loss of appetite. Her physical examination revealed that she had splenomegaly but no hepatomegaly. A STAT complete blood count was ordered.

■ Laboratory Data
RBC 3.82×10^{12}/L
Hematocrit 29%
Hemoglobin 9.5 g/dL
WBC 1.51×10^9/L
Platelets 55×10^9/L
MCV 74 fL
MCH 25 pg
MCHC 33 g/dL

■ Leukocyte Differential
Band neutrophils 3%
Segmented neutrophils 32%
Eosinophils 2%
Monocytes 8%
Lymphocytes 55%

Decreased platelets were noted on the peripheral blood smear; 2+ anisocytosis and slight hypochromia also were noted on the smear; and 1+ toxic granulation was noted in the granulocytic leukocytes.

A follow-up bone marrow examination revealed trilineage hematopoiesis with full maturation of all three cell lines. The myeloid:erythroid ratio was normal. A few histiocytes were seen. These cells exhibited abundant pale basophilic cytoplasm and fibrillar cytoplasmic inclusions.

■ Questions
1. What type of disorder is suggested by the blood and bone marrow observations?

2. What specific disorders would be included in the differential diagnosis?
3. Is a particular population more likely to suffer from this disease?
4. What is the etiology of the disease?

■ Discussion
1. The presence of histiocytes with abundant basophilic cytoplasm suggests a storage disease.
2. Niemann-Pick and Gaucher disease are classified as storage diseases.
3. Yes. Gaucher disease is one of the most common cellular storage disease in the world, particularly in the Ashkenazi Jewish population. This genetic condition exhibits a carrier frequency of 1:15 in Ashkenazi Jews with four to five gene mutations.
4. Gaucher disease is usually a genetically caused cellular lysosomal storage disease. A deficiency of the lysosomal enzyme, β-glucocerebrosidase, causes the patient's histiocytes to become filled with glucocerebroside remnants. These remnants give the cytoplasm the appearance of crinkled paper.

DIAGNOSIS: Gaucher Disease

CASE 15.7

A 6-year-old boy was taken to the emergency department by his mother because of a high fever. The fever began about 10 days before. Physical examination revealed a temperature of 102°F (38.9°C). A complete blood count, urinalysis, and blood culture were ordered STAT. Oral antibiotic therapy was begun. The patient was subsequently discharged home.

■ Laboratory Data
RBC 3.53×10^{12}/L
Hemoglobin 11.5 g/dL
Hematocrit 33%
WBC 7.0×10^9/L
Platelet count 175.0×10^9/L

■ Leukocyte Differential
Band neutrophils 10%
Segmented neutrophils 60%
Lymphocytes 27%
Monocytes 3%

Platelet distribution was slightly decreased. RBC morphology was within normal limits. Results of the urinalysis were normal. The blood culture exhibited no growth after appropriate incubation.

■ Follow-Up
The next day, the patient's mother brought him back to the emergency department, reporting an elevated temperature 103°F (39.4°C). A repeat complete blood count and urinalysis were ordered STAT. Serological assays for *B. burgdorferi*,

(continued)

E. chaffeensis, and the HGE agent as well as polymerase chain reaction (PCR) for the causative agents of human ehrlichiosis were ordered. The patient was admitted to the hospital.

■ **Laboratory Data**
RBC 2.90×10^{12}/L
Hemoglobin 9.5 g/dL
Hematocrit 27%
WBC 10.0×10^9/L
Platelet count 175.0×10^9/L

■ **Leukocyte Differential**
Band neutrophils 10%
Segmented neutrophils 59%
Lymphocytes 21%
Monocytes 10%

Platelet distribution was slightly decreased. RBC morphology was within normal limits.

Subsequent serology specimens reported that the acute polyclonal (indirect fluorescent antibody [IFA]) for *E. equi* was nonspecific. The convalescent specimen obtained 23 days later was positive (titer of 1:320). Five months later, the IFA for *E. equi* was positive for IgG (1:264), but the IgM component was less than 1:20. IgM and IgG titers for *E. chaffeensis* were negative.

■ **Questions**
1. Which serological assays were significant in establishing a diagnosis?
2. Is this confirmation of HGE?
3. Is HGE more common in children than adults?

■ **Discussion**
1. The diagnosis of HGE was established serologically by the positive PCR for HGE agent, the presence of an elevated IFA to *E. equi*, and an increase in the IFA *E. equi* titer between the acute and convalescent specimens.
2. Yes. The confirmed case definition of HGE includes a fourfold rise in antibody titer or seroconversion between acute and convalescent specimens.
3. Unlike Lyme disease, another tickborne infectious disease, HGE is less common in children than in adults. Among confirmed cases, rates of Ehrlichiosis in Connecticut, children who were 9 years old or younger had the lowest rate of confirmed cases compared to Lyme disease where disease rates are highest in this age group. Very few cases of pediatric HGE are diagnosed in individuals younger than 20 years of age.

DIAGNOSIS: **Human Granulocytic Ehrlichiosis (HGE)**

1. Leukocytosis can be caused by
   A. increased movement of immature cells out of the bone marrow's proliferative compartment
   B. increased mobilization of granulocytes from the maturation-storage compartment
   C. increased movement of granulocytes from the marginating pool to the circulating pool
   D. all of the above
2. Neutrophilia can be related to a variety of conditions or disorders. Select the appropriate conditions.
   A. Surgery
   B. Burns
   C. Stress
   D. All of the above
3. Charcot-Leyden crystals can be found in _____ of patients with active eosinophilic inflammation.
   A. sputum
   B. tissues
   C. stool
   D. all of the above

4. Monocytosis can be observed in
   A. tuberculosis
   B. fever of unknown origin
   C. rheumatoid arthritis
   D. all of the above
5. Neutropenia can be observed in
   A. bone marrow injury
   B. nutritional deficiency
   C. increased destruction and utilization
   D. all of the above

Questions 6 through 9: Match the following abnormalities with the appropriate characteristic.
   A. Gigantic peroxidase-positive deposits.
   B. Precipitated mucopolysaccharides.
   C. Döhle body–like inclusions.
   D. Single or multiple pale-blue staining inclusions.
6. _____ Alder-Reilly inclusions
7. _____ Chédiak-Higashi syndrome
8. _____ Döhle body inclusions
9. _____ May-Hegglin anomaly

(continued)

REVIEW QUESTIONS (continued)

Questions 10 through 12: Match the following abnormalities with the appropriate characteristic.

 A. Dark blue-black precipitates of RNA.
 B. Five or more nuclear segments.
 C. Failure of the nucleus to segment.
 D. Precipitated mucopolysaccharides.

10. _____ Pelger-Huët anomaly
11. _____ Toxic granulation
12. _____ Hypersegmentation

Questions 13 through 16: Match the following abnormalities with the appropriate condition.

 A. Associated with a deficiency of vitamin B_{12} or folic acid
 B. Associated with frequent infections in children or young adults
 C. May be related to a maturational arrest in some acute infections
 D. Associated with viral infections and burns

13. _____ Chédiak-Higashi syndrome
14. _____ Döhle bodies
15. _____ Pelger-Huët anomaly
16. _____ Hypersegmentation

Questions 17 through 21: Select the appropriate cell type involved in the following disorders.

 A. Neutrophilic series
 B. Monocytic-macrophage series

17. _____ Gaucher disease
18. _____ Niemann-Pick disease
19. _____ Chédiak-Higashi syndrome
20. _____ Chronic granulomatous disease
21. _____ Lazy leukocyte syndrome

22. In the United States, human diseases caused by *Ehrlichia* species can be caused by
 A. *E. chaffeensis*
 B. *E. ewingii*
 C. *E. phagocytophilia* (similar or identical to)
 D. all of the above

23. Ehrlichiosis is transmitted by _____.
 A. mosquitoes
 B. ticks
 C. rats
 D. cats

24. Gaucher cells have
 A. wrinkled cytoplasm
 B. one to three nuclei
 C. a deficiency of β-glucocerebrosidase
 D. all of the above

BIBLIOGRAPHY

Bakken JS, et al. Human granulocytic ehrlichiosis in the Upper Midwest United States, *JAMA*, 272(3):212–218, 1994.

Barenfanger J, et al. Identifying human ehrlichiosis, *Lab Med*, 27(6):372–374, 1996.

Beutler E. Gaucher's disease, *N Engl J Med*, 325(19):1354–1359, 1991.

Centers for Disease Control and Prevention (CDC). Human ehrlichiosis in the United States (www.cdc.gov). Retrieved October 16, 2003.

Dannenberg AM Jr. Macrophages and monocytes. In: Spivak JL (ed.). *Fundamentals of Clinical Hematology*, Hagerstown, MD: Harper & Row, 1980:137–153.

Figueroa ML, et al. A less costly regimen of alglucerase to treat Gaucher's disease, *N Engl J Med*, 327(23):1632–1636, 1992.

Francis GE, et al. DNA strand breakage and ADP-ribosyl transferase mediated DNA ligation during stimulation of human bone marrow cells by granulocyte-macrophage colony stimulating activity, *Leuk Res*, 8(3):407–415, 1984.

Grabowski GA, et al. Enzyme therapy in type I Gaucher disease: Comparative efficacy of mannose-terminated glucocerebrosidase from natural and recombinant sources, *Ann Intern Med*, 122(1):33–39, 1995.

Hartmann LC, et al. Granulocyte colony-stimulating factor in severe chemotherapy-induced afebrile neutropenia, *N Engl J Med*, 336(25):1776–1785, 1997.

Hellmann A. Production of colony stimulating activity in mixed mononuclear cell culture, *Br J Haematol*, 45:245–249, 1980.

Howard J. Myeloid series abnormalities: Neutrophilia, *Lab Med*, 14(3):147–151, 1983.

Koepke JA (Ed). *Leukocyte Differential Counting, Tentative Standard H20-T*. Villanova, PA: National Committee for Clinical Laboratory Standards (NCCLS), 1982.

Lopker A, et al. Stereoselective muscarinic acetylcholine and opiate receptors in human phagocytic leukocytes, *Biochem Pharmacol*, 29:1361–1365, 1980.

Markell EK, et al. *Medical Parasitology*, Philadelphia, PA: Saunders, 1986:314.

O'Connor BH. *A Color Atlas and Instruction Manual of Peripheral Blood Morphology*, Baltimore, MD: Williams & Wilkins, 1984.

Raphael SS. *Lynch's Medical Laboratory Technology*, 4th ed., Philadelphia, PA: Saunders, 1983:653–692.

Robinson SH, Reich PR. *Hematology: Pathophysiological Basis for Clinical Practice*, 3rd ed., Boston: Little, Brown & Co., 1993.

Sidransky E, Ginns EI. Clinical heterogeneity among patients with Gaucher's disease, *JAMA*, 269(9):1154–1157, 1993.

Stein RB. Granulocytosis and granulocytic leukemoid reactions. In: Koepke J (ed.). *Laboratory Hematology*, Edinburgh, UK: Churchill-Livingstone, 1984:153–187.

Tsan M-F. Neutrophils. In: Spivak JL (ed.). *Fundamentals of Clinical Hematology*, Hagerstown, MD: Harper & Row, 1980:109–117.

Wynn TE. Letters to the editor, *Lab Med*, 15(4):276–277, 1984.

Zigmond SH, Lauffenburger DA. Assays of leukocyte chemotaxis, *Annu Rev Med*, 137:149–155, 1986.

CHAPTER 16

Leukocytes: Lymphocytes and Plasma Cells

Anatomical origin and development of lymphocytes

- Briefly describe the role of lymphocytes and plasma cells in the body defense mechanism against disease.
- Name and locate the two primary and three secondary lymphoid tissues.
- Identify the anatomical sites populated by T cells and B cells.
- Explain the importance of lymphocyte recirculation.
- Cite the percentage of T and B cells found in the peripheral circulation of adults.
- State the major type and percentage of leukocytes found in 6-month-old infants.
- Compare the normal percentages and quantities of lymphocytes at different ages ranging from birth to adulthood.

Morphological characteristics of normal lymphocytes

- Compare the characteristics, such as chromatin patterns, of the three major developmental stages of lymphocyte maturation.
- Discuss the morphological abnormalities of variant lymphocytes.

- State at least three conditions associated with specific lymphocytic abnormalities that may be seen in peripheral blood.

Functions and membrane characteristics of lymphocytes

- Describe the major function of T, B, and natural killer (NK) cells.
- Describe the major lymphocytic membrane characteristics.
- Name several applications of lymphocyte subset testing.
- Briefly describe the production of monoclonal antibodies.
- Briefly describe membrane marker development in T cells.
- Name four cytokines or chemokines produced by T cells.

Plasma cell development and maturation

- Describe the pathways of plasma cell development.
- Identify the maturational characteristics of plasma cells.
- Describe the appearance and cytoplasmic contents of Russell bodies, Mott cells, and flame cells.

ANATOMICAL ORIGIN AND DEVELOPMENT OF LYMPHOCYTES

In addition to the activities of the granulocytes, monocytes, and macrophages (discussed in Chapter 14), the lymphocytes and plasma cells cooperate in defending the body against disease through recognition of foreign **antigens** and **antibody** production.

Sites of Lymphocytic Development

During embryonic development, lymphocytes arise from the pluripotent, precursor cells of the yolk sac and liver. Later in fetal development and throughout the life cycle, the bone marrow becomes the sole provider of hematopoietic stem cells. Cells under the influence of hematopoietic growth factors interleukin-1 (IL-1) and IL-6, differentiate into the lymphoid stem cell. Continued cellular development of the lymphoid precursors and proliferation occur as the cells travel to specific microenvironments. Hematopoietic growth factors play an important role in differentiation into the pathway of the pre-B cell or prothymocyte. The majority of cells differentiate into either **T lymphocytes** or **B lymphocytes**. The plasma cell is the fully differentiated B cell.

Primary Lymphoid Tissue

In humans, both the bone marrow and the thymus are classified as primary or central lymphoid tissues (Fig. 16.1) and are active in lymphopoiesis. Stem cells that migrate to the thymus proliferate and differentiate under the influence of specific cytokines. These cells acquire thymus-dependent characteristics to become **immunocompetent** (able to function in the immune response) T lymphocytes. It is believed that the bone marrow functions as the bursal equivalent in humans. It is from the term **bursa** that the B lymphocytes derive their name. Most of the cells produced in the primary sites die before leaving; only a small percentage migrate to the secondary tissues.

Secondary Lymphoid Tissue

The secondary lymphoid tissues include the lymph nodes (Fig. 16.2), spleen, and Peyer patches in the intestine (see Fig. 16.1). Proliferation of the T and B lymphocytes in the secondary or peripheral lymphoid tissues is primarily dependent on antigenic stimulation. The T lymphocytes or T cells (Fig. 16.3) are located in

1. Perifollicular and paracortical regions of the lymph node
2. Medullary cords of the lymph nodes

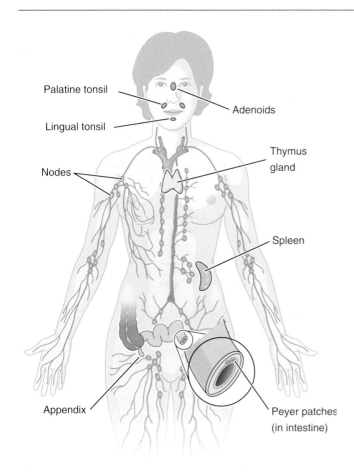

Palatine tonsil

Lingual tonsil

Nodes

Adenoids

Thymus gland

Spleen

Appendix

Peyer patches (in intestine)

FIGURE 16.1 Location of lymphoid tissue. (Reprinted with permission from Cohen BJ, Taylor JJ. *Memmler's The Human Body in Health and Disease*, 11th ed, Baltimore, MD: Wolters Kluwer Health, 2009.)

3. Periarteriolar regions of the spleen
4. Thoracic duct of the circulatory system

The B lymphocytes or B cells (see Fig. 16.3) multiply and populate these sites:

1. Follicular and medullary areas (germinal centers) of the lymph nodes
2. Primary follicles and red pulp of the spleen
3. Follicular regions of gut-associated lymphoid tissue (GALT)
4. Medullary cords of the lymph nodes

Lymphocyte Physiology

The mature T lymphocyte survives for several months or years, whereas the average life span of the B lymphocytes is only a few days. Lymphocyte lifespan disorders involving dysregulation of the apoptotic pathway include chronic lymphocytic leukemia (CLL) and autoimmune lymphoproliferative syndrome (ALPS).

The pool of peripheral lymphocytes is closely regulated and remains relatively constant in the absence of disease.

The size of the lymphocyte pool is of crucial importance to the adaptive immune system. This pool of cells must be as diverse as possible, but the physical space that the cells occupy is limited. Waves of T-cell clonal expansions and contractions are usually due to external stimuli, for example, infections. During a primary immune response, the antigen-specific T-cell population may increase 1,000-fold, but less than 10% of these new cells will survive in the memory pool. Shortly after the peak of the immune response, both antigen-presenting cells (APCs) and antigen-activated T cells die in large numbers as the immune response wanes. The numbers of T lymphocytes both in secondary lymphoid organs and in the circulation are kept under strict control. This process is called homeostatic proliferation, which occurs when lymphopenia occurs.

Lymphocytes move freely between the blood and lymphoid tissues. This activity, referred to as **lymphocyte recirculation**, enables lymphocytes to come in contact with processed foreign antigens and to disseminate antigen-sensitized memory cells throughout the lymphoid system. Lymphocytes recirculate back to the blood via the major lymphatic ducts (see Fig. 16.4).

Lymphocytes enter the lymph node from the blood circulation via arterioles and capillaries to reach the specialized postcapillary venules. From the venule, the lymphocytes enter the node and either remain in the node or pass through the node and return to the circulating blood.

Lymphatic fluid, lymphocytes, and antigens from certain body sites enter the lymph node through the afferent lymphatic duct and exit through the efferent lymphatic duct. The lymphatic system consists of widely distributed lymph nodes and lymphatic vessels. The right lymphatic duct drains the heart, lungs, part of the diaphragm, the right upper part of the body, and the right side of the head and neck. The thoracic duct drains the rest of the body.

Lymphatic fluid returns to the venous blood circulation. Fluid and lymphocytes leaving the lymph node move into the medullary lymphatic sinuses and then to the efferent lymphatic duct, which in turn collects in the major lymphatic ducts. The principal return is into the left or right brachiocephalic vein or into one of the two veins that unite to form it, the left subclavian or left internal jugular vein.

Normal Reference Values

At any one time, approximately 5% of the total body lymphocyte mass is present in the circulating blood. Sixty to eighty percent of the blood lymphocyte pool in adults is composed of T lymphocytes and approximately 20% is composed of B lymphocytes. Total blood lymphocyte levels vary considerably with age (Table 16.1). Lymphocytes represent 31% of the total leukocytes present at birth; within a few days of birth, lymphocytes are the dominant type of leukocyte in the circulation. Most of the cells are T lymphocytes. In adults, lymphocytes represent approximately 34% of the total circulation of leukocytes, or 2.5×10^9/L.

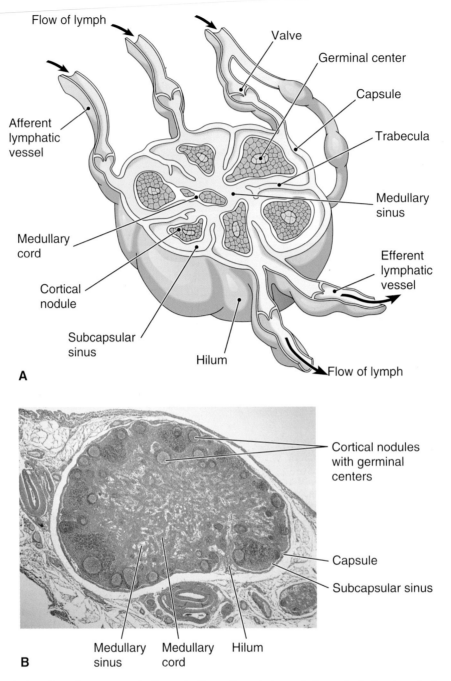

FIGURE 16.2 Structure of a lymph node. **A:** *Arrows* indicate the flow of lymph through the node. **B:** Section of a lymph node as seen under the microscope (low power). (A: Reprinted with permission from Cohen BJ, Taylor JJ. *Memmler's The Human Body in Health and Disease*, 11th ed, Baltimore, MD: Wolters Kluwer Health, 2009; B: Reprinted with permission from Cormack DH. *Essential Histology*, 2nd ed, Philadelphia, PA: Lippincott Williams & Wilkins, 2001.)

Determining Absolute Lymphocyte Values

The **absolute** number of lymphocytes is the total number of lymphocytes compared with the total number of leukocytes. The **relative** number of lymphocytes is the percentage of lymphocytes as determined by a differential blood smear enumeration of leukocytes (see Chapter 17).

MORPHOLOGICAL CHARACTERISTICS OF NORMAL LYMPHOCYTES

The stages of lymphocyte development (see Fig. 16.5) are the **lymphoblast, prolymphocyte,** and **mature lymphocyte.** The morphological characteristics of these cells on a peripheral blood smear when stained with Wright stain are summarized in Table 16.2.

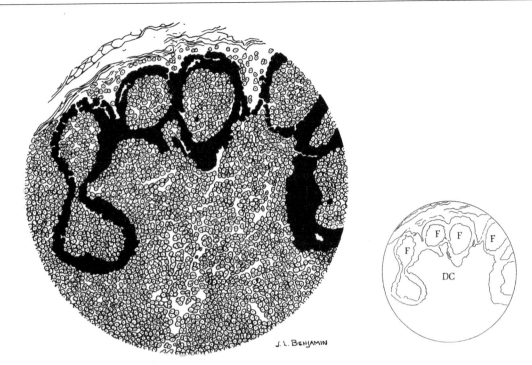

FIGURE 16.3 T cell and B cell areas in the lymph node. The lymphocytes of the outer cortex are mainly arranged in lymphoid follicles (F), which are the major sites of B-lymphocyte localization and proliferation. The deep cortical zone (DC), or paracortex, is composed mainly of T lymphocytes that are never arranged in follicles. The number of cortical follicles and the depth of the deep cortical zone vary according to the immunological state of each lymph node and in each individual person.

Under normal conditions, only mature lymphocytes are found in the peripheral blood. Mature cells can be classified as either large or small. Although T and B cells cannot be distinguished by routine Romanowsky-type staining of blood smears, most small lymphocytes are T cells and most large lymphocytes are B cells.

Maturational Stages

Lymphoblast

The lymphoblast (see Fig. 16.6) is the first morphologically identifiable cell of the lymphocytic maturational series in the bone marrow. The overall size ranges from 15 to 20 μm, with a nuclear-cytoplasmic (N:C) ratio of 4:1.

The nuclear shape is either round or oval. One or two nucleoli may be present. The chromatin pattern is delicate looking. The small amount of cytoplasm is medium blue and may have a darker-blue border. No granules are present.

Prolymphocyte

The second stage in the maturational development of the lymphocyte is the prolymphocyte (see Fig. 16.7). This cell may be seen in the bone marrow, thymus, and secondary lymphoid tissues. The overall size is usually about the same (15 to 18 μm) as the lymphoblast. The N:C ratio ranges from 4:1 to 3:1.

The nuclear shape is usually oval or slightly indented. The number of nucleoli varies from none to one. The chromatin pattern is slightly condensed. The small amount of cytoplasm is medium blue with a thin, darker blue rim. A few azurophilic granules may be present.

Mature Lymphocyte

Mature lymphocytes (see Fig. 16.8) range in size from large (17 to 20 μm) in younger cells to small (6 to 9 μm) in older cells. The N:C ratio ranges from 2:1 in younger cells to 4:1 to 3:1 in older cells.

The nucleus is round or oval and may have an indentation (cleft). Nucleoli are not visible. The chromatin pattern is dense and appears clumped. The cytoplasm is light sky blue and very scanty. A few azurophilic granules may be present. Erythrocytes in late stages of nucleated development should not be confused with mature lymphocytes (see Fig. 16.9).

General Variations in Lymphocyte Morphology

Variant lymphocytes may be referred to by several names, including atypical lymphocytes, Downey cells, reactive or transformed lymphocytes, lymphocytoid or plasmacytoid lymphocytes, and virocytes.

The term **variant** denotes that a lymphocyte is not normal but does not further classify a lymphocyte. Healthy persons may have up to 5% or 6% of variant lymphocytes. These represent morphological evidence of a normal immune mechanism. Variant lymphocytes can be found in increased numbers in disorders such as infectious mononucleosis, viral pneumonia, and viral hepatitis.

The morphology of variant lymphocytes differs (see Fig. 16.10), and several distinct types have been described, including the classic but obsolete grouping of lymphocytes seen in infectious mononucleosis, the Downey classification. Variant lymphocytes can embrace all transitional changes from mature unstimulated lymphocytes to immunoblasts to

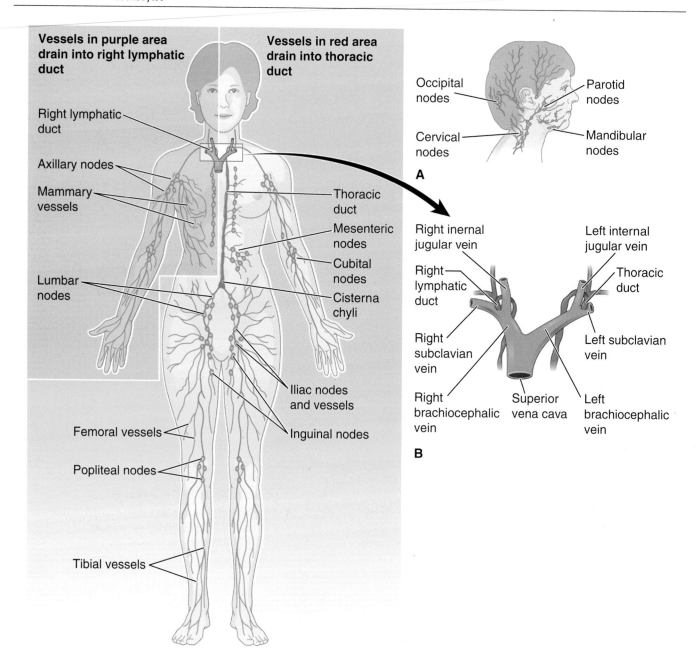

FIGURE 16.4 Vessels and nodes of the lymphatic system. **A:** Lymph nodes and vessels of the head. **B:** Drainage of right lymphatic duct and thoracic duct into subclavian veins. (Reprinted with permission from Cohen BJ, Taylor JJ. *Memmler's The Human Body in Health and Disease*, 11th ed, Baltimore, MD: Wolters Kluwer Health, 2009.)

TABLE 16.1	Average Lymphocyte Values in Peripheral Blood	
Age	**Total White Cell Count**	**Lymphocytes Percentage**
Birth	18.1×10^9/L	31
6 months	11.9×10^9/L	61
10 years	8.1×10^9/L	38
21 years and older	7.4×10^9/L	34

Source: Dallman PR. Blood-forming tissues. In: Rudolph AM (ed.) *Pediatrics,* 16 ed, New York, NY: Appleton-Centry-Crofts, 1977:1178.

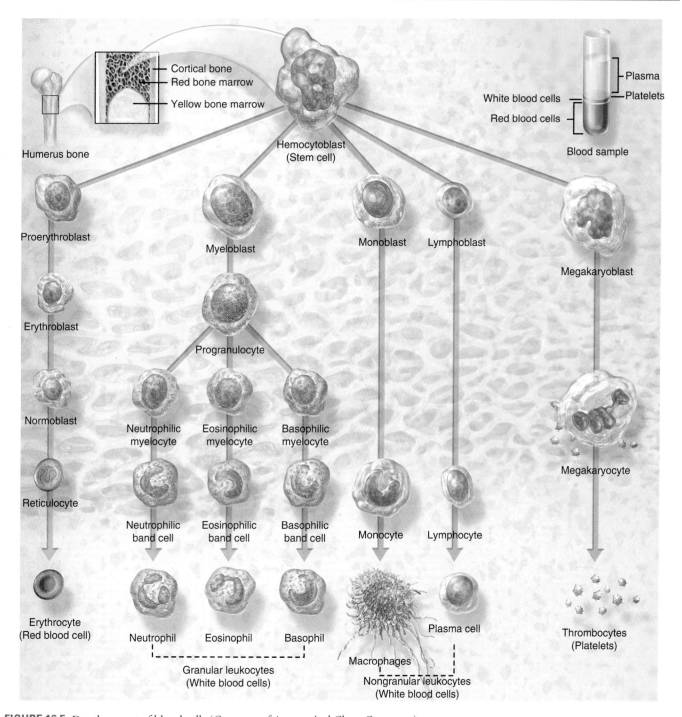

FIGURE 16.5 Development of blood cells (Courtesy of Anatomical Chart Company).

plasma cells (discussed later in this chapter). These lymphocytes represent stimulated lymphocytes that have increased DNA and RNA activity. Similarities between some variant lymphocytes and lymphoblasts can lead to difficulties in identification. The formation of distinctive nucleoli characterizes the immunoblast, the further transformation of which produces plasma cells or small sensitized committed lymphocytes called **memory cells**.

The general characteristics of **variant** lymphocytes include the following:

1. Usually the overall size is increased (16 to 30 μm).
2. The nucleus may be enlarged.
3. The nuclear shape may be lobulated or resemble the nucleus of a monocyte (**monocytoid**) with clefts or notching and may be folded.
4. Chromatin patterns vary from fine patterns to a coarsely granular appearance.
5. One to three nucleoli may be present.
6. The cytoplasm is frequently abundant and often foamy or vacuolated.

TABLE 16.2	Comparative Characteristics of Lymphocytes		
Lymphoblast	**Lymphocyte**	**Prolymphocyte**	**Mature**
Size	15–20 mm	15–18 μm	Small, 6–9 μm Large, 17–20 μm
N:C ratio	4:1	4:1 to 3:1	Small, 4:1 to 3:1 Large, 2:1
Nucleus			
Nuclear shape	Round or oval	Oval, slightly indented	Round or oval; may have clefts
Nucleoli	1 or 2	0 or 1	Absent
Chromatin	Delicate	Slightly condensed	Dense and clumped
Cytoplasm			
Granules	None	May have a few azurophilic granules	Few azurophilic granules may be present
Amount	Small	Small	Very scanty
Color	Medium blue, may have a darker blue border	Medium blue with a thin rim of darker blue	Light blue

7. Cytoplasmic color may range from gray to light blue or intensely blue.
8. Granules may be present.

Specific Lymphocyte Morphological Variations

A variety of abnormal lymphocytes or lymphocyte-like cells are associated with specific disorders. They include the following.

Binucleated Lymphocytes

These cells can be seen in viral infections. If more than 5% of the lymphocytes are binucleated, it is suggestive of either lymphocytic leukemia or leukosarcoma (the hematological spread of lymphosarcoma).

Rieder Cells

Rieder cells are similar to normal lymphocytes except that the nucleus is notched, lobulated, and cloverleaf-like. They

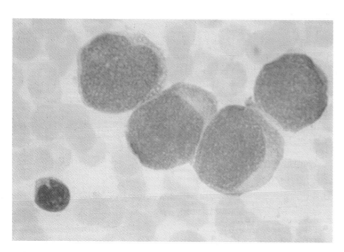

FIGURE 16.6 Lymphoblastic cell. (Reprinted with permission from Anderson SC. *Anderson's Atlas of Hematology*, Philadelphia, PA: Wolters Kluwer Health/Lippincott Williams & Wilkins, Copyright 2003.)

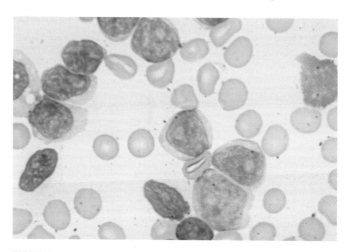

FIGURE 16.7 Prolymphocyte. (Reprinted with permission from Anderson SC. *Anderson's Atlas of Hematology*, Philadelphia, PA: Wolters Kluwer Health/Lippincott Williams & Wilkins, Copyright 2003.)

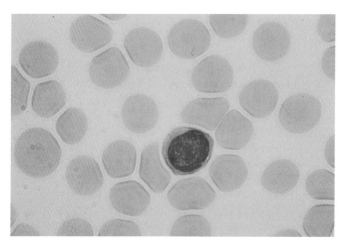

FIGURE 16.8 Mature lymphocyte. (Reprinted with permission from Anderson SC. *Anderson's Atlas of Hematology*, Philadelphia, PA: Wolters Kluwer Health/Lippincott Williams & Wilkins, Copyright 2003.)

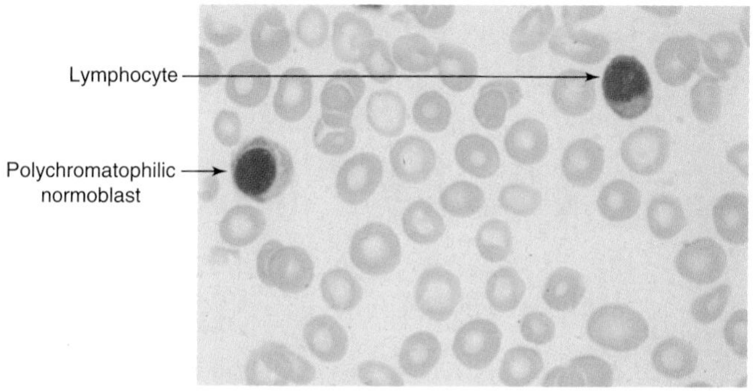

FIGURE 16.9 Late polychromatophilic normoblast, lymphocyte. (Reprinted with permission from Anderson SC. *Anderson's Atlas of Hematology*, Philadelphia, PA: Wolters Kluwer Health/Lippincott Williams & Wilkins, Copyright 2003.)

occur in CLL (discussed in Chapter 20) or can be artificially produced through blood smear preparation.

Vacuolated Lymphocytes

Vacuolated lymphocytes are frequently associated with Niemann-Pick disease, Tay-Sachs disease, Hurler syndrome, and Burkitt lymphoma. Vacuoles can also be seen in variant lymphocytes and as a reaction to viral infections, radiation, and chemotherapy.

Smudge Cells

Smudge cells (see Fig. 16.11) are a natural artifact produced in the preparation of a blood smear. They represent the bare nuclei of lymphocytes and neutrophils. Increased fragility of cells contributes to the increased percentage of smudge cells. Some laboratories enumerate smudge cells as a percentage of the total 100 leukocytes in a differential leukocyte count. Smudge cells are seen in increased proportions in lymphocytosis, particularly CLL.

CHARACTERISTICS OF LYMPHOCYTES

Major Lymphocyte Categories and Functions

Several major categories of lymphocytes are recognized as functionally active. These categories are the **T cells, B cells**, and **natural killer** (**NK**) lymphocytes.

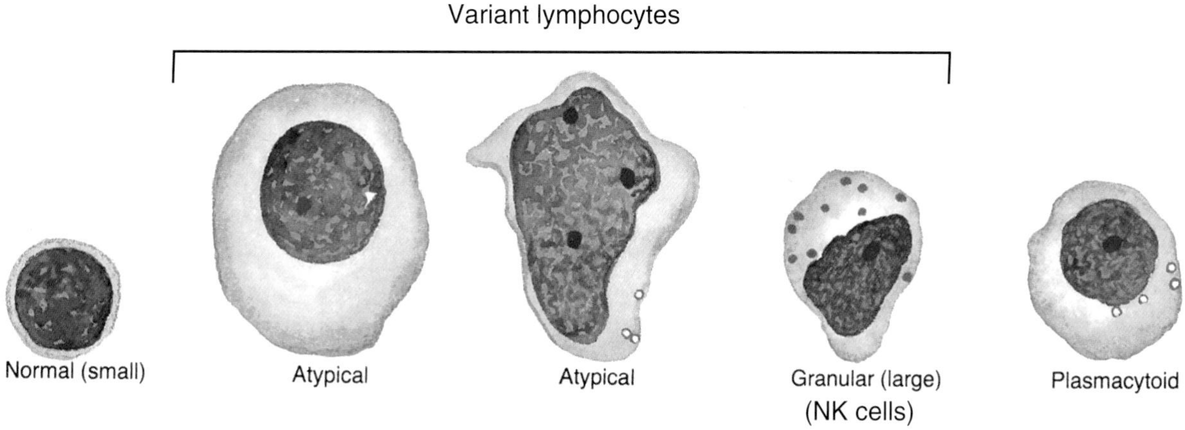

Variant lymphocytes

Normal (small)   Atypical   Atypical   Granular (large) (NK cells)   Plasmacytoid

FIGURE 16.10 Lymphocyte morphology. The term "variant lymphocytes" covers atypical lymphocytes and large granular lymphocytes. Atypical lymphocytes are large and exhibit deep blue to pale gray cytoplasm; they are seen in benign reactive processes. Large granular lymphocytes are medium-to-large lymphoid cells with some pink cytoplasmic granules. They are suppressor T lymphocytes, some with NK function, and may be increased in benign or malignant disorders. Plasmacytoid lymphocytes have abundant blue cytoplasm and are seen in some reactive disorders. (Reprinted with permission from Rubin R, Strayer DS. *Rubin's Pathology: Clinicopathologic Foundations of Medicine*, 5th ed, Philadelphia, PA: Lippincott Williams & Wilkins, 2008.)

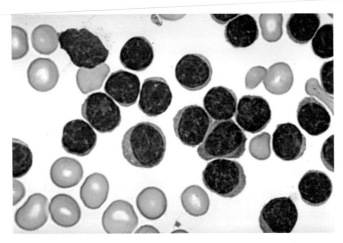

FIGURE 16.11 Chronic lymphocytic leukemia. A smear of peripheral blood shows numerous small- to medium-sized lymphocytes. A smudge cell is seen at the upper left. (Reprinted with permission from Rubin E, Farber JL. *Pathology*, 3rd ed, Philadelphia, PA: Lippincott Williams & Wilkins, 1999.)

T Lymphocytes

T cells are responsible for cellular immune responses and are involved in the regulation of antibody reactions by either helping or suppressing the activation of B lymphocytes. Sensitized T lymphocytes protect humans against infection by mediating intracellular pathogens that are viral, bacterial, fungal, or protozoan. These cells are responsible for chronic rejection in organ transplantation.

B Lymphocytes

B cells serve as the primary source of cells responsible for humoral (antibody) responses. Participation of B cells in the humoral immune response is accomplished by their transformation into plasma cells, with subsequent synthesis and secretion of immune antibodies (immunoglobulins). Stimulation of B cells to produce antibodies is a complex process, usually requiring interactions among macrophages (that phagocytize, process, and present antigens to T cells), T cells, and B cells. B lymphocytes aid in body defense against encapsulated bacteria such as streptococci. The condition of hyperacute rejection of transplanted organs is mediated by the B cell.

Natural Killer Lymphocytes

NK cells were discovered more than 30 years ago. Today, these cells are recognized as a unique and important part of the immune system with roles in infectious disease and tumor surveillance.

NK cells, derived from CD34+ hematopoietic progenitor cells, belong to the innate immune system. Unlike T or B lymphocytes of the adaptive or antigen-specific immune system, NK cells do not rearrange T-cell receptor or immunoglobulin genes from their germline configuration.

NK cells outnumber B cells in the circulation by a 3:1 ratio and with newly discovered functional complexity that indicates a very important role in host defense. NK cells are believed to be relatively short-lived, but at any one time, there are likely more than 2 billion of them circulating in an adult.

On a Wright-stained peripheral blood smear, NK cells vary morphologically from typical lymphocytes and appear as large lymphocytes with characteristic azurophilic granules in the cytoplasm.

The total population of human NK cells is phenotypically and functionally heterogeneous. Two immunophenotypically distinct subsets of NK cells, CD56^{bright} and CD56^{dim}, are found in the peripheral blood. CD56^{dim} cells produce more cytotoxic granules and are more effective in antibody-dependent cellular cytotoxicity (ADCC) and natural antibody–independent cytotoxicity than CD56^{bright} cells. By comparison, CD56^{bright} cells stimulated by monocyte-derived cytokines produce more interferon gamma (IFN-γ), GM-CSF, IL-10, and IL-13 which has a role in the immune response. Functionally, the production of interferon gamma (IFN-γ) is considered the prototypic NK-cell cytokine which shapes the Th1 immune response, activates APCs to upregulate MHC class I expression, activates macrophage killing of obligate intracellular pathogens, and has antiproliferative effects on viral and malignant-transformed cells.

Monoclonal Antibodies

Monoclonal antibodies to cell surface antigens now provide a method of classifying and identifying specific cellular membrane characteristics. This technique is one application of laser technology (see Chapter 27). Monoclonal antibodies are produced by a complex process of fusing two cell types: a plasma cell derived from a malignant tumor and a lymphocyte activated by a specific antigen. The fusion products are incubated until enough cells exist to permit testing for antibody production. The resultant monoclonal reagent, an antibody specific for an activated lymphocyte, is finally tested for specificity. The process of producing monoclonal antibodies takes 3 to 6 months to complete.

In practical terms, surface markers are used to identify and enumerate various subclasses of T lymphocytes and other lymphocytes. Variations exist in the concentration of most marker antigens on the cell surface. The evaluation of surface membrane markers is useful in certain applications such as establishing lymphocyte maturity, identifying disorders of lymphocytes (e.g., acquired immunodeficiency syndrome [AIDS]), classifying leukemias (see Chapter 19), and monitoring patients receiving immunosuppressive therapy.

Major Lymphocyte Membrane Characteristics and Development

The naming of the surface membrane antigen is identified with a monoclonal antibody. The relationship between lymphocyte phenotype (expressed surface membrane marker) and the subset is presented in Table 16.3. Cells of the immune system have specialized receptors on their membrane surfaces for eliciting an immune response. Before 1979, human

TABLE 16.3	Cell Differentiation Antigens Distribution
Antigen Cluster Designation	**Cell Differentiation Antigens Distribution**
CD2	78%–88% T cells, NK cells
CD3	68%–82% mature T cells
CD4	35%–55% mature T cells, monocytes
CD5	65%–79% T cells, B-cell subset
CD7	75% T cells and NK cells
CD8	20%–36% mature T cells
CD10 (CALLA)	90% of common ALLs, granulocytes, immature B cells
CD19	5%–15% B cells
CD20	5%–15% B cells
CD21	5%–15% mature B cells, dendritic cells
CD22	5%–15% B cells
CD34	Bone marrow progenitor cells, TdT+ cells, some acute leukemias

Adapted with permission from Turgeon M. *Immunology and Serology in Laboratory Medicine,* 4th ed, St. Louis, MO: Mosby, 2006:63.

lymphocytes could be classified as T cells, which regulate antibody production and directly kill certain cells (effector cells), and B cells, which produce antibodies.

The development of T and B lymphocytes is traditionally separated into sequential phases of antigen-independent and antigen-dependent maturational phases. Lymphocyte development in the thymus and bursal equivalent are antigen independent. Antigen-dependent maturation involves exposure of the T or B cell to a specific antigen, resulting in the expression of surface receptor molecules that can recognize the foreign antigen on representation. Lymphocytes in the peripheral lymphoid organs, including the lymph nodes, spleen, and other lymphoid tissues, remain in a resting state until they are stimulated to undergo antigen-dependent development.

T Cells

Maturation of T cells (see Fig. 16.12) is recognized by the presence of surface membrane markers. Early T and B cells share the enzymes TDT, CD9, and CD10, which are lost during maturation. However, these markers, particularly CD9 and CD10, are used to identify the lineage of immature T cells. Other surface markers are acquired during maturation. Some of these markers will be lost during maturation. The two characteristic markers of T lymphocytes, CD4 and CD8, are the hallmark markers of the mature lymphocyte subset.

In 1986, two subsets of activated CD4 T lymphocytes have been identified: Th1 and Th2. These subsets differ from each other in their pattern of cytokine production and their functions. Th1 cells are regarded as critical for immunity to intracellular microorganisms; Th2 cells are critical for immunity to many extracellular pathogens, including helminth parasites. Abnormal activation of Th1 is associated with most organ-specific autoimmune diseases; Th2 cells are associated with asthma and allergic inflammatory diseases.

Today at least four distinct CD4 T-cell subsets have been demonstrated to exist: Th1, Th2, Th17, and induced regulatory T (iTreg) cells.

CD4 T cells play a central role in immunity. The functions of CD4 T cells include

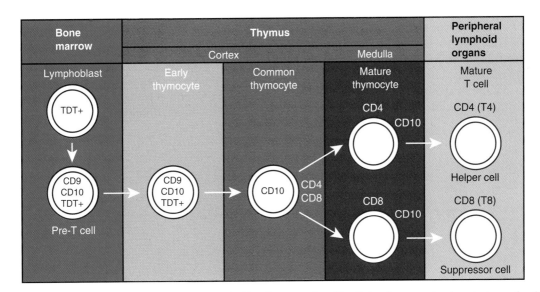

FIGURE 16.12 Examples of surface marker antigens present in T-cell maturation. T-cell development (antigen independent) in the thymus is divided into early thymocyte, common thymocyte, and mature thymocyte. Some of the surface membrane markers are depicted here. CD4 (T4) and CD8 (T8) are the hallmark markers of the lymphocyte subset.

TABLE 16.4	Characteristics of CD4 T Cells	
Subset	Major Activities	Representative Cytokines Produced
Th1	Autoimmunity Intracellular pathogen defense	IFN-α, IL-2, IL-10
Th2	Extracellular parasites defense Active in asthma and allergic reactions	IL-4, IL-5, IL-10, IL-13, IL-25
Th17	Autoimmunity Extracellular bacteria defense Fungi defense	IL-10, IL-17a, IL-17f, IL-21, IL-22
iTreg	Regulation of immune responses Immune tolerance Lymphocyte homeostasis	IL-10, IL-35, TGFβ

IFN-α, interferon gamma; TGFβ, transforming growth factor beta.

- Helping B lymphocytes make antibodies
- Inducing macrophages to develop enhanced microbicidal activity
- Recruiting neutrophils, eosinophils, and basophils to sites of inflammation or infection
- Producing cytokines and chemokines to integrate immune responses

Th 17 cells are recognized as playing a critical function in protection against microbial challenges, especially extracellular bacteria and fungi. See Table 16.4 for a summary of the four major sets of CD4 T cells.

B Cells

Certain immunological characteristics are associated with B cells (Table 16.5). The early pre-B cell is terminal deoxynucleotidyl transferase (TDT)-positive and expresses HLA-DR, CD19, and usually common ALL antigen (CALLA [CD10]). The first unique feature that identifies pre-B cells is the appearance of immunoglobulin chains in the cytoplasm.

Immunoglobulins consist of light and heavy molecular weight chains. The heavy chain (μ) of IgM is synthesized first and characterizes the pre-B cell. Other markers include TDT, CD19, CD20, CALLA, and HLA-DR. In the next stage of maturation, the early or immature B cell has cytoplasmic (cIg) and surface immunoglobulin (sIg) in the form of complete heavy and light chain molecules of IgM. The surface-bound IgM is structurally different from the IgM molecules that normally circulate in the plasma. Receptors for complement proteins and the Fc (fragment, crystallizable) portion of an immunoglobulin (IgG) also appear. All of this occurs while the cells reside in the bone marrow, before antigen stimulation.

The mature B cell produces two types of surface immunoglobulin, IgM and IgD. When activated, B cells undergo clonal expansion, producing daughter cells that retain the same antibody idiotype (antigen-binding region). Some daughter cells become memory cells and retain the small mature B-cell morphology and phenotype; others continue development into a short-lived antibody-secreting cell, the plasma cell.

TABLE 16.5	Cell Surface (CD) Molecules Expressed by B Cells	
CD 19	CD 23
CD20	CD24
CD21	CD40
CD22	CD72
	CD79a, b

Functional Testing of Lymphocytes

Tests of T-lymphocyte function measure mediator production. Soluble mediators (**cytokines**) are secreted by monocytes, lymphocytes, or neutrophils, providing the language for cell-to-cell communication. Important cytokines are as follows:

1. **Migration inhibition factor** (**MIF**): affects macrophage migration during delayed hypersensitivity reactions
2. **IL-2** (**T-cell growth factor**): major factor stimulating T-cell proliferation
3. **Chemotactic factor**: attracts granulocytes to affected areas
4. **IL-1**: released by macrophages and activates helper T cells

PLASMA CELL DEVELOPMENT AND MATURATION

The function of plasma cells is the synthesis and excretion of immunoglobulins (antibodies). Plasma cells are not normally found in the circulating blood but are found in the bone marrow in concentrations that do not normally exceed 2%. Plasma cells arise as the end stage of B-cell differentiation into a large activated plasma cell.

Plasma Cell Development

The pathway (see Fig. 16.13) from the B lymphocyte to the antibody-synthesizing plasma cell occurs when the B cell is antigenically stimulated and undergoes blast transformation. The immune antibody response begins when individual B lymphocytes encounter an antigen that binds to their specific immunoglobulin surface receptors. After receiving an appropriate second signal provided by interaction (see Fig. 16.14) with helper T cells, these antigen-binding B cells undergo blast cell transformation and proliferation to generate a clone of mature plasma cells that secrete a specific type of antibody.

Maturational Morphology

Mature B Cell (After Blast Transformation)

The overall size is 8 to 20 μm. The nucleus may be round or oval and may be *eccentrically placed* (not in the middle of the cell). The chromatin may be arranged in a fine pattern. The cytoplasm is nongranular, is moderate in amount, and has a mottled blue color.

Plasmacytoid Lymphocytes

The overall size is 15 to 25 μm. The round or oval nucleus is eccentrically placed. The chromatin is coarse and irregularly spaced. Nucleoli may be visible. Usually, the cytoplasm is a distinctive dark blue with a lighter staining area, the **hof**, next

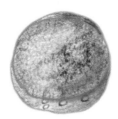

Plasmablast

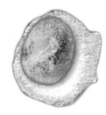

Proplasmacyte

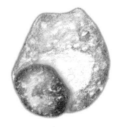

Plasma cell

FIGURE 16.13 Plasma cells drawing. (Reprinted with permission from Anderson SC. *Anderson's Atlas of Hematology*, Philadelphia, PA: Wolters Kluwer Health/Lippincott Williams & Wilkins, Copyright 2003.)

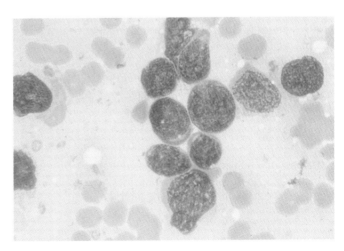

FIGURE 16.14 Plasmablast. (Reprinted with permission from Anderson SC. *Anderson's Atlas of Hematology*, Philadelphia, PA: Wolters Kluwer Health/Lippincott Williams & Wilkins, Copyright 2003.)

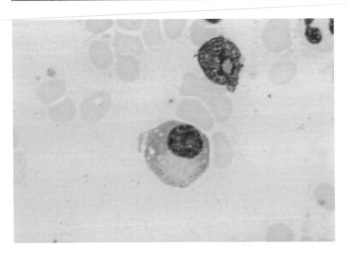

FIGURE 16.15 Plasma cells. (Reprinted with permission from Anderson SC. *Anderson's Atlas of Hematology*, Philadelphia, PA: Wolters Kluwer Health/Lippincott Williams & Wilkins, Copyright 2003.)

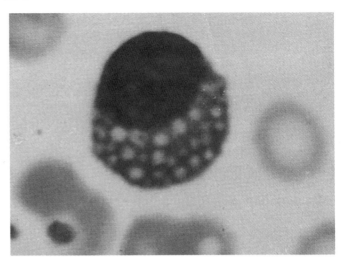

FIGURE 16.16 Mott cell (Russell bodies). (Reprinted with permission from O'Connor BH. *A Color Atlas and Instruction Manual of Peripheral Blood Morphology*, Baltimore, MD: Williams & Wilkins, 1984.)

to the nucleus. The hof represents the area containing the Golgi apparatus.

Plasma Cell

The mature plasma cell (see Fig. 16.15) is not normally found in peripheral blood; however, 1% or 2% of plasma cell–like lymphocytes may be encountered under stress conditions. The overall cell size is 14 to 20 μm. The nucleus is small and eccentrically located. More than one nucleus may be seen in a cell. The chromatin is condensed and has a cartwheel configuration.

Although the cytoplasm is dark blue, the hof area is usually visible. The cell has a well-developed, rough endoplasmic reticulum, which is characteristic of a cell producing proteins for export. The distinctive dark-blue cytoplasm is indicative of active synthesis and secretion of proteins (antibodies). The cytoplasm is oval in outline and abundant. Granules are absent, but vacuoles are common. Cytoplasmic inclusions can include Russell bodies, acidophilic refractile globules that represent gamma globulin (protein) secretions. Other forms of plasma cells, usually associated with abnormal conditions, are as follows:

1. **Grape** or **Mott cells**, in which the cytoplasm is completely filled with Russell bodies (see Fig. 16.16)
2. **Flame cells**, in which the cytoplasm stains a bright-red color and contains increased quantities of glycogen or intracellular deposits of amorphous matter

Plasma Cell Disorders

Although plasma cells are not normally found in the peripheral blood, an increase in these cells can be seen in a variety of nonmalignant disorders:

1. Viral disorders (e.g., rubella, chickenpox, mumps, and infectious mononucleosis)
2. Allergic conditions
3. Chronic infections
4. Collagen diseases

In plasma cell dyscrasias, the plasma cells may be greatly increased or may completely infiltrate the bone marrow, as in, for example, Waldenström macroglobulinemia and multiple myeloma (discussed in Chapter 20).

CHAPTER HIGHLIGHTS

Anatomical Origin and Development of Lymphocytes

Lymphocytes and plasma cells represent the blood cells primarily concerned with antigen recognition and antibody production. Following embryonic and fetal development, the bone marrow becomes the sole provider of undifferentiated stem cells. Further development and proliferation of these cells continue in the primary tissues—the bone marrow and thymus—and the secondary tissues—the lymph nodes, spleen, and GALT. In the primary tissues, the lymphocytes differentiate into one of the major categories of lymphocytes: T cells or B cells.

Lymphocytes, mostly of the T type, move freely between the blood and lymphoid tissues. The process of recirculation is important in the dissemination of immunological information. At any one time, approximately 5% of the total body lymphocyte mass is present in the circulating blood. In newborn infants, lymphocytes, mostly T cells, represent 90% of the total peripheral leukocytes, whereas the adult has an average of 35% lymphocytes in the circulating blood, with a distribution of 60% to 80% T cells and 20% B cells.

Morphological Characteristics of Normal Lymphocytes

The stages of lymphocyte development are the lymphoblast, the prolymphocyte, and the mature lymphocyte. When lymphocytes are stained with Wright stain, their maturational characteristics are generally consistent with those seen in other leukocytes.

Lymphocytes can assume variant morphological features. As many as 5% to 6% of variant lymphocytes can be found in healthy persons; however, an increase in these forms is associated with a variety of disorders. Some of the disorders that can produce an increase in variant lymphocytes are infectious mononucleosis, viral hepatitis, and viral pneumonia.

Functions and Membr ane Characteristics of Lymphocytes

The categories of lymphocytes that are recognized as functionally active are T cells, B cells, and NK cells. T lymphocytes are responsible for cellular immune responses and in either helping or suppressing the activation of B lymphocytes. B lymphocytes serve as the primary source of cells responsible for humoral immune (antibody) responses. NK lymphocytes lack the mature surface markers of T and B cells. These cells destroy target cells through the nonphagocytic process referred to as a cytotoxic reaction.

All cells of the immune system have specialized receptors on their membrane surfaces. Functional testing may be used to evaluate the response of lymphocytes to mitogens.

Plasma Cell Development and Maturation

Plasma cells are not normally found in the circulating blood but can be seen in nonmalignant or malignant disorders. Plasma cells arise from stimulated B lymphocytes. Abnormal forms of the plasma cell include Russell body inclusions, grape cells, and flame cells.

A few plasma cells can be seen in the circulating blood in severe chronic infections or viral disorders. Increased numbers of plasma cells are associated with malignant conditions, such as multiple myeloma.

REVIEW QUESTIONS

Questions 1 through 6: Match the following anatomical structures with the appropriate anatomical category. An answer can be used more than once.

1. _____ Lymph nodes
2. _____ Liver
3. _____ Spleen
4. _____ Red bone marrow
5. _____ Thymus
6. _____ Peyer patches of the intestine
   A. Primary lymphoid tissue
   B. Secondary lymphoid tissue
   C. Not a lymphoid tissue

7. T cells are found in the:
   A. perifollicular areas of the lymph nodes
   B. paracortex regions of the lymph nodes
   C. periarteriolar regions of the spleen
   D. all of the above

8. A major site of B-lymphocyte localization and proliferation is
   A. lymphoid follicles
   B. deep cortical zone
   C. paracortex
   D. all of the above

9. The process of lymphocyte recirculation is important in
   A. antibody production
   B. lymphocyte proliferation
   C. dissemination of antigen-sensitized memory cells
   D. commitment of lymphocytes to T and B cells

10. T lymphocytes constitute _____% of the blood lymphocyte pool in adults.
    A. 0–20
    B. 20–40
    C. 40–60
    D. 60–80

11. Lymphocytes represent approximately _____% of the total circulating leukocytes in adults.
    A. 15
    B. 35
    C. 55
    D. 75

12. The percentage of lymphocytes as compared with the other types of leukocytes in the peripheral blood _____ as humans age.
    A. increases
    B. decreases
    C. remains the same

13. If a patient has a total leukocyte count of 20×10^9/L and a 50% lymphocyte count on the differential count, the absolute lymphocyte value is _____ $\times 10^9$/L.
    A. 1
    B. 5
    C. 10
    D. 15

Questions 14 through 18: Complete the following statements with answers A, B, or C.

(continued)

14. As a lymphocyte matures, the nuclear-cytoplasmic ratio _____.

15. As a lymphocyte matures, the overall size _____.

16. As a lymphocyte matures, the number of nucleoli _____.

17. As a lymphocyte matures, the chromatin clumping _____.

18. As a lymphocyte matures, the quantity of cytoplasm _____.
   A. increases
   B. decreases
   C. remains about the same

19. The most characteristic morphological features of variant lymphocytes include
   A. increased overall size, possibly one to three nucleoli, and abundant cytoplasm
   B. increased overall size, round nucleus, and increased granulation in the cytoplasm
   C. segmented nucleus, light-blue cytoplasm, and no nucleoli
   D. enlarged nucleus, six to eight nucleoli, and dark-blue cytoplasm

Questions 20 through 23: Match the following using an answer only once.

20. _____ Rieder cells
21. _____ Vacuolated lymphocytes
22. _____ Crystalline inclusions
23. _____ Smudge cells
   A. Niemann-Pick disease and Burkitt lymphoma
   B. CLL
   C. Leukosarcoma
   D. Natural artifact

24. T cells are
   A. lymphocytes
   B. monocytes
   C. helper or suppressor types
   D. both A and C

25. B cells are
   A. lymphocytes
   B. associated with antigen recognition
   C. found in the thymus and bone marrow
   D. all of the above

26. NK cells are classified as
   A. macrophages
   B. monocytes
   C. effector lymphocytes
   D. K-type lymphocytes

27. Which of the following statements is (are) true of T cells?
   A. Responsible for humoral responses
   B. Responsible for cellular immune responses
   C. Responsible for chronic rejection in organ transplantation
   D. Both B and C

28. Which of the following statements is (are) true of B cells?
   A. Responsible for antibody responses
   B. Protect against intracellular pathogens
   C. Responsible for chronic rejection in transplantation
   D. Both A and B

29. An abnormal plasma cell with red-staining cytoplasm is a
   A. Russell body
   B. Mott cell
   C. grape cell
   D. flame cell

BIBLIOGRAPHY

Beck JW, Davies JE. *Medical Parasitology*, 2nd ed, St. Louis, MO: Mosby, 1976:58–61.

Caligiuri MA. Human natural killer cells, *Blood* 2008;112(5):,461–469.

Caligiuri MA, Blaser BW. Natural killer cells: development, receptor biology, and their role in cancer immunotherapy, *The Hematologists* 2008;5(1):7.

Giovannetti A, Stifano AG, Pierdominici M. Evaluating T cell homeostasis in the biomedical laboratory, *MedLab Mag*, 2008;(3):26–28.

Henry JB. *Clinical Diagnosis and Management*, 17th ed, Philadelphia, PA: Saunders, 1984:824–827, 1049, 1286, 1290–1291.

Koepke JA, et al. *Reference Leukocyte Differential Count (Proportional) and Evaluation of Instrumental Methods H20-A*, Villanova, PA: NCCLS, 1992.

LeBien TW, Tedder TF. B lymphocytes: how they develop and function, *Blood*, 2008; 112(5):1570–1580.

Sigma Diagnostics, *Monoclonal Antibodies*, St. Louis, MO: 1985.

Reisfeld RA. Memory T cells: death by acquisition, *Blood*, 2007;109(6):2269–2270.

Seif AE, et al. Identifying autoimmune lymphoproliferative syndrome in children with Evans syndrome: a multi-institutional study, *Blood*, 115(11):2142–2145, 2010.

Zhang X, Jianjua Y. Target recognition-induced NK-cell responses, *Blood*, 115(11):2119–2120, 2010.

Zhu J, Paul, WE. CD4 T cells: fates, functions, and faults, *Blood*, 112(5):1557–1569, 2008.

CHAPTER 17

Leukocytes: Nonmalignant Lymphocytic Disorders

Lymphocytosis

- Define the term lymphocytosis.
- Name at least three disorders associated with lymphocytosis.

Disorders associated with lymphocytosis

- Describe the etiology, epidemiology, clinical signs and symptoms, and laboratory data for at least two disorders associated with lymphocytosis.

Lymphocytopenia

- Define the term lymphocytopenia.
- Name at least three disorders associated with lymphocytopenia.

Immune disorders associated with lymphocytopenia

- Describe the etiology, epidemiology, clinical signs and symptoms, and laboratory data for at least two disorders associated with lymphocytosis.

Case studies

- Apply the laboratory data to the stated case studies and discuss the implications of these cases to the study of hematology.

CHARACTERISTICS OF LYMPHOCYTES

The normal range for lymphocytes in an adult is 22% to 40%, with absolute values of 1.2 to 3.4×10^9/L. The following is a sample calculation of the absolute lymphocyte count:

Absolute number = total leukocyte count × relative % of lymphocytes

Total leukocyte count = 25.0×10^9/L
Relative number of lymphocytes = 76%
Absolute number = 19.0×10^9/L

A value less than the normal reference range is called **lymphocytopenia.** When the blood lymphocyte count increases above the upper limit of the reference range, the condition is referred to as **lymphocytosis.**

Disorders of lymphocytes (Table 17.1) are frequently encountered in the clinical laboratory. Many of these nonmalignant disorders result from viral or bacterial infections. Examples of viral diseases include infectious mononucleosis, cytomegalovirus (CMV) infection, and acquired immunodeficiency syndrome (AIDS). Bacterial diseases associated with lymphocytic disorders can include whooping cough. The parasitic infection toxoplasmosis, although rarer than viral and bacterial causes, can also display lymphocytic involvement. In addition, conditions such as drug-induced (immunological) hypersensitivity reactions elicit lymphocytic proliferative reactions that simulate or even surpass the lymphocytosis observed in infectious mononucleosis (Table 17.2).

LYMPHOCYTOSIS

Lymphocytosis is natural and normal in infants and children up to approximately 10 years old, with total lymphocyte counts as high as 9×10^9/L. This increase probably results from the limited production of adrenal corticosteroid hormones during this period of the life cycle. This limited production of hormones may underlie the lymphocytosis seen in later childhood in conditions such as malnutrition and scurvy.

Lymphocytosis is not a common nonspecific response to inflammation as is neutrophilia. In adolescence and adulthood, nonmalignant conditions associated with an absolute lymphocytosis include

1. Acute viral infections (e.g., infectious mononucleosis, infectious hepatitis, posttransfusion syndrome, CMV infection, and infectious lymphocytosis)
2. Some bacterial infections (e.g., *Bordetella pertussis* infection [whooping cough] and brucellosis)
3. Parasitic infections (e.g., toxoplasmosis)
4. Drug reactions (e.g., *p*-aminosalicylic acid hypersensitivity and phenytoin hypersensitivity)
5. Uncommon causes (e.g., tertiary and congenital syphilis and smallpox)

Malignant conditions that produce lymphocytosis (discussed in Chapter 20) include

1. Lymphocytic leukemia (acute and chronic forms)
2. The leukemic phase of lymphomas
3. Waldenström macroglobulinemia
4. Cancer

TABLE 17.1	Examples of Nonmalignant Disorders of Lymphocytes	
Disorder	**Etiology**	**Laboratory Data**
Viral disorders		
Infectious mononucleosis	EBV	Lymphocytosis
		Variant lymphocytes
		Increased titer of heterophil antibodies
Infectious lymphocytosis	Coxsackie group	Lymphocytosis
		Negative for heterophil antibodies
CMV infection	Herpes group—CMV	Slight lymphocytosis
		Variant lymphocytes
		Negative for heterophil antibodies
		Positive for ANA, RA, and CMV nonspecific antibodies
AIDS	HIV	Leukopenia
		Lymphocytopenia
		Abnormality of T-cell subsets
Bacterial disorders		
Whooping cough	*Bordetella pertussis*	Significant lymphocytosis
		Rare lymphoblasts
		All antibodies negative
Parasitic disorders		
Toxoplasmosis	*Toxoplasma gondii*	Variant lymphocytes
		Negative for heterophil antibodies
		Positive for *Toxoplasma* antibodies
Autoimmune disorders		
Systemic lupus erythematosus	Autoimmune	Positive LE cell preparation
		Positive for ANA antibodies
		Lymphocyte subset abnormalities

ANA, antinuclear antibodies; RA, rheumatoid factor antibodies; CMV, cytomegalovirus; AIDS, acquired immunodeficiency syndrome; HIV, human immunodeficiency virus.

DISORDERS ASSOCIATED WITH LYMPHOCYTOSIS

Infectious Mononucleosis

Infectious mononucleosis is usually an acute, benign, and self-limiting lymphoproliferative condition caused by Epstein-Barr virus (EBV). EBV is also the cause of Burkitt lymphoma, a malignant tumor of the lymphoid tissue occurring mainly in African children; nasopharyngeal carcinoma; and neoplasms of the thymus, parotid gland, and supraglottic larynx.

Etiology

EBV was first discovered in 1964 as the cause of infectious mononucleosis. EBV is widely disseminated. It is estimated that 95% of the world's population is exposed to the virus, making it the most ubiquitous virus known.

EBV is a human herpes DNA virus. In infectious mononucleosis, the virus infects B lymphocytes, but the variant lymphocytes produced in response to the virus and seen in microscopic examination of the peripheral blood have T-cell characteristics. One of the habitats of the persisting viral genome in hosts with a latent infection is the B lymphocyte of the lymphoreticular system and the epithelial cell of the oropharynx (Fig. 17.1).

TABLE 17.2	Causes of Lymphocytosis	
Lymphocytosis Associated with Atypical Lymphocytes		
% of White Cells That Are Atypical Lymphocytes		
>20%	**<20%**	**Lymphocytosis Associated with Small Mature Lymphocytes**
Infectious mononucleosis Infectious hepatitis Posttransfusion syndrome CMV infection p-Aminosalicylic acid (PAS) Phenytoin (Dilantin) and mephenytoin (Mesantoin) hypersensitivity	Mumps,[a] varicella,[a] rubeola, rubella, atypical pneumonia, herpes simplex, herpes zoster, roseola infantum, influenza,[a] other viral illnesses, tuberculosis,[a] rickettsialpox, brucellosis,[a] toxoplasmosis[a] Radiation	Infectious lymphocytosis Pertussis
	Agranulocytosis	
	Lead intoxication	
	Stress	
	Leukemias and lymphomas[a]	

[a]Higher counts of atypical lymphocytes are occasionally found.

Epidemiology

Although EBV appears to be transmitted primarily by close contact with infectious oropharyngeal secretions, the virus has been reported to be transmitted by blood transfusion and transplacental routes. Under ordinary conditions, transmission of EBV through transfusion or transplacental exposure is unlikely.

The frequency of **seronegativity** is nearly 100% in early infancy and declines with increasing age, more or less rapidly depending on socioeconomic conditions, to less than 10% in young adults. After primary exposure, a person is considered to be immune and generally no longer susceptible to overt reinfection. In Western society, primary exposure to EBV occurs in two waves. Approximately half the population is exposed to the virus before the age of 5 years; a second wave of seroconversion occurs during late adolescence (15 to 24 years old). Approximately 90% of adult patients demonstrate antibodies to the virus.

Individuals at risk include those who lack antibodies to the virus. EBV is only a minor problem for immunocompetent persons, but it can become a major problem for immunologically compromised patients. In immunosuppressed patients, the incidence of EBV infection ranges from 35% to 47%. Blood transfusion from an immune donor to a nonimmune recipient may produce a primary infection in the recipient known as infectious mononucleosis postperfusion syndrome. Infectious mononucleosis or infectious mononucleosis-like illness following blood transfusion may often be caused by a concomitant CMV infection rather than EBV.

A low percentage of patients experience symptomatic reactivation. Reactivation of latent infection has been implicated in a persistent illness referred to as the EBV-associated fatigue syndrome, but this phenomenon is not universally accepted.

In adolescents, clinically apparent infectious mononucleosis has an estimated frequency of 45/100,000 (Fig. 17.2). In immunosuppressed patients, the incidence of EBV infection ranges from 35% to 47%. As occurs with other herpesviruses, there is a carrier state after primary infection.

Clinical Signs and Symptoms

The majority of individuals seroconvert without any signs and symptoms of disease. In children younger than 5 years of age, infection is either asymptomatic or frequently characterized by mild, poorly defined signs and symptoms. Although anyone can suffer from this viral disorder, it is typically manifested in young adults.

The incubation period of infectious mononucleosis is from 10 to 50 days; once the disease is fully developed, it lasts for 1 to 4 weeks. Clinical manifestations include extreme fatigue, malaise, sore throat, fever, and cervical lymphadenopathy. Splenomegaly occurs in about 50% of patients, although the incidence of splenic rupture is low. When rupture occurs, however, mortality is significant. Jaundice is infrequent, although the most common complication is hepatitis. A smaller percentage of patients develop hepatomegaly or splenomegaly and hepatomegaly. Because abnormal liver function is more significant in EBV-induced

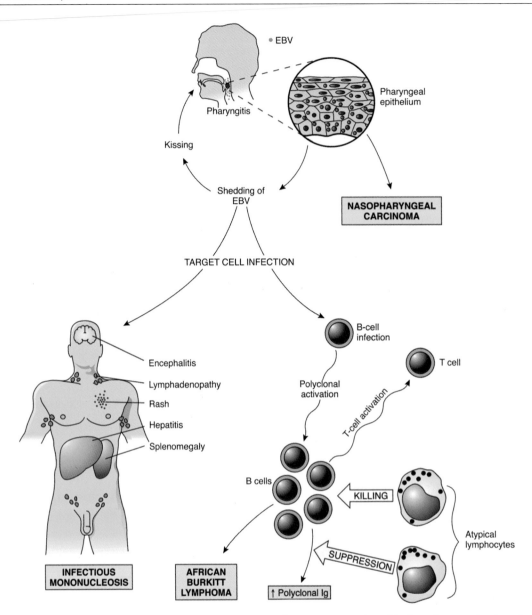

FIGURE 17.1 Role of EBV in infectious mononucleosis, nasopharyngeal carcinoma, and Burkitt lymphoma. EBV invades and replicates within the salivary glands or pharyngeal epithelium and is shed into the saliva and respiratory secretions. In some people, the virus transforms pharyngeal epithelial cells, leading to nasopharyngeal carcinoma. In people who are not immune from childhood exposure, EBV causes infectious mononucleosis. EBV infects B lymphocytes, which undergo polyclonal activation. These B cells stimulate the production of atypical lymphocytes, which kill virally infected B cells and suppress the production of immunoglobulins. Some infected B cells are transformed into immature malignant lymphocytes of Burkitt lymphoma. (Reprinted with permission from Rubin E, Farber JL. *Pathology*, 3rd ed, Philadelphia, PA: Lippincott Williams & Wilkins, 1999.)

infectious mononucleosis than in CMV-associated mononucleosis, EBV must be considered in the differential diagnosis of hepatitis. A significant number of patients with infectious mononucleosis do not manifest classic signs and symptoms.

Laboratory Data

Laboratory testing is necessary to establish or confirm a diagnosis of infectious mononucleosis. Hematological studies reveal leukocyte counts ranging from 10 to 20 × 10^9/L in approximately two thirds of patients; about 10% of the patients with this disorder demonstrate **leukopenia.** A differential leukocyte count may initially disclose

neutrophilia, although mononuclear cells usually predominate as the disorder develops. Typical relative lymphocyte counts range from 60% to 90%, with 5% to 30% variant lymphocytes. These variant lymphocytes (Fig. 17.3) exhibit diverse morphological features and persist for 1 to 2 months in some patients and as long as 4 to 6 months in others. In the past, the now obsolete Downey Classification (Table 17.3) was used to describe variant lymphocytes.

If the classic signs and symptoms of infectious mononucleosis are absent, a diagnosis of infectious mononucleosis is more difficult to make. The diagnosis may be established by antibody testing. The antibodies present in patients with

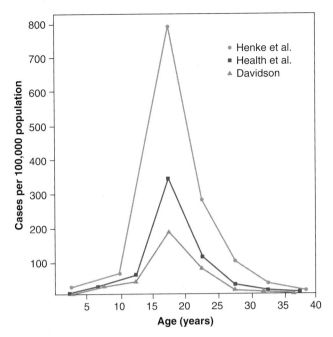

FIGURE 17.2 Incidence by age of infectious mononucleosis in three large studies.

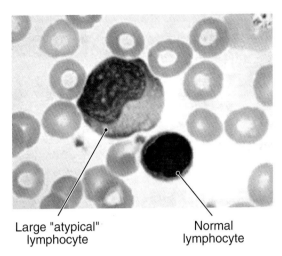

FIGURE 17.3 The blood in infectious mononucleosis. The large "atypical" lymphocyte is characteristic. (Reprinted with permission from McConnell TH. *The Nature of Disease Pathology for the Health Professions*, Philadelphia, PA: Lippincott Williams & Wilkins, 2007.)

infectious mononucleosis are heterophil and EBV antibodies. Heterophil antibodies comprise a broad class of antibody. They are defined as antibodies that are stimulated by one antigen and react with an entirely unrelated surface antigen present on cells from different mammalian species. Heterophil antibodies may be present in normal individuals in low concentrations (titers), but a titer of 1:56 or greater is clinically significant in patients suspected to have infectious mononucleosis. Rapid slide tests (see Chapter 26) that use the principle of agglutination of horse erythrocytes are available. The use of horse erythrocytes appears to increase the sensitivity of the test.

Within the adult population, 10% to 20% of individuals with acute infectious mononucleosis do not produce the associated heterophil antibody. The pediatric population is of particular concern because more than 50% of children younger than 4 years of age with infectious mononucleosis are heterophil negative.

TABLE 17.3	Descriptive Features of the Classic Downey Classification of Lymphocytes Seen in Infectious Mononucleosis
Type I	
Nucleus	May be irregularly shaped
Cytoplasm	Usually many cytoplasmic vacuoles Dark blue (basophilic)
Type II	
Nucleus	Chromatin is coarse and clumped
Cytoplasm	Increased amount Dark blue (basophilic) around the periphery or in a radial pattern A few cytoplasmic vacuoles
Type III[a]	
Nucleus	Nucleoli usually visible Enlarged in size
Cytoplasm	Dark blue (basophilic)

[a]This cell resembles an immature lymphocyte.

TABLE 17.4	Characteristic Antibody Formation in Infectious Mononucleosis					
	VCA IgM	VCA IgG	EA-D	EA-R	EBNA IgG	Heterophil
No previous exposure	−	−	−	−	−	−
Recent (acute) infection	+	+	±	−	−	+
Past infection (convalescent) period	−	+	−	−	+	−
Reactivation of latent infection	±	+	+	±	+	±

VCA, viral capsid antigen; EA-D, early antigen (diffuse); EA-R, early antigen (restricted); EBNA, Epstein-Barr nuclear antigen; IgG, immunoglobulin G.

For patients with diagnostically inconclusive infectious mononucleosis, a more definitive assessment of immune status may be obtained through an EBV serological panel. Candidates for EBV serology include those who do not exhibit the classic symptoms, those who are heterophil negative, and those who are immunosuppressed.

EBV-infected B lymphocytes express a variety of new antigens encoded by the virus (Fig. 17.4). Infection with EBV results in the expression of viral capsid antigen (VCA), early antigen (EA), and nuclear antigen (NA), with corresponding antibody responses. Assays for immunoglobulin M (IgM) and G (IgG) antibodies to these EBV antigens are available. EBV-specific serological studies (Table 17.4) are beneficial in defining immune status, and the time of antibody appearance may be indicative of the stage of disease (Fig. 17.1). This can provide important information for both the diagnosis and the management of EBV-associated disease.

Anti-i can be a clinically significant antibody in infectious mononucleosis. This antibody can be the cause of hemolytic anemia.

Cytomegalovirus Infection

Etiology

The first descriptive report of histological changes characteristic of the changes now associated with CMV infection was originally published in 1904. In 1956 and 1957, CMV was isolated in the laboratory. In 1966, actual isolation of the virus following a blood transfusion was noted.

Human CMV is classified as a member of the herpes family of viruses. There are currently five recognized human herpesviruses: herpes simplex I, herpes simplex II, varicella-zoster virus, EBV, and CMV. All the herpesviruses are relatively large, enveloped DNA viruses that undergo a replicative cycle involving DNA expression and nucleocapsid assembly within the nucleus. The viral structure gains an envelope when the virus buds through the nuclear membrane that is altered to contain specific viral proteins.

Although the herpes family produces diverse clinical diseases, the viruses share the basic characteristic of being cell associated. The requirements for cell association vary, but all five viruses may spread from cell to cell, presumably via intercellular bridges, and in the presence of antibody in the extracellular phase. This common characteristic may play a role in the ability of the virus to produce subclinical infections that can be reactivated under appropriate stimuli.

Epidemiology

CMV is a ubiquitous human viral pathogen and is endemic worldwide. Dissemination of the virus can occur by oral, respiratory, and venereal routes. It can also be transmitted parenterally by organ transplantation or via the transfusion

FIGURE 17.4 Antibody response to acute infection with EBV. VCA, virus capsid antigen; HA, heterophil antibody; EA, early antigen; EBNA, EBV nuclear antigen. (Source: Henle W, Henle G. Seroepidemiology of the virus. In: *Epstein M, Achong B* (eds.). The *Epstein-Barr virus*. Berlin: Springer-Verlag, 1979:61–78; and Tomkinson B, Sullivan J. Epstein-Barr virus infection and mononucleosis. In: Gorbach S, Bartlett J, Blacklow N (eds.). *Infectious Diseases*, Philadelphia, PA: WB Saunders, 1991:1348–1356.)

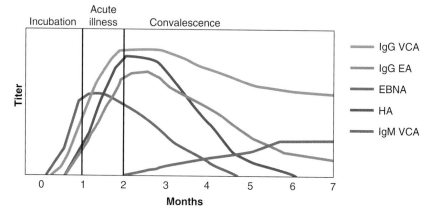

of fresh blood. Transmission of CMV appears to require close intimate contact with secretions or excretions (primarily urine, respiratory secretions, tears, feces, and genital secretions) of infected persons. The most likely mode of acquisition is via a venereal route through contact with infectious virus in body secretions.

The virus can be present in blood, urine, and breast milk. For more than 15 years, it has been recognized that transfusion of blood from healthy asymptomatic blood donors is occasionally followed by active CMV infection in the recipient. There is strong evidence to incriminate peripheral blood leukocytes and transplanted tissues as sources of CMV.

Although fatal infections have been reported in children with leukemia and premature infants with a birth weight less than 1,200 g, the incidence of primary infections during childhood is low. The rate of exposure to the virus, however, may be accelerated during the first years of life in toddlers and children in day care centers. During adolescence, the infection rate rises significantly. By adulthood, most individuals have experienced asymptomatic contact with CMV. Because CMV can persist latently, active infections may develop under a variety of conditions, such as pregnancy, immunosuppression, and subsequent to organ or bone marrow transplantation. Active CMV infection is a major cause of morbidity and often mortality in patients with AIDS.

CMV can exist as a latent infection and is characterized by periods of reactivation. In addition, CMV is one of the most important causes of congenital viral infections in the United States. Primary and recurrent maternal CMV infection can be transmitted in utero.

Healthcare professionals are one of the groups becoming increasingly concerned about the risks associated with exposure to CMV. Nosocomial transmission from patients to healthcare workers has not been documented, but observance of good personal hygiene and handwashing offer the best measures for preventing transmission.

Clinical Signs and Symptoms

Acquired CMV infection is usually asymptomatic and can persist in the host as a chronic or latent infection. In the majority of patients, CMV infection is asymptomatic. Occasionally, a self-limited, heterophil-negative, mononucleosis-like syndrome results. The symptoms include a sore throat and fever, chills, profound malaise, and myalgia. Lymphadenopathy and splenomegaly may be observed. Infections occurring in healthy immunocompetent individuals usually result in seroconversion. Virus may be excreted in the urine during both primary and recurrent CMV infection; it can persist sporadically for months or years.

Persons experiencing acquired infection, reinfection with the same or different strains of CMV, or reactivation of a latent infection can excrete the virus in titers as high as 10^6 infective units per mL in the urine and/or saliva for weeks or months.

Healthy adults and children usually experience CMV infection without serious complications. Infrequent complications of CMV infection in previously healthy individuals,

however, include interstitial pneumonitis, hepatitis, Guillain-Barré syndrome, meningoencephalitis, myocarditis, thrombocytopenia, and hemolytic anemia.

CMV infection, however, can be life threatening in immunosuppressed patients. Infections in these patients may result in disseminated multisystem involvement including pneumonitis, hepatitis, gastrointestinal ulceration, arthralgias, meningoencephalitis, and retinitis. Interstitial pneumonitis, frequently associated with CMV infection, is a major cause of death following allogeneic bone marrow transplantation. In premature infants, acquired CMV infection can result in atypical lymphocytosis, hepatosplenomegaly, pneumonia, or death.

Transfusion-acquired CMV infections may cause not only mononucleosis-like syndrome but also hepatitis and an increased risk of rejection of transplanted organs.

The classic congenital CMV syndrome is manifested by a high incidence of neurological symptoms as well as neuromuscular disorders, jaundice, hepatomegaly, and splenomegaly. Congenitally infected newborns, especially those who acquire CMV during a maternal primary infection, are more prone to develop severe cytomegalic inclusion disease (CID).

Laboratory Data

In patients with CMV infection, hematological examination of the blood usually reveals a characteristic leukocytosis. A slight lymphocytosis with more than 20% variant lymphocytes is common. Clinical chemistry assays may demonstrate abnormal liver function. Another assessment of the presence of infection is the demonstration of inclusion bodies in leukocytes in urinary sediment.

The incidence of viral exposure and subsequent antibody formation (seropositivity) varies greatly, depending on the socioeconomic status and living conditions of the population surveyed. The prevalence of CMV antibody varies with age and geographical location but ranges from 40% to 100%.

A definitive diagnosis, however, can only be made by isolating the virus from urine or blood samples or by demonstrating CMV-specific IgM or increasing CMV-specific IgG antibody titers. Serological methods to detect the presence of IgM antibodies can aid in the diagnosis of primary infection. Detection of CMV-specific IgM can represent primary infection or rare reactivation of infection. False-positive results, however, can occur because of the presence of other antibodies such as rheumatoid factor. Although results of tests for heterophil, EBV, and *Toxoplasma* antibodies are generally negative, elevated concentrations (titers) of several antibodies may occur. These include antinuclear antibody (ANA), rheumatoid factor antibody (RA), and nonspecific cold agglutinins.

Toxoplasmosis

Etiology

The microorganism *Toxoplasma gondii* causes toxoplasmosis. *Toxoplasma* was recently recognized as a tissue Coccidia.

Epidemiology

Toxoplasmosis is a widespread disease that occurs in humans and animals. *T. gondii* was first discovered in a North African rodent and has been observed in numerous birds and mammals around the world, including humans. It is a parasite of cosmopolitan distribution that is able to develop in a wide variety of vertebrate hosts. Human infections are common in many parts of the world. The incidence rates vary from place to place, for unknown reasons. The highest recorded rate (93%) was found in Parisian women who prefer undercooked or raw meat, and there is a 50% rate of occurrence in their children.

The definitive host is the house cat and certain other *Felidae*. Domestic cats as a source of the disease produce oocysts that are present in their feces. Accidental ingestion of oocysts by humans and animals, including the cat, produces a proliferative infection in the body tissues. Feces-contaminated food, water, and hands; inadequately cooked infected meat; and raw milk can be important sources of human infection.

The hazard of transfusion-transmitted toxoplasmosis has been recently recognized in connection with the transfusion of leukocyte concentrates. Patients at risk are those who are receiving immunosuppressive agents or corticosteroids.

All mammals, including humans, can transmit the infection transplacentally. Transplacental transmission usually takes place in the course of an acute but inapparent or undiagnosed maternal infection. New evidence indicates that the number of infants born in the United States each year with congenital *T. gondii* infection is considerably higher than the 3,000 previously estimated. It is estimated that 6 of every 1,000 pregnant women in the United States will acquire primary infection with *Toxoplasma* during a 9-month gestation. Approximately 45% of women who acquire the infection for the first time and who are not treated will give birth to congenitally infected infants. Consequently, the expected incidence of congenital toxoplasmosis is 2.7/1,000 live births.

Clinical Signs and Symptoms

In adults and children other than newborn babies, the disease is usually asymptomatic. A generalized infection probably occurs. Although spontaneous recovery follows acute febrile disease, the organism can localize and multiply in any organ of the body or the circulatory system.

In acquired infection, symptoms are frequently mild if they are observable at all. The disease may resemble infectious mononucleosis, with chills, fever, headache, lymphadenopathy, and extreme fatigue. A chronic form of toxoplasmic lymphadenopathy has been described. *T. gondii* presents a special problem in immunosuppressed or otherwise compromised hosts, who can develop reactivation of a latent toxoplasmosis. This has been observed in patients with either Hodgkin or non-Hodgkin lymphomas as well as in recipients of organ transplants. Reactivation of cerebral toxoplasmosis is not uncommon in patients with AIDS. Primary infection may be promoted by immunosuppression.

Congenital toxoplasmosis infection can result in central nervous system malformation or prenatal mortality. Many infants who are serologically positive at birth fail to display neurological, ophthalmic, or generalized illness at birth. In as many as 75% of the congenitally infected newborns who are not serologically diagnosed at birth, the disease remains dormant, only to be discovered when other symptoms such as chorioretinitis, unilateral blindness, and severe neurological sequelae become apparent.

Laboratory Data

Both clinical and laboratory findings in this disease resemble infectious mononucleosis. An increased number of variant lymphocytes can be seen on a peripheral blood smear. The diagnosis is established by serologically demonstrating significant elevations of *Toxoplasma* antibodies. Antibodies are demonstrable within the first 2 weeks after infection, rise to high levels early in the infection, and fall slightly but persist at an elevated level for many months before declining to low levels after many years.

Because *T. gondii* is difficult to culture, diagnosis must be supported by serological methods. Diagnosis can be established by biopsy, necropsy, or intraperitoneal inoculation into mice.

Infectious Lymphocytosis

Acute infectious lymphocytosis is a poorly defined benign condition.

Etiology

Infectious lymphocytosis is caused by a virus, probably a member of the Coxsackie group.

Epidemiology

Infectious lymphocytosis is usually a mild disorder occurring in epidemics. Children are the most common victims. A chronic form of infectious lymphocytosis has also been observed in children.

Clinical Signs and Symptoms

An incubation period of 10 to 21 days is typical. Symptoms can include vomiting, fever, abdominal discomfort, central nervous system involvement, rashes, upper respiratory distress, and diarrhea. Some patients may be asymptomatic or have symptoms that mimic infectious mononucleosis. The spleen and liver are rarely enlarged. Lymphadenopathy is also rare or minimal, if present.

Children with the chronic form of infectious lymphocytosis usually have a history of recurrent upper respiratory tract infections. In addition, enlargement of the tonsils, lymph nodes, and spleen is usually manifested.

Laboratory Data

Leukocytosis with lymphocytosis characterizes this disease. It may precede clinical manifestations of the disease with leukocyte counts of 20 to 50×10^9/L. Differential peripheral blood counts reveal up to 95% small, mature, normal-appearing lymphocytes. These lymphocytes are probably of T-cell origin. No lymphoblasts are present. An increase in eosinophils may be noted. Results of heterophil and EBV antibody tests are negative.

The illness and leukocytosis usually subside within 3 to 5 weeks. A moderate lymphocytosis, however, may persist for as long as 3 months.

In children with the chronic form of infectious lymphocytosis, the leukocyte count ranges from 10 to 25 × 10⁹/L, with a predominance of normal-appearing lymphocytes. Other leukocytic alterations are minimal.

Bordetella Pertussis (Haemophilus Pertussis) Infection

Etiology

Whooping cough is caused by *B. pertussis*, a bacterial organism that produces inflammation of the entire respiratory tract.

Epidemiology

This illness occurs primarily in unimmunized children.

Clinical Signs and Symptoms

Following an incubation period of 2 weeks, symptoms become evident. Characteristically, symptoms include a cough and cold accompanied by pain in the neck and chest. A sputum-producing cough with pain over the trachea and bronchi characteristically emerges.

Laboratory Data

The total leukocyte count can be increased to as high as 100×10^9/L, with an absolute lymphocyte value of as high as 50×10^9/L. The absolute lymphocyte value is usually 15 to 40×10^9/L. These leukocyte and lymphocyte values are major laboratory findings and may be present if the characteristic cough has not yet developed or is mild enough to be missed during physical examination.

Lymphocytosis is most evident during the first 3 weeks of illness and then decreases. Lymphocytosis is caused by the release of lymphocytosis-promoting factor (LPF) from *B. pertussis*. This factor causes an increased mobilization of lymphocytes from lymphoid organs, followed by inhibition of recirculation of lymphocytes from blood into the lymph flow.

On a peripheral blood smear, the lymphocytes are small and mature, with only a rare occurrence of lymphoblasts. A definitive diagnosis can be made on isolation of the bacteria.

LYMPHOCYTOPENIA

Lymphocytopenia is generally defined as less than 3.0×10^9/L lymphocytes in adults or less than 1.5×10^9/L lymphocytes in children. A decrease in lymphocytes is a common response to stress and to the administration of corticosteroids, or it may be seen in healthy persons with no apparent cause. Transient relative lymphocytopenia is generally associated with conditions resulting in granulocytosis. Pathological conditions that exhibit absolute lymphocytopenia are related to decreased production, mechanical loss, increased destruction, and various functional abnormalities. These conditions may be caused by immune deficiency disorders, physical agents (e.g., radiation exposure), or cytotoxic drugs.

IMMUNE DISORDERS ASSOCIATED WITH LYMPHOCYTOPENIA

Immune disorders may be caused by defects in the numbers or functional properties of lymphocytes and may be congenital or acquired. These conditions are usually classified as either T-cell or B-cell disorders. Some of the less common disorders involve both T and B cells.

DiGeorge Syndrome

A number of T- and B-cell defects involve the alteration of some lymphocyte subpopulations. Patients with **DiGeorge syndrome** exhibit a decrease in total T lymphocytes coupled with an increased ratio of helper to suppressor cells. In AIDS, a reversed phenotypic helper-to-suppressor ratio due to a decrease in helper cells is observed. A decrease in total T cells and a lack of, or reduced, suppressor cell population are among the immunological changes observed in active systemic lupus erythematosus (SLE).

Acquired Immunodeficiency Syndrome (HIV/AIDS)

The human immunodeficiency virus (HIV) (Fig. 17.5) is the predominant virus responsible for AIDS. Although

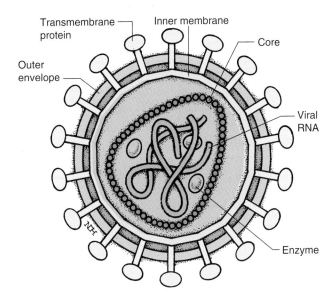

FIGURE 17.5 HIV virus. (Reprinted with permission from *Stedman's Medical Dictionary*, 28th ed. Baltimore, MA: Lippincott Williams & Wilkins, 2006.)

HIV was recently recognized, it is tentatively concluded that HIV-1 has infected humans for more than 20 but less than 100 years.

Etiology

At the beginning of the 1980s, no infectious retroviruses had been found in humans, and many believed that no human retroviruses would be found. Despite this skepticism, however, the first human retrovirus, human T lymphotrophic virus type I (HTLV-I), was isolated in 1980 and HTLV-II was isolated in 1982.

In 1983, researchers at the Pasteur Institute in Paris isolated a retrovirus from a homosexual man with lymphadenopathy. The virus was named the lymphadenopathy-associated virus, but the researchers were unable to prove that this agent caused AIDS. The American research team headed by Dr. Robert Gallo also isolated the same class of virus, which they labeled HTLV-III. In 1984, the Gallo team was able to demonstrate conclusively through virological and epidemiological evidence that it was the cause of AIDS. When it was demonstrated that LAV and HTLV-III were the same virus, an international commission changed the name of the virus to HIV, to eliminate confusion caused by two names for the same entity and to acknowledge that the virus does cause AIDS.

In addition to the original HIV-1, a second AIDS-causing virus, HIV type 2 (HIV-2), was identified in 1985. In evolutionary terms, the two viruses are related and have a similar overall structure. The pathogenic potential of HIV-2, however, is not as well established as that of HIV-1.

HIV has a significant preference for the helper/inducer subset of T lymphocytes. These cells, however, are not the only cells that have CD4 antigen embedded in their membrane. Macrophages, as many as 40% of the peripheral blood monocytes, and cells in the lymph nodes, skin, and other organs also express measurable amounts of CD4 and can be infected by HIV. In addition, approximately 5% of the B lymphocytes may express CD4 and be susceptible to HIV infection.

Although some cells do not produce detectable amounts of CD4, they do contain low levels of messenger RNA encoding the CD4 protein, which indicates that they do produce some CD4. These cell types include certain cells of the brain, **glial cells**, a variety of malignant brain tumor cells, and some cells derived from cancers of the bowel. In addition, cells of the gastrointestinal system do not produce appreciable amounts of CD4, but gut cells, called **chromaffin cells**, do sometimes appear to be infected by HIV in vivo. This suggests that gastrointestinal infection may be what leads to the AIDS-associated weight loss and emaciation known in Africa as slim disease.

Epidemiology

AIDS has become a major cause of morbidity and mortality worldwide. The number of people living with HIV infection continues to increase steadily. According to the World Health Organization, United Nations Children's Fund, UNAIDS

(2009), the number of people living with HIV worldwide continued to grow in 2008, reaching an estimated 33.4 million (31.1 to 35.8 million). The total number of people living with the virus in 2008 was roughly threefold higher than in 1990. The latest epidemiological data indicate that globally the spread of HIV appears to have peaked in 1996, when 3.5 million (3.2 to 3.8 million) new HIV infections occurred. In 2008, the estimated number of new HIV infections was approximately 30% lower than at the epidemic's peak 12 years earlier. The epidemic appears to have stabilized in most regions, although prevalence continues to increase in Eastern Europe and Central Asia and in other parts of Asia due to a high rate of new HIV infections. Sub-Saharan Africa remains the most heavily affected region, accounting for 71% of all new HIV infections in 2008.

The latest data reported by the Centers for Disease Control (CDC) indicate that more than 25 years into the AIDS epidemic, HIV infection continues to exact a tremendous toll in the United States. Recent data indicate that African Americans and gay and bisexual men of all races continue to be most severely affected. The largest population living with HIV (45%) comprises men who have sex with men (MSM), followed by persons infected through high-risk heterosexual contact (27%), those infected through injection drug use (22%), and those who were exposed through both male-to-male sexual contact and injection drug use (5%).

HIV transmission from mother to child during pregnancy, labor and delivery, or breast-feeding is called perinatal transmission. Research published in 1994 showed that zidovudine (ZDV) given to pregnant women infected with HIV and their newborns reduced the risk for this type of HIV transmission. Since then, the testing of pregnant women and treatment for those who are infected have resulted in a dramatic decline in the number of children perinatally infected with HIV. However, much work remains to be done: about 100 to 200 infants in the United States are infected with HIV annually. Many of these infections involve women who were not tested early enough in pregnancy or who did not receive prevention services.

Perinatal HIV transmission is the most common route of HIV infection in children and is now the source of almost all AIDS cases in children in the United States. Most of the children with AIDS are members of minority races/ethnicities.

Clinical Signs and Symptoms

Early Stages

The early phase of the natural history of HIV-1 infection may last from many months to many years after the initiation of infection (Fig. 17.6). Typically, patients in the early stages of HIV-1 infection either are completely asymptomatic or show mild, chronic lymphadenopathy.

An unknown number of infected patients experience a brief, infectious mononucleosis-like or flu-like illness with fever, malaise, and possibly a skin rash. Neurological complaints may also be reported. These symptoms parallel the first wave of HIV replications and develop at about the time antibodies produced by the body against HIV-1 can first be

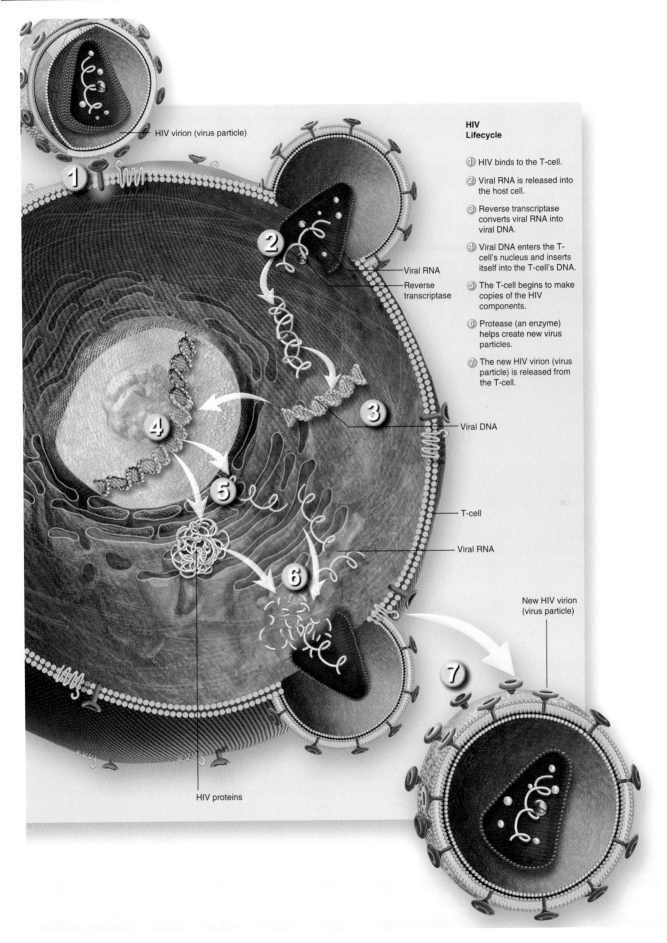

HIV virion (virus particle)

**HIV
Lifecycle**

1 HIV binds to the T-cell.

2 Viral RNA is released into the host cell.

3 Reverse transcriptase converts viral RNA into viral DNA.

4 Viral DNA enters the T-cell's nucleus and inserts itself into the T-cell's DNA.

5 The T-cell begins to make copies of the HIV components.

6 Protease (an enzyme) helps create new virus particles.

7 The new HIV virion (virus particle) is released from the T-cell.

Viral RNA

Reverse transcriptase

Viral DNA

T-cell

Viral RNA

New HIV virion (virus particle)

HIV proteins

FIGURE 17.6 HIV life cycle.

detected. This is usually between 2 weeks and 3 months after acquiring the infection, rarely later.

Following the early phase of HIV infection and any clinically manifested signs and symptoms, a person may remain symptom-free for years.

Late Phase

Untreated HIV causes a predictable, progressive derangement of immune function, and AIDS is just one late manifestation of that process. From 2 to 10 years after acquiring HIV-1 infection, replication of the virus flares again and the infection enters its final stage. An average of 8 or 9 years may pass before AIDS is fully developed. The virus behaves differently, depending on the kind of host cell and the cell's own level of mitotic activity. In T cells, however, the virus can lie dormant indefinitely but it can destroy the host cell in a burst of replication. HIV grows continuously but slowly in macrophages/monocytes. This saves the cell from destruction but probably alters its function.

Clinical symptoms of the later phase of HIV-1 infection include extreme weight loss, fever, and multiple secondary infections. The end stage of fulminant AIDS is characterized by the occurrence of neoplasms and opportunistic infections. Lethal *Pneumocystis carinii* pneumonia is a hallmark of AIDS. Other opportunistic infections, for example, CMV, however, are frequent and may exist concurrently. Cryptosporidiosis and *Histoplasma capsulatum* infection are being recognized with increasing frequency. The most frequent malignancy observed is an aggressive, invasive variant of **Kaposi sarcoma**, discovered in many patients at autopsy. Malignant B-cell lymphomas are also being more commonly recognized in patients with HIV/AIDS or at high risk for HIV/AIDS. Because certain lymphomas can develop quite early, it is hypothesized that B-cell hyperactivity plays a role in their development. Lymphomas and other cancers that appear late in HIV-1 disease could also stem from the failure of the compromised immune system to recognize and destroy cancer cells.

Disease Progression

Although a large enough dose of the right strain of HIV can cause AIDS on its own, cofactors can influence the progression of untreated disease. One is debilitation; for example, patients weakened by a medical condition existing before HIV infection occurred may progress toward AIDS more quickly than others. Stimulation of the immune system in response to later infections may also hasten disease progression. Other pathogenic microorganisms such as a herpesvirus, called human B-cell lymphotropic virus (HBLV) or human herpesvirus 6 (HHV-6), can interact with HIV-1 in a way that may increase the severity of HIV infection.

Laboratory Data

Laboratory evaluation of HIV-1–infected patients consists of an assessment of cellular and humoral components. Screening of blood donors and patients at risk is usually by serological methods. In patients who have developed the signs and symptoms of AIDS, assessment of the number of lymphocytes and their function becomes important.

Both leukopenia and lymphocytopenia exist in AIDS patients. The number of circulating lymphocytes is severely decreased. The common denominator of the disease is a deficiency of a specific subset of thymus-derived (CD4+) lymphocytes. This abnormality (reversal of the ratio of helper-to-suppressor lymphocytes [i.e., CD4+:CD8+ cells]) has become synonymous with AIDS. Normally, this ratio is 2:1 in heterosexuals and 1.5:1 in homosexuals. In patients with AIDS, it is less than 0.5:1. T-lymphocyte subset distribution is altered, with a decrease in the helper/inducer T cells and increase in suppressor/cytotoxic T cells. The absolute decrease in CD4+ cells, however, does not result from an absolute increase in CD8+ cells. This abnormality exists in the lymph nodes and in circulating T lymphocytes. Although characteristic, a diminished T4:T8 ratio is not diagnostic of HIV/AIDS because it can be observed in patients with other types of acute viral infections. In non-AIDS patients, the lymphocyte ratio reverts to normal after recovery from the viral infection.

The progressive decline of CD4+ cells leads to a general decline in immune function. It is the primary underlying factor in determining the clinical progression of AIDS. The main host of HHV-6 is the B cell but this virus can also infect CD4+ cells. If these lymphocytes are simultaneously infected by HIV-1, HHV-6 can stimulate the virus, which further impairs the immune system and promotes disease progression.

Total leukocyte and absolute lymphocyte concentrations need to be assessed periodically. Enumeration of lymphocyte subsets is usually performed by flow-cell cytometry (see Chapter 27). A decreased lymphocyte proliferative response to soluble antigens and mitogens, such as a diminished response to pokeweed mitogen (PWM), exists in this disorder.

Serological Markers

Detection of Viral Antigen

Following initial infection, the body mounts a vigorous immune response against viremia. Immunological activities include the production of different types of antibodies against HIV. Some antibodies neutralize it, others prevent it from binding to cells, and others stimulate cytotoxic cells to attack HIV-infected cells.

The time and sequence of the appearance and disappearance of antibodies specific for the serologically important antigen of HIV-1 during the course of infection are variable. A window of seronegativity exists from the time of initial infection until 6 or 12 weeks or longer thereafter. With enzyme immunoassay methods based on defined HIV-1 proteins produced by recombinant DNA methods, antibodies specific for glycoprotein (gp) 41 are detectable for weeks or months before assays specific for protein (p) 24 can detect antibodies. The appearance of antibodies specific for p24, however, has been shown in several studies to precede that of anti-gp41 when serum specimens are tested by Western blot analysis. This discrepancy in the sequence of antibody appearance is believed to be owing to the greater sensitivity of the Western blot technique compared to viral lysate-based enzyme immunoassays used for the detection of anti-p24. Antibodies to gp41 persist throughout the course of infection. Antibodies specific for p24 not only rise to detectable levels after gp41 is detectable but also can disappear unpredictably and abruptly in a short period.

Increased production of core antigen is believed to be associated with a burst of viral replication and host cell lysis. The disappearance of antibody directed against p24 has been demonstrated to occur concomitantly with an increase in the concentration of core antigen in the serum. This parallel activity may be caused by the sequestration of antibody in immune complexes, and the sudden decrease in anti-p24 is considered to be a grave prognostic sign in HIV-1–infected patients.

Antibodies to HIV-1

Antibodies to HIV-1 appear after a lag period of approximately 6 weeks between the time of infection and a detectable antibody response. Because of this, some virus-positive, antibody-negative individuals are undetected during initial screening assays.

In addition to positive test results for HIV antibody in 85% to 90% of patients, increased antibody titers to viruses such as CMV, EBV, hepatitis A and B, and *T. gondii* as well as circulating immune (antigen-antibody) complexes can be found. Currently, blood samples from donors that are initially reactive in HIV antibody testing are rechecked in duplicate to rule out technical errors. If on repeat testing, the result on one or more of the duplicate tests is positive, the specimen is considered repeatedly reactive. If the specimen is from a unit of blood, it is not used for transfusion. To rule out false-positive results, it is necessary to confirm repeatedly reactive test results by an alternate protocol.

Other Immune Changes

A variety of other immune changes occur. These ancillary findings include polyclonal hypergammaglobulinemia and elevated levels of interferon α, α-1 thymosin, and β-microglobulin. Reduced levels of interleukin-1 or interleukin-2 have also been noted.

Systemic Lupus Erythematosus

Etiology, Signs, and Symptoms

SLE is a classic model of autoimmune disease that can affect practically every organ of the body. SLE is a systematic rheumatic disorder, a name commonly used for the disorders of the joints, connective tissues, and collagen-vascular disorders. SLE occurs primarily in adolescent and young adult females and may be present for years before a diagnosis is made. This disorder is eight times more common in female than in male patients.

Clinical symptoms include fever, weight loss, malaise, arthralgia (joint pain), arthritis (inflammation of the joints),

and the characteristic erythematosus (butterfly) rash over the bridge of the nose. Drugs can produce an SLE-like syndrome. Those that have been implicated include hydralazine, procainamide, and isoniazid. In rare cases, drugs such as contraceptives, anticonvulsants, and phenothiazines have been suspected of producing symptoms.

Deterioration of the renal system is a usual consequence of the high levels of immune complexes in the blood that are deposited in tissues such as the kidneys. As the kidneys degenerate, the urinary sediment is typical of **acute nephritis** and later **chronic glomerulonephritis**. Although the disease can be rapidly fatal, it usually follows a chronic and irregular course, with periods of remission.

Laboratory Data

The laboratory findings in SLE are numerous. These tests include the classic, but now obsolete, LE cell preparation, testing for circulating antibodies, various antibody tests, and tests for lymphocyte subset abnormalities.

LE Cell Preparation

The classic but now outdated test for lupus is the LE cell test. An LE cell is either a normal segmented neutrophil or another phagocytic cell with the engulfed homogeneous and swollen nucleus of either a neutrophil or a lymphocyte.

Antibody Tests

Antibodies to DNA commonly occur in the systemic rheumatic disorders. The ANA procedure is a valuable screening tool for SLE and has virtually replaced the LE cell test because of its wider range of reactivity with NAs, greater sensitivity, and quality control characteristics. ANA refers to many different antibodies produced against a variety of antigens within the cell nucleus. These antigens are present on nucleic acid molecules (DNA and RNA) or proteins (histones and nonhistones) and on determinants consisting of both nucleic acid and protein molecules.

Some of these antibodies are directed against the double-stranded helical DNA (native DNA or DS-DNA). High titers of DS-DNA are seen primarily in SLE and parallel disease activity closely. Some antibodies are directed at the determinants of single-stranded DNA (SS-DNA). ANA testing may be by fluorescent antibody technique or by radioimmunoassay (RIA). In the fluorescent technique, a substrate that contains only DS-DNA is used. Antibody titers are frequently performed. Titers of 1:32 or greater indicate a substantial amount of antibody in an autoimmune response.

A positive ANA test result may be found in diseases other than SLE, in healthy persons, in the elderly, in those with other chronic diseases, and in some patients receiving specific drug therapy. A negative ANA test result virtually eliminates SLE as a possible diagnosis if the patient is not being treated. Other antibodies, such as anti-Sm, are present in only 25% to 30% of all patients with SLE but are considered a marker for SLE. Patients with drug-induced SLE have a high incidence of antibodies to histones.

Lymphocytotoxic antibodies with predominant specificity for T lymphocytes may also be detected. These antibodies are able to lyse T lymphocytes in the presence of complement and antibodies coating the peripheral blood T cells. This can interfere with certain functional activities of T lymphocytes.

Lymphocyte Subsets

Disturbances of the lymphocyte subsets are major immunological features of SLE. Among the T-cell subsets, a lack of, or reduced, generalized suppressor T-cell function or hyperproduction of helper T cells occurs. Among B cells, hyperactivity with corresponding enhancement of serum antibodies and autoantibodies, particularly IgG, and subsequent formation of pathogenic circulating immune complexes that lead to renal disease takes place.

CHAPTER HIGHLIGHTS

The normal range for lymphocytes in an adult is 22% to 40%, with absolute values of 1.1 to 4.4×10^9/L. When there is an increase in the blood lymphocyte concentration greater than the upper normal limit, the condition is referred to as **lymphocytosis**. A decrease to less than the normal limit is called **lymphocytopenia**.

Lymphocytosis

Lymphocytosis is natural and normal in infants and children up to approximately 10 years old, with total lymphocyte counts as high as 9.0×10^9/L. In adolescence and adulthood, nonmalignant conditions associated with an absolute lymphocytosis include acute viral infections (e.g., infectious mononucleosis) and some bacterial infections (e.g., whooping cough and brucellosis). Malignant conditions that produce lymphocytosis include cancer, lymphocytic leukemia (acute and chronic forms), the leukemic phase of lymphomas, and Waldenström macroglobulinemia.

Disorders Associated with Lymphocytosis

Infectious mononucleosis is caused by EBV. This same virus is associated with Burkitt lymphoma, a malignant tumor of the lymphoid tissue occurring mainly in African children. EBV is a human herpesvirus that has been isolated with increasing regularity.

Acute infectious lymphocytosis is a poorly defined benign condition caused by a virus, probably a member of the Coxsackie group. This is usually a mild disorder occurring in epidemics, with children being the most common victims.

CMV, a herpes family virus, can cause congenital infections in the newborn. The clinical syndrome resembles infectious mononucleosis.

Whooping cough is an infection caused by *B. pertussis,* a bacterial organism that produces inflammation of the entire respiratory tract. This is an illness that occurs primarily in children who have not been immunized.

Toxoplasmosis is an infection produced by the protozoa *T. gondii.* Both the clinical and the laboratory findings resemble those of infectious mononucleosis.

Lymphocytopenia

Lymphocytopenia is generally defined as less than 3.0×10^9/L lymphocytes in adults or less than 1.5×10^9/L lymphocytes in children. A decrease in lymphocytes is a common response to stress and to the administration of corticosteroids or may be seen in healthy persons with no apparent cause. Specific categories of lymphocyte disturbances include immune deficiency disorders.

Immune Disorders Associated with Lymphocytopenia

Immune deficiency disorders may be caused by defects in the quality (defects) or quantity (deficiencies) of lymphocytes and may be congenital or acquired. These conditions are usually classified as either T-cell or B-cell disorders. Some of the less common disorders involve both T and B cells.

AIDS is a contemporary example of leukopenia and lymphocytopenia. The number of circulating T lymphocytes is severely decreased. A decreased lymphocyte proliferative response to soluble antigens and mitogens exists in this disorder. This condition additionally demonstrates defective natural killer cell activity. T-lymphocyte subset distribution is also altered, with a decrease in the helper/inducer T cells and an increase in the number of suppressor/cytotoxic T cells.

SLE is a collagen-vascular disorder. It occurs most frequently in young adult females. A characteristic manifestation of SLE is a butterfly rash over the bridge of the nose. The renal system usually deteriorates because of high levels of immune complexes in the blood. Testing for ANA is the most significant screening in SLE.

CASE STUDIES

CASE 17.1

A female college freshman complaining of extreme fatigue, headaches, and a sore throat was seen by the college physician. A routine physical examination revealed that the patient had puffiness around the eyes, swollen lymph nodes (lymphadenopathy), slight splenomegaly, and pharyngitis. A complete blood count, urinalysis, and mononucleosis screening test were ordered.

(continued)

■ Laboratory Data

The blood count demonstrated normal values for erythrocytes and hemoglobin; however, the total leukocyte count was $13.5 \times 10^9/L$. The percentage of lymphocytes on the differential smear was 56%. Many variant forms of lymphocytes (25%) were seen, including cells with convoluted nuclei and highly vacuolated cytoplasm. The result of urinalysis was normal. The result of the mononucleosis screening test was negative.

The physician prescribed medication for the patient's headache and bed rest. A follow-up appointment was scheduled for 10 days later.

■ Questions

1. What was this patient's absolute lymphocyte count? Is this considered normal?
2. What is the most probable diagnosis of this disorder?
3. If repeat testing were performed on the patient after 10 days, could any of the results vary?
4. Discuss the antibodies that could occur in this condition.
5. Why are increased variant lymphocytes produced in this disorder?

■ Discussion

1. The patient's absolute lymphocyte count is $7.83 \times 10^9/L$. This represents a value higher than normal; hence, lymphocytosis is present.
2. The age and physical findings in this patient are highly suggestive of infectious mononucleosis. The laboratory findings of normal erythrocyte parameters and an increase in variant lymphocytes further support the diagnosis of mononucleosis. However, the absence of a positive heterophil screening test precludes a definitive diagnosis of infectious mononucleosis.
3. The heterophil antibody test usually becomes positive within 3 weeks after the initial symptoms.
4. Heterophil antibodies are the antibodies normally encountered in infectious mononucleosis. Rare cases of infectious mononucleosis have been described as heterophil negative. The clinical manifestations of infectious mononucleosis are present in these patients, but the heterophil test result remains negative for weeks after the onset. An Epstein-Barr antibody test may be helpful in distinguishing these cases from syndromes caused by other agents such as CMV or *Toxoplasma*. Occasionally, unusual antibodies occur in cases of infectious mononucleosis. Some of them may produce false-positive results for ANA, rheumatoid factor, and syphilis. Anti-i can also be encountered in acquired hemolytic anemias subsequent to infectious mononucleosis.
5. Several types of nonneoplastic disorders, such as systemic infection, diffuse inflammation, viral infections, and autoimmune disease, can produce transient lymphocytosis. This lymphocytosis results from either an increased production, a release of cells from peripheral lymphatic tissue, or both. If the normal proliferation and mobilization of lymphocytes from the lymph nodes and spleen are augmented by significant stimulation from other factors, increased numbers of variant lymphocytes can be seen in the peripheral blood. Lymphocytosis associated with infectious mononucleosis results from preferential infection of B cells by EBV. This infection results in a short burst of B-cell proliferation and mobilization, which produces the transient rise in the number of B cells with the variant lymphocyte structure. The altered membrane of the B cells further induces a prolonged proliferation response in T cells.

DIAGNOSIS: Infectious Mononucleosis

CASE 17.2

A 6-year-old boy was taken to the emergency department by his parents. The child had been having extreme difficulty in breathing for the past several days and had been experiencing diarrhea for the past 24 hours. There was no history of illness or infections.

Physical examination revealed that the child was severely dehydrated, had an elevated temperature, and had swollen lymph nodes (lymphadenopathy). The physician on duty ordered a complete blood count, serum electrolyte determination, urinalysis, infectious mononucleosis screening test, and a chest radiograph.

■ Laboratory Data

The boy's blood count was normal, except for the leukocytes. The total leukocyte count was $28 \times 10^9/L$, with 78% of leukocytes being lymphocytes. Most of the lymphocytes were small and normal in appearance. The serum electrolytes were consistent with a mild state of dehydration. The result of the urinalysis was normal, and the infectious mononucleosis screening test result was negative. The chest radiograph displayed mild congestion in the upper quadrant of the lungs.

■ Questions

1. What is the possible etiology of this disorder?
2. What other laboratory tests can assist in making a definitive diagnosis?
3. What mechanism is responsible for the lymphocytosis?
4. What is the expected duration of this condition?

■ Discussion

1. Pediatric patients with lymphocytosis, respiratory distress, and diarrhea are usually prime candidates for infectious lymphocytosis caused by bacterial or viral agents. Leukocytosis with a concurrent lymphocytosis can be caused by alterations in lymphocyte recirculation or abnormalities in lymphocyte turnover. Disorders

(continued)

producing this type of abnormality can include *B. pertussis,* certain viral infections, systemic infection, diffuse inflammation, autoimmune disease, immunoproliferative disorders, and some medications.

2. Laboratory tests that can assist in making a definitive diagnosis include microbiological culture for *B. pertussis* or viral cultures. A culture was positive for *B. pertussis.*

3. In healthy persons, the rate of the entry and exit of lymphocytes from the blood is relatively constant. This balance can be disrupted by bacterial or viral agents, such as *B. pertussis* and adenoviruses, or by medications such as heparin and dextran. If disruption of lymphocyte recirculation occurs because the lymphocytes are unable to recognize and attach to the endothelial venules in the lymph nodes, the number of lymphocytes in the blood circulation rapidly increases. However, the normal morphology of the lymphocytes is not altered.

4. In cases of acute infectious lymphocytosis, the elevated peripheral blood lymphocyte count may persist for 2 or 3 weeks and then begin to decline. Frequently, transient eosinophilia is noted during the period of lymphocyte decline.

DIAGNOSIS: *B. pertussis* Infection Producing an Infectious Lymphocytosis

CASE 17.3

A 5-year-old girl was taken to the pediatrician by her mother because of recurrent high fevers over the past few days. Physical examination revealed a light-colored rash but no other abnormalities. The child was referred to the clinic for a complete blood count.

▪ Laboratory Data

The complete blood count revealed normal erythrocyte parameters; however, the total leukocyte count was 4.0×10^9/L. The differential count revealed a lymphocyte count of 40%; all of the lymphocytes were mature and small.

▪ Questions

1. Are the leukocyte count and differential count normal?
2. What is the probable etiology of this disorder?
3. What is the mechanism of this disorder?

▪ Discussion

1. The total leukocyte count and percentage of lymphocytes are slightly below normal for a child of this age.
2. Mild lymphopenias can occur in some types of viral diseases, such as measles, varicella, and polio. The most common worldwide cause of lymphopenia is malnutrition. Other congenital defects caused by disturbed

maturation of T or B cells are rare, and related disorders usually appear in early childhood.

3. Some severe viral infections produce a noticeable decrease in B cells. These alterations are caused by the ability of the virus to infect and destroy B cells. Because B cells constitute only a small percentage of circulating lymphocytes in children, the decrease in circulating lymphocytes is not dramatic.

DIAGNOSIS: Measles

CASE 17.4

A 27-year-old white woman sought medical attention because of persisting pain in her wrists and ankles and an unexplained skin irritation of the face. On physical examination, swelling of the joints of the hands and ankles was evident, along with erythema of the skin over the bridge of the nose and the upper cheeks. The patient had a slightly elevated temperature. The following laboratory tests were ordered: a complete blood count, urinalysis, and rheumatoid arthritis screening test.

▪ Laboratory Data

The hemoglobin and hematocrit were normal, with a total leukocyte count of 7.0×10^9/L. The differential count was as follows: segmented neutrophils 80%, bands 1%, lymphocytes 17%, monocytes 1%, and eosinophils 1%. The morphology of the erythrocytes, leukocytes, and platelets was normal. The gross and microscopic urinalysis results were normal. A positive result was obtained for the rheumatoid arthritis screening test. An ANA screening test was ordered; the results were positive.

▪ Questions

1. What is the most probable diagnosis in this case?
2. What is the principle of the ANA test?

▪ Discussion

1. The patient's symptoms are all highly suggestive of a collagen-type disease, such as one of the rheumatoid disorders. However, both a positive LE test result and a positive ANA test result are highly suggestive of SLE.
2. Antibodies to DNA with high titers of DS-DNA are seen primarily in SLE. ANA testing may be by fluorescent antibody technique or by RIA. In the fluorescent technique, a substrate that contains only DS-DNA is used. Titers of 1:32 or greater indicate a substantial amount of antibody.

DIAGNOSIS: Systemic Lupus Erythematosus

REVIEW QUESTIONS

1. Lymphocytopenia means a
   A. total increase in leukocytes
   B. total increase in lymphocytes
   C. total increase in the absolute value or percentage of lymphocytes
   D. total decrease in lymphocytes

2. The helper subset of T lymphocytes is _____ in AIDS.
   A. increased
   B. decreased
   C. not altered

Questions 3 through 8: Match the following disorders with either A or B.
   A. Lymphocytosis
   B. Lymphocytopenia

3. _____ Radiation exposure
4. _____ Infectious mononucleosis
5. _____ Cytotoxic drugs
6. _____ Whooping cough
7. _____ Immune deficiency disorders
8. _____ Toxoplasmosis

9. Which of the following characterizes infectious mononucleosis?
   A. Etiology: EBV
   B. A T-cell disorder
   C. A greater incidence in Africa
   D. Nonheterophil antibodies

10. The laboratory findings in infectious mononucleosis are generally characterized by
    A. an increase in variant lymphocytes
    B. a heterophil titer less than 1:56
    C. no agglutination of the patient's serum with horse erythrocytes
    D. all of the above

11. Which of the following characterizes infectious lymphocytosis?
    A. An adult disorder
    B. Leukocytopenia in the early stages
    C. Lymphocyte differential counts over 95%
    D. Lymphoblasts on the peripheral blood smear

12. Which of the following are characteristics of CMV infection?
    A. Etiology: a herpes family virus
    B. Lymphocytopenia
    C. A positive heterophil test result
    D. Both A and B

13. AIDS is caused by
    A. a herpes family virus
    B. CMV
    C. HIV-1
    D. EBV

14. Which of the following generally characterize(s) toxoplasmosis?
    A. Symptoms may resemble infectious mononucleosis
    B. Occurrence in pregnant women who own cats
    C. Etiology: parasitic
    D. All of the above

15. Which antibody test has replaced the LE cell preparation in the diagnosis of SLE?
    A. Rheumatoid arthritis factor
    B. ANA test
    C. Complement fixation test
    D. Antibody Smith test

BIBLIOGRAPHY

Ascherio A, et al. Epstein-Barr virus antibodies and risk of multiple sclerosis: A prospective study, *JAMA*, 286(24):3083, 2001.

Bowden R, et al. Cytomegalovirus immune globulin and seronegative blood products to prevent primary cytomegalovirus infection after marrow transplantation, *N Engl J Med*, 314:1006–1010, 1986.

Brown KA. Nonmalignant disorders of lymphocytes, *Clin Lab Sci*, 10(6):329–335, 1997.

Bruce-Chwatt LJ. Transfusion associated parasitic infections. In: Dodd R (ed.). *Infection, Immunity, and Blood Transfusion*, New York, NY: Wiley–Liss, 1985:101–125.

Centers for Disease Control and Prevention. Mother-to-Child (Perinatal) HIV Transmission and Prevention, Oct 2007 Retrieved www.cdc.gov January 4, 2010.

Fleischer GR. Epstein-Barr virus. In: Belshe M (ed.). *Textbook of Human Virology*, Littleton, MA: PSG Publishing, 1984:490–558.

Hall SM. The diagnosis of toxoplasmosis, *Br Med J*, 289:570–571, 1984.

Kinney JS, et al. Cytomegaloviral infection and disease, *J Infect Dis*, 151:772–774, 1985.

Lennette ET, Henle W. Epstein-Barr virus infections: Clinical and serologic features, *Lab Manage*, 25:23–28, 1987.

Mandell GE (ed.). *Principles and Practices of Infectious Disease*, 2nd ed, New York, NY: Wiley, 1985.

Markell EK, et al. *Medical Parasitology*, 6th ed, Philadelphia, PA: Saunders, 1986:112–117, 131–138.

Steinbrook R. The AIDS epidemic in 2004, *N Engl J Med*, 351(2):115–117, 2004.

World Health Organization United Nations Children's Fund. HIV/AIDS-2009. Retrieved January 10, 2010.

CHAPTER 18

Characteristics of Leukemias, Lymphomas, and Myelomas

OBJECTIVES

Comparison of leukemia, lymphoma, and myeloma
- Define and compare the characteristics of leukemia, lymphoma, and myeloma.

Forms of leukemia
- Describe the terms acute and chronic leukemia.

Classification of leukemias
- List the traditional forms of the major types of leukemias.

Prognosis and treatment
- Compare the early treatment of leukemias and lymphomas with current therapy.

Factors related to the occurrence of leukemia
- Describe the role of oncogenes in leukemias and lymphomas.
- Describe the effects of ionizing radiation on the incidence of leukemia.
- Name one chemical that is correlated with an increased incidence of leukemia.

- Name several occupations that are associated with a higher-than-normal risk of hematological malignancies.
- Name one genetic defect that is correlated with an increased incidence of leukemia.
- Explain the significance of the discovery of the human T-cell leukemia virus (HTLV) family and describe associated disorders.

Demographic distribution of leukemia and lymphomas
- Describe the variations in the incidence of leukemia in different ethnic and racial groups.
- Correlate patient age to the overall incidence of various leukemias.
- Describe the overall differences between the incidence of leukemia in female and male patients.

Leukemia vaccines
- Explain the role of vaccines in treatment and/or prevention of leukemias.

Although the symptoms of leukemia had been reported since the time of Hippocrates, Virchow was the first to recognize leukemia as a distinct clinical disorder between 1839 and 1845. He named this disorder **leukemia** because of the white appearance of the blood from patients with fever, weakness, and **lymphadenopathy**. Virchow originally divided the leukemias into two classes, those with and those without lymphadenopathy. Now, sophisticated classification systems including molecular diagnostics of leukemias and **lymphomas** exist.

COMPARISON OF LEUKEMIAS, LYMPHOMAS, AND MYELOMAS

Leukemia, lymphomas, and myelomas are neoplastic proliferative diseases (neoplasms).

Leukemia is a disease, usually of leukocytes, in the blood and bone marrow. Lymphoma is a general term for malignancy that starts in the lymph system, mainly the lymph nodes. The two main types of lymphomas are Hodgkin lym-

phoma and non-Hodgkin lymphoma. Myeloma is a form of cancer of the plasma cells. In myeloma, the cells overgrow, forming a mass or tumor that is located in the bone marrow (see Table 18.1).

FORMS OF LEUKEMIA

The clinical symptoms, maturity of the affected cells, and total leukocyte count determine whether a leukemia is classified as **acute** or **chronic**. Acute leukemias are characterized by symptoms of short duration, many immature cell forms in the bone marrow and/or peripheral blood, and an elevated total leukocyte count. Chronic leukemias have symptoms of long duration, mostly mature cell forms in the bone marrow and/or peripheral blood, and total leukocyte counts that range from extremely elevated to lower than normal. The prognosis of survival in untreated acute forms is from several weeks to several months, compared with the untreated chronic forms, which can have a prognosis of survival ranging from months to many years after diagnosis.

TABLE 18.1 Comparative Features of Leukemias and Lymphomas			
	Leukemias	**Lymphomas**	**Myelomas**
Basic characteristic	Overproduction of various types of immature or mature leukocytes in the bone marrow and/ or peripheral blood, in most types of leukemias	Solid malignant tumors of the lymph nodes	Overproduction of plasma cells in the bone marrow with concurrent production of abnormal proteins
Cell type	Usually involves leukocytes of the myelogenous or lymphocytic cell types	Lymphocyte is the distinctive cell type. Reed-Sternberg cells are diagnostic of Hodgkin-type lymphoma.	Plasma cells
Site of malignant cells	Malignant cells freely trespass the blood-brain barrier	Malignant cells are initially confined to the organs containing mononuclear phagocyte cells such as the lymph nodes, spleen, liver, and bone marrow.	Plasma cells form a mass or tumor that is located in the bone marrow.
Notes		Lymphomas can spill over into the circulating blood and present a leukemic-appearing picture on a peripheral blood smear.	

CLASSIFICATIONS OF LEUKEMIAS

Although Virchow divided leukemias into two groups based on the presence of lymphadenopathy, different forms of leukemia were later classified according to the predominant blood cell morphological and cytochemical result and clinical criteria by the French-American-British (FAB) classification. This system has been enhanced with molecular information by the World Health Organization (WHO).

French-American-British Classification

Using the FAB system, leukemias are separated into three broad leukocyte groups:

- Myelogenous
- Monocytic
- Lymphocytic

When this information is coupled with the degree of cell maturity, the traditional classifications of the major types of leukocytic leukemias can be classified as acute or chronic according to the leukocyte groups, for example, acute or chronic myelogenous, acute or chronic monocytic, acute or chronic myelomonocytic, acute or chronic lymphocytic leukemia (CLL).

More uncommon forms of leukocytic leukemia are acute undifferentiated (stem cell), eosinophilic, and basophilic. Overproliferation of the erythrocytic and megakaryocytic cell lines, either solely or in conjunction with abnormalities of the leukocytic line, also exists.

World Health Organization Classification

The newest fourth edition (2008) of the WHO classification stratifies neoplasms primarily according to lineage: myeloid, lymphoid, and histiocytic/dendritic cell. Classifications are based on morphology but combine this information with immunophenotyping and genetic studies of peripheral blood, bone marrow, and lymph node samples.

Precursor neoplasms, for example, acute myeloid leukemias, lymphoblastic lymphomas/leukemias, acute leukemias of ambiguous lineage, and blastic plasmacytoid dendritic neoplasms, are considered separately from more mature neoplasms, for example, myeloproliferative neoplasms, myelodysplastic/myeloproliferative neoplasms, myelodysplastic

TABLE 18.2	Potential Predisposing Factors for the Development of Leukemias and Lymphomas
Chemicals	Benzene, hydrocarbons, hair dyes
Environmental	Ionizing radiation, insecticides, herbicides, and fungicides
Drugs	Alkylating agents, chloramphenicol
Viruses	Herpes virus (EBV)
	Human immunodeficiency virus (HIV)
	Human T-cell leukemia virus (HTLV-1)
Genetic syndromes	Down syndrome
	Fanconi anemia
Hematologic conditions	Myelodysplastic syndromes

syndromes, mature (peripheral) B-cell and T/NK neoplasms, Hodgkin lymphoma, and histiocyte/dendritic-cell neoplasms.

The mature myeloid neoplasms are stratified according to biological features as well as by genetic features. With mature lymphoid neoplasms, the diseases are listed according to clinical presentation and, to some extent, according to the stage of differentiation.

PROGNOSIS AND TREATMENT

Untreated leukemias and lymphomas are ultimately fatal. Radiation therapy in the 1920s provided the first type of curative intervention. The first effective drug therapy, adrenoglucocorticosteroids and antifolate agents, was discovered in the late 1940s. Modern drugs, which are more effective against malignant cells and are less toxic to the patient, have had a significant impact on the longevity of patients with many forms of leukemia and lymphoma. In the recent past, drugs directed at treatment at the molecular level have been successfully introduced, for example, chronic myelogenous leukemia (CML). Effective treatment requires selecting the proper mode and method of treatment. The time of administration of treatment can also have an effect (refer to Chapter 27 for applications of flow cell cytometry). Specific treatment requires prompt and accurate diagnosis and classification of the disorder by the clinical laboratory.

FACTORS RELATED TO THE OCCURRENCE OF LEUKEMIA

Leukemia is a clonal disease that develops subsequent to the malignant transformation of one or more normal hematopoietic progenitor cells. It appears likely that mutation and the altered expression of specific genes cause this transformation. Leukemic stem cells are capable of proliferation and

self-renewal, which gives rise to one or more dominant clones of cells that eventually fill the bone marrow and suppress normal hematopoiesis.

Although the majority of cases of acute leukemia have no identifiable cause, many agents or factors have been implicated in the occurrence of leukemias and lymphomas (see Table 18.2). These factors include

1. Genetic and immunological factors
2. Occupational exposure
3. Environmental exposure
4. Chemical and drug exposure
5. Genetic abnormalities and associations
6. Viral agents
7. Secondary causes

Genetic and Immunological Factors

Mutations in a single gene are found in many cases of leukemia; larger changes in one or more chromosomes are also common. Several types of chromosomal changes may be found:

- *Translocations* are the most common type of DNA change that can lead to leukemia. A translocation means that a part of one chromosome breaks off and becomes attached to a different chromosome. The point at which the break occurs can affect nearby genes—for example, it can turn on oncogenes or turn off genes that would normally help a cell to mature.
- *Deletions* occur when part of a chromosome is lost. This may result in the cell losing a gene that helped keep its growth in check, for example, a tumor suppressor gene.
- *Inversions* occur when part of a chromosome gets turned around, so it is now in reverse order. This can result in the loss of a gene (or genes) because the cell can no longer read its instructions in protein translation.

■ *Addition* means that an extra chromosome or part of a chromosome is gained. This can lead to too many copies of certain genes within the cell. This can be a problem if one or more of these genes are oncogenes.

Each time a cell prepares to divide into new daughter cells, it must make a new copy of the DNA in its chromosomes. Cancers can be caused by DNA mutations that turn on oncogenes or turn off tumorsuppressor genes. For example, changes in certain genes such as FLT3, c-KIT, and RAS are commonly found in acute myelogenous leukemias (AMLs).

Oncogenes

A single oncogene produced through mutation in a target cell is not sufficient to convert these cells into full-blown cancer cells. Cancer cells typically carry multiple genetic changes that act together. Cancer-predisposing genes may act in several ways:

1. They may affect the rate at which exogenous precarcinogens are metabolized to actively carcinogenic forms that can damage the cellular genome directly.
2. Some genes may affect a host's ability to repair resulting damage to DNA.
3. Predisposing genes may alter the immune system's ability to recognize and wipe out incipient tumors.
4. Some genes may affect the function of the apparatus responsible for the regulation of normal cell growth and associated proliferation of tissue.

Relatively few cancer-predisposing genes have been described. An absence of functional alleles at specific loci, however, allows the genesis of a malignant process.

Malignant proliferation of cells is related to genes. Cancer often begins when a carcinogenic agent, such as a chemical or ionizing radiation, damages the DNA of a critical gene in a cell. The mutant cell multiplies and the succeeding generations of cells aggregate to form a malignant tumor.

Protooncogenes

Protooncogenes act as central regulators of growth in normal cells and are antecedents of oncogenes. Not one of the protooncogenes, however, has yet been linked to genes that are thought to increase the risk of cancer. The rare involvement of these genes in the cancer process is a consequence of somatic mutations that take place in specific target tissues and convert these genes into oncogenic alleles. Because oncogenic alleles arise somatically, they cannot be used to explain genetic susceptibilities to cancer that exist at the moment of conception.

The genetic targets of carcinogens are known to be oncogenes. Oncogenes have been associated with various tumor types that stem in large part from preexisting genes present in the normal human genome. Therefore, oncogenes are considered to be altered versions of normal genes. In the course of a lifetime, a variety of mutations can convert a normal gene into a malignant oncogene. Once an oncogene is activated by mutation, it promotes excessive or inappropriate

TABLE 18.3	Oncogenes Formed by Somatic Mutation of Normal Genetic Loci
Oncogene	**Disorder**
Abl	Chronic myelogenous leukemia
Myc	Burkitt lymphoma
Ras type	Variety of tumors

cell proliferation. Oncogenes have been detected in approximately 15% to 20% of a variety of human tumors and appear to be responsible for specifying many of the malignant traits of these cells. More than 30 distinct oncogenes, some of which are associated with specific tumor types, have been identified (Table 18.3). Each gene has the ability to evoke many of the phenotypes characteristic of cancer cells.

Tumor-Suppressing Genes

A very different class of cancer genes has been discovered recently. These tumor-suppressing genes appear to regulate the proliferation of cell growth in normal cells. When this type of gene is inactivated, a block to proliferation is removed and cells begin a program of deregulated growth, or the genetically depleted cell itself may proliferate uncontrollably. Thus, tumor-suppressing genes are referred to as antioncogenes and their discovery will in time lead to the reformulation of ideas about how the growth of normal cells is regulated.

There is much speculation as to how tumor-suppressing genes operate in normal tissue. It is known that normal cells exert a negative growth influence on each other within a tissue. Normal cells also secrete factors that are negative regulators of their own growth and that of adjacent cells. Diffusible factors may also be released by normal cells to induce the end-stage differentiation of other cells in the immediate environment. Examples of such factors include

1. β-Interferon
2. Tumor growth factor
3. Tumor necrosis factor

Normal gene products appear to prevent malignant transformation in some way. It is speculated that normal cells have receptors able to detect the presence of these growth-inhibiting and differentiation-inducing factors, which allows the receptors to process the signals of negative growth and respond with appropriate modulation of growth. Genes may specify proteins that are necessary to detect and also respond to the negative regulators of growth. If this process becomes dysfunctional owing to inactivation or the absence of a critical component such as the loss of chromosomal loci, a cell may continue to respond to mitogenic stimulation but lose its ability to respond to negative feedback to cease proliferation.

Animal experiments suggest that humans carry a repertoire of genes, each of which is involved in the negative regulation of the growth of specific cell types. Somatic inactivation of these genes may be involved in the initiation of tumor cell growth or the transformation of benign tumors into malignant ones. The somatic inactivation of tumor-suppressing genes may be as important to carcinogenesis as the somatic activation of oncogenes.

Immunological Surveillance

Immunologists regard the immune response as a means of diagnosing and treating malignancy. Although no single satisfactory explanation exists to explain the success of tumors in escaping the immune rejection process, it is believed that early clones of neoplastic cells are eliminated by the immune response. The functions of normal antitumor mechanisms and the failure of these mechanisms in the pathogenesis of cancer are incompletely understood at the present time.

Occupational Exposure

Ionizing radiation is an example of an occupational factor associated with an increased incidence of leukemia. Historically, Madame Curie and her daughter, Irene, both probably died from radiation-induced leukemia. The survivors of Hiroshima had a radiation dose–related increase in the incidence of leukemia. Before the use of protective measures, radiologists were found to have leukemia 10 times more frequently than the general population. The acute and chronic forms of myelogenous leukemia are most frequently associated with radiation.

Environmental Exposure

The possible risks of leukemia from exposure to lower levels of radiation, for example, radiation therapy, x-rays, or CT scans, are not well-defined. Exposure of a fetus to radiation within the first months of development may carry an increased risk of leukemia, but the extent of the risk is not clear and is likely to be small.

Exposure to high levels of radiation is a risk factor for acute leukemias. Japanese atomic bomb survivors had a greatly increased risk of developing acute leukemia, usually within 6 to 8 years after exposure.

Chemical and Drug Exposure

Occupational exposure to chemicals is also highly correlated with an increased incidence of leukemia. Prolonged exposure to the chemical benzene is known to increase the probability of various forms of cancer, including leukemia. Benzene is an organic solvent used in oil refineries, chemical plants, shoe manufacturing, and gasoline-related industries. It is also present in cigarette smoke, some glues, cleaning products, detergents, art supplies, and paint strippers. Chemical exposure is more strongly linked to an increased risk of AML than to acute lymphoblastic leukemia (ALL). The occupations

TABLE 18.4	**Occupations Related to a Higher-Than-Average Risk of Malignancy in Hematologically Related Sites**
Occupation	**Site**
Chemist	Lymphatic system
Petrochemical worker	Blood
Radiologist	Bone marrow
Rubber industry worker	Blood
Woodworker	Lymphatic system

associated with job-related death caused by a higher-than-average risk of malignancy in the hematopoietic system are presented in Table 18.4.

Patients getting intensive treatment to suppress their immune function, for example, organ transplant patients, have an increased risk of certain cancers, such as lymphoma and ALL.

An increased risk of secondary leukemia due to platinum-based treatment for ovarian cancer has been documented among women who received platinum-based combination chemotherapy. The relative risk increases with the cumulative dose of platinum administered and the duration of therapy.

Genetic Abnormalities and Associations

Cytogenetic abnormalities are now associated with many varieties of leukemia. Studies of twins have shown that if leukemia develops in one twin, then the other has one chance in five of leukemia development, usually within the first year of life. Many doctors feel the increased risk among identical twins may be due to leukemia cells being passed from one fetus to the other while still in the womb. Siblings of children with leukemia have a slightly increased chance (two to four times normal) of getting leukemia but the overall risk is low.

The link between certain genetic abnormalities and leukemia is consistent with a germinal or somatic mutation in a stem cell line, and the increased incidence of lymphomas in congenital, acquired, and drug-induced immunosuppression is consistent with the failure of normal immune mechanisms or antigen overstimulation with a loss of normal feedback control.

Down Syndrome

Down syndrome (DS) is the most common human aneuploidy. Children with DS, or constitutional trisomy 21, show a spectrum of clinical anomalies, commonly demonstrating macrocytosis, abnormal platelet counts, and an increased incidence of leukemia. DS children have greatly increased rates of ALL and acute megakaryoblastic leukemia (AMKL). DS newborns present with transient myeloproliferative disorder (TMD), a preleukemic form of AMKL.

The natural history of leukemia in children with Down syndrome suggests that trisomy 21 directly and functionally contributes to the malignant transformation of hematopoietic cells. TMD and DS-AMKL patients almost always have acquired and clonal mutation in exon 2 of the X-linked *GATA*1 gene, which codes for the GATA1 transcription factor. The mutation results in exclusive synthesis of a truncated protein (GATA1s) and suggested that both trisomy 21 and GATA1 mutations contribute to hematopoietic abnormalities.

Children with DS are 20 times more likely to have ALL develop than children without this genetic disorder. The incidence of acute megakaryocytic leukemia is 500-fold higher than the general population. TMD, a clonal disease characterized by immature megakaryoblasts in the fetal liver and peripheral blood, occurs in 4% to 10% of infants with Down syndrome. Most cases of TMD spontaneously disappear but it is regarded as a preleukemic syndrome. Approximately 20% of children with TMD develop AMKL within 4 years.

Genetic Abnormalities

The most common translocation in adults with CML and some adults with ALL is known as the Philadelphia chromosome, which is a swapping of DNA (translocation) between chromosomes 9 and 22, abbreviated as t(9;22). It occurs in about 25% to 30% of adult leukemia cases. Other, less common translocations are those between chromosomes 4 and 11, abbreviated as t(4;11), or 8 and 14, abbreviated as t(8;14).

Other chromosome changes such as *deletions* and *inversions* (the rearrangement of the DNA within part of a chromosome) are less common.

Viral Agents

Certain viral infections, for example, Epstein-Barr virus (EBV), most often causes infectious mononucleosis ("mono") in the United States. In Africa, the virus has been linked to Burkitt lymphoma, as well as to a form of acute lymphocytic leukemia. Infection with the human T-cell lymphoma/leukemia virus-1 (HTLV-1) can cause a rare type of T-cell acute lymphocytic leukemia. Most cases occur in Japan and the Caribbean area. This disease is not common in the United States.

Viral Characteristics

The incidence of cancers such as lymphoma is significantly increased (10,000 times greater than expected) in patients who have human immunodeficiency virus (HIV). Other specific viruses have been found to be associated with the development of disorders, including leukemias and lymphomas. These viruses can be separated epidemiologically into two groups:

1. Those that are ubiquitous, such as the EBV
2. Those that have a higher incidence in certain populations, for example, HIV

A variety of RNA and DNA viruses have been associated with human malignancies. Some viral agents have clear causative roles, such as EBV and certain papillomaviruses, that are the etiological agents in Burkitt lymphoma and cervical carcinoma, respectively.

Viral oncogenes are carried by viruses into target cells, where they become firmly established. Clonal descendants then carry the viral genes that maintain the malignant phenotype of the cell clones.

Epstein-Barr Virus

The association of DNA-related EBV with Burkitt lymphoma was the first recognized link between a specific virus and a human malignant disease. Burkitt lymphoma represents a well-characterized epidemiological entity in equatorial Africa and is found less frequently elsewhere. In nonendemic areas, such as Europe and the United States, it has been shown that only 15% to 18% of the Burkitt type of malignant lymphomas in children are associated with EBV. Among adolescents in Western countries, EBV is the etiological agent in the nonmalignant disorder infectious mononucleosis.

Human T-Cell Leukemia Viruses

The first member of the HTLV family of viruses (HTLV- I) was isolated in 1980. Since this discovery, an enormous amount of accumulated data has established this viral family as the etiological agent of unusually aggressive forms of adult T-cell leukemia or lymphoma. HTLV is the first RNA tumor virus (retrovirus) known to occur in humans.

HTLV-I was the first retrovirus to be isolated from patients suffering from aggressive T-cell cancers with skin involvement. Cases do occur in the United States but they are unusual. HIV is the etiological agent in acquired immunodeficiency syndrome (AIDS). This virus is now believed to be only distantly related to HTLV-I and HTLV-II and is recognized as the clinical entity characterized by helper T-cell depletion and immunodeficiency.

HIV belongs to the retrovirus group. Retroviruses carry a single, positive-stranded RNA and use a special enzyme, called **reverse transcriptase**, to convert viral RNA into DNA. This reverses the normal process of transcription where DNA is converted to RNA—hence, the term **retrovirus.**

Secondary Causes of Leukemias

Children and adults treated for other cancers with certain chemotherapy drugs have a higher risk of getting a second cancer, usually AML, later in life. Drugs such as alkylating agents, for example, cyclophosphamide and chlorambucil, and epipodophyllotoxins, for example, etoposide and teniposide, have been linked to a higher risk of leukemia. These leukemias usually develop within 5 to 10 years of treatment and can be difficult to treat.

Secondary AML may develop in patients:

■ With a hematologic disorder (e.g., severe congenital neutropenia)
■ With an inherited disease (e.g., Fanconi anemia)

■ With myelodysplastic syndrome for at least 3 months
■ Who have been treated with leukemogenic agents, often for an unrelated neoplasm

AML can be expected to develop in 3% to 10% of patients with Hodgkin disease, non-Hodgkin lymphoma, multiple myeloma, and breast or ovarian cancer who receive alkylating agents as therapy. A second distinct subtype of therapy-induced AML has been identified as a complication of treatment with certain regimens of topoisomerase II inhibitors (e.g., epipodophyllotoxins).

Secondary cancer is an important complication of the treatment of childhood leukemia. The occurrence of secondary acute myeloid leukemia (AML) after successful treatment for a variety of malignancies, for example, acute monoblastic leukemia, generally carries a poor prognosis.

A case of donor-derived acute promyelocytic leukemia has been reported in a liver transplant patient 2 years after transplantation. The leukemic clone had genetic and phenotypic markers of the donor. The research findings indicate that leukemic transformation of donor myeloid cells that resided in the transplanted liver occurred in the transplant recipient.

DEMOGRAPHIC DISTRIBUTION OF LEUKEMIA AND LYMPHOMAS

Leukemias, lymphomas, and multiple myelomas represent almost 10% of the cancer deaths in the United States. Lymphomas are diagnosed most frequently. The majority of cases of lymphoma are of the non-Hodgkin type (see Table 18.5A and B).

The overall occurrence of leukemia can be correlated with a variety of factors, including ethnic origin, race, age, and gender. Although the number of new cases of leukemia, lymphoma, and myeloma diagnosed each year has slightly increased, deaths from neoplasms have decreased in recent years. This decrease in deaths may be due to many factors, including early detection and more effective treatments.

Ethnic Origin and Race

Although leukemia occurs worldwide, the highest incidence is in the Scandinavian countries and Israel, whereas the lowest incidence is in Japan and Chile.

In adult whites, CLL accounts for more than 20% of the new cases of leukemia, but among Asians it is rare. ALL is slightly more common among white children than among African American and Asian American children. Myeloma is about twice as common among African Americans as among whites.

Age has a significant correlation with the various types of leukemias. Leukemia in very young infants (younger than 18 months of age) is generally of a myelogenous nature. Leukemia is the most commonly diagnosed cancer and leading

TABLE 18.5A	Estimated Ranked Hematopoietic Neoplastic Diagnoses Annually in the United States	
Type of Cancer		**New Cases**
Lymphoma		±60,000
Non-Hodgkin lymphoma		±53,000
Hodgkin lymphoma		±7,500
Leukemias		±30,500
Acute myeloid leukemia		±10,500
Chronic lymphocytic leukemia		±7,000
Chronic myeloid leukemia		±4,250
Acute lymphoblastic leukemia		±3,700
Other types of leukemias		±5,000
Multiple myeloma		±14,500

TABLE 18.5B	Estimated Ranked Hematopoietic Neoplastic Deaths Annually in the United States	
Lymphoma		±25,000
Non-Hodgkin lymphoma		±24,000
Hodgkin disease		±1,500
Leukemias		±22,000
Acute myeloid leukemia		±8,000
Chronic lymphocytic leukemia		±4,500
Other types of leukemias		±7,000
Chronic myeloid leukemia		±2,000
Acute lymphoblastic leukemia		±1,500
Multiple myeloma		±11,000

cause of death in children aged 0 to 19 years. The distribution rate of pediatric leukemias (see Table 18.6) demonstrates that the

■ Highest incidence rate is found among children aged 1 to 4 years
■ Highest death rate is found among children aged 15 to 19 years

Children (ages 0 to 14 years) who develop leukemia in three out of four cases are diagnosed with acute lymphoblastic leukemia (ALL). Most of the remaining cases are AML. Chronic leukemias are rare in children.

TABLE 18.6	Age-Adjusted Invasive Cancer Incidence Rates and 95% Confidence Intervals for Ages 0–19 by International Classification of Childhood Cancer (ICCC) Group and Subgroup, and Age, United States[a]		

		Age	
Cancer Types		0–14	0–19
All ICCC Groups Combined		148.4	165.4
I. Leukemias, myeloproliferative, and myelodysplastic diseases		47.1	42.7
(a) Lymphoid leukemias		36.0	31.0
(b) Acute myeloid leukemias		6.9	7.3
(c) Chronic myeloproliferative diseases		1.3	1.7
(d) Myelodysplastic syndrome and other myeloproliferative diseases		1.4	1.4
(e) Unspecified and other specified leukemias		1.4	1.3
II. Lymphomas and reticuloendothelial neoplasms		16.2	25.2
(a) Hodgkin lymphomas		5.8	12.6
(b) Non-Hodgkin lymphomas (except Burkitt lymphoma)		6.3	8.9
(c) Burkitt lymphoma		2.5	2.4
(d) Miscellaneous lymphoreticular neoplasms		1.3	1.1
(e) Unspecified lymphomas		~	0.3

[a]Rates are per 1,000,000 persons and are age adjusted to the 2000 U.S. standard population (19 age groups – Census P25–1130). (Adapted from Centers for Disease Control and Prevention (CDC) www.cdc.gov retrieved January 10, 2010.)

Of patients diagnosed with ALL, about one out of three will be adults. Persons older than 60 years of age are more likely to develop CLL than other types of leukemias. The myelogenous leukemias, both acute and chronic forms, have a peak incidence among young and middle-aged adults.

Age is the most significant risk factor for developing myeloma. People under age 45 rarely develop the disease. Those aged 67 years or older are at greatest risk of developing this neoplasm.

Over the past 25 years, there have been significant improvements in the 5-year relative survival rates for many childhood cancers, particularly ALL. The death statistics for ALL demonstrate that about three out of four instances will be in adults.

Gender

Most forms of leukemia are diagnosed more frequently in American males than in females regardless of race or age, except among children younger than 18 months of age. ALL is slightly more common in boys than in girls. AML occurs equally among boys and girls of all races.

The gender differences tend to be most dramatic in adults with CLL, in which the male-female ratio is 2:1. According to the *U.S. Cancer Statistics* published by the Centers for Disease Control and Prevention, more adult males than adult females are diagnosed with non-Hodgkin lymphoma than

Hodgkin lymphoma. Adult males outnumber adult females with the diagnosis of myeloma as well.

Men are more likely than women to develop myeloma.

Leukemia Vaccines

The majority of patients with leukemia can achieve clinical complete remission following high-dose chemotherapy, but they frequently relapse. To cure leukemia, eradication of minimal residual disease (MRD) is essential. Research being conducted by the U.S. National Institutes of Health suggests that a vaccine could help to reduce the risk of relapse in some patients who are treated for CML with the drug, imatinib mesylate. The vaccine being tested is prepared from cancer cells blasted with radiation to stop them from being cancerous. Tumor immunotherapy such as this in the form of a vaccine holds great promise in controlling or even eradicating MRD and may provide an alternative treatment modality to conventional chemotherapy for cancer patients, including patients with hematopoietic disorders.

CHAPTER HIGHLIGHTS

Leukemias are neoplastic proliferative diseases that are characterized by an overproduction of immature or mature cells of various leukocyte types in the bone marrow and/or blood. Lymphomas are similar to leukemias, but lymphomas are solid tumors of lymph nodes and associated tissues or bone marrow.

The clinical symptoms, the maturity of the affected cells, and the total leukocyte count determine whether a leukemia will be classified as **acute** or **chronic**. Acute leukemias are characterized as having symptoms of short duration, many immature cell forms in the bone marrow and/or peripheral blood, and an elevated total leukocyte count. Chronic leukemias have symptoms of long duration, mostly mature cell forms in the bone marrow and/or peripheral blood, and total leukocyte counts that range from extremely elevated to less than normal. The prognosis of survival in untreated acute

forms is from several weeks to several months, compared with the untreated chronic forms, which can have a prognosis of survival ranging from months to many years after diagnosis.

The commonly encountered types of leukemias are separated into three broad groupings by cell type: **myelogenous, monocytic,** and **lymphocytic.**

Untreated leukemias and lymphomas are ultimately fatal. Specific treatment requires accurate diagnosis and classification of the disorder by the clinical laboratory.

The occurrence of leukemias and lymphomas has been related to a variety of factors. These factors include genetic conditions, environmental exposure, and viral agents.

REVIEW QUESTIONS

1. A definition of a leukemia could include
   A. an overproduction of leukocytes
   B. solid, malignant tumors of the lymph nodes
   C. malignant cells trespass the blood-brain barrier
   D. both A and C
2. Descriptive terms for most lymphomas can include
   A. a nonneoplastic proliferative disease
   B. a solid malignant tumor of the lymph nodes
   C. a lymphocytopenia
   D. freely trespassing the blood-brain barrier
3. An acute leukemia can be described as being
   A. of short duration with many mature leukocyte forms in the peripheral blood
   B. of short duration with many immature leukocyte forms in the peripheral blood
   C. of short duration with little alteration of the leukocytes of the peripheral blood
   D. of long duration with many mature leukocyte forms in the peripheral blood
4. The etiological agents of leukemias can include
   A. ionizing radiation
   B. certain infectious agents
   C. chemical exposure to benzene
   D. all of the above
5. HIV is associated with
   A. hairy cell leukemia
   B. Sézary cell syndrome
   C. AIDS
   D. leukemia
6. Cancer-predisposing genes may act by
   A. affecting the rate at which exogenous precarcinogens are metabolized to actively carcinogenic forms
   B. affecting the host's ability to repair resulting damage to DNA
   C. altering the immune system's ability to recognize and wipe out incipient tumors
   D. all of the above
7. The incidence of leukemia is higher in
   A. Scandinavian versus Japanese populations
   B. American blacks versus American whites
   C. chronic forms in children versus chronic forms in adults
   D. acute forms in older adults versus acute forms in children

BIBLIOGRAPHY

Alford KA, et al. Perturbed hematopoiesis in the Tc1 mouse model of Down syndrome, *Blood*, 115(14), 2928-2937, 2010.

Chan MP, Weissman IL, Park CY. Cancer stem cells: on the verge of clinical translation, *Labmedicine*, 39(11):679–686, 2008.

DeThe G, et al. Viruses as risk factors or causes of human leukemias and lymphomas? *Leuk Res,* 9(6):691–696, 1985.

Malinge S, Izraeli S, Crispino JD. Insights into the manifestations, outcomes, and mechanisms of leukemogenesis in Down syndrome, *Blood*, 113(12):2619–2628, 2009.

Miller RW. The features in common among persons at high risk of leukemia. In: Levin DL (ed.). *Cancer Epidemiology in the USA and USSR.* Bethesda, MD: National Cancer Institute, 1980:125–127.

Neri G. Some questions on the significance of chromosome alterations in leukemias and lymphomas: A review, *Am J Med Genet*, 18:471–481, 1984.

Stevens W, et al. Leukemia in Utah and radioactive fallout from the Nevada test site: A case–control study, *JAMA*, 264(5):585–591, 1990.

Swerdlow SH, et al (ed.). *WHO Classification of Tumours of Haematopoietic and Lymphoid Tissues*, Lyon, France: IARC, 2008.

Wing S, et al. Mortality among workers at Oak Ridge National Laboratory, *JAMA*, 265(11):1397–1408, 1991.

General characteristics
■ Describe the general characteristics of leukemias.

Categories
■ Name and briefly describe the classification of leukemias according to the French-American-British (FAB) and World Health Organization (WHO) systems.

Acute myeloid leukemias
■ List and name the various types of acute leukemias, including the FAB nomenclature.
■ Describe the clinical symptoms and laboratory findings, including peripheral blood morphology, of acute leukemias.
■ Explain some of the general features of other forms of acute leukemia.

Acute lymphoblastic leukemia
■ Describe the clinical symptoms, laboratory findings, and special identification techniques in acute lymphoblastic leukemia (ALL).

Cytogenetic analysis
■ Explain the chromosomal alterations that may be observed in various myeloid and lymphoblastic leukemias.

Chemical methods of cellular identification
■ Explain the principle and purpose of the Sudan black B stain, myeloperoxidase (MPO), and the periodic acid-Schiff test.
■ Compare the two common esterase procedures in terms of their purposes.

Monoclonal antibodies
■ Describe the utility of monoclonal antibodies in differentiating between various leukemias.

Life-threatening emergencies
■ Name and describe five life-threatening emergencies.

Treatment options
■ Name and explain three treatment options.

Future trends
■ Discuss future trends in the treatment of leukemia.

Case studies
■ Apply the laboratory data to the stated case studies and discuss the implications of these cases to the study of hematology.

INTRODUCTION

Each type of leukemia, acute or chronic, has unique characteristics. This chapter presents the general characteristics, classification, clinical symptoms, laboratory data, and treatment of various types of acute leukemias.

Acute myeloid leukemia (AML) must be distinguished from acute lymphoblastic leukemia (ALL), myelodysplastic syndrome (MDS), or AML arising in the presence of MDS, because therapeutic strategies and the prognosis vary considerably for these diseases.

EPIDEMIOLOGY OF ACUTE LEUKEMIAS

According to the National Cancer Institute, there were an estimated 44,790 new cases of leukemia and an estimated 21,870 deaths from leukemia in the United States in 2009. As a group, the acute leukemias are characterized by the presence of blasts and immature leukocytes in the peripheral blood and bone marrow. Anemia is usually present. Anemia can be caused by bleeding and the replacement of normal marrow elements by leukemic blasts. Although the total leukocyte count is usually elevated, some patients may demonstrate normal or decreased leukocyte counts. Thrombocytopenia is also usually present in patients with acute leukemia.

AML (also called acute myelogenous leukemia, acute non-lymphocytic leukemia, or ANLL) remains a lethal disorder, which kills the majority of afflicted adults. Nearly 70% of adult patients with acute leukemia ultimately die of infection. The median survival time for an untreated patient with acute leukemia is 3 months. Ninety percent of children and approximately sixty to seventy percent of adults achieve at least one remission. More than 25% of adults with AML can be expected to survive three or more years and may be cured. Remission rates are inversely related to age. Patients who are older than age 55 to 65 when diagnosed with AML, with a few exceptions, have challenging odds for long-term survival because of poor chemotherapeutic tolerance and inherent disease resistance.

MORPHOLOGY	CLASSIFICATION	NUCLEUS	NUCLEOLUS	CHROMATIN	CYTOPLASM
	L1 ACUTE LYMPHOBLASTIC (principally pediatric)	Uniformly round, small	Single, indistinct	Slightly reticulated with perinucleolar clumping	Scant, blue
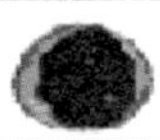	L2 LYMPHOBLASTIC (principally adult)	Irregular	Single to several, indistinct	Fine	Moderate, pale
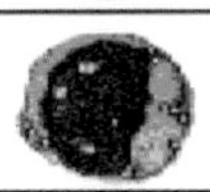	L3 BURKITT-TYPE	Round to oval	Two to five	Coarse with clear parachromatin	Moderate blue, prominently vacuolated
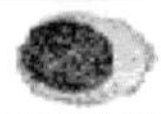	M0 MYELOBLASTIC (minimally differentiated)	Round to oval	Single to multiple, distinct	Fine to coarse	Scant, non-granulated
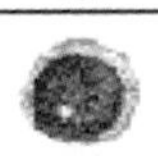	M1 MYELOBLASTIC (without maturation)	Round to oval	Single to multiple, distinct	Fine	Scant, variably granulated
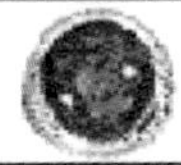	M2 MYELOBLASTIC (with maturation)	Round to oval	Single to multiple, distinct	Fine	Moderate azurophilic granules with or without Auer rods
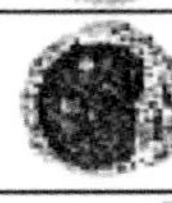	M3 MYELOCYTIC	Round to indented to lobed, "cottage-loaf"	Single to multiple, (granules may obscure)	Fine	Prominent azurophilic granules and/or multiple Auer rods
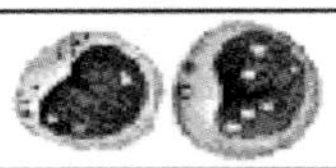	M4 MYELOMONOBLASTIC (biphasic M1 and M5)	Round to indented, folded	Single to multiple, distinct	Fine	Moderate, blue to gray, may be granulated
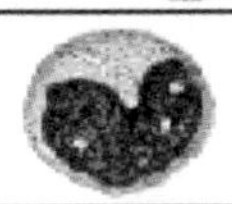	M5 MONOBLASTIC	Round to indented, folded	Single to multiple, distinct	Variable, lacy or ropy	Scant to moderate, gray-blue, dustlike lavender granules
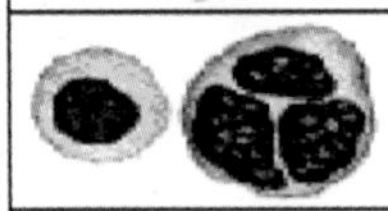	M6 ERYTHROBLASTIC	Single to bizarre multinucleated, multilobed	Single to multiple, distinct	Open "megaloblastoid"	Abundant, red to blue
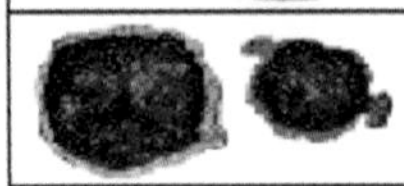	M7 MEGAKARYOBLASTIC	Round to oval	Single to multiple, distinct	Slightly to moderately reticulated	Scant to moderate, gray-blue, with blebbing

FIGURE 19.1 Acute leukemia: FAB classification. (Reprinted with permission from Rubin E, Farber JL. *Pathology*, 3rd ed, Philadelphia, PA: Lippincott Williams & Wilkins, 1999.)

PROGNOSIS OF ACUTE LEUKEMIAS

Modern treatment methods have produced a high rate of survival in children but the only significant progress in treatment for the last three decades has been confined mostly to younger rather than the majority of patients who are older. The best time to achieve the longest remission and possible cure of acute leukemia via maximum cell kill is when the disease is first diagnosed. Because treatment regimens vary, accurate diagnosis of the acute types of leukemias is critically important. Cytogenetic analysis and cell surface antigens provide some of the strongest prognostic information. The progenitor cell antigen CD34 and the P-glycoprotein, if expressed, predict an inferior outcome. AML associated with an internal tandem duplication of the FLT3 gene also predicts an inferior outcome.

FRENCH-AMERICAN-BRITISH AND WORLD HEALTH ORGANIZATION CATEGORIES

French-American-Brititsh (FAB) Classification

In 1976, a group of seven French, American, and British hematologists proposed a system of nomenclature, the French-American-British (FAB) cooperative classification system (Fig. 19.1). This FAB classification is based on the morphological characteristics of Wright-stained cells in peripheral blood or bone marrow and cytochemical staining of blasts. Since its introduction, the FAB classification (Table 19.1) that divides acute leukemias into two major divisions—AMLs and ALLs—has been widely accepted internationally.

The FAB system groups AMLs into subtypes (M0 through M7); ALL into three categories (L1 through L3). This system is based on the type of cell from which the leukemia developed and the maturity of cells. Classifications are based largely on how the leukemia cells look under the microscope after routine staining. In a revision of the original criteria, more than 30% blasts in the marrow suffice for the diagnosis of acute leukemia in any of the categories.

World Health Organization (WHO) Organization Classfication

In comparison to the older morphologically based FAB system, there is now increased recognition of the importance of genetic events in the classification and treatment of AML. The underlying rationale behind the **World Health Organization (WHO)** classification uses all available information—morphology, cytochemistry, immunophenotype, genetics, and clinical features—to define clinically significant disease entities.

Accurate classification of leukemias is essential in guiding therapy and provides useful prognostic information. In AML characterized by recurrent chromosome translocation—t(5;17)(q22;q12); t(8;21) (q22;q2) and inv 16(p13q22)—patients generally have a favorable prognosis. In comparison, leukemias with complex karyotypes, partial deletions or loss of chromosome, are frequently characterized by multilineage dysplasia and an unfavorable response to therapy.

GENERAL CHARACTERISTICS OF ACUTE MYELOID LEUKEMIAS

AML is the most common leukemia subtype with an estimated 13,000 new diagnoses yearly in the United States (Fig. 19.2). AML is a genetically heterogeneous clonal disorder characterized by a maturation block and the accumulation of acquired somatic genetic alterations in hematopoietic progenitor cells that alter normal mechanisms of self-renewal, proliferation, and differentiation. AML has been recognized as a heterogeneous disorder. Classification of AML subtypes is clinically relevant because particular abnormalities are associated with distinct clinical behavior—prognosis is favorable or unfavorable response to treatment.

The 2008 WHO classification of myeloid neoplasms is complex but it does continue to include categories that resemble the previous FAB classificatios of AML (Box 19.1),

myeloproliferative neoplasms (see Chapter 21), MDSs (see Chapter 22), and myelodysplastic/myeloproliferative neoplasms. These myeloid neoplasms have common features including

Neoplastic diseases in which a clonal abnormal stem cell overtakes normal marrow elements and fills the marrow with abnormal hematopoiesis

Abnormal hematopoiesis that may be effective, ineffective, or blastic

Genetic Differences

Although AML blasts evolve from common myeloid precursors, the subtypes differ in terms of the particular myeloid lineage involved and the degree of leukemic cell differentiation. In the movement beyond morphologic classification of AML to genetic classification, two major subgroups of AML have emerged, patients with disruptions of

■ FLT3 gene
■ Core-binding factor (CBF) complex

The FTL3 gene encodes a type III receptor tyrosine kinase. Upon activation, FLT3 exerts positive effects on a multitude of downstream pathways. FLT3 tyrosine kinase can be involved in leukemogenesis by a number of different genetic mechanisms. FLT3 is known to be mutated in up to 30% of patients with AML.

The CBF complex is a transcription factor complex critical for regulation of hematopoiesis and normal myeloid development. Disruptions of the CBF complex, t(8;21) (q22;q22)

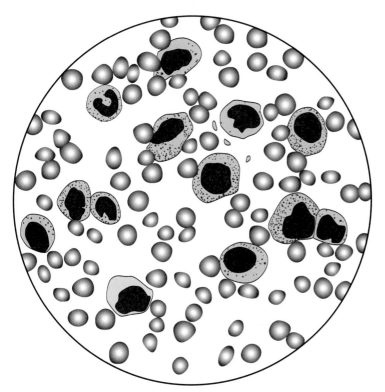

FIGURE 19.2 Acute myeloid leukemia. Increased numbers of immature cells are seen in acute leukemias. The predominating cells in this peripheral blood smear are myeloblasts and promyelocytes. The number of platelets (thrombocytes) is severely decreased. (Simulates magnification 1,000×.)

TABLE 19.1   The FAB Classification System

M0 myeloid	Undifferentiated blasts, AML—not otherwise categorized
M1 myeloid	Blasts and promyelocytes predominate without further maturation of myeloid cells
M2 myeloid	Myeloid cells demonstrate maturation beyond the blast and promyelocyte stage
M3 promyelocytic	Promyelocytes predominate in the bone marrow
M4 myelomonocytic	Both myeloid and monocytic cells are present to the extent of at least 20% of the total leukocytes
M5 monocytic	Most cells are monocytic; two subtypes (a and b) are recognized, one characterized by large blasts in bone marrow and peripheral blood, the other (differentiated type) by monoblasts, promonocytes, and monocytes
M6 erythroleukemia	Also known as Di Guglielmo syndrome; abnormal proliferation of both erythroid and granulocytic precursors; may include abnormal megakaryocytic and monocytic proliferations
M7 megakaryocytic	Large and small megakaryoblasts with a high nuclear-cytoplasmic ratio; pale, agranular cytoplasm
L1 homogeneous	One population of cells within the case; small cells predominant; nuclear shape is regular with an occasional cleft; chromatin pattern is homogeneous and nucleoli are rarely visible; cytoplasm is moderately basophilic
L2 heterogeneous	Large cells with an irregular nuclear shape; clefts in the nucleus are common; one or more large nucleoli are visible; cytoplasm varies in color
L3 Burkitt lymphoma type	Cells are large and homogeneous in size; nuclear shape is round or oval; one to three prominent nucleoli; cytoplasm is deeply basophilic with vacuoles often prominent

or inv (16) (p13q22/t(16,16) (p13;q22), constitute AML subgroups with favorable prognosis.

The two major subgroups of genetic disruptions in AML can demonstrate interaction in initiating and maintaining the leukemic clone.

Micro-RNAs

Micro-RNA expression is associated with cytogenetics, molecular and morphological alterations, and clinical outcomes in AML. Micro-RNAs are naturally occurring 19- to 25-nucleotide RNAs cleaved from 70 to 100 nucleotide precursors that hybridize to complementary mRNA targets and either lead to their degradation or inhibit their translation of the corresponding proteins. Recently, micro-RNAs have been

shown to be a new class of genes altered in several human malignancies and play an active role in malignant transformation, for example, hematologic malignancies. Micro-RNA signatures are capable of distinguishing between different leukemias, for example, AML and ALL, and also between cytogenetic subtypes of AML.

Acute Myeloid Leukemia

AML is characterized by an increase in the number of immature cells in the bone marrow and arrest in their maturation. This condition frequently results in hematopoietic insufficiency with or without leukocytosis. The subtype M0 consists of undifferentiated myeloid blasts (Fig. 19.3). The unique characteristic of M1 to M4 is the possession

World Health Organization Classification of Acute Myeloid Leukemia

Examples of World Health Organization Acute Myelogenous Leukemia (AML)[a] categories that are similar to FAB Categories

ACUTE MYELOID LEUKEMIA WITH CERTAIN GENETIC ABNORMALITIES

AML with t(8;21)
AML with inv(16)or t(16;16)
AML with t(9;11)
APL with t(15;17)

ACUTE MYELOID LEUKEMIA, NOT OTHERWISE SPECIFIED

AML with minimal differentiation
AML without maturation
AML with maturation
Acute myelomonocytic leukemia
Acute monoblastic/monocytic leukemia
Acute erythroid leukemia
Acute megakaryoblastic leukemia
Acute basophilic leukemia

ACUTE LEUKEMIAS OF AMBIGUOUS LINEAGE

Acute undifferentiated leukemia
Mixed phenotype acute leukemia with t(9;22)
Mixed phenotype acute leukemia with t(v;11q23)
Mixed phenotype acute leukemia, B lymphocytes-myeloid cells
Mixed phenotype acute leukemia, T-myeloid

Source: "How is Acute Myeloid Leukemia (AML) Classified?" www.cancer.org. Retrieved July 13, 2010.
[a]The 2008 World Health Organization. *Classification of Tumors of the Hematopoietic and Lymphoid Tissues*, 4th ed, Lyon: France contains all of the classifications.

of granulocytic differentiation with varying degrees of maturation. M4 represents a combination of myeloid and monocytic leukemias. M5 is the designated category for monocytic leukemias with additional subcategories. The M6 category is reserved for erythroleukemias, an abnormality of both erythrocytic and myeloid cell lines. M7 is the designation for megakaryocytic leukemias. Monoclonal antibodies are helpful in the classification of acute leukemias (Table 19.2).

FAB M0

FAB M0 is synonymous with the WHO classification of AML not otherwise categorized (Fig. 19.3). This category encompasses those cases (approximately 5% of cases of

adults with AML) that do not fulfill criteria for inclusion in other established groups. Patients are classified in this group based on morphological and cytochemical features of the leukemic cells and the degree of maturation. AML, minimally differentiated, has no evidence of myeloid differentiation. The myeloid nature of the blasts is demonstrated by immunological markers and/or ultrastructural studies. Immunophenotyping is essential. Evidence of bone marrow failure is characterized by anemia, neutropenia, and thrombocytopenia. There may be leukocytosis with a significantly increased number of blasts.

Among the acute forms of myeloid leukemia, some forms are more common than others. When a population of 358 untreated patients, children and adults, with AML were classified, FAB M2 represented approximately 45% of the cases and FAB M4 represented 19% of the cases. Together these two types comprised the majority of the cases. The least common varieties were FAB M3 and FAB M5b.

Acute Myeloid Leukemia (FAB M1)

The WHO synonym for this condition is acute myeloblastic leukemia without maturation. This form of leukemia is the most common type of leukemia in children younger than 18 months of age, but it typically occurs in middle-aged adults with a median age of 46 years. The typical male:female ratio of FAB M1 is 1:1. The median survival time is 3.5 months after diagnosis.

Clinical Signs and Symptoms

FAB M1 is characterized by either a rapid or gradual onset that may resemble an acute infection. The patient may have a history of fever, infections, fatigue, and bleeding episodes. Physical examination may reveal tenderness of the bones, particularly the ribs and sternum; ulcerated mucous membranes; petechiae; and purpura. Additional physical findings may include hepatomegaly, splenomegaly, and lymphadenopathy; however, approximately 50% of patients exhibit no organomegaly or lymphadenopathy.

Cellular infiltration of organs is less prominent in AML compared with ALL. Occasional localized tumor masses consisting of myeloblasts may arise in bone or soft tissues in patients with AML. In these tumors, the presence of large quantities of the enzyme MPO produces a green appearance if the tissue is cut. This type of tumor is referred to as a **chloroma**. In some cases, the appearance of these tumors is an early sign of AML.

Laboratory Data

Anemia and thrombocytopenia are present in approximately 85% of all AMLs. Leukocytosis is encountered in more than one third of patients, and the total leukocyte count is usually greater than 100×10^9/L.

The peripheral blood smear does not usually exhibit many immature erythrocytes, which are more common in other forms of acute leukemia. If severe disruption of

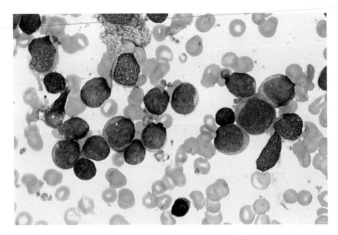

FIGURE 19.3 Acute myeloid leukemia M0. (Reprinted with permission from McClatchey KD. *Clinical Laboratory Medicine*, 2nd ed, Philadelphia, PA: Lippincott Williams & Wilkins, 2002.)

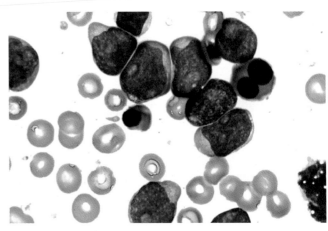

FIGURE 19.4 Acute myeloid leukemia M1. (Reprinted with permission from McClatchey KD. *Clinical Laboratory Medicine*, 2nd ed, Philadelphia, PA: Lippincott Williams & Wilkins, 2002.)

erythrocyte development does occur and many immature forms are present, the leukemia is possibly an erythroleukemia (FAB M6).

The outstanding feature of the peripheral blood smear (Fig. 19.4) and bone marrow is the predominance of myeloblasts. These blasts usually have a regular cytoplasmic outline and may contain slender, red-staining Auer rods in the cytoplasm. The nuclear chromatin is very fine and homogeneous. Three to five nucleoli are usually evident. Some differential development of the myeloid cell line may be noted. Depending on the type, some promyelocytes may be present. Agranular or hypogranular segmented neutrophils may be seen (acquired Pelger-Huët anomaly). Abnormal eosinophils may also be seen. Monocytes usually constitute less than 1% of the nucleated cells in the peripheral blood.

Acute Myeloid Leukemia (FAB M2)

The WHO synonym for this disease is acute myeloblastic leukemia with maturation. The FAB M2 form of leukemia typically occurs in middle-aged persons. The median age of occurrence is 48 years; however, approximately 40% of cases occur in individuals 60 years or older. The approximate

TABLE 19.2	Examples of Monoclonal Antibody Classification of Acute Leukemias
Myeloid lineage	CD13, CD3, CD15, MPO, CD117
T-cell lineage	CD2, CD3, CD5, CD7
B-cell lineage	CD19, CD20, CD22, CD79a
Megakaryoblastic	CD41, CD61

male:female ratio is 1.6:1. The median survival time is 8.5 months.

Clinical Signs and Symptoms

Hemorrhagic manifestations such as easy bruising, epistaxis, gingival bleeding, and petechiae are common initial symptoms. Hepatomegaly, splenomegaly, and lymphadenopathy are seen infrequently.

Laboratory Data

Anemia and thrombocytopenia are present in most cases. Leukocytosis is commonly seen, with rare patients having total leukocyte counts exceeding 300×10^9/L.

Myeloblasts predominate on peripheral blood smears (Fig. 19.5). The nuclei are usually round or oval with one or more prominent nucleoli and fine reticular chromatin. The cytoplasm is basophilic with a variable number of azurophilic granules. Auer rods are commonly seen. Maturation of the granulocytic cell line is also observed.

Acute Promyelocytic Leukemia (FAB M3)

In acute promyelocytic leukemia (APL), the median age of occurrence is 38 years, with a median survival of approximately 16 months. The approximate male:female ratio is 2:1.

Since the introduction of all-trans retinoic acid (ATRA) in the treatment and optimization of the ATRA-based regimens, the complete remission rate has reached greater than 90%, and 5-year disease-free survival is greater than 90%. This treatment regimen is the first model of molecular target-based induction of differentiation and apoptosis, ahead of targeting therapy with imatinib mesylate for CML.

Clinical Signs and Symptoms

Fatigue and symptoms of bleeding such as bruising, hematuria, and petechiae are common. Hepatomegaly, splenomegaly, and lymphadenopathy are seen infrequently. M3

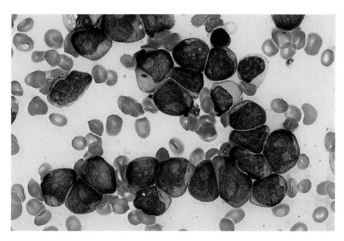

FIGURE 19.5 Acute myeloid leukemia M2 with numerous single Auer rods. (Reprinted with permission from McClatchey KD. *Clinical Laboratory Medicine*, 2nd ed, Philadelphia, PA: Lippincott Williams & Wilkins, 2002.)

appears to be the most aggressive of acute leukemia with a severe bleeding tendency and a fatal course, if untreated, of only weeks.

Laboratory Data

Laboratory findings may be similar to those of the FAB M2 type. Anemia and thrombocytopenia are present in most cases. Total leukocyte counts range from conditions of leukopenia to leukocytosis. Leukopenia is seen frequently. Promyelocytes are the predominating cell type (Fig. 19.6). The promyelocytes may be hypergranular, microgranular, or hypogranular variations. Coarsely granular promyelocytes with dumbbell-shaped or bilobed nuclei may be seen. The nuclear chromatin is finely reticular and the cells often lack nucleoli. Myeloblasts and cells at the myelocyte level of development may also be present and contain many small Auer rods. An increased incidence of disseminated intravascular coagulation (DIC) (see Chapter 24) is common.

Cytogenetically, M3 is characterized by a balanced reciprocal translocation between chromosomes 15 and 17, which results in the fusion between PML gene and retinoic acid receptor α (RARα).

Microgranular (hypogranular) variant of acute promyelocytic leukemia (aPML-M3v) (Fig. 19.7) accounts for 20% to 30% of aPML. It is impossible to diagnose aPML-M3v with modern testing because the leukemic cells do not show the hypergranular cytoplasm and dysplastic changes of the nucleus as seen in typical cases of aPML. Morphologically, the tumor cells resemble monoblasts with few, fine cytoplasmic granules and bilobed and irregular nuclei. Only rare cells exhibit Auer rods. The presence of the PML/RARα gene is essential for the diagnosis of aPML because more than 95% of AML-M3 cases have the PML/RARα fusion protein. The need to identify the PML/RARα gene fusion product is essential for the clinical management of these patients and the potential to achieve 3-year disease-free survival rates.

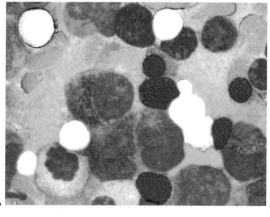

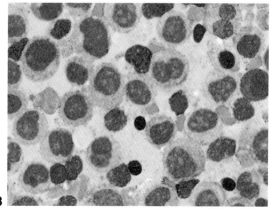

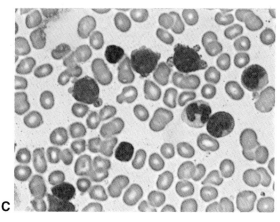

FIGURE 19.6 Acute promyelocytic FAB M3. Subtypes **A:** Classic M3. **B:** Microgranular variant (M_3v). **C:** Hyperbasophilic variant. (Reprinted with permission from Greer JP, et al. *Wintrobe's Clinical Hematology*, 11th ed, Philadelphia, PA: Lippincott Williams & Wilkins, 2004.)

Acute Myelomonocytic Leukemia (FAB M4)

The WHO synonym is acute myelomonocytic leukemia. This form of leukemia may also be referred to as **Naegeli-type** monocytic leukemia. Occurrence of this form of leukemia is uncommon in children and young adults. The highest frequency of occurrence is in adults older than 50 years of age. The average male:female ratio is 1.4:1. Most forms of myelomonocytic leukemia are of the acute form, with the average length of survival being approximately 8 months.

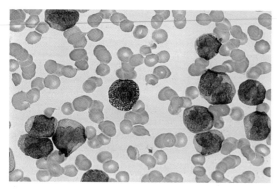

FIGURE 19.7 Acute myeloid leukemia M3 variant (hypogranular acute promyelocytic leukemia). (Reprinted with permission from McClatchey KD. *Clinical Laboratory Medicine*, 2nd ed, Philadelphia, PA: Lippincott Williams & Wilkins, 2002.)

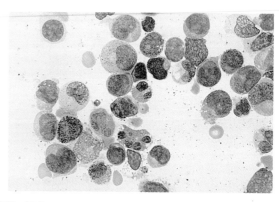

FIGURE 19.9 Wright-stained bone marrow with myeloblasts, monoblasts, and abnormal eosinophils with large basophilic granules. (Reprinted with permission from Greer JP, et al. *Wintrobe's Clinical Hematology*, 11th ed, Philadelphia, PA: Lippincott Williams & Wilkins, 2004.)

Juvenile myelomonocytic leukemia (JMML) is a rare malignant disease in children that accounts for less than 3% of all childhood hematologic malignancies. Treatment of JMML has no curative therapy except for stem cell transplantation.

Clinical Signs and Symptoms

Symptoms of this form of leukemia are similar to those of other forms of acute leukemia. Fatigue, fever, and bleeding manifestations are common. Pharyngitis may be observed. Hepatomegaly and splenomegaly are seen in about one third of patients. Gingival hyperplasia due to leukemic infiltration may be noted.

Patients with FAB M4 or FAB M5 leukemia or ALL (predominantly of the T-cell type) with hyperleukocytosis (an excessive increase in the total leukocyte count) are at risk of leukostasis development. **Leukostasis** refers to a pathological finding of slightly dilated, thin-walled vessels filled with leukemic cells. The brain and lungs are the most commonly involved organs. Symptoms of leukostasis are headache, visual impairment, and shortness of breath.

Laboratory Data

In FAB M4 (Fig. 19.8) proliferation of granulocytes and monocytes is characteristic. Anemia and thrombocytopenia are present. The total leukocyte count varies from leukopenia to leukocytosis. The total leukocyte count rarely exceeds 100×10^9/L. In many patients, the absolute monocyte count reaches or exceeds 5×10^9/L in the peripheral blood.

On a peripheral blood smear, early myeloid cells predominate, but approximately 20% of the cellular elements are monocytes. The blasts may have indented and convoluted nuclei as in monocytes. The number of nucleoli averages from three to five. Auer rods may be present. Promyelocytes are often present but do not predominate. Agranular and hypogranular neutrophils may be seen, and an acquired pseudo–Pelger-Huët anomaly may be noted. The number of platelets is usually reduced. Erythrocytic precursors are not usually seen. DIC can be observed.

A variant of FAB M4 is FABM4 Eo. A bone marrow aspiration (Fig. 19.9) reveals myeloblasts and monoblasts along with abnormal eosinophils.

Acute Monocytic Leukemia (FAB M5)

Pure monocytic leukemia is uncommon and comprises less than 15% of all leukemias. Two forms, FAB M5a (Fig. 19.10) and FAB M5b (Fig. 19.11), have been distinguished. The WHO synonyms are acute monoblastic leukemia (FAB M5a) and acute monocytic leukemia (FAB M5b), respectively.

The FAB M5a form is most common in young adults (median age, 16 years); the FAB M5b form has a peak occurrence characteristically during middle age (median age, 49 years). The male:female ratio is about 0.7:1 in the M5A form and is approximately 1.8:1 in the M5B form. Because this form of acute leukemia is very resistant to therapy, the life expectancy is short, ranging from 5 to 8 months depending on the type.

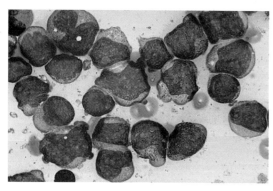

FIGURE 19.8 Acute myeloid leukemia M4. (Reprinted with permission from McClatchey KD. *Clinical Laboratory Medicine*, 2nd ed, Philadelphia, PA: Lippincott Williams & Wilkins, 2002.)

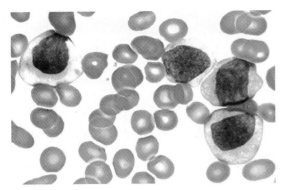

FIGURE 19.10 Acute monocytic leukemia M5a. (Reprinted with permission from McClatchey KD. *Clinical Laboratory Medicine*, 2nd ed, Philadelphia, PA: Lippincott Williams & Wilkins, 2002.)

Clinical Signs and Symptoms

The onset of this form of leukemia is dramatic, with headaches and fevers being the chief complaints. Typical symptoms of monocytic leukemia additionally include fatigue, weight loss, and bleeding from the mouth or nose. Physical examination frequently reveals gingival (mouth and gums) hyperplasia, as in myelomonocytic leukemia; pallor; and skin lesions. Enlargement of the lymph nodes and spleen is uncommon. Extramedullary masses may be seen in about one third of patients.

Laboratory Data

As in other forms of acute leukemia, anemia and thrombocytopenia are usually evident. The total leukocyte count ranges from 15 to 100×10^9/L. Peripheral blood smears (Fig. 19.12) normally exhibit a high proportion of blast forms. Monocytes and promonocytes constitute 25% to 75% of the nucleated cells. Blasts frequently have a muddy or smoggy gray-blue cytoplasm containing tiny granules, and pseudopods are common. The nucleus has a reticular granular chromatin pattern and may contain from one to five large nucleoli. A few immature erythrocytes may be seen occasionally.

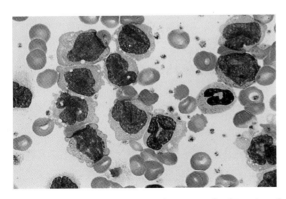

FIGURE 19.11 Acute monocytic leukemia M5b. (Reprinted with permission from McClatchey KD. *Clinical Laboratory Medicine*, 2nd ed, Philadelphia, PA: Lippincott Williams & Wilkins, 2002.)

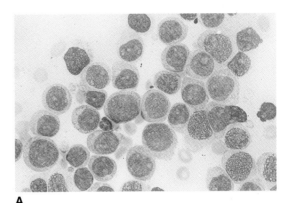

A

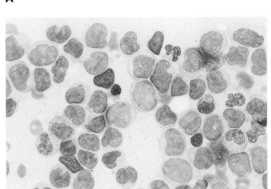

B

FIGURE 19.12 Acute monocytic leukemia (FAB M5). **A:** FAB M5a. **B:** FAB M5b. (Reprinted with permission from Greer JP, et al. *Wintrobe's Clinical Hematology*, 11th ed, Philadelphia, PA: Lippincott Williams & Wilkins, 2004.)

Erythroleukemia (FAB M6)

The WHO synonym for FAB M6a and M6b is acute erythroid leukemia. This form of leukemia, also referred to as erythemic myelosis or Di Guglielmo syndrome represents a proliferation of both immature granulocytic and erythrocytic cell types (Fig. 19.13). This form of leukemia is usually acute. The median age of occurrence is 54 years; usually, more than half of patients are older than 50 years. The male:female ratio is 1.4:1. The average length of survival is 11 months.

Clinical Signs and Symptoms

A common presenting symptom is a bleeding manifestation. Hepatomegaly, splenomegaly, and lymphadenopathy are infrequently observed.

Laboratory Data

Blast cells of erythroid and myeloid origin are found in both the bone marrow and the peripheral blood. Erythroblasts on blood smears typically have an irregular outline with a high nuclear-cytoplasmic ratio. Some of the blasts exhibit the intense blue color associated with rubriblasts. Blasts of myeloid origin may have Auer rods (Fig. 19.14). Promyelocytes may also be present as well as monocytes and promonocytes.

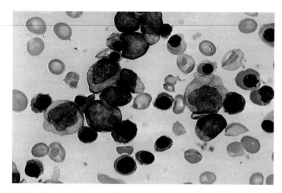

FIGURE 19.13 Acute myelogenous leukemia M6. (Reprinted with permission from McClatchey KD. *Clinical Laboratory Medicine*, 2nd ed, Philadelphia, PA: Lippincott Williams & Wilkins, 2002.)

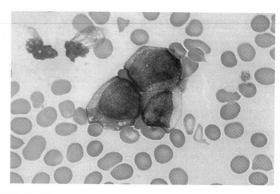

FIGURE 19.15 Acute leukemia M7. (Reprinted with permission from McClatchey KD. *Clinical Laboratory Medicine*, 2nd ed, Philadelphia, PA: Lippincott Williams & Wilkins, 2002.)

Selected Examples of Unusual Forms

Eosinophilic Leukemia

Eosinophilic leukemia is rare, although it can be indistinguishable from reactive eosinophilia or chronic myeloid leukemia (CML). If eosinophilic leukemia is present, it is usually acute. Death generally occurs within 1 year. Tissue infiltration and cardiac failure have been described in this form of leukemia. Signs and symptoms include a chronic cough, pulmonary infiltration by leukocytes, and central nervous system (CNS) involvement.

Twenty percent of patients demonstrate anemia and thrombocytopenia. Leukocytosis with total leukocyte counts of 50 to 200 × 10⁹/L may exist. A few patients may have absolute eosinophil counts greater than 100 × 10⁹/L. On peripheral blood smears, more than 60% of the leukocytes can be eosinophils. These cells are usually mature with segmented nuclei; however, the granules may not have the typical appearance of eosinophils. The granules may not stain uniformly, and some of the granules may appear empty. In the terminal phases of this leukemia, blasts may constitute

80% of the nucleated cells. Abnormal eosinophils are often present in small numbers in all leukemias.

Basophilic Leukemia

Basophilic leukemia (mast cell leukemia) is the rarest form of all leukemias. Frequently, an infiltration of mast cells in large numbers into affected skin is observed. Patients with this form of leukemia generally exhibit leukocytosis, with total leukocyte counts exceeding 30 × 10⁹/L. Peripheral blood smears can demonstrate greater than 50% basophils in this disorder.

Acute megakaryoblastic leukemia FAB M7

The WHO synonym is acute megakaryoblastic leukemia. In this form of acute leukemia, 50% or more of the blasts are of megakaryocyte lineage (Fig. 19.15). Acute megakaryocytic leukemia occurs in children and adults. It comprises approximately 3% to 5% of cases of AML.

Clinical Signs and Symptoms

Organomegaly is infrequent except in children. Radiographic evidence of bone lytic lesions has been observed in children.

Laboratory Data

Cytopenia is usually present, particularly thrombocytopenia. Dysplastic features in the neutrophils and platelets may be present. There is no unique chromosomal abnormality associated with this form of AML. Immunophenotyping reveals that megakaryoblasts express one or more of the platelet glycoprotein: CD41 or CD61. Blasts are negative with anti-MPO antibody.

Prognosis is usually poor, particularly in infants.

EPIDEMIOLOGY OF ACUTE LYMPHOBLASTIC LEUKEMIA

ALL is the most common cancer in children, representing 23% of cancer diagnoses among children younger than 15 years of age. It occurs in about one of every 29,000 children in the

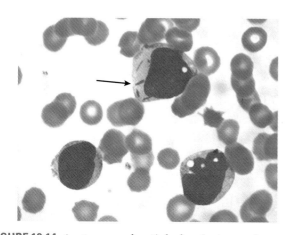

FIGURE 19.14 Acute promyelocytic leukemia. Auer rods are prominent (*arrow*). (Reprinted with permission from Rubin R, Strayer DS. *Rubin's Pathology: Clinicopathologic Foundations of Medicine*, 5th ed, Philadelphia, PA: Lippincott Williams & Wilkins, 2008.)

United States each year. ALL has a bimodal age distribution, peaking in children between 3 and 5 years of age and again in persons older than 65 years. Pediatric ALL occurs slightly more often in boys than in girls and in white children more often than in black children.

PROGNOSIS OF ACUTE LYMPHOBLASTIC LEUKEMIA

The improvement in survival for children with ALL over the past 35 years is one of the great success stories of cancer treatment. In the 1960s, less than 5% of children with ALL survived for more than 5 years. Today, about 85% of children with ALL live 5 years or more and 78.1% 10 years. Treatment of adults with ALL has lagged behind the results of treatment achieved with children.

CLASSIFICATIONS OF ACUTE LYMPHOBLASTIC LEUKEMIA

ALL is divided into

■ FAB L1 (children)
■ L2 (older children and adults)
■ L3 (patients with leukemia secondary to Burkitt lymphoma)

The three subtypes are differentiated based on morphology, including cell size, prominence of nucleoli, and the amount and appearance of cytoplasm (Table 19.3). Altered regulation of the cell cycle and apoptosis are well-established events in the process of neoplastic transformation. ALL cell lines and circulating leukemic cells from pediatric patients possess different regulatory mechanisms.

It is generally accepted that T-cell acute lymphoblastic leukemia (T-ALL) results from the malignant transformation of normal developing T cells in the thymus, the so-called thymocytes. In children, more than 85% of ALLs are of the L1 subtype. T-ALL represents only about 15% of pediatric

ALL cases. T-ALL represents 15% of childhood and 25% of adult ALL. The remainder of ALL patients have proliferating B lymphocytes.

The WHO classification that is synonymous with the FAB L1 and L2 classification is precursor B lymphoblastic leukemia/lymphoblastic lymphoma (precursor B-cell ALL)/precursor T lymphoblastic leukemia/lymphoblastic lymphoma (precursor T-cell ALL). Precursor B-cell acute lymphoblastic leukemia (B-ALL) is a neoplasm of lymphoblasts committed to the B-cell lineage. Precursor T-cell acute lymphoblastic leukemia (T-ALL) is a neoplasm of lymphoblasts committed to the T-cell lineage.

CHARACTERISTICS OF ACUTE LYMPHOBLASTIC LEUKEMIA

Clinical Signs and Symptoms

The history of symptoms in ALL can vary from a few days to a few weeks. Symptoms can include fatigue, fever, infection, headache, nausea, and vomiting. Bone and joint pain related to the replacement of normal hematopoietic elements is common. Pain in the extremities, particularly the legs, is produced by an infiltration of leukemic cells into the tissues. Physical examination may reveal petechiae or other evidence of hemorrhage and pallor. Gastrointestinal hemorrhage and hematuria are less common findings. Lymphadenopathy and hepatomegaly are present in 75% of patients. Leukemic meningitis and cranial nerve palsies caused by nerve infiltration by leukemic blasts are quite common. Leukemic cells can infiltrate many areas of the body (Fig. 19.16). Nephropathy may be present but is usually precipitated later by therapy that lyses the abundant leukocytes.

Laboratory Data

The total leukocyte count is elevated in 60% to 70% of patients, with total leukocyte counts ranging from 50 to 100 × 10^9/L. Less than 15% of patients have extreme

TABLE 19.3	**Morphological Classification and Characteristics of ALL**			
FAB Type	**Morphological Classification and Characteristics**			
	Size of Blasts	**Nuclear Shape**	**Nucleoli**	**Cytoplasm**
L1	Small	Indistinct	Scant	Invisible
L2	Large, heterogeneous	Indented, prominent	Large, abundant	Moderately clefted
L3	Large	Regular oval to round	Prominent, basophilic	Prominent, vacuoles

ALL, acute lymphocytic leukemia; FAB, French-American-British Cooperative Group Classification.

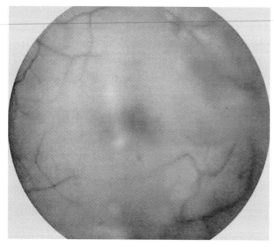

FIGURE 19.16 Leukemic cells in the vitreous of a boy with relapse of ALL. (Reprinted with permission from Tasman W, Jaeger E. *The Wills Eye Hospital Atlas of Clinical Ophthalmology*, 2nd ed, Philadelphia, PA: Lippincott Williams & Wilkins, 2001.)

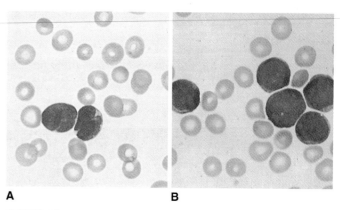

A   **B**

FIGURE 19.18 Acute leukemia. **A:** L1 lymphoblastic leukemia. **B:** L2 lymphoblastic leukemia, peripheral blood. (Reprinted with permission from Greer Courtesy of Greer JP, et al. *Wintrobe's Clinical Hematology*, 11th ed, Philadelphia, PA: Lippincott Williams & Wilkins, 2004.)

leukocytosis with a total leukocyte count of more than 100×10^9/L. In only approximately 25% of patients is a leukocytopenia present.

Peripheral blood smears (Fig. 19.17) show a predominance of blast cells in about 50% of patients. In addition to blasts, the peripheral blood is usually composed of close to 100% lymphoblasts, lymphocytes, and smudge cells. The blast forms have one or two nucleoli in the nucleus, and Auer rods are absent from the cytoplasm. These blasts have a high

nuclear-cytoplasmic ratio. The shape of the nucleus is usually round rather than indented or twisted. In addition, blood smears reveal a granulocytopenia, although some immature granulocytes are often seen in the blood as a response to leukemic replacement of the bone marrow. In the FAB L2 variety (Fig. 19.18), the lymphoblasts may have indented nuclei and frequently show mature cells of the myeloid type. Early forms of erythrocytes and megakaryocytes are absent in all forms of this type of leukemia. The presence of anemia, owing to decreased red cell production and blood loss, and severe thrombocytopenia are remarkable on peripheral smears.

Patients may develop meningeal leukemia following prolonged remission without evidence of abnormalities in the peripheral blood or bone marrow. In adults, ALL (Fig. 19.19) is differentiated from lymphosarcoma by the presence of poorly differentiated lymphocytes, which may have prominent nucleoli.

Special Identification Techniques

Surface markers, proteins on the cell membrane that can be detected with immunologic reagents, are extremely helpful in differentiating ALL (Fig. 19.20). Different proteins are expressed at different stages of maturation, which allows them to be used as markers of both cell lineage and maturation (Table 19.4). Terminal deoxynucleotidyl transferase (TdT) is an intracellular enzyme that catalyzes the nonspecific incorporation of nucleotides into DNA. TdT(+) lymphoblasts are found in the bone marrow and blood of the majority of patients with ALL of T- and B-cell lineage, except in some cases of B-cell ALL, and are believed to occur in a small number of patients with AML. TdT is also present in most cases of lymphoblastic lymphoma and in about one third of patients with CML in blast crisis. In the latter patients, this surface marker is a predictor of favorable response to treatment.

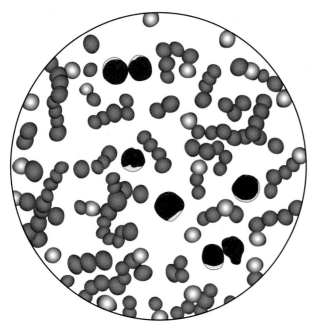

FIGURE 19.17 Acute lymphoblastic leukemia. Increased numbers of immature cells are seen in acute leukemias. The predominating cell in this peripheral blood smear is the lymphoblast. Blood platelets (thrombocytes) are completely absent from this field of the smear. (Simulates magnification 1,000×.)

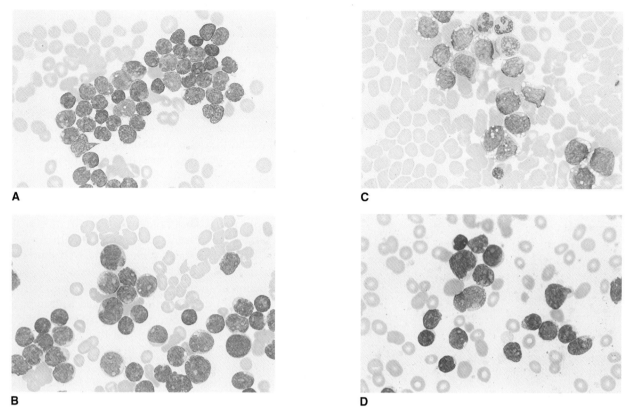

FIGURE 19.19 Acute lymphoblastic leukemia (ALL). **A:** FAB L1. **B:** FAB L2. **C:** FAB L3. **D:** ALL with cytoplasmic granules, bone marrow. (Reprinted with permission from Greer JP, et al. *Wintrobe's Clinical Hematology*, 11th ed, Philadelphia, PA: Lippincott Williams & Wilkins, 2004.)

The common ALL antigen (cALLA) is found on the surface of lymphoblasts in 70% of patients with ALL. CD 20 expression is associated with inferior survival in adults with ALL.

Treatment

Treatment regimens differ for Philadelphia (Ph) chromosome positive and negative ALL. Ph chromosome stems from a reciprocal translocation between chromosomes 9 and 22. Genetically, this translocation places upstream domains from the BCR gene from chromosome 22 in juxtaposition with the downstream tyrosine kinase domains of Abl, from chromosome 9. Although Ph chromosome is found in virtually all cases of CML, approximately 5% of pediatric and 25% of adult ALL patients demonstrate the Ph chromosome.

First- and second-generation ABL kinase inhibitors have become front-line therapy in cases of Ph chromosome–positive ALL. Incorporating imatinib mesylate, an inhibitor of the bcr-abl tyrosine kinase, into the hyper-Cytoxan (cyclophosphamide), vincristine, adriamycin (doxorubicin), dexamethasone (hyper-CVAD) regimen for adult ALL with t(9;22) has improved the patient outcomes compared to a regimen with imatinib mesylate.

MIXED LINEAGE LEUKEMIA

A new drug-resistant form of childhood leukemia may exist. This form, mixed lineage leukemia (MLL), has been established to be a distinct disease and not a subtype of the prevalent ALLs. Using DNA microarray technology, gene profiles of more than 12,000 genes established that about 1,000 genes were underexpressed and about 200 were expressed at higher levels in MLL when compared to ALL. This gene expression signature distinguishes MLL from classic ALL.

CYTOGENETIC ANALYSIS

Cytogenetic Analysis in Acute Myeloid Leukemia

Cytogenetic studies are important because two thirds of patients diagnosed with AML or ALL and 90% of patients with secondary leukemia will have leukemic blasts showing clonal chromosomal abnormalities. Chromosomal abnormalities differ between AML and ALL and among the various subtypes. Immunophenotyping and cytogenetic analyses assist in risk stratification and provide information that has important clinical, prognostic, and treatment implications. Not only can a patient's response to therapy and survival be

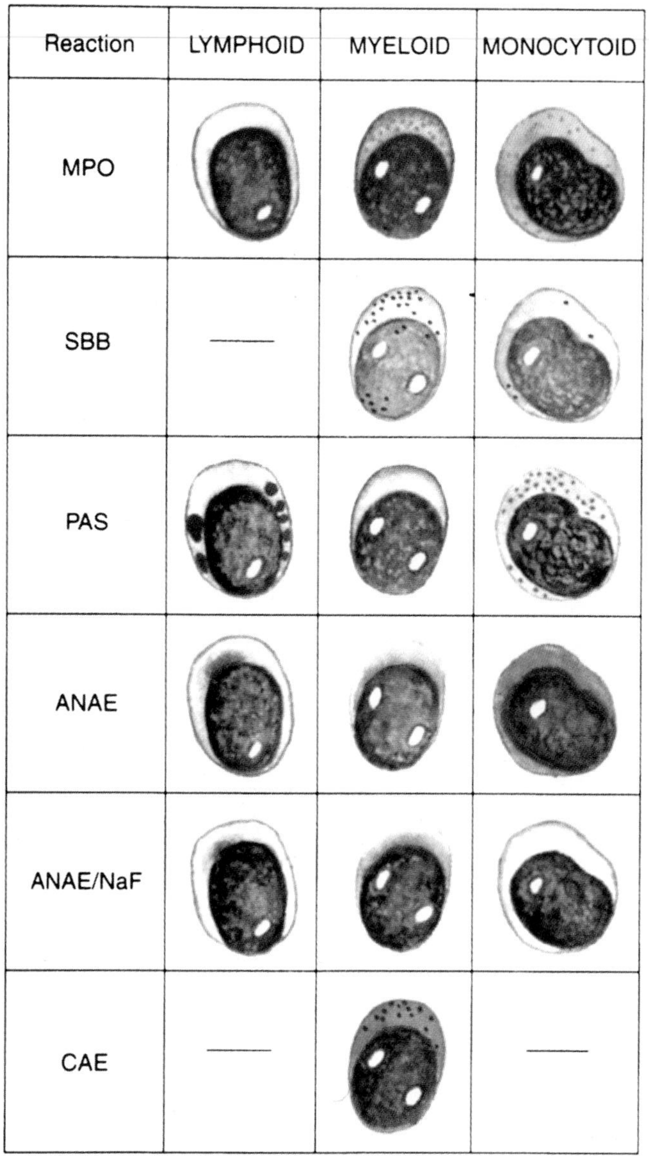

Reaction	LYMPHOID	MYELOID	MONOCYTOID
MPO			
SBB	—		
PAS			
ANAE			
ANAE/NaF			
CAE	—		—

FIGURE 19.20 Acute lymphoblastic, myeloblastic, and monocytic leukemias: cytochemical stains. PAS, periodic acid-Schiff; CAE, chloracetate esterase; SBB, Sudan black B; MPO, myeloperoxidase; NaF, sodium fluoride; ANAE, alphanapthol acetate esterase (with and without fluoride inhibition). (Reprinted with permission from Rubin E, Farber JL. *Pathology*, 3rd ed, Philadelphia, PA: Lippincott Williams & Wilkins, 1999.)

correlated with the karyotype and gene rearrangement of malignant cells but diagnosed patients can be monitored for remission and relapse (minimal residual disease) using chromosomal and molecular analysis.

Since the initial observation of the Ph chromosome, a number of other recurring chromosome abnormalities (such as gains and losses of entire chromosomes, deletions, translocations, and inversions) have been described in human leukemias and lymphomas, including AML, ALL, and non-Hodgkin lymphomas. Analysis of chromosome morphology (karyotyping) and specific banding patterns of individual chromosomes (refer to Figures 3.4 and 3.5 in Chapter 3) have been particularly

useful in terms of identifying the type of acute leukemia. The most consistent and specific chromosomal abnormalities that are found in human leukemia cells are translocations (Table 19.5). These alterations are found in leukocytes but not in other somatic (body) cells. Examples of chromosomal translocations and gene rearrangements consistently associated with specific hematological malignancies are given in Table 19.6. Abnormal gene rearrangements result from chromosomal abnormalities that are usually the consequence of chromosomal translocations and involve cellular oncogenes. Activation of normal cellular oncogenes by translocation-induced gene rearrangement is an important part of the process of malignant transformation.

Cytogenetic analysis of leukemic blasts has resulted in the identification of nonrandom clonal chromosomal aberration in a large percentage of patients with AML. Some of these lesions correlated with specific FAB subtypes. The importance of specific cytogenetic lesions as powerful determinants of the therapeutic response suggests that the mechanisms of transformation associated with these lesions are likely to influence directly the sensitivity of the leukemic blasts to therapeutic agents. An example is the highly successful therapeutic use of the differentiation-inducing agent all-trans retinoic acid. All-trans retinoic acid targets the chimeric protein encoded by the t(15;17) translocation associated with acute promyelocytic leukemlia.

The BCR/ABL t(9;22), translocation qualitative assay by RT-PCR should be ordered to screen patients suspected of ALL or CML for the presence of the bcr/abl transcript. This assay can be used to distinguish between the major and minor transcripts. The major transcript characterized by the p210 fusion gene product is typically detected in CML. The minor transcript, characterized by the p190 fusion gene product, is typically detected in ALL. The bcr/abl quantitative assay is intended for monitoring for genetic recurrence and minimal residual disease.

Cytogenetics in Acute Lymphoblastic Leukemia

About half of patients with lymphoblastic leukemia have abnormal karyotypes. Structural changes in ALL include t(9;22), t(4;11), t(8;14), t(8;22), t(2;8), and the Ph1 chromosome. Gains in chromosome 21 and losses in chromosome 7, 9, or 20 have all been cited. Although no consistent markers have been associated with L1 and L2 types of ALL, the t(8;14) alteration is commonly seen in the L3 type of ALL with Burkitt lymphoma morphology and other abnormalities of chromosome 14.

Patients with more than 50 chromosomes in their leukemic cells have the longest survival; patients with an abnormal karyotype have somewhat shorter survival times; and those with a t(4;11), t(9;22), or t(8;14) do relatively poorly.

PRINCIPLES OF SPECIAL CYTOCHEMICAL STAINS

Special cytochemical stains (Fig. 19.20) can be used as supplementary sources of information in the identification

TABLE 19.4	Immunological Markers in Acute Lymphoblastic Leukemia						
Type	FAB	TdT	CALLA	CD7	CD19	HLA-DR	SIg
Precursor B-cell ALL	L1, L2	+	0	0	+	+	0
Common ALL	L1, L2	+	+	0	+	+	0
Pre–B-cell ALL	L1, L2	+	+	0	+	+	0
B-cell ALL	L3	0	0ᵃ	0	+	+	+
T-cell ALL	L1, L2	+	0ᵃ	+	0	0	0
Null cell ALL	L1, L2	+	0	0	0	+	0

ᵃSome cases are positive.
TdT, terminal deoxynucleotidyl transferase; CD, cluster designation; CALLA, common ALL antigen; SIg, surface immunoglobulin; +, positive; 0, negative.

and differentiation of leukemias. Cytochemistry is the application of biochemical stains to blood and bone marrow cells. These stains reflect the chemical composition of cells through the use of color reactions, without damaging the cell to the point at which the cell itself can no longer be recognized. Cytochemical stains include

Sudan black B
MPO
Periodic acid-Schiff (PAS)
Naphthol AS-D chloroacetate (NASDCA) esterase
Alpha-naphthyl acetate-butyrate esterase with fluoride inhibition
Leukocyte alkaline phosphatase (LAP)
Acid phosphatase with or without tartaric acid inhibition

Sudan Black B Stain

The Sudan stains, such as Sudan black B, are substances belonging to a series of lipid-soluble pigments that detect cellular lipids. Hematopoietic cells contain finely dispersed cytoplasmic lipids as well as complex lipids, such as lipoproteins, in the cell membrane and in the membranes of the mitochondria and other organelles. These lipids are not identifiable in Wright-stained smears. However, when lipid-containing blood or bone marrow cells are stained with a solution containing Sudan black B, this lipophilic dye leaves the solvent because the pigment is more soluble in the lipids than in the solvent. On microscopic exami-

TABLE 19.5	Example of Chromosomal Translocation: t(9q+;22q−)
Code	**Meaning**
t	The translocation of chromosomal material from one chromosome to another nonhomologous chromosome
9;22	The numbers of the 22 pairs of autosomal chromosomes or pair of sex chromosomes that are involved in the translocation
Q	The lower portion (arm) of a chromosome involved in the translocation
P	The upper portion (arm) of a chromosome
±	The chromosome that *gained* the extra chromosomal material followed by the chromosome that lost the chromosomal material; these symbols may be absent

TABLE 19.6	Examples of Chromosomal Translocations Consistently Associated With Hematological Malignant Disease	
Disorder		**Translocation**
CML, ALL, AML		t(9;22) (q34;q11)
AML (FAB M2)		t(8;21) (q22;q22)
AML (FAB M3)		t(15;17) (q22;q21)
Burkitt lymphoma,		t(8;14) (q24;q32)
ALL (FAB M3)		t(8;22) (q24;q11)
		t(2;8) (p11;q24)
Lymphoma (follicular)		t(14;18) (q32;q21)
CLL, multiple myeloma		t(11;14) (q13;32)
T-cell leukemia/lymphoma		t(8;14) (q24;q11)
		t(10;14) (q23;q11)

CML, chronic myeloid leukemia; ALL, acute lymphoblastic leukemia; AML, acute myeloid leukemia; FAB, French-American-British classification; CLL, chronic lymphocytic leukemia.

nation, the concentrated pigment produces a black color in positive reactions.

Positive staining reactions are associated with the granulocytic leukocytes. The intensity of staining becomes more pronounced as the neutrophilic granulocytes mature. In this procedure, the monocytic cell line displays variable reactions, and the lymphocytic cell line is negative (Table 19.7).

This procedure is helpful in differentiating AML from ALL. In the FAB M1 variant of acute leukemia, intensely positive groups of particles may be localized in the Golgi region of the cell. Auer rods also demonstrate a strong sudanophilic reaction. Acute monocytic leukemia cells may display scattered positive granulation, and lymphocytes and their precursors are usually negative.

Myeloperoxidase Stain

Peroxidase enzymes are relatively rare in animal tissues; however, they are very common in plant tissues. In humans, peroxidases are found in the microbodies of liver and kidney cells and in the granules of myeloid and monocytoid cells.

MPO is located in the primary, azurophilic granules. However, primitive blasts that are committed to the myeloid cell line demonstrate MPO activity in areas such as the endoplasmic reticulum and the Golgi region. Positive peroxidase reactions produce a black precipitate, depending on the procedure.

A positive reaction pattern in early cells may appear as dots or rod-type structures, referred to as phi bodies. Cells of the myeloid series exhibit positive reactions that intensify as the cells mature, whereas cells in the monocytic cell line display a less intense positive reaction that is characterized by fine granular deposits scattered throughout the cell. Other cell types demonstrate negative reactions. MPO reactions (Table 19.8) and Sudan black B reactions frequently parallel each other.

This procedure is useful in differentiating acute myeloid and acute monocytic leukemia from ALL. Although MPO and Sudan black B reactions are usually parallel, rare cases can deviate from this pattern. Occasionally, an MPO-negative reaction may be associated with a Sudan black B–positive reaction, or an MPO-positive reaction with a Sudan black B–negative reaction. Examples of exceptional reactions include negative evidence of MPO in some persons who are in preleukemic states or suffering from severe infections and cases of positive reaction of lymphocytes in persons with hairy cell leukemia (leukemic reticuloendotheliosis). A condition of hereditary decreases in MPO also exists.

Periodic Acid-Schiff Stain

The PAS reaction is important in carbohydrate histochemistry. Positive staining reactions indicate the presence of glycogen, a polymer of glucose, and other 1,2-glycol–containing carbohydrates. Mature neutrophils contain high levels of cytoplasmic glycogen, which is physiologically related to the high energy needs of neutrophils in phagocytosis.

TABLE 19.7	Sudan Black B Reactions
Cell Type	**Reaction**
Positive reactions	
Granulocytic cells (neutrophils and eosinophils)	Become increasingly positive (sudanophilic) as they mature
Myeloblasts	May have a few, small granules in the Golgi region
Promyelocyte	Increased granulation
Neutrophilic myelocytes	Granules concentrated near the nucleus or rim of the cytoplasm
Metamyelocytes, bands, and segmented neutrophils	Strongly positive
Eosinophils at all stages	Granules react positively at the periphery of the granule
Monocytes and precursors	May have granules scattered over the entire cell
Variable reactions	
Basophils	
Negative reactions (Sudanophobic)	
Lymphocytes and lymphocytic precursors	
Megakaryocytes and thrombocytes (platelets)	
Erythrocytes	
Erythroblasts may display a few granules that represent mitochondrial phospholipid components	

The PAS stain involves a two-step procedure. The first step is an oxidation reaction with periodic acid, in which hydroxy groups on adjacent carbon atoms are oxidized to aldehydes. The second step is the demonstration of the resulting dialdehydes formed, using Schiff's reagent. A basic fuchsin dye in the Schiff's reagent produces a color ranging from magenta to purple, depending on the percentage of fuchsin dye in the solution. The color produced is at the site of the oxidizable carbohydrates. Several classes of carbohydrates produce positive reactions: monosaccharides, polysaccharides, glycoproteins, and mucoproteins.

The PAS reaction is strongly positive in neutrophilic granulocytes except blast forms, immature and mature platelets, and erythrocytes in erythroleukemia (FAB M6).

The usefulness of this procedure is in establishing the negative characteristics of myeloblastic and monoblastic leukemias from lymphoblastic leukemias (Table 19.9).

TABLE 19.8	**Myeloperoxidase Reactions**
Cell Type	**Reaction**
Positive reactions	
Neutrophilic granulocytes except blast forms	Strongly positive
Eosinophils	Positive
Monocytes except blast forms	Positive, but reaction is faint with few granules
Negative reactions	
Basophils	
Lymphocytic cell series	
Plasma cell series	
Erythrocytic cell series	

Esterase Stains

Esterases are a very diverse group of enzymes. Perhaps the most significant property of these enzymes is that their natural substrates are esters of carboxylic acids. The esterase enzymes are capable of hydrolyzing aliphatic and aromatic ester bonds. Many esterases have a low substrate specific-

ity and are referred to as nonspecific esterases. Those with high substrate specificity are given specific names, such as chloroacetate esterase. Several types of esterase enzyme reactions can be used in leukocytes to differentiate neutrophilic granulocytes and earlier forms from monocytic cell lines.

If a NASDCA substrate is enzymatically hydrolyzed by a cell's specific chloroacetate esterase, a free naphthol compound is liberated. This compound is then coupled with a diazonium salt to form a highly colored deposit at the sites of enzyme activity. Positive reactions are observable in cells of granulocytic lineage. This enzyme has occasionally been observed in promonocytes and mature monocytes. Monoblasts are negative. The reactions with this enzymatic substrate, with the exception of the FAB M1 class of AML, which is invariably negative for NASDCA, are similar to those with both Sudan black B and MPO stains but appear later in cellular development, usually at the differentiated myeloblast/progranulocyte stage (Box 19.2).

The nonspecific esterase enzymes alpha-naphthyl acetate and butyrate esterase are used clinically to recognize cells of monocytic origin. If the enzyme is of monocytic origin, it is inhibited by sodium fluoride; however, no sodium fluoride inhibition of enzyme occurs if the enzyme is of granulocytic or lymphocytic origin. This reaction also liberates a free naphthol compound from alpha-naphthyl acetate substrate. The naphthol compound couples with a diazonium salt, as

TABLE 19.9	**Periodic Acid-Schiff (PAS) Reactions**	
Cell Type	**Reaction**
Positive reactions[a]	
Neutrophilic granulocytes except blast forms	Strongly positive
Megakaryoblasts in malignant or proliferative disease; both blasts and megakaryocytes are strongly positive	Strongly positive
Erythrocytes in erythroleukemia (FAB M6)	Strongly to moderately positive
Variable reactions	
Eosinophils, basophils	Granules are negative; cytoplasm may contain faintly positive (PAS) granules
Monocytes	Faint pink cytoplasm, with or without granules
Lymphocytes	May contain a few pink or red granules
Thrombocytes	Intense pink or red
Megakaryocytes	Diffuse pink or red; may have coarse red granules
Lymphoblasts (leukemic)	30% to 40% may show strong coarse or block-like positivity
Negative reactions	
Erythrocytic series	Negative
Myeloblasts and monoblasts	Faint diffuse reaction may be occasionally observed

[a]Appear as a diffuse pink or large red aggregate of particles.

Esterase Staining Reactions

NAPHTHOL AS-D CHLOROACETATE ESTERASE

POSITIVE REACTIONS[a]
Promyelocyte
Myelocyte
Metamyelocyte
Bands and segmented neutrophils

NEGATIVE REACTIONS
Myeloblasts (variable)
Monoblasts (uniformly negative)
Promonocytes and monocytes[b]

ALPHA-NAPHTHYL ESTERASE (pH 7.6)

POSITIVE REACTIONS
Monocytes
Histiocytes
Segmented neutrophils (rare)
Mature lymphocytes (rare)
Megakaryoblasts
Erythroblasts

NEGATIVE REACTION (WITH SODIUM FLUORIDE INCUBATION)
Monocytes
[a]Reaction becomes more intense with maturation.
[b]Occasionally weakly positive.

in the previous enzyme reaction, to form a black deposit at the sites of enzyme activity.

Alpha-naphthyl acetate esterase, unlike NASDCA esterase, is strongly positive for monocytes, weakly positive or negative for granulocytes, and positive for other cell types.

Phosphatase Stains

The phosphatase enzymes are widely distributed in mammalian tissue. As a group, these enzymes liberate orthophosphate from organic phosphates. The two major classifications, based on pH, are alkaline and acid phosphatase. Microscopic determinations of these enzymes are based on methods that produce a visible precipitate of the organic phosphates hydrolyzed by these enzymes.

Alkaline Phosphatase

Chapter 26 contains a discussion of this cytochemical staining procedure and its clinical applications.

Acid Phosphatase

Acid phosphatase is one of many acid hydrolases that have been demonstrated in lysosomes. The acid phosphatases and other

lysosomal enzymes appear to be formed in the endoplasmic reticulum of cells that are metabolically active. These enzymes are then packaged into primary lysosomes in the Golgi apparatus and later take part in intracellular digestive processes.

Using a naphthol AS-B1 phosphoric acid and fast garnet dye procedure, a maroon pigment is precipitated at the cellular sites of acid phosphatase activity. Most leukocytes exhibit a positive reaction in varying degrees (Table 19.10) to this test. However, monocytes demonstrate a more intense positive reaction than do neutrophils. Although lymphocytes display little activity, T cells do exhibit intense positivity in the Golgi region, whereas B cells may be positive or negative. For this reason, the procedure is useful in differentiating subgroups of ALL.

An additional tartaric acid inhibition study may be conducted. Most of the acid phosphatase isoenzyme is inhibited by L-tartaric acid. However, the cells in hairy cell leukemia (leukemic reticuloendotheliosis), Sézary syndrome, and some T-cell ALLs are tartrate resistant.

TABLE 19.10 Monoclonal Antibodies Used in Leukemia and Lymphoma Identification

Cluster	Cell Type
CD1a	T
CD2	T
CD3	T
CD4	T
CD5	T
CD7	T
CD8	T
CD10	B
CD11b	M/G
CD11c	M/G precursors
CD13	G/M (most G, some M)
CD14	M, some G
CD19	B
CD20	B
CD21	B
CD22	B
CD25	T
CD33	G
CD41	Megakaryocytes and platelets
CD42b	Megakaryocytes and platelets
CD45	Various cells

CD, cluster designation; M, monocytes; G, granulocytes; T, T lymphocyte; B, B lymphocyte.

MONOCLONAL ANTIBODIES

Immunophenotyping

Immunophenotyping by flow cytometry will confirm the diagnosis of leukemia or establish a diagnosis in questionable cases. In addition to the surface membrane markers discussed previously, it is important to realize the role of monoclonal antibodies (Table 19.10) in supplementary differential testing in the various leukemias and lymphomas (Table 19.11).

During the past decade, considerable progress has been made in the identification and characterization of surface membrane antigens that are expressed by human leukemic cells. The majority of patients with ALL express surface antigens characteristic of normal B-lymphocyte lineage cells; smaller numbers express antigens of T cells. The use of immunological surface membrane markers has improved diagnostic accuracy. Rapid identification of the T-cell leukemias is important clinically because the prognosis is generally worse and therapy is difficult if delayed. Immunophenotyping by flow cytometry will confirm the diagnosis of leukemia or establish the diagnosis in questionable cases.

Granulocytes and monocytes can be effectively identified by using an anti-MPO antibody. MPO is expressed in cells of the neutrophilic and eosinophilic series and some monocytes. Other antibodies that can be useful are CD15, CD45RO, and CD43. The KP-1 epitope of CD68 and lysozyme react with other myeloid and monocytes/macrophage cells; the PG-M1 epitope is mostly restricted to latter cells.

Megakaryocytes can be identified in tissue sections by their positivity with factor VIII, CD42b, CD61m, CD31, and anti-LAT. These markers are more strongly expressed in mature megakaryocytes but can be used to identify immature cells.

Lymphoid

The most useful antibodies are those directed at CD20 (B cells) and CD3 (T cells) membrane markers. Precursor B cells express TdT, CD9, and CD 79a positive in early B-cell precursors, hematogones. In all, blasts are positive CD34 and TdT.

In addition, blasts CD34, TdT, and CD117 are expressed by immature cells and can be valuable in assessing the proportion of blasts present in a bone marrow biopsy. Residual blasts in posttreatment samples minimal residual disease.

CD68 is expressed throughout the monocytic differentiation, usually more intensely in macrophages than in monocytes.

Acute erythroleukemia can be identified by the antihemoglobin or antiglycophorin A immunostain.

Factor VIII/CD42b/CD61/CD31/anti-LAT is useful for the diagnosis of megakaryoblastic leukemia.

All TdT- and CD34-positive cells are present in almost all T- and most B-cell ALLs.

B-Lineage Markers

CD79a is more frequently present than is CD20 in precursor B-ALL. CD10 is positive in the majority of cases of precursor B-cell ALL and is rare in T-ALL. TdT and CD99 are usually negative in mature B-cell ALL.

T-Lineage Markers

CD3 with TdT identifies cases of T-cell ALL. Other T-cell antibodies—CD2, CD5, CD7, and CD1a—can be used in selected cases.

B Cell Markers

B-cell maturation (Fig. 19.21) is divided into the early pre-B, pre-B, and mature B-cell stages. The specific surface marker beginning with pre-B cell is CD19. The mature B cell is identifiable by the presence of surface immunoglobulin (SIg).

TABLE 19.11 Cytochemical Reactions in Selected Leukemias						
FAB Class	SB	MP	PAS	NASDCA	(α) NA (7.6)	Acid Phos
M1 myeloid	+	+	−	−	−	−
M2 myeloid	++	++	−	+	−	−
M4 myelomonocytic	±	±	−	±	++	−
M5 monocytic	±	±	++	−	++	−
M6 erythrocytic	−	−	+	+	+++	−
M7 megakaryocytic	−	(+)[a]	+	+	+++	−
L1 or L2 (T-ALL)	−	−	±	−	−	(++)[b]

[a]Test is performed on unfixed preparation.
[b]The reactivity must be focal or Golgi in nature.
SB, Sudan black B; MP, myeloperoxidase; NASDCA, naphthol AS-D chloroacetate esterase; (α) NA, alpha-naphthyl acetate esterase; Acid Phos, acid phosphatase; PAS, periodic acid-Schiff.
Note: Negative reactions for all tests, except for the PAS, indicate common acute lymphoblastic leukemia, pre-B or B-cell lymphoblastic leukemia, or unclassified acute lymphoblastic leukemia.

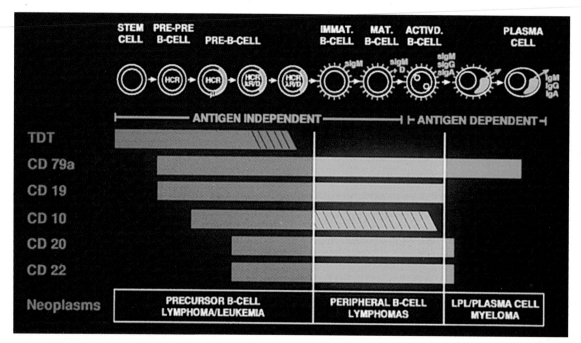

FIGURE 19.21 B-cell maturation. (From Jaffe ES, et al. *Tumours of Haematopoietic and Lymphoid Tissues.* Lyon, France: IARC, 2001:121. With permission from Elaine S. Jaffe, M.D. Chief, Hematopathology Section, Lab of Pathology, National Cancer Institute, Bethesda, MD.)

The immunological classification of ALL is based on potentially identifying cells in one of the preceding stages. Before the availability of specific B-cell monoclonal antisera against CD19 and CD20, many cases of ALL were incorrectly classified. The CD21 marker reacts with cells from patients suffering from B-cell chronic lymphocytic leukemia (B-CLL), B-cell lymphomas, B-cell leukemias excluding ALL, T-CLL Sézary syndrome, AML, and CML in blast crisis.

Other Surface Membrane Markers

Other surface membrane markers are widely distributed among plasma cells, some bone marrow cells, and some B-cell malignancies. The HLA-DR surface marker is found in various cells. In addition, some surface markers such as CD11b, CD11c, CD13, and CD14 are unique to granulocytes and monocytes.

LIFE-THREATENING EMERGENCIES

The most common life-threatening emergencies confronting patients with acute leukemia are
Infection
Bleeding
Leukemic infiltration of organs
Metabolic abnormalities
Hyperleukocytosis

Infection

Chemotherapy produces a decrease in leukocytes and nonintact mucous membranes. When these natural body defenses are compromised, the risk of infection is increased.

Bleeding

Bleeding can be the consequence of decreased platelets, leukemic infiltration of a tissue or organ, DIC, or other abnormal conditions (such as vitamin K deficiency). A decrease in platelets develops from leukemic infiltration of the marrow. A patient with a platelet count less than 20×10^{12}/L is at risk of bleeding if a lesion is present.

DIC (discussed in Chapter 24) is commonly present in patients who have AML. Leukemic patients with sepsis also can develop DIC. DIC can be mediated by the release of leukemic cell factors (e.g., procoagulants and fibrinolytic agents).

Leukemic Infiltration of Organs

Infiltration of organs with leukocyte or extramedullary involvement is more commonly seen in patients with ALL. Common sites of extramedullary involvement include the CNS, lymph nodes, spleen, liver, and testes. Skin involvement (leukemia cutis) or gingival infiltration is seen in approximately 10% of patients with AML.

Metabolic Abnormalities

Metabolic abnormalities may relate to the effects of products released from the leukemic cells. Tumor lysis may result in metabolic abnormalities after the initiation of treatment. Metabolic abnormalities include hyperuricemia and hypocalcemia, although these are rarely found at initial presentation.

Hyperleukocytosis

Patients with very high blast counts, most commonly patients suffering from AML who have greater than $50,000 \times 10^9$/L in the peripheral blood, are affected by hyperleukocytosis. The condition of hyperleukocytosis refers to clumping of leukemic cells in the vasculature of the lungs and brain. The condition frequently results in hypoxia, dyspnea, confusion, and coma and may be fatal.

Treatment Options

Refinements in the diagnosis of subtypes of leukemia and advances in therapeutic approaches have improved the outlook for leukemia patients (Table 19.12). Over the last decade, major advances have been made in the description of mechanisms related to leukemogenesis, particularly protein tyrosine kinase. This has led to the development of small molecules that specifically inhibit the abnormally activated kinase. The first such targeted therapy is imatinib mesylate, an inhibitor of the BCR-ABL fusion gene found in more than 90% of patients with Philadelphia-positive (Ph⁺) CML and in 20% to 30% of patients with (Ph⁺) ALL.

AML in older adults is a biologically and clinically distinct entity. It is known that leukemic cells in older patients are intrinsically resistant to standard chemotherapy. These patients need more effective and less toxic therapeutic options.

The primary objective of treating patients with acute leukemia is to induce remission and subsequently to prevent relapse. Remission is traditionally defined morphologically by the presence of fewer than 5% blasts in bone marrow together with the reduction of the number of immature cells in the peripheral blood.

Some genes are associated with treatment responses. Classic multidrug resistance (governed by the MDR1 gene) is associated with the expression of the membrane marker P-glycoprotein. This molecule transports antileukemic drugs (e.g., anthracyclines and etoposide) out of the plasma membrane, so that high levels of expression of MDR1 have been associated with reduced intracellu-

lar concentrations of chemotherapeutic agents in tumor cells.

Other genes involved in the mechanisms of resistance to chemotherapy and serving as predictors of treatment response are MRP, which codes for multidrug-resistance-associated protein; a transporter of the glutathione complex; and LRP, which encodes the lung resistance protein. Although the molecular pathways leading to the development of drug resistance in patients with AML remain largely unknown, drugs that reverse or abrogate resistance are being developed. Phase III studies of competitive inhibitors of P-glycoprotein (e.g., cyclosporine and its analogues) have recently been initiated.

Chemotherapy

Cytotoxic chemotherapy for acute leukemia patients is very intense. Most patients with AML and ALL will achieve remission, but high relapse rates exist.

Therapy is divided into two phases: induction therapy and postremission therapy. The major causes of morbidity and mortality during induction and postremission therapy are infection and hemorrhage.

Induction Phase of Therapy

Induction therapy consists of administration of multiple drugs aimed at inducing a complete remission or producing an absence of overt leukemia in the bone marrow or at other sites (Box 19.3).

Induction therapy for AML consists of a combination of a cytosine analog (cytarabine, Ara-C) and an anthracycline (idarubicin or daunorubicin). The complete response rate is 50% to 70%. Patients with an aggressive type of AML may

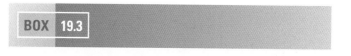

BOX 19.3

Adverse Prognostic Factors

FACTORS USED TO PREDICT A POOR RESPONSE TO INDUCTION CHEMOTHERAPY
Unfavorable karyotype
Age >60 years
Secondary AML
Existing disabilities
Features of multidrug resistance
Peripheral blood leukocyte count $>20,000 \times 10^9$/L

FACTORS USED TO PREDICT A RELAPSE
Unfavorable karyotype
Age >60 years
Delayed response to induction chemotherapy
Features of multidrug resistance
Peripheral blood leukocyte count $>20,000 \times 10^9$/L
Female gender
AML, acute myeloid leukemia.

TABLE 19.12	Favorable Prognostic Factors in Acute Leukemia
Acute myeloid leukemia	
Cytogenetic factors (patients aged 16–59 y)	
t(15;17)	
t(8;21)	
inv(16)/t(16:16)	
Acute lymphoblastic leukemia	
Children aged 1–10 y	

be treated with more aggressive therapy, including very high doses of cytarabine (HIDAC) alone or in combination with amsacrine, mitoxantrone, or etoposide.

Once remission is achieved, intensive treatment of patients with AML is essential to prevent a relapse.

Allogenic stem cell transplant from an HLA-matched related or unrelated donor is the only chance for a cure. Postremission therapy for AML yields a median leukemia-free duration of 12 to 18 months, with approximately 20% to 25% of these patients being cured of their disease.

Relapse

When treatment fails in patients with AML, the available options are determined by age, duration of the first remission, and cytogenetic findings, among other factors. Patients with favorable cytogenetic characteristics—t(15;17), t(8;21), or inv(16) mutation—who were in remission for more than 1 year before relapse have an approximately 20% chance of survival after subsequent therapy. For children and younger adults who have a first relapse or who do not have a complete response to first-line induction therapy, the recommended option is marrow-ablative (high-dose) cytotoxic treatment followed by hematopoietic stem cell transplantation, including autografts or allografts from genotypically HLA-matched related donors or phenotypically HLA-matched unrelated donors. Patients older than 60 years with adequate organ function are usually offered induction chemotherapy and have a 50% chance of remission.

Treatment of acute promyelocytic leukemia (APL) differs significantly from the standard therapy for other types of AML. Induction therapy for APL includes all-trans retinoic acid (ATRA) combined with standard therapy. Arsenic trioxide may also be included.

Induction therapy for ALL differs from therapy for AML, which uses two medications administered over 1 week. Induction therapy for ALL consists of a complex schedule of multiple drugs administered over 2 to 4 weeks. Medications can include anthracyclines, vincristine, corticosteroids, cytarabine, L-asparaginase, cyclophosphamide, or methotrexate. Unlike AML, postremission therapy for adults with ALL involves weeks to months of chemotherapy in combination with prophylactic treatment of the CNS. Chemotherapy with irradiation of the brain is used to prevent or treat leukemic infiltration of the CNS.

The postremission phase of therapy is aimed at preventing relapse. Postremission therapy is initiated approximately 4 to 8 weeks after induction chemotherapy has ended, once the patient has recovered from the side effects of therapy and his or her blood counts have begun to normalize. Postremission therapy for ALL consists of two parts: consolidation or intensification therapy in which multiple chemotherapeutic agents are administered over a 1- to 2-week period each month for 3 to 4 months, followed by maintenance therapy. This phase includes administration of daily oral doses of 6-mercaptopurine with weekly infusions of methotrexate. Maintenance treatment usually lasts for approximately 2 years. The long-term survival rate after maintenance therapy is approximately 30% to 40%.

Stem Cell Transplant

AMLs and ALLs are treatable by stem cell transplantation. Progenitor blood cells are considered to be pluripotent because they have the ability to evolve into different types of cells, for example, granulocytes, lymphocytes, etc. Some progenitor cells circulate in the blood stream and are called peripheral blood stem cells (PBSCs). PBSCs are found in much smaller quantities in the circulating blood than in the bone marrow but are becoming a popular mode of allogenic transplantation. The CD34 antigen identifies a population of stem cells that can reconstitute hematopoiesis after myeloablative chemotherapy.

Future Trends Vaccines

Vaccines for cancer, including AML, are under investigation. An ongoing clinical trial of peptide vaccines, derived from proteins called proteinase 3 (PR1) and Wilm tumor-1 (WT1), that can elicit highly active immunity against leukemia cells and induce remission has been reported to be successful in early trials with AML patients. The vaccine is intended to offset the accumulation of immature leukocytes in the bone marrow because of chromosomal translocations that cause activation of growth regulatory proteins and unregulated cell proliferation.

The proteins in the peptide vaccines are produced in large amounts by cells of MDS, AML, and CML patients. The peptides are combined with an "adjuvant" called Montanide to make the vaccines, and the vaccines are given with GM-CSF (sargramostim). Both Montanide and sargramostim help the immune system respond to the vaccines. The vaccines then activate the immune system to make specialized cells that search out and kill the MDS, AML, and CML cells containing the two proteins.

CHAPTER HIGHLIGHTS

General Characteristics

Acute leukemias are characterized by the presence of blast and immature cells in peripheral blood and bone marrow. The majority of adult patients will die of infection in a relatively short time after diagnosis. The best time to achieve the longest remission is when the disease is first diagnosed.

In addition to the traditional system of classification for leukemias, a new nomenclature for acute leukemias has been proposed. This system, the FAB system, classifies cells on the basis of their appearance and classifies the acute leukemias in AML and ALL types.

Acute Myeloid (Myeloid) Leukemias

Some forms of myeloid leukemia are more common than others. Each type has distinctive characteristics, clinical signs and symptoms, and laboratory features.

Acute Lymphoblastic Leukemia

This is the predominant type of leukemia in children 2 to 10 years old. ALL is divided into three FAB categories: FAB L1, FAB L2, and FAB L3. Cellular identification techniques include surface marker analysis.

Mixed Lineage Leukemia

A new drug-resistant form of all may exist, MLL.

Cytogenetic Analysis

Demonstration of chromosomal alterations and molecular pathology can be valuable in the diagnosis and treatment of patients with leukemias. At least half of patients demonstrate some type of chromosomal abnormality. Certain chromosomal abnormalities and gene rearrange-ments are consistently associated with specific hematological malignancies.

Methods of Cellular Identification

Supplementary testing in the acute leukemias is important because they typically have more than 20% to 30% blast cells. Cytochemical staining of peripheral blood and bone marrow smears is the most common supplementary test.

Monoclonal Antibodies

Monoclonal antibodies have become increasingly important in the study of leukemias and lymphomas. Other surface membrane markers are widely distributed among plasma cells, some bone marrow cells, and some B-cell malignancies.

Life-Threatening Emergencies

Infection, bleeding, leukemic infiltration of organs, metabolic abnormalities, and hyperleukocytosis can all constitute life-threatening emergencies.

Treatment Options

Chemotherapy and stem cell transplantation are treatment options.

CASE STUDIES

Future Trends

New monoclonal drugs and vaccines hold promise for more effective treatments of leukemia.

CASE 1

An 8-year-old white girl had been complaining of fatigue and had experienced night sweats for several weeks. Her mother took her to the pediatrician when she noted that the child was beginning to look pale and had some unexplained large bruises.

Physical examination revealed that the mucous membranes were pale. Hepatomegaly was present, but lymphadenopathy was absent. The physician ordered a routine complete blood count (CBC) and urinalysis.

■ Laboratory Data

The erythrocytes and hemoglobin were severely decreased. The total leukocyte count was 110×10^9/L. The leukocyte distribution on the differential counts was as follows:

Blast cells 53%
Promyelocytes 12%
Myelocytes 8%
Metamyelocytes 6%
Bands 4%
Segmented neutrophils 10%
Lymphocytes 7%

Auer rods were seen in many of the blast cells. The thrombocyte distribution was severely diminished on the peripheral blood smear. The result of urinalysis was normal.

Follow-up cytochemical staining demonstrated that the blast cells were positive for Sudan black B, with a variable number of moderate and coarse black granules. The PAS stain was negative. A bone marrow aspiration revealed hyperproliferation of the granulocytic precursors.

■ Questions

1. What is the most probable diagnosis in this case?
2. What types of supplementary testing could be done to establish the diagnosis?
3. What is the prognosis in such a case?

(continued)

■ **Discussion**

1. Although children are more frequently afflicted with ALL, the presence of increased numbers of immature granulocytes on the peripheral blood smear in conjunction with the blast forms suggest a myeloid leukemia. The absence of lymphadenopathy and the presence of hepatomegaly are consistent with the physical findings in AML.

2. In addition to the Sudan black B and peroxidase cytochemical stains, which were positive, cytogenetic studies to determine any chromosomal translocations or alterations may be helpful in establishing a diagnosis. A translocation of a portion of the long arm of chromosome 8 to chromosome 21, t(8;21), is seen only in leukemia of the FAB M2 type. The t(8;21) alteration is the most frequent chromosomal alteration in children.

3. The complete chromosomal analysis on this patient demonstrated not only a t(8;21) alteration but also the loss of a sex chromosome. This karyotype is predictive of a grave prognosis.

DIAGNOSIS: Acute Myeloid (FAB M2) Leukemia

CASE 2

A 12-year-old white boy had a sudden onset of fatigue, which increased. He had been diagnosed at birth as having Down syndrome and mental retardation.

Physical examination revealed that the patient had the physical abnormalities associated with Down syndrome, pale mucous membranes, and slight splenomegaly. No lymphadenopathy or hepatomegaly was present. The physician ordered a CBC and urinalysis.

■ **Laboratory Data**

The erythrocytes and hemoglobin were severely decreased. The total leukocyte count was 255×10^9/L. Distribution of the leukocytes on differential smear was as follows:

Blast cells 82%
Promyelocytes 2%
Myelocytes 2%
Metamyelocytes 1%
Segmented neutrophils 7%
Lymphocytes 6%

The distribution of platelets was significantly decreased. Auer rods were noted in many of the blast forms. The urinalysis was normal.

Follow-up cytochemical staining revealed that some blasts were positive for Sudan black B and for NASDCA esterase without inhibition by sodium fluoride. Negative results were obtained with alpha-naphthyl acetate esterase (monocytic esterase), PAS, and acid phosphatase.

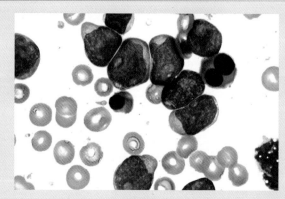

(Reprinted with permission from McClatchey KD, *Clinical Laboratory Medicine*, 2nd Ed, Philadelphia: Lippincott Williams & Wilkins, 2002.)

■ **Questions**

1. What is the most probable diagnosis?
2. What supporting laboratory tests would be helpful?
3. Does this patient have any special circumstances that are often correlated with leukemia?

■ **Discussion**

1. The presence of a severe leukocytosis and blast cells with Auer rods is diagnostic of an AML. However, additional testing of blood and bone marrow is needed to confirm a diagnosis.

2. In addition to the cytochemical stains that were ordered, a peroxidase stain could be performed. The results of a peroxidase staining procedure should roughly parallel the results of the Sudan black B stain. Cytogenetic analysis might be of additional value in differentiating between FAB M1 and M2 types.

3. The incidence of acute leukemias among persons with Down syndrome is about 20 times that in the general population. Several other congenital disorders, such as Fanconi anemia, are also known to be associated with a higher incidence of acute leukemia. Karyotypes of persons with Down syndrome and other congenital disorders show a high frequency of chromosome breaks that may be responsible for malignant transformations.

DIAGNOSIS: Acute Myeloid (FAB M1) Leukemia

CASE 3

A 38-year-old white woman had been referred to her family physician after seeing her dentist. She had gone to the dentist because she had been suffering from swollen, bleeding gums for several weeks. Physical examination revealed that the patient was pale and febrile and had hepatomegaly,

(continued)

CASE STUDIES *(continued)*

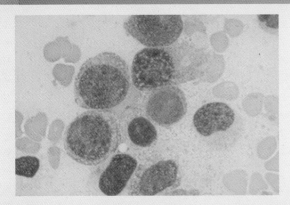

(Reprinted with permission from Anderson, SC, *Anderson's Atlas of Hematology*, Wolters Kluwer Health/Lippincott Williams & Wilkins Copyright 2003.)

splenomegaly, and lymphadenopathy. Her physician sent her to the clinic laboratory directly from his office for a CBC. On receipt of the results, the family physician admitted her to the hospital and requested a hematological consultation.

■ Laboratory Data

The CBC revealed a moderate decrease in erythrocytes and hemoglobin. The total leukocyte count was 32×10^9/L. The leukocyte distribution was as follows:

Blast forms 89%
Promonocytes 6%
Monocytes 4%
Lymphocytes 1%

The distribution of platelets was significantly decreased. Subsequent hematological study showed a platelet count of 0.12×10^{12}/L. Bone marrow aspiration revealed a predominance of immature and abnormal monocytes. No increase in granulocyte precursors was noted. The cytochemical findings were as follows: Sudan black B, slightly positive; NASDCA, blue granulation over the nucleus and cytoplasm of the majority of cells; alpha-naphthyl esterase, initially positive, but negative after incubation with sodium fluoride; and PAS reaction, negative.

■ Questions

1. What is the most probable type of leukemia in this case?
2. Would you expect the blasts to have any distinctive morphological features?
3. What are the cytogenetic findings in this type of leukemia?

■ Discussion

1. Pure monocytic leukemia is rare. Because this form of leukemia has a peak incidence after middle age, the patient's age is consistent with the peak incidence period. The rather abrupt physical finding of bleeding from the mouth and gums is also consistent with either acute monocytic or acute myelomonocytic leukemia. The supplementary cytochemical test results are consistent with a monocytic leukemia rather than a mixed myelomonocytic or other form of granulocytic leukemia. Additional analysis of the patient's karyotype might be valuable.

2. Monoblasts can also have the Auer rods that are characteristic of myeloblasts. The nuclei of monoblasts are frequently convoluted and twisted rather than being evenly rounded, as in most other blast forms. The cytoplasm might additionally have a smoggy blue-gray appearance. The cytoplasmic membrane is fragile and can be slightly irregular in shape.

3. In the FAB M5 type of leukemia, a chromosomal alteration of t(9;11) has been demonstrated.

DIAGNOSIS: Acute Monocytic (FAB M5) Leukemia

CASE 4

A 60-year-old white male bank manager saw his physician because he had been experiencing severe pain in his abdomen and back. He had also experienced frequent nausea for the past few weeks. These symptoms were very disturbing to the patient because he worked out regularly and was very health conscious. He neither smoked nor consumed alcohol. Physical examination revealed no abnormalities.

The patient's physician ordered a CBC and urinalysis. A radiographic examination of the lower back was also ordered.

■ Laboratory Data

Both the erythrocytes and the hemoglobin levels were below normal limits. The total leukocyte count was 185×10^9/L. Distribution of the leukocytes was as follows:

Blast cells 45%
Promyelocytes 4%
Myelocytes 10%

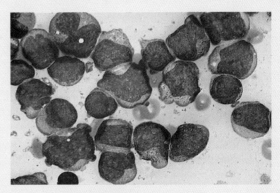

(Reprinted with permission from McClatchey KD, *Clinical Laboratory Medicine*, 2nd Ed, Philadelphia, PA: Lippincott Williams & Wilkins, 2002.)

(continued)

Metamyelocytes 3%
Bands 3%
Segmented neutrophils 5%
Monocytes 13%
Promonocytes 10%
Lymphocytes 7%

Platelet distribution was within the lower range of normal on the peripheral blood smear. The urinalysis revealed a small amount of protein.

■ **Questions**
1. On the basis of the peripheral blood smear, what is the probable diagnosis in this case?
2. What additional tests are needed to establish a diagnosis?
3. What type of leukemia does this patient have, and what is the probable prognosis?

■ **Discussion**
1. The presence of granulocytic precursors and monocytic precursors along with blast forms is suggestive of a mixed myelocytic-monocytic leukemia.
2. Cytochemical staining is particularly helpful in establishing a diagnosis. In this case, it gave the following results: 98 blast cells were positive for Sudan black B stain, with few to many black granules; blast cells were negative for PAS; 73 blasts showed a few reddish granules (monocytic esterase) in the combined esterase test; 5 blasts had a few fine blue granules with the granulocytic esterase test; and 4 blasts with both red and blue granules appeared on the monocytic and granulocytic esterase tests.
3. On the basis of the peripheral blood smear morphological appearance and the cytochemical staining results, a diagnosis of acute myelomonocytic (FAB M4) leukemia was established. It is basically a granulocytic leukemia, which usually runs an acute, fulminant course and carries a life expectancy of less than 1 year.

DIAGNOSIS: Acute Myelomonocytic (FAB M4) Leukemia

CASE 5

A 3-year-old black girl was taken to the emergency department by her mother because of an elevated temperature that could not be controlled by aspirin. The mother also reported that her daughter had been crying, pulling at her ear, and complaining of a sore throat for the past several days.

Physical examination revealed a well-nourished but listless child. The tympanic membrane was inflamed. The child had both lymphadenopathy and hepatosplenomegaly. The emergency department physician ordered a STAT CBC.

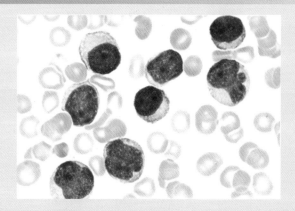

(Reprinted with permission from Rubin R, Strayer DS. *Rubin's Pathology: Clinicopathologic Foundations of Medicine*, 5th ed., Philadelphia, PA: Lippincott Williams & Wilkins, 2008.)

■ **Laboratory Data**
The child's erythrocyte count and hemoglobin level were substantially below normal. The total leukocyte count was 66.0×10^9/L. Leukocyte distribution on the differential smear was as follows:

Blast forms 76%
Prolymphocytes 12%
Lymphocytes 12%

The blast cells had one to two nucleoli and a high nuclear-cytoplasmic ratio. The nuclear shape of the blasts was round, and no Auer rods were seen in the cellular cytoplasm. The number of platelets (thrombocytes) was severely decreased.

Subsequent cytochemical examination revealed a strongly positive PAS reaction on the bone marrow lymphoblasts. The Sudan black B and esterase cytochemical stains were negative. Additional immunological testing revealed that the lymphoblasts exhibited a common ALL surface marker phenotype.

■ **Questions**
1. What is the most probable diagnosis in this case?
2. What additional tests could be done?
3. What is the prognosis?

■ **Discussion**
1. The predominant type of leukemia in children from ages 2 to 10 years is lymphoblastic leukemia. Peripheral smears in these cases show a predominance of blasts. The morphological appearance of the blasts is consistent with lymphoblasts rather than other types of blasts. These findings are consistent with a probable diagnosis of ALL.
2. Common ALL antigen is found on the surface of lymphoblasts of 70% of patients with ALL. Cytogenetic analysis would be of little value in a case such as this.

(continued)

CASE STUDIES *(continued)*

An additional PAS cytochemical stain may be valuable because PAS-positive particles are frequently found in lymphoblasts, sometimes in large quantities. This feature is important in differentiating between lymphoblasts and myeloblasts or monoblasts.

3. Although meningeal leukemia is frequently encountered in childhood ALL, remission rates for children are high. Approximately 90% of children achieve at least one remission. According to current statistics, approximately 50% of children with ALL will live at least 5 years.

DIAGNOSIS: Acute Lymphoblastic (FAB L1) Leukemia

CASE 6

A 12-year-old white girl was brought by her mother to see the pediatrician. She was complaining of joint pain, jaw pain, and tiredness. No bleeding was noted. She had no history of infectious disease exposure or recent immunizations.

Physical examination revealed that the child had an enlarged liver and spleen. A CBC, urinalysis, and urine culture were ordered.

■ Laboratory Data

RBC 2.61×10^{12}/L
Hematocrit 25%
Hemoglobin 8.0 g/dL
WBC 28.0×10^9/L
Platelets 57×10^9/L

■ Leukocyte Differential

Segmented neutrophils 5%
Lymphocytes 5%
Mononuclear cells 90%

Decreased platelets were noted on the peripheral blood smear; 2+ anisocytosis and slight hypochromia also were noted on the smear. The urinalysis was normal. The urine culture was negative.

A follow-up bone marrow examination and serum uric acid were ordered. The bone marrow revealed numerous immature, mononuclear cells. Subsequent partial immunophenotyping results were

Nuclear Tdt Positive
HLA-DR Positive
CD 10 (CALLA) Positive
CD 19 Positive
CD 34 Positive

The follow-up serum uric acid was elevated.

■ Questions

1. Based on the laboratory findings, what is the most likely diagnosis in this case?
2. What is the significance of the follow-up bone marrow examination and phenotyping?
3. What is the prognosis for a patient with this immunophenotyping?

■ Discussion

1. Based on the history, physical findings, and preliminary laboratory findings, ALL is a strong consideration.
2. This patient was diagnosed with common (L1) ALL. The presence of specific cluster designations (CDs) confirmed the diagnosis.
3. The prognosis is excellent. In fact, after initial treatment that achieved remission in 4 weeks and follow-up consolidation and maintenance therapy over a 2-year period, the patient returned to good health. Three years after diagnosis, she was well and needed no further therapy.

DIAGNOSIS: Acute Lymphoblastic Leukemia

REVIEW QUESTIONS

1. Which of the following are typical characteristics of an acute leukemia?
   A. Replacement of normal marrow elements by leukocytic blasts and bleeding episodes
   B. Blasts and immature leukocyte forms in the peripheral blood and anemia
   C. Leukocytosis
   D. All of the above

Questions 2 through 5: Match the following types of acute leukemia with their FAB classifications.

2. _____ Myeloid and monocytic
3. _____ Monocytic
4. _____ Myeloid without maturation
5. _____ Lymphoblastic (one cell population)

(continued)

A. M1
B. M4
C. M5
D. L1

6. Characteristics of FAB M1 include
   A. leukocytosis with maturation of the myeloid cell line in the peripheral blood
   B. leukocytosis with maturation of the lymphocytic cell line in the peripheral blood
   C. leukocytosis without maturation of the myeloid cell line in the peripheral blood
   D. leukocytosis with many mature leukocytes in the peripheral blood

7. The incidence of FAB M1 is
   A. high in children younger than 18 months of age
   B. high in children between 1.5 and 12 years of age
   C. high in middle-aged adults
   D. both A and C

Questions 8 through 12: Match the following predominant peripheral blood cell morphological appearances with the FAB classifications.
8. _____ A mixture of myeloid and monocytic blasts
9. _____ Blasts of the monocytic type
10. _____ Many coarsely granular promyelocytes with dumbbell-shaped or bilobed nuclei
11. _____ Myeloblasts, promyelocytes, and myelocytes
12. _____ Immature leukocytic and erythrocytic cell types
    A. FAB M2
    B. FAB M3
    C. FAB M4
    D. FAB M6
    E. FAB M5

Questions 13 through 15: Match the FAB classifications with the correct descriptive term.
13. _____ Leukemia secondary to Burkitt lymphoma
14. _____ Childhood lymphoblastic leukemia
15. _____ Older children and adults
    A. FAB M1
    B. FAB L1
    C. FAB L2
    D. FAB L3

16. Chloromas are associated with
    A. FAB M1
    B. FAB M3
    C. FAB M4
    D. FAB M5

17. A common characteristic of ALL is
    A. bone and joint pain
    B. many blast cells with Auer rods

C. leukocytopenia
D. a leukemia of older persons

Questions 18 through 20: Match one of the following chromosomal alterations with the appropriate FAB type.
18. _____ t(15q+;17q−)
19. _____ t(8q−;21q+)
20. _____ t(9;22)
    A. FAB M2
    B. FAB M3
    C. FAB ALL

Questions 21 through 23: Match one of the following cytochemical stains with the appropriate constituent.
21. _____ Sudan black B
22. _____ Myeloperoxidase
23. _____ PAS
    A. Glycogen
    B. Enzymes
    C. Lipids

24. The Sudan black B cytochemical stain differentiates
    A. acute myeloid from ALL
    B. acute monocytic from AML
    C. myeloid leukemia from a leukemoid reaction
    D. acute myeloid from acute myelomonocytic leukemia

25. Myeloperoxidase differentiates
    A. acute myeloid from chronic myelocytic leukemia
    B. acute myeloid and acute monocytic from ALL
    C. acute myelomonocytic from acute monocytic leukemia
    D. acute lymphoblastic from acute monocytic leukemia

26. The PAS reaction is
    A. positive in the neutrophilic granulocytes, except blasts
    B. positive in a block-like pattern in some lymphoblasts
    C. negative in megakaryoblasts
    D. negative in myelocytes

27. Esterase (naphthol AS-D chloracetate) differentiates
    A. granulocytic (promyelocytic to segmented neutrophils) from the monocytic cell line
    B. promyelocytes from myelocytes
    C. monoblasts from myeloblasts
    D. metamyelocytes from myelocytes

28. In the nonspecific esterase (alpha-naphthyl acetate) staining reaction, the cells of monocytic origin are
    A. strongly positive
    B. positive initially and positive after sodium fluoride incubation
    C. positive initially and negative after sodium fluoride incubation
    D. negative

(continued)

29. Specific nature B-cell surface marker(s) membrane is
  A. CD 79a
  B. CD19
  C. CD 20
  D. all of the above

30. Patients with AML have a good prognosis if
  A. Less than 45 years of age
  B. Over rods are present in blast cells
  C. Ph chromosome
  D. all of the above

BIBLIOGRAPHY

Bacher U, et al. A comparative study of molecular mutations in 381 patients with myelodysplastic syndrome and in 4130 patients with acute myeloid leukemia, *Haematologica*, 92(6):744–752, 2007.

Bell A, et al. Use of cytochemistry and FAB classification in leukemia and other pathological states, *Am J Med Technol*, 47(6):437–470, 1981.

Bonci D, et al. Blocking the APRIL circuit enhances acute myeloid leukemia cell chemosensitivity, *Haematologica*, 93(12):1899–1902.

Cascavilla N, et al. Philadelphia chromosome and BCR/ABL positive early T acute lymphoblastic leukemia (ALL) preceding B-lineage (CD10+) ALL, *Hematol J*, 4(Suppl 2):119, 2003.

Cazzaniga G, Biondi A. Molecular monitoring of childhood acute lymphoblastic leukemia using antigen receptor gene rearrangements and quantitative polymerase chain reaction technology, *Haematologica*, 90(3):382–390, 2005.

Chalandon U, Schwaller J. Targeting mutated protein tyrosine kinases and their signaling pathways in hematologic malignancies, *Haematologica*, 90(7):949–968, 2005.

Cochran DL. Unique features of acute promyelocytic leukemia, *Clin Lab Sci*, 10(6):315–319, 1997.

Cox CV, et al. Characterization of a progenitor cell population in childhood T-cell acute lymphoblastic leukemia. *Blood*, 109(2):674–682, 2007.

de Vries ACH, et al. Role of mutation independent constitutive activation of FLT 3 in juvenile myelomonocytic leukemia, *Haematologica*, 92(11):1557–1560, 2007.

DeThe G, et al. Viruses as risk factors or causes of human leukemias and lymphomas? *Leuk Res*, 9(6):691–696, 1985.

Döhner K, Döhner H. Molecular characterization of acute myeloid leukemia, *Haematologica*, 93(7):976, 2008.

Flotho C, et al. A set of genes that regulate cell proliferation predicts treatment outcome in childhood acute lymphoblastic leukemia, *Blood*, 110(4):1271–1277, 2007.

Gallo R. Human T-cell leukemia (lymphotropic) retroviruses and their causative role in T-cell malignancies and acquired immune deficiency syndrome, *Cancer*, 55(10):2317–2323, 1985.

Gallo RC. The human T cell leukemia/lymphotropic retroviruses (HTLV) family: Past, present and future, *Can Res Suppl*, 45:4524–4533, 1985.

Ghaith F, et al. Molecular genetic detection of P53, T(1:19), MLL gene rearrangement and cyclin D1 gene expression in acute lymphoblastic leukemia, *Hematol J*, 4(Suppl 2):115, 2003.

Griffin JD. Surface marker analysis of acute myeloblastic leukemia. In: Bloomfield CD (ed.). *Chronic and Acute Leukemias in Adults*, Boston, MA: Martinus Nijhoff, 1985:113–137.

Gupta P. Granulocyte colony-stimulating factor in children with acute lymphoblastic leukemia, *N Engl J Med*, 337(18):1320, 1997.

Hassane DC, et al. Discovery of agents that eradicate leukemia stem cells using an in silico screen of public gene expression data, *Blood*, 111:5654–5662, 2008.

Hershey DW. Detection of minimal residual diseases in childhood leukemia with the polymerase chain reaction, *N Engl J Med*, 324(11):772–773, 1991.

Hess, CE. Acute Lymphoblastic Leukemia (ALL). www.healthsystem.virginia.edu. Retrieved Nov 30, 2008.

Iacobucci I, et al. Identification of different Ikaros cDNA transcripts in Philadelphia-positive adult lymphoblastic leukemia by a high-throughput capillary electrophoresis sizing method, *Haematologica*, 93(12):1814–1821, 2008.

Jaffe ES, et al. *Tumours of Haematopoietic Tissues*, Lyon, France: IARC, 2001.

Jeha S, et al. Prognostic significance of CD20 expression in childhood B-cell precursor acute lymphoblastic leukemia, *Blood*, 108(10):3302–3304, 2006.

Korycka AK, Robak T. The interaction of new purine nucleoside analogues with signal transduction inhibitors (ST1571 and R115777) on myeloid progenitor cells in vitro, *Hematol J*, 4(Suppl 2):20, 2003.

Kroschinsky FP, et al. Cup-like acute myeloid leukemia: new disease or artifical phenomenon? *Haematologica*, 93(2), 283–286, 2008.

Li Z, et al. Gene expression-based classification and regulatory networks of pediatric acute lymphoblastic leukemia, *Blood*, 114(20):4486–4493, 2009.

Lo-Coco F, et al. Prognostic impact of genetic characterization in the GIMEMA LAM99P multicenter study for newly diagnosed acute myeloid leukemia, *Hematologica*, 93(7):1017–1024, 2008.

Lowenberg B. Post-remission treatment of acute myeloid leukemia, *N Engl J Med*, 332(4):260–262, 1995.

Lowenberg B, et al. Acute myeloid leukemia, *N Engl J Med*, 341(14):1051–1066, 1999.

Malfuson J, et al. Risk factors and decision criteria for intensive chemotherapy in older patients with acute myeloid leukemia, *Haematologica*, 93(12):1806–1813, 2008.

Mead AJ, et al. FLT3 tyrosine kinase domain mutations are biologically distinct from and have a significantly more favorable prognosis than FLT3 internal tanem duplications in patients with acute myeloid leukemia, *Blood*, 110:1262–1270, 2007.

Mittal P, Meehan KR. The acute leukemias, *Hosp Phys*, 37(5):37–44, 2001.

Mulligan CG, et al. BCR-ABL 1 lymphoblastic leukemia is characterized by the deletion of Ikaros, *Nature*, 453:110–114, 2008.

Musgrave BL, et al. Expression of death receptors and associated regulatory proteins in pediatric acute lymphocytic leukemia, *Hematol J,* 4(Suppl 2):20, 2003.

OBrien S. Ask the hematologist, *ASH News,* 7(1):5, 2010.

Olsen RJ. Acute leukemia immunohistochemistry: a systematic diagnostic approach, *Arch Pathol Lab Med,* 132:462–475, 2008.

Orazi A, O'Malley DP. Bone marrow immunohistochemistry, *Adv Lab Admin,* 12(1):22–24, 2003.

Paietta E, Wiernik PH. Acute versus chronic leukemic cells: Is phenotyping a good prognostic indicator, *Diagn Med,* 12:20–34, 1984.

Pedraza MA, et al. Acute leukemias: Ultrastructural, cytochemical, and immunologic diagnostic approaches, *Lab Med,* 14(1):45–49, 1983.

Penchansky L, Krause JR. Flow cytochemical study of acute leukemia of childhood with the Technicon H-1, *Lab Med,* 22(3):184–190, 1991.

Pui CH, et al. Human granulocyte colony-stimulating factor after induction chemotherapy in children with acute lymphoblastic leukemia, *N Engl J Med,* 336(25):1781–1788, 1997.

Radmacher MD, et al. MicroRNAs in Acute Myeloid Leukemia, *Hematologist: ASH News Rep,* 5(6):5, 2008.

Reed JC. Bcl-2-family proteins and hematologic malignances: history and future prospects, *Blood,* 111:3322–3330, 2008.

Rowley JD. Consistent chromosome abnormalities in human leukemia and lymphoma, *Can Invest,* 1(3):267–280, 1983.

Santamaria C, et al. The relevance of preferentially expressed antigen of melanoma (PRAME) as a maker of disease activity and prognosis in acute promyelocytic leukemia, *Haematologica,* 93:1797–1805, 2008.

Sekeres MA. Treatment of older adults with acute myeloid leukemia: state of the art and current perspectives, *Haematologica,* 93(12):1769–1772, 2008.

Staal FJT, Langerak, AW. Signaling pathways involved in the development of T-cell acute lymphoblastic leukemia, *Haematologica,* 93(4):493–496, 2008.

Stanley M, et al. Classification of 358 cases of acute myeloid leukemia by FAB criteria: Analysis of clinical and morphologic features. In: Bloomfield CD (ed.). *Chronic and Acute Leukemias in Adults,* Boston, MA: Martinus Nijhoff, 1985:147–173.

Starkweather W, Searcy RL. New stabilized staining procedures for classification of specific acute leukemia subgroups, *Am Clin Prod Rev,* 2(8):10–15, 1987.

Starkweather WH, et al. A systemic approach to the cytochemical classification of acute leukemia, *Lab Perspect,* 5:2–7, 1985.

Stone RM. Older AML patients:fit for what? *Blood,* 108(10):3233, 2006.

Tallman MS, et al. All-*trans*-retinoic acid in acute promyelocytic leukemia, *N Engl J Med,* 337(15):1021–1028, 1997.

Wang Z, Chen Z. Acute promyelocytic leukemia: from highly fatal to highly curable, *Blood,* 111:2505–2515, 2008.

Welte K, Riehm H. Granulocyte colony-stimulating factor in children with acute lymphoblastic leukemia, *N Engl J Med,* 337(18):1320, 1997.

Williams, DA. A new mechanism of leukemia drug resistance? *NEJM,* 357:1, 2007.

Windebank KP, et al. Acute megakaryocytic leukemia (M7) in children, *Mayo Clin Proc,* 64:1339–1351, 1989.

Wouters BJ, et al. A decade of genome-wide gene expression profiling in acute myeloid leukemia: flashback and prospects, *Blood,* 113(2):291–298, 2009.

Yanada M, et al. Karyotype at diagnosis is the major prognostic factor predicting relapse-free survival for patients with Philadelphia chromosome-positive acute lymphoblastic leukemia treated with imatinib-combined chemotherapy, *Haematologica,* 93(2):287–290, 2008.

Lymphoid and Plasma Cell Neoplasms

Chronic leukemias

- Describe the general characteristics, including clinical symptoms and laboratory data, of chronic lymphocytic leukemia (CLL).
- Explain the usefulness of chromosome analysis and molecular analysis in the diagnosis and prognosis of CLL.

Plasma cell neoplasms

- Describe the general characteristics and laboratory data in multiple myeloma.
- Describe the general characteristics and laboratory data in Waldenström macroglobulinemia (WM).

Lymphomas

- Describe the relationship between leukemias and lymphomas.
- Explain the characteristics of lymphomas and their relationship to clinical hematology.
- Describe some of the characteristics of Hodgkin disease.

Case studies

- Apply the laboratory data to the case studies and discuss the implications of these cases to the study of hematology.

MATURE B-CELL NEOPLASMS

The World Health Organization (WHO) Classification of Tumours of the Haematopoietic and Lymphoid Tissues, fourth edition, has enhanced the classification of lymphoid neoplasms by including immunophenotypic features and genetic abnormalities to define different disorders. This chapter focuses on selected examples of the disorders of the mature B-cell neoplasm classification:

- CLL/small lymphocytic lymphoma (SLL)
- B-cell prolymphocytic leukemia
- Hairy cell leukemia (vHCL)
- Plasma cell neoplasms

CHRONIC LYMPHOCYTIC LEUKEMIA/SMALL LYMPHOCYTIC LYMPHOMA

Chronic leukemias are generally characterized by the presence of leukocytosis with an increased number of mature lymphocytes, lymphocytosis, on a peripheral blood film. For example, malignant lymphoproliferative disorders (Table 20.1) are characterized by an accumulation of lymphocytes.

Both CLL and SLL are neoplasms composed of small B lymphocytes in the peripheral blood, bone marrow, spleen, and lymph nodes, mixed with prolymphocytes and paraimmunoblasts forming proliferation centers in tissue infiltrates. In contrast to CLL, SLL is used for nonleukemic patients with the tissue morphology and immunophenotype of CLL.

Epidemiology

CLL is the most common form of leukemia in adults in Western countries but it is very rare in far Eastern countries. CLL/SLL accounts for almost 7% of non-Hodgkin lymphomas (NHLs) in biopsies.

The median age of onset is 65 years. This form of leukemia is rare before age 20 and uncommon before age 50. But it is now diagnosed more often in younger persons. More males than females (1.5 to 2.1:1) are afflicted by the disorder.

CLL has the highest genetic predisposition of all hematologic neoplasms. A family predisposition can be documented in 5% to 10% of patients with CLL. The overall risk is two to seven times greater in first-degree relatives of CLL patients.

Etiology

Classic CLL is usually a B-cell disorder. Mature B-cell neoplasms are clonal proliferations of B cells at various stages of differentiation ranging from naïve B cells to mature plasma cells. Mature B-cell neoplasms (Box 20.1) comprise more than 90% of lymphoid neoplasms worldwide.

B-CLL is a biologically and clinically heterogeneous hematologic malignancy characterized by a gradually progressive accumulation of morphologically mature B lymphocytes in the blood, bone marrow, and lymphatic tissues. More than 90% of CLL cells are nondividing and arrested at G_0 or G_1 phase of the cell cycle. These cells are characterized as CD5+ CD19+ CD23+ monoclonal B cells.

An excess of B cells is more likely to be a result of decreased apoptosis and deregulation of cell cycle control than of an increased proliferation rate. CLL cells are very resistant to

TABLE 20.1	Classification of Lymphoproliferative Disorders
Type	**Alternate Names**
Acute lymphoblastic leukemia	
Chronic lymphocytic leukemia	
B cell	
T cell	
Prolymphocytic leukemia	
Hairy cell leukemia	Leukemic reticuloendotheliosis
Plasma cell leukemia	Leukemic phase of multiple myeloma
Sézary syndrome	Leukemic phase of mycosis fungoides
Non-Hodgkin lymphoma	
Large granular lymphocytosis[a]	
Reactive lymphocytosis[a]	

[a]These disorders usually have a benign clinical course.

apoptosis. The antiapoptotic BCL2 gene is reported to be overexpressed in 65% to 70% of B-cell CLLs.

Cytogenetics

CLL is heterogeneous at the clinical, cellular, and molecular levels. Chromosomal alterations occur in approximately 80% of CLL cases; these alterations include the 13q deletion, the 11q deletion, trisomy of chromosome 12, and the 17p deletion. The high rate of recurrence of the same chromosomal abnormalities suggests that these abnormalities may affect a common pathway.

Cytogenetic studies have demonstrated clonal chromosome abnormalities in about 80% of patients with B-cell CLL by fluorescence in situ hybridization (FISH) testing. Based on gene expression profiling of 18 genes using microarray technology, five distinct cytogenetically defined CLL subtypes have been identified. The most consistent finding is an extra chromosome 12 (trisomy 12), which is present in approximately 50% of patients. A translocation of chromosomes 8 and 14 is also associated with B-cell CLL. Chromosome abnormalities can be found in T-CLL and adult T-cell leukemia. A variety of chromosomal abnormalities are found, the most consistent being trisomy 7. In non-T and non-B types, a translocation of chromosomes 9 and 22 may be observed. Immunologically, B cells display the classic surface immunoglobulin (SIg) marker. In addition, B cells can be identified by monoclonal antibodies as expressing CD19, CD20 or CD24, and CD5 markers.

Another technique that can be valuable in CLL includes the polymerase chain reaction (PCR). This procedure reveals the nature of a lymphoid neoplasm and detects residual disease, which can lead to relapse of the disease. PCR produces multiple copies of a scarce sequence of DNA by using recombinant DNA methods.

Molecular genetics has two major applications in the analysis of chronic lymphoid malignancies:

- Demonstration of the clonal nature of a population of lymphoid cells
- Detection of pathogenetically important rearrangements, for example, clonal IG or TCR gene rearrangements, that are useful in diagnosis of CLL

Molecular genetic detection of genomic rearrangements may not only assist with the diagnosis but can also provide important prognostic information. Many of these rearrangements can act as molecular markers for the detection of low levels of residual disease.

BOX 20.1

Examples of World Health Organization of Mature B-Cell Neoplasms

- Chronic lymphocytic leukemia/small lymphocytic leukemia
- B-cell prolymphocytic leukemia
- Hairy cell leukemia
- Plasma cell myeloma
- Monoclonal gammopathy of undetermined significance (MGUS)
- Primary amyloidosis
- Heavy chain diseases
- Burkitt lymphoma/leukemia

Molecular Genetics

Variable Region Genes

New knowledge regarding the biology of CLL has demonstrated that approximately 50% to 70% of CLL cases undergo immunoglobulin variable region genes (IgV_H) hypermutation. The IgV_H mutational status is important in determining the prognosis of patients with CLL.

Patients with mutated CLL have a better prognosis than those with unmutated CLL, at least for those with a low stage. Cases can be divided into two subgroups on the basis of the presence or absence of somatic mutations in the specific immunoglobulin heavy-chain variable-region (IgV_H) genes used by the leukemic cells. The mutation status of the immunoglobulin variable (V) gene segments allows for differentiation between mutated and unmutated CLL, with low or high risk for disease progression, respectively. Mutations in these genes are somehow closely linked to the clinical courses. Patients whose leukemic B cells express IgV_H have a better survival rate (e.g., 24-year survival) compared with patients who lack such mutations (e.g., 6- to 8-year survival).

The leukemic cells from patients with few or no IgV_H mutations more frequently have cytogenetic changes that forecast a poor clinical outcome (e.g., a 11q22-23 deletion, a 17p deletion, trisomy 12, or p53 dysfunction). Patients with biologically significant numbers of IgV_H mutations more frequently have chromosomal changes associated with a benign course of the disease (e.g., a 13q14 deletion).

Zeta-chain–Associated Protein 70

Another signaling associated molecule, the zeta-chain–associated protein 70 (ZAP-70), was recently discovered to be differentially expressed in the CLL subgroup without IgV_H mutation that had poor outcomes. ZAP-70, an enzyme normally expressed in T lymphocytes, is critical for the activation of T cells by antigen. The expression of this T-lineage gene in CLL cells is surprising but has been confirmed by research studies. Inappropriate expression of ZAP-70 in CLL may alter the action of another protein tyrosine kinase, Syk, found in B lymphocytes.

Thymidine Kinase

Another new finding is the correlation of the serum value of thymidine kinase with IgVH gene mutational status and also with disease progression. DNA microarray has demonstrated that CLL exhibits a characteristic gene expression profile closely related to memory B cells and independent of the presence of IgVH mutations.

CD38

Expression of CD38, a membrane protein that marks cellular activation and maturation and that has signaling activity, often correlates with the presence of IgV_H mutations. CD38 surface expression on the malignant cell is now viewed as an independent marker of a patient's clinical outcome. CD38+ B-CLL patients are characterized by a more advanced disease stage, lesser responsiveness to chemotherapy, and shorter survival times than CD38-negative patients.

MicroRNA

MicroRNA (miRNA) expression profiles can be used to distinguish normal B cells from malignant B cells in CLL patients. A unique microRNA signature is associated with prognostic factors and disease progression in CLL. Mutations in microRNA transcripts are common and can have functional importance.

MicroRNAs regulate the expression of protein-coding genes and can act as oncogenes, tumor suppressors, or both. Alterations in CLL affect the following:

■ Evasion of apoptosis
■ Self-sufficiency in growth
■ Stimulation of angiogenesis and dissemination

Evasion of apoptosis is associated with overexpression of the antiapoptotic protein bcl2. BCL2 is responsible for maintaining the delicate homeostasis between proliferation and apoptosis and promotes cell survival by inhibiting cell death. MicroRNAs are major direct negative regulators of the bcl2 antiapoptotic protein and indirect activators of the intrinsic apoptotic program leading to apoptotic peptidase activating factor.

Myeloid cell leukemia-1 (Mcl-1) is an antiapoptotic member of the bcl2 protein family. Increased Mcl-1 expression is associated with failure to achieve remission after treatment with fludarabine and chlorambucil in patients with CLL. Mcl-1 expression may be useful in predicting poor response to chemoimmunotherapy.

Note that patients with lymphadenopathy, splenomegaly, and pancytopenia with an atypical lymphocyte population may have an acquired mutation in a gene that is crucial to cellular apoptosis. If the somatic mutation is in the expression of FAS, the diagnosis may be autoimmune lymphoproliferative syndrome (ALPS). ALPS is a disorder of abnormal lymphocyte survival due to dysregulation of the FAS apoptotic pathway. This defective apoptosis leads to chronic lymphoproliferations, autoimmune disorder, for example, primarily autoimmune cytopenias.

Self-sufficiency in Growth

Self-sufficiency in growth demonstrates that normal cells require growth stimuli compared to cancer cells that are capable of generating their own growth signals without having to rely on mitogens in the surrounding environment in order to actively proliferate.

Stimulation of Angiogenesis and Dissemination

This is characteristic of the marrow and lymph nodes of patients with CLL. Patients show a high degree of tissue neovascularization.

Staging and Prognosis

CLL has a variable clinical course. Clinical staging systems (Rai and Binet) for assessing prognosis in CLL were developed in the early 1980s, based on easily obtainable biological and clinical parameters.

The staging classification is

0   Bone marrow and blood lymphocytosis
I   Lymphocytosis with enlarged nodes
II Lymphocytosis with enlarged spleen or liver or both
III Lymphocytosis with anemia
IV Lymphocytosis with thrombocytopenia

Most patients with CLL now have Rai stage 0 or I disease at diagnosis. Patients with early-stage disease are a heterogeneous group: approximately 30% to 50% will have accelerated disease progression, and the remainder may live for decades and possibly never require therapy. Prognosis is roughly related to the extent of organ infiltration at the time of diagnosis.

At present, in addition to Binet stages, the mutational status of the V_H genes, molecular markers such as ZAP-70 and CD38, and chromosomal aberrations 11q−, 13q−, 17p−, and +12 are used to predict survival. The average survival times for untreated patients are related to each stage as follows: 0, 150 months; I, 101 months; II, 71 months; III, 19 months; and IV, 19 months. Elderly patients, treated and untreated, survive from 3 to 5 years on average. The principal cause of death is usually infection, although 25% of CLL patients die of causes unrelated to the disorder because of older age. The high risk of infection in patients with CLL is the result of altered humoral (antibody) immunity caused by suppression of immunoglobulin synthesis that leads to hypogammaglobulinemia. Autoimmune disease may also develop; autoimmune hemolytic anemia develops in approximately one third of patients.

Since the introduction of clinical stages, there has been a continuous effort to identify new prognostic factors in CLL (Table 20.2). Parameters with demonstrated independent prognostic value include the

■ Number of lymphocytes in the peripheral blood
■ Degree of bone marrow infiltration
■ Proportion of abnormal lymphoid cells in the peripheral blood
■ Lymphocyte doubling time
■ Immunoglobulin heavy-chain variable-region gene mutation status
■ Cytogenetic abnormalities assessed by fluorescent in situ hybridization
■ Z-chain–associated protein kinase-70 protein expression

These characteristics can identify patients with early-stage disease who are at high risk for early disease progression.

Poor-risk patients are characterized by advanced clinical stage, short lymphocyte doubling time, unmutated immunoglobulin heavy gene (IgV_H) status, distinct genomic aberrations, ZAP70 and CD38 expression, and an elevated serum thymidine kinase levels.

Clinical Signs and Symptoms

The typical patient with CLL is asymptomatic, and the disease is usually discovered at the time of a routine physical examination. The disease is typically suggested by abnormal findings discovered on a complete blood count (CBC) for the evaluation of an unrelated illness. Common symptoms include malaise, low-grade fever, and night sweats. Other symptoms may be weakness, fatigue, anorexia, and weight loss. Physical examination usually reveals cervical and supraclavicular adenopathy. Hepatosplenomegaly is also frequently present.

TABLE 20.2	Factors With Prognostic Significance in Chronic Lymphocytic Leukemia		
Factor		**Low Risk**	**High Risk**
Clinical stage			
Binet		A	B,C
Rai		0	I, II, III, IV
Bone marrow infiltration			
Biopsy		Nondiffuse pattern	Diffuse pattern
Aspirate		<80% lymphocytes	>80% lymphocytes
WBC ($\times 10^9$/L)		<50	>50
Prolymphocytes in peripheral blood (%)		<10	>10
Lymphocyte doubling time		<12 months	>12 months
β-2-microglobulin		Normal	Increased
CD38 expression		<30%	>30%
IgV_H genes		Mutated	Unmutated

Laboratory Data

Normal bone marrow elements get crowded out because of the excessive lymphoid production and packing of the marrow space by malignant lymphocytes. This infiltration by the leukemic clone results in anemia, thrombocytopenia, and neutropenia.

Although leukocytosis may be observed, it is less pronounced than in chronic myelogenous leukemia. Total leukocyte counts can range from 30 to 200×10^9 L. In one third of patients, the total leukocyte count is greater than 100×10^9/L.

Absolute lymphocytosis is a usual finding. The International Workshop on CLL report requires that the lymphocytosis must be present for at least 3 months. In addition, the International Workshop allows for a diagnosis of CLL with a lower lymphocyte count in patients with cytopenias or disease-related symptoms. In the absence of extramedullary tissue involvement, there must be $\geq 5 \times 10^9$/L monoclonal lymphocytes with a CLL phenotype in the peripheral blood.

Peripheral blood smears (Figs. 20.1–20.3) commonly exhibit up to 80% or 90% small lymphocytes. Many of these cells have an overmature look because of the hypercondensed nuclear chromatin pattern. An occasional large lymphoblast may be noted. Smudge cells are highly characteristic. Both the granulocytes and the platelets are normal.

Other mild to severe immunological dysfunction typifies the disease. Serum electrophoresis studies usually show hypogammaglobulinemia.

Treatment Options

Previously, patients with CLL were only treated for palliative reasons, but numerous new treatment options are now available for the treatment of CLL. Allogeneic hematopoietic stem cell transplantation (alloHSCT) is the only potentially curative treatment available for patients with B-cell CLL.

Decision to Treat

The decision to treat a patient depends on the stage of the disease, the presence of symptoms, and the disease activity. Only patients in Rai III and IV, or Binet C stages should be treated. Patients in early stages of CLL should only be treated if symptoms associated with the disease occur (e.g., threatening complications from spleen or liver enlargement and lymphomas that can produce compression of the large abdominal vessels). High disease activity is defined by a lymphocyte doubling time of less than 6 months or by rapidly growing lymphomas. High disease actually is also an indication to treat in the early stages of the disease.

Original Treatments

Historically, the first-line treatment of CLL in the 1960s consisted of alkylating agents, for example, chlorambucil and cyclophosphamide. This produced a response in up to 70% of patients but did not improve survival. Complete remissions are rare and partial remissions are of short duration. Nucleoside (purine) analogues, for example, fludarabine, pentostatin, and Cladribine, that were popular in the 1980s demonstrated a higher response rates than alkylating agents and to provide for longer progression-free survival. Treatment with purine analogues alone does not appear to improve survival. The main adverse reactions to purine analogues are myelosuppression and lymphocytopenia.

Purine analogues in combination with other cytotoxic drugs (alkylators) were introduced as a treatment strategy in the 1990s. An estimated 35% of patients achieved a complete remission. The most common side effects of these fludarabine combinations are severe infections.

Newer Treatments

Newer treatment chemoimmunotherapy was introduced in 2000. This strategy incorporates the use of monoclonal antibodies to chemotherapy. This strategy appears to provide for a first time–observed survival benefit but is not considered curative. Chronic lymphocytic leukemia patients with p53 pathway dysfunction have poor responses to conventional chemoimmunotherapy and short survival. Monoclonal antibodies (e.g., anti-CD20 monoclonal antibody [rituximab] or anti-CD52 [alemtuzumab]) bind to CLL cells by reacting with surface antigens. This results in the destruction of CLL cells by apoptosis, complement activation, or antibody-mediated cellular cytotoxicity. Depending on the rituximab regimen, partial remission rates of short duration occur in 50% to 70% of patients. If the total peripheral leukocyte count is high, dangerous side effects can occur because of release of cytokines from the leukemic cells or agglutination of leukemic cells in small blood vessels. Recently, fludarabine, cyclophosphamide, and rituximab (FCR) combination therapy has produced the largest proportion of complete responses ever reported in CLL patients. FCR may become the new "gold standard" for CLL therapy.

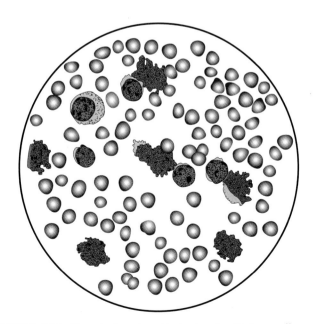

FIGURE 20.1 Chronic lymphocytic leukemia. Mature cells predominate in the chronic leukemias. In this blood smear, a typical increase in the number of smudge cells is seen. (Simulates magnification 1,000×.)

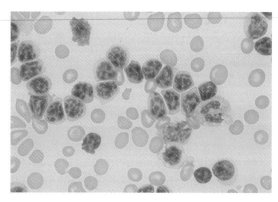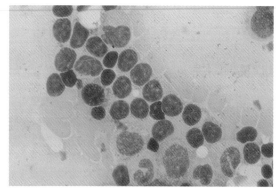

FIGURE 20.2 Two slides showing chronic lymphocytic leukemia. (Reprinted with permission from Anderson S, Poulsen K. *Anderson's Atlas of Hematology*, Philadelphia, PA: Lippincott Williams & Wilkins, 2003.)

CD52+ is expressed by normal T and B lymphocytes and almost all CLL cells. Anti-CD52 has been used primarily in patients who have had a relapse and, in some cases, as postremission consolidation therapy. This humanized monoclonal antibody has produced significant responses in patients with residual disease after chemotherapy. Bone marrow disease was eradicated more frequently than nodal disease, and molecular remissions were achieved. Because the action of alemtuzumab is limited by bulky lymph nodes, some researchers have hypothesized that activity may be greater with less extensive disease. Monoclonal antibodies have a different mechanism of action than cytotoxic chemotherapeutic agents. They play a significant role in attainment of MRD negativity and eradication of MRD up to 20% of patients with refractory disease. Regimens consisting of combinations of fludarabine with monoclonal antibodies (e.g., rituximab and alemtuzumab) are highly promising treatments to achieve complete molecular remission.

MicroRNA may potentially be used in therapy for CLL. In the future, patient-specific therapeutic drugs may be designed for CLL patients harboring abnormalities in miRNA expression in their malignant cells. miRNAs are potential targets for therapy as well, as knocking down overexpression of miRNAs and inducing expression of silenced miRNAs in cancer cells may contribute to selective tumor killing. Loss of miRNA expression in CLL patients may selectively suppress proapoptotic pathways, providing such malignancies with a survival advantage.

Myeloablative high-dose chemotherapy, with subsequent autologous or allogeneic stem cell transplant (SCT), an experimental treatment, is the most intensive form of chemoimmunotherapy for CLL. This approach combines all available regimens of antileukemic treatment.

Minimal Residual Disease

PCR-based and flow cytometry–based assays are used to assess MRD in CLL. Real-time PCR has become common for quantification by PCR.

HAIRY CELL LEUKEMIA

HCL is an uncommon chronic lymphoproliferative disorder of the B-lymphocyte type. This mature B-cell malignancy is diagnosed based on clinical features, morphology, and phenotyping and generally treated with curative intent.

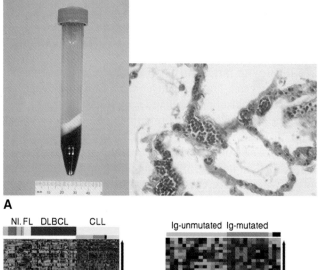
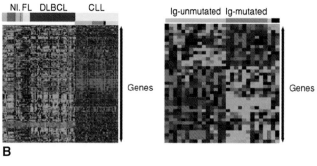

A

B

FIGURE 20.3 **A:** Hyperleukocytosis (**left**). An elevated leukocyte concentration in a centrifuged peripheral blood specimen from a patient with T-cell acute lymphoblastic leukemia (**right**). Pulmonary alveolar capillaries expanded by leukocyte aggregates indicative of leukostasis in a patient with acute myeloid leukemia. **B:** Microarray analysis in chronic lymphocytic leukemia (CLL) (**left**); the expression of C247 signature genes (**right**). Differentiation of CLL patients into those with or without mutations of the Ig V gene by the expressions of 56 genes and Ig Immunoglobulins. (Reprinted with permission from Greer JP, et al. *Wintrobe's Clinical Hematology*, 11th ed, Philadelphia, PA: Lippincott Williams & Wilkins, 2004.)

HCL is much more common in males than in females. It has been suggested that a locus on the X chromosome might be involved in HCL. It usually affects patients older than 30 years of age.

Initial patient symptoms include fatigue, anemia, leukocytopenia, thrombocytopenia, splenomegaly, and marrow fibrosis. Pancytopenia is common. Bleeding and infection can be present. The bone marrow may become fibrotic; therefore, bone marrow aspirates frequently are unsuccessful (a dry tap). Treatment with interferon may have a positive effect on bone marrow fibrosis.

Diagnosis of HCL includes morphological appearance of the lymphocytes, cytochemical staining, and immunocytological characterization by flow cytometry.

HCL is so named because of the appearance of fine, hair-like, irregular cytoplasmic projections that are characteristic of lymphocytes (Fig. 20.4) in this disease. Cytoplasmic projections are not always obvious in HCL and in some cases (e.g., artifactually in other lymphoid neoplasms or reactive cells) are not specific for HCL.

Morphologically, HCLs are large with moderately large nuclei. Sometimes the slate-blue cytoplasm is vacuolated. The nucleus is frequently oval or slightly clefted and may be convoluted with a homogeneous chromatin pattern. The cytochemical features of HCL include a strong acid phosphatase reaction that is not inhibited by tartaric acid or tartrate-resistant acid phosphatase (TRAP) stain. TRAP positivity can vary with disease progression. In addition, following interferon therapy, enzyme activity in the hairy cell may be TRAP negative.

The immunological markers include CD19+, CD20+, CD22+, CD24+, and CD25+ reactivity to the monoclonal antibody that recognizes the interleukin-2 (Tac) receptor. In addition, the cells display strong SIg.

The clinical course of HCL is more benign than many forms of leukemia. In most cases, it is controllable with traditional chemotherapy, cladribine. In a small clinical trial, 70% of HCL patients whose diseases were resistant to conventional chemotherapy experienced remission when treated with anti-CD22 recombinant immunotoxin (BL22).

Patients frequently live more than a decade after diagnosis. The greatest risk of death is from infection.

Hairy Cell Leukemia Variant

A variant form of HCL, hairy cell leukemia variant (vHCL), was discovered in 1980. In addition, much rarer variants, Japanese variant and blastic variant, exist. vHCL is a more aggressive type of HCL and has different morphological characteristics than typical HCL.

vHCL cells are smaller than the typical HCL cell with a central round nucleus, prominent nucleoli, a larger nuclear-cytoplasmic ratio, and basophilic cytoplasm with occasional cytoplasmic projections. vHCL may present with morphologic features intermediate between hairy cells and prolymphocytes.

Differential diagnosis of vHCL from typical HCL can be made by cytochemical staining (TRAP) and immunophenotyping using flow cytometry. vHCL has a poor prognosis.

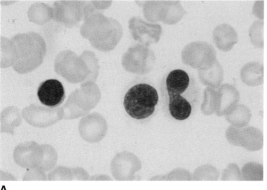

A

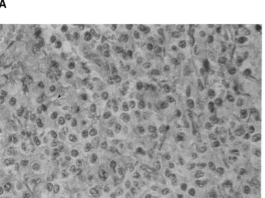

C

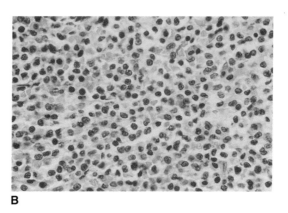

B

FIGURE 20.4 Hairy cell leukemia. **A:** Peripheral blood. **B:** Bone marrow (H&E stain). **C:** Spleen (H&E stain). (Reprinted with permission from Handin RI, et al. *Blood Principles and Practice of Hematology*, 2nd ed, Philadelphia, PA: Lippincott Williams & Wilkins, 2003.)

PROLYMPHOCYTIC LEUKEMIA

B-cell prolymphocytic leukemia represents a malignancy of B prolymphocytes affecting blood, bone marrow, and spleen. Prolymphocytic leukemia is characterized by a large number of small lymphocytes with scant cytoplasm and the immature features of prolymphocytes in the peripheral blood. The leukocytosis can exceed 100×10^9/L. Prolymphocytes must exceed 55% of lymphoid cells in the peripheral blood.

Most patients have a disease of B-cell origin and demonstrate immunological markers CD19+, CD20+, CD24+, or CD22+. In addition, the cells display strong SIg. Cases of transformed CLL, CLL with increased prolymphocytes, and lymphoid proliferations with a relatively similar morphology but carrying the t(11;14) translocation are excluded.

This leukemia progresses rapidly with a variable prognosis.

MULTIPLE MYELOMA (PLASMA CELL MYELOMA)

Multiple myeloma is a malignant bone marrow–based, plasma cell neoplasm associated with abnormal protein production. **Plasma cell leukemia** is an increased number of plasma cells in the peripheral blood and should be considered a form of multiple myeloma and not a separate entity.

Epidemiology

Multiple myeloma accounts for approximately 1% of all types of malignant diseases and about 10% of hematological malignancies. It usually evolves from an asymptomatic premalignant stage of clonal plasma cell proliferation called "monoclonal gammopathy of undetermined significance (MGUS)."

MGUS is present in more than 3% of the population above the age of 50 years and progresses to myeloma or related malignancy at a rate of 1% per year. The onset of this disorder is between the ages of 40 and 70 years, with a peak incidence in the seventh decade of life. Myeloma is not found in children and rarely in adults who are less than 30 year of age.

Plasma cell myeloma is more common in men than women (1.4:1). It occurs twice as frequently in African Americans as in whites.

Etiology

In multiple myeloma, typically, the bone marrow is involved, but the disorder may involve other tissues as well. The etiology is unknown; however, radiation may be a factor, and the possibility of a viral cause has been suggested. The likelihood of a genetic factor in some cases is supported by well-documented reports of 23 familial clusters with multiple myeloma.

Chromosomal abnormalities are found in at least half of patients with multiple myeloma. Numerous changes and structural abnormalities, including giant chromosomes, translocations, and deletions, have been noted; however, the abnormalities are limited to the plasma cells.

Clinical Signs and Symptoms

Symptoms of multiple myeloma include bone pain (typically in the back or chest) that is present at the time of diagnosis in more than two thirds of patients, weakness, and fatigue. Weight loss and night sweats are not prominent until the disease is advanced. Abnormal bleeding may be a prominent feature. In some patients, the major symptoms result from acute infection, renal insufficiency, hypercalcemia, or amyloidosis. In addition to the conclusive laboratory findings, including bone marrow examination results, approximately 90% of patients suffer from broadly disseminated destruction of the skeleton (Fig. 20.5).

This disorder runs a progressive course, and most patients die in 1 to 3 years. The major causes of death are infection and renal insufficiency. Several factors contribute to the immunocompromised state. Multiple myeloma leads to a compensatory decrease in synthesis and increase in catabolism of normal immunoglobulins. As the tumor burden increases, the antibody response becomes more impaired and the degree of humoral immunosuppression increases. Complement activity is also deficient in patients with multiple myeloma. As the disease progresses, granulocytopenia may develop as a result of bone marrow failure. Treatment with corticosteroids results in transient T-cell sequestration, diminished synthesis of immunoglobulins, and decreased adherence and degranulation of neutrophils. As a result of cytotoxic chemotherapy, there is a variable decrease in the numbers and function of T cells, B cells, and granulocytes.

Laboratory Data

Anemia is present at the time of diagnosis in approximately two thirds of patients. Increased plasma volume caused by monoclonal protein commonly produces hypervolemia. The leukocyte count can be normal, although about one third of patients have leukopenia. Relative lymphocytosis is usually present. Sometimes eosinophilia is noted. In rare cases in the terminal stages, plasmablasts and plasma cells (Fig. 20.6) may amount to 50% of the leukocytes in the peripheral blood. Rouleaux formation (discussed in Chapter 6) on peripheral blood smears is common.

Bleeding is common. Platelet abnormalities, impaired aggregation of platelets, and interference with platelet function by the abnormal monoclonal protein contribute to bleeding. Inhibitors of coagulation factors and thrombocytopenia from marrow infiltration of plasma cells or chemotherapy may also contribute to bleeding. Some patients have a tendency toward thrombosis, which may be manifested by a shortened coagulation time, increased fibrinogen, and increased factor VIII.

Electrophoresis of serum usually demonstrates the overproduction of IgM (19S) antibodies. Electrophoresis (Figs. 20.7 and 20.8) of the serum or urine reveals tall sharp peaks on the densitometer tracing; a dense localized band is seen in 75% of myeloma cases. A monoclonal serum protein is detected in 91% of patients. The type of antibody is IgG

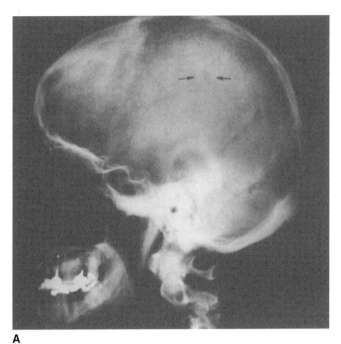
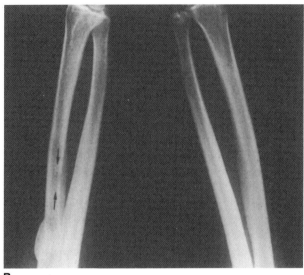

FIGURE 20.5 Lesions in multiple myeloma. **A:** A single osteolytic lesion is detectable in this skull radiograph and exhibits a "punched-out" appearance. **B:** Another osteolytic lesion is detectable in the tibia.

in the majority of patients. Less frequently IgA is seen, and rarely IgD is demonstrated.

Growing clinical acceptance of a serum free light chain assay has all but eliminated urine tests for Bence-Jones protein in the identification of MM. Monoclonal free light chains can occur either as part of an intact monoclonal immunoglobulin or as a single product. Usually, these free light kappa and lambda chains are bounded to the heavy chain of the immunoglobulin. Plasma cells also produce always an amount of free light chains that were secreted as monomer (kappa) or dimer (lambda). Until recently, it was not possible to detect the free light chains in the serum. A nephelometric respectably turbidimetric quantification of free kappa and light chain has been introduced. Up to 20% of MM cases have free light chain-only disease in which light chains in the serum and/or urine are the only immunochemical abnormality found.

Treatment

Multiple myeloma is incurable with conventional chemotherapy.

Melphalan-based high-dose chemotherapy with hematopoietic stem cell support increases the rate of complete remission and extends event-free and overall survival. Many patients still experience relapse, and options for salvage therapy are limited. Patients with myeloma who experience relapse after high-dose chemotherapy have few therapeutic options.

Thalidomide, lenalidomide, and bortezomib are novel agents that first demonstrated efficacy in treating relapsed and refractory MM, but they are now all being utilized as treatment for newly diagnosed disease. Angiogenesis is

important in tumor progression. The immunomodulatory drug thalidomide can inhibit angiogenesis and induce apoptosis of established neovasculature in experimental models. For this reason, angiogenesis-inhibiting drugs (e.g., thalidomide) may be useful for treating cancers that depend on neovascularization.

Thalidomide is active against advanced myeloma. It can induce significant and durable responses in some patients with multiple myeloma, including those who relapse after high-dose chemotherapy. Thalidomide combined with melphalan and prednisone for the elderly nontransplant candidate with newly diagnosed MM is superior to melphalan and prednisone and to melphalan. Autologous stem cell transplantation is now recommended for young patients as part of the initial therapy or at time of the disease progression. The median duration of response after the newer chemotherapeutic protocols and ASCT does not exceed 3 years, and almost all patients relapse.

A new twist in myeloma treatment is directed at reversing renal complications. One of the severe and common complications of MM is renal failure. The underlying etiology is cast nephropathy, also known as myeloma kidney, in more than two thirds of myeloma-associated renal diseases. Renal cast nephropathy represents a potentially reversible form of renal failure. Early identification and treatment may prevent the progression to end-stage kidney failure commonly seen in cast nephropathy. By decreasing the circulation levels of monoclonal light chain, cytoreductive therapies are mainstays of treatment.

Increased bone marrow vascularity imparts a poor prognosis in myeloma. High-dose therapy with supporting autologous stem cell transplantation remains a controversial

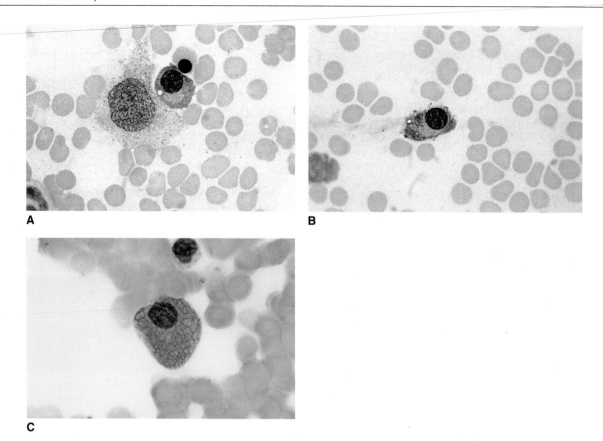

FIGURE 20.6 Various appearances of plasma cells in a smear of normal bone marrow. A prominent pale paranuclear zone and cytoplasmic vacuoles are seen in (**A**) and (**B**). The cytoplasm in (**C**) has a reticular appearance. The other cells in (**A**) are a nonphagocytic reticular cell and a late polychromatic erythroblast. (Reprinted with permission from Mills SE. *Histology For Pathologists*, 3rd ed, Philadelphia, PA: Lippincott Williams & Wilkins, 2007.)

treatment for cancer. In multiple myeloma, first-line regimens incorporating high-dose therapy yield higher remission rates than do conventional-dose treatment.

WALDENSTRÖM PRIMARY MACROGLOBULINEMIA (LYMPHOPLASMACYTIC LYMPHOMA)

Epidemiology

The condition of WM has an age-specific incidence. It is most commonly found in older men; the median age of onset varies between 63 and 68 years of age. Onset is usually insidious. The incidence of WM is higher among whites.

Prognostic factors include the patient's age, β_2-microglobulin level, monoclonal protein level, hemoglobin concentration, and platelet count. The reported median survival of patients with WM ranges between 5 and 10 years from the time of diagnosis.

Etiology

WM is a B-cell neoplasm characterized by lymphoplasmoproliferative disorder with infiltration of the bone marrow and a monoclonal immunoglobulin M (IgM) protein. This malignant lymphocyte–plasma cell proliferative disorder is associated with the production of abnormally large amounts of gamma globulin of the 19S or IgM type. The basic abnormality in this macroglobulinemia is uncontrolled proliferation of lymphocyte and plasma cells.

Clinical Signs and Symptoms

The symptoms of WM are due to the extent of tumor infiltration and to elevated IgM levels in the blood circulation. Symptoms include weakness, fatigue attributable to anemia, and bleeding. Bone pain is virtually nonexistent. About one fourth of patients with WM have neurological abnormalities. The incidence of infection is twice the normal rate. Patients usually suffer from chronic anemia and bleeding episodes. Thrombocytopenia and hyperviscosity may also contribute to the bleeding disorder.

Laboratory Data

The most consistent feature of the bone marrow or lymph nodes of WM patients is the presence of pleomorphic B-lineage cells at different stages of maturation, such as small lymphocytes, lymphoplasmacytoid cells (abundant basophilic cytoplasm but lymphocyte-like nuclei), and plasma cells. Bone marrow mast cells of WM patients overexpress the CD40 ligand (CD154), which is a potent inducer of B-cell

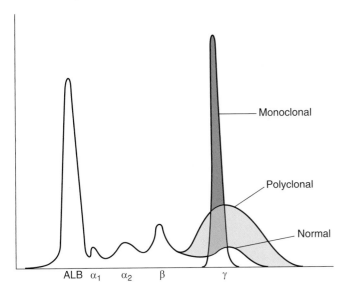

FIGURE 20.7 Abnormal serum protein electrophoretic patterns contrasted with a normal pattern. Polyclonal hypergamma-globulinemia, characteristic of benign reactive processes, shows a broad-based increase in immunoglobulins, owing to immuno-globulin secretion by a myriad of reactive plasma cells. Monoclo-nal gammopathy of unknown significance (MGUS) or plasma cell neoplasia shows a narrow peak, or spike, owing to the homogene-ity of the immunoglobulin molecules secreted by a single clone of aberrant plasma cells. ALB, albumin. (Reprinted with permission from Rubin R, Strayer DS. *Rubin's Pathology: Clinicopathologic Foundations of Medicine*, 5th ed, Philadelphia, PA: Lippincott Wil-liams & Wilkins, 2008.)

expansion. The lymphocyte–plasma cells vary morphologi-cally, ranging from small lymphocytes to obvious plasma cells (Fig. 20.9). Their cytoplasm is frequently ragged and may contain periodic acid-Schiff (PAS)-positive material that is probably identical to the circulating macroglobulin.

The total leukocyte count is usually normal, with an abso-lute lymphocytosis. Moderate to severe degrees of anemia are frequently observed on peripheral blood smears as well as rouleaux formation. The patient's plasma volume may be greatly increased, and the ESR is increased. Platelet counts are usually normal. Bleeding caused by abnormalities in platelet adhesiveness and prothrombin time may be seen, and the values of factor VIII may be low.

Characteristically, blood samples are described as having **hyperviscosity**. Detecting monoclonal gammopathies usually involves serum protein electrophoresis (SPEP) and immu-noelectrophoresis (IEP) to test both serum and urine. Addi-tionally, **cryoglobulins** can be detected in the patient's serum. Cryoglobulins are proteins that precipitate or gel when cooled to 0°C and dissolve when heated. In most cases, monoclonal cryoglobulins are IgM or IgG.

Treatment

Therapy is postponed for asymptomatic patients, and pro-gressive anemia is the most common indication for initiation of treatment. Main therapeutic options include alkylating

agents, nucleoside analogues, and rituximab. Novel agents, for example, vortezomib show promise as a targeted therapy option in WM.

LYMPHOMAS

Relationship Between Lymphomas and Leukemias

The term lymphoproliferative disorder includes the vari-ous forms of leukemias and malignant lymphomas that are of lymphoreticular origin. The neoplastic cells of leukemia and lymphoma have an intimate relationship. Frequently, the neoplastic cells of these two disorders are identical (Table 20.3).

Characteristics

The lymphomas are a group of closely related disorders that are characterized by the overproliferation of one or more types of cells of the lymphoid system such as lymphoreticu-lar stem cells, lymphocytes, reticulum cells, and histiocytes. During the progression of the disease, the malignant cells may spill into the blood circulation. This spillover may pro-duce a leukemic phase of the disease. Such transitions to a leukemic phase are rare in disorders such as Hodgkin dis-ease but are common in the well-differentiated lymphocytic lymphomas.

Malignant lymphoma expresses itself as a disorder of the lymph nodes. It is characterized by the infiltration of abnor-mal lymphocytes and destruction of the normal architecture of the node. This results in the invasion and destruction of the lymph node capsule and subcapsular sinuses, and the infiltration of the pericapsular fat by large numbers of the cells that destroyed the architecture of the lymph nodes. Eventually, this disorder progresses to all of the lymphoid tissues of the gastrointestinal tract.

Categories

Lymphomas have been described in all races and ethnic groups. The gender distribution of these disorders is approxi-mately equal. The major forms of malignant lymphomas are divided into Hodgkin and non-Hodgkin types. The NHLs account for more than two thirds of all lymphomas and more than 75% of the fatalities due to lymphoma. Rare forms of lymphoma include Burkitt lymphoma and mycosis fungoi-des, a variant of Sézary syndrome, which demonstrates skin involvement.

Diagnosis and subclassification of lymphoma have changed dramatically over time. The two contemporary classification systems are the Revised European-Ameri-can Lymphoma Classification (REAL classification) and the World Health Organization (WHO) Classification of Tumours of the Haematopoietic and Lymphoid Tissues, fourth edition. The REAL and WHO classifications, which

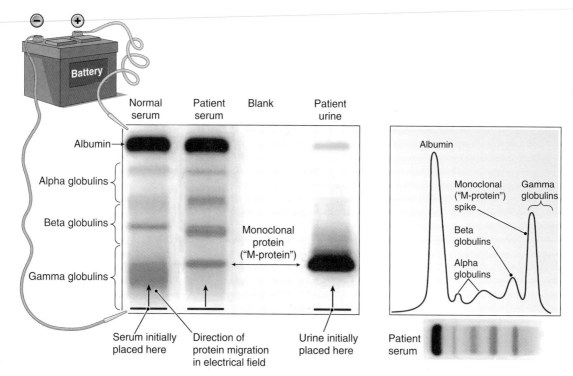

FIGURE 20.8 Protein electrophoresis in plasma cell disease. Serum or urine is placed at one end of a strip of gel, across which an electrical current is applied. Most proteins have a negative charge and migrate toward the positive pole at various speeds according to their molecular weight and charge. The serum on the left shows a narrow band in the gamma globulin region. Serum protein has spilled into urine, which demonstrates a matching band. In the scan of patient serum on the right, the height of the tracing is proportional to the amount of protein stained in each band. Monoclonal protein appears as a tall, narrow (monoclonal) "M-protein." (Reprinted with permission from McConnell TH. *The Nature of Disease Pathology for the Health Professions*, Philadelphia, PA: Lippincott Williams & Wilkins, 2007.)

include approximately 30 different abnormalities, include entities defined by a combination of morphological, immunophenotypical, genetic, and clinical features (see Box 20.2; Tables 20.4 and 20.5). The importance of the various features differs depending on the different types of lymphomas.

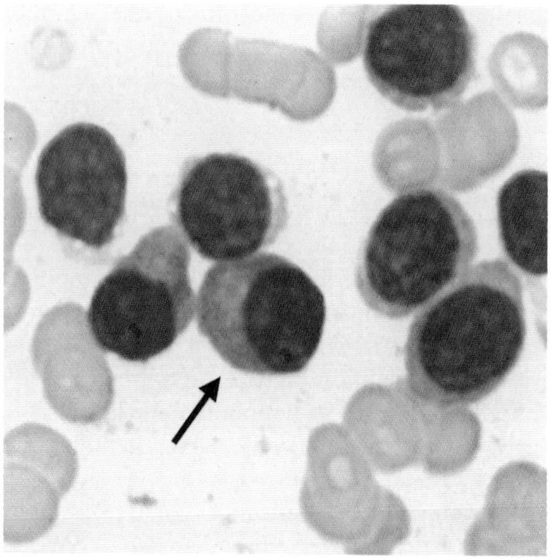

The REAL and WHO classifications include Hodgkin disease and NHL. The term Hodgkin lymphoma is preferred because of recent discoveries establishing the origin of the Reed-Sternberg cell in almost all cases of Hodgkin

FIGURE 20.9 Waldenström. Bone marrow aspirate showing malignant cells with lymphoid and plasmacytoid morphology. (Reprinted with permission from Greer JP, et al. *Wintrobe's Clinical Hematology*, 11th ed, Philadelphia, PA: Lippincott Williams & Wilkins, 2004.)

TABLE 20.3	Relationship of Leukemias and Lymphomas
Leukemia Type	**Solid Tumor Counterpart**
Stem cell leukemia	Lymphoma, undifferentiated
Acute lymphoblastic leukemia	Lymphoma, poorly differentiated; lymphocytic
Chronic lymphocytic leukemia	Lymphoma, well differentiated; lymphocytic
Monocytic leukemia	Reticulum cell sarcoma
Acute myelogenous leukemia	Chloroma granulocytic
Plasma cell leukemia	Myeloma

Examples of Common Lymphoid Neoplasms

B-CELL NEOPLASMS

Precursor B-cell neoplasm
- Precursor B-lymphoblastic leukemia/lymphoma (precursor B-cell acute lymphoblastic leukemia)

Mature (peripheral) B-cell neoplasms with leukemic presentation
- Chronic lymphocytic leukemia/B-cell SLL
- B-cell prolymphocytic leukemia
- Hairy cell leukemia
- Plasma cell neoplasms

Mature (peripheral) B-cell neoplasms node based
- Diffuse large B-cell lymphoma
- Burkitt lymphoma/leukemia

T- AND NK-CELL NEOPLASMS

Precursor T-cell neoplasm
- Precursor T-lymphoblastic leukemia/lymphoma (precursor T-cell acute lymphoblastic leukemia)

Mature (peripheral) T-cell neoplasms with leukemic presentation
- T-cell prolymphocytic leukemia
- Adult T-cell lymphoma/leukemia (HTLV 1+)
- Mycosis fungoides/Sézary syndrome

HODGKIN LYMPHOMA (HODGKIN DISEASE)
- Nodular lymphocyte predominant Hodgkin lymphoma
- Classical Hodgkin lymphoma

disease as the B lymphocytes. The WHO classification also includes plasma cell neoplasms within the category of B-cell neoplasms. Separate sections of the WHO classification include immunodeficiency-associated lymphoproliferative disorders, acute myeloid leukemias, myelodysplastic syndromes, and chronic myeloproliferative disorders.

Within the group of NHLs, lymphoblastic neoplasms are separated from mature B- and T-cell neoplasms. Both the mature B- and T-cell neoplasms are subclassified into those that are

- Predominantly disseminated or leukemic at presentation
- Primarily extranodal
- Predominantly lymph node–based entities

As advances are made in hematopathology, changes will be incorporated into the WHO classification system. Precise diagnostic subclassification is important to administer effective therapy.

Pathophysiology

Although the etiology of most lymphomas is unknown, the potential role of a virus in the pathogenesis of lymphomas is strongly suspected. In humans, the development of B cells in the bone marrow is initiated by the assembly of genes for the variable regions of the heavy and light chains of antibodies in B-cell progenitors, mediated by a process called V(D)J recombination. In this process, the DNA located between the rearranging gene elements is deleted from the chromosome (or sometimes inverted). Distinct gene rearrangements equip each B cell with individual molecular clonal markers—an essential feature for the analysis of B-cell lymphomas. The expression antibody as an antigen receptor on the surface of B cells is critically important for the development and survival of B cells. In development, the cells go through an ordered program of V(D)J rearrangements in which the only surviving cells are those that have acquired heavy- and light-chain variable-region genes that can be translated into protein because they preserve the correct reading frame (in-frame rearrangements). Cells with out-of-frame V(D)J rearrangements die by programmed cell death, apoptosis.

TABLE 20.4	Immunohistological Features of Selected B-Cell Neoplasms					
	Surface Membrane	Marker				
Type of Neoplasm	SIg	CD5	CD10	CD23	CD43	
Chronic lymphocytic leukemia	+	+	–	+	+	
Hairy cell leukemia	+	–	–	–	+	
Burkitt lymphoma	+	–	+	–	–	

SIg, surface immunoglobulin.
Source: Handin RI, et al. (eds). *Blood: Principles and Practice of Hematology*, 2nd ed, Philadelphia, PA: Lippincott Williams & Wilkins, 2003:75.

TABLE 20.5	Genetic Features of Selected B-Cell Neoplasms	
Type of Neoplasm	**Chromosomal Abnormality**	**Ig Genes**
Chronic lymphocytic leukemia	Trisomy 12; 13q	R, U (50%), M (50%)
Hairy cell leukemia	None known	R,M
Burkitt lymphoma	t(8;14)m t(2;8)	R,M
	t(8;22); c-myc; EBV ≃/+	
Lymphoplasmacytic lymphoma	t(9;14)	R,M
	del 6 (q23)	
Diffuse large B-cell lymphoma	t(8;14), 3q;	R,M
	BCL2, myc, BCL6	

Ig, immunoglobulin genes; R, rearranged; M, mutated, U, unmutated; EBV, Epstein-Barr virus.
Source: Handin RI, et al. (eds). *Blood: Principles and Practice of Hematology*, 2nd ed, Philadelphia, PA: Lippincott Williams & Wilkins, 2003:75.

In mature B cells, the expression of an antigen receptor is also essential for cellular survival because induced deletion of the receptor in vivo leads to rapid cell death.

Naïve B cells that recognize an antigen with their membrane-bound antibody collect in the germinal center of secondary lymphoid organs: lymph nodes, spleen, and mucosa-associated lymphoid tissue (MALT).

Most mature B-cell lymphomas, including Hodgkin lymphomas, develop as a result of malignant transformation of germinal center or postgerminal center B cells.

Most types of non-Hodgkin B-cell lymphomas and Hodgkin lymphomas in humans are derived from germinal center or postgerminal center B cells. In both normal B-cell development and B-cell tumors is the dependence on the expression of antigen receptor for survival and growth of the B cells, with the remarkable exception of Reed-Sternberg cells in classic Hodgkin disease. The germinal center has a central role in both normal B-cell differentiation and the genesis of B-cell tumors, the latter because of the unique combination of genetic changes and intense cellular proliferation that characterized B-cell differentiation in this microenvironment. The benefit of the germinal center reaction is that the defense against pathogens outweighs the increased risk of malignant transformation of the responding cells.

Precursors of Hodgkin Disease and B-Cell Lymphomas

Cytogenetic studies now suggest that Reed-Sternberg cells arise from a single clone, a common B-cell precursor located in a germinal center. Reed-Sternberg cells are a defining feature of Hodgkin disease, but less than 1% of cells in a sample of Hodgkin disease tissue are Reed-Sternberg cells. Immunoglobulin gene rearrangements in Reed-Sternberg cells strongly suggest a B-cell origin of Reed-Sternberg cells, but it is imaginable that Reed-Sternberg cells could represent transformed macrophages or dendritic cells with anomalous recombination of their germ line immunoglobulin genes.

Hodgkin Disease

Although the etiology of Hodgkin disease remains questionable, it has long been suspected that the cause is an infectious agent with a long latent period. Hodgkin disease has an age-related incidence, with one peak occurring in the period from 25 to 35 years of age and a second peak after 50 years of age. Sixty percent of adults afflicted with the disease are male, as are 80% of children who have the disease.

In the early stages of the disease, both the total leukocyte count and the result of differential examination of leukocytes from peripheral blood are normal. However, as the disease advances, a neutrophilia with total leukocyte counts of 15 to 25×10^9/L develops. Neutrophilia, varying degrees of eosinophilia, and monocytosis become apparent on peripheral smears as the disease progresses. In the later stages of the disorder, most patients develop lymphocytopenia and thrombocytopenia.

Hodgkin disease is characterized by the presence of **Reed-Sternberg cells** (Fig. 20.10) in the lymph nodes. The nodes and other lymphoid tissue are often infiltrated with lymphocytes, reticulum cells, fibrocytes, plasma cells, monocytes, and eosinophils. Fibrosis and necrosis are frequent findings.

Hodgkin disease (Fig. 20.11) is considered a distinct clinical entity. A diagnosis is made primarily by examination of sections of lymph nodes. There are no unique phenotypic characteristics and there are no specific genotypic findings or chromosomal abnormalities that can substitute for the diagnostically important histopathological features.

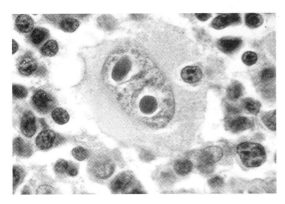

FIGURE 20.10 Reed-Sternberg cell typical of Hodgkin disease. (Reprinted with permission from Rubin E, Farber JL. *Pathology*, 3rd ed, Philadelphia, PA: Lippincott Williams & Wilkins, 1999.)

Hodgkin disease is characterized by a persistent defect in the cellular immunity with abnormalities in T lymphocytes, IL-2 production, and increased sensitivity to suppressor monocytes and normal T suppressor cells.

The cellular origin of the Reed-Sternberg cell is unknown, but Reed-Sternberg cells have been shown to function as stimulatory cells in many lymphocyte reactions, as accessory cells in mitogen-induced T-cell proliferation, and as antigen-presenting cells in HLA-DR–restricted, antigen-specific T-cell activation.

Although little is known about the karyotypic pattern of Hodgkin disease, it is clear that the involvement of specific chromosomes in numerical and structural abnormalities is nonrandom. **Aneuploidy**, or a deviation from the diploid number of chromosomes, resulting from the gain or loss of chromosomes or from polyploids is a characteristic feature of Hodgkin disease. Hyperdiploidy is observed in the majority of Hodgkin disease tumors that have an abnormal karyotype. A gain of chromosomes 1, 2, 5, 12, and 21 is a recurring numerical abnormality; structural rearrangements involving chromosome 1 are frequently observed.

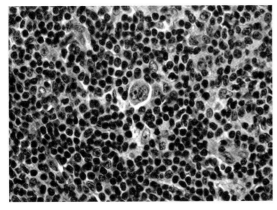

FIGURE 20.11 Hodgkin lymphocyte–rich "classic" Hodgkin disease. The background is primarily lymphocytes with Reed-Sternberg cells. (Reprinted with permission from Greer JP, et al. *Wintrobe's Clinical Hematology*, 11th ed. Philadelphia, PA: Lippincott Williams & Wilkins, 2004.)

Non-Hodgkin Lymphoma

The most frequent type of NHL (Fig. 20.12) is diffuse large B-cell lymphoma, which accounts for approximately 40% of new cases of lymphoma. More than half of patients with diffuse large B-cell lymphoma are older than 60 years of age.

Three different types of diffuse large B-cell lymphomas can be defined based on gene expression subgroups:

1. Germinal center, B-cell–like lymphoma that expresses high levels of genes characteristic of germinal center, B-cell–like lymal germinal center B cells
2. Activated B-cell–like lymphoma, which expresses genes characteristic of mitogenically activated blood B cells
3. New subgroup, type 3 diffuse large B-cell lymphoma, which has a heterogeneous gene expression that suggests it includes more than one subtype of lymphoma

Prognosis

In the early stages of Hodgkin disease, extended field irradiation only was previously the standard therapy. Relapse occurred in approximately one third of patients. Today, combined modality treatment with abbreviated chemotherapy and limited irradiation has reduced the relapse rate, but radiation therapy increases the risks of a second cancer.

Zevalin is the first and only radioimmunoconjugate (RIC) to be approved by the U.S. Food and Drug Administration (FDA) for the treatment of CD20-positive relapsed or refractory, low-grade, follicular, or transformed B-cell NHL, including rituximab-refractory follicular NHL. The toxicity of this treatment is primarily hematological. Approximately 20% of patients require transfusions of platelets and red blood cells (RBCs). Severe neutropenia, thrombocytopenia, and anemia occur in up to 30% of treated patients. Documented remissions range from 3 to 5+ years following treatment.

The treatment of advanced Hodgkin disease was improved considerably with the introduction of combination chemotherapy—initially mechlorethamine, vincristine, procarbazine, and prednisone (MOPP) and later the ABV form of doxorubicin, bleomycin, vinblastine, and dacarbazine (ABVD). Patients receiving these therapies have a 20% to 25% relapse rate. Escalated doses of first-line chemotherapy and consolidation radiation therapy have lowered the relapse rate but without improvement in survival.

Prognostic Factors

1. Histological type, tumor size, number of involved lymph nodes and extranodal sites, presence or absence of systemic symptoms, ESR, lactic dehydrogenase (LDH), albumin, β-2-microglobulin, and alkaline phosphatase, hemoglobin, clinical state, and presence or absence of involvement of bone marrow, inguinal lymph nodes, or both are prognostic indicators. Characteristics of the patient include age, gender, and the presence or absence of lymphocytopenia.

FIGURE 20.12 Lymphomas. **A:** Non-Hodgkin lymphoma. **B:** Reactive adenitis in a child. **C:** Mixed large and small lymphocytes in a patient with Hodgkin disease. **D:** Large B-cell lymphoma. (Reprinted with permission from Greer JP, et al. *Wintrobe's Clinical Hematology*, 11th ed. Philadelphia, PA: Lippincott Williams & Wilkins, 2004.)

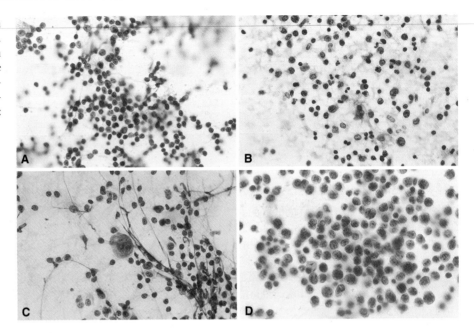

2. Other biological features are important prognostic factors in Hodgkin disease and include the serum level of soluble CD30 (an antigen expressed by Reed-Sternberg cells), the number of activated cytotoxic T cells, and the presence or absence of CD15 (an antigen expressed by Reed-Sternberg cells in some variant of Hodgkin disease).

Germinal center, B-cell–like large-cell lymphoma has the best prognosis with a 60% 5-year patient survival rate after anthracycline-based chemotherapy. It exhibited two oncogenic events not seen in the other subgroups: t(14;18) translocation of the BCL2 gene and amplification of the c-rel locus on chromosome 2p. Patients in the type 3 subgroup had a survival rate of 39%; those in the activated B-cell–like subgroup had the poorest prognosis, with a survival rate of 35%.

Treatment

The outcome of treatment for advanced Hodgkin lymphomas has improved dramatically over the past two decades. Cure rates of more than 70% are now possible with a hybrid regimen of mechlorethamine, vincristine, procarbazine, prednisone, doxorubicin, bleomycin, vinblastine (MOPP-ABV); a regimen of doxorubicin, bleomycin, vinblastine, and dacarbazine (ABVD); or a regimen of bleomycin, etoposide, doxorubicin, cyclophosphamide, vincristine, procarbazine, and prednisone (BEACOPP). Radiation therapy has been suggested as beneficial only for patients who have achieved partial remission after chemotherapy.

The standard treatment for patients with diffuse large B-cell lymphoma is cyclophosphamide, doxorubicin, vincristine, and prednisone (CHOP). Rituximab, a chimeric IgG1 monoclonal antibody against the CD20 B-cell antigen, has therapeutic activity in diffuse large B-cell lymphoma. The addition of rituximab to the CHOP regimen increases the complete response rate and prolongs event-free and overall survival in elderly patients with diffuse large B-cell lymphomas compared with CHOP alone without a clinically significant increase in toxicity.

Characteristics of Other Forms

In NHL, Reed-Sternberg cells are absent. The infiltrating cells may be of one type or may have a mixed cell population of lymphocytes, histiocytes, eosinophils, and some plasma cells.

Cytogenetic Analysis

The chromosomal anomalies that have been observed in hematological malignant disease include structural rearrangement as translocations and deletions and numerical abnormalities with respect to structural rearrangements. Analysis of DNA sequences, located at the chromosomal breakpoint of several of the recurring translocations in leukemias or lymphomas, has revealed that the genes located at these sites are protooncogenes. As a result of the genetic mutation induced by the chromosomal rearrangement, the function of the gene is altered, thereby converting the gene to an oncogene.

The best examples are the translocations observed in Burkitt lymphoma and chronic myelogenous leukemia. In Burkitt lymphoma, one of three translocations is usually observed. These translocations involve the *Myc* oncogene normally located on chromosome 8 and either chromosome 14, 2, or 22. These are the sites of the immunoglobulin heavy chain [t(8;14)], kappa light chain [t(2;8)], and lambda light chain [t(8;22)] genes, respectively. In these translocations, *Myc* oncogene is juxtaposed with the DNA sequence of the immunoglobulin genes, resulting in the unregulated transcriptional activity of the *Myc* gene.

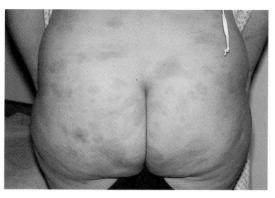

FIGURE 20.13 Mycosis fungoides (cutaneous T-cell lymphoma). Lesions have characteristic "smudgy," poorly defined patches and plaques in a typical location. (Reprinted with permission from Goodheart HP. *Goodheart's Photoguide of Common Skin Disorders*, 2nd ed. Philadelphia, PA: Lippincott Williams & Wilkins, 2003.)

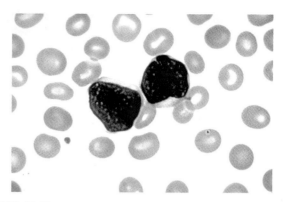

FIGURE 20.15 Sézary cells. Two circulating neoplastic T-helper cells with irregular nuclei and a thin rim of cytoplasm are seen. (Reprinted with permission from Rubin E, Farber JL. *Pathology*, 3rd ed, Philadelphia, PA: Lippincott Williams & Wilkins, 1999.)

Mature T-Cell and NK-Cell Neoplasms

Mature T-cell neoplasms are derived from mature or postthymic T cells. Because NK cells are closely related and share some immunophenotypical and functional properties with T cells, these two classes of neoplasms are considered together (Tables 20.6 and 20.7).

CHAPTER HIGHLIGHTS

Lymphoid Neoplasms

The World Health Organization (WHO) Classification of Tumours of the Haematopoietic and Lymphoid Tissues, fourth edition, has enhanced the classification of lymphoid neoplasms by including immunophenotypic features and genetic abnormalities to define different disorders. Disorders of the mature B-cell neoplasm classification include CLL/SLL,

Sézary Syndrome

The leukemic phase of cutaneous T-cell lymphoma, **mycosis fungoides** (Fig. 20.13), is called Sézary syndrome. Diagnosis of Sézary syndrome is dependent on the primary diagnosis of mycosis fungoides in a skin biopsy. Adults between 40 and 60 years old are most frequently afflicted with skin lesions that progress to the tumor stage. In peripheral blood, the disease is characterized by the presence of abnormal circulating lymphocytes, **Sézary cells**.

A Sézary cell (Figs. 20.14 and 20.15) is typically the size of a small lymphocyte and has a dark-staining, clumped, nuclear chromatin pattern. The distinctive folded, groove-like chromatin pattern is described as **cerebriform**. Mature T lymphocytes in Sézary display a phenotype with reactivity for CD2, CD3, CD4, and CD5.

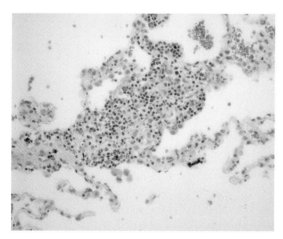

FIGURE 20.14 Mycosis fungoides with focal interstitial infiltration by small lymphocytes. (Reprinted with permission from Cagle PT. *Color Atlas and Text of Pulmonary Pathology*, Philadelphia, PA: Lippincott Williams & Wilkins, 2005.)

TABLE 20.6	Immunohistological Features of Selected T-Cell Neoplasms			
	Surface Membrane Markers			
Type of Neoplasm	CD3	CD4	CD5	CD8
T-PLL	+	±	−	−/+
T-LGL	+	−	−	+
Mycosis fungoides/Sézary syndrome	+	+	+	−

T-PLL, T-cell prolymphocytic leukemia/lymphoma; T-LGL, T-cell large granular lymphocytic leukemia; +, >90%; ±, >50%; ˜/+, <50%; ˜/+, <10%. *Source*: Handin RI, et al. (eds). *Blood: Principles and Practice of Hematology*, 2nd ed, Philadelphia, PA: Lippincott Williams & Wilkins, 2003.

TABLE 20.7	Genetic Features and Epstein-Barr Virus Status in Selected T-cell Neoplasms	
Type of Neoplasm	**Genetic Abnormality**	**EBV Status**
T-PLL	inv 14, trisomy 8q	–
T-LGL	None known	–
Mycosis fungoides/Sézary syndrome	None known	–

EBV, Epstein-Barr virus; T-PLL, T-cell prolymphocytic leukemia/lymphoma; T-LGL, T-cell large granular lymphocytic leukemia.
Source: Handin RI, et al (eds). *Blood: Principles and Practice of Hematology*, 2nd ed, Philadelphia, PA: Lippincott Williams & Wilkins, 2003.

B-cell prolymphocytic leukemia, HCL, and plasma cell neoplasms. CLL is the most common form of leukemia in adults in Western countries. CLL/SLL accounts for almost 7% of NHLs in biopsies.

Plasma Cell Neoplasms

Multiple myeloma is a malignant plasma cell disease, typically of the bone marrow. Plasma cell leukemia is considered to be a form of multiple myeloma, not a separate entity; however, increased numbers of plasma cells are found in the peripheral blood rather than in the bone marrow. The etiology of multiple myeloma is unknown. The outstanding laboratory characteristics include the presence of Bence Jones protein in the urine and an abnormal serum and/or urinary electrophoretic pattern.

WM is a malignant lymphocyte–plasma cell proliferative disorder with abnormally large amounts of the gamma globulin type (19S or IgM). Abnormal serum electrophoresis patterns and the presence of cryoglobulin are characteristic.

Lymphomas

Lymphomas are closely related to leukemias. Frequently, the neoplastic cells of leukemia and lymphoma are identical. Initially, lymphomas are confined to the lymph nodes, but they may spillover into the blood in the leukemic phase. Lymphomas are commonly divided into the Hodgkin and non-Hodgkin types. The presence or absence of Reed-Sternberg cells is critical in establishing a diagnosis. Cytogenetic analysis is valuable in identifying Burkitt lymphoma and some other malignant lymphomas.

CASE STUDIES

CASE 20.1

A 58-year-old female medical records librarian was admitted to the hospital for minor elective surgery. Although the patient had been complaining of general malaise and fatigue, she suspected that it was a work-related problem rather than a physical problem. Physical examination revealed that she had both cervical and supraclavicular lymphadenopathy.

■ Laboratory Data
Her preoperative blood count revealed that her erythrocytes and hemoglobin were within normal ranges; however, her total leukocyte count was 26.5×10^9/L. The distribution of leukocytes was as follows:

Bands 6%
Segmented neutrophils 18%
Lymphocytes 75%
Monocytes 1%

Some variant lymphocytes and smudge-type cells were present. The distribution of platelets was normal.

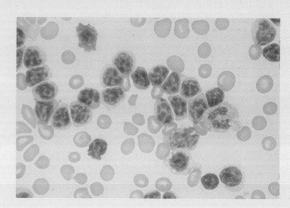

(Reprinted with permission from Anderson S, Poulsen K. *Anderson's Atlas of Hematology*, Philadelphia, PA: Lippincott Williams & Wilkins, 2003.)

(continued)

Follow-up laboratory tests included an infectious mononucleosis screen, with negative results. Bone marrow examination revealed lymphocytic infiltration of approximately 50% of the cells in the marrow.

■ Questions

1. What could be the possible explanation for the leukocytosis and concurrent lymphocytosis?
2. What further testing could be done to establish a diagnosis?
3. What is the patient's prognosis?

■ Discussion

1. Persons older than 50 years of age with leukocytosis and lymphocytosis may be suffering from the early stages of CLL. The lymphadenopathy further suggests a lymphoproliferative disorder.
2. A lymph node biopsy could be performed to study the architecture of the node. This examination would be helpful in differentiating a lymphocytic lymphoma from CLL. Electron microscope studies may be of additional value in demonstrating the ultrastructure of the lymphocytes. Patients with CLL frequently have lymphocytes that vary from normal. Cytogenetic analysis might also be useful. The existence of a trisomy 12 would be helpful in establishing the patient's prognosis.
3. The majority of these patients usually survive for at least 10 years after diagnosis if the karyotype is normal. However, a patient with an abnormal karyotype would have a graver prognosis. The general prognosis in CLL is much more favorable than in other forms of leukemia. Some patients survive for more than 30 years, although the median survival time is from 4 to 6 years.

DIAGNOSIS: Chronic Lymphocytic Leukemia

CASE 20.2

A 58-year-old male college professor saw his family physician because of increasing fatigue and weakness. He also reported pain in his lower back and arms when he walked. Physical examination revealed that the man had pale mucous membranes and hepatosplenomegaly. The physician ordered a CBC and urinalysis. A follow-up appointment was scheduled for the following week.

■ Laboratory Data

The CBC revealed that the patient had anemia. His leukocyte count and differential count were normal, except for a rouleaux (rolled coin) appearance of the RBCs. The result of urinalysis was normal. The patient was called and it was requested that he returns to the laboratory for additional tests. The physician ordered the following tests: ESR, kidney screening profile, liver blood profile, and radiographic skeletal survey, with the following results: ESR, 50 mm/hour; normal kidney profile; and normal liver profile

except for increased globular protein. The skeletal survey indicated bone lesions in various sites.

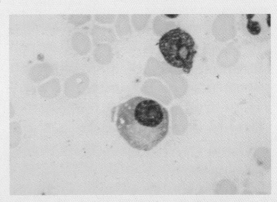

(Reprinted with permission from Anderson S, Poulsen K. *Anderson's Atlas of Hematology*, Philadelphia, PA: Lippincott Williams & Wilkins, 2003.)

■ Questions

1. What follow-up laboratory tests might be ordered to assist in establishing a definitive diagnosis?
2. What type of leukocyte disorder could be present?
3. What is the nature of the protein found in the urine?
4. What is the most significant laboratory finding in this disorder?

■ Discussion

1. In this case, further investigation of the increased ESR and increased serum globular protein was ordered. A serum electrophoresis and immunoelectrophoresis revealed the presence of an abnormal protein, a 7S immunoglobulin. Bence Jones protein was identified in the urine. Subsequent bone marrow examination revealed a remarkable increase in plasma cells.
2. Although an increase in proteins, specifically immunoglobulins, is responsible for the elevated ESR, an absence of cells related to antibody production is frequently noted in this disorder. However, a bone marrow examination would reveal an overproliferation of plasma cells. In rare cases, a leukemic form of myeloma, called **plasma cell leukemia**, develops. In these cases, some plasma cells may be seen in the peripheral blood.
3. Bence Jones protein precipitates when heated to 56°C, dissolves when heated to boiling, and reprecipitates with cooling. On electrophoresis, this protein will reflect its monoclonal nature and appear in the beta or gamma region.
4. Although metastatic carcinoma involving the liver can produce bone marrow plasmacytosis, the presence of increased plasma cells is significant in establishing the diagnosis. Laboratory tests, particularly serum and urine electrophoresis, are important adjuncts.

DIAGNOSIS: Multiple Myeloma

(continued)

CASE 20.3

A 70-year-old woman with a diagnosis of refractory multiple myeloma and diabetes was admitted to the hospital because of bleeding caused by pancytopenia.

■ **Laboratory Data**

Hemoglobin 6.0 g/dL
Hematocrit 20%
Total leukocyte count 4.1×10^9/L

■ **Leukocyte Differential**

Plasma cells 25%
Segmented neutrophils 26%
Immature granulocytes 13%
Lymphocytes (variant forms noted) 36%

■ **Other Test Results**

Urinalysis Positive for blood and positive for protein
Blood culture Negative
Immunoelectrophoresis Decreased IgG
Complement assay Decreased

■ **Questions**

1. Why does this patient have immunocompetency?
2. Why does the patient have granulocytopenia?
3. Could this patient have an infection?

■ **Discussion**

1. Patients who have multiple myeloma experience a compensatory decrease in the synthesis and an increase in catabolism of normal immunoglobulins. As the tumor burden increases, the patient's antibody response becomes more challenged and the degree of antibody (humoral) immunity increases. Complement levels are also decreased.
2. In multiple myeloma, granulocytopenia may develop as a result of bone marrow failure.
3. Yes. A dysfunctional immune system can contribute to the development of an infection. In cases of pancytopenia, cellular immunity is impaired. Infections associated with chemotherapy-induced granulocytopenia have become more common. Because this patient also has diabetes, she may have altered cellular immunity. Microorganisms that can be threatening are *Pseudomonas aeruginosa*, *Klebsiella pneumoniae*, *Staphlococcus. aureus*, mycobacteria, and fungi (e.g., candida or cryptococcus).

DIAGNOSIS: **Multiple Myeloma**

CASE 20.4

A 75-year-old man was referred to a multispecialty group practice for evaluation of a chronic lymphoproliferative disorder.

■ **Laboratory Data**

Hemoglobin 9.0 g/dL
Hematocrit 32%
RBC count 2.9×10^{12}/L
Total leukocyte count 7.5×10^9/L
Total platelet count 150×10^{12}/L

The peripheral blood smear revealed lymphocytic-looking leukocytes with cytoplasmic projections, prominent nucleoli, and overall smaller cell size.

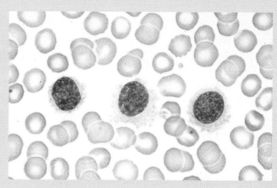

(Reprinted with permission from Rubin R, Strayer DS. *Rubin's Pathology: Clinicopathologic Foundations of Medicine*, 5th ed, Philadelphia, PA: Lippincott Williams & Wilkins, 2008.)

■ **Follow-up**

TRAP stain was negative.

■ **Questions**

1. What is this patient's diagnosis?
2. What follow-up tests are needed to confirm a diagnosis?
3. Is this a classic example of a lymphoproliferative disorder?

■ **Discussion**

1. The category of this patient's abnormality is a chronic, malignant lymphoproliferative disorder. Based on the morphological appearance of the lymphocyte-like cells in the peripheral blood, the possibility of HCL exists. However, a typical HCL would be expected to be positive for TRAP.
2. Flow cytometry studies of immunophenotyping of cell surface membrane markers are important. In this case, CD25 (interleukin-2 receptor) and CD11c markers were

(continued)

negative. In a classic case of HCL, these markers would be expected to be positive.

3. No. Typical HCL would display a positive reaction with TRAP staining as well as CD25 and CD11c markers. These findings were not present in this patient. However, based on the overall compilation of findings, a diagnosis of hairy cell variant (vHCL) was established.

DIAGNOSIS: Hairy Cell Leukemia-Variant (vHCL)

CASE 20.5

A 60-year-old man sought medical advice after suffering from fatigue, upper abdominal pain, and a 20-lb weight loss over the past 9 months. Physical examination revealed a distended abdomen with massive splenomegaly and moderate hepatomegaly. There was no evidence of lymphadenopathy.

■ Laboratory Data
Hemoglobin 10.0 g/dL
Hematocrit 33%
Total RBC count 4.0×10^{12}/L
Total WBC count 120.0×10^{9}/L
Total platelet count 153×10^{9}/L

Erythrocyte Indices
MCV 90 fL
MCH 25 pq
MCHC 33 g/dL

Peripheral Blood Smear Examination
Mononuclear cells 65%
Segmented neutrophils 5%
Lymphocytes (prolymphocytes) 30%
Decreased platelets were noted

■ Questions
1. What is the most abnormal laboratory finding?
2. From what type of abnormality is the patient suffering?
3. What other laboratory assays would aid in establishing a diagnosis of this man's condition?

■ Discussion
1. Both the total leukocyte (WBC) count and the presence of a large number of mononuclear cells are suggestive of a leukemic condition.
2. The patient is certainly suffering from a lymphoproliferative condition. The most likely diagnosis would be lymphocytic leukemia.
3. Cytochemical staining (e.g., TRAP stain) and immunophenotyping using flow cytometry would be valuable. In this case, the patient was TRAP negative. The patient's lymphocytes were positive for CD19, CD20, CD24, or CD22. In addition, the cells display strong SIg.

DIAGNOSIS: Prolymphocytic Leukemia

CASE 20.6

An 80-year-old man, a native of the Dominican Republic, was transferred from a rural community hospital to a Boston teaching hospital because of multiorgan failure. At admission, he was weak and lethargic. He exhibited severe lymphadenopathy.

■ Laboratory Data
Hemoglobin 8.2 g/dL
Hematocrit 22%
Total RBC count 3.0×10^{12}/L
Total WBC count 14.0×10^{9}/L

Peripheral blood smear examination revealed many lymphocytes (62%) and many variant lymphocytes with prominent nuclear lobation as well as a few nucleated RBCs. The number of platelets was slightly decreased. The erythrocytes were microcytic and hypochromic.

Total bilirubin 5.3 mg/dL (reference range, <1.5 mg/dL)

■ Questions
1. From what type of abnormalities is he suffering?
2. What could be the cause of his abnormal findings?
3. What steps must be taken to establish a diagnosis?

■ Discussion
1. His lymphadenopathy on physical examination, lymphocytosis on peripheral blood smear, and increased total serum bilirubin are all abnormal findings.
2. Lymphadenopathy can be manifested in infectious diseases, autoimmune disorders, granulomatous disease, drug hypersensitivity reactions, and malignant diseases (e.g., solid tumors and lymphomas).
3. It is important to distinguish between a benign lymphocytosis caused by infection and a primary lymphoproliferative disorder. Flow cytometry studies of this patient's bone marrow demonstrated a predominant population of CD3-positive (dim expression) and CD4-positive T cells. Cells were negative for the pan-T-cell antigens CD7 and CD5. Dim expression of CD3 and lack of one or more pan-T-cell antigens indicate the presence of an abnormal T-cell population, which suggests a T-cell neoplasm. Other findings were CD4+, CD2+, CD1a+, and terminal deoxynucleotidyl transferase (TdT)-positive.

Because of the patient's history of living in the Caribbean, he was tested for HTLV-I and HTLV-II. His results were positive.

DIAGNOSIS: Adult T-Cell Leukemia-Lymphoma, HTLV-I Associated

REVIEW QUESTIONS

1. The most common form of chronic leukemia in Western countries is
   A. myelogenous
   B. lymphocytic
   C. monocytic
   D. eosinophilic

2. The median survival time of patients with CLL, compared with patients with chronic monocytic leukemia, is
   A. not significantly different
   B. shorter
   C. longer
   D. shorter, if the patient is female

3. CLL is classically a
   A. T-cell disorder
   B. B-cell disorder
   C. null cell disorder
   D. disorder of the young

4. CLL symptoms frequently include
   A. weight loss, anemia, and extreme leukocytosis
   B. absolute lymphocytosis, edema, and splenic infarction
   C. absolute lymphocytosis, malaise, and low-grade fever
   D. neutrophilia, splenomegaly, and anemia

5. Characteristics of malignant lymphoma typically include
   A. overproliferation of neutrophils
   B. overproliferation of lymphocytes
   C. lymph node involvement
   D. both B and C

6. Hodgkin disease
   A. is characterized by neutrophilia in the early stages of the disease
   B. occurs more frequently in females than males
   C. is a lymphoma, characterized by Reed-Sternberg cells, and occurs more frequently in females than in males
   D. is a lymphoma, characterized by Reed-Sternberg cells, and occurs more frequently in males than in females

7. Rare forms of lymphoma include
   A. Hodgkin and non-Hodgkin lymphoma
   B. Burkitt lymphoma and mycosis fungoides
   C. Hodgkin and non-Hodgkin lymphoma and Burkitt lymphoma
   D. Non-Hodgkin lymphoma and mycosis fungoides

8. Multiple myeloma is a disorder of
   A. T lymphocytes
   B. megakaryocytes
   C. plasma cells
   D. the lymph nodes

9. The abnormal protein frequently found in the urine of persons with multiple myeloma is
   A. albumin
   B. globulin
   C. IgG
   D. Bence Jones

10. WM is characterized by increased levels of
    A. IgG
    B. IgM
    C. IgD
    D. IgA

11. Which cluster designations are positive in typical HCL?
    A. CD25 CD11c, CD19, CD20
    B. CD25 CD11c, CD19, CD10
    C. CD25 CD11c, CD10, CD5
    D. CD25 CD22, CD19, CD20

BIBLIOGRAPHY

Attal M, et al. Maintenance therapy with thalidomide improves survival in patients with multiple myeloma, *Blood*, 108(10):3289–3294, 2006.

Awan FT, et al. Mcl-1 expression predicts progression-free survival in chronic lymphocytic leukemia patients treated with pentostatin, cyclophosphamide, and rituximab, *Blood*, 113(3):535–537, 2009.

Ayliffe MJ, et al. Demonstration of changes in plasma cell subsets in multiple myeloma, *Haematologica*, 92(08):1135–1138, 2007.

Baskar S, et al. A human monoclonal antibody drug and target discovery platform for B-cell chronic lymphocytic leukemia based on allogeneic hematopoietic stem cell transplantation and phage display, *Blood*, 114(20):4494–4502, 2009.

Bench AJ, et al. Molecular genetic analysis of haematological malignancies II: mature lymphoid neoplasms, *Int J Lab Hematol*, 29(4):229–260, 2007.

Binet J-L, et al. Perspectives on the use of new diagnostic tools in the treatment of chronic lymphocytic leukemia, *Blood*, 107(3):859–861, 2006.

Burger JA. Fledgling prognostic markers in CLL, *Blood*, 110(12):3820–3821, 2007.

Caligaris-Cappio F. IG genes and hairy cell leukemia, *Blood*, 114(21):4610, 2009.

Calin GA, Croce CM. Chronic lymphocytic leukemia: interplay between noncoding RNAs and protein-coding genes, *Blood*, 114(23):4761–4770, 2009.

Calin GA, et al. A microRNA signature associated with prognosis and progression in chronic lymphocytic leukenia, *N Eng J Med*, 353(17):1793–1801, 2005.

Cazin B. First line treatment of CLL: New approaches. In: *New Treatment Approaches for Chronic Lymphoproliferative Disorders and Lymphoma*. Satellite symposium presentation at the 8th Congress of the European Hematology Association, Lyon, France June 12, 2003.

Child JA, et al. High-dose chemotherapy with hematopoietic stem-cell rescue for multiple myeloma, *N Engl J Med*, 348(19):1875–1883, 2003.

Coifier B, et al. CHOP chemotherapy plus rituximab compared with CHOP alone in elderly patients with diffuse large-B-cell lymphoma, *N Engl J Med*, 346(4):235–241, 2002.

Crespo M, et al. ZAP-70 expression as a surrogate for immunoglobulin-variable-region mutations in chronic lymphocytic leukemia, *N Engl J Med*, 348(18):1764–1775, 2003.

Cuneo A, et al. Chronic lymphocytic leukemia with 6Q shows distinct hematological features and intermediate prognosis, *Hematol J*, 4(Suppl 2):32, 2003.

DeVita VT. Hodgkin's disease—Clinical trials and travails, *N Engl J Med*, 348(24):2375–2376, 2003.

Dicker F, et al. CD154 induces p73 to overcome the resistance to apoptosis of chronic lymphocytic leukemia cells lacking functional p53, *Blood*, 108(10):3450–3457, 2006.

Diehl V, et al. Standard and increased-dose BEACOPP chemotherapy compared with COPP-ABVD for advanced Hodgkin's disease, *N Engl J Med*, 348(24):2386–2395, 2003.

Duerig J, et al. Gene expression profiling in CD38+ versus CD38–B cell chronic lymphocytic leukemia [Abstract]. Annual Meeting of the American Society of Hematology, Philadelphia, PA, December 2002.

Engert A. MAb Campath® and Fludara® in combination: Exciting potential. Satellite symposium presentation at the 8th Congress of the European Hematology Association, Lyon, France, June 12, 2003.

Evans PAS. Recent aspects of t(14;18) detection and quantification. In: *Educational Book of the 8th Congress of the European Hematology Association*, Lyon, France: 2003:187–190.

Fermé C, et al. Chemotherapy plus involved-field radiation in early-stage Hodgkin's Disease, *N Eng J Med*, 357(19):1916–1927, 2007.

Fermé C. Hodgkin's lymphoma: Place of radiation therapy. In: *Educational Book of the 8th Congress of the European Hematology Association*, Lyon, France: 2003:212–217.

Fernàndez V, et al. Gene expression profile and genomic changes in disease progression of early-stage chronic lymphocytic leukemia, *Haematologica*, 93(1):132–136, 2008.

Ferry JA. Lymphoma classification. In: *Current Concepts in Clinical Pathology*, Boston: Department of Pathology, Massachusetts General Hospital and Harvard Medical School, 2003:45–61.

Foss FM, et al. Case 10–2003: A 72-year-old man with rapidly progressive leukemia, rash, and multiorgan failure, *N Engl J Med*, 348(13):1267–1275, 2003.

Foubister V. Genes pointing the way in lymphoma prognosis, *CAP Today*, 16(9):30–32, 2002.

Fröhling S, et al. Cytogenetics and age are major determinants of outcome in intensively treated acute myeloid leukemia patients older than 60 years: results from AMLSG trail AML HD98-B, *Blood*, 108(10):3280–3288, 2006.

Ghielmini M. Follicular lymphoma: chemotherapy and/or antibodies? *Blood*, 108(10):3235, 2006.

Hallaert DYH. c-Abl kinase inhibitors overcome CD40-mediated drug resistance in CLL: implications for therapeutic targeting of chemoresistant niches, *Blood*, 112(13):5141–5149, 2008.

Hallek M. Chemo-immunotherapy of CLL. In: *Educational Book of the 8th Congress of the European Hematology Association*, Lyon, France: 2003:175–179.

Hamblin TJ. CLL, how many diseases? In: *Educational Book of the 8th Congress of the European Hematology Association*, Lyon, France: 2003:183–186.

Hasenclever D, Diehl V. A prognostic score for advanced Hodgkin's disease, *N Engl J Med*, 339(21):1506–1513, 1998.

Hooker A, Gregson L. Hematology no. H-4 2002, *Am Soc Clin Pathol Tech Sample*, 2002:17–20.

Jaffe ES, et al. Classification of lymphoid neoplasms: the microscope as a tool for disease discovery, *Blood*, 112(12):4384–4399, 2008.

Kater AP, et al. Cellular immune therapy for chronic lymphocytic leukemia, *Blood*, 110(8):2811–2818, 2007.

Kay NE (Chair). A symposium on chronic lymphocytic leukemia. Annual Meeting of the American Society of Hematology, Philadelphia, PA, December 2002.

Kay NE. Treatment and evaluation of CLL: a complicated affair, *Blood*, 107(3):848, 2006.

Kohlmann A, et al. Gene expression profiles of distinct cytogenetic CLL subtypes [Abstract]. Annual Meeting of the American Society of Hematology, Philadelphia, PA, December 2002.

Kreitman RJ, et al. Soluble CD22, a new test which correlates with disease status in B-cell leukemia and lymphoma [Abstract]. Annual Meeting of the American Society of Hematology, Philadelphia, PA, December 2002.

Kroger N. diagnosis and montoring of monoclonal gammopathies by serum free light chain assay, *MedLab Magazine*, Issue One, 2009.

Kyle RA, Rajkumar SV. Multiple myeloma, *Blood*, 111(6):2962–2972, 2007.

Lambert MP. Childhood ITP: knowing when to worry? *Blood*, 114(23):4758–4759, 2009.

Lee RV, et al. B-cell lymphoma with intermediate- to high-grade features and different immunophenotypic profiles involving separate anatomic sites with a good response to R-CHOP, *Labmedicine*, 40(2):79–86, 2009.

Lin P, Medeiros LJ. High-grade B-cell lymphoma/leukemia associated with t(14;18) and 8q24/MYC rearrangement: a neoplasm of germinal center immunophenotype with poor prognosis, *Haematologica*, 92(10):1297–1301, 2007.

Mayr C, et al. Chromosomal translocations are associated with poor prognosis in chronic lymphocytic leukemia, *Blood*, 107(2):742–751, 2006.

Mileshkin L, et al. Patients with multiple myeloma treated with thalidomide: evaluation of clinical parameters, cytokines, angiogenic markers, mast cells and narrow CD57+ cytotoxic T cells as predictors of outcome, *Haematologica*, 92(08):1075–1082, 2007.

Molina A. Zevalin™ in NHL: A new approach in the treatment of NHL. Satellite symposium presentation at the 8th Congress of the European Hematology Association, Lyon, France, June 12, 2003.

Montserrat E, et al. Redefining prognostic elements in chronic lymphocytic leukemia. In: *Educational Book of the 8th Congress of the European Hematology Association*, Lyon, France: 2003:180–182.

Oberlin O. Hodgkin's lymphoma in children. In: *Educational Book of the 8th Congress of the European Hematology Association*, Lyon, France: 2003: 218–221.

O'Brien S. MAb Campath® as consolidation therapy. Satellite symposium presentation at the 8th Congress of the European Hematology Association, Lyon, France, June 12, 2003.

Pearson M, Rowley JD. The relation of oncogenetics in leukemia and lymphoma, *Annu Rev Med*, 36:471–483, 1985.

Qian J, et al. Myeloma cell line-derived, pooled heat shock proteins as a universal vaccine for immunotherapy of multiple myeloma, *Blood*, 114(18):3880–3889, 2009.

Rai KR, Chiorazzi N. Determining the clinical course and outcome in chronic lymphocytic leukemia, *N Engl J Med*, 348(18):1797–1799, 2003.

Rogoski RR. Serum free light chain assays: detecting plasma cell disorders, *MLO*, 41(7):10–21, 2009.

Rosenwald A. Bridging molecular pathology and clinics in lymphoma. In: *Educational Book of the 8th Congress of the European Hematology Association*, Lyon, France: 2003:208–211.

Rozman C, Montserrat E. Chronic lymphocytic leukemia, *N Engl J Med*, 333(16):1052–1057, 1995.

Sales G. Histological transformation in follicular lymphoma. In: *Educational Book of the 8th Congress of the European Hematology Association*, Lyon, France: 2003:195–197.

San-Miguel JF, et al. Thalidomide and new drugs for treatment of multiple myeloma. In: *Educational Book of the 8th Congress of the European Hematology Association*, Lyon, France: 2003:201–207.

San-Miguel JF, et al. Incorporating novel agents into upfront myeloma therapy, *N Eng J Med*, 2008;359:906–917.

Sanders PW. A new twist in myeloma treatment, *Blood*, 107(2):413–414, 2006.

Saven A. Treatment of hairy-cell leukemia, *N Engl J Med*, 345(20):1500, 2001.

Siegal D, et al. Serum free light chain analysis for diagnosis, monitoring, and prognosis of monoclonal gammopathies, *Labmedicine*, 40(6):363–367, 2009.

Steingrimsdottir H, et al. Monoclonal gammopathy: natural history studied with a retrospective approach, *Haematologica*, 92(08):1131–1134, 2007.

Teachey DT. Somatic ALPS: a FAScinating condition, *Blood*, 115(25):5125–5126, 2010.

Urba WJ, Longo DL. Hodgkin's disease, *N Engl J Med*, 326(10):678–687, 1992.

Vanura K, et al. Autoimmune conditions and chronic infections in chronic lymphocytic leukemia patients at diagnosis are associated with unmutated IgV_H genes, *Haematologica*, 93(12):1912–1916, 2008.

Vijay A, Gertz MA. Waldenström macroglobulinemia, *Blood*, 109(12):5096–5103, 2007.

Williams H, Crawford DH. Epstein-Barr virus: the impact of scientific advances on clinical practice, *Blood*, 107(3):862–869, 2006.

Zent CS. Time to test CLL p53 function, *Blood*, 115(21):4154, 2010.

CHAPTER **21**

Myeloproliferative Neoplasms

OBJECTIVES

General characteristics and classification

- Name the diseases classified as myeloproliferative neoplasms (MPNs).
- Differentiate and compare the peripheral blood characteristics of these disorders.
- Briefly describe the common abnormalities of hemostasis and coagulation in MPNs.
- Report the general prognostic features of MPNs.
- Briefly explain general treatment approaches to MPNs.

Chronic myelogenous leukemia

- Name the subtypes of chronic myelogenous leukemia (CML).
- Describe the epidemiology of CML.
- Explain the pathophysiology of this leukemia.
- Delineate the usefulness of detection of genetic alterations in CML.
- Compare the clinical signs and symptoms of this leukemia in the three phases of chronic myelogenous leukemia.
- Describe the cellular aspects of CML.
- Explain the application of cytochemistry in the diagnosis of CML compared to a leukemoid reaction.
- Characterize modes of treatment and prognostic features in CML.

Polycythemia vera

- State the other names that might be used to refer to polycythemia vera (PV).
- Describe the epidemiology of PV.
- Name the most striking feature of PV.
- Identify unique genetic abnormality in PV.
- Describe the clinical signs and symptoms of PV.
- List criteria for establishing a diagnosis of PV.
- Compare the characteristics of PV and other types of polycythemias.
- Explain the factors that influence prognosis.
- Name the control and treatment methods in PV.

Primary myelofibrosis

- State the other name for primary myelofibrosis.
- Briefly describe the epidemiology of primary myelofibrosis.
- Name the predominant clinical manifestation in primary myelofibrosis.
- Describe the pathophysiology of primary myelofibrosis.
- Define and describe the consequences of dysmegakaryocytopoiesis.
- Briefly characterize the genetic mutation profile of primary myelofibrosis.
- Delineate the clinical signs and symptoms of primary myelofibrosis.
- Name the cellular components of a leukoblastic peripheral blood picture.
- Describe the life span prognosis in primary myelofibrosis.
- Explain the treatment approach to primary myelofibrosis.

Essential thrombocythemia

- List and describe the major criteria and other findings for the diagnosis of essential thrombocythemia.
- Describe the epidemiology of essential thrombocythemia.
- Outline the major features of essential thrombocythemia.
- Explain the most common disorders in patients with essential thrombocythemia.
- State the classic laboratory findings in essential thrombocythemia.
- Discuss platelet function findings in essential thrombocythemia.
- Compare the bone marrow architecture of essential thrombocythemia with other MPNs.
- Review the relationship between essential thrombocythemia and PV. Report the treatment approach to essential thrombocythemia.

Case studies

- Apply the laboratory data to the stated case studies and discuss the implications of these cases to the study of hematology.

GENERAL CHARACTERISTICS OF MYELOPROLIFERATIVE NEOPLASMS

The MPNs (Box 21.1) are interrelated clonal hematopoietic stem cell disorders characterized by excessive proliferation of one or more mature myeloid cell lines, for example, granulocytes, erythrocytes, megakaryocytes, or mast cells. The discovery of mutations in crucial genes distinguishes MPNs from other neoplasms. Molecular analysis is now incorporated into the diagnosis workup of MPNs. Research molecular advances were capped by the discovery of the JAK2, Janus kinase 2 (JAK2V617F mutation). This discovery allowed for refinement of the classification of MPNs.

Initially, an MPN is characterized by hypercellularity of the bone marrow with effective hematopoietic maturation and increased numbers of granulocytes, red blood cells, and/or platelets in the peripheral blood. One type of MPN may evolve into another type during the course of the disease. All the types of MPNs may evolve into acute leukemia.

All of the MPNs involve dysregulation at the multipotent hematopoietic stem cell (CD34), with one or more of the following shared features:

1. Cytogenetic abnormalities
2. Overproduction of one or more types of blood cells with dominance of a transformed clone
3. Hypercellular marrow or marrow fibrosis
4. Thrombotic and/or hemorrhagic bleeding
5. Extramedullary hematopoiesis
6. Transformation to acute leukemia

MPNs are divided into the following:

1. CML
2. Polycythemia vera
3. Primary myelofibrosis (also known as agnogenic myeloid metaplasia or myelofibrosis with myeloid metaplasia)
4. Essential thrombocytosis or essential thrombocythemia

Relationship of the Myeloproliferative Neoplasms

MPNs are primarily neoplasms of adults between 50 and 70 years of age, but some subtypes occur in children. MPNs have overlapping clinical features.

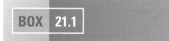

BOX 21.1

Major Categories of MPNs

Chronic myelogenous leukemia, BCR-ABL positive (CML)
Polycythemia vera (PV)
Essential thrombocytosis thrombocythemia (ET)
Primary myelofibrosis

Major changes in the new World Health Organization 2008 classification scheme include

1. The inclusion of JAK2 and MPL mutations as clonal markers for the diagnosis of PV, essential thrombocytosis or essential thrombocythemia (ET), and primary myelofibrosis (PM)
2. Minimization of the role of red cell mass measurement for the diagnosis of PV
3. Lowering of the platelet count cutoff level for a diagnosis of ET from 600 to 450×10^9 L

Variation in the pattern of cellular proliferation and differentiation can be explained by the clonal mutation of pluripotent stem cells with different lineage potentials. Features that distinguish one category from another are presented in Table 21.1.

Common Disorders of Hemostasis and Coagulation

Patients with an MPN suffer from various mild disorders of hemostasis or coagulation. An abnormal coagulation mechanism is believed to be related to a low-grade, possibly secondary form of disseminated intravascular coagulation (DIC), a chronic state of abnormal blood coagulation that occurs even after treatment to reduce the platelet count. Coagulation abnormalities include a prolonged activated partial thromboplastin time (APTT) and a significantly decreased level of factor V. In many patients, the levels of D-dimer, thrombin-antithrombin III complex, and plasmin-alpha 2-plasmin inhibitor complex are higher than normal.

Patients with an MPN commonly exhibit thrombotic phenomena. This is believed to be associated with an increase in circulating platelets affecting the arterial and venous circulation. In rare cases, the initial manifestation of MPN can be gangrene of the extremities. Numerical and morphological characteristics of the megakaryopoiesis differ in each category of MPN. A triad of qualitative platelet defects (abolished second-wave epinephrine aggregation, increased adenosine diphosphate [ADP] aggregation threshold, and significantly reduced adenosine triphosphate [ATP] secretion during collagen-induced aggregation) seems to be a good diagnostic marker of MPN with thrombocytosis.

In addition, arachidonate metabolism is frequently deranged in patients with MPN. The change in thromboxane formation in essential thrombocythemia and PV could be one of the factors responsible for the different incidences of thrombotic and hemorrhagic complications in these diseases. When arachidonic acid metabolism in patients with an MPN was evaluated, the generation of thromboxane B_2 was found to be significantly reduced and inversely correlated with the platelet count in patients with essential thrombocythemia. PV patients showed an increased formation of this metabolite of arachidonic acid. The generation of prostaglandin E2 and 6-keto-prostaglandin $F_{1\alpha}$ was significantly reduced in patients with CML.

TABLE 21.1	Comparative Peripheral Blood Characteristics of MPNs			
	CML	PM	PV	ET
Erythrocytes × 10^{12}/L	Decreased	Decreased	Extremely increased	Normal
Leukocytes × 10^9/L	Extremely increased	Variable	Increased	Normal
Platelets × 10^9/L	Moderately increased	Variable	Moderately increased	Extremely increased
Teardrop-shaped erythrocytes	None	Extremely increased	None	None
Leukocyte alkaline phosphate score	Decreased	Variable	Extremely increased	Normal/increased
Marrow fibrosis	Variable	Very increased	None	None
Ph[1] chromosome	Positive	Negative	Negative	Negative

CML, chronic myelogenous leukemia; PM, primary myelofibrosis; PV, polycythemia vera; ET, essential thrombocythemia.

Prognosis and Treatment

Acute leukemic transformation in primary myelofibrosis generally has an insidious presentation, contrasting with its abrupt onset in most patients with PV or essential thrombocythemia. Approximately two thirds of patients whose illness transforms into acute leukemia develop myelogenous leukemia; the remaining one third develop lymphoblastic leukemia. Median survival time from diagnosis of the acute transformation averages only 3 months.

Molecular therapy for CML has revolutionized treatment at the molecular level. Ongoing clinical trials are directed at molecular therapy for other MPNs. Cytogenetic and molecular changes after interferon therapy are apparent in patients with CML, as manifested by a change in the Philadelphia (Ph[1]) chromosome and *BCR-ABL* gene, respectively.

Data to date suggest that interferon alfa may be a new and effective drug for the treatment of MPNs. The mechanism of action of interferon is not completely understood. This biological agent, either alone or in combination with other antineoplastic treatment, represents the classic therapeutic approach for the treatment of these disorders.

CHRONIC MYELOGENOUS LEUKEMIA

CML is an MPN that originates in an abnormal pluripotent bone marrow stem cell and is consistently associated with the *BCR-ABL* 1 fusion gene located in the Philadelphia chromosome. CML and chronic lymphocytic leukemia (CLL) (see Chapter 20) are the other principal types of chronic leukemias.

Epidemiology

Ninety-five percent of patients with CML have the common type. Other forms, for example, chronic neutrophilic leukemia, are extremely rare.

This CML is predominantly a leukemia of middle-aged adults. The median age at diagnosis is in the fifth and sixth decades of life. Males have a slightly greater rate of disease occurrence. The incidence of CML in Western countries is estimated to be approximately 2 per 100,000 persons annually and accounts for 15% of leukemias in adults (all age groups included). Five to ten percent of patients have a history of excessive radiation exposure.

Pathophysiology

CML is a clonal proliferative disorder of the pluripotent hematopoietic progenitor cell that results in a disordered proliferation of cells. An excessive increase in mostly mature myeloid cells in the peripheral blood is the hallmark of the initial (chronic) phase of CML. The disorderly expansion of myeloid progenitor cells appears to result from alterations in their proliferative capacity and a shift in the balance between self-renewal and differentiation, increasing the number of progenitor cells and reducing the pool of stem cells. Stem cells become part of the proliferating compartment, causing the neoplastic cell population to expand exponentially in later maturational compartments, where they may also be less responsive to growth-regulatory signals from cytokines or the bone marrow microenvironment. In addition, defective adherence of immature hematopoietic CML progenitors to marrow stromal elements may facilitate their release into the blood. The suppression of pathways of apoptosis has been implicated in the pathogenesis of CML.

CML is characterized by a chronic, indolent disease course that frequently transforms into a terminal, acute blast crisis phase. An accelerated phase, when patients become refractive to traditional therapy, may precede the acute phase. Some patients may enter the phase of blast transformation abruptly.

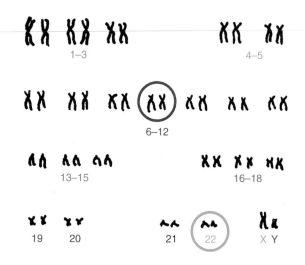

FIGURE 21.1 Philadelphia chromosome. This chromosomal aberration represents a translocation of the long arm of chromosome 22 to the long arm of chromosome 9.

Cytogenetics

The Ph[1] chromosome (Fig. 21.1), the first aberrant chromosome described in a malignant disorder, was discussed by Nowell and Hungerford in 1960. In 1973, it was shown to result from the reciprocal translocation of DNA between chromosomes 9 and 22. The Ph[1] chromosome is the first demonstrable hematological change in more than 90% of CML patients and is present in myelogenous and erythroid precursors as well as megakaryocytes. It is usually not found in normal lymphocytes.

The majority of Ph[1]-positive patients have the typical t(9;22) translations. The reciprocal translocation t(9;22) generates two novel fusion genes: BCR-ABL on the derivative 22q- (Philadelphia) chromosome and ABL-BCR on chromosome 9q+. The ABL gene product is a protein tyrosine kinase (TK), and the fusion protein bcr-abl has constitutive kinase activity that deregulates signal transduction pathways, causing abnormal cell cycling, inhibition of apoptosis, and increased proliferation of cells. Seventy-five to eighty percent of patients in a blast crisis of CML develop other chromosome aberrations in addition to the Ph[1] chromosome. The most common abnormalities are a duplication of the Ph[1] chromosome and trisomy 8. Nonrandom clonal changes found in 80% of patients, in addition to trisomy 8, include +19 and loss of the Y chromosome.

The t(9;22) translocation can also be found in 3% to 5% of children and adults with acute myelogenous (FAB M1) leukemia and in about 5% of children and 10% to 25% of adults with acute lymphoblastic (FAB L1 and L2 types) leukemia.

Genetic Alterations

CML is the best-characterized leukemia at a molecular level. Patients with CML and acute lymphoblastic leukemia express the BCR gene rearrangement (Fig. 21.2), which is the molecular counterpart of the Ph[1] chromosome. These

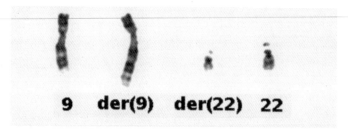

FIGURE 21.2 Chronic myelogenous leukemia. The Philadelphia chromosome der(22) is shown. (Reprinted with permission from Rubin R, Strayer DS. *Rubin's Pathology: Clinicopathologic Foundations of Medicine*, 5th ed, Philadelphia, PA: Lippincott Williams & Wilkins, 2008.)

reciprocal translocations involve the relocation and fusion of the protooncogene c-ABL on the distal arm of chromosome 9 to a break in the newly identified genetic locus of chromosome 22, known as BCR (breakpoint cluster region). The significance of the presence of the Ph[1] chromosome is possibly related to amplification of the BCR/ABL fusion gene product. The BCR-ABL fusion gene is transcribed into a chimeric mRNA transcript, which is in turn translated into a fusion protein with abnormal structure and function. The BCR/ABL fusion gene, mRNA, and protein are diagnostic markers of CML at the molecular level (Fig. 21.3).

Evidence of the role of *mRNA* transcripts as central mediators of myeloid proliferation and transformation in CML stems from experiments with models of tumor developmentThese transcripts cause factor-independent and leukemogenic cell growth in hematopoietic cell lines and can generate in mice a syndrome that closely resembles human CML. abl proteins are nonreceptor TKs that have important roles in signal transduction and the regulation of cell growth. Various structural alterations of ABL and BCR genes facilitate the leukemogenic transformation.

Clinical Signs and Symptoms
The clinical course of CML can be characterized by three separate progressive phases. (Table 21.2).

Initial Phase

The onset of the early, initial phase (chronic phase) of CML is insidious and may last from 3 to 5 years. Most cases (85%) are diagnosed in this phase. Signs and symptoms can include progressive fatigue and malaise, low-grade fever, anorexia, weight loss, and bone pain. Night sweats and fever, associated with an increased metabolism caused by granulocytic cell turnover, may occur. Physical examination usually reveals splenic enlargement. Splenic infarction is common because of the abnormal overproduction and accumulation of granulocyte precursors in the bone marrow, spleen, and blood. These infarcts in the spleen may produce left upper quadrant pain. Any organ may eventually be infiltrated with myeloid elements. Extramyeloid masses in areas other than the spleen and liver, however, are uncommon findings in the chronic phase. On fresh incision, extramyeloid masses appear green, presumably because of the presence of the myeloid enzyme myeloperoxidase. These greenish tumors have been called **chloromas**.

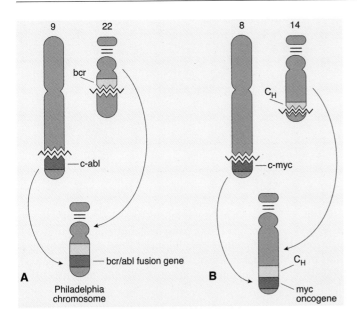

FIGURE 21.3 Oncogene activation by chromosomal translocation. A: Chronic myelogenous leukemia. Breaks at the ends of the long arms of chromosomes 9 and 22 allow reciprocal translocations to occur. The c-abl protooncogene on chromosome 9 is translocated to the breakpoint region (bcr) of chromosome 22. The result is the Philadelphia chromosome, which contains a new fusion gene coding for a hybrid oncogenic protein (bcr-abl), presumably involved in the pathogenesis of chronic myelogenous leukemia. B: Burkitt lymphoma. In this disorder, chromosomal breaks involve the long arms of chromosomes 8 and 14. The c-myc gene on chromosome 8 is translocated to a region on chromosome 14 adjacent to the gene coding for the constant region of an immunoglobulin heavy chain (CH). The expression of c-myc is enhanced by its association with the promoter/enhancer regions of the actively transcribed immunoglobulin genes. (Reprinted with permission from Rubin E, Farber JL. *Pathology*, 3rd ed, Philadelphia, PA: Lippincott Williams & Wilkins, 1999.)

Accelerated Phase

A transitional, accelerated period may precede blast transformation. This transition is heralded by an increase in splenomegaly, a rising peripheral blood leukocyte count, an increased percentage of basophils, worsening anemia, and thrombocytopenia.

Blast Crisis (Acute)

In the past, CML virtually always progressed to blast crisis. Treatment today slows down blast crisis in most patients and possibly presents it in some. The most recent WHO definition proposes a blast count of 20% in analogy to the definition of acute myelogenous leukemia. Patients with 20% to 29% blasts, currently classified as accelerated phase, had a significantly better prognosis than patients with more than 30% blasts.

About three fourths of patients eventually enter a gradual transformation to a blast crisis. The blast crisis phase is characterized by the appearance of primitive blast cells similar to those seen in acute leukemia. The blast phase is defined by the presence of 30% or more leukemic cells in peripheral blood or marrow or the presence of extramedullary infiltrates of blast cells. Acute-phase CML is hematologically and clinically indistinguishable from acute leukemia. In one third of cases, the blasts have a lymphoid morphology and express lymphoid markers such as terminal deoxynucleotidyl transferase (TdT) or CD10 (common acute lymphoblastic leukemia antigen). The remaining two thirds of cases have a phenotype similar to that of acute myeloblastic leukemia and form a heterogeneous group. Making a distinction between the two is important because patients whose leukemia is in the lymphoid blast phase respond to treatment with regimens that are active against acute lymphoid leukemia.

Excessive bleeding or bruising as well as fevers may be manifested in the later stage of CML. Complications are frequent in conjunction with the blast crisis. Bleeding complications are related to thrombocytopenia, impaired platelet function, and low intraplatelet concentrations of beta-thromboglobulin and platelet factor 4 (PF4).

Laboratory Data

Cellular Components

The chronic leukemias are usually characterized by the presence of leukocytosis. In the case of CML, the degree of leukocytosis is extreme. In addition, CML can also be identified by the presence of the entire spectrum of immature and mature myelogenous cells in the blood and marrow.

Anemia is a common finding. The total leukocyte count is usually greater than 50×10^9/L and may exceed 300×10^9/L. Peripheral blood smears (Figs. 21.4 and 21.5) demonstrate increased numbers of mature granulocytic forms, such as segmented neutrophils and band forms, and smaller numbers of immature forms. Myeloblasts rarely exceed 5% of the nucleated cells. Eosinophils and basophils may also be increased. Thrombocytosis may be observed in 40% of patients, although thrombocytopenia often ensues. Nucleated erythrocytes and red blood cells exhibiting anisocytosis and basophilic stippling can be seen.

TABLE 21.2	Typical Phases of Chronic Myelogenous Leukemia	
Phase	**Approximate Length of Phase**	**Treatment Status**[a]
Initial (chronic)	2–5 yrs	Highly treatable
Accelerated	6–18 mo	Resistance develops
Blast crisis (acute)	3–4 mo	Generally unresponsive

[a]Treated with chemotherapy.

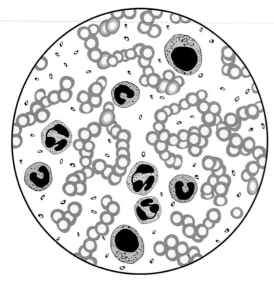

FIGURE 21.4 Chronic myelogenous leukemia. Most of the cells in this field are mature granulocytes (band forms and segmented neutrophils). An increased number of platelets (thrombocytes) is also seen in this field of the smear. (Simulates magnification 1,000×.)

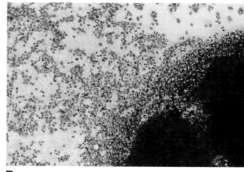

FIGURE 21.5 Characteristic peripheral blood smear of chronic myelogenous leukemia shows basophilia and granulocytosis with neutrophils and immature granulocytes. (Reprinted with permission from McClatchey KD. *Clinical Laboratory Medicine*, 2nd ed, Philadelphia, PA: Lippincott Williams & Wilkins, 2002.)

Patients experiencing the terminal phase of CML may enter a blast crisis, which is indistinguishable from acute myelogenous leukemia, particularly the FAB M2 type. Approximately 30% of patients have cytological features of CLL.

Examination of a bone marrow (Fig. 21.6) biopsy specimen reveals hypercellularity with prominent granulocytic hyperplasia. An increased number of myeloid cells in the intermediate stage is seen. The myeloid-erythroid (M:E) ratio can be as high as 25:1. The bone marrow may become fibrotic late in the disease and may be mistaken for primary myelofibrosis.

Cytochemistry

Cytochemical studies are used less frequently for chronic leukemias than for acute leukemias. In special cases, however, these stains may be of diagnostic value. The leukocyte alkaline phosphatase (LAP) procedure is used to differentiate between CML and a **leukemoid reaction**. A leukemoid reaction is produced by a severe infection or inflammation and frequently resembles leukemia on bone marrow or blood smears. In CML, the LAP score is decreased as compared with a leukemoid reaction, in which a high score is usual. An increased LAP score may be encountered in CML because of subsequent secondary infections or inflammation. Additionally, during remission phases of CML, the LAP score may return to normal limits.

In the LAP (see Chapter 26) or neutrophilic alkaline phosphatase (NAP) reaction, a solution of naphthol AS-MX phosphate alkaline and either fast blue RR or fast red violet LB salt is incubated with a microscopic smear of peripheral blood or bone marrow. Positive reactions are indicated by the deposition of blue or violet pigment at the cellular sites of alkaline phosphate activity within either band form or segmented neutrophils.

Following staining, 100 bands or segmented neutrophils are counted. Each cell is rated according to the distribution

FIGURE 21.6 Chronic myelogenous leukemia. A: Peripheral blood. B: Bone marrow. (Reprinted with permission Handin RI, et al. *Blood: Principles and Practice of Hematology*, 2th ed, Philadelphia, PA: Lippincott Williams & Wilkins, 2003.)

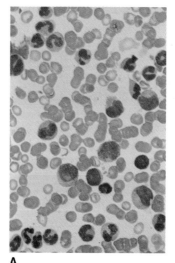

A

B

and intensity of staining. The possible range is 0 to 400, although the normal range is from 20 to 100. Increased scores are associated with leukemoid reactions, severe bacterial infections, and PV. Decreased scores can be found in viral infections and CML.

Cytogenetic Studies

Cytogenetic studies are the standard diagnostic test for CML. Other diagnostic procedures include genomic polymerase chain reaction (PCR) and Southern blot analysis that can determine the exact breakpoints of DNA fusion products. Reverse-transcriptase PCR (RT-PCR) and Northern blot analysis allow detection of *BCR-ABL* transcripts at the RNA level. The BCR-ABL protein can be demonstrated by using antibodies against the N-terminal region of BCR and the C-terminal region of *abl* in immunoprecipitation or Western blot analysis.

Detecting gene rearrangements involving the *BCR* and c-*ABL* genes is clinically useful for

1. Confirmation of Ph[1]-positive cases of CML
2. Diagnosis of Ph[1]-negative cases of CML
3. Diagnosis of CML presenting in blast crisis
4. Monitoring of patients with CML during and after therapy for detection of minimal residual disease

5. Confirmation of remission
6. Early detection of relapse

Prognosis and Treatment

Because chronic-phase CML is highly responsive to treatment, many patients experience at least one remission. These remissions can last from several weeks to months, with 60% of patients becoming asymptomatic. Imatinib (Gleevec, Novartis Pharmaceuticals, Basel, Switzerland) is a selective inhibitor of the BCR-ABL TK, which occupies the ATP-binding site of several TK molecules (*bcr-abl* oncoprotein) and prevents phosphorylation of substrates that are involved in regulating the cell cycle. The TKs are ABL, BCR/ABL, AARG, PDGF-R α and β, and c-KIT.

The introduction of imatinib has fundamentally altered the management of patients with CML in chronic phase (Fig. 21.7). It is recommended as the best single agent for newly diagnosed patients who are not eligible for initial treatment by allogeneic stem cell transplantation. There is no consensus on whether imatinib should be administered alone or in conjunction with IFN-α, cytarabine, hydroxyurea, or arsenic trioxide. Imatinib now seems to be the initial treatment of choice for patients with CML who do not have a suitable bone marrow donor or who are not candidates for transplantation. It is now widely

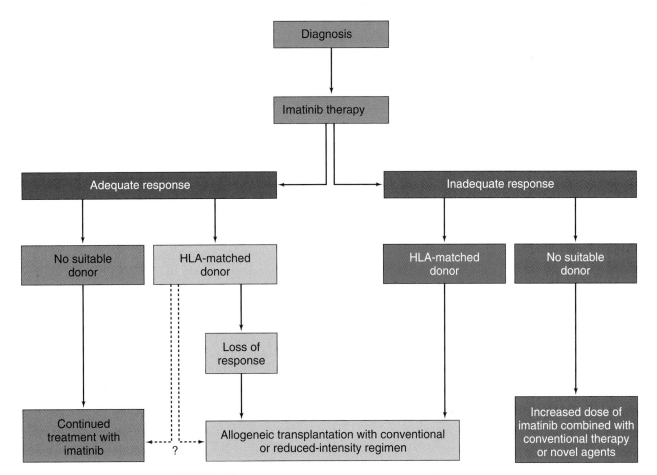

FIGURE 21.7 Algorithm for treating chronic myeloid leukemia.

accepted that imatinib mesylate (previously ST1571) is the best single agent for managing newly diagnosed patients with CML in chronic phase who are not clearly candidates for allogeneic stem cell transplantation. Primary resistance to imatinib seems to be rare in chronic-phase patients, but the majority of advanced-phase patients become resistant to imatinib.

Constitutive activation of these TKs documents in CML, Ph + ALL, and myeloproliferative disorders is due to chromosomal rearrangement. Although imatinib is effective in Ph pos leukemias, relapses do occur mainly as a result to the outgrowth of leukemic subclones with imatinib-resistant BCR-ABL mutations. The median survival time from the time of diagnosis is approximately 1 year in patients lacking Ph[1]. Those patients with Ph[1] have a better prognosis, with a median survival time of 3 to 4 years. After progression to the blast crisis phase, the prognosis is poor, with patient survival time usually being less than 6 months. Molecular techniques (e.g., PCR of BCR-ABL, RNA transcripts) can guide therapy by distinguishing patients who are doing well with imatinib from those who will experience relapse and thus require alternative therapy (e.g., stem cell transplantation). In the future, gene expression microarray studies might help predict responders to a specific therapy.

Imatinib mesylate has largely supplanted allogeneic hematopoietic stem cell transplantation as first-line therapy for CML. Many CML patients eventually undergo stem cell transplantation raising a question of whether prior therapy impacts transplantation success. Survival rates are high among chronic-phase patients receiving imatinib mesylate. Hematological response may be associated with symptomatic improvement in CML.

In patients with CML who achieve complete cytogenetic remission (CCR) with interferon alpha (IFN-α), the duration of remission has been previously correlated with the *BCR-ABL* mRNA transcript level measured by quantitative (Q-)PCR in blood.

Interferon therapy leads to a reduction in the number of Ph[1] chromosome and positive cells, but additional chromosomal anomalies may be induced by interferon directly or may arise at random and gain a proliferative advantage during interferon therapy. The role and importance of most of these anomalies are not known. In terms of both safety and effectiveness, it has been established that treatment with interferon alfa is an appropriate method of inducing complete hematological remission in early, chronic-phase, Ph[1] chromosome–positive CML. Combined treatment with interferon alfa and cytarabine may have further benefit, and many view it as the gold standard of therapy. However, none of these approaches induce molecular remission (the elimination of BCR-ABL transcripts detectable by PCR assay). Allogeneic stem cell transplantation has been considered the only curative treatment for CML.

Based on the toxicity of stem cell transplantation and the associated risk of death with age, transplantation is an option for approximately 40% of patients with CML.

Previously, five principal prognostic factors were identified for survival after stem cell transplantation: the donor type (sibling vs. unrelated donor), the recipient's age, the stage of disease, the gender of the donor and the recipient (same or different), and the interval from diagnosis to transplantation. These factors are being reconsidered in view of the development of less-intensive transplantation regimens and the introduction of imatinib mesylate, a well-tolerated oral agent that was first administered in clinical trials in June 1998 in the United States and approved by the U.S. Food and Drug Administration on May 10, 2001.

Minimal Residual Disease

Patient monitoring at the cytogenetic and molecular level is crucial for identifying the disease stage and progression as well as response to therapy. In general, patients who achieve CCR may be monitored just by RT-PCR on peripheral blood, but marrow cytogenetics should still be checked at intervals and in the face of rising blood BCR-*ABL mRNA* transcript levels.

Not only is the detection of the BCR-ABL gene translocation a diagnostic tool, but it is also useful for assessment of patients regarding therapy with either stem cell transplantation or interferon alfa and for evaluating the efficacy of treatment by monitoring residual disease. PCR has become the diagnostic test of choice for monitoring residual leukemia. Cytogenetic relapse usually precedes hematological relapse, and early detection of a relapse can trigger effective salvage therapy.

Cytogenetic response correlates with increased survival, and patients show a decrease in the presence of Ph chromosomes by classic karyotyping of bone marrow cells. This method is able to detect 1 Ph-positive cell in 25 to 30 normal cells (3% to 4% sensitivity) but cannot detect minimal residual disease in peripheral blood. Fluorescence in situ hybridization (FISH) can detect BCR/ABL-positive cells with a sensitivity of 1 in 200 to 500 normal cells in either bone marrow or peripheral blood (Fig. 21.8). Another increase in sensitivity is achieved with real time PCR, which uses primer-amplified DNA to detect the *BCR/ABL* fusion at the RNA level and evaluates the ratio of BCR-ABL mRNA transcripts in bone marrow or peripheral blood. RT-PCR can detect one leukemic cell in 10^3 to 10^4 normal cells. An even more sensitive variation of this technique is a two-step nested real time PCR, using two rounds of RT-PCR. It is able to detect bcr/abl transcripts in 1 of 10^6 cells without quantifying the level of transcripts. Nested RT-PCR is useful when other test results (including real time PCR,) become negative. In clinical practice, Taqman (Applied Biosystems TaqMan Foster City, California) or LightCycler (LightCycler, Roche Diagnostics Corp. Indianapolis, Indiana), real time PCR,is now largely replacing the nonquantitative real time PCR, approach, although levels that are undetectable by real time PCR,sometimes need to be validated by two-step nested real time PCR.

Prognostic Significance of Cytogenetic and Molecular Responses

Currently, the gold standard for evaluating patient response to treatment is conventional cytogenetic analysis. Molecular response is emerging as a key endpoint for clinical trials (Fig. 21.8) and may become a key clinical management tool.

It has been established that—particularly for patients treated with IFN-α, the first biological agent capable of inducing a significant number of cytogenic remissions in CML—the degree of tumor load reduction during therapy is an important prognostic factor.

Three different levels of response can be differentiated. The hematological response is achieved with the normalization of peripheral blood counts and absence of signs and symptoms of disease. The cytogenetic responses established on the basis of the proportion of residual Ph-positive metaphases are defined as complete (0% of metaphases), partial (1% to 33%), minor (34% to 66%), or minimal (67% to 99%). A major response represents the sum of the complete and partial cytogenetic responses. Molecular remission is traditionally defined on the basis of the detection of residual BCR-aABL mRNA transcripts by qualitative RT-PCR.

Resistance in Chronic Myelogenous Leukemia

Resistance has been observed in a proportion of patients after variable periods of imatinib monotherapy. Patients in the chronic phase have responded to imatinib therapy for more than 2 years, but most responding patients in blast crisis may experience relapse early despite continued therapy. Clinical mechanisms of imatinib resistance can be divided into two groups: (1) reactivation of BCR-ABL with continuing dependence on BCR-ABL signaling and (2) remaining inhibition but BCR-ABL signaling is bypassed by alternative signaling pathways. In the latter case, resistance may be caused by the evolution of the disease with occurrence of novel numeric or structural cytogenetic aberrations [e.g., trisomy 8, iso(17q)], which lead to BCR-ABL –independent proliferation of leukemic cells.

The development of imatinib resistance presents new therapeutic challenges. The fact that BCR-ABL is active in many imatinib-resistant patients suggests that the chimeric oncoprotein remains a rational drug target. Knowledge of the mutations should permit the development of an assay to detect drug-resistant clones before clinical relapse occurs.

Leukemia-Specific Targets

Leukemia-specific targets may involve leukemia-specific peptides that mediate a graft versus leukemia effect. In CML, the only unique amino acid is the one formed by the novel codons at the b2-a2 or b3-ae junctions in the bcr-abl proteins. Evidence produced by mass spectrometry validates

Leukemic Burden	Response	
10^{13}	hematologic remission	
10^{12}		
2 logs $\quad$ 10^{11}	cytogenic remission	Ph positive 0%
10^{10}		
4 logs $\quad$ 10^{9}	molecular remission	PCR positive
10^{8}		
10^{7}		
10^{6}		
10^{5}	molecular remission	PCR negative
10^{4}		
10^{3}		
10^{2}		
10^{1}		
10		
0		

FIGURE 21.8 Schematic illustration of therapeutic response of CML patients on cytogenetic and molecular level. (*Source:* Saglio G. *Measuring molecular response in CML: Problems and significance, 8th EHA Congress,* June 2003).

that CML cells do express this leukemia-specific peptide and human T cells can kill fresh CML cells in an HLA-restricted peptide specific manner. This makes it possible to design CML-specific oligopeptides that are presented in conjunction with HLA class I or class II molecules that may be immunogenic in humans. Vaccination of a small number of patients with junction-specific peptides has produced a partial or complete hematological response in patients with CML. The vaccinated patients developed delayed-type hypersensitivity reactions and a CD4+ lymphocyte proliferative response. This approach to treatment may be valuable in suppressing proliferation of leukemia cells in patients with minimal residual disease.

When CML patients harbor minimal residual disease, an approach is to try to induce immunity to antigens known to be overexpressed in leukemia cells. Human cytotoxic T cells (CTLs) can kill Ph-positive CD34+ progenitor cells. The use of CTLs directed against the Pr-1 component of proteinase 3 is also promising. Proteinase 3 is a serine protease that is induced during cell differentiation and stored in azurophilic granules. It is overexpressed in myeloid leukemias. The development of CML could be caused by selective deletion of a Pr-specific CTL clone; this supports the theory that breaking specific tolerance could be a valuable treatment approach for patients with minimal residual disease.

Allogeneic Bone Marrow Transplantation

A long-standing and universally accepted therapy for CML is allogeneic stem cell transplantation (allo-SCT). Allo-SCT achieves its curative potential via at least two mechanisms:

1. Myeloablation induced by high-dose chemoradiotherapy
2. Allo-immune graft versus leukemia (GvL) effect mediated by donor T lymphocytes

Infusion of donor T cells at a time of minimal residual disease may be required within the first year of transplant. Newer understanding of the alloimmune effect has led to the development of reduced intensity conditioning for transplantation that focuses on immunosuppression of the host rather than myeloablation. Engraftment of donor hematopoietic cells can take place without necessarily eradicating all the host population of cells. Despite the benefits, allo-SCT is a procedure with a considerable procedural-related mortality and chronic morbidity (e.g., chronic graft versus host disease for some long-term survivors).

POLYCYTHEMIA VERA, ESSENTIAL THROMBOCYTOSIS (ESSENTIAL THROMBOCYTHEMIA), AND PRIMARY MYELOFIBROIS

Polycythemia vera (PV), essential thrombocytosis or essential thrombocythemia (ET), and primary myelofibrosis (PM) were identified as pathogenetically related myeloproliferative disorders in 1951. Subsequently, PV, ET, and PM were identified as clonal disorders of multipotent hematopoietic progenitors. In 2005, a somatic activating mutation in Janus kinase (JAK2) nonreceptor TK (JAK2V617F) was identified in most patients with PV and in a significant proportion of patients with ET and PM. Subsequently, additional mutations in JAK-STAT pathway in some patients with JAK2V617F-MPN suggested that constitutive activation of this signaling pathway is a unifying feature of these disorders. JAK2 is a nonreceptor protein located on the cytoplasmic inside of the cell membrane that functions to transfer signals from the cell surface to the nucleus. JAK2V617F mutation is an important marker to segregate patients with high RBC, hemoglobin, and hematocrits into those with PV and those without this disorder. The V617F mutation causes the substitution of phenylalanine for valine at position 617 of the Janus kinase (JAK)2 gene (JAK2). This mutation is often present in PV, ET, and IM. The m molecular basis is unclear but this serves as the research foundation for development of small molecule inhibitors of JAK2.

POLYCYTHEMIA VERA

Sir William Osler first described polycythemia rubra vera (PV) in 1910. The clinical description was that of a patient with engorged veins, plethora, and an elevated red blood cell count. Leukocytosis and thrombocythemia were recognized as additional features. In 1951, Dameshek added PV to the classification of MPNs. PV is a rather common disease, and the main differential diagnosis is that of reactive erythrocytosis due to hypoxia.

Epidemiology

PV has an incidence of 2.3 per 100,000 people. The median age at diagnosis is approximately 60 years, with a slight male predominance. Exposure to radiation, benzene, and petroleum refineries seems to increase risk.

Etiology

PV is a clonal stem cell disorder characterized by hyperproliferation of the erythroid, myeloid, and megakaryocytic lineages. The molecular pathogenesis of this disease remains unknown. The cDNA for polycythemia rubra vera-1 (PV-1), a novel hematopoietic receptor, was recently cloned by virtue of its overexpression in patients with PV. Northern blot analysis showed that PV-1 is highly expressed in normal human bone marrow and to a much lesser degree in fetal liver.

Pathophysiology

Although PV is a clonal hematopoietic progenitor cell disorder with trilineage hyperplasia, the most constant and striking feature is erythroid hyperplasia of the bone marrow. This very slow evolution of the malignant erythroid clone leads to overexpansion of the red cell mass, hypervolemia, and splenomegalic red cell pooling. These consequences eventually cause generalized marrow hyperplasia with subsequent increases in the quantity of all three cell lines.

Abnormalities in PV erythroid progenitors are expressed at the level of both the colony-forming unit-erythroid (CFU-E) and burst-forming unit-erythroid (BFU-E), which suggests multiple changes in the erythroid progenitors. A shift in the cell compartment may occur in PV. Interleukin-3 (IL-3) stimulates trilineage hematopoiesis, but a striking hypersensitivity of PV BFU-E to recombinant IL-3 has been noted. This may be a major factor in the pathogenesis of increased erythropoiesis without increased erythropoietin concentrations.

In addition, the manganese and zinc contents of the physiologically active erythrocytic microelements demonstrate disturbances in erythrocytes of the peripheral venous blood in patients with PV. These changes indicate the neoplastic character of proliferation of bone marrow cells in PV.

Karyotype

Chromosomal disorders are found in only approximately 15% of patients, but there is no common chromosomal abnormality as is found in CML. A newly described gene, PV-1 gene, has been described in neutrophils of patients with PV, but the significance of this gene is as yet uncertain.

During the first 10 years of disease, approximately one fourth of patients demonstrate an abnormal clone; after more than 10 years, greater than three fourths of patients exhibit an abnormal clone. Patients with a chromosomally abnormal clone at the time of diagnosis have a poorer chance of survival than those exhibiting a normal karyotype in metaphase cells. Cytogenetic results do not predict evolution of the disease but do provide clues to the hematological phenotype, duration of the disease, and consequences of myelosuppressive therapy.

Clinical Signs and Symptoms

Plethora is the hallmark of PV. Splenomegaly is a commonly found sign of disease; it occurs in more than three fourths of patients. Reversible, moderate hypertension frequently occurs as the result of the expanded blood volume. An increased total blood volume (hypervolemia) occurs in PV and in disorders such as congestive heart failure, primary aldosteronism, and Cushing syndrome, and as a result of overtransfusion of donor blood.

Neurological symptoms are reported by 50% to 80% of patients. Symptoms such as headaches, dizziness, paresthesias, and sight alterations are frequently related to hyperviscosity and respond immediately to a reduction of cell counts, except in ictus patients. Other neurological symptoms seem to result from an associated coagulopathy.

The most serious complications are arterial and venous complications (vascular accidents) and the transition to acute leukemia. PV, sickle cell anemia, sickle cell–hemoglobin

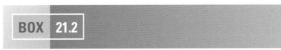

BOX 21.2

Diagnostic Criteria for Polycythemia Vera

MAJOR CRITERIA

1. Hemoglobin >18.5 g/dL in males, 16.5 g/dL in females or other evidence of increased red cell volume
2. Presence of JAK2V617F or other functionally similar mutations, e.g., JAK2 exon 12 mutation

MINOR CRITERIA

1. Hypercellular bone marrow with prominent granulocytic, erythrocytic, and megakaryocytic proliferation
2. Decreases serum erythropoietin levels
3. Endogenous erythroid colony formation in vitro

C disease, and essential thrombocythemia are the major disorders of formed blood elements causing stroke. Hemorrhagic phenomena are frequent among patients with digestive manifestations, including gastrointestinal hemorrhage, abdominal pain, or portal vein thrombosis, or thrombosis of the suprahepatic vein. In addition, thrombophlebitis with pulmonary embolism is a common complication of PV and often is unrecognized.

Severe psychotic depression is rare in patients with PV. In venography-documented Budd-Chiari syndrome, the underlying diseases include PV. The criteria for the diagnosis of PV are presented in Box 21.2.

Laboratory Data

An increased erythrocyte cell count, packed cell volume, and hemoglobin with normal erythrocytic indices are characteristic of PV. Red cell proliferation is thought to be independent of endogenous erythropoietin, and hence, serum levels of erythropoietin are usually decreased. A genetic alteration of the erythropoietin receptor is thought to create a loss of regulatory function and abnormal erythroid proliferation. Plasma levels of thrombopoietin (the growth factor for megakaryocyte production of platelets) are elevated or normal, implying a loss of the normal negative feedback mechanism.

Peak polycythemic values are a hemoglobin of approximately 20.6 g/dL, a microhematocrit of approximately 80%, a total leukocyte (white blood cell [WBC]) count of 28,000 × 10^9/L, and a platelet count of 1,400 × 10^9/L.

In patients with PV, as in those with the other diseases, the red blood cell distribution width (RDW) tends to be higher than normal. The RDW transiently increases following administration of a myelosuppressive agent, corresponding to the transition period from microcytes to normal blood cells. The RDW is even higher during polycythemic periods than during the myelofibrotic period. This may be associated with hematopoietic abnormality caused by extramedullary hematopoiesis. RDW seems to reflect accurately the pathological status of PV.

Not all patients with an elevated red cell count have PV. Various tumors are known to result in an elevated red cell mass. Renal cell carcinomas and hepatomas are the tumors most noted for creating erythrocytosis. Some produce exogenous erythropoietin. The most common secondary cause of erythrocytosis is cigarette smoking. Smokers have elevated plasma levels of carbon monoxide. Carbon monoxide displaces oxygen from red cell hemoglobin, resulting in tissue hypoxia and an elevated drive to red cell production. Smokers' erythrocytosis is most commonly distinguished from true PV by the observation that patients usually have normal values for leukocytes and platelets. The mean corpuscular volume is usually within normal limits (patients with PV usually have a low mean corpuscular volume because of marrow depletion of iron resulting in microcytic red cells). Serum erythropoietin levels are normal or elevated because of an increased red cell production. The serum erythropoietin level can often be used to distinguish this from PV.

An elevated hematocrit above the level of 50% or greater in the absence of dehydration is highly suggestive of the diagnosis, and a hematocrit greater than 60% for men or 56% for women is consistent with an elevated red cell mass. The oxygen saturation should be normal and if the patient is a smoker, the carboxyhemoglobin level should also be normal.

Lymphocyte populations in patients with PV demonstrate an altered CD4/CD8 ratio, mainly because of a decreased CD8 subpopulation. Increased lymphocyte activity has also been observed. Interleukin-2 (IL-2) production is significantly higher; the lymphoproliferative response both to phytohemagglutinin and IL-2 is also greater in lymphocytes from PV patients. These observations suggest that patients may also suffer from an altered lymphoid lineage.

The bone marrow is hypercellular (Fig. 21.9) with increased production of all three cell lines, especially the red cell series. Some investigators believe that a bone marrow examination is not necessary for diagnosis. Others believe that the bone marrow histology should be examined and cytogenetic analysis for the *BCR-ABL* mutation should be performed. An occasional patient with CML can present with erythrocytosis, although this is distinctly unusual.

Abnormalities of Hemostasis and Coagulation

Patients with PV frequently demonstrate a complex of hemorheological disorders (high blood viscosity at different rates of deviation, intensified red blood cell aggregation, and decreased deformability of these cells) and hemocoagulation disorders.

Complications of PV include thrombosis and paradoxical hemorrhage. The thrombosis seems to be related to the height of the red cell volume with a subsequent increase in blood viscosity. Whole blood viscosity pursues a rather linear rate of rise, and most physicians prefer to keep the patient's hematocrit below 45%. Increased whole blood viscosity contributes to vascular occlusions and reversible lesions, including cerebral and myocardial infarction, as well as shortness of breath and hot flushes, probably caused by circulatory disturbance. Patients with a blood viscosity higher than twice the normal mean value may be in danger of vascular occlusion. A correlation has been revealed among the parameters of red blood cell rheological properties, hemostasis, and disease severity.

In some cases, disorders in the rheological phenomena of red blood cells are a triggering mechanism in the development of the DIC syndrome.

In the chronic phase of PV, patients with thrombohemorrhagic complications have higher platelet counts, more severe platelet aggregation defects, and increased plasma levels of beta thromboglobulin and fibrinopeptide A compared with patients who do not have complications. However, thrombohemorrhagic complications are not predictable by changes in these parameters in individual patients during the chronic disease phase.

The plasma level of tissue plasminogen activator antigen (t-PA-Ag) is significantly decreased in patients with PV compared with healthy individuals. In contrast, patients with spurious polycythemia and secondary polycythemia exhibit significantly increased concentrations of t-PA-Ag. There is no significant difference in t-PA-Ag levels in polycythemic patients with or without thromboembolic disease.

Other Laboratory Assays

Erythropoietin excretion in the urine is decreased in PV, in contrast to the other kinds of polycythemias. Radioimmunoassay of erythropoietin has been used to distinguish between PV and other forms of erythrocytosis.

Laboratory findings that support a diagnosis of PV compared with other forms of polycythemia are an absence of hemosiderin from the bone marrow and an increased

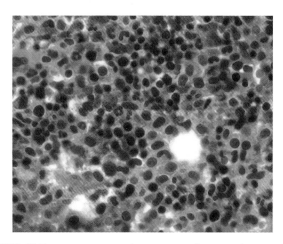

FIGURE 21.9 Bone marrow clot section of PV in the proliferative stage showing hypercellular marrow with marked erythroid hyperplasia. (McClatchey KD. *Clinical Laboratory Medicine*, 2nd ed, Philadelphia, PA: Lippincott Williams & Wilkins, 2002.)

LAP score. In addition, hyperuricemia and hyperuricosuria are present in more than half of PV patients at diagnosis because of excess nucleic acid degradation. The level of uric acid parallels increases in severity of PV as the disease progresses.

Thrombocytosis also seems to be related to both the risk of thrombosis and hemorrhage. The level of thrombocytosis seems to be related, and most hematologists prefer to keep the platelet count below 400,000. Qualitative abnormalities of platelets also might contribute to PV complications. Abnormalities in platelet responsiveness to naturally occurring platelet inhibitors such as prostaglandins, increased levels of thromboxanes (inducers of platelet aggregation), and abnormal levels of naturally occurring anticoagulants (proteins C and S and antithrombin III) have occasionally been reported and could also contribute to thrombosis.

A comparison of the laboratory findings in PV and other forms of polycythemia is presented in Table 21.3.

Treatment

Phlebotomy

Primary control of PV is achieved by therapeutic phlebotomy (Fig. 21.10). The aim of phlebotomy is to produce an iron deficiency that then limits red blood cell production. This may be performed by the removal of units of whole blood or by large-volume erythrocytapheresis using a cell separator. Cytapheresis produces a long-lasting reduction of red blood cell volume (microhematocrit), hemoglobin, and erythrocyte counts as well as the immediate disappearance or reduction of clinical symptoms.

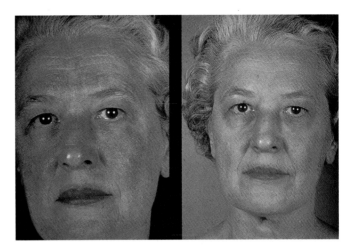

FIGURE 21.10 Adult woman with PV showing marked reduction in facial rubor after phlebotomy. (Reprinted with permission from Gold DH, Weingeist TA. *Color Atlas of the Eye in Systemic Disease*, Baltimore, MD: Lippincott Williams & Wilkins, 2001.)

The evolution of PV is favorably altered by therapeutic phlebotomy and chemotherapeutic cytoreduction, which are often performed simultaneously.

Chemotherapy

The mainstay of cytoreduction of the platelet count is drug therapy. Phosphorous 32 (P32) is effective as a treatment in reducing red cell and platelet proliferation but at the expense of an excess rate of the development of acute leukemia. Chlorambucil also produces an increased rate of acute leukemia. Neither are current therapeutic options.

TABLE 21.3	A Summary of Significant Differences Between Polycythemia Vera and Other Types of Polycythemias	
	Polycythemia Vera	**Other Types**
Total blood volume	Increased	Normal or decreased
Total leukocytes	Increased	Normal
Immature red blood cells	Occasional	None
Platelets	Increased	Normal
LAP stain	Increased	Normal
Erythrocyte sedimentation rate	Decreased	Normal
Serum iron	Decreased	Normal or increased
Erythropoietin	Decreased or absent	Normal or increased
Blood histamine	Increased	Normal
Unsaturated vitamin B_{12}–binding capacity	Increased	Normal
Basophil count	Increased	Normal
Hyperuricemia	Present or absent	Normal
Hyperuricosuria	Present or absent	Normal

Anagrelide (Agrylin, Bristol-Myers Squibb, New York) is a relatively new addition to the therapeutic arsenal. Anagrelide is a prostaglandin synthetase inhibitor that also inhibits megakaryocyte production of platelets and has little effect on red cell production. There is no effect on myelopoiesis.

Interferon has also been used to control marrow overproduction but causes a high risk of flu-like symptoms, myalgia, fatigue, and fever.

Prognosis and Complications

The median survival time for untreated symptomatic patients after diagnosis is 6 to 18 months. With treatment, the median survival is more than 10 years.

Certain prognostic factors and treatment strategies have an effect on survival. The clinical course of most patients is characterized by a low rate of acute leukemia and a high rate (~40%) of thromboembolic complications. Myelofibrosis develops in some patients. A high initial hemoglobin concentration in peripheral blood and the use of any myelosuppressive therapy are associated with an increased risk of leukemic transformation.

PRIMARY MYELOFIBROSIS

Primary myelofibrosis is characterized by systemic bone marrow fibrosis and extramedullary hematopoiesis. Secondary myelofibrosis is caused by infiltrative disorders, including malignancies and infections, or exposure to chemical toxins or irradiation.

Epidemiology

Patients with myelofibrosis may undergo temporary or permanent transition to PV or may convert to CML. Approximately one fifth of patients with PV develop myelofibrosis.

Primary myelofibrosis is uncommon, with the number of new cases estimated at 1,000 to 2,000 per year in the United States or an overall rate of 2 per 100,000 worldwide. The incidence of myelofibrosis, however, is known to be increased after exposure to irradiation and chemicals such as benzene.

Although there have been a few reports of patients in the pediatric population, the majority of patients with primary myelofibrosis are in their late 50s, 60s, and 70s. It is also more common in the white population, and men and women are equally affected.

Pathophysiology

Primary myelofibrosis is a clonal disorder of the multipotential progenitor cell compartment. The blood-marrow barrier is disrupted early in the course of myelofibrosis, so that blast cells and committed stem cells such as colony-forming unit-granulocyte-macrophage (CFU-GM), BFU-E,

and colony-forming unit-megakaryocyte (CFU-Meg) cells escape into the circulating blood in large numbers.

Sclerosis of the bone develops in about half of patients. However, myelofibrosis, the predominant clinical manifestation, occurs secondarily and is not a component of the abnormal clonal proliferation. The process of fibrosis ensues from proliferation of fibroblasts and increased collagen production in reaction to the abnormal clone of hematopoietic cells. Fibrosis is probably the result of a product secreted by megakaryocytes.

If the constituents of the hematopoietic microenvironment (myeloid stroma) are examined microscopically, an overall increase, particularly in so-called undifferentiated (primitive pluripotent) and also in transitional (fibroblastic) reticular cells and myofibroblasts, can be observed. Undifferentiated and transitional reticular cells as well as myofibroblasts seem to form an integral part of the hematopoietic microenvironment and are assumed to play an important role in the evolution of disease-specific myelofibrosis. In addition, the evolution of medullary fibrosis is thought to be associated with the striking predominance of large, atypical, possibly overaged and hyperpolyploid megakaryocytes, but not with an increase in precursor cells.

Dysmegakaryocytopoiesis leading to an overproduction of defective platelets is the most constant feature of myelofibrosis. Research findings imply that the significant increase in circulating progenitor cells of the megakaryocyte lineage may be generated by extramedullary, probably splenic hematopoiesis. One abnormality of the megakaryopoiesis in bone marrow tissue, however, is pronounced pleomorphism of the megakaryocytic cell line consisting of giant forms, micromegakaryocytes, and naked (pyknotic) nuclei. Another maturational abnormality is the dissociation of nuclear-cytoplasmic maturation, including the amount of dense granules, and the development of the demarcation membrane system as well as the occurrence of emperipolesis (i.e., internalization of hematopoietic cells) already in immature or megakaryoblastic elements. A striking variety in the appearance of dense granules of the alpha type also frequently exists. Thrombocytes show giant forms with either hypertrophy of the open canalicular system or an abundance of dense granules and beta glycogen accumulation. Other remarkable features include a focal sponge-like proliferation of the open canalicular system in many of the large platelets and giant and fused granules of the alpha and osmiophilic type. These abnormalities in megakaryocytes and thrombocytes may have certain functional implications (e.g., hemorrhage and thrombosis) that are often encountered out of proportion to the platelet counts in this disorder.

In addition, those anomalies indicate a disorganization of megakaryopoiesis, which may contribute to the abnormal release of factors (platelet-derived growth factor and PF4) predominantly involved in the process of myelofibrosis. It has been postulated that platelet-derived growth factor and PF4 are involved in the imbalance of the mechanism of medullary stroma maintenance, which triggers the bone marrow myelofibrotic process. A relationship between the presence of myelofibrosis and abnormal levels of beta thromboglobulin, PF4, and mitogenic activity in platelet-poor plasma and platelet extracts has been observed in patients with primary myelofibrosis.

Karyotype

Approximately 40% of patients acquire recurrent cytogenetic abnormalities and nearly 80% acquire nonspecific aberrations. Several chromosomal abnormalities are overrepresented in patients with myelofibrosis. These alterations involve the long arm of chromosome 1; monosomy and partial deletion of chromosomes 5, 7, 9, 11, and 13; loss of Y chromosome; and trisomy of 8, 9, and 21. Partial trisomy 1q is a karyotypic change detectable in unstimulated peripheral blood cell cultures or bone marrow cultures, which suggests that partial trisomy 1q is a primary chromosome aberration in myelofibrosis and is relevant to the pathogenesis of this disorder.

Karyotypic changes occur as secondary events during the multistep process of leukemogenesis. Therefore, changes such as t(5;17) may represent a therapy-induced abnormality nonrandomly related to the terminal phase of myeloid disorders.

Clinical Signs and Symptoms

Patients with myelofibrosis usually exhibit progressive anemia, splenomegaly, and marrow fibrosis. Splenomegaly and some hepatomegaly are caused by extramedullary hematopoiesis. Patients may note easy bruising or bleeding resulting from thrombocytopenia, abnormal platelet function, or both. About one third of patients manifest purpura. More than 40% of patients have osteosclerosis with accompanying bone pain, malaise, and leukocytosis. A mild degree of jaundice, abdominal fullness, dyspepsia, or weight loss may be manifested in some patients. Portal hypertension may be evident.

In a rare case, one patient presented with a breast mass. Excision biopsy of the mass revealed extramedullary hematopoiesis, as did histopathological examination of the liver and the spleen. This type of presentation demonstrates the complementary character of both diagnostic modalities and the resemblance to lymphoma of the breast, although the findings are too nonspecific to rule out breast carcinoma. Knowledge of the clinical history and histopathology is necessary to make the proper diagnosis. Another rare presentation occurred in a patient with cutaneous extramedullary hematopoiesis. The skin lesions appeared as multiple papules and nodules on the trunk. Histological examination of a lesion showed all three components of the hematopoietic tissue, that is, myeloid, erythroid, and megakaryocytic series.

Cellular Alterations

Hematological findings (Box 21.3) are variable and nonuniform, but blood morphology provides the best clues to

Diagnosis of Primary Myelofibrosis[a]

MAJOR CRITERIA
1. Megakaryocytic proliferation with abnormal morphology, usually accompanied by reticulin and/or collagen fibrosis
2. Not meeting the criteria for other MPNs
3. Evidence of JAK2V617F or other related mutations

MINOR CRITERIA
1. Leukoerythroblastosis
2. Anemia
3. Increased serum lactic dehydrogenase (LDH) levels
4. Splenomegaly

[a]Diagnosis requires meeting all three major and two minor criteria.

diagnosis. The leukoerythroblastic picture of teardrop-shaped erythrocytes, nucleated erythrocytes, and immature myeloid cells is classic for myelofibrosis. Leukocytosis, mild anemia, thrombocytosis, and panhyperplasia in the marrow are characteristic in the early stages. Extramedullary hematopoiesis, peripheral cytopenias (i.e., anemia, leukopenia, or thrombocytopenia), and myelofibrosis, with or without osteosclerosis, reflect the changes seen in the later stages. Transitions among the different types of MPNs and termination in acute leukemia or marrow failure are common.

Erythrocytes

Mild anemia caused by ineffective erythropoiesis (Fig. 21.11), decreased red blood cell survival, and overt hemolysis may occur. Polychromatophilia and an elevated reticulocyte count in the absence of erythropoietic stress provide an important clue to diagnosis because they signify a breakdown in marrow ultrastructure.

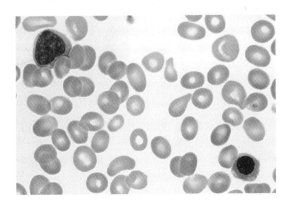

FIGURE 21.11 Typical peripheral blood smear of chronic primary myelofibrosis with leukoerythroblastosis and teardrop red blood cells. (Reprinted with permission from McClatchey KD. *Clinical Laboratory Medicine,* 2nd ed, Philadelphia, PA: Lippincott Williams & Wilkins, 2002.)

Leukocytes

In approximately 50% of patients, the total leukocyte (WBC) count is increased. Most patients have total WBC counts less than 30×10^9/L, but the total WBC count can be as high as 100×10^9/L. A high WBC count (neutrophilia) and immature granulocytes on peripheral blood smears including blasts can create a picture that can be confused with leukemia.

Platelets

The concentration of platelets is variable, but giant dysplastic platelets and fragments of megakaryocytes can be seen. Thrombocytosis gradually progresses to thrombocytopenia. As myelofibrosis progresses, the entire morphological picture of myelophthisis (infiltrative myelopathy) unfolds: teardrop-shaped erythrocytes, nucleated erythrocytes, early granulocytic forms, bizarre platelets, and megakaryocyte fragments.

Bone Marrow

The bone marrow is hypocellular and becomes fibrotic with an associated decrease in hematopoiesis. Bone marrow aspiration is unsuccessful in nearly 90% of patients because reticulin and collagen fibrosis lock in the marrow content, causing a dry tap. A bone marrow biopsy shows fibrosis, generally with increased numbers of megakaryocytes.

Prognosis

The median survival time ranges from 4.3 to 5.0 years. In patients with primary myelofibrosis, hemoglobin concentration, platelet count, and the presence of osteomyelosclerosis have been identified as factors with prognostic significance. Patients with a hemoglobin concentration less than 10 g/dL have a significantly shorter survival time than those with a hemoglobin concentration greater than or equal to 10 g/dL. A platelet count less than 100×10^9/L also implies a significantly shorter survival time and is of prognostic significance within the first 6 months of diagnosis. Patients with osteomyelosclerosis, as demonstrated on radiograph of the skeleton, have a significantly better prognosis compared to those without osteomyelosclerosis. The presence of osteomyelosclerosis emerges as a favorable parameter at 3 and 5 years. Using these three parameters and spleen size, a prognostic scoring system has been designed; it categorizes patients into three prognostic groups with highly different survival times (low-risk group, 69 months; intermediate-risk group, 33 months; high-risk group, 4 months).

In addition, major thromboembolic complications that contribute to shortened survival times are seen in approximately one fifth of patients.

Treatment

Asymptomatic patients require no treatment. Treatment of myelofibrosis can consist of periodic transfusions of packed red blood cells, androgens, cytotoxic agents, and platelet reduction by plateletpheresis. Administration of prophylactic antibiotics may also be considered. Recombinant interferon alfa may be efficacious when used in the cellular (i.e., proliferative) phase but less so when the marrow is fibrotic or osteosclerotic. Moderate doses of radiation therapy to the spleen have been effective in controlling symptoms. However, clinical improvement after irradiation is a slow, gradual process.

Splenectomy may be appropriate in some circumstances (e.g., massively enlarged spleen). Splenectomy in patients with myelofibrosis is associated with an operative mortality rate of 13.4%, an early morbidity rate of 45.3%, and a late morbidity rate of 16.3%. Almost all patients with portal hypertension and painful splenomegaly, but only about half of those with thrombopenia and anemia, have experienced relief of symptoms or signs after splenectomy. There is no evidence that splenectomy affects survival in myelofibrosis. Splenectomy in patients with advanced myelofibrosis is a palliative procedure that carries a substantial risk.

ESSENTIAL THROMBOCYTOSIS/ESSENTIAL THROMBOCYTHEMIA

Essential or primary thrombocythemia is characterized by a significant increase in circulating platelets, usually in excess of $1,000 \times 10^9$/L. Elevated platelet counts may be encountered as a reactive phenomenon, secondary to a variety of systemic conditions, or they may represent essential thrombocythemia, a primary disorder of the bone marrow.

Diagnostic Characteristics

The diagnosis of essential thrombocythemia is difficult and relies on the exclusion of other myeloproliferative states and nonhematological illnesses associated with an increased concentration of platelets. Major criteria and ancillary findings manifested in essential thrombocythemia are presented in Box 21.4.

BOX 21.4

Criteria for Diagnosis of Essential Thrombocytosis/Essential Thrombocythemia[a]

1. Persistent elevation of platelets ($<450 \times 10^{12}$ L) in peripheral blood
2. Significant increase (hyperplasia) of megakaryocytes in the bone marrow
3. Not meeting criteria of other MPNs
4. Demonstration of JAK2V617F or related mutation, or in the absence of JAK2V617F, no evidence for reactive thormbocytosis, e.g., inflammation

[a]Diagnosis requires all four criteria.

Epidemiology

Essential or primary thrombocythemia (essential thrombocytosis) is the least common MPN. Essential thrombocythemia occurs most frequently among persons in the fifth and sixth decades of life. Men and women are equally affected.

Pathophysiology

Essential thrombocythemia is a clonal disorder of multipotential cell origin and belongs to the MPNs that include PV, CML, and primary myelofibrosis. This rare disorder includes a mucocutaneous hemorrhagic diathesis and thromboembolic events. Both thrombocytosis and platelet dysfunction can be responsible for the thrombohemorrhagic phenomena exhibited by patients with this disease. However, qualitative platelet abnormalities rather than thrombocytosis are believed to be the main cause of thromboembolic events.

Karyotype

At least three fourths of patients have a normal karyotype. The balance of patients demonstrates variable chromosomal abnormalities, with aneuploidy being the most common.

Clinical Signs and Symptoms

Thrombotic or bleeding problems are the most commonly seen disorders in patients with thrombocythemia. Patients typically manifest easy bruising, nosebleeds, or gastrointestinal bleeding.

Splenomegaly is found in less than half of patients. Neurological manifestations, however, are frequent and are caused by obstruction of the cerebral microvasculature. Cerebral ischemia and digital ischemia or even gangrene relent or respond completely to a reduction of platelet levels. In addition, unexplained hematomas are common.

A benign form free of hemorrhagic or thrombotic presentation can be observed in a subset of patients aged from 15 to 25 years.

Laboratory Findings

Cellular Abnormalities

The classic laboratory finding in essential thrombocythemia is a significantly elevated peripheral blood platelet count. The number of platelets in the circulating blood is usually in excess of $1,000 \times 10^9$/L, with a minimum of 600×10^9/L. Platelet morphology reveals a normal discoid-shaped cell; bleeding time is normal. In addition, pseudohyperkalemia may result during the preparation of serum. Potassium from platelets is not released during the aggregation phase but during the degranulation phase of the coagulation process.

Peripheral blood erythrocytes are frequently hypochromic and microcytic. If splenic atrophy is present, abnormal erythrocyte morphology includes target cells, Howell-Jolly bodies, nucleated erythrocytes, and acanthocytes. The total concentration of leukocytes is elevated in about 50% of patients but seldom exceeds 40×10^9/L. The LAP value is normal or increased. Concentrations of vitamin B_{12} and uric acid are usually increased.

Platelet Function

In patients with thrombocythemia, the mean extent of aggregation induced by epinephrine, collagen, or ADP is significantly lower than in normal controls. In more than half of patients with thrombocythemia, the platelet-rich plasma does not respond to epinephrine. The total calcium content of platelets is also significantly lower.

Bone Marrow

Bone marrow morphology in essential thrombocythemia (Fig. 21.12) is similar to the architecture seen in PV and CML with associated extreme thrombocytosis. However, significant differences are observable between the marrow findings in MPN and those in extreme reactive thrombocytosis. These differences include the numbers of megakaryocytes, the presence or absence of megakaryocyte clusters, stainable iron, cellularity, and reticulin content.

In addition to increased marrow cellularity (hyperplasia), megakaryocytic hyperplasia is striking. This conspicuous megakaryocytic proliferation also manifests polyploidy of the nuclei, giant forms, and clusters.

Relationship of Thrombocythemia and PV

The seminal events responsible for initiating thrombocythemia and PV clones are unknown. Both clonal disorders are marked by a low-grade hyperproliferation of two

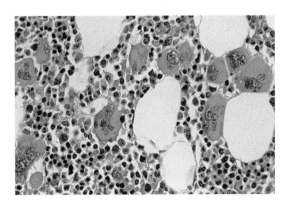

FIGURE 21.12 Bone marrow biopsy of essential thrombocythemia with megakaryocytic hyperplasia. The megakaryocytes are clustering and show characteristic morphology: large size and hyperlobated nuclei. (Reprinted with permission from McClatchey KD. *Clinical Laboratory Medicine*, 2nd ed, Philadelphia, PA: Lippincott Williams & Wilkins, 2002.)

committed stem cell lines plus a significant stimulation of a third cell line. These two disorders are differentiated by a single characteristic—the absence of an expanded red blood cell mass in thrombocythemia.

The mutant stem cell in both disorders has a predisposition to undergo transformation to either myelofibrosis or acute leukemia. The similarities in the natural history of these MPNs suggest that they both begin as very similar, pluripotent stem cell disorders expressed differently only at the colony-forming cell level.

Treatment

The course of the disease is rather benign and resembles that of PV. It may evolve into another form of MPN and in some cases into acute leukemia.

Hemapheresis has been used in a variety of clinical states, primarily for its ability to remove an offending component, likely to be either plasma or cellular elements. Therapeutic hemapheresis is useful in certain clinical conditions, but judicious application should be considered.

Alkylating agents and radioactive phosphorous (^{32}P) are effective treatments, but these agents are associated with an increased risk of leukemia and other neoplasms.

Although treatment of the symptomatic patient with platelet-lowering agents or antiplatelet drugs may be indicated and effective, the role of therapy in the asymptomatic individual remains highly controversial. No remarkable advances have been made in the treatment of MPNs except for the development of an antiplatelet drug, anagrelide. This agent seems to be highly effective in controlling thrombocytosis. The relative merit of this agent compared with interferon alfa, and the impact of this agent on the survival time and on the quality of life of patients with MPNs, have yet to be defined.

CHAPTER HIGHLIGHTS

General Characteristics and Classification

MPNs are interrelated clonal abnormalities resulting in an excessive proliferation of various phenotypically normal mature cells. Classifications of MPNs include CML, PV, primary myelofibrosis (or agnogenic myeloid metaplasia), and essential thrombocythemia.

No environmental causes of MPNs have been identified; however, it has been suggested that a genetic susceptibility may exist. The dysfunction appears to be a loss of regulatory signals that control the production of mature cells.

Patients with an MPN suffer from various mild disorders of hemostasis or coagulation such as DIC. Patients with an MPN commonly exhibit thrombotic phenomena. Many patients with a form of MPN progress to acute leukemia. Interferon may be a new and effective drug for the treatment of the MPNs. This biological agent, either alone or in combination with other antineoplastic treatment, may represent a new therapeutic approach for these disorders.

Chronic Myelogenous Leukemia

CML is one of the most common forms of chronic leukemia. The disease course is characterized by a chronic, indolent stage that frequently transforms into a terminal, acute blast crisis phase. An accelerated phase, when patients become refractive to traditional therapy, may precede the acute phase. The Philadelphia chromosome, Ph[1], was the first aberrant chromosome described in a malignant disorder. It results from the reciprocal translocation of DNA between chromosomes 9 and 22. It is the first demonstrable hematological change in more than 90% of CML patients and is present in myelogenous and erythroid precursors as well as megakaryocytes. Patients with CML or acute lymphoblastic leukemia express the BCR gene rearrangement, which is the molecular counterpart of the Ph[1] chromosome.

The clinical course of CML can be characterized by three separate progressive phases. The onset of the early, initial phase (chronic phase) of CML is insidious and may last from 2 to 3 years. A transitional, accelerated period may precede blast transformation. About three fourths of patients eventually enter a gradual transformation to a blast crisis, which is characterized by the appearance of primitive blast cells similar to those seen in acute leukemia.

The chronic leukemias are usually characterized by the presence of leukocytosis. In CML, the degree of leukocytosis is extreme. CML can also be identified by the presence of the entire spectrum of immature and mature myelogenous cells in the blood and marrow. The total leukocyte count is usually greater than 50×10^9/L and may exceed 300×10^9/L. Bone marrow biopsy reveals hypercellularity with prominent granulocytic hyperplasia.

Because chronic-phase CML is highly responsive to newer treatment, many patients experience at least one remission. After progression to the blast crisis phase, the prognosis is poor, with the patient surviving usually less than 6 months.

Polycythemia Vera

PV is distinguished from the other kinds of MPN by the remarkable increases in red blood cell mass and total blood volume. PV occurs gradually over many decades. The mean age at diagnosis ranges from 60 to 65 years. The most serious complications are vascular accidents and the transition to acute leukemia.

PV is a clonal MPN of the pluripotent hematopoietic stem cell, with an unknown etiology. Although it is a clonal hematopoietic stem cell disorder with trilineage hyperplasia, the most constant and striking feature is erythroid hyperplasia of the bone marrow. Abnormalities in PV erythroid progenitors are expressed at the level of both the CFU-E and BFU-E, which suggests multiple changes in the erythroid progenitors. A shift in the stem cell compartment may occur. IL-3 stimulates trilineage hematopoiesis, but a striking hypersensitivity of polycythemia BFU-E to recombinant IL-3 has been noted. This may be a major factor in the pathogenesis of increased erythropoiesis without increased erythropoietin concentrations.

PV is considered to be a chronic disease with a 10- to 20-year life expectancy after diagnosis. Certain prognostic factors and treatment strategies have an effect on survival. Primary control is achieved by phlebotomy. Recombinant interferon alfa, a natural product with growth-inhibiting capabilities, was recently demonstrated for the first time to have significant therapeutic efficacy in controlling the red blood cell mass in patients with PV. The striking advantage in the use of this drug is the presumed absence of antileukemic effect.

Primary myelofibrosis

Primary myelofibrosis is a clonal disorder of the multipotential progenitor cell compartment. The blood-marrow barrier is disrupted early in the course of myelofibrosis so that blast cells and committed stem cells such as CFU-GM, BFU-E, and CFU-Meg escape into the circulating blood in large numbers. Sclerosis of the bone develops in about half of patients. However, myelofibrosis, the predominant clinical manifestation, occurs secondarily and is not a component of the abnormal clonal proliferation. The process of fibrosis ensues from the proliferation of fibroblasts and increased collagen production in reaction to the abnormal clone of hematopoietic cells. Dysmegakaryocytopoiesis leading to an overproduction of defective platelets is the most constant feature of myelofibrosis.

Essential Thrombocythemia

Essential or primary thrombocythemia (essential thrombocytosis) is characterized by a significant increase in circulating platelets, usually in excess of $1,000 \times 10^9$/L. The diagnosis of essential thrombocythemia is difficult and relies on the exclusion of other myeloproliferative states and nonhematological illnesses associated with an increased concentration of platelets.

Essential thrombocythemia is a clonal disorder of multipotential stem cell origin and belongs to the MPNs that include PV, CML, and primary myelofibrosis. It is a rare disorder.

Thrombotic or bleeding problems are the most commonly seen disorders in patients with thrombocythemia.

CASE STUDIES

CASE 21.1

A 51-year-old white male construction worker was taken to the emergency department by a fellow worker after injuring his wrist at work. On physical examination, an elevated blood pressure was noted. No other abnormalities were found. The patient reported that he had been diagnosed as suffering from hypertension about 5 years ago. The emergency department physician ordered a routine blood count (CBC), urinalysis, and radiograph of the wrist.

■ Laboratory Data
Hemoglobin 21.5 g/dL
Hematocrit 64%
Erythrocyte count 9.2×10^{12}/L
Total leukocyte count 14.0×10^9/L

An increase in neutrophilic bands and segmented neutrophils was observed as well as an increase in the number of thrombocytes. The erythrocytic indices were all within the normal range.

Follow-up testing revealed a total blood volume of 79 mL/kg (normal: adult males, 61.5 ± 8.5 mL/kg of body weight; adult females, 59.0 ± 5 mL/kg) and a total red cell volume of 48 mL/kg (normal: 20 to 36 mL/kg of body weight). A urinary erythropoietin assay revealed the absence of measurable erythropoietin in the urine.

■ Questions
1. What quantitative cellular abnormalities were revealed by laboratory testing?

2. What do the laboratory data suggest in this case?
3. Name other tests that would support a differential diagnosis of PV.

■ Discussion
1. The erythrocyte count, hematocrit, and hemoglobin were all extremely elevated. The total leukocyte count was slightly elevated and the platelet count was also increased.
2. An increased total blood volume (hypervolemia) occurs in disorders such as congestive heart failure, primary aldosteronism, Cushing syndrome, and PV as well as after an overtransfusion of donor blood. This patient's increased total blood volume is undoubtedly producing his hypertension. Additionally, an increased erythrocyte count, hematocrit, and hemoglobin with normal erythrocytic indices are suggestive of polycythemia. A red cell volume greater than 36 mL/kg in males and 32 mL/kg in females is considered to be in the polycythemic range. The absence of erythropoietin in this patient's urine further suggests that the patient has PV.
3. Further testing that would differentiate PV from other forms of polycythemia would be

LAP score
Erythrocyte sedimentation rate
Serum iron determination
Blood histamine assay
Vitamin B_{12}–binding capacity

(continued)

Basophil count
Examination of the bone marrow for hemosiderin

DIAGNOSIS: Polycythemia Vera, Hypertension

CASE 21.2

A 64-year-old white man saw his physician because he was experiencing pain in the shoulders and wrists since returning from his winter home in Florida 6 weeks before. Physical examination revealed that the patient was pale but otherwise in good health. The physician sent the patient to the outpatient laboratory for a CBC and prescribed an analgesic for the joint discomfort.

■ Laboratory Data

The patient's erythrocytes and hemoglobin were moderately decreased. His total leukocyte count was 68×10^9/L. The leukocyte distribution was as follows:

Promyelocytes 1%
Myelocytes 8%
Metamyelocytes 15%
Bands 35%
Segmented neutrophils 25%
Lymphocytes 14%
Monocytes 2%

Some immature erythrocytes were noted, and the number of platelets was increased. A subsequent bone marrow examination revealed both granulocytic and megakaryocytic overproliferation. Cytochemistry staining resulted in the following LAP scores:

Patient 6
Control 43

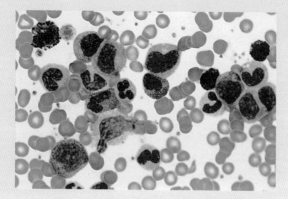

(Reprinted with permission from McClatchey KD. *Clinical Laboratory Medicine,* 2nd ed, Philadelphia, PA: Lippincott Williams & Wilkins, 2002.)

■ Questions

1. What is the most probable diagnosis in this case?
2. Would any additional tests be valuable?

3. Why did this patient exhibit a thrombocytosis on the peripheral blood smear?

■ Discussion

1. Based on the findings of a leukocytosis, many immature and mature granulocytic forms, and a severely diminished LAP score, a diagnosis of CML can be established.
2. Cytogenetic analysis would be valuable in confirming the other test results. Approximately 85% of patients with CML carry Ph[1]. CML patients can be subdivided into Ph[1]-positive and Ph[1]-negative types. Ph[1]-negative patients with CML are correlated with a shorter survival time, lower leukocyte and platelet counts, and a younger age of incidence.
3. Thrombocytosis is common in patients with CML. Frequently, the platelet count reaches into the millions. Thrombotic and hemorrhagic tendencies may complicate the clinical course of this type of leukemia.

DIAGNOSIS: Chronic Myelogenous (Granulocytic) Leukemia

CASE 21.3

A 55-year-old white man was taken by the local volunteer ambulance service to the hospital emergency department. His chief complaint was severe pain in the abdomen and diarrhea for the past 3 days. Physical examination revealed extensive abdominal distention, fresh blood in the stool, an elevated oral temperature, decreased blood pressure, and a rapid pulse. The physician admitted the patient and ordered a STAT CBC and serum electrolyte determinations. An intravenous physiological saline solution was started after the blood had been drawn for examination. A full-body computed tomography (CT) scan was scheduled for the next morning because a conventional lower gastrointestinal radiographic series was contraindicated owing to the fresh bleeding.

■ Laboratory Data

The patient's erythrocyte and hemoglobin parameters were within normal range; however, the total leukocyte count was 63×10^9/L. The leukocyte differential results were as follows:

Blast forms 2%
Promyelocytes 5%
Myelocytes 13%
Metamyelocytes 20%
Bands 20%
Segmented neutrophils 35%
Lymphocytes 4%
Monocytes 1%

(continued)

The platelet estimate from the differential smear indicated a slightly increased number. The serum electrolyte values indicated a state of dehydration.

Additional Clinical Data

The patient's temperature remained elevated during the night of admission. A broad-spectrum antibiotic was added to the intravenous infusion. The patient's blood pressure became unstable during the night. A repeat CBC was ordered the next morning. At that time, the leukocyte count had risen to 118×10^9/L with essentially the same differential distribution of leukocytes. At 10 AM, the laboratory was notified that the patient had died and an autopsy had been requested.

The autopsy revealed that the patient had a mesenteric thrombosis, and acute peritonitis had subsequently developed.

Questions

1. What disorder is suggested by the peripheral blood film?
2. What other hematological test could differentiate between various types of leukocytosis?

Discussion

1. CMLs and leukemoid reactions are indistinguishable on a peripheral blood smear. The sudden elevation of the total leukocyte count and the significant increase (to the left) of granulocytic precursors could have suggested a serious infection with or without an underlying leukemic state.
2. The LAP test is of diagnostic importance in distinguishing between CML and a leukemoid reaction. The LAP score is high in leukemoid reactions and usually low in the CMLs.

DIAGNOSIS: Leukemoid Reaction

CASE 21.4

A 58-year-old man went to see his family physician because of a 3-month history of dizziness. On physical examination, he had a flushed appearance. He had splenomegaly but no hepatomegaly. A CBC was ordered.

Laboratory Data

RBC 5.82×10^{12}/L
Hematocrit 58%
Hemoglobin 20 g/dL
WBC 17.4×10^9/L
Platelets 855×10^9/L

A follow-up bone marrow examination revealed a hypercellular marrow with trilineage hyperplasia and giant megakaryocytes. The Prussian blue iron stain demonstrated absent iron stores.

Questions

1. Based on the laboratory data, what is the suggested diagnosis for this patient?
2. What is the most common therapeutic approach in this disorder?
3. What is the most common cause of death in this disorder?

Discussion

1. A significant increase in red blood cells, WBCs, and platelets is a classic finding in the MPN PV. This disorder differs from secondary polycythemia because the leukocytes and platelets, not just the red blood cells, are also increased. Essential thrombocythemia and PV can be difficult to distinguish because the peripheral blood and bone marrow manifestations in the two diseases are similar.
2. Therapeutic phlebotomy is the most common therapeutic approach to PV, but it is the single most important factor in the increased risk of thrombosis. Chemotherapy aimed at reducing the proliferation of cells increases the risk of secondary acute leukemia.
3. Circulatory disturbances secondary to decreased blood flow, hemorrhage, or thrombosis are the most frequent causes of death in a patient with PV. Cerebral thrombosis presents a high risk of death.

DIAGNOSIS: Polycythemia Vera

CASE 21.5

A 21-year-old male athlete visited the sports medicine clinic after noting that his knee was swollen. He had no history of recent injuries. He reported having frequent, bilateral nose bleeds, bleeding from his gums when brushing his teeth, and some blood in the stool. The attending orthopedic surgeon ordered a CBC and CAT scan of the swollen knee.

Laboratory Data

RBC 4.40×10^{12}/L
Hematocrit 43%
Hemoglobin 14.8 g/dL
WBC 12.5×10^9/L
Platelets 955×10^9/L

The CAT scan of his knee revealed a large effusion, which was bloody when tapped.

Questions

1. What is the probable diagnosis, based on the patient's history?
2. Based on the initial and follow-up studies, how does this disease presentation differ from PV?
3. Is this thrombocytosis a reactive thrombosis?

(continued)

■ **Discussion**

1. The significantly increased platelet count and slightly decreased red blood cell parameters are an indication of a probable hematological problem. Follow-up bone marrow and platelet aggregation studies were ordered.

The follow-up bone marrow exhibited a hypercellular marrow. The Prussian blue iron stain demonstrated normal marrow iron stores. The platelet aggregation studies were grossly abnormal.

2. In contrast to PV, this patient has normal bone marrow iron stores.

3. No. Reactive thrombocytosis is associated with acute or chronic inflammatory conditions, acute hemorrhage, and a variety of other conditions. The patient had no medical history suggestive of these causes of his thrombocytosis. The diagnosis of essential (primary) thrombocythemia is one of exclusion.

DIAGNOSIS: Essential (primary) Thrombocythemia

REVIEW QUESTIONS

1. MPNs are characterized by all of the following except
   A. clonal disorders
   B. they may evolve into acute leukemia
   C. initial increase of immature cells
   D. increased production of mature cells

2. In CML, the total leukocyte (WBC) count is
   A. extremely increased
   B. slightly increased
   C. extremely variable
   D. usually normal

3. Primary myelofibrosis differs from other types of MPN in which of the following ways?
   A. Ph[1] chromosome is present
   B. Marrow fibrosis is greatly increased
   C. LAP score is increased
   D. Platelet count is increased

4. Which of the following is a remarkable characteristic of PV compared with other types of MPNs?
   A. Extremely increased erythrocyte mass
   B. Extremely increased leukocyte count
   C. Extremely increased platelet count
   D. Teardrop-shaped erythrocytes

5. Which of the following is a predominant feature of essential thrombocythemia compared with other types of MPNs?
   A. Variable number of platelets
   B. Moderately increased number of platelets
   C. Extremely increased number of platelets
   D. Increased marrow fibrosis

6. In MPN, the test results of disorders of hemostasis and coagulation that are most likely to be abnormal are
   A. decreased platelet count, increased APTT, and increased factor V level
   B. increased APTT, decreased factor V level, and increased concentration of antithrombin III in many

   C. decreased APTT, decreased factor V level, and increased concentration of D-dimers
   D. decreased concentration of D-dimers, decreased concentration of antithrombin III, and increased concentration of plasmin-alpha 2-plasmin inhibitor complex

7. Interferon alfa has been shown to
   A. stimulate trilineage cell proliferation
   B. suppress proliferation of hematopoietic progenitor cells
   C. subdue erythropoiesis only
   D. suppress megakaryocytopoiesis only

8. A leukemia of long duration that affects the neutrophilic granulocytes is referred to as
   A. acute lymphoblastic leukemia
   B. acute myelogenous leukemia
   C. acute monocytic leukemia
   D. CML

9. The alkaline phosphatase cytochemical staining reaction is used to differentiate between
   A. chronic lymphoblastic leukemia and acute myelogenous leukemia
   B. acute lymphoblastic leukemia and acute myelogenous leukemia
   C. CML and severe bacterial infections
   D. leukemoid reactions and severe bacterial infections

10. Patients with the initial phase of CML are prone to
    A. weight gain, edema, and fatigue
    B. edema, anemia, and splenic infarction
    C. low-grade fevers, night sweats, and splenic infarction
    D. prominent lymphadenopathy and night sweats

(continued)

11. The total leukocyte count in CML usually is _____ × 10^9/L.
    A. normal
    B. <25
    C. <50
    D. >50

12. The Philadelphia chromosome is typically associated with
    A. acute myelogenous leukemia
    B. leukemoid reactions
    C. acute lymphoblastic leukemia
    D. CML

13. Patients with PV suffer from
    A. leukemic infiltration
    B. bone marrow fibrosis
    C. hypervolemia
    D. anemia

14. In PV, cytogenetic results do not predict/provide
    A. duration of the disease
    B. consequences of myelosuppressive therapy
    C. clues to hematological phenotype
    D. evolution of the disease

15. Hyperviscosity can produce
    A. anemia
    B. dizziness
    C. hemorrhages
    D. psychotic depression

16. The major criteria for diagnosis of PV include all of the following except
    A. increased red blood cell mass
    B. presence of JAK2V617F
    C. hypercellular bone marrow
    D. splenomegaly

17. Increased blood viscosity in patients with PV can cause a dangerous condition of
    A. hot flushes
    B. shortness of breath
    C. high RDW
    D. vascular occlusion

18. The level of erythropoietin in the urine is _____ in patients with PV compared with other kinds of polycythemia.
    A. increased
    B. the same
    C. variable
    D. decreased

19. Patients with PV demonstrate a(n) _____ of hemosiderin in the bone marrow.
    A. absence
    B. normal amount
    C. slightly increased amount
    D. extremely increased amount

20. Treated patients with PV have a _____ life expectancy after diagnosis.
    A. 1- to 6-month
    B. 6- to 12-month
    C. 1- to 5-year
    D. more than 10-year

21. The primary treatment for PV is
    A. therapeutic phlebotomy
    B. myelosuppressive agents
    C. radioactive phosphorus
    D. low-dose busulfan

22. Primary myelofibrosis is also called
    A. essential thrombocythemia
    B. CML
    C. PV
    D. agnogenic myeloid metaplasia

23. The incidence of primary myelofibrosis is known to increase after exposure to
    A. sunshine
    B. benzene
    C. antibiotics
    D. interferon

24. The predominant clinical manifestation of primary myelofibrosis is
    A. anemia
    B. splenomegaly
    C. medullary fibrosis
    D. all of the above

25. The most constant feature of primary myelofibrosis is
    A. dyserythropoiesis
    B. dysleukopoiesis
    C. dysmegakaryocytopoiesis
    D. trilineage maturational disruption

26. A leukoerythroblastic picture includes all of the following except
    A. teardrop-shaped erythrocytes
    B. nucleated erythrocytes
    C. immature lymphocytes
    D. immature myeloid cells

27. The median survival time for patients with primary myelofibrosis is approximately _____ year(s).
    A. 1
    B. 3
    C. 5
    D. 10

28. The least common form of MPN is
    A. PV
    B. CML
    C. primary myelofibrosis
    D. essential thrombocythemia

(continued)

29. A major criterion for the diagnosis of essential thrombocythemia is
A. absence of Ph[1] chromosome
B. increased red blood cell mass
C. mild neutrophilia in peripheral blood
D. persistent increase of platelets in peripheral blood

30. The most common disorder in patients with essential thrombocythemia is
A. neurological manifestations
B. thrombotic or bleeding problems
C. abnormal karyotype
D. anemia

31. The bone marrow architecture in essential thrombocythemia is similar to the architecture seen in
A. erythroid hyperplasia
B. leukocyte hyperplasia
C. CML
D. lymphocytic leukemia

BIBLIOGRAPHY

Apperly J. Allografting for chronic myeloid leukemia in the Glivec era, *Hemato J,* 4 Suppl 3. In: *Educational Book of the 8th Congress of the European Hematology Association.* Lyon: France, 2003:11–14.

Bowers GR (ed.). Polycythemia rubra vera, *CDH Oncol,* 7(7):1–6, 2003.

Campbell PJ, Green AR. The myeloproliferative disorders, *N Eng J Med,* 355(23):2452–2466, 2006.

Clark M. Chronic myelomonocytic leukemia transforming into acute myelogenous leukemia, *Lab Med,* 40(1):19–21, 2009.

Conley CL. Polycythemia vera, *JAMA,* 263(18):2481–2483, 1990.

Crisan D, Carr ER. BCR/*abl* gene rearrangement in chronic myelogenous leukemia and acute leukemias, *Lab Med,* 23(11):730–735, 1992.

Drucker BJ. Translation of the Philadelphia chromosome into therapy for CML, *Blood,* 112(13):4808–4817, 2008.

Drucker BJ, et al. Five year follow-up of patients receiving imatinib for chronic myeloid leukemia, *N Engl J Med,* 355(23):2408–2417, 2006.

Drucker BJ, et al. Efficacy and safety of a specific inhibitor of the BCR-ABL tyrosine kinase in chronic myeloid leukemia, *N Engl J Med,* 344(14): 1031–1037, 2001.

Fabarius A, et al. Dynamics of cytogenetic aberrations in Philadelphia chromosome positive and negative hematopoiesis during dasatinib therapy of chronic myeloid leukemia patients after imatinib failure, *Haematologica,* 92(06):834–837, 2007.

Faderl S, et al. The biology of chronic myeloid leukemia, *N Engl J Med,* 341(3):164–172, 1999.

Fischer T. Beyond CML—New horizons for Imatinib. In: *Imatinib—Impact on CML Management and Beyond, 8th EHA Congress,* Lyon, France: 2003.

Gilliland DG, et al. Clonality in myeloproliferative disorders: Analysis by means of the polymerase chain reaction, *Proc Natl Acad Sci USA,* 88(15):6848–6852, 1991.

Goldman J. Novel treatment approaches. In: *The Educational Book of the 8th EHA Congress,* Lyon, France: 2003:21–24.

Goldman JM. Practical considerations to optimize outcome for patients with CML in chronic phase. In: *Imatinib—Impact on CML Management and Beyond, 8th EHA Congress,* Lyon, France: 2003.

Guilhot F, et al. Interferon alfa-2b combined with cytarabine versus interferon alone in chronic myelogenous leukemia, *N Engl J Med,* 337(4):223–228, 1997.

Hehlmann R, Saussele S. Treatment of chronic myeloid leukemia in blast crisis, *Haematologica,* 93(12):1765–1768, 2008.

Hochhaus A. Molecular response and resistance to Imatinib (Glivec®). In: *Education Book of the 8th EHA Congress,* Lyon, France: 2003:15–20.

Hochhaus A. Perspectives on managing resistance in CML. In: *Imatinib—Impact on CML Management and Beyond, 8th EHA Congress,* Lyon, France: 2003.

Kantarjian HM, et al. Long-term survival benefit and improved complete cytogenetic and molecular response rates with imatinib mesylate in Philadelphia chromosome-positive chronic-phase chronic myeloid leukemia after failure of interferon-α, *Blood,* 104(7): 1979–1988, 2006.

Kantarjian H, et al. Nilotinib in imatinib-resistant CML and Philadelphia chromosome-positive ALL, *N Eng J Med,* 354(24): 2542–2551, 2006.

Kralovics R, et al. A gain-of-function mutation of JAK2 in myeloproliferative disorders, *N Eng J Med,* 352(17):1779–1790, 2005.

Klippel S, et al. Biochemical characterization of PV-1, a novel hematopoietic cell surface receptor, which is overexpressed in polycythemia rubra vera, *Blood,* 100(7):2441–2448, 2002.

Lee SJ, et al. impact of prior imatinib mesylate on the outcome of hematopoietic cell transplantation for chronic myeloid leukemia, *Blood,* 112(8):3500–3507, 2008.

Levine RL, Gilliland G. Myeloproliferative disorders, *Blood,* 112(6): 2190–2198, 2008.

Martinelli G, et al. New tyrosine kinase inhibitors in chronic myeloid leukemia, *Haematologica,* (90)4:534–541, 2005.

Marsh GM, et al. Mortality patterns among petroleum refinery and chemical plant workers, *Am J Ind Med,* 19(1):29–42, 1991.

Mertens F, et al. Karyotypic patterns in chronic myeloproliferative disorders: Report on 74 cases and review of the literature, *Leukemia,* 5(3):214–220, 1991.

Mumprecht S, et al. Imatinib mesylate selectively impairs expansion of memory cytotoxic T cells without affecting the control of primary viral infections, *Blood,* 108(10):3406–3413, 2006.

O'Brien SG, et al. Imatinib compared with interferon and low-dose cytarabine for newly diagnosed chronic-phase chronic myeloid leukemia, *N Engl J Med,* 348(11):994–1004, 2003.

Palandri F, et al. Chronic myeloid leukemia in blast crisis treated with imatinib 600 mg: outcome of the patients alive after a 6-year follow-up, *Haematologica,* 93(12):1792, 2008.

Peggs K, Mackinnon S. Imatinib mesylate—The new gold standard for treatment of chronic myeloid leukemia, *N Engl J Med*, 348(11): 1048–1050, 2003.

Quintás-Cardama A, Cortes J. Molecular biology of *bcr-abl1*-positive chronic myeloid leukemia, *Blood*, 113(80);1619–1630, 2009.

Randolph T. JAK2: The next BCR/ABL among the myeloproliferative disorders (MPN)? *ACLS Today*, 22(5):5–11, 2008.

Rowe JM. Closing the gap in CML, *Blood*, 109(6):2271, 2007.

Saglio G. Measuring molecular response in CML: Problems and significance. In: *Imatinib—Impact on CML Management and Beyond, 8th EHA Congress*, Lyon, France: 2003.

Schaich M, et al. Prognosis of acute myeloid leukemia patients up to 60 years of age exhibiting trisomy 8 within a non-complex karotype: individual patient data-based meta-analysis of the German acute myeloid leukemia intergroup, *Haematologica*, 92(06): 763–770, 2007.

Schiffer CA. BCR-ABL tyrosine kinase inhibitors for chronic myelogenous leukemia, *N Eng J Med*, 357(3):258–265, 2007.

Schwartz R. A molecular star in the wars against cancer, *N Engl J Med*, 347(7):462–463, 2002.

Scott LM, et al. JAK2 exon 12 mutations in polycythemia vera and idiopathic erythrocytosis, *N Eng J Med*, 356(5):459–468, 2007.

Smyth MJ. Imatinib mesylate – uncovering a fast track to adaptive immunity, *N Eng J Med*, 354(21):2282–2284, 2006.

Stuart BJ, Viera AJ. Polycythemia vera, *Am Fam Physician* 69: 2139–2144, 2146, 2004.

Talpaz M. Dasatinib in imatinib-resistant Philadelphia chromosome-positive leukemias, *N Eng J Med*, 354(24):2531–2540, 2006.

Temerinac S, et al. Cloning of PV-1, a novel member of the uPAR receptor superfamily, which is overexpressed in polycythemia rubra vera, *Blood*, 95(8):2569–2576, 2000.

Myelodysplastic Syndromes and Myelodysplastic/Myeloproliferative Neoplasms

Classification
- Describe the comparative characteristics of the French-American-British (FAB) and World Health Organization (WHO) classification of myelodysplastic syndromes (MDSs) and myelodysplastic/myeloproliferative neoplasms (MPNs).

Pathophysiology
- Explain the pathophysiology of MDSs.

Etiology
- Explain the causes or predisposing factors of primary and secondary MDSs.

Epidemiology
- Describe the age and gender distribution of MDSs.

Chromosomal abnormalities
- Briefly describe the causes, types, and consequences of chromosomal abnormalities in MDSs.
- List the incidence of chromosomal abnormalities.
- Describe the relationship of karyotype to prognosis in MDSs.

Clinical signs and symptoms
- Explain the clinical signs and symptoms of MDSs.

Laboratory manifestations
- Itemize the cellular alterations, with an emphasis on the prominent features and additional hematological features in MDSs.
- Compare the laboratory features of specific types of MDSs.
- Calculate the percentage of myeloblasts in the bone marrow.

Myelodysplastic syndromes/myeloproliferative neoplasms
- Describe the unique features and laboratory characteristics of chronic myelomonocytic leukemia (CMML).

Treatment
- Explain the forms of treatment and supportive care for the MDSs.

Prognosis
- Discuss factors that can affect prognosis in the MDSs, including FAB classification and karyotype.
- Compare the parameters used in the International Scale for Prognosis.

Case studies
- Apply the laboratory data to the case studies and discuss the implications of these cases to the study of hematology.

CLASSIFICATION

Since the original development of the FAB classification for MDS (Table 22.1), the WHO has developed a newer classification of MDSs and myelodysplastic/myeloproliferative neoplasms (MDS/MPNs). The most recent WHO revision of Tumors and Hematopoietic and Lymphoid Tissues was published in 2008 (Table 22.2).

Myelodysplastic Syndromes

MDS is characterized by the simultaneous proliferation and apoptosis of hematopoietic cells that lead to a normal or hypercellular bone marrow biopsy and peripheral blood cytopenia(s). These disorders are among the most challenging of the myeloid neoplasms to both diagnose and classify (Box 22.1).

Myelodysplastic/myeloproliferative neoplasms

The MDS/MPN classification (Box 22.2) includes clonal myeloid neoplasms that at initial presentation have some clinical, laboratory, or morphologic findings that support a diagnosis of MDS and other findings that are more consistent with MPN (see Chapter 21). Patients placed in this category, for example, (CMML), usually demonstrate a hypercellular bone marrow because of proliferation of one or more cell lines.

TABLE 22.1	Traditional FAB Cooperative Group Classification of MDSs				
Subtype	Peripheral Blood Monocytes (×10^9/L)	Ring Sideroblasts (%)	Blast Cells (%)		Auer Bodies in Marrow
			Peripheral Blood	Bone Marrow	
RA	No	<15	<1	<5	No
RARS	No	>15	<1	<5	No
RAEB	No	No	>5	5–20	No
CMML	>1,000	No	<5	<20	No
RAEB-T	No	No	<5	20–30	Yes or no

RA, refractory anemia; RARSs, refractory anemia with ring sideroblasts; RAEB, refractory anemia with excess of blasts; CMML, chronic myelomonocytic leukemia; RAEB-T, refractory anemia with excess of blasts in transition.

PATHOPHYSIOLOGY

The MDS and MDS/myeloproliferative disorders (MPDs) are a heterogeneous group of clonal disorders of the bone marrow. The clonal nature of MDS is supported by research studies, even in the absence of detectable cytogenetic abnormalities.

Isoenzyme and cytogenetic analyses suggest that the pathogenesis of these clonal disorders is a multistep process beginning with the destabilization of the multipotential progenitor cell, causing proliferation of a divergent clone of genetically unstable pluripotential stem cells that produce morphologically variable but clonally related progeny. This type of aberration becomes permanent when the acquisition of a clonal chromosome abnormality exists.

If the cell abnormality persists, additional subclones with recurrent chromosome abnormalities emerge. This precedes either failure of effective hematopoiesis or acute transformation (clonal escape) to acute myelogenous leukemia (AML) or both. Hematopoiesis is dysplastic because of inefficient maturation of a slowly expanding or sometimes stable population of blood cell precursors.

MYELODYSPLASTIC SYNDROME

The MDSs are classified into various types of refractory anemias (RAs), unclassified myelodysplastic syndrome, childhood MDS and MDS associated with isolated del(5q). The specific subtypes include

TABLE 22.2	WHO Criteria MDSs	
MDS Subtype	Peripheral Blood	Bone Marrow
Refractory anemia (RA)[a]	Anemia	Unilineage dysplasia ≥ 10% in one myeloid line
	<1% blasts	<5% blasts
		<15% ring sideroblasts
Refractory anemia with ring sideroblasts (RARS)	Anemia	Erythroid dysplasia *only* ≥15% ring sideroblasts
	No blasts	<5% blasts
Refractory cytopenias with multilineage dysplasia (RCMD)	Cytopenias	Dysplasia in ≥10% of cells in 2 myeloid cell lines
	No or rare blasts	No Auer rods
	<1 × 10^9/L monocytes	<5% blasts in marrow
	No Auer rods	No Auer rods
		± 15% ring sideroblasts
Refractory anemia with excess blasts, type 1 (RAEB-1)	Cytopenias	Unilineage or multilineage dysplasia
	<5% blasts	5% to 9% blasts

(continued)

TABLE 22.2	WHO Criteria MDSs *(Continued)*	
MDS Subtype	**Peripheral Blood**	**Bone Marrow**
	No Auer rods	No Auer rods
	$<1 \times 10^9$/L monocytes	
Refractory anemia with excess blasts, type 2 (RAEB-2)	Cytopenias	Unilineage or multilineage dysplasia
	<5% to 19% blasts	10%–19% blasts
	Auer rods ± <1 × 10⁹/L monocytes	Auer rods ±
MDS associated with isolated del (5q)	Anemia	<5% blasts
	Normal or elevated platelet count	Anemia, hypolobulated megakaryocytic anemia isolated 5q31 chromosome deletion
	<1% blasts	
Childhood MDS, including refractory cytopenia of childhood (provisional)	Pancytopenia	< 5% marrow red blood cell blasts
		usually hyptocellular marrow
MDS, unclassifiable (MDS, U)	Cytopenias	Does not fit other categories
	≤1% blasts	Dysplasia and <5% blasts
		If no dysplasia, MDS-associated karyotype

MDS, myelodysplastic syndrome.
ᵃThis category is refractory cytopenias with unilineage dysplasia (RCUD) refractory anemia. The category includes refractory anemia, refractory neutropenia, and refractory thrombocytopenia.

■ Refractory cytopenias with unilineage dysplasia, grouping RA, refractory neutropenia, and refractory thrombocytopenia
■ Refractory anemia with ring sideroblasts (RARSs)
■ Refractory cytopenia with multilineage dysplasia (RCMD)
■ Refractory anemia with excess of blasts (RAEB-1 and RAEB-2)

■ MDS associated with isolated del(5q)
■ Childhood MDS, including refractory cytopenia of childhood (provisional)
■ Myelodysplastic syndrome-unclassified (MDS-U)

Etiology

Primary or de novo MDS occurs without a known history of chemotherapy or radiation exposure. Secondary MDS can sometimes be directly related to a known agent. Certain risk factors may be possible etiologies for developing MDS. These factors include

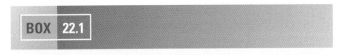

Myelodysplastic syndromes (MDSs)

■ Refractory cytopenia with unilineage dysplasia

Refractory anemia
Refractory neutropenia
Refractory thrombocytopenia

■ Refractory anemia with ring sideroblasts (RARSs)
■ Refractory cytopenia with multilineage dysplasia (RCMD)
■ Refractory anemia with excess blasts (RAEBs)
■ MDS with isolated del(5q)
■ Myelodysplastic syndrome, unclassifiable (MDS,U)
■ Childhood MDS

Provisionally refractory cytopenia of childhood

Myelodysplastic/myeloproliferative Neoplasms (MDS/MPNs)

Chronic myelomonocytic leukemia
Atypical chronic myeloid leukemia
Juvenile myelomonocytic leukemia
Myelomonocytic/Myeloproliferative neoplasms, unclassifiable

■ *Age.* Population studies in England have found that the crude incidence increases from 0.5 per 100,000 people younger than age 50 years to 89 per 100,000 people 80 years of age or older.

■ *Genetic predisposition.* Familial syndromes have been reported but are rare. Fanconi anemia, Shwachman-Diamond syndrome, and Diamond-Blackfan syndrome are associated with an increased risk of MDS.

■ *Environmental exposures.* Particularly with benzene and possibly other industrial solvents.

■ *Prior therapy.* The greatest incidence of MDS follows combined chemotherapy and radiation therapy. It should also be noted that secondary MDS precedes AML as a late consequence of chemotherapy or radiation therapy or both in many treated patients. For alkylating agents, the risk of developing a secondary MDS or AML starts with the end of therapy and peaks at 4 years, with a plateau at 10 years. For epipodophyllotoxins, the latency period to development of MDS/AML is almost always less than 5 years, with a shorter latency of transition from MDS to AML.

Examples of diseases that precede MDS include ovarian carcinoma treated with alkylating agents (10% to 15% of MDS cases), Hodgkin disease treated with combined therapy (8% to 10% of MDS cases), and multiple myeloma (approximately 15% of MDS cases). One theory to explain the induction of MDS and perhaps eventual AML is that alkylating agents induce DNA cross-linkages, which because of unequal crossing-over may place DNA in juxtaposition to certain oncogenes. The oncogenes may then become activated and lead to the development of a malignant clone of bone marrow cells, which develops into MDS.

■ *Other factors.* Abuse of prescription or over-the-counter drugs may also be causative of MDS. Although no firm relationship has been established to date, drugs such as analgesics, tranquilizers, and nonsteroidal anti-inflammatory drugs may eventually be linked to the pathogenesis of MDS (sideroblastic anemia).

Epidemiology

MDS is rare in childhood. The adult form usually occurs in persons older than 50 years of age (most patients are 60 to 75 years old). MDS is more common in males.

The incidence of MDS is still unknown but is probably similar to that of acute leukemia. There are estimated to be at least 1,500 to 2,000 cases annually in the United States. The prevalence of MDS, however, may be as high as 1:500 in individuals older than 55 years of age.

Chromosomal Abnormalities

Karyotype differences exist between primary (de novo) and secondary MDSs and may be observed on initial bone marrow observation or during evolution of the disease. Clonal cytogenetic abnormalities are observed in about 50% of MDS cases. Some chromosomal alterations seem to be consistently involved in the pathogenetic mechanisms of secondary leukemia and MDS.

Clonal chromosomal anomalies may be observed during initial bone marrow analysis or seen as the result of karyotypic evolution during disease progression. These abnormalities may be monosomic or trisomic in nature and may involve partial or total chromosomal alterations. Most chromosomes display a recurrent loss of chromosomal material rather than the translocations or inversions commonly found in AML. In many instances, the cytogenetic abnormalities become complex and involve more than one chromosome. Complex karyotypes (≥3 abnormalities) typically include chromosomes 5 and 7.

Characteristic karyotype anomalies involve mainly chromosomes 5, 7, and 8. These same chromosomes are known to carry different oncogenes. The most frequent alterations are in the marker chromosomes: 5 (monosomy or 5q−), 7 (monosomy, partial loss of the long arm, 7q−, rearrangement), and 8 (trisomy or rearrangement). Other implicated chromosomes are 1, 3 (monosomy), 4 (monosomy), 9, 12, 17, 20 (20 q−), and 21 as well as the Y chromosome (loss).

The most frequent abnormalities in children are trisomy 8, monosomy 7, and deletions involving the long arms of chromosomes 20 and X. In children with MDS, an abnormality like monosomy 7 is typical and probably indicates an unfavorable prognosis.

Consequences

Chromosomal alterations, mostly of the deleted type, are assumed to play a specific role in the genesis of MDS. These abnormalities are perhaps reflections of an alteration of oncogene function and alterations of production of growth factors and their receptors that may lead to proliferation of the abnormal clone. Some theories suggest that abnormalities in the production of growth factors or receptors relate to the development of MDS.

In primary MDS, abnormal growth of the granulocyte-macrophage precursor, colony-forming unit–granulocyte-macrophage (CFU-GM), occurs in approximately 79% of patients and clonal chromosome abnormalities occur in an average of 34% of patients.

Relationship of Karyotype to Prognosis

Survival of patients with MDS is better for those with normal chromosomal patterns. Both single-chromosome anomalies and multiple cytogenetic changes are significant. Sequential cytogenetic studies demonstrate that most patients whose conditions transform to acute leukemia exhibit a karyotypic evolution. The existence of monosomy 5 or monosomy 7 can be useful in identifying patients in whom acute leukemia will probably develop.

The occurrence of trisomy 11 in MDS and in AML suggests that this abnormality can be specifically associated with the subsequent development of AML. Patients with a long-arm deletion of chromosome 20 (20q−) usually have intractable dysplastic syndromes, and many progress to leukemia.

Although de novo and secondary MDSs share certain clinical and cytogenetic features, more than 20% of patients with de novo MDS have a normal karyotype, and nearly all these patients survive beyond 5 years. In contrast, secondary MDS is frequently associated with clonal chromosome abnormalities, and overt leukemia generally occurs within 1 year.

Clinical Signs and Symptoms

A history of infections, bleeding, weight loss, or cardiovascular symptoms may be reported by a patient. Infections are caused by dysfunctional granulocytic neutrophils or absolute granulocytopenia. Hemorrhages can occur because of decreased or dysfunctional platelets. Anemia is a common initial presenting symptom. A paucity of other physical symptoms is usually present.

Neutrophilic dermatosis has occurred occasionally in MDS patients. In these patients, biopsy specimens of skin lesions showed significant infiltration by neutrophils with nuclear anomalies, that is, hyposegmentation (pseudo–Pelger-Huët anomaly) or hypersegmentation.

Laboratory Manifestations

Cellular Abnormalities

Anemia, low platelet count, and low total leukocyte count, usually with an absolute neutropenia, are commonly present. Peripheral blood smears frequently exhibit red blood cell (RBC) abnormalities and large dysfunctional platelets. MDS is characteristically manifested by pancytopenia in the peripheral blood, dysplasia of two or three cell lines that may initially be in just one cell line, and a low leukemic blast count in the bone marrow and peripheral blood. Pancytopenia occurs in more than 50% of patients.

Some categorical characteristics of MDS types are overlapping. The hematopoietic disorders comprising MDS also share some common features with the early phases of myeloproliferative diseases, especially AML. However, the bone marrow of many pancytopenic patients may reveal acute leukemia, de novo or from other causes, including MDS. In addition, pancytopenia may represent an aplastic anemia. Distinguishing between MDS and aplastic anemia can be difficult, because both of these disorders can have similar clinical and morphological features (see Chapter 9 for a discussion of aplastic anemia). MDS must also be differentiated from secondary anemias (e.g., vitamin B$_{12}$ deficiency).

Patients with aggressive subtypes of MDS (i.e., RAEB) frequently have thrombocytopenia and neutropenia, and their marrow demonstrates dysmegakaryocytopoiesis and dysgranulocytopoiesis as compared to the more benign subtypes (i.e., RA and RARS). In addition, leukemic transformation most frequently comes from the aggressive subtypes.

Children with a primary MDS can have clinical and laboratory features of juvenile chronic myeloid leukemia. Some pediatric patients could be considered to have either the monosomy 7 syndrome or juvenile chronic myeloid leukemia, indicating that these two entities are not mutually exclusive. In these patients, abnormal frequencies of hematopoietic progenitors or differentiation patterns in culture or both can occur. Abnormalities often affect the erythroid and the granulopoietic lineages, predominantly abnormal-appearing macrophage colonies. Clinical outcomes are poor, with rapid transformation to AML in most patients.

Summary of Cell Line Abnormalities

Erythrocyte Abnormalities

Erythroid abnormalities of blood and bone marrow are common because MDS is dominated by ineffective hematopoiesis. Islands of erythroid hyperplasia with erythroblastic deformities can be seen in the bone marrow. The megaloblastic changes (e.g., nuclear-cytoplasmic dyssynchrony) often are similar to those of nutritional megaloblastic anemias. Erythroblasts (rubriblasts) may be multinucleated, fragmented, or misshaped. Abnormal nuclear shapes include indentations, lobes, or an irregular outline. Cytoplasmic staining is often uneven, and the cell margins may be ragged or indistinct and may display punctate basophilic stippling.

About one fourth of patients with RA demonstrate ring sideroblasts similar to those of sideroblastic anemias in the bone marrow. Ring sideroblasts are scarce in megaloblastic anemias. Patients with RARS usually present with a dual population of red cells: a minor one that is hypochromic and microcytic, often displaying basophilic stippling, and a major one that is macrocytic with a high mean corpuscular volume and megaloblastoid changes. An occasional nucleated RBC may be seen in the peripheral blood.

Leukocyte Abnormalities

Abnormalities of the myeloid series are generally more subtle than those of dyserythropoiesis. Neutrophils are often agranular or hypogranular. Precursor marrow myelocytes may also lack secondary granules. A dense rim of basophilia may occur at the cell periphery. Primary granules may be absent from promyelocytes.

Myelocytes and promyelocytes can have central, round nuclei. Nuclear anomalies include the pseudo–Pelger-Huët anomaly and the twinning deformity. The twinning deformity involves two discrete segmented strands in a tetraploid cell, which also produces an abnormally large cell. Hypersegmentation may also be seen. Peripheral blood and bone marrow neutrophils have similar anomalies.

Low lymphocyte counts in bone marrow can be observed. A significant decrease of CD3-defined pan T lymphocytes in peripheral blood can be exhibited. This reduction is primarily confined to the CD4-defined helper subset, but there can be a relative increase in the CD8-defined suppressor subpopulation. As a result, the ratio of CD4-CD8 lymphocytes is reversed. Consequently, abnormalities of cell-mediated immunity function can occur.

Platelet Abnormalities

The megakaryocyte population may be decreased, normal, or increased. Micromegakaryocytes, mononuclear megakaryocytes, multiple small separated nuclei, and giant granules can be seen in the peripheral blood. Large bizarre platelets are a frequent finding in the peripheral blood. A distinct subpopulation of platelets in MDS, which by phase-contrast microscopic examination seem to have a balloon-shaped bulge of the cell membrane, has been observed. Increased numbers of these atypical platelets can be observed in the majority of patients with MDS. Normal platelet morphology may be observed in patients with RARS. The number of atypical platelets is negatively correlated with the peripheral platelet counts in MDS. The atypical platelets most likely reflect maturation disturbances of megakaryocytopoiesis. Unless associated with recent cytotoxic therapy, an increased value (>1%) in a cytopenic patient would suggest a diagnosis of MDS.

Additional Hematological Features

Numerous morphological features have been observed in the bone marrow and peripheral blood of patients with MDS. In addition, a subtle morphological feature, **internuclear bridging (INB)**, was recently recognized in MDS. The occurrence of INB in MDS suggests an underlying abnormality of mitotic division that could explain the impaired production of hematopoietic cells, the cytogenetic changes of addition and deletion, and the stepwise disease progression and cytogenetic progression characteristic of MDS. Lack of awareness that INB occurs in MDS may cause a confusion of MDS with congenital dyserythropoietic anemia type I, a congenital process also characterized by INB.

Intracellular alkaline phosphatase activities in peripheral neutrophils are decreased in MDS compared with healthy controls. The measurement of intracellular alkaline phosphatase activity is useful for supporting a diagnosis of MDS.

Lymphoid agglutination or cell clusters of blast cells are also seen in biopsy specimens from patients with MDS.

Features of Selected Types of Myelodysplastic Syndromes

Refractory anemia (RA), one of the refractory cytopenias with unilineage dysplasia, is the mildest form of all types of MDS. Approximately 20% of patients have this type of MDS. Most patients exhibit pancytopenia. The percentage of reticulocytes and the total peripheral red blood count are typically decreased. Peripheral erythrocytes have a tendency to be macrocytic. Decreased hemoglobin levels are caused by an impaired release of erythrocytes from the bone marrow. The total peripheral blood leukocyte and platelet counts are either normal or decreased. Some neutrophils are agranular or tetraploid. Giant platelets are common. The level of bone marrow storage iron is increased.

Refractory anemia with ring sideroblasts (RARSs) is similar to RA but differs because of the presence of ring sideroblasts (Figs. 22.1 and 22.2). Ring sideroblasts, which exceed 15% of the nucleated erythroid cells of the bone marrow, are formed when iron deposits encircle the nuclei of erythroid precursors. Over time, the number of dysplastic sideroblasts and the medullary iron levels increase in parallel, and serum ferritin levels steadily rise. A small number of patients eventually develop hemochromatosis. In these patients, the incidence of HLA-A3 is significantly higher (71%) than in the general population,

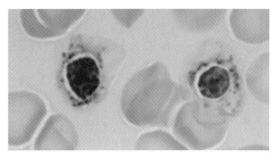

FIGURE 22.1 Ring sideroblasts. The large granules with stainable iron, termed diserosomes, appear in the abnormal erythroblasts surrounding the nucleus of the cells like a ring. Prussian blue stain. (Reprinted with permission from Handin RI, et al. *Blood: Principles and Practice of Hematology*, 2nd ed, Philadelphia, PA: Lippincott Williams & Wilkins, 2003).

which suggests that patients in this subgroup inherited a gene for hemochromatosis and later acquired a mutant one for RARS.

The percentage of reticulocytes and the total peripheral RBC count are typically decreased, although few patients manifest leukocytopenia or thrombocytopenia. Erythroid dimorphism is present, with macrocytosis predominating.

It is important to note that RARS is not related etiologically to congenital forms of sideroblastic anemia or to acquired, secondary sideroblastic anemias.

Refractory anemia with excess blasts (RAEB-1 and RAEB-2) is the first MDS type to demonstrate an overt classic relationship to AML, that is, an elevated percentage of type I and type II myeloblasts in the bone marrow and the presence of myeloblasts in the circulating blood. RAEB is the most frequent of the MDS types, representing 40% to 50% of all new cases.

Dyserythropoiesis, dysgranulocytopoiesis, and dysmegakaryocytopoiesis are common. Anemia is usually macrocytic and often dimorphic, and oval macrocytes may be present. A variable number of ring sideroblasts are also present. Granulocytic abnormalities can include pseudo–Pelger-Huët anomaly, ring-shaped nuclei, and agranular or hypergranu-

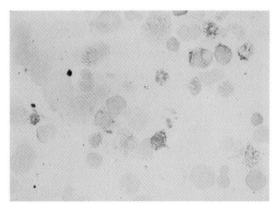

FIGURE 22.2 Refractory anemia with ring sideroblasts (Prussian blue stain ×1250). (Reprinted with permission from Greer JP, et al. *Wintrobe's Clinical Hematology*, Philadelphia, PA: Lippincott Williams & Wilkins, 2004).

lar forms. About half of RAEB patients exhibit giant platelets and micromegakaryocytes.

The percentage of reticulocytes and the total peripheral RBC count, white blood cell (WBC) count, and platelet count are typically decreased. The presence of cytopenias and dyspoiesis distinguishes RAEB from chronic myelogenous leukemia.

MYELODYSPLASTIC/MYELOPROLIFERATIVE NEOPLASMS

Characteristics of the MDS/MPNs, for example, CMML, include an increased number of cells in the peripheral blood that may be morphologically and/or functionally abnormal. The blast percentage in the bone marrow and blood is always less than 20%. Laboratory findings vary between having characteristics of MDS and MPN. Patients with the BCR-ABL1 fusion gene or rearrangements of PDGFRA should not be included in this category, nor should CMML patients with PDGFRB rearrangements be included.

Patients with refractory anemia with ring sideroblasts and thrombocytosis are provisionally included in this category as MDS/MPD, unclassifiable. The majority of these patients demonstrate a mutation JAK2 V617F. The threshold of platelets in this category has been lowered from 600×10^9/L to 450×10^9/L. Other laboratory characteristics include anemia and rig sideroblasts in the bone marrow and morphologically abnormal megakaryoctes that are similar to essential thrombocythemia and primary myelofibrosis (see Chapter 21).

Chronic Myelomonocytic Leukemia

Chronic myelomonocytic leukemia (CMML) is a clonal hematologic malignancy that is characterized by features of both an MPN and an MDS (Box 22.3). This form of myelomonocytic leukemia is much less frequent than the acute variety.

Diagnosis of CMML, according to the FAB classification criteria, distinguishes between two forms, CMML-1 and CMML-2 (see Box 22.4). One shows only an increase of mature monocytes, and it has no relationship to the type that transforms into AML. It is considered a reactive monocytosis. The other form, in addition to an increase of mature monocytes, shows an increase of a few monoblasts and promonocytes. This is considered to be a true CMML and usually quickly develops into the M4 or M5 forms of leukemia (AML). The clinical symptoms closely resemble those of subacute myelogenous leukemia.

Pathophysiology

Dyshematopoiesis of all three cell lines is present. The percentage of reticulocytes, the total peripheral RBC count, and the platelet count are typically decreased, although the total peripheral WBC count may be normal or slightly decreased.

BOX 22.3

Characteristics of Chronic Myelomonocytic Leukemia

- Persistent peripheral blood monocytosis ($>1 \times 10^{-9}$/L)
- Less than 20% myeloblasts, nonblasts, and promonocytes in the blood and bone marrow
- Absence of Philadelphia (Ph) chromosome or BCR-ABL1 fusion gene
- No evidence of PDGFRA or PDGFRB mutation
- Dysplasia in one or more myeloid cell lines
- In the absence of dysplasia,

    diagnosis of CMML is supported by evidence of an acquired, clonal cytogenetic or molecular genetic abnormality, or
    monocytosis for at least 3 months and exclusion of all other causes of monocytosis.

Laboratory Data

Peripheral blood smears usually demonstrate a persistent monocyte count greater than 1×10^9/L (Fig. 22.3). This is the hallmark of CMML (Box 22.5). Neutrophilia is commonly observed, with morphological abnormalities being present. Neutrophil precursors (promyelocytes and myelocytes) usually account for less than 10% of the leukocytes.

The bone marrow is hypercellular in more than 75% of patients. Granulocytic proliferation can be striking. An increase in erythroid precursors may be seen as well.

Cytochemical and immunophenotyping of peripheral blood and bone marrow aspirates are strongly recommended (see Table 22.3). Immunophenotyping has been useful in detecting early transformation to acute leukemia. The peripheral blood and bone marrow usually express the expected myelomonocytic antigens, for example, CD13 and CD33. An increased percentage of CD34+ cells has been associated with transformation (Fig. 22.4).

BOX 22.4

Cytochemical Staining in CMML

Alpha naphthyl acetate esterase
Alpha naphthyl butyrate esterase
Napthol-ASD-chloroacetate esterase

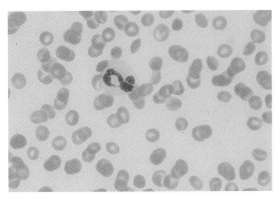

FIGURE 22.3 Anemia with excess blasts (RAEB-1 and RAEB-2). (Reprinted with permission from Anderson SC. *Anderson's Atlas of Hematology*, Philadelphia, PA: Wolters Kluwer Health/Lippincott Williams & Wilkins, Copyright 2003.)

TABLE 22.3	Characteristics of Chronic Myelomonocytic Leukemia
	Blasts[a]
CMML-1	Peripheral blood <5%
	Bone marrow <10%
CMML-2	Peripheral blood 5%–19%
	Bone marrow 10%–19%
	or
	Presence of Auer rods irrespective of the percentage of promonocytes and blasts

[a]Including promonocytes.

Other Classifications

Atypical chronic myeloid leukemia (BCR-ABL1negative), juvenile myelomonocytic leukemia (JMML), and MDS/MPN, unclassifiable (MDS/MPN, U), are the other, less frequent classifications in the myelodysplastic/myeloproliferative category.

1. Atypical chronic myeloid leukemia (BCR-ABL1negative). This category exhibits features of both myelodysplastic and myeloproliferative disorders at the time of diagnosis. It is characterized by leukocytosis with a majority of neutrophils. Multilineage dysplasia is common.
2. Juvenile myelomonocytic leukemia. JMML is a disorder of childhood. It is characterized by the proliferation of granulocytic and monocytic lineages. Blasts and promonocytes account for less than 20% of peripheral blood cells and bone marrow aspirates. Erythroid and megakaryocytic abnormalities are frequently preset. The BCR-ABL1 mutation is absent but mutations of genes of the RAS/MAPK pathway are characteristic.
3. Myelodysplastic/myeloproliferative neoplasm, unclassifiable. This neoplasm meets the definition of MDS/MPN but does not meet the criteria for CMML or the other classification in this category.

TREATMENT STRATEGIES

General treatment for MDS and MPN is RBC or platelet transfusion to control anemia or bleeding. Vitamins or other drugs may also be given as a supplement. Chemotherapy and biological therapy are being tested in clinical trials. Biological therapy is sometimes called biological response modifier therapy or immunotherapy. Bone marrow transplantation is a newer treatment approach.

The choice of treatment depends on the type of MDS as well as the patient's age and overall health. Standard protocol treatment may be considered because of its effectiveness in patients in the past, but most patients with MDS are not

BOX 22.5

Prominent Hematological Findings in MDSs

Dyserythropoiesis
Sideroblasts
Multinuclearity
Howell-Jolly bodies and nuclear fragments
Basophilic stippling
Uneven cytoplasmic staining
Anisocytosis and poikilocytosis
Dysgranulocytopoiesis
Hypogranulation
Pseudo–Pelger–Huët anomaly
Hypersegmentation
Dysmegakaryopoiesis
Micromegakaryocytes
Abnormal segmentation (hyposegmentation or hypersegmentation)
Giant platelets

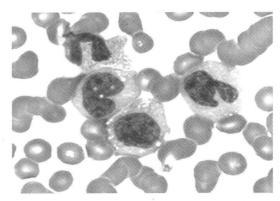

FIGURE 22.4 Chronic Myelomonocytic Leukemia (CCML). (Reprinted with permission from Anderson SC. *Anderson's Atlas of Hematology*, Philadelphia, PA: Wolters Kluwer Health/Lippincott Williams & Wilkins, Copyright 2003.)

cured with standard therapy. Participation in a clinical trial of an experimental drug may be a better option.

If a patient has MDS with no previous history of disease (de novo presentation), treatment may take the form of one of the following:

1. Supportive care to relieve symptoms of the disease, such as anemia or bleeding
2. Immunotherapy (e.g., granulocyte colony–stimulating factor [G-CSF], granulocyte-macrophage colony–stimulating factors [GM-CSF], and erythropoietin)
3. Chemotherapy (e.g., idarubicin, mitoxantrone, cytosine, and daunorubicin)
4. Allogeneic bone marrow/stem cell transplantation.

Patients with secondary MDS or those who were previously diagnosed with MDS and treated will probably receive treatment to relieve symptoms of the disease (e.g., anemia or bleeding). Participation in a clinical trial of chemotherapy or biological therapy may also be an option (www.clinicaltrials.gov).

Treatment considerations must weigh the risk of therapy versus the risk of problems associated with existing cytopenias as well as the likelihood and imminence of leukemic transformation. Patients whose disease is more severe or getting worse more quickly may be treated with chemotherapy.

In patients with AML transforming from MDS, the clinical responses to the standard therapy are poor. The greatly decreased hematopoiesis in these patients is considered responsible for their clinical picture. Leukemia-associated inhibitory activity, which inhibits human GM progenitors, may be responsible for the suppression of normal granulocytopoiesis in some patients. In addition, the profound derangement of normal hematopoietic capability in these cases may be because of multiple complex factors. Although MDS is rare in children, these represent some of the most difficult dyscrasias to treat. Children treated for MDS respond poorly to conventional chemotherapy. Infrequently, children may achieve remission with intensive therapy and allogeneic bone marrow transplantation.

RELATIONSHIP OF KARYOTYPE TO PROGNOSIS

MDS patients with multiple karyotypic anomalies have a shorter survival time (average, 8 months) than do patients with single anomalies (average, 18 months) or those with a normal karyotype (average, 36 months). Transformation to AML can be observed in approximately 25% of patients with a normal karyotype, an average of 40% of patients with single anomalies, and 50% of patients with multiple changes. Therefore, an unstable karyotype can be associated with a poor prognosis.

Patients with MDS and patients with AML share certain specific karyotypes. Patients with unfavorable karyotypes have similarly short survival times. Patients with diploid karyotypes survive significantly longer but with relatively minor differences between patients with various diagnoses. Classification of patients with excess myeloblasts in the marrow might more appropriately be based on cytogenetics than on the distinction between MDS and AML.

The absence of cytogenetically normal cells indicates a poor prognosis with frequent progression to AML, which is resistant to chemotherapy. Progression to AML depends not only on chromosomal abnormalities but also on FAB subtype. Patients with monosomy 7, del(7q), trisomy 8, or i(17q), have shorter survival times, more frequent progression to leukemia, and less response to treatment with 13-*cis* retinoic acid than patients with del(20q) or t(2;11).

Prognosis

One of the most widely used prognostic systems for MDS patients is the International Prognostic Scoring System (IPSS; Table 22.4). This system separates patients into four distinct subgroups based solely on

1. The percentage of bone marrow blasts
2. Cytogenetics
3. The number of cytopenic cell lines, that is, RBC, WBC, or platelets

A score of 0 represents low risk, intermediate-1 has a score of 0.5 to 1, intermediate-2 has a score of 1.5 to 2.0, and high risk is ≥2.5. Patients with fewer bone marrow blasts and cytopenias and with better cytogenetics (normal, 5q, 20q, Y)

TABLE 22.4	International Prognostic Scoring System				
	Score				
Prognostic variables	0	0.5	1	1.5	2
% blasts in bone marrow	<5%	5%–10%		11%–19%	20%–30%[a]
Karyotype	Normal, -Y, del(5q), del(20q)	Other Chromosomal abnormalities	≥3 abnormalities or chromosome 7 anomalies		
Number of cytopenic[b] cell lines (RBC, WBC, platelets)	None	1	2–3		

[a]Recognized as AML by WHO.
[b]Hemoglobin < 10g/dL; neutrophils < 1.8 × 10⁹/L; platelets < 100 × 10⁹/L.

have a prolonged median survival, whereas those with more blasts and cytopenias and worse cytogenetics (complex or abnormalities of chromosome 7) have a shorter survival.

Survival is generally good for patients with RA and RARS and intermediate for those with RAEB and CMML. In most FAB groups, deaths caused by the complications of bone marrow failure are more common than those caused by transformation to AML. Complications of bone marrow failure, including infections and hemorrhage, are major causes of death. The overall rate of 0.96 infection per patient-year is slightly lower than rates for multiple myeloma and hairy cell leukemia. Patients with RAEB are at particularly high risk, as are patients who are neutropenic or receiving immunosuppressive therapy.

The median survival time for all patients with MDS is about 2 years. In the types of MDS with 5% to 30% or more bone marrow blasts, the risk of progression to AML is high, especially in childhood, and usually leads to death.

The median survival is 20 to 40 months. Progression to AML occurs in about 15% to 30% of patients. The percentage of peripheral blood and bone marrow blasts is the most important factor in determining survival. CMML develops at a median age of 66 years, and the male-female ratio is 2.4:1. CMML is preceded by an MDS of a different subtype in about one fourth of patients and is transformed into acute leukemia in onefourth.

CHAPTER HIGHLIGHTS

Terminology

The FAB group established a classification for MDS in 1982. There have been many terms for MDS, which resulted in an inconsistent terminology used among clinicians and the erroneous impression that all the disorders classified under the MDS umbrella progressed to acute leukemia as the major cause of death. A second category, MDS/MPNs, is also included in this chapter.

Pathophysiology

The MDSs and MDS/MPNs are a heterogeneous group of clonal disorders of the bone marrow. Analyses suggest that the pathogenesis of MDS is a multistep process beginning with the destabilization of the multipotential stem cell, causing proliferation of a divergent clone of genetically unstable pluripotential stem cells that produce morphologically variable but clonally related progeny. Hematopoiesis is dysplastic because of inefficient maturation of a slowly expanding or sometimes of a stable population of blood cell precursors.

Etiology

The etiology of primary MDS is unknown. Secondary MDS can sometimes be directly related to a known agent. The greatest incidence of MDS follows combined chemotherapy and radiation therapy. Chemical agents that have been implicated in MDS include alkylating agents and phenylbutazone. Environmental mutagens might also be involved in primary MDS. In addition, some predisposing factors for MDS may be genetic.

Epidemiology

MDS is rare in childhood. It occurs mainly in older individuals and is more common in males. It is estimated that at least 1,500 to 2,000 cases of MDS are diagnosed annually in the United States. The prevalence of MDS, however, may be as high as 1:500 in individuals older than 55 years of age.

Chromosomal Abnormalities

Chromosomal abnormalities have been observed in a significant proportion of patients with MDS. Karyotype differences exist between primary (de novo) and secondary MDS and may be observed on initial bone marrow observation or during evolution of the disease. The cause of de novo MDS resulting from genetically unstable pluripotential stem cells is unclear. Secondary MDS frequently results from exposures to alkylating agents or radiation. Abuse of prescription or over-the-counter drugs may also be causative in MDS. Chromosome abnormalities may be monosomic or trisomic in nature and involve partial or total chromosomal alterations. Most chromosomes display a recurrent loss of chromosomal material rather than the translocations or inversions commonly found in AML. In many instances, the cytogenetic abnormalities become complex and involve more than one chromosome. Characteristic karyotype anomalies involve mainly chromosomes 5, 7, and 8. The most frequent abnormalities in children with MDS are trisomy 8, monosomy 7, and deletions involving the long arms of chromosomes 20 and X.

Forty to ninety percent of patients with MDS have chromosomal abnormalities. Different rates of occurrence exist between de novo and secondary MDS. The majority of patients with de novo MDS have recurrent chromosomal defects, with alterations of chromosomes 5, 7, and 8 being seen in one third to one half of patients. In secondary MDS and AML, chromosomal abnormalities are more frequent in patients with a history of multiple myeloma or macroglobulinemia and myeloproliferative disorders. Survival of patients with MDS is better for those with normal chromosomal patterns.

Clinical Signs and Symptoms

A history of infections, bleeding, weight loss, or cardiovascular symptoms may be reported. Anemia is a common initial presenting symptom.

Laboratory Manifestations

MDS is characteristically manifested by pancytopenia in the peripheral blood, dysplasia of two or three cell lines that may initially be in just one cell line, and a low leukemic blast count in the bone marrow and peripheral blood. Pancytopenia occurs in more than 50% of patients.

Treatment

Treatment considerations in MDS must weigh the risk of therapy against the risk of problems associated with existing cytopenias as well as the likelihood and imminence of leukemic transformation. In patients with acute leukemia transforming from MDS, the clinical responses to the standard therapy are poor. Although MDS is rare in children, these represent some of the most difficult dyscrasias to treat. Children treated for MDS respond poorly to conventional chemotherapy.

Prognosis

Survival is generally good for patients with RA and RARS. The median survival time for all patients with MDS is approximately 2 years. MDS patients with multiple karyotypic anomalies have a shorter survival time (average, 8 months) than patients with single anomalies (average, 18 months) or those with a normal karyotype (average, 36 months).

CASE STUDIES

CASE 22.1

An elderly white woman with a history of anemia visited her primary care provider because of increasing shortness of breath, dizziness, and severe fatigue. She had no history of prior treatment with drugs or exposure to lead or other toxins. Her physician ordered a CBC.

■ **Laboratory Data**

RBC 3.52×10^{12}/L
Hematocrit 37%
Hemoglobin 12.4 g/dL
WBC 8.4×10^9/L
Platelets 275×10^9/L

The peripheral blood smear demonstrated 3+ polychromatophilia, coarse basophilic stippling, occasional Pappenheimer bodies, and occasional hyposegmented neutrophils. Ten nucleated RBCs were seen per hundred leukocytes counted on the peripheral blood differential. Significant thrombocytopenia with occasional giant platelets were also noted.

Follow-Up Laboratory Data
Reticulocyte count 4.3%

Bone Marrow Examination
The bone marrow was hypercellular with erythroid hyperplasia. The RBC precursors exhibited an abnormal growth (dysplastic) pattern with nuclear:cytoplasmic asynchrony. Many binuclear rubricytes were observed. More than 15% of the metarubricytes were sideroblasts.

■ **Questions**
1. What are sideroblasts?
2. What do sideroblasts represent?
3. What is the most probable diagnosis in this case?

■ **Discussion**
1. Sideroblasts are erythrocytes with iron particles within the cytoplasm.
2. Sideroblasts represent defective heme synthesis and an overload of iron in developing erythroid precursors.
3. Sideroblasts are the hallmark of a myelodysplastic disorder. In this case, dyspoiesis of various blood cell

lines is characteristic as is the presence of abnormal metarubricytes and Pappenheimer bodies. Hyposegmentation of the neutrophils (Pelger-Huët anomaly) can be observed in myelodysplasia or acute leukemias. Karyotyping would further support the diagnosis.

DIAGNOSIS: Refractory Anemia with Ring Sideroblasts

CASE 22.2

A 26-year-old white man, with a history of colitis 20 years earlier, visited his family practitioner because of fatigue. He is taking medication for hypertension (Captopril) and carbonic anhydrase inhibitor for glaucoma. He states that he drinks 1 to 2 beers a day. He had a cold several weeks ago and has not felt well since then. He has no lifestyle risk factors. His physical examination revealed bruises in unusual locations (e.g., inside his thigh) with no report of any injury. He has scattered petechiae.

■ **Laboratory Data**
RBC 2.47×10^{12}/L
Hematocrit 24%
Hemoglobin 7.7 g/dL
WBC 4.4×10^9/L
Platelets 10×10^9/L
MCV 96 fL

The peripheral blood smear exhibited macrocytic, hypochromic red blood cells. A few hyposegmented neutrophils were observed.

■ **Follow-Up Laboratory Data**
Reticulocyte count 0.3%
Bone marrow examination revealed a hypercellular marrow with dysplasia of the hematopoietic cells. The Prussian blue stain was positive for iron.

■ **Questions**
1. What is the cause of his elevated MCV?
2. What is the significance of the hypercellular bone marrow?
3. What could be the potential cause of this patient's anemia?

(continued)

CASE STUDIES *(continued)*

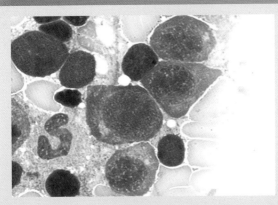

(Reprinted with permission from Anderson SC, *Anderson's, Atlas of Hematology*, Philadelphia, PA: Wolters Kluwer Health, Lippincott Williams & Wilkins, 2003, Copyright 2003.)

■ Discussion

1. With the presence of an increased MCV, it is unlikely that this patient has iron deficiency anemia. An elevated MCV could be caused by liver damage (e.g., alcohol abuse) or a vitamin deficiency. His history of colitis could be the cause.
2. A hypercellular bone marrow would rule out aplastic anemia as the cause of the patient's anemia. In addition, the presence of iron in the bone marrow further confirms the absence of iron deficiency anemia.
3. The medications that are being taken by the patient are known to have the potential to cause bone marrow suppression. No other evidence supports a virally induced aplastic anemia or the presence of leukemia.

DIAGNOSIS: MDS

REVIEW QUESTIONS

1. Patients with some variety of MDS are at increased risk of developing
   A. acute lymphoblastic leukemia
   B. AML
   C. chronic lymphocytic leukemia
   D. chronic myelogenous leukemia
2. Which of the following agents has not been supported by scientific research as being associated with the development of secondary MDS?
   A. Alkylating agents
   B. Organic solvents
   C. Insecticides
   D. Both B and C
3. An increased incidence of MDSs is seen in
   A. males younger than 55 years of age
   B. females younger than 55 years of age
   C. males older than 55 years of age
   D. females older than 55 years of age
4. The most frequently involved chromosomes in adults with MDS are
   A. 1, 5, and 7
   B. 3, 5, and 8
   C. 5, 7, and 8
   D. 8, 12, and 13
5. The most frequent chromosomal abnormalities in children with MDS include all of the following except
   A. trisomy 8
   B. monosomy 7
   C. deletion of long arm of chromosome 20
   D. all of the above

6. The incidence of chromosomal abnormality in adults with MDS is
   A. 5% to 15%
   B. 15% to 25%
   C. 25% to 60%
   D. 40% to 90%
7. The karyotype associated with a high probability of transforming to AML is
   A. monosomy 5
   B. monosomy 7
   C. trisomy 11
   D. both A and B
8. Patients with MDSs commonly suffer from _____ initially.
   A. a rash
   B. anemia
   C. visual disturbances
   D. vertigo

Questions 9 through 11: Match the type of myelodysplastic syndrome with the appropriate description.
9. Refractory anemia (RA)
10. Refractory anemia with ring sideroblasts (RARS)
11. Refractory anemia with excess blasts, type 1 (RAEB-1)
   A. anemia, no blasts
   B. anemia, less than 1% blasts
   C. cytopenia(s), less than 5% blasts, no Auer rods
12. In young patients, the therapy of choice for MDSs involves
   A. vitamins
   B. allogeneic bone marrow transplantation
   C. cytotoxic drugs
   D. colony-stimulating growth factors

BIBLIOGRAPHY

Bennett JM, et al. Acute myeloid leukemia and other myelopathic disorders following treatment with alkylating agents, *Hematol Pathol*, 1(2):99–104, 1987.

Borbenyi Z, et al. Factors influencing leukemic transformation in myelodysplastic syndrome, *Orv Hetil*, 131(23):1231–1236, 1239, 1240, 1990.

Brent BJ, Nandedkar M. Vular and oral lesions in a 34-year old woman, *Labmedicine*, 36(10):644–646, 2005.

Estey EH, et al. Karyotype is prognostically more important than the FAB system's distinction between myelodysplastic syndrome and acute myelogenous leukemia, *Hematol Pathol*, 1(4):203–208, 1987.

Heaney ML, Golde DW. Myelodysplasia, *N Engl J Med*, 340(21):1649–1660, 1999.

Leone G. Therapy-related leukemia and myelodysplasia: susceptibiity and incidence, *Hemotologica*, 92(10):1389–1398, 2007.

List A, et al. Lenalidomide in the myelodysplastic syndrome with chromosome 5q deletion, *N Eng J Med*, 355(14):1456–1465, 2006.

List A, et al. Efficacy of lenalidomide in the myelodysplastic syndromes, *N Eng J Med*, 352(6):549–557, 2005.

Malcovatti L, et al. Prognostic factors and life expectancy in myelodysplastic syndromes classified according to WHO criteria: a basis for clinical decision making, *J Clin Oncol*, 23(30):7594–7603, 2005.

Mufti GJ, et al. Diagnosis and classification of myelodysplastice syndrome: international working group on morphology of myelodysplastic syndrome (IWGM-MDS) consensus proposals for the definition and enumeration of myeloblasts and ring sideroblasts, *Haematologica*, 93(11):1712–1717, 2008.

Nimer SD. Myelodysplastic syndromes, *Blood*, 111(10):4841–4851, May 2008.

Rappaport ES, et al. Myelodysplastic syndrome: Identification in the routine hematology laboratory, *South Med J*, 80(8):969–974, 1987.

Seo IS, Li CY. Myelodysplastic syndrome: Diagnostic implications of cytochemical and immunocytochemical studies, *Mayo Clin Proc*, 68(1):47–53, 1993.

Sridhar K, et al. Relationship of differential gene expression profiles in CD34+ myelodysplastic syndrome marrow cells to disease subtype and progression, *Blood*, 114(23):4847–4858, 2009.

Suciu S, et al. Results of chromosome studies and their relation to morphology, course, and prognosis in 120 patients with de novo myelodysplastic syndrome, *Cancer Genet Cytogenet*, 44(1):15–26, 1990.

Turgeon ML. Myelodysplastic syndromes, *Guthrie J*, 61(4):149–159, 1992.

Principles and Disorders of Hemostasis and Thrombosis

CHAPTER **23**

Principles of Hemostasis and Thrombosis

OBJECTIVES

Overview of hemostasis and thrombosis
- Describe the components of bleeding and clotting mechanisms.

Blood vasculature: structure and function
- Describe and compare the histological features of the tissues of the arteries and veins.
- Name the blood vessels that constitute the microcirculation and compare their size and other features with those of arteries and veins.
- Define the term **vasoconstriction**.
- Explain how vasoconstriction participates in hemostasis.
- Describe the metabolic activity of the endothelium and its role in hemostasis.
- Outline the general process of hemostasis in small vessels that contributes to the maintenance of vascular integrity.

The megakaryocytic cell series
- Define the term **endoreduplication** and relate this process to megakaryocytic development.
- List and explain the three functions of thrombopoietin or thrombopoietin-like cytokines.
- Describe the morphological features of the mature stages of development in the megakaryocyte series.
- Describe the process of formation of platelets from a megakaryocyte.
- List the ultrastructural components and cytoplasmic constituents of a mature platelet and describe the overall function of each.
- Explain the life span activities of a mature platelet.
- Explain the function of platelets in response to vascular damage.
- Define generally the terms **platelet adhesion** and **platelet aggregation**.
- Explain the events that take place during platelet adhesion, including the substances produced.

- Explain the events that take place during platelet aggregation.
- List substances that promote and substances that inhibit some aspect of platelet aggregation.
- Briefly describe the process of platelet plug consolidation and stabilization.

Blood coagulation factors
- Explain the procedure for naming the coagulation factors.
- List the principal coagulation factors.
- Name the three groupings of coagulation factors and describe their similarities.
- Describe the individual functional characteristics of each of the coagulation factors.
- Name the four basic phases of blood coagulation.
- Describe the sequence of events in the extrinsic pathway.
- Describe the sequence of events in the intrinsic pathway.
- Describe the sequence of events in the coagulation pathway.
- Name and explain the principles of the laboratory tests that are used in assessing blood coagulation factors.

Normal protective mechanisms against thrombosis
- Explain the effect of normal blood flow and the removal of substances from the circulation on protecting the body from thrombosis.
- Describe the activities of antithrombin III (AT-III) as a normal body defense mechanism.
- Name the two heparin-dependent thrombin inhibitors and describe their role as part of the natural anticoagulant system.
- Describe the functions of protein C and protein S.
- Explain the activities of the cellular proteases and the role of specific body cells in the production of coagulation factors and cofactors.
- Name and describe the assay techniques that can be used for the detection of fibrin split products.

OVERVIEW OF HEMOSTASIS AND THROMBOSIS

The maintenance of circulatory hemostasis is achieved through the process of balancing bleeding (hemorrhage) and clotting (thrombosis). Hemostasis, the arresting of bleeding, depends on several components. The four major components are the vascular system, platelets (thrombocytes), blood coagulation factors, and fibrinolysis and ultimate tissue repair. Three other, less important, components are the complement and kinin systems as well as serine protease inhibitors. Functionally, several processes are involved in hemostasis following injury to a small blood vessel:

1. Blood vessel spasm
2. Formation of a platelet plug
3. Contact among damaged blood vessel, blood platelet, and coagulation proteins
4. Development of a blood clot around the injury
5. Fibrinolytic removal of excess hemostatic material to reestablish vascular integrity

BLOOD VASCULATURE: STRUCTURE AND FUNCTION

Arteries and Veins

Arteries are the distributing vessels that leave the heart, and veins are the collecting vessels that return to the heart. Arteries have the thickest walls of the vascular system. Although variations in the size (Fig. 23.1A) and type of vessel exist, the tissue (Fig. 23.1B) in a vessel wall is divided into three coats or tunics. These coats are the tunica intima, tunica media, and tunica adventitia. The tunica intima forms the smooth glistening surface of endothelium that lines the lumen (inner tubular cavity) of all blood and lymphatic vessels and the heart. The simple squamous epithelium that lines these vessels is referred to as endothelium. The tunica intima consists of a single layer of endothelial cells thickened by a subendothelial connective tissue layer containing elastic fibers. The tunica media, the thickest coat, is composed of smooth muscle and elastic fibers. The tunica adventitia consists of fibrous connective tissue that contains autonomic nerve endings and the vasa vasorum, small networks of blood vessels that supply nutrients to the tissues of the wall.

Veins are larger and have a more irregular lumen than arteries. In comparison with arteries, veins are relatively thin-walled with a weaker middle coat. Elastin fibers are usually found only in larger veins, and there are fewer nerves distributed to the veins than to the arteries.

Arterioles and Venules

Arteries branch extensively to form a tree of ever-smaller vessels. Arterioles are the microscopic continuation of arteries that give off branches called metarterioles, which in turn join the capillaries. The walls become thinner as the arterioles approach the capillaries, with the wall of a very small arteriole consisting only of an endothelial lining and some smooth muscle surrounded by a small amount of connective tissue.

The microscopically sized veins are referred to as venules. Venules connect the capillaries to the veins.

Capillaries

The capillaries, arterioles, and venules constitute the major vessels of the microcirculation. As a unit, the microcirculation functions as the link between the arterial and venous circulation. Blood passes from the arterial to the venous system via the capillaries. Capillaries are the thinnest walled and most numerous of the blood vessels. Sinusoids, which are specialized types of capillaries, are found in locations such as the bone marrow, spleen, and liver.

Capillaries are small structures consisting of a supportive basement membrane to which a single layer of endothelium is tightly anchored. The basement membrane, immediately adjacent to the endothelium, is composed of a diffuse network of small fibers that support the endothelium and act as a barrier against particulate material that may gain access to the extravascular space. Collagen bands also offer structural support to the microvascular unit. Unlike the vessels of the arterial and venous systems, capillaries are composed of only one cell layer of simple squamous epithelium, which permits a more rapid rate of transport of materials between blood and tissue. Electron microscope examination of the

FIGURE 23.1. Blood vasculature. **A:** Size of vessels. **B:** Tissue zones.

Structure	Aorta	Artery	Arteriole	Precapillary sphincter	Capillary	Venule	Vein	Vena cava
Diameter of lumen	25 mm	4 mm	30 μm	35 μm	8 μm	20 μm	5 mm	20 mm

A

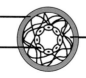

Tunica adventitia or tunica externa (fibrous connective tissue)

Tunica intima or tunica interna (endothelium)

Tunica media (smooth muscle and elastic fibers)

B

endothelium demonstrates organelles such as mitochondria, ribosomes, and endoplasmic reticulum.

VASCULATURE PHYSIOLOGY

The Role of Vasoconstriction in Hemostasis

Vascular injury to a large or medium-size artery or vein requires rapid surgical intervention to prevent exsanguination. When a smaller vessel, such as an arteriole, venule, or capillary, is injured, contraction occurs to control bleeding. This contraction of the blood vessel wall is called **vasoconstriction**.

Vasoconstriction is a short-lived reflex reaction of the smooth muscle in the vessel wall produced by the sympathetic branches of the autonomic nervous system. This narrowing, or **stenosis**, of the lumen of the blood vessel decreases the flow of blood in the injured vessel and surrounding vascular bed and may be sufficient to close severed capillaries.

The Role of the Endothelium

The endothelium contains connective tissues such as collagen and elastin. This connective tissue matrix regulates the permeability of the inner vessel wall and provides the principal stimulus to thrombosis following injury to a blood vessel. The endothelium is highly active metabolically and is involved in the clotting process by producing or storing clotting components (discussed in detail in a later section of this chapter). It is also rich with plasminogen activator, which, if appropriately stimulated, is released and activates plasminogen, which ensures rapid lysis of fibrin clots. Additionally, the endothelium elaborates prostacyclin, which is synthesized by the endothelium from prostaglandin precursors and strongly inhibits platelet aggregation and adhesion.

Minimal interactions leading to platelet activation or clot formation occur between the circulating blood and intact endothelial surfaces. However, disrupted endothelial cells release thromboplastic substances that can initiate coagulation. Collagen, in particular, initiates contact activation of factor XII, thereby initiating blood coagulation.

The endothelium forms a biological interface between circulating blood elements and all the various tissues of the body. It is strategically situated to monitor systemic as well as locally generated stimuli and to adaptively alter its functional state. This adaptive process typically proceeds without notice, contributing to normal homeostasis. The presence of a unique organelle discovered by Weibel and Palade in 1964 turned out to be an important marker to identify authentic endothelial cells. This organelle, called Weibel-Palade body (WPB) represents the storage granule for von Willebrand factor, a molecule mediating platelet adhesion. A receptor for leukocytes (P selectin) was found in WPB membrane. Secretion of these organelles provides a rapid method for activated endothelium to become adhesive for platelets and leukocytes.

Nonadaptive changes in endothelial structure and function, provoked by pathophysiological stimuli, can result in localized, acute, and chronic alterations in the interactions of endothelium with the cellular and macromolecular components of circulating blood and of the blood vessel wall. These alterations can include

- Enhanced permeability to (and subsequent oxidative modification of) plasma lipoproteins
- Hyperadhesiveness for blood leukocytes
- Functional imbalances in local prothrombotic and antithrombotic factors, growth simulators and inhibitors, and vasoactive (dilator, constrictor) substances (Tables 23.1 and 23.2)

TABLE 23.1	Endothelial Prothrombotic-Antithrombotic Balance[a]
Prothrombotic	**Antithrombotic**
Platelet-activating factor	Prostacyclin
Tissue factor	Thrombomodulin
von Willebrand factor	Tissue plasminogen activator
Plasminogen activator	Urokinase
Inhibitor-1	Heparin-like molecules
Other coagulation factors	
Synthesis of factor V	
Binding of factors V, IXa, Xa	
Activation factor XII	

[a]These various endothelial-associated factors and functions contribute to a dynamic physiological antagonism or "balance" that determines the status of local hemostatic/thrombotic activity.

TABLE 23.2	Endothelial Vasoconstrictor-Vasodilator Balance

Constrictor	Dilator
Endothelin-I	Prostacyclin
Angiotensin-II	Nitric oxide
Vasoconstrictor	Other "EDRF-like" substances
Prostaglandins	

These various endothelial-generated substances contribute to the local regulation of vascular tone through their effects on smooth muscle contractility.

TABLE 23.3	Endothelial Functions

Angiogenesis	Synthesis of stromal components
Coagulation	Vascular tone regulation
Inflammation	Special metabolic functions[a]
Immune responses	

[a]Transporting molecules from the vascular lumen to the subendothelium, producing angiotensin-converting enzyme, and binding lipoproteins, high-density lipoproteins, and low-density lipoproteins.

The endothelium is involved in the metabolism and clearance of molecules such as serotonin, angiotensin, and bradykinin that affect blood pressure regulation, the movement of fluid across the endothelium, and inflammation. With respect to blood coagulation, one of the basic characteristics of normal, intact endothelium is its nonreactivity with platelets and inability to initiate surface contact activation of clotting factor XII (Table 23.3).

The Endothelins

In 1985, a family of peptides, named the endothelins, was isolated and identified. The three members of the family—endothelin-1, endothelin-2, and endothelin-3—are produced in a variety of tissues, where they act as modulators of vasomotor tone, cell proliferation, and hormone production.

Endothelin-1 is the only family member produced in endothelial cells and is also produced in vascular smooth muscle cells. It is not stored in secretory granules within endothelial cells. Stimuli such as hypoxia, ischemia, or shear stress induce the mRNA and synthesis and secretion of endothelin-1 within minutes. The half-life is approximately 4 to 7 minutes.

Endothelin-2 is produced predominantly within the kidney and intestine, with smaller amounts produced in the myocardium, placenta, and uterus. The cells of origin are not clear. Endothelin-2 has no unique physiological functions as compared with endothelin-1.

Endothelin-3, like endothelin-1, circulates in the plasma, but its source is not known. Endothelin-3 has been found in high concentrations in the brain and may regulate important functions, such as proliferation and development in neurons and astrocytes. It also is found throughout the gastrointestinal tract and in the lung and kidney.

All three endothelins bind to two types of receptors (A and B) on the cells of many mammalian species, including humans. Endothelin-A receptors are expressed abundantly on vascular smooth muscle cells and cardiac myocytes. These receptors mediate the vasoconstrictor action of endothelin-1, although endothelin-B receptors may contribute to this action in some vascular beds. Type B receptors are expressed predominately on endothelial cells and to a much lesser extent on vascular smooth muscle cells. Endothelin-B receptors bind endothelin-1 and endothelin-3 with similar affinity.

Endothelial Dysfunction

Manifestations, collectively termed **endothelial dysfunction**, play an important role in the initiation, progression, and clinical complications of various forms of inflammatory and degenerative vascular diseases. Various stimuli of endothelial dysfunction have been identified, including immunoregulatory substances such as tumor necrosis factor (TNF) and interleukin-1 (IL-1), viral infection and transformation, bacterial toxins, and cholesterol and oxidatively modified lipoproteins.

Disruption of the endothelium directly activates all four components of hemostasis. After this event, the following events take place:

1. Initially, rapid vasoconstriction for up to 30 minutes reduces blood flow and promotes contact activation of platelets and coagulation factors.
2. In the second phase, platelets adhere immediately to the exposed subendothelial connective tissue, particularly collagen. The aggregated platelets enhance sustained vasoconstriction by releasing thromboxane A_2 and vasoactive amines, including serotonin and epinephrine.
3. In the third phase, coagulation is initiated through both the **intrinsic** and **extrinsic** systems.
4. Finally, fibrinolysis occurs following the release of tissue plasminogen activators (t-PAs) from the vascular wall. Fibrinolytic removal of excess hemostatic material is necessary to reestablish vascular integrity.

Maintenance of Vascular Integrity

Vascular integrity or the resistance to vessel disruption requires three essential factors. These factors are circulating functional platelets, adrenocorticosteroids, and ascorbic acid. A lack of these factors produces fragility of the vessels, which makes them prone to disruption. Maintenance of vascular integrity through the hemostatic process depends on the events previously described. The importance of these reactions varies with vessel size (e.g., capillaries seal easily because of vasoconstriction). The integrity of arterioles and venules depends on vasoconstriction, the formation of a plug of fused platelets over the injury, and the formation of a fibrin clot. Arteries, because of their thick walls, are the most resistant to bleeding; however, hemorrhage from these vessels is the most dangerous. Vasoconstriction is of ultimate importance in damaged arteries. Veins, which contain 70% of the blood volume, may rupture with a slight increase in hydrostatic pressure.

THE MEGAKARYOCYTIC CELL SERIES

Mature platelets (thrombocytes) (Fig. 23.2), metabolically active cell fragments, are the second critical component in the maintenance of hemostasis. These anuclear cells circulate in the peripheral blood after being produced from the cytoplasm of bone marrow **megakaryocytes**, the largest cells found in the bone marrow.

General Characteristics of Megakaryocytic Development

Bone marrow megakaryocytes Figure 23.3 are derived from pluripotential stem cells. The sequence of development from megakaryocytes to platelets is thought to progress from the proliferation of progenitors to polyploidization, that is, nuclear endoreduplication, and finally to cytoplasmic maturation and the formation of platelets.

There appears to be a complex relationship between the circulating platelet mass and the number, ploidy, and size of megakaryocytes, but the sensing mechanisms that regulate platelet production have not yet been identified. Recently, the gene for the human mpl protein was cloned and found to be expressed selectively in megakaryocytic cells. It was then found that antisense oligonucleotides that block the synthesis of human mpl protein inhibit the formation of megakaryocyte colonies but not of erythroid or granulocyte-macrophage colonies in vitro. This orphan receptor of unknown function might be the receptor for thrombopoietin. The protein may act synergistically with other growth factors during the proliferation state. It is not known whether further hormonal stimulation is needed for cytoplasmic maturation or platelet release.

Megakaryocytopoiesis proceeds initially through a phase characterized by mitotic division of a progenitor cell, followed by a wave of nuclear endoreduplication. **Endoreduplication** is the process in which chromosomal material (DNA) and the other events of mitosis occur *without* subsequent division of the cytoplasmic membrane into identical daughter cells. Recognizable megakaryocytes have ploidy values of $4n$, $8n$, $16n$, and $32n$. The maturation of megakaryocytes from immature, largely non–DNA-synthesizing cells to morphologically iden-

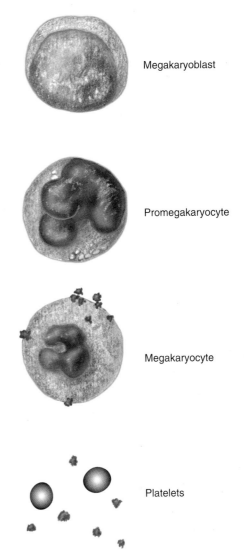

FIGURE 23.2. Normal megakaryocytic series. (Reprinted with permission from Anderson SC. *Anderson's Atlas of Hematology*, Philadelphia, PA: Wolters Kluwer Health/Lippincott Williams & Wilkins, Copyright 2003.)

tifiable megakaryocytes involves processes such as the appearance of cytoplasmic organelles, the acquisition of membrane antigens and glycoproteins, and the release of platelets.

Thrombopoietin, the hormone thought to stimulate the production and maturation of megakaryocytes, which in turn produce platelets, has recently been purified and cloned. Thrombopoietin activity results from several different cytokines: erythropoietin, IL-3, and granulocyte-macrophage colony-stimulating factor (GM-CSF). These substances have been shown to be able to increase megakaryocyte size, maturational stage, and ploidy.

The Developmental Sequence of Platelets
Early Development

Two classes of progenitors have been identified: the burst-forming-unit megakaryocyte (BFU-M) and the colony-forming-unit megakaryocyte (CFU-M). The BFU-M

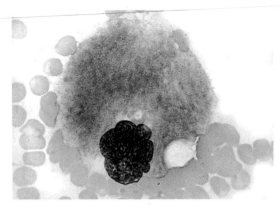

FIGURE 23.3. Granular megakaryocyte from an MGG-stained normal bone marrow smear. (Reprinted with permission from Mills SE. *Histology for Pathologists*, 3rd ed, Philadelphia, PA: Lippincott Williams & Wilkins, 2007.)

is the most primitive progenitor cell committed to megakaryocyte lineage.

The next stage of megakaryocyte development is a small, mononuclear marrow cell (Fig. 23.4) that expresses platelet-specific phenotypic markers but is not morphologically identifiable as a megakaryocyte. These transitional cells represent 5% of marrow megakaryocyte elements. Some transitional immature megakaryocyte cells may be capable of cellular division, but most are nonproliferating while actively undergoing endomitosis.

Megakaryocytes

The final stage of megakaryocyte development is the morphologically identifiable megakaryocyte (Fig. 23.5). These cells are readily recognizable in the marrow because of their large size and lobulated nuclei. These cells are polyploid (Table 23.4).

Megakaryocytes are the largest bone marrow cells, ranging up to 160 μm in size. The nuclear-cytoplasmic (N:C) ratio can be as high as 1:12. Nucleoli are no longer visible. A

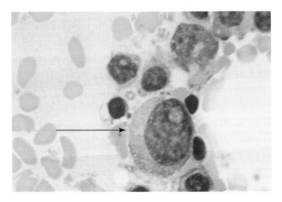

FIGURE 23.4. Megakaryoblast. (Reprinted with permission from Anderson SC. *Anderson's Atlas of Hematology*, Philadelphia, PA: Wolters Kluwer Health/Lippincott Williams & Wilkins, Copyright 2003.)

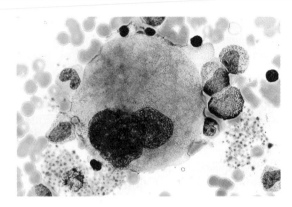

FIGURE 23.5. Megakaryocyte.

distinctive feature of the megakaryocyte is that it is **multilobular**, not multinucleated. The fully mature lobes of the megakaryocyte shed platelets from the cytoplasm on completion of maturation. Platelet formation begins with the initial appearance of a pink color in the basophilic cytoplasm of the megakaryocyte and increased granularity.

Mature Platelets

Platelets have an average diameter of 2 to 4 μm, with younger platelets being larger than older ones. In contrast to megakaryocytes, platelets have no nucleus. The cytoplasm is light blue, with evenly dispersed, fine red-purple granules.

TABLE 23.4	Developmental Characteristics of Mature Megakaryocytic Cells	
	Megakaryocyte	**Platelet**
Size	30–160 μm	2–4 μm
Nuclear-cytoplasmic ratio	1:1–1:12	
Nucleus		
Shape	Lobulated (two or more lobes)	(Anuclear)
Chromatin color	Blue-purple	—
Chromatin clumping	Granular	—
Nucleoli	Not visible	—
Cytoplasm		
Color	Pinkish blue	Light-blue fragments
Shape	Occasional pseudopods Irregular border	
Amount	Abundant	
Granules	Abundant near the borders of the cytoplasm	Scattered

An inactive or unstimulated platelet circulates as a thin, smooth-surfaced disc. This discoid shape is maintained by the microtubular cytoskeleton beneath the cytoplasmic membrane.

Platelets circulate at the center of the flowing bloodstream through endothelium-lined blood vessels without interacting with other platelets or with the vessel wall. Platelets are extremely sensitive cells and may respond to minimal stimulation by forming pseudopods that spontaneously retract. Stronger stimulation causes platelets to become sticky without losing their discoid shape; however, changes in shape to an irregular sphere with spiny pseudopods will occur with additional stimulation. This alteration in cellular shape is triggered by an increase in the level of cytoplasmic calcium. Such changes in shape accompanied by internal cellular contractions can result in the release of many of the internal organelles. A loss of viability is associated with this change to a spiny sphere.

Cellular Ultrastructure of a Mature Platelet

Examination of a platelet with an electron microscope reveals a variety of structures. These structures are fundamental to the functioning of the platelet.

The Glycocalyx

Ultrastructure examination of the platelet (Fig. 23.6) reveals that the cellular membrane is surrounded externally by a fluffy coat or **glycocalyx**. This glycocalyx is unique among the cellular components of the blood. It is composed of

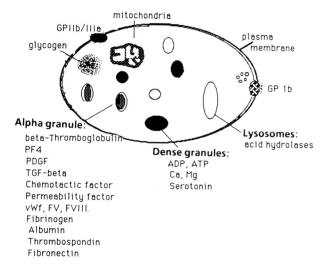

FIGURE 23.6. Platelet with its inventory of granular content. ADP, adenosine diphosphate; ATP, adenosine triphosphate; FV, factor V; GPIb, platelet surface glycoprotein Ib; PDGF, platelet-derived growth factor; PF4, platelet factor 4; TGF-β, transforming growth factor-β; vWf, von Willebrand factor. (Reprinted with permission from Koopman WJ, Moreland LW. *Arthritis and Allied Conditions: A Textbook of Rheumatology*, 15th ed, Philadelphia, PA: Lippincott Williams & Wilkins, 2005.)

plasma proteins and carbohydrate molecules that are related to the coagulation, complement, and fibrinolytic systems. The glycoprotein receptors of the glycocalyx mediate the membrane contact reactions of platelet adherence, change of cellular shape, internal contraction, and aggregation.

Cytoplasmic Membrane

Adjacent to the glycocalyx is the cytoplasmic membrane whose chemical composition and physical structure are described in Chapter 3. Extending through the plasma membrane and into the interior of the platelet is an open canalicular or surface-connecting system. It is this system that forms the invaginated, sponge-like portion of the cell that provides an expanded reactive surface to which plasma clotting factors are selectively adsorbed. Contact activation of the membrane phospholipids also generates procoagulant activity and arachidonic acid to the blood-clotting process. The cytoplasmic membrane and open canalicular membrane system articulate with the dense tubular system that is not surface connected.

Although the canaliculi penetrate the cytoplasm in a random manner, they are generally in close proximity to granules and other organelles. Therefore, products released by the granules or cytoplasm can be transported to the exterior environment through the canaliculi. In addition to the movement of extracellular materials against the concentration gradient through the canaliculi, phagocytosis is also likely to occur through these channels. Additionally, the channels of the open canalicular system and dense tubular system appear to constitute the calcium-regulating mechanism of the cell.

Microfilaments and Microtubules

Directly beneath the cell membrane is a series of submembrane filaments and microtubules that form the cellular cytoskeleton. In addition to providing the structure for maintaining the circulating discoid shape of the cell, the cytoskeleton also maintains the position of the organelles. A secondary system of microfilaments is functional in internal organization and secretion of blood coagulation products, such as fibrinogen. The microfilaments interact with the dense tubular system in sequestering calcium, which initially causes centralization of internal organelles. These subcellular and cytoplasmic filaments make up the contractile system (sol gel zone) of the platelet.

Granules

Three different types of storage granules related to hemostasis are present in the mature platelet. These granules are **alpha granules**, **dense** or **delta granules**, and **lysosomes**. The alpha granules are the most abundant. Alpha granules contain heparin-neutralizing platelet factor 4 (PF 4), beta-thromboglobulin, platelet-derived growth factor, platelet fibrinogen, fibronectin, von Willebrand factor (vWF), and thrombospondin. Dense bodies, named because of their appearance when viewed by electron microscopy, contain serotonin, adenosine diphosphate (ADP), adenosine triphosphate (ATP), and calcium. Lysosomes, the third type of granule, store hydrolase enzymes. Extrusion of the contents of these storage granules requires internal, cellular contraction. Secretions from the granules are released into the open canalicular system.

Other Cytoplasmic Constituents

In addition to containing substantial quantities of the contractile proteins, including actomyosin (thrombosthenin), myosin, and filamin, the cytoplasm of the platelet contains glycogen and enzymes of the glycolytic and hexose pathways. Energy for metabolic activities and cellular contraction is derived from aerobic metabolism in the mitochondria and anaerobic glycolysis–utilizing glycogen stores. The platelet is a very high-energy cell with a metabolic rate 10 times that of an erythrocyte. Based on energy availability and endogenous constituents, the platelet is effectively equipped to fulfill the role of protecting the body against vascular trauma.

Platelet Kinetics, Life Span, and Normal Values

An average megakaryocyte produces about 1,000 to 2,000 platelets. Marrow transit time, or the maturation period of the megakaryocyte, is approximately 5 days.

It is believed that platelets initially enter the spleen, where they remain for 2 days. Following this period, platelets are in either the circulating blood or the active splenic pool. At all times, approximately two thirds of the total number of platelets are in the systemic circulation, while the remaining one third exist as a pool of platelets in the spleen that freely exchange with the general circulation. A normal person has an average of 250×10^9/L (range, 150×10^9/L to 450×10^9/L) platelets in the systemic circulation. Platelet turnover or effective thrombopoiesis averages 350×10^9/L $\pm 4.3 \times 10^9$/L/day.

The life span of a mature platelet is 9.0 days $\pm$ 1 day. At the end of their life span, platelets are phagocytized by the liver and spleen and other tissues of the mononuclear phagocytic system.

PLATELET FUNCTION IN HEMOSTASIS

Platelets normally move freely through the lumen of blood vessels as components of the circulatory system. Maintenance of normal vascular integrity involves nourishment of the endothelium by some platelet constituents or the actual incorporation of platelets into the vessel wall. This process requires less than 10% of the platelets normally in the circulating blood. For hemostasis to occur, platelets not only must be present in normal quantities but also must function properly. This section discusses the hemostatic functions of platelets, including platelet adherence and aggregation.

Overall Functions of Platelets

Following damage to the endothelium of a blood vessel, a series of events occur, including adhesion to the injured vessel, shape change, aggregation, and secretion. Each structural and functional change is accompanied by a series

of biochemical reactions that occur during the process of platelet activation. The platelet plasma membrane is the focus of interactions between extracellular and intracellular environments. Agonists that lead to platelet activation are varied and include a nucleotide (ADP), lipids (thromboxane A_2, platelet-activating factor), a structural protein (collagen), and a proteolytic enzyme (thrombin).

One of the distinct activities associated with platelet activity in response to vascular damage is the continued maintenance of vascular integrity by the rapid adherence of platelets to exposed endothelium. In addition, platelets spread, become activated, and form large aggregates. Formation of a platelet plug initially arrests bleeding.

The adherence and aggregation of platelets at the sites of vascular damage allow for the release of molecules involved in hemostasis and wound healing and provide a membrane surface for the assembly of coagulation enzymes that lead to fibrin formation. Vascular healing is promoted by stimulating the migration and proliferation of endothelial cells and medial smooth muscle cells through the release of the mitogen, platelet-derived growth factor.

Platelet Adhesion

If vascular injury exposes the endothelial surface and underlying collagen (Fig. 23.7), platelets *adhere* to the subendothelial collagen fibers, spread pseudopods along the surface, and clump together (**aggregate**). Platelet adhesion to subendothelial connective tissues, especially collagen, occurs within 1 to 2 minutes after a break in the endothelium.

Epinephrine and serotonin promote vasoconstriction. ADP increases the adhesiveness of platelets. Considerable evidence indicates that the adhesion and aggregation of platelets are mediated by the binding of large soluble macromolecules to distinct glycoprotein receptors anchored in the platelet membrane. This increase in adhesiveness causes circulating platelets to adhere to those already attached to the collagen. The result is a cohesive platelet mass that rapidly increases in size to form a platelet plug.

The transformation of the platelet from a disc to a sphere with pseudopods produces surface membrane reorganization. Internal contraction of the platelet results in release of granular contents of the alpha and dense granules and the lysosomal contents. This process resembles the secretory activities of other cells.

Platelets adhere at sites of mechanical vascular injury and then undergo activation and express functional glycoprotein IIb/IIIa receptors (also referred to as integrin alpha$_{IIb}$beta$_3$) for circulating adhesive ligand proteins (primarily fibrinogen). These functional glycoprotein IIb/IIIa receptors mediate the recruitment of local platelets by forming fibrinogen bridges between platelets—a process called platelet cohesion. Although functional glycoprotein IIb/IIIa receptors bind with other circulating adhesive molecules in plasma (including vWF, fibronectin, vitronectin, and thrombospondin), fibrinogen is the predominant ligand because of its rela-

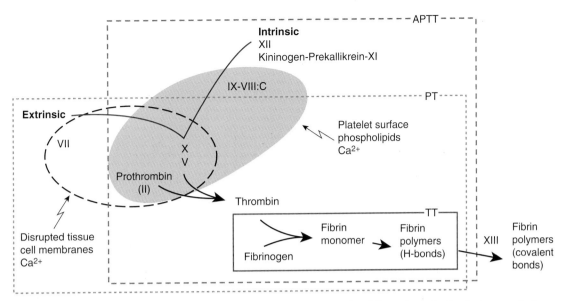

FIGURE 23.7. Coagulation mechanisms. *Shaded areas* ("platelet surface phospholipids") enclose the intrinsic coagulation reactions that occur on the surface membranes of platelets. *Dashed lines* enclose the extrinsic coagulation reactions that occur on disrupted tissue cell phospholipoprotein membranes intruded into the circulation. aPTT, activated partial thromboplastin time; PT, prothrombin time; TT, thrombin time.

tively high concentration. The peptide recognition sequence arginine-glycine-aspartic acid present in these different adhesive molecules mediates binding with expressed glycoprotein IIb/IIIa receptors. Glycoprotein IIb/IIIa is specific for platelets. Platelet recruitment depends almost exclusively on the final phase of glycoprotein IIb/IIIa–dependent platelet cohesion. Glycoprotein IIb/IIIa is the most abundant platelet membrane protein (with approximately 50,000 receptors per platelet).

Platelet Aggregation

Platelet aggregation is the gold standard test to determine platelet function. Platelet aggregation in vivo is a much more complex and dynamic process than previously thought. Over the last decade, it has become clear that platelet aggregation represents a multistep adhesion process involving distinct receptors and adhesive ligands, with the contribution of individual receptor-ligand interactions to the aggregation process dependent on the prevailing blood flow conditions. It is now believed that three distinct mechanisms can initiate platelet aggregation.

A variety of agents are capable of producing in vitro platelet aggregation, an energy-dependent process. These agents include particulate material such as collagen, proteolytic enzymes such as thrombin, and biological amines such as epinephrine and serotonin.

It is believed that bridges formed by fibrinogen in the presence of calcium produce a sticky surface on platelets. This results in aggregation. If these aggregates are reinforced by fibrin, they are referred to as a thrombus.

Aggregation of platelets by at least one pathway can be blocked by substances such as prostaglandin E (PGE), adenosine, and nonsteroidal anti-inflammatory agents (e.g., aspirin). Aspirin, including aspirin-containing products such as AlkaSeltzer, induces a long-lasting functional defect in platelets (Fig. 23.8). It is clinically detectable as a prolongation of bleeding time. The mechanism of aspirin appears to be primarily, if not exclusively, the permanent inactivation of prostaglandin G/H synthase, which catalyzes the first step in the synthesis of the prostaglandins, the conversion of arachidonate to prostaglandin H_2. Reduced formation of various eicosanoids (thromboxane A_2, prostaglandin E_2, and prostacyclin) in various tissues probably accounts for the variety of pharmacological effects of aspirin that form the basis of its therapeutic use and its toxicity.

Because platelets lack the biosynthetic mechanisms needed to synthesize new protein, the defect induced by aspirin cannot be repaired during their life span (approximately 8 to 10 days). Therefore, after treatment with aspirin is stopped, cyclooxygenase activity recovers slowly, as a function of platelet turnover. This explains the apparent paradox of how a drug with a 20-minute half-life in the systemic circulation can be fully effective as an antiplatelet agent when administered once daily.

Because of the permanent nature of aspirin-induced inactivation of platelet prostaglandin G/H synthase, the inhibitory effect of repeated daily doses less than 100 mg is cumulative. Daily administration of 30 to 50 mg of aspirin results in virtually complete suppression of platelet thromboxane biosynthesis after 7 to 10 days. These changes in platelet biochemistry are associated with maximal inhibition

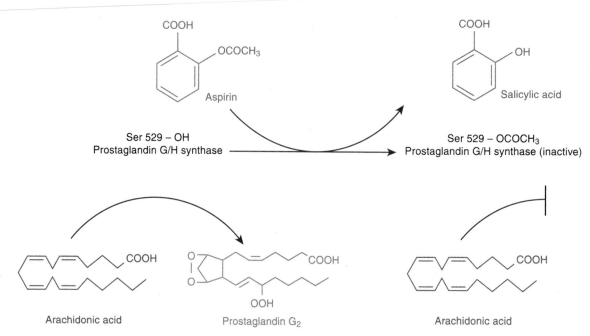

FIGURE 23.8. Mechanism of the antiplatelet action of aspirin. Aspirin acetylates the hydroxyl group of a serine residue at position 529 (Ser529) in the polypeptide chain of human platelet prostaglandin G/H synthase, resulting in the inactivation of cyclooxygenase catalytic activity. Aspirin-induced blockade of prostaglandin synthesis results in decreased biosynthesis of prostaglandin H_2 and thromboxane A_2. (Reprinted with permission from Patrono C. Aspirin as an antiplatelet drug, *N Engl J Med*, 330(18):1288, 1994. Copyright© 1994 Massachusetts Medical Society. All rights reserved.)

of thromboxane-dependent platelet aggregation, and prolongation of the bleeding time accounts for the antithrombotic effects of aspirin.

Qualitative platelet disorders can be attributed to adhesion, aggregation, or secretion defects. Release defects are the largest group of platelet function disorders. This condition is caused by abnormalities of signal transductase from membranes, abnormal internal metabolic pathways, or abnormal release mechanisms.

Platelet Plug Consolidation and Stabilization

The permanently anchored platelet plug requires additional consolidation and stabilization. Fibrinogen, under the influence of small amounts of thrombin, provides the basis for

this consolidation and stabilization. This process involves the precipitation of polymerized fibrin around each platelet. The result is a fibrin clot that produces an irreversible platelet plug (Box 23.1).

Laboratory Assessment of Platelets

A platelet count is a fundamental component in the evaluation of a patient. Examination of the peripheral blood smear for platelet number and morphology is critical because many clinical clues may be obtained from an evaluation of platelet quantity and morphology.

Quantitative Determination of Platelets

The circulating platelet count can be accurately determined in a blood sample using an electronic particle counter (see Chapter 27). Examination of a stained blood film provides a rapid estimate of platelet numbers. Normally, there are 8 to 20 platelets per 100× (oil) immersion field in a properly prepared smear (where the erythrocytes barely touch or just overlap). At least 10 different fields should be carefully examined for platelet estimation. The average number (e.g., 14) can be multiplied by a factor of 20,000 to arrive at an approximation of the quantitative platelet concentration. If an average number of 14 platelets is multiplied by 20,000, the approximate platelet concentration would be 280,000 or 280 × 10^9/L. Although the estimation of platelets from a blood smear does *not* replace an actual quantitative measurement, it should be done as a cross-check of the quantitative measurement.

Laboratory Assessment of Platelet Function

Peripheral blood smear
Platelet count
Template bleeding time
Petechiometer
Platelet aggregation
  Adenosine diphosphate (ADP)
  Epinephrine
  Collagen
  Ristocetin
  Arachidonate
  Thrombin
Platelet lumiaggregation (release)
Platelet antibodies (IgM and IgG)
Platelet membrane glycoproteins (flow cytometry)
Platelet factor IV
(Beta)-thromboglobulin
Thromboxanes

Qualitative Assessment of Platelets

If a platelet count is normal but a patient has a suggestive bleeding history, an assessment of platelet function should be conducted. Methods of evaluation (Box 23.2) include bleeding time, aggregating agents, and lumiaggregation.

Bleeding Time With and Without Aspirin

The bleeding time test (see Chapter 26) is an in vivo measurement of platelet adhesion and aggregation on locally injured vascular subendothelium. This test provides an estimate of the integrity of the platelet plug and thereby measures the interaction between the capillaries and platelets. Platelet adhesiveness is the process of the sticking of platelets to the vessel wall, whereas platelet aggregation is the sticking or clumping of platelets to each other. The bleeding time reflects these aspects of platelet function.

As the platelet count drops below 100×10^9/L, the bleeding time increases progressively from a normal of 3 to 8 minutes to more than 30 minutes. A prolonged bleeding time in a patient with a platelet count greater than 100×10^9/L indicates either impaired platelet function or a defect of subendothelial factor. Results between 8 and 11 minutes are usually not clinically significant.

The antiplatelet effects of aspirin are owing to the inhibition of thromboxane A_2 synthesis, a potent mediator of platelet aggregation and vasoconstriction. The onset of the effect of aspirin is rapid. Platelet inhibition is measurable within 60 minutes. The effects of aspirin last for the duration of the life span of the platelet, approximately 7 to 10 days.

With borderline results, the aspirin tolerance test is often useful and is repeated 2 hours after aspirin challenge.

Clot Retraction

The contractile abilities of platelets also result in the contraction of formed clots. Clot retraction reflects the number and quality of platelets, fibrinogen concentration, fibrinolytic activity, and packed red cell volume. Because the fibrin clot enmeshes the cellular elements of the blood, primarily erythrocytes, the degree of clot retraction is limited to the extent that fibrin contracts by the volume of erythrocytes (hematocrit). Therefore, the smaller the hematocrit, the greater the degree of clot retraction.

The degree of clot retraction is directly proportional to the number of platelets and inversely proportional to the hematocrit and the level of the blood coagulation factor fibrinogen. When clot dissolution (fibrinolysis) is very active, the fibrin clot may be dissolved almost as quickly as it is formed, and clot retraction is impaired.

Platelet Aggregation

Most platelet aggregation procedures (see Chapter 27) are based on some variation of Born method. Agents such as ADP, collagen, epinephrine, snake venom, thrombin, and ristocetin can be used to aggregate platelets. The principle of the test is that platelet-rich plasma is treated with a known aggregating agent. If aggregated, cloudiness or turbidity can be measured using a spectrophotometer. Depending on the type of aggregating agent used, a curve that can be used to assess platelet function is obtained.

In vivo, platelets participate in primary hemostasis by first adhering and then aggregating at the site of an injured blood vessel. Platelet aggregation is a contributing factor to subacute stent thrombosis. Patients undergoing a stent procedure are monitored to assess the effect of using aspirin and clopidogrel, a prodrug whose active metabolite selectively inhibits ADP-dependent platelet aggregation. In vitro, platelet aggregation assays use various platelet activators to identify abnormal platelet function and to monitor antiplatelet drug therapy. ADP, collagen, epinephrine, ristocetin, and arachidonic acid are reagents commonly used to induce platelet aggregation.

The platelet aggregation procedure is performed on a turbidimetric aggregometer as first described by Born. Changes in aggregation are recorded as platelet-rich plasma and aggregating reagents are stirred together in a cuvette. The aggregometer serves as a standardized spectrophotometer. As aggregation proceeds, more light passes through the sample.

Epinephrine is usually used in two doses, as is ADP. A monophasic curve is elicited with ADP. A biphasic curve is usually elicited with epinephrine. Ristocetin and arachidonic acid also usually induce a monophasic curve. Lumiaggregation is an extension of aggregation.

For more than 20 years, ristocetin cofactor (RCo) assay (which measures vWF) mediated agglutination of platelets in the presence of the antibiotic, ristocetin, and has been the most commonly used assay for the measurement of the functional activity of vWF. Recently, a collagen-binding enzyme-linked immunosorbent assay (ELISA) has been introduced as an alternative procedure. Circulating plasma vWF antigen is a marker of generalized endothelial dysfunction.

Platelet Adhesion

Platelet adhesion in vivo occurs as platelets attach either to a damaged vessel wall or to each other. Methods of in vitro analysis rely on the adherence of platelets to glass surfaces. The amount of adherence of platelets in a blood sample to a glass surface can be measured by counting the number of platelets before and after exposure to glass beads. The reliability of this methodology has been questioned; therefore, use of the method is not universal.

Antiplatelet Antibody Assays

Antibodies against platelets may appear in the plasma of patients in certain clinical conditions, although it may be difficult to demonstrate these antibodies in cases of immune thrombocytopenia. Available techniques can include complement fixation methods, lysis of chromium 51–labeled platelets, assays of platelet-bound immunoglobulins, and competitive inhibition assays.

BLOOD COAGULATION FACTORS

Bleeding from small blood vessels may be stopped by vasoconstriction and the formation of a platelet plug, but the formation of a clot (thrombus) usually occurs as part of the normal process of hemostasis. The soluble blood coagulation factors are critical components in the formation of a thrombus.

Hepatic cells are the principal site of the synthesis of coagulation factors. However, other cells, such as endothelial cells, also play an important role in the normal process of hemostasis and thrombosis. Classically, the coagulation factors have been described as reacting in a cascading sequence. Modifications of this sequence are now known to occur as the blood factors interact to form the final insoluble gelatinous thrombus.

Basic Concepts of Blood Coagulation

Blood coagulation is a sequential process of chemical reactions involving plasma proteins, phospholipids, and calcium ions. Most of the circulating factors (Table 23.5) that participate in the coagulation process are designated by Roman numerals. The activated form of an enzymatic factor appears as a Roman numeral followed by the suffix -a, whereas the inactive enzymatic factors, zymogens, are indicated by the Roman numeral alone. For example, factor II, prothrombin, is designated as factor II; however, in the active state, it is IIa, thrombin. Nonenzymatic factors have no such designations. The Roman numeral designation does *not* indicate the sequence of reactions in the clotting process. For example, factor X precedes factor II in the coagulation pathway.

Common Characteristics of Coagulation Factors

Proteins that are clotting factors have four characteristics in common. These characteristics are as follows:

1. A deficiency of the factor generally produces a bleeding tendency disorder with the exception of factor XII, prekallikrein (Fletcher factor), and high–molecular-weight kininogen (HMWK; Fitzgerald factor).
2. The physical and chemical characteristics of the factor are known.
3. The synthesis of the factor is independent of other proteins.
4. The factor can be assayed in the laboratory.

To develop an understanding of the theory of coagulation and the underlying principles of related laboratory procedures, it is helpful to compare the characteristics (Table 23.6) of various coagulation factors. Three groups of factors exist: the fibrinogen group, the prothrombin group, and the contact group.

The **fibrinogen group** consists of factors I, V, VIII, and XIII. These factors are consumed during the process of coagulation. Factors V and VIII are known to decrease during blood storage in vitro. These factors are known to increase during pregnancy, in the presence of conditions of inflammation, and subsequent to the use of oral contraceptive drugs.

The **prothrombin group** consists of factors II, VII, IX, and X. All these factors are dependent on vitamin K during their synthesis. Vitamin K is available to the body through dietary sources and intestinal bacterial production. This group is inhibited by warfarin. This group is considered to be stable and remains well preserved in stored plasma.

The **contact group** consists of factors XI, XII, prekallikrein (Fletcher factor), and HMWK (Fitzgerald factor). These factors are involved in the intrinsic coagulation pathway. They are moderately stable and are not consumed during coagulation.

Characteristics of Individual Factors

Each of the individual coagulation factors has some unique characteristics. These characteristics include the following:

Factor I (Fibrinogen)

Fibrinogen is a large, stable globulin protein (molecular weight, 341,000). It is the precursor of fibrin, which forms the resulting clot. When fibrinogen is exposed to thrombin, two peptides split from the fibrinogen molecule, leaving a fibrin monomer. These monomers aggregate together to form the final polymerized fibrin clot product.

Fibrinogenthrombin → fibrin monomers → fibrin clot.

Factor II (Prothrombin)

Prothrombin is a stable protein (molecular weight, 63,000). In the presence of ionized calcium, prothrombin is converted to thrombin by the enzymatic action of thromboplastin from both extrinsic and intrinsic sources. Prothrombin has a half-life of almost 3 days with 70% consumption during clotting.

TABLE 23.5	Proteins in Blood Coagulation	
Factor	Name	Alternate Terms
Coagulation Factors		
I	Fibrinogen	
II	Prothrombin	
V	Proaccelerin	Labile factor, Ac globulin
VII	Proconvertin	Stabile factor, SPCA
VIII	AHF	AHG, antihemophilic factor A
IX	PTC	Christmas factor, antihemophilic factor B
X	Stuart factor	Stuart-Prower factor
XI	Plasma thromboplastin antecedent	PTA, antihemophilic factor C
XII	Hageman factor	Glass or contact factor
XIII	Fibrin-stabilizing factor	FSF
Others	*Prekallikrein*	*Fletcher factor*
	HMW kininogen	HMW kininogen, Fitzgerald factor
	vWF	Factor VIII–related antigen
	Fibronectin	
	Antithrombin III	
	Heparin cofactor II	
	Protein C	
	Protein S	

SPCA, serum prothrombin conversion accelerator; AHF, antihemophilic factor; AHG, antihemophilic globulin; PTC, plasma thromboplastin component; PTA, plasma thromboplastin antecedent, FSF, fibrin-stabilizing factor; HMW, high–molecular-weight kininogen; vWF, von Willebrand factor.

$$\text{Prothrombin} + Ca^{2+}\text{extrinsic or intrinsic thromboplastin} \rightarrow \text{thrombin}$$

Factor IIa (Thrombin)

Thrombin (molecular weight, 40,000) is the activated form of prothrombin, which is normally found as an inert precursor in the circulation. This proteolytic enzyme, which interacts with fibrinogen, is also a potent platelet-aggregating substance. A large quantity of thrombin is consumed during the process of converting fibrinogen to fibrin. A unit of thrombin will coagulate 1 mL of a standard fibrinogen solution in 15 seconds at 28°C.

$$\text{Fibrinogenthrombin} \rightarrow \text{fibrin monomer} + \text{peptides}$$

Tissue Thromboplastin (Formerly Factor III)

Tissue thromboplastin is the term given to any nonplasma substance containing lipoprotein complex from tissues. These tissues can be from the brain, lung, vascular endothelium, liver, placenta, or kidneys; these tissue types are capable of converting prothrombin to thrombin.

Ionized Calcium (Formerly Factor IV)

The term *ionized calcium* has replaced the term factor IV. Ionized calcium is necessary for the activation of thromboplastin and for the conversion of prothrombin to thrombin. Ionized calcium is the physiologically active form of calcium in the human body, and only small amounts are needed for blood coagulation. A calcium deficiency would not be expressed as a coagulation dysfunction, except in cases of massive transfusion.

Factor V (Proaccelerin)

Factor V is an extremely labile globulin protein. It deteriorates rapidly, having a half-life of 16 hours. Factor V is consumed in the clotting process and is essential to the later stages of thromboplastin formation.

Factor VII (Proconvertin)

Factor VII, a beta-globulin, is not an essential component of the intrinsic thromboplastin-generating mechanism. It is not destroyed or consumed in clotting and is found in both plasma and serum, even in serum left at room temperature for up to 3 days. The action of factor VII is the activation

TABLE 23.6	Characteristics of Coagulation Factors		
	Group		
Characteristic	**I**[a]	**II**[b]	**III**[c]
Molecular weight	High	Low	?
Plasma	Present	Present	Present
Serum	Absent	Present, except II	Present
Absorption (BaSO$_4$)	No	Yes	None or partial
Destruction	Thrombin, plasmin		
Stability	Factors V, VIII unstable	Heat stable	Stable
Increase	Inflammation, pregnancy, stress and fear, oral contraceptives	Pregnancy, oral contraceptives	
Decrease		Oral anticoagulants	

[a]Group I: fibrinogen group (factors I, V, VIII, XIII)
[b]Group II: prothrombin group (factors II, VII, IX, X)
[c]Group III: contact group (factor XI, XII, Fletcher factor, Fitzgerald factor)

of tissue thromboplastin and the acceleration of the production of thrombin from prothrombin. This factor is reduced by vitamin K antagonists.

Factor VIII (Antihemophilic Factor)

This factor, an acute-phase reactant, is consumed during the clotting process and is not found in serum. Factor VIII is extremely labile, with a 50% loss within 12 hours at 4°C in vitro and a similar 50% loss in vivo within 8 to 12 hours after transfusion. In addition, factor VIII can be falsely decreased in the presence of lupus anticoagulant (LA).

Factor VIII can be subdivided into various functional components. The total molecule, consisting of both a high–molecular-weight fraction and a low–molecular-weight fraction, is described by the nomenclature VIII/vWF. Factor VIII/vWF consists of two major moieties. The high–molecular-weight moiety consists of the vWF, VIIIR:RCo, and VIIIR:Ag components. The low–molecular-weight moiety consists of the VIII:C and VIIIC:Ag components.

Factor VIII:C has procoagulant activity as measured by clotting assay techniques. Factor VIII/vWF multimers form ionic bonds with factor VIII:C and transport VIII:C in the circulation.

Factor VIIIC:Ag is a procoagulant antigen as measured by immunological techniques using antibodies for factor VIII:C. Factor VIIIR:Ag is a related factor VIII antigen that has been identified using immunological techniques employing heterologous antibodies to VIII/vWF.

Factor VIIIR:RCo demonstrates ristocetin cofactor activity, which is required for the aggregation of human platelets induced by the antibiotic ristocetin.

Factor VIII/vWF is factor VIII-vWF. Endothelial cells are known to synthesize and secrete VIII/vWF multimers.

Factor IX (Plasma Thromboplastin Component)

Factor IX is a stable protein factor that is neither consumed during clotting nor destroyed by aging at 4°C for 2 weeks. It is an essential component of the intrinsic thromboplastin-generating system, where it influences the amount rather than the rate of thromboplastin formation.

Factor X (Stuart Factor)

This alpha-globulin is a relatively stable factor that is not consumed during clotting. Together with factor V, factor X in the presence of calcium ions forms the final common pathway through which the products of both the extrinsic and intrinsic thromboplastin-generating systems merge to form the ultimate thromboplastin that converts prothrombin to thrombin. The activity of factor X appears to be related to factor VII.

Factor XI (Plasma Thromboplastin Antecedent)

Factor XI, a beta-globulin, can be found in serum because it is only partially consumed during the clotting process. This factor is essential to the intrinsic thromboplastin-generating mechanism.

Factor XII (Hageman Factor)

Factor XII is a stable factor that is not consumed during the coagulation process. Adsorption of factor XII and kininogen (with bound prekallikrein and factor XI) to negatively charged surfaces such as glass or subendothelium (collagen) exposed by blood vessel injury initiates the intrinsic coagulation pathway. Surface absorption alters and partially activates factor XII to factor XIIa by exposing an active enzyme (protease) site. Because of a feedback mechanism, kallikrein (activated Fletcher factor) cleaves partially activated factor XIIa molecules adsorbed onto the subendothelium to produce a more kinetically effective form of XIIa.

Factor XIII (Fibrin-Stabilizing Factor)

Fibrin-stabilizing factor in the presence of ionized calcium produces a stabilized fibrin clot.

Fine fibrin clotsfactor XIII + calcium ions
→ stable fibrin clot

The Mechanism of Coagulation

Many chemical reactions occur in hemostasis, from the initial stimulus that triggered bleeding to the final formation of a stable clot. To understand the process more easily, portions of the normal coagulation sequence are artificially segregated into smaller sections such as the extrinsic and intrinsic pathways. These pathways are not actual physiological pathways of hemostasis but allow for the grouping of factor defects and the focusing of laboratory assays.

The initiation of the coagulation process may occur via one of two pathways: the extrinsic pathway and the intrinsic pathway. Regardless of the initiating pathway, the two pathways converge into a final common pathway. The outcome of this process is the conversion of circulating insoluble coagulation factors into a gelatinous fibrin clot with entrapped blood cells, a blood clot. As repair of damaged tissue takes place, the clot is lysed and the particulate matter is removed by the mononuclear phagocytic system.

Coagulation Pathways

Initiation of clotting begins with either the extrinsic or the intrinsic pathway. Factor X activation is the point of convergence. Factor X can be activated by either of the two pathways and subsequently catalyzes the conversion of prothrombin to thrombin.

The Extrinsic Coagulation Pathway

The extrinsic pathway (Fig. 23.9) is initiated by the entry of tissue thromboplastin into the circulating blood. Tissue thromboplastin is derived from phospholipoproteins and organelle membranes from disrupted tissue cells. These membrane lipoproteins, termed **tissue factors**, are normally extrinsic to the circulation. Platelet phospholipids are not necessary for activation of the extrinsic pathway because tissue factor supplies its own phospholipids.

Factor VII binds to these phospholipids in the tissue cell membranes and is activated to factor VIIa, a potent enzyme capable of activating factor X to Xa in the presence of ionized calcium. The activity of the tissue factor–factor VII complex seems to be largely dependent on the concentration of tissue thromboplastin. The proteolytic cleavage of factor VIIa by

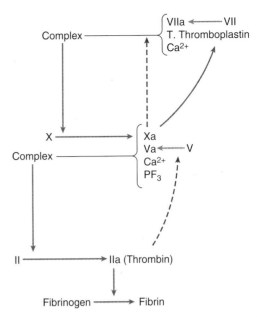

FIGURE 23.9. Extrinsic pathway of coagulation. PF_3, platelet factor 3.

factor Xa results in inactivation of factor VIIa. Factor VII participates *only* in the extrinsic pathway. Membranes that enter the circulation also provide a surface for the attachment and activation of factors II and V. The final step is the conversion of fibrinogen to fibrin by thrombin.

The Intrinsic Coagulation Pathway

The intrinsic pathway (Fig. 23.10) involves the contact activation factors prekallikrein, HMWK, factor XII, and factor XI. These factors interact on a surface to activate factor IX to IXa. Factor IXa reacts with factor VIII, PF 3, and calcium to activate factor X to Xa. In the presence of factor V, factor Xa activates prothrombin (factor II) to thrombin, which in turn converts fibrinogen to fibrin.

Strong negatively charged solids that can participate in the activation of factor XII include glass and kaolin in vitro as well as elastin, collagen, platelet surfaces, kallikrein, plasmin, and high–molecular-weight kininogen in vivo. Collagen exposed by blood vessel injury greatly influences the rate of reaction.

Factor XIIa interacts in a feedback loop to convert prekallikrein to additional kallikrein. This reaction is facilitated by the action of HMWK. In the absence of prekallikrein, factor XIIa is generated more slowly.

Ionized calcium plays an important role in the activation of certain coagulation factors in the intrinsic pathway. Calcium is not required for the activation of factor XII, prekallikrein, or factor XI but is necessary for the activation of factor IX by factor XIa.

Final Common Pathway

Once factor X is activated to Xa, the extrinsic and intrinsic pathways enter a common pathway. Factor II, prothrombin, is activated to thrombin (factor IIa), which normally circulates in the blood as an inactive factor.

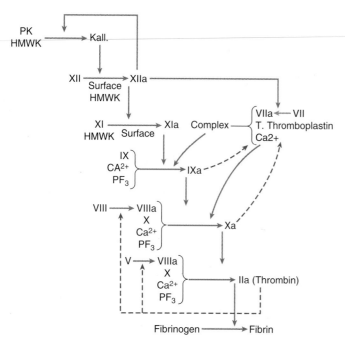

FIGURE 23.10. Intrinsic pathway of coagulation. PK HMWK, prekallikrein, high–molecular-weight kininogen; Kall., kallikrein; PF$_3$, platelet factor 3.

Following the activation of factor Xa, it remains platelet bound and activates factor V. The complex of factors Xa and Va on the platelet surface is formed near platelet-bound factor II molecules. In turn, the platelet-bound Xa/Va complex cleaves factor II into thrombin, factor IIa. The stage is accelerated by factor V and ionized calcium.

Fibrin Formation

Clotting is the visible result of the conversion of plasma fibrinogen into a stable fibrin clot. Thrombin plays a major role in converting factor XIII to XIIIa and in converting fibrinogen to fibrin. Fibrin formation occurs in three phases: proteolysis, polymerization, and stabilization.

Initially, thrombin, a protease enzyme, cleaves fibrinogen, which results in a fibrin monomer, fibrinopeptide A, and fibrinopeptide B fragments. In the second step, the fibrin monomers spontaneously polymerize end-to-end due to hydrogen bonding. Finally, the fibrin monomers are linked covalently by factor XIIIa into fibrin polymers. These polymers form a meshy network, and the final fibrin solution is converted to a gel when more than 25% of the fibrinogen is converted to fibrin.

Factor XIII is converted to the active form, factor XIIIa, in two steps. In the first step, thrombin cleaves a peptide from each of the two alpha chains of factor XIII with formation of an inactive intermediate form of factor XIII. In the second step, calcium ions cause factor XIII to dissociate, forming factor XIIIa.

Fibrinogen is normally present in the plasma as a soluble molecule. Subsequent to the action of thrombin, fibrinogen is transformed into fibrin, an insoluble gel. This conversion of fibrinogen to a cross-linked gel occurs in several stages.

Factor XIIIa introduces peptide bonds within the polymerized fibrin network. This cross-linking makes the fibrin more elastic and less susceptible to lysis by fibrinolytic agents.

Fibrin forms a loose covering over the injured area, reinforces the platelet plug, and closes off the wound. After a short period, the clot begins to retract and becomes smaller and more dense. This retraction process is thought to be caused by the action of platelets trapped along with erythrocytes and leukocytes in the clot. As the fibrin filaments gather around the aggregated platelets, the platelets send out cytoplasmic processes that attach to the fibrin and pull the fibers closer together. When a clot forms in a test tube, clot retraction can be observed (refer to the procedure in Chapter 26). The fluid squeezed from this clot is **serum**.

Thrombin-Mediated Reactions

Numerous pathways exist that ultimately lead to the generation of thrombin and consequently fibrin formation following vascular injury. The categories of essential thrombin bioregulation of hemostasis are

1. Procoagulant
2. Coagulation inhibitor
3. Tissue repair

Procoagulant

Acting as a procoagulant, thrombin induces platelet activation and aggregation. In addition, thrombin activates cofactor VIII to VIIIa, converts fibrinogen to fibrin, and activates factor XIII to XIIIa. It converts prothrombin to thrombin via autocatalysis.

Coagulation Inhibitor

The coagulation inhibition activity displayed by thrombin is the binding of AT-III to inhibit serine proteases and binding to thrombomodulin to activate protein C. In addition, the other activity in this category is the promotion of endothelial cell release of t-PA.

Tissue Repair

Thrombin mediates tissue repair by inducing cellular chemotaxis and stimulation of proliferation of smooth muscle and endothelial cells.

Fibrinolysis

Fibrin clots are temporary structures that seal off a damaged area until healing can take place. Fibrinolysis is the physiological process that removes insoluble fibrin deposits by enzymatic digestion of the stabilized fibrin polymers. As healing occurs, the clots themselves are dissolved by plasmin.

Plasmin digests fibrin and fibrinogen by hydrolysis to produce progressively smaller fragments. This slow-acting process gradually dissolves away the clot as tissue repair is taking place, with the particulate matter being phagocytized by the mononuclear phagocytic system.

Components of the Plasma Fibrinolytic System

PLASMINOGEN ACTIVATORS
Endogenous
    Tissue-type plasminogen activator (t-PA)
    Urokinase
Exogenous
    Streptokinase
    Acyl-plasminogen streptokinase activator complex (APSAC)

PLASMINOGEN INHIBITORS
Alpha-2 plasmin inhibitor
Tissue plasminogen activator inhibitor

Inactive **plasminogen** circulates in the plasma until an injury occurs. The activators of plasminogen consist of endogenous and exogenous groups (Box 23.3). Plasminogen activation to plasmin is the result of the activity of a number of proteolytic enzymes. These enzymes, the kinases, are referred to as the **plasminogen activators**. Plasminogen activators are found in various sites, such as the vascular endothelium or lysosomal granules, and biological fluids. At least two forms of tissue activators have been described: those that seem related to urokinase, a urinary activator of plasminogen, and those unrelated to urokinase. The activators unrelated to urokinase include thrombin, bacterial products such as streptokinase from beta-hemolytic streptococci, and staphylokinase. Plasma activators of plasminogen include plasma kallikrein, activated plasma thromboplastin antecedents (factor XI), and activated Hageman factor (factor XIIa).

It is estimated that 1.5 million Americans have a heart attack each year. Most are caused by clots that cut off blood flow to the heart muscle. Tissue-type plasminogen activator (t-PA) is present in minute quantities in the vascular endothelium. When t-PA encounters a blood clot, t-PA transforms plasminogen to plasmin, and plasmin then degrades the clot's fibrin network. As a result of biotechnology (recombinant DNA), a synthetic tissue-type plasminogen has been developed and is used clinically to treat postmyocardial infarction and pulmonary emboli. t-PA is considered by many to be more specific and twice as effective as streptokinase in dissolving clots and has caused fewer side effects.

Through its lysis of fibrin or fibrinogen, plasmin is responsible for forming degradation or fibrin split products consisting of intermediate fragments X and Y, and fragments D and E. These fragments exert an antithrombin effect, inhibit the hemostasis system through interference with fibrin monomer polymerization, and interfere with platelet aggregation.

Small amounts of plasmin become trapped in the clot. The specificity of plasmin ensures that clot dissolution occurs without widespread proteolysis of other proteins. Plasmin also activates the complement system, liberates kinins from kininogen, and can hydrolyze coagulation factors V, VIII, and XII. Further clot formation is impeded by antiplasmins and naturally occurring inhibitors, some of which prevent the activation of plasminogen. The naturally occurring inhibitors include AT-III, alpha-2 macroglobulin inhibitor, and alpha-1 antitrypsin. Plasmin is not normally found in plasma because it is neutralized by an excess of inhibitors.

Other Systems and Inhibitors

Two other systems and proteases inhibitors have an effect on hemostasis and coagulation. The two adjunct systems are

1. Kinin system
2. Complement system

Kinin System
This system is activated by both the coagulation and fibrinolytic systems. Fletcher factor (prekallikrein) and Fitzgerald factor (HMWK) are also needed to enhance or amplify the contact factors involved in the intrinsic system. Factor XIIa in the presence of HMWK converts prekallikrein to kallikrein. Kallikrein feeds back to accelerate the conversion of factor XII to XIIa, which accelerates the intrinsic system processes. Activation of factor XII acts as the common path between many components of the hemostatic mechanism, including the fibrinolytic system, the kinin system, and the complement system.

Complement System
Complement facilitates cell membrane lysis of antibody-coated target cells. Two independent pathways of complement activation, the classic and alternate pathways, can occur along with a common cytolytic pathway.

Plasmin activates complement by cleaving C3 into C3a and C3b. C1 esterase inhibitor inactivates complement and also has a role in hemostasis.

Protease Inhibitors
Because the fibrinolytic system is activated when the coagulation cascade is activated, extra fibrin is degraded and eliminated along with some coagulation factors. Enzymes such as plasmin and kallikrein still circulate until they are eliminated by various mechanisms: liver hepatocytes, mononuclear phagocytic cells, or serine protease inhibitors present in the plasma. Serine protease inhibitors attach to various enzymes and inactivate them. Serine protease inhibitors include

1. α-Antiplasmin
2. α-Antitrypsin
3. α-Macroglobulin
4. AT-III
5. C1 esterase inhibitor

6. Protein C inhibitor
7. Protein S inhibitor

Laboratory Assessment of Blood Coagulation Factors

The intrinsic and extrinsic pathways are now thought to function in an interrelated manner in vivo, and previously established in vitro methods are valid to screen for abnormalities.

■ Preoperative screening tests usually include a bleeding time, platelet count, activated partial thromboplastin time (aPTT), and prothrombin time (PT).

A variety of laboratory procedures (see Chapter 26) are valuable in assessing coagulation factors. General procedures include

■ aPTT
■ PT
■ Thrombin time
■ Quantitative fibrinogen concentration assay

More specialized or classic procedures include fibrin split products test, mixing study, specific factor assays, and the various tests for inhibitors and circulating anticoagulants.

The Activated Partial Thromboplastin Time

The **aPTT** procedure measures the time required to generate thrombin and fibrin polymers via the intrinsic and common pathways. In the aPTT assay, calcium ions and phospholipids that substitute for platelet phospholipids are added to blood plasma. In vitro, the activation of factor XII to XIIa, prekallikrein to kallikrein, and factor XI to XIa occurs on the negatively charged glass surface. The generation of fibrin is the end point.

The aPTT assay reflects the activity of prekallikrein, HMWK, and factors XII, XI, IX, VIII, X, V, II, and I. aPTT may be prolonged because of a factor decrease, such as fibrinogen (factor I), or the presence of circulating anticoagulants.

The reference range for aPTT is less than 35 seconds (depending on the activator used).

Mixing Study

A mixing study can be used in the case of a prolonged aPTT. The principle of the mixing study relies on a 1:1 mix of a normal patient plasma added to the patient's test plasma. The aPTT is repeated, and if the results are normal, it suggests a coagulation factor deficiency. If there is no correction of the patient's aPTT, the presence of an inhibitor is suggested.

Anti-Xa

The Chromogenic anti-Xa method for monitoring low–molecular-weight heparin and unfractionated heparin is another assay. This automated assay can replace the aPTT for monitoring unfractionated heparin because it eliminates the variability seen with aPTT results. Some advantages of the anti-Xa heparin assay compared to the aPTT are

■ Unaffected by underfilled blood collection tubes
■ Not susceptible to interference from elevated concentrations of factor VIII or fibrinogen from acute-phase reactions
■ Not influenced by factor deficiencies (possible exception is AT deficiency)
■ No need to establish an aPTT therapeutic range

Some disadvantages of the anti-Xa heparin assay compared to the aPTT are

■ High cost
■ Processing of specimen within 1 hour to avoid heparin neutralization from PF4
■ Questionable therapeutic range limitations
■ No safety and effectiveness data on outcomes for managing therapy

Prothrombin Time

The PT procedure evaluates the generation of thrombin and the formation of fibrin via the extrinsic and common pathway. Thromboplastin reagent is used for this assay. Thromboplastin can be prepared by various methods: tissue extraction of rabbit brain or lung, tissue culture, and molecular methods. Thromboplastin reagent is a mixture of tissue factor, phospholipid, and calcium ions and is used to initiate clotting measure as the PT. Thromboplastin forms complexes with and activates factor VII. This provides surfaces for the attachment and activation of factors X, V, and II. Thromboplastin, derived from tissues that supply phospholipoprotein, and calcium are added to the blood plasma. The time required for the fibrin clot to form is measured.

Reference ranges are from 10 to 13 seconds. Prolonged results can indicate a deficiency of one or more factors in the extrinsic pathway: factors VII, X, V, and II or I. Prolonged values will be seen if an oral anticoagulant such as coumarin or a coumarin-containing substance (e.g., rat poison) is ingested.

Carriers of a point mutation in the prothrombin gene, Prothrombin 20210 discovered in 1996, demonstration increased prothrombin activity. There is no screening test for this mutation, but it can be investigated using molecular techniques if clinical signs and symptoms are suggestive of a defect.

International Normalized Ratio

Because thromboplastins are produced using different methods and from different sources, the sensitivity of an individual thromboplastin to another can vary greatly between and within lots. Variance can even occur within a single batch depending on shelf time of the reagent. The more sensitive the thromboplastin reagent, the longer the resulting PT; the less sensitive the reagent, the shorter the resulting PT.

To help standardize the difference in sensitivity in individual thromboplastin reagents and the effect on PT assays, two approaches have been developed to standardize results. The first was the International Sensitivity Index (ISI) and the second was the International Normalized Ratio (INR). The INR was developed to incorporate the ISI values and attempt to make prothrombin results uniformly useable.

The ISI is a calibration parameter that defines the responsiveness of the reagent relative to a World Health Organization (WHO) International Reference Preparation, which by definition has an ISI of 1.0. A manufacturer assigns an ISI to each commercial batch of reagent after comparing each batch to a "working reference" reagent preparation. This working reference has been calibrated against internationally accepted standard reference preparations that have an ISI value of 1.0. Theoretically, the more sensitive thromboplastin has ISI less than 1.0, and less sensitive reagents have an index that is greater than 1.0. The ISI value is critical for calculation of the INR, because the ISI value is the exponent in the formula. Small errors in the ISI value may affect the calculated INR substantially.

INR use has been recommended for monitoring oral anticoagulant therapy. It is important to emphasize that the INR is not a new laboratory test. It is simply a mathematical calculation that corrects for the variability in PT results caused by variable sensitivities (ISI) of the thromboplastin agents used by laboratories.

$$INR = \left(\frac{PT \text{ patient}}{\text{mean normal PT}} \right)^{ISI}$$

PTR (prothrombin time ratio) is the patient's observed PT (in seconds) divided by each laboratory's calculated mean normal PT (in seconds). A target INR range of 2.0 to 3.0 is recommended for most indications (e.g., treatment or prophylaxis of deep venous thrombosis [DVT], or prevention of further clotting in patients who have had a myocardial infarction). An INR of 2.5 to 3.5 is recommended for patients with prosthetic heart valves. When the INR is used to guide anticoagulant therapy, there are fewer bleeding events. There is also a trend toward fewer thromboembolic complications. The target INR for pulmonary embolism (PE) treatment is 3.0 for the duration of anticoagulation. Periods of treatment have also lengthened: first-time DVT patients are treated for 3 to 6 months and first-time PE patients are treated for 6 to 12 months with warfarin. Anticoagulation is called treatment, but it really constitutes secondary prevention of recurrent PE.

Three regimens are currently used for oral anticoagulant therapy: low-intensity, fixed-dose therapy (usually 1.0 to 2.0 mg/day); moderate-intensity therapy (PT ratio, approximately 1.3 to 1.5; INR, 2.0 to 3.0); and high-intensity therapy (PT ratio, approximately 1.5 to 1.8; INR, 2.5 to 3.5). INR is used only for patients receiving stable, orally administered anticoagulant therapy. It does not substantially contribute to the diagnosis or the treatment of patients whose PT is prolonged for other reasons.

Some patients do not respond to warfarin. As a result, their INR does not change as the dosage is increased. A hepatic cytochrome P450 is central to metabolism of drug molecules resulting in clinical implications.

Specialized Assays for Coagulation Factors

These assays are usually conducted by specialized coagulation laboratories:

1. One-stage quantitative assay for factors II, V, VII, and X. This assay uses aged serum and absorbed plasma in the PT. Aged serum contains factors VII, IX, X, and XII. Absorbed plasma contains factors V, VIII, XI, and XIII. The PT is conducted using specific factor-deficient plasma with specific dilutions of patient plasma. The percentage of factor activity is plotted to construct an activity curve.
2. One-stage quantitative assay for factors VIII, IX, XI, and XII. This procedure is based on the aPTT assay. It is based on the results of patient plasma to correct specific factor-deficient plasma. The results are expressed in percent activity on an activity curve.
3. Factor VIII antibodies in hemophiliacs. An ELISA technique that uses the binding of antibodies in the plasma to solid-phase antigen, which is subsequently detected by a human polyclonal IgG labeled with the alkaline phosphatase-p-nitrophenyl phosphate substrate system.

Anticoagulants

Most clinical laboratories are accustomed to monitoring patients who are receiving warfarin (Coumadin) or heparin anticoagulant therapy. In addition to these traditional therapies, new anticoagulants are joining the list of drugs in use and may be encountered in US laboratories.

Traditional Anticoagulants

Warfarin

The traditional oral anticoagulant is warfarin (Coumadin). Warfarin drugs are vitamin K antagonists that interfere with the normal synthesis of factors II, VII, IX, and X as well as proteins C and S. These drugs cause incomplete coagulation because they lack calcium-binding sites and cannot form enzyme substrate complexes. Thus, these factors are unable to function as procoagulants or anticoagulants.

Biological activity is significantly decreased, as revealed by the PT. The onset of action of most warfarin derivatives is between 8 and 12 hours. The maximum effect occurs in approximately 36 hours, and the duration of action is approximately 72 hours.

The PT, used to adjust the dose of oral anticoagulants, should be reported according to the INR, not the PT ratio or the PT expressed in seconds. The INR is essentially a corrected PT that adjusts for the several dozen assays used in North America and Europe.

Oral anticoagulant therapy monitoring in patients with lupus inhibitors has presented problems for some laboratories. The PT can be prolonged in patients with antiphospholipid antibody syndrome for a variety of reasons:

1. Antibodies produced in this syndrome are directed toward phospholipid-binding proteins including prothrombin
2. LA or inhibitor interferes with the phospholipid in the in vitro assays of PT and aPTT

Heparin

Heparin anticoagulation is the mainstay of immediate therapy for acute PE. Heparin has no anticoagulant activity of its own but acts as an anticoagulant by accelerating the binding of antithrombin to target enzymes (e.g., thrombin and factor Xa). Heparin is termed an antithrombin because it helps to prevent new thrombus formation and buys time for endogenous fibrinolytic mechanisms to lyse the clot.

Heparin can cause bleeding, thrombocytopenia, and osteopenia. Before initiating heparin, patients should be screened for clinical evidence of active bleeding. The baseline laboratory evaluation should include complete blood count (CBC), platelets, PTT, PT, stool analysis for occult blood, and urine dipstick for hematuria.

Heparin anticoagulation is used during percutaneous transluminal coronary angioplasty (PTCA) and cardiopulmonary bypass (CPB) to prevent clot formation.

The activated clotting time (ACT) has been used for more than 25 years to assess the degree of anticoagulation in heparinized patients. Typically, ACTs are monitored to establish a minimum target ACT to ensure adequate anticoagulation. The ACT was one of the first coagulation tests to be offered at the point care, for example, operating room, cardiac catherization, or hemodialysis, and other interventional procedures that require large doses of heparin. Typically, the ACT is measured prior to and immediately after heparinization. Subsequent testing is performed to ensure that adequate anticoagulation continues or additional heparin is administered.

Low–Molecular-Weight Heparin

Low–molecular-weight heparin (LMWH), a new family of compounds produced by the controlled fragmentation of heparin, is available for clinical use. These LMWHs (e.g., tinzaparin [Innohep], dalteparin [Fragmin], and enoxaparin [Lovenox]) react with the regulatory protein AT-III to inhibit activated factor X (factor Xa) but not thrombin (factor IIa).

Unfractionated heparin, by contrast, is active against both procoagulants. LMWH is less capable than standard heparin to activate resting platelets so that they release platelet factor 4, and it binds less well to platelet factor 4. The only accepted method of monitoring LMWH is by a chromogenic assay based on the inhibition of factor Xa. This method has been automated in coagulation instrumentation capable of conducting chromogenic assays.

LMWH peaks at about 4 hours after subcutaneous injection. At peak therapeutic levels, laboratory assay values should be 0.5 to 1.1 IU/mL for patients who receive the drug twice a day and 1.0 to 2.0 IU/mL for those receiving one dose a day.

Other Antithrombin-Dependent Inhibitors

Danaparoid (Orgaran)

Danaparoid is a mixture of heparinoids which only accelerates the binding of factor Xa to antithrombin and possesses no anticoagulant activity of its own. It is monitored by chromogenic assay.

Fondaparinux (Arixtra)

Fondaparinux is a synthetic pentasaccharide that accelerates the binding of antithrombin to activated factor Xa. It has no antithrombin activity. Although this drug usually does not require monitoring, it is recommended that it be assayed by a system based on the inhibition of factor Xa, if monitoring is needed.

Direct Thrombin Inhibitors

Two new types of drugs are direct thrombin inhibitors. These drugs are

1. Hiruden, lepirudin (Refludan)
2. Argatroban

Lepirudin, a recombinant product, has the same anticoagulant activity as Hiruden, which is produced by medicinal leech. These drugs act as direct thrombin inhibitors by blocking both the active site and the substrate binding site on the thrombin molecule. Lepirudin levels can be monitored by the aPTT, ECARIN clotting time, or a chromogenic assay based on the inhibition of thrombin. The aPTT is the most widely used method of monitoring patients. The target range for anticoagulation is 1.5 to 2.5 times the baseline aPTT. Among the disadvantages of this medication is the need to monitor patients with a laboratory assay.

Argatroban binds to thrombin directly and acts as an anticoagulant by blocking the active site on the thrombin molecule. This drug is monitored by the aPTT. The therapeutic level is 1.5 to 3.0 greater than the baseline aPTT. Disadvantages of this medication include no know inhibitor to reverse the anticoagulant effect, the need for administration by continuous intravenous infusion, and the need for monitoring by laboratory assay.

New Thromboplastins

The new types of thromboplastins for measuring the PT are mixtures of phospholipids and recombinantly derived human tissue factor. Because the new thromboplastins are more sensitive (typical ISI, 1.0) than the traditional North American ones (ISIs, 1.8 to 3.0), the PTs for patients with inherited or acquired deficiencies of coagulation factors will be much more prolonged with use of the new reagents, although normal values may change minimally. However, the therapeutic range (in seconds) of the PTs in patients receiving orally administered anticoagulant agents is wider with the sensitive thromboplastins than with the traditional ones. The INR, however, will be the same, as will the recommended ranges of the INR for intensity of anticoagulation.

Recombinant thromboplastin has the following advantages:

1. It is made from a human protein, not from the protein of a different species.
2. The material is pure, and the concentration can be readily adjusted, unlike currently available rabbit brain thromboplastins. Adjustment will minimize variation between different lots of the reagent; thus, the normal and therapeutic ranges of the PT will remain the same.
3. The reagent is free of contamination with noxious viruses because it is a recombinant product.
4. When the ISI is approximately 1.0, the PTs will be the same as those obtained with use of the World Health Organization reference thromboplastin. Therefore, the PT ratio (PT of patient/mean normal PT) will be the same as the INR.
5. The new reagents are more sensitive to mild deficiencies of coagulation factors than are the traditional thromboplastins. Patients with hemostatically adequate levels of coagulation factors II, V, VII, or X (30% to 40% of mean normal activity) will have INRs of 1.4 or less.

Assays for Fibrin Formation

Fibrinogen Levels

Fibrinogen assays are useful in detecting deficiencies of fibrinogen and alterations in the conversion of fibrinogen to fibrin. Fibrinogen can be quantitated by various methods including precipitation or denaturation methods, turbidimetric or fibrin clot density method, coagulable protein assays, immunological assays, and the modified thrombin time. The normal value of 200 to 400 mg/dL may be decreased in liver disease or the consumption of fibrinogen owing to accelerated intravascular clotting. Fibrinogen titers may be useful. The normal titer of fibrinogen is 1:128 to 1:256; a titer less than 1:64 is abnormal.

Thrombin Time

The thrombin time test determines the rate of thrombin-induced cleavage of fibrinogen to fibrin monomers and the subsequent polymerization of hydrogen-bonded fibrin polymers to form an insoluble fibrin clot. The normal value is less than 20 seconds. Prolonged results will be seen if the fibrinogen concentration is less than 100 mg/dL. Abnormal results will also be encountered in the presence of thrombin inhibitors or substances that interfere with fibrin formation (e.g., heparin, fibrin degradation products), or high concentrations of immunoglobulins that interfere with fibrin monomer polymerization such as in cases of multiple myeloma.

Reptilase Time

This assay is similar to the thrombin time. The difference is that the clotting sequence is initiated with the snake venom enzyme, reptilase, which is thrombin-like in nature and hydrolyzes fibrinopeptide A from the intact fibrinogen molecule. In contrast to thrombin, which hydrolyzes

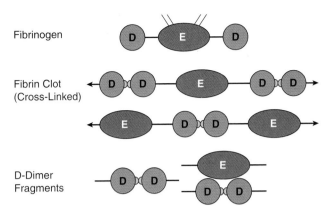

FIGURE 23.11. Basic structures of fibrinogen, cross-linked fibrin clot, and the D-dimer.

fibrinopeptide A and B from fibrinogen, reptilase is not inhibited by heparin. This assay is used to screen for dysfibrinogenemia, a coagulation disorder caused by a variety of acquired or inherited structural abnormalities in the fibrinogen molecule. In the inherited form, family members will exhibit assay abnormalities. In comparison, patients with the acquired form of dysfibrinogenemia will not have affected family members and will exhibit abnormal liver function tests.

D-Dimer Testing

The D-dimer (Fig. 23.11) is a specific fragment generated from two cross-linked fibrin molecules after a clot has formed. For D-dimers to be formed, three major hemostatic stages must be functioning:

1. Coagulation to form the clot
2. Covalent cross-linking of fibrin by activated factor XIII
3. Fibrinolysis to dissolve the fibrin clot into smaller fragment

All three of these stages require adequate formation of thrombin. Following the formation of a clot, the fibrinolytic system is activated to regulate plasmin formation. Plasmin degrades the fibrin clot into smaller specific fibrin fragments of which some or all contain the D-dimer epitope. On activation of the fibrinolytic system, D-dimer fragments are released from the clot and circulate in the blood.

Laboratory assay of D-dimers has been established to help in the diagnosis of disseminated intravascular coagulation (DIC) and DVT-PE. The qualitative and semiquantitative D-dimer assays are useful in the confirmation of DIC. The rapid, sensitive quantitative D-dimer assay has been developed to help exclude DVT and PE. The presence of D-dimers suggests that a coagulation-fibrinolytic process is taking place but does not confirm that a thrombus has formed.

Assays used in the clinical laboratory to measure the D-dimer fragment can be divided into the following:

1. Qualitative (semiquantitative)
2. Quantitative

Qualitative assays (e.g., traditional latex agglutination) are manual methods in which the end point is detected visually. Because of ease of use and low cost, these methods have been widely adopted. Because of the potential for user variability and less than ideal sensitivity, these assays are gradually being replaced with newer, more sensitive automated quantitative assays.

Newer automated methods are based on monoclonal antibodies and microscopic latex-light scattering methodology. Quantitative D-dimer assays may be referred to by the synonyms of immunoturbidimetric, microlatex immunoassay, or turbidimetric assays. In 1997, the first sensitive automated quantitative assay was approved by the U.S. Food and Drug Administration (the STA Liatest D-DI assay, Diagnostica Stago, Parsippany, New Jersy). Now several assays are on the market that use immunoturbidimetric technology.

The negative predictive value of the automated assays is excellent. D-dimers are present in many patients with ongoing disease processes or who have undergone an invasive procedure, but these patients do not need to be suffering from DVT or PE. In addition, the quantitative D-dimer assay should not be used in patients receiving anticoagulant therapy (e.g., warfarin or heparin), because they will have decreased circulating D-dimers and can generate a falsely low value (Box 23.4 for conditions that can generate falsely decreased or falsely elevated D-dimer values). It is more important to eliminate falsely decreased values than falsely elevated ones.

NORMAL PROTECTIVE MECHANISMS AGAINST THROMBOSIS

In the blood circulation, the predisposition to thrombosis depends on the balance between procoagulant and anticoagulant factors. Several important biological activities normally protect the body against thrombosis. These activities include the following:

1. The normal flow of blood
2. The removal of activated clotting factors and particulate material

3. Natural anticoagulant systems known to be operative in vivo:
   A. AT-III
   B. Heparin cofactor II (HC-II)
   C. Protein C and its cofactor, protein S
4. Cellular regulators

Normal Blood Flow

The normal flow of blood prevents the accumulation of procoagulant material. This mechanism reduces the chance of local fibrin formation.

Removal of Activated Clotting Factors and Particulate Material

Another normal mechanism against inappropriate thrombosis is the removal from the blood of activated clotting factors by hepatocytes. This process, along with the naturally occurring inhibitors, limits intravascular clotting and fibrinolysis by inactivation of such factors as XIa, IXa, Xa, and IIa. Removal of particulate material by the cells of the mononuclear phagocytic system is also important in preventing the initiation of coagulation.

The Natural Anticoagulant Systems

The in vivo existence of natural anticoagulant systems is essential to prevent thrombosis. These natural anticoagulant systems include AT-III, HC-II, and protein C and its cofactor, protein S. AT-III and HC-II are serine protease inhibitors. When activated, protein C is capable of degrading activated factors V (Va) and VIII (VIIIa) in the presence of the cofactor protein S.

Antithrombin III

AT-III is considered the major inhibitor of coagulation. AT-III is one of the serpin superfamily of *ser*ine *p*roteinase *in*hibitors that also includes alpha-1 antitrypsin, C1 inhibitor, alpha-2 antiplasmin, HC-II, and plasminogen activator inhibitor.

AT-III is an alpha-2 globulin glycoprotein that circulates in the plasma. It is synthesized by hepatocytes, megakaryocytes, and vascular endothelium. AT-III is the principal physiological inhibitor of thrombin that slowly and irreversibly inhibits thrombin by forming a stable one-to-one complex with thrombin. This complex is devoid of any thrombotic or antithrombotic activity. AT-III is also the principal physiological inhibitor of factor Xa. In addition, it is known to inhibit factors IXa, XIa, and XIIa.

AT-III is normally a slow inhibitor, but in the presence of heparin, it rapidly inhibits activated serine proteases such as activated factors II, IX, X, XI, and XII. The binding of AT-III and thrombin is increased 1,000-fold or greater in the presence of heparin. Initially, AT-III was designated heparin cofactor. The enhancement of the activity of AT-III is considered to be the primary mechanism of heparin's anticoagulation effects. Normally, AT-III accounts for the majority of the thrombin inhibitory activity in plasma. The concentration of AT-III at the endothelial surface is rate limiting for inactivation of thrombin and factor Xa when the plasma level of AT-III falls below 50%.

AT-III is rapidly removed from the circulation following one-to-one binding with an activated coagulation factor. The half-life of AT-III in plasma is approximately 70 hours.

Heparin Cofactor

Heparin is produced endogenously by mast cells, and heparin-like molecules are found in the endothelium. Two heparin-dependent thrombin inhibitors are present in human plasma: AT-III heparin cofactor and HC-II, previously referred to as heparin cofactor A. The inhibitory activity of HC-II is accelerated by heparin. The inhibition of thrombin by HC-II is not limited to the activity of thrombin or fibrinogen; also inhibited are thrombin-induced platelet aggregation and release. In addition to thrombin, HC-II inhibits chymotrypsin. It does not significantly inhibit blood coagulation factors IXa, Xa, and XIa or plasmin.

Protein C

Protein C and protein S are involved in one of the major natural anticoagulation systems in the body. Deficiency and alteration in either protein have been clearly associated with predisposition to thrombosis.

Protein C, a vitamin K–dependent plasma protein synthesized in the liver, represents a natural anticoagulant formed in response to thrombin generation. Protein C circulates in the blood as a **zymogen**, an inactive precursor form. The majority of plasma protein C exists as a two-chain zymogen (molecular weight, 62,000) before activation. A single-chain form and a minor beta form have also been demonstrated.

Protein C requires proteolytic cleavage to become active (Fig. 23.12). It is converted by thrombin to its enzymatically active form. All forms can be activated. Thrombin activates protein C in the presence of the endothelial cell–associated lipoprotein cofactor **thrombomodulin**. This reaction converts the zymogen form into the serine protease, activated protein C (APC). Thrombin activation of protein C is also enhanced by activated factor V, although considerably less efficiently.

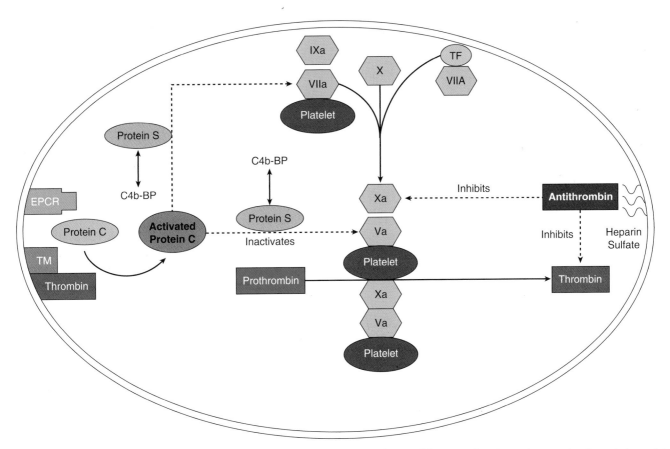

FIGURE 23.12. Schematic depiction of pathways that generate factor Xa, thrombin, and the natural anticoagulant mechanisms that regulate the activity of these enzymes. Factor X can be activated by the extrinsic pathway (factor VIIIa-tissue factor [TF]) or the intrinsic pathway (factor IXa/VIIIa–activated cell surface complex). Factor Xa binds to factor Va on activated platelets and mediates the conversion of prothrombin to thrombin under physiological conditions. Thrombin and factor Xa are inactivated by antithrombin bound to heparan sulfate molecules associated with the vascular endothelium. Protein C is activated by thrombin bound to thrombomodulin (TM) and endothelial cell protein C receptor (EPCR). Once evolved, APC functions as a potent anticoagulant by inactivating factors VIIIa and Va. Protein S enhances the binding of APC to phospholipid-containing membranes and accelerates the inactivation of factors VIIIa and Va. The complement component, C4b-binding protein (C4b-BP), forms complexes with protein S, which results in a reduction of its functional activity.

The protein C anticoagulant pathway is recognized as a major blood coagulation regulatory mechanism. APC is a potent plasma anticoagulant. Once activated, APC—in the presence of its cofactor protein S (S)—proteolytically cleaves factors Va (V-Vi) and VIIIa (VIII-VIIIi). This cleavage dramatically decreases the conversion of prothrombin to thrombin and is one of the regulatory feedback mechanisms of coagulation. Thrombin thus acts not only as a procoagulant but also activates natural anticoagulation.

Protein C requires a second vitamin K–dependent factor, protein S, to function as an anticoagulant. APC is also believed to promote fibrinolysis by neutralizing the inhibitor of t-PA. t-PA inhibitor (t-PA-I) functions by inhibiting t-PA, an enzyme responsible for the conversion of plasminogen to plasmin.

Protein C is involved in each stage of the anticoagulant pathway. This pathway can be divided into three stages:

1. Protein C activation
2. Expression of APC anticoagulant activity
3. Inhibition of APC

Protein C can be activated by thrombin, but the rate of activation is too slow to be physiologically relevant. Thrombomodulin (Table 23.7) is expressed in a functional form on the surface of the vascular endothelium. Rapid protein C activation occurs when thrombin binds to thrombomodulin. The interaction of thrombin with thrombomodulin is characterized by the formation of a reversible, high-affinity complex between thrombin and thrombomodulin. Protein C is inhibited slowly in human plasma. An identified plasma protease inhibitor may be the major mechanism for the clearance of APC, but it has been demonstrated to have a half-life of approximately 8 minutes. Direct cell-mediated clearance of APC cannot be excluded as an important secondary mechanism.

The normal plasma concentration of protein C is 4 to 5 μg/mL. Many cases of familial thrombotic disease (e.g., DVT) associated with decreased levels of protein C have been described in the past decade. In addition, their production is impaired in vitamin K deficiency, liver disease, and warfarin therapy.

Oral anticoagulants can reduce the levels of protein C and protein S. Protein C levels decrease dramatically in patients with DIC. Patients with impaired liver function or those in the postoperative period may also experience decreased levels of protein C.

Laboratory Findings

The ability to detect decreased protein C activity depends on the type of assay used (Table 23.8). Plasma is evaluated for LA before performing the protein C assay to be sure that LA is not the cause of thrombosis. The plasma concentration of purified protein C is 4 μg/mL.

Laboratory diagnosis of protein C and protein S deficiency involves functional and antigenic assays. Diagnosis of a deficiency is best made using functional assays for screening and a combination of functional and antigenic assays for confirmation and characterization of the deficiency.

Protein C Testing

Functional protein C assays can be either clot based or chromogenic. The clot-based method involves a snake venom that specifically activates protein C. The resulting APC inhibits factors Va and VIIIa, thus prolonging the aPTT of a system in which all the coagulation factors are constantly present and in excess.

TABLE 23.7	**Properties of Thrombomodulin**
Molecular weight	~74,000, single chain
Cellular location	Endothelium
Function	Accelerates protein C activation by thrombin
Mechanism	Forms 1:1 complex with thrombin; functions as a cofactor
Role of Ca^{2+} in protein C activation	Ca^{2+} is required
Role of Ca^{2+} in complex formation between thrombin and thrombomodulin	Ca^{2+} is not required
Control of protein C activation	Thrombin can be inhibited by AT-III when bound to thrombomodulin
Other functions of thrombomodulin	Reduces thrombin's ability to clot fibrinogen, activate factor V, and trigger platelet activation
Vitamin K dependent	No
AT-III, antithromboplastin III.	

Source: Esmon CT. *The Protein C Anticoagulant Pathway*, Miami, FL: Baxter Healthcare, 1990.

TABLE 23.8	General Assay Types for Determination of Protein C in Plasma
Antigenic	Measures amount of material present Does not measure function
Chromogenic	Measures some but not all functions
Clotting	Measures all functions of the protein C molecule

Chromogenic protein C assay involves the same venom to activate protein C. The quantity of APC formed is measured by its amidolytic activity on a specific chromogenic substrate.

Antigenic protein C can be assessed by ELISA or Laurell technologies, which have been well defined.

Factor V (Leiden)

APC resistance, a hypercoagulable condition discovered in 1993, is associated with a point mutation in the factor V gene (factor V [Leiden]). The mutation results in the replacement of Arg506 with Gln(Q) in the factor V protein. This mutation slows the inactivation of factor Va by APC causing a hypercoagulable state. The presence of factor V (Leiden) is the most common cause of inherited thrombophilia. It accounts for 20% to 50% of cases.

Factor V (Leiden) (Russell viper venom–based screening test) is a simple functional clotting test intended for screening of resistance to APC in plasma from individuals with the factor V (Leiden) defect.

Protein S

Protein S is another vitamin K–dependent plasma protein that is an essential cofactor for APC to express an anticoagulant effect. Protein S does not require proteolytic modification to function but it can be regulated by proteolysis.

Protein S circulates to C4b-binding protein (C4b-BP) in two forms, free and bound, in a ratio of 40% free to 60% bound. Only the free protein molecule supports the functional activity. Elevation of C4b-binding protein (which is an acute-phase reactant protein) results in an acquired decrease of free protein S.

Relevant properties and functions of protein S are summarized in Table 23.9. Basic science research studies suggest that free, functional protein S forms a one-to-one complex with APC on synthetic membrane surfaces, which increases the affinity of APC for membrane surfaces approximately 10-fold.

Protein S increases the rate of inactivation of factor Va by APC by enhancing the binding of APC to phospholipids, thereby stimulating the inactivation of factor Va. Protein S

TABLE 23.9	Protein S Structure, Function, and Regulation
Protein S structure	Single chain, Mr = 69,000 Accelerates factor Va and factor VIIIa inactivation by APC (functions as a cofactor)
Vitamin K dependent	Yes
Binds to membranes	Yes: forms a 1:1 complex with APC on membrane surfaces
Forms in plasma	Free and in reversible complex with C4b-binding protein
Regulation	Inactivated by thrombin; not active when complexed to C4b-binding protein

Source: Esmon T. *The Protein C Anticoagulant Pathway*, Miami, FL: Baxter Health Care, 1990.

has been found within platelets, suggesting that these cells may also be responsible for limiting coagulation by the protein S–enhanced inactivation of factors Va and VIIIa by APC. Similar interactions occurring in vivo may be localized on the surface of platelets, peripheral blood cells, and endothelial cells. An increase in APC mediated by thrombin necessitates an increase in protein S levels to attain maximum protein C activity.

Protein S Testing

The principle of a protein S functional assay is based on the cofactor activity of protein S, which enhances the anticoagulation action of APC. This enhancement is reflected by the prolongation of the clotting time of a system enriched with factor Va, which is a physiological substrate of APC.

Like antigenic protein C, antigenic protein S can be measured by ELISA or Laurell technologies. More recently, a rapid technology has been developed involving agglutination of antibody-coated microlatex particles. This agglutination is read spectrophotometrically.

Both total and free protein S antigens can be assessed by these techniques. The measurement of free (versus total) forms of protein S is done on 25% polyethylene glycol–treated plasma.

The association of C4b-binding protein and protein S necessitates C4b-binding protein evaluation to exclude acquired free protein S deficiency. C4b-binding protein can be measured by the Laurell technique or microlatex agglutination.

Cellular Regulators

Cellular activities related to thrombosis are becoming recognized as essential to the maintenance of hemostasis and thrombosis.

Cellular Proteases

Plasma contains, in addition to plasmin, are another powerful mechanism to limit the formation or spread of clotting and the reliquefication of clots. This mechanism consists of the cellular proteases derived from the lysosomes of granulocytes that may be trapped within a thrombus. These proteases block the activation or action of plasmin. A cellular protease of particular interest is alpha-2 plasmin inhibitor, which rapidly neutralizes the fibrinolytic properties of plasmin.

Cells That Regulate Coagulation

Synthesis of blood coagulation proteins was once thought to be the domain of the hepatic cells; however, it is now known that other cells are capable of synthesizing some of the coagulation factors and cofactors. Monocytes and macrophages have been demonstrated to synthesize factor VII. Platelets and endothelial cells are now known to be the principal components in the initiation, propagation, and suppression of hemostasis and thrombosis.

Platelets store and release HMWK, vWF, and factor V, all of which are involved in clot formation. Endothelial cells are known to synthesize vWF, factor VIII, factor V, HMWK, and protein S.

The production of protein S cofactor by endothelial cells is believed to play a significant regulatory role in the initiation, propagation, and suppression of hemostasis and thrombosis. Endothelial cells synthesize and secrete protein S and internalize this molecule in a dynamic manner. Once low levels of APC are formed by thrombin on the endothelial surface, it may be in proximity to protein S (receptor), resulting in the formation of an active, stable inactivator complex for factors VIIIa and Va.

MODERN VIEW OF HEMOSTASIS

Since the mid-1960s, a variety of key components of the coagulation system (e.g., protein C pathway) and other hemostasis-related factors (e.g., protein Z) have been discovered. Historically, the intrinsic pathway was considered to be the most important pathway. One major weakness of this pathway has been that this pathway could not correctly explain the questionable or even nonexistent role of HMWK, prekallikrein, and factor XII (Hageman factor) in the initiation of coagulation.

Recently, tissue factor and factor VIIa in the extrinsic pathway have been demonstrated to be the major pathway for activation of coagulation. It has also been discovered that thrombin has a far more important role as an activator and an inhibitor. Thrombin is

■ The key enzyme in the conversion of soluble fibrinogen into fibrin
■ Required for the activation of the protein C system, which downregulates hemostasis
■ Required for the activation of thrombin-activatable fibrinolysis inhibitor (TAFI), which is involved in the downregulation of the fibrinolytic process

The cumulative result of new discoveries in coagulation has led to the development of alternative schematic representations of the pathways that better represent the normal in vivo process of coagulation.

CHAPTER HIGHLIGHTS

Blood Vasculature: Structure and Function

Arteries have the thickest walls of the vascular system. Veins are larger and have a more irregular lumen than the arteries. In comparison to arteries, veins are relatively thin walled with a weaker middle coat. Arterioles are the microscopic continuation of arteries. Microscopically sized veins are referred to as venules. Venules connect the capillaries to the veins. Blood passes from the arterial to the venous system via the capillaries. Capillaries are the thinnest walled and most numerous of the blood vessels.

Vascular injury to a large or medium-size artery or vein requires rapid surgical intervention to prevent exsanguination. When a smaller blood vessel is injured, contraction occurs to control bleeding. This contraction of the blood vessel wall is called **vasoconstriction**.

The endothelium is involved in the metabolism and clearance of molecules such as serotonin, angiotensin, and bradykinin that affect blood pressure regulation, the movement of fluid across the endothelium, and inflammation. With respect to blood coagulation, one of the basic characteristics of normal, intact endothelium is its nonreactivity with platelets and inability to initiate surface contact activation of clotting factor XII. Endothelin-1 is the only family member produced in endothelial cells. Endothelin-2 has no unique physiological functions compared with endothelin-1. Endothelin-3, like endothelin-1, circulates in the plasma, but its source is not known. Endothelium is highly active metabolically and is involved in the clotting process by producing or storing clotting components. It is also rich with plasminogen activator, which, if appropriately stimulated, is released and activates plasminogen, which ensures rapid lysis of fibrin clots. Additionally, the endothelium elaborates prostacyclin, which is synthesized by the endothelium from prostaglandin precursors and strongly inhibits platelet aggregation and adhesion.

Minimal interactions leading to platelet activation or clot formation occur between the circulating blood and intact endothelial surfaces. However, disrupted endothelial cells release thromboplastic substances that can initiate coagulation. Collagen, in particular, initiates contact activation of factor XII, thereby initiating blood coagulation. Disruption of the endothelium directly activates all four components of hemostasis.

The Megakaryocytic Cell Series

Mature platelets (thrombocytes), metabolically active cell fragments, are the second critical component in the maintenance of hemostasis. These anuclear cells circulate in the peripheral blood after being produced from the cytoplasm of bone marrow **megakaryocytes**, the largest cells found in the bone marrow.

Bone marrow megakaryocytes are derived from pluripotential stem cells. The sequence of development from megakaryocytes to platelets is thought to progress from the proliferation of progenitors to polyploidization, that is, nuclear endoreduplication, and finally to cytoplasmic maturation and the formation of platelets.

Platelet Kinetics, Life Span, and Normal Values

An average megakaryocyte produces approximately 1,000 to 2,000 platelets. Marrow transit time, or the maturation period of the megakaryocyte, is approximately 5 days.

It is believed that platelets initially enter the spleen where they remain for 2 days. Following this period, platelets are in either the circulating blood or the active splenic pool. At all times, approximately two thirds of the total number of platelets are in the systemic circulation, whereas the remaining one third exist as a pool of platelets in the spleen that freely exchange with the general circulation. A normal person has an average of 250×10^9/L (range, 150×10^9/L to 450×10^9/L) platelets in the systemic circulation. Platelet turnover or effective thrombopoiesis averages 350×10^9/L $\pm$ 4.3 $\times$ 10^9/L/day.

The life span of a mature platelet is 9 days $\pm$ 1 day. At the end of their life span, platelets are phagocytized by the liver and spleen and other tissues of the mononuclear phagocytic system.

Platelets normally move freely through the lumen of blood vessels as components of the circulatory system. For hemostasis to occur, platelets not only must be present in normal quantities but also must function properly. Following damage to the endothelium of a blood vessel, a series of events occur, including adhesion to the injured vessel, shape change, aggregation, and secretion. Each structural and functional change is accompanied by a series of biochemical reactions that occur during the process of platelet activation. The platelet plasma membrane is the focus of interactions between extracellular and intracellular environments. Agonists that lead to platelet activation are varied and include a nucleotide (ADP), lipids (thromboxane A_2, platelet-activating factor), a structural protein (collagen), and a proteolytic enzyme (thrombin).

A platelet count is a fundamental component in the evaluation of a patient. Examination of the peripheral blood smear for platelet number and morphology is critical because many clinical clues may be obtained from an evaluation of platelet quantity and morphology. If a platelet count is normal but a patient has a suggestive bleeding history, an assessment of platelet function should be conducted.

Blood Coagulation Factors

Bleeding from small blood vessels may be stopped by vasoconstriction and the formation of a platelet plug, but the formation of a clot (thrombus) usually occurs as part of the normal process of hemostasis. The soluble blood coagulation factors are critical components in the formation of a thrombus.

Blood coagulation is a sequential process of chemical reactions involving plasma proteins, phospholipids, and calcium ions.

The **prothrombin group** consists of factors II, VII, IX, and X. All these factors are dependent on vitamin K during their synthesis. The **contact group** consists of factors XI, XII, prekallikrein (Fletcher factor), and HMWK (Fitzgerald factor). These factors are involved in the intrinsic coagulation pathway. Each of the individual coagulation factors has some unique characteristics.

The initiation of the coagulation process may occur via one of two pathways: the extrinsic pathway and the intrinsic pathway. Regardless of the initiating pathway, the two pathways converge into a final common pathway. The outcome of this process is the conversion of circulating insoluble coagulation factors into a gelatinous fibrin clot with entrapped blood cells, a blood clot. As repair of damaged tissue takes place, the clot is lysed and the particulate matter is removed by the mononuclear phagocytic system.

The intrinsic and extrinsic pathways are now thought to function in an interrelated manner in vivo, and previously established in vitro methods are valid to screen for abnormalities. A variety of laboratory procedures are valuable in assessing coagulation factors. General procedures include the aPTT, the PT, the thrombin time, and quantitative fibrinogen concentration assay. More specialized or classic procedures can be performed in special circumstances.

Normal Protective Mechanisms Against Thrombosis

In the blood circulation, the predisposition to thrombosis depends on the balance between procoagulant and anticoagulant factors. The normal flow of blood prevents the accumulation of procoagulant material. This mechanism reduces the chance of local fibrin formation. Another normal mechanism against inappropriate thrombosis is the removal from the blood of activated clotting factors by hepatocytes. This process, along with the naturally occurring inhibitors, limits intravascular clotting and fibrinolysis by inactivation of such factors as XIa, IXa, Xa, and IIa. Removal of particulate material by the cells of the mononuclear phagocytic system is also important in preventing the initiation of coagulation.

The in vivo existence of natural anticoagulant systems is essential to prevent thrombosis. These natural anticoagulant systems include AT-III, HC-II, and protein C and its cofactor, protein S. AT-III and HC-II are serine protease inhibitors. When activated, protein C is capable of degrading activated factors V (Va) and VIII (VIIIa) in the presence of the cofactor protein S.

Modern View of Hemostasis

In addition to other discoveries, thrombin has been found to have a far more important role as an activator and inhibitor than previously thought.

REVIEW QUESTIONS

1. Normal hemostasis depends on all of the following *except*
   A. an intact vascular system
   B. inadequate numbers of platelets
   C. appropriate coagulation factors
   D. fibrinolysis

Questions 2 through 6: The sequence of events following injury to a small blood vessel is (2) _____ to (3) _____ to (4) _____ to (5) _____ to (6) _____.
   A. Contact between damaged blood vessel, blood platelets, and coagulation proteins
   B. Formation of a platelet plug
   C. Fibrinolysis and reestablishment of vascular integrity
   D. Development of a blood clot around the injury
   E. Blood vessel spasm (vasoconstriction)

7. Which blood vessels have the thickest walls?
   A. Veins
   B. Arteries
   C. Capillaries
   D. Arterioles

8. All blood and lymphatic vessels are lined with
   A. endothelium
   B. nerve endings
   C. stratified epithelial cells
   D. simple squamous epithelium

9. Blood passes from the arterial to the venous system via
   A. arterioles
   B. capillaries
   C. veins
   D. arteries

10. The initiating stimulus to blood coagulation following injury to a blood vessel is
   A. contact activation with collagen
   B. vasoconstriction
   C. stenosis
   D. release of serotonin

11. Endothelium is involved in the metabolism and clearance of molecules such as
   A. serotonin
   B. angiotensin
   C. bradykinin
   D. all of the above

12. Which of the following is *not* correct?
   A. Vasoconstriction reduces blood flow and promotes contact activation of platelets and coagulation factors
   B. Platelets adhere to exposed endothelial connective tissues
   C. Aggregation of platelets releases thromboxane A_2 and vasoactive amines (serotonin and epinephrine)
   D. None of the above

13. Which of the following is (are) true of endoreduplication?
   A. Duplicates DNA without cell division
   B. Results in cells with ploidy values of $4n$, $8n$, $16n$, and $32n$
   C. Is unique to the megakaryocytic type of blood cell
   D. All of the above

14. Which of the following is (are) true of thrombopoietin?

(continued)

A. Thought to stimulate the production and maturation of megakaryocytes

B. Is influenced by various cytokines, which increase megakaryocyte size

C. Is influenced by various cytokines, which impact maturational stage and ploidy

D. All of the above

15. Which of the following is *not* a characteristic of platelets?
   A. The presence of a nucleus
   B. Size of 2 to 4 μm
   C. Cytoplasm is light blue with fine red-purple granules
   D. A discoid shape as an inactive cell

16. The cellular ultrastructural component(s) unique to the platelet is (are)
   A. Cytoplasmic membrane
   B. Glycocalyx
   C. Mitochondria
   D. Microtubules

17. Choose the incorrect statement regarding storage granules related to hemostasis in the mature platelet.
   A. Alpha-granules contain platelet factor 4, beta-thromboglobulin, and platelet-derived growth factor
   B. Alpha-granules contain platelet fibrinogen and von Willebrand factor
   C. Dense bodies contain serotonin and ADP
   D. Lysosomes contain actomyosin, myosin, and filamin

18. At all times, approximately _____ of the total number of platelets are in the systemic circulation.
   A. one fourth
   B. one third
   C. one half
   D. two thirds

19. The reference range of platelets in the systemic circulation is
   A. 50 to 150×10^9/L
   B. 100 to 200×10^9/L
   C. 150 to 350×10^9/L
   D. 150 to 450×10^9/L

20. The functions of platelets in response to vascular damage include
   A. maintenance of vascular integrity by sealing minor defects of the endothelium
   B. formation of a platelet plug
   C. promotion of fibrinolysis
   D. all of the above

Questions 21 and 22: If vascular injury exposes the endothelial surface and underlying collagen, platelets (21) _____ to the collagen fibers and (22) _____.
   A. adhere
   B. aggregate

23. Agents that are capable of aggregating platelets include
   A. collagen
   B. thrombin
   C. serotonin
   D. all of the above

24. Examination of a Wright-stained peripheral blood smear provides an estimate of platelet numbers. Using 100× (oil) immersion in the areas of erythrocytes just touching each other, the upper limit of the number of platelets seen per field should not exceed
   A. 10 to 15
   B. 15 to 20
   C. 20 to 25
   D. 25 to 30

25. If 10 platelets are seen per oil immersion field, what is the approximate platelet count?
   A. 50×10^9/L
   B. 100×10^9/L
   C. 150×10^9/L
   D. 200×10^9/L

26. Aspirin ingestion has the following hemostatic effect in a normal person.
   A. Prolongs the bleeding time
   B. Prolongs the clotting time
   C. Inhibits factor VIII
   D. Has no effect

27. The bleeding time test measures
   A. the ability of platelets to stick together
   B. platelet adhesion and aggregation on locally injured vascular subendothelium
   C. the quantity and quality of platelets
   D. antibodies against platelets

28. The clot retraction test is
   A. a visible reaction to the activation of platelet actomyosin (thrombosthenin)
   B. a reflection of the quantity and quality of platelets and other factors
   C. a measurement of the ability of platelets to stick to glass
   D. a measurement of the cloudiness of blood

Questions 29 through 31: Match the following.

29. _____ Fibrinogen group
30. _____ Prothrombin group
31. _____ Contact group
   A. Factors II, VII, IX, and X
   B. Factors I, V, VIII, and XIII
   C. Factors XI, XII, prekallikrein, and high–molecular-weight kininogen

32. The fibrinogen group of coagulation factors is
   A. known to increase during pregnancy
   B. known to increase in conditions of inflammation

(continued)

C. known to increase subsequent to the use of oral contraceptives

D. all of the above

33. The prothrombin group of coagulation factors is
    A. dependent on vitamin K for production
    B. considered to be stable
    C. well preserved in stored plasma
    D. all of the above

34. Warfarin acts by
    A. neutralizing the effects of thrombin
    B. interfering with fibrin monomer formation
    C. acting as a vitamin K antagonist
    D. inducing hypercoagulation

Questions 35 through 38: Match the name of the coagulation factor with the appropriate symbolic designation.

35. _____ Thrombin
36. _____ Tissue thromboplastin
37. _____ Antihemophilic factor
38. _____ Hageman factor
    A. III
    B. XII
    C. VIII
    D. IIa

Questions 39 through 42: Arrange the four stages of coagulation in their proper sequence.

39. _____
40. _____
41. _____
42. _____
    A. Fibrinolysis
    B. Formation of thrombin from prothrombin
    C. Generation of plasma thromboplastin
    D. Formation of fibrin from fibrinogen

43. The extrinsic pathway of coagulation is triggered by the entry of _____ into the circulation.
    A. membrane lipoproteins (phospholipoproteins)
    B. tissue thromboplastin
    C. Ca^{2+}
    D. factor VII

44. The intrinsic pathway of coagulation begins with the activation of _____ in the early stage.
    A. factor II
    B. factor I
    C. factor XII
    D. factor V

45. The final common pathway of the intrinsic-extrinsic pathway is
    A. factor X activation
    B. factor II activation
    C. factor I activation.
    D. factor XIII activation.

46. Prothrombin to thrombin conversion is accelerated by
    A. a complex of activated factors IX and VII
    B. factor V and ionized calcium
    C. a complex of phospholipids and factor VII
    D. a complex of activated factors X and V

47. Fibrinogen is converted to fibrin monomers by
    A. prothrombin
    B. thrombin
    C. calcium ions
    D. factor XIIIa

48. The inactive plasminogen is activated to _____ by proteolytic enzymes.
    A. prothrombin
    B. plasmin
    C. plasma kallikrein
    D. plasma thromboplastin antecedent

49. Which of the following statements are true of the fibrinolytic system?
    A. Plasmin digests fibrin and fibrinogen
    B. The active enzyme of the system is plasmin
    C. Inactive plasminogen circulates in the plasma until an injury occurs
    D. All of the above

50. If a pediatric preoperative patient has a family history of bleeding but has never had a bleeding episode herself, what test should be included in a coagulation profile in addition to the PT, aPTT, and platelet count?
    A. Lee-White clotting time
    B. Clot retraction
    C. Bleeding time
    D. Fibrin split products

51. A patient with a severe decrease in factor X activity would demonstrate normal
    A. aPTT
    B. PT
    C. thrombin time
    D. bleeding time

52. Neither the aPTT nor the PT detects a deficiency of
    A. platelet factor 3
    B. factor VII
    C. factor VIII
    D. factor IX

53. The function of thromboplastin in the prothrombin test is to provide _____ to the assay.
    A. kaolin
    B. fibrinogen
    C. phospholipoprotein
    D. thrombin

54. An abnormally prolonged aPTT may indicate
    A. a severe depletion of fibrinogen
    B. the presence of a circulating anticoagulant
    C. factor VIII deficiency
    D. all of the above

(continued)

55. If a child ingested rat poison, which of the following tests should be performed to test the effect of the poison on the child's coagulation mechanism?
  A. aPTT
  B. PT
  C. Fibrinogen assay
  D. Thrombin time

56. Which of the following conditions can cause an increased thrombin time?
  A. Fibrin split products
  B. High concentrations of immunoglobulins
  C. Heparin therapy
  D. All of the above

57. Heparin inhibits the clotting of blood by neutralizing the effect of
  A. thrombin
  B. calcium ions
  C. platelets
  D. factor VIII

58. A patient has a prolonged aPTT and a normal PT. The aPTT is not corrected by factor VIII–deficient plasma but is corrected by factor IX–deficient plasma. In which factor does the patient appear to be deficient?
  A. Factor II
  B. Factor V
  C. Factor VIII
  D. Factor IX

59. The normal protective mechanisms against thrombosis include
  A. the flow of blood
  B. the action of antithrombin III.
  C. protein C and protein S
  D. all of the above

60. If heparin therapy is initiated in a patient, a decreased anticoagulant response can be caused by decreased levels of
  A. platelet factor 3
  B. platelet factor 4
  C. antithrombin III
  D. factor XIII

61. Which of the following is (are) characteristic of protein C?
  A. It is not vitamin K dependent
  B. It is formed in response to thrombin generation
  C. It inactivates factors Va and VIIIa
  D. Both B and C

62. Which of the following characteristics is (are) true of protein S?
  A. It is a cofactor of protein C
  B. It increases the rate of inactivation of factor Va
  C. It enhances the binding of APC to phospholipids
  D. All of the above

63. Antithrombin III is the principal physiological inhibitor of
  A. thrombin
  B. factor Xa
  C. factor XIa
  D. both A and B

64. Which of the following is not correct regarding cellular proteases?
  A. They block the activation or action of plasmin
  B. They include alpha-2 inhibitor
  C. They rapidly neutralize the fibrinolytic properties of plasmin
  D. They participate in clot formation

BIBLIOGRAPHY

Babich V, et al. Selective release of molecules from Weibel-Palade bodies during a lingering kiss, *Blood*, 111(11):5282–5290, 2008.

Baudhuin LM. Warfarin pharmacogenetics: ready for clinical utility? *Clin Lab Sci*, 22(3):151–155, 2009.

Beyer LK, Santrach PJ. The basics of rapid coagulation, *Adv Lab*, 14(10):52–58, 2005.

Bick RL. Oral anticoagulants in thromboembolic disease, *Lab Med*, 26(3):188–193, 1995.

Bode AP, et al. *Evaluation of Platelet Function*, Beaumont, TX: Helena Laboratories, 1993.

Byrne KM, et al. Platelets: key player in hemostasis, *Adv Med Lab Prof*, 18–21, 2006.

Carrol JJ. Role of endothelial cells in coagulation, *Adv Med Lab Prof*, 8(1):10–18, 1996.

Castellone D. Anticoagulation: Heparin, Coumadin and beyond, *Adv Admin Lab*, 11(10):82–90, 2002.

Castellone D. Fundamentals of coagulation testing, *Adv Admin Lab*, 10(2):47–51, 2001.

Castellone D. Reflections in coagulation, *Adv Admin Lab*, 11(12):17–20, 2002.

Castellone D. INR's impact on coagulation, *Adv Admin Lab*, 14(5):36–44, 2005.

Castellone D. Clinical decision support systems in coagulation, *Adv Lab*, 62–66, 2005.

Castellone D. Progress continues in coagulation, *Adv Med Lab Prof*, 18–29, 2006.

Castellone D. Will this patient bleed? *Adv Med Lab Prof*, 18–25, 2007.

Chandler WL. For warfarin monitoring in patients with lupus inhibitors, review PT method, *CAP TODAY*, 17(1):18, 2003.

Cohen A, Rosen MH. *Handbook of Microscopic Anatomy for the Health Sciences*, St. Louis, MO: Mosby, 1975:45–46.

Colman RW. Platelet receptors, *Hematol Oncol Clin North Am*, 4(1):27–42, 1990.

Creager JG. *Human Anatomy and Physiology,* Belmont, CA: Wadsworth, 1983:431–435, 468–469.

D'Angelo A, et al. Comparison of mean normal prothrombin time with PT of fresh normal pooled plasma or of a lyophilized control plasma (R82A) as denominator to express PT results: Collaborative Study of the International Federation of Clinical Chemistry, *Clin Chem,* 43(11): 2169–2174, 1997.

deFouw NJ, et al. The cofactor role of protein S in the acceleration of whole blood clot lysis by activated protein C in vitro, *Blood,* 67(4):1189–1192, 1986.

Esmon CT. *The Protein C Anticoagulant Pathway,* Miami, FL: Baxter Healthcare, 1990.

Fair DS, et al. Human endothelial cells synthesize protein S, *Blood,* 67(4):1168–1171, 1986.

FDP News, Research Triangle Park, NC: Wellcome Diagnostics, 1984:1(2).

FDP News, Research Triangle Park, NC: Wellcome Diagnostics, 1984:1(3).

Francis CW, Marder VJ. Concepts of clot lysis, *Annu Rev Med,* 37: 187–204, 1986.

Frenette PS. Adhesion molecules—Part II: Blood vessels and blood cells, *N Engl J Med,* 335(1):43–45, 1996.

Gewirtz AM, Hoffman R. Human megakaryocyte production, *Hematol Oncol Clin North Am,* 4(1):43–64, 1990.

Gimbrone M. Endothelium in health and disease. In: *Intensive Review of Internal Medicine,* Boston, MA: Harvard University, 1995:891–900.

Ginsburg D. The von Willebrand factor gene and genetics of von Willebrand's disease, *Mayo Clin Proc,* 66:506–515, 1991.

Glassberg H, Kim KY. *Antiplatelet Therapy,* Philadelphia, PA: Temple University Press, 2002.

Gralnick HR, et al. Platelet von Willebrand factor, *Mayo Clin Proc,* 66:634–640, 1991.

Greenberg CS, et al. Cleavage of blood coagulation factor XIII and fibrinogen by thrombin during in vitro clotting, *J Clin Invest,* 75:1463–1470, 1985.

Hassell KL. A practical guide to hypercoagulability testing, *Int Med,* 17(7):55–60, 1996.

Hillis LB. Low molecular weight heparins, *Adv Med Lab Prof,* 32–34, 1997.

Hole JW. *Human Anatomy and Physiology,* 3rd ed, Dubuque, IA: Wm. C. Brown, 1984:672–673.

Hopkins S. Recent advances in hemostasis & thrombosis, *Adv Lab,* 42–47, 2006.

Hui SKR, Mast AE. D-Dimer, *Clin Lab News,* 10–12, 2009.

Jackson SP. The growing complexity of platelet aggregation, *Blood,* 109(12):5087–5095, 2007.

Jandl JH. *Blood,* Boston, MA: Little, Brown & Co., 1987:1147–1150.

Johns CS. Platelet function testing: Evolution or revolution? *Adv Med Lab Prof,* 14(2):19–23, 2002.

Kitchens CS. Vascular aspects of hemostasis. In: Hirsch T (ed.). *Coagulation Education,* Miami, FL: American Dade, 1983:99–105.

Kjeldsen J, et al. Biological variation of International Normalized Ratio for prothrombin times, and consequences in monitoring oral anticoagulant therapy: Computer simulation of serial measurements with goal-setting for analytical quality, *Clin Chem,* 43(11):2175–2182, 1997.

Koepke JA. Von Willebrand profile, *Med Lab Observ,* 28(3):16, 1996.

Lehman CM, Frank EL. Laboratory monitoring of heparin therapy: partial thromboplastin time or anti-Xa assay? *Labmedicine,* 40(1):47–51.

Leung L, Nachman R. Molecular mechanisms of platelet aggregation, *Annu Rev Med,* 37:179–186, 1986.

Levin ER. Mechanisms of disease, *N Engl J Med,* 333(6):356–363, 1995.

Lollar P. The association of factor VIII with von Willebrand factor, *Mayo Clin Proc,* 66:524–534. 1991.

Marlar RA. D-dimer: Establishing a laboratory assay for ruling out venous thrombosis, *Med Lab Observ,* 34(11):28–32, 2002.

Marlar RA. The value of D-dimer testing, *Adv Admin Lab,* 12(1): 52–55, 2003.

Marques MB. Testing for genetic predisposition to venous thrombosis, *Med Lab Observ,* 34(1):8–13, 2002.

McEver RP. The clinical significance of platelet membrane glycoproteins, *Hematol Oncol Clin North Am,* 4(1):87–105, 1990.

McGlasson L. Oral anticoagulants, *Clin Lab Sci,* 17(2), 107–112, 2004.

McGlinchey K. Sophistication in coagulation platforms, *Adv Med Lab Prof,* 20–24, 2008.

McMorran BJ, et al. Platelets kill intraerythrocytic malarial parasites and mediate survival to infection, *Science,* 323:797–800, 2009.

Migaud-Fressart MB, et al. An updated view of the haemostasis process, *Clin Lab Int,* 27(4):22–24, 2003.

Miller JL. Blood coagulation and fibrinolysis. In: Henry JB (ed.). *Clinical Diagnosis and Management by Laboratory Methods,* 18th ed, Philadelphia, PA: Saunders, 1991:738–739.

Montgomery KA. New parameters in hematology, coagulation, *Adv Lab,* 18(24):86, 2006.

O'Connor BH. *A Color Atlas and Instruction Manual of Peripheral Blood Cell Morphology,* Baltimore, MD: Williams & Wilkins, 1984:101–112.

Ogedegbe H, St. Hill H. Specialized tests for hemostasis, *Med Lab Observ,* 35(12):10–13, 2003.

Palareti G, et al. D-dimer testing to determine the duration of anticoagulation therapy, *N Engl J Med,* 355(17):1780–1789, 2006.

Plaut D. D-dimer applications in the ED, *Adv Lab,* 14(4):46–49, 2005.

Plaut D, Shearer C. The power of D-dimer in the ED, *Adv Lab,* 15(2):56–60, 2006.

Patrono C. Aspirin as an antiplatelet drug, *N Engl J Med,* 330(18): 1287–1294, 1994.

Riley RS, et al. A review in hemostasis testing, part 1, *Adv Lab,* 13(9):80–90, 2004.

Sanfelippo MJ. The new anticoagulants, *Adv Lab Prof,* 15(2):9–11.

Smith TJ. Progressive methods in coagulation, *Adv Lab,* 44–49, 2006.

Statland BE (ed.). Skin bleeding time test, *Med Lab Observ,* 15(10):14, 1985.

Taylor SL. Explorations of the D-dimer, *Adv Lab,* 54–60, 2004.

The Le D, et al. The International Normalized Ratio (INR) for monitoring warfarin therapy: Reliability and relation to other monitoring methods, *Ann Intern Med,* 120(7):552–558, 1994.

Thomas CL (ed.). *Taber's Cyclopedic Medical Dictionary,* 13th ed, Philadelphia, PA: FA. Davis, 1977:173.

Titus K. Identity crisis persists—which D-dimer? *CAP TODAY,* 17(1):1–18, 2003.

Van De Graft K. *Concepts of Human Anatomy and Physiology,* Dubuque, IA: Wm. C. Brown, 1986:618.

Wagner DD, Frenette PS. The vessel wall and its interactions, *Blood,* 111:5271–5281, 2008.

Warkentin TE, Arnold DM. "Spare-spleen-uximab" for chronic ITP, *Blood,* 112(4):925–926, 2008.

Warwick R, Williams PL (eds.). *Gray's Anatomy,* 35th British ed, Philadelphia, PA: Saunders, 1973:590–593.

Wheater PR, et al. *Functional Histology,* Edinburgh: Churchill-Livingstone, 1979:76–86.

Disorders of Hemostasis and Thrombosis

Vascular disorders

- Define the term **purpura** and describe various vascular conditions that can produce this condition.

Abnormal platelet morphology

- Name and compare four types of disorders in which abnormal platelet morphology can be observed.

Quantitative platelet disorders

- Cite at least two symptoms of thrombocytopenia.
- List the three major mechanisms that produce thrombocytopenias.
- Summarize the major characteristics of each of the three thrombocytopenic categories, including examples of disorders within each of the categories or subcategories.
- List and summarize the characteristics of the two categories of thrombocytosis, including examples of disorders within each category.

Qualitative characteristics of platelets: thrombocytopathy

- Compare the four categories of platelet dysfunctions, including examples of disorders within each category.

Bleeding disorders related to blood clotting factors

- Give examples and describe conditions that contribute to the defective production of blood coagulation factors.

- Describe the physiology of the destruction and consumption of coagulation factors, including the role of factor VIII, protein C, and thrombin in the process of fibrinolysis.
- Compare the laboratory test results in conditions of disseminated intravascular coagulation (DIC) and fibrinolysis.
- Name and describe the factors that contribute to the pathological inhibition of coagulation.

The hypercoagulable state

- Explain the role of vascular damage and blood flow in the hypercoagulable state.
- Detail how platelets contribute to hypercoagulation.
- Describe the activity of blood coagulation factors in increasing the tendency toward thrombosis.
- Describe the relationship between impaired fibrinolysis and protein C, antithrombin III, and plasminogen.
- Describe the laboratory assessments that illustrate the condition of hypercoagulation.

Case studies

- Apply the laboratory data to the stated case studies and discuss the implications of these cases to the study of hematology.

VASCULAR DISORDERS

Disorders of the microcirculation, platelets, or plasma proteins may cause abnormal bleeding. Abnormal bleeding involving the loss of red blood cells from the microcirculation expresses itself as the condition of **purpura**, which is characterized by hemorrhages into the skin, mucous membranes, and internal organs.

Purpura may be produced by a variety of vascular abnormalities. These abnormalities include the following:

1. Purpura associated with direct endothelial cell damage. The overall action of endothelins, a family of peptides, is to increase blood pressure and vascular tone. Endothelial damage may result from physical or chemical injury to the tissue caused by microbial agents such as in rickettsial disease or immunological antibody-mediated injury.

Bacterial toxins produce de-endothelialization induced by an endotoxin. Antibody vascular injury, vasculitis, may be induced by drug reactions, insect bites, or the activation of complement.

2. Purpura associated with an inherited disease of the connective tissue. Alterations of the vascular supportive framework can occur in disorders such as diabetes.

3. Purpura associated with decreased mechanical strength of the microcirculation. Decreased strength can be seen in conditions such as scurvy and amyloidosis.

4. Purpura associated with mechanical disruption of small venules. The principal cause of this type of purpura is increased intraluminal pressure. This condition can be observed around the ankles with prolonged standing and may be caused by the presence of abnormal proteins in macroglobulinemias or hyperviscosity disorders.

5. Purpura associated with microthrombi (small clots). This type of disorder is associated with abnormal intravascular coagulation conditions.

6. Purpura associated with vascular malignancy. Purpura of this origin is observed in Kaposi sarcoma and vascular tumors.

ABNORMAL PLATELET MORPHOLOGY

When examining a peripheral blood smear for platelets, the morphology of the platelets should be observed. Abnormal variations in size should be noted. Disorders of platelet size include the following:

1. Wiskott-Aldrich syndrome, which demonstrates the smallest platelets seen

2. May-Hegglin anomaly, which is characterized by the presence of large platelets and the presence of Döhle-like bodies (see Chapter 15) in the granulocytic leukocytes

3. Alport syndrome, a disorder that exhibits giant platelets and thrombocytopenia

4. Bernard-Soulier syndrome, which demonstrates the largest platelets seen and is also referred to as giant platelet syndrome. In this disorder, it has been demonstrated that the giant platelets are probably an artifact of the slide preparation. Actual measurement of the platelets reveals that their mean platelet volume (MPV) is normal

QUANTITATIVE PLATELET DISORDERS

The normal range of circulating platelets is $150 \times 10^9/L$ to $450 \times 10^9/L$. When the quantity of platelets decreases to levels below this range, a condition of thrombocytopenia exists. If the quantity of platelets increases, thrombocytosis is the result. Disorders of platelets can be classified as quantitative (thrombocytopenia or thrombocytosis) or qualitative (thrombocytopathy).

Thrombocytopenia

A correlation exists between severe thrombocytopenia and spontaneous clinical bleeding. If platelets are absent or severely decreased below $100 \times 10^9/L$, clinical symptoms usually include the presence of **petechiae** or **purpura**. Petechiae appear as small, purplish hemorrhagic spots on the skin or mucous membranes; purpura is characterized by extensive areas of red or dark-purple discoloration.

Thrombocytopenia can result from a wide variety of conditions, such as after the use of extracorporeal circulation in cardiac bypass surgery or in alcoholic liver disease. Heparin-induced thrombocytopenia (HIT) and associated thrombotic events, relatively common side effects of heparin therapy, can cause substantial morbidity and mortality. Thrombocytopenia in itself rarely poses a threat to affected patients, but disorders associated with it—which include deep venous thrombosis, **disseminated intravascular coagu-**

lation (DIC), pulmonary embolism, cerebral thrombosis, myocardial infarction, and ischemic injury to the legs or arms—can produce severe morbidity and mortality. Serum from patients with HIT contains immunoglobulin G (IgG) that, in the presence of small amounts of heparin, activates normal platelets and causes them to aggregate and release the contents of their granules, including serotonin. Platelet-activating antibodies are specific not for heparin but for complexes formed between heparin and platelet factor 4, a heparin-binding protein normally found in the alpha-granules of platelets. IgG and IgM also react with endothelial cells coated with platelet factor 4 (Fig. 24.1). This suggests a mechanism of antibody-mediated vascular injury that could predispose a patient to thrombosis or DIC when challenged with heparin. To prevent these complications, it has become standard medical practice to monitor platelet counts in patients receiving heparin for any extended period.

Most thrombocytopenic conditions can be classified into major categories. These categories are

1. Disorders of production

2. Disorders of destruction, including decreased megakaryocytopoiesis and ineffective platelet production, and disorders of utilization

3. Disorders of platelet distribution and dilution

Disorders of Production

Decreased production of platelets may be caused by hypoproliferation of the megakaryocytic cell line or ineffective thrombopoiesis caused by acquired conditions or hereditary factors (Box 24.1). A hypoproliferative state frequently affects other normal cell lines of the bone marrow and platelets. Thrombocytopenia owing to hypoproliferation can result from acquired damage to hematopoietic cells of the bone marrow caused by factors such as irradiation, drugs (e.g., chloramphenicol and chemotherapeutic agents), chemicals (e.g., insecticides), and alcohol. Infiltration of the bone marrow by malignant cells in the conditions of metastatic cancer, leukemia, and Hodgkin disease can produce a hypoproliferative state. Hypoproliferation may also result from nonmalignant conditions, such as infections, lupus erythematosus, granulomatous disease such as **sarcoidosis**, and idiopathic causes.

Ineffective thrombopoiesis may result in decreased platelet production. Thrombocytopenias of this type may be the manifestation of a nutritional disorder, such as a deficiency of vitamin B_{12} or folic acid. In these megaloblastic anemias caused by deficiencies of vitamin B_{12} or folic acid, the defect in thymidine and DNA synthesis affects megakaryocytes and causes decreased or ineffective thrombopoiesis. Another disorder related to ineffective thrombopoiesis is iron deficiency anemia, which usually results in a decrease in megakaryocyte size and the suppression of megakaryocyte endoproliferation and size. Hereditary thrombocytopenias include Fanconi syndrome, constitutional aplastic anemia and its variants, ameiosis thrombocytopenia (TAR syndrome), X-linked amegakaryocytic thrombocytopenia, Wiskott-Aldrich syndrome, May-Hegglin anomaly, and hereditary macrothrombocytopenia (e.g., Alport syndrome).

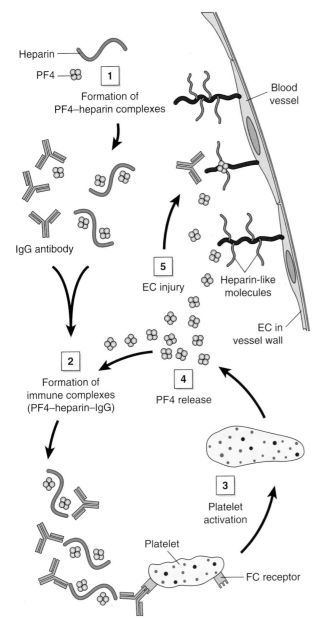

FIGURE 24.1. Proposed explanation for the presence of both thrombocytopenia and thrombosis in heparin-sensitive patients who are treated with heparin. Researchers believe that injected heparin reacts with platelet factor 4 (PF4) that is normally present on the surface of endothelial cells or released in small quantities from circulating platelets to form PF4-heparin complexes (*1*). Specific IgG antibodies react with these conjugates to form immune complexes (*2*) that bond to Fc receptors on circulating platelets. Fc-mediated platelet activation (*3*) releases PF4 from alpha-granules in platelets (*4*). Newly released PF4 binds to additional heparin, and the antibody forms more immune complexes, establishing a cycle of platelet activation. PF4 released in excess of the amount that can be neutralized by available heparin binds to heparin-like molecules (glycosaminoglycans) on the surface of endothelial cells (ECs) to provide targets for antibody binding. This process leads to immune-mediated EC injury (*5*) and heightens the risk of thrombosis and disseminated intravascular coagulation. (Adapted with permission from Aster RH. Heparin-induced thrombocytopenia and thrombosis, *N Engl J Med*, 332(20):1375, 1995. Copyright© 1995 Massachusetts Medical Society. All rights reserved.)

Hereditary Platelet Function Defects

ADHESION DEFECTS
Bernard-Soulier syndrome
Impaired adhesion to collagen

AGGREGATION DEFECTS: PRIMARY
Glanzmann thrombasthenia
Essential athrombia

AGGREGATION DEFECTS: SECONDARY
Storage pool diseases
Aspirin-like defects
Release reaction defects

ISOLATED PLATELET FACTOR III DEFICIENCY

SEVERE COAGULATION FACTOR DEFICIENCIES
Afibrinogenemia
Factor VIII: C deficiency
Factor IX: C deficiency

Disorders of Destruction or Utilization

Increased destruction or utilization of platelets may result from a number of mechanisms.

Destruction Caused by Immune Mechanisms, Antigens, Antibodies, or Complement

Drugs

Drugs or foreign substances can produce platelet destruction. These drugs include quinidine, sulfonamide derivatives, heroin, morphine, and snake venom. Sulfonamide derivative reactions involve the interaction of platelet antigens with drug antibodies. Morphine reactions involve the activation of complement.

Bacterial Sepsis

Bacterial sepsis causes increased destruction of platelets because of the attachment of platelets to bacterial antigen–antibody immune complexes. Certain microbial antigens may attach initially to platelets followed by specific antibodies to the microorganism. This mechanism has been reported to cause the thrombocytopenia that frequently complicates the *Plasmodium falciparum* type of malaria. Thrombocytopenia occurs within 1 to 3 weeks following viral infections (e.g., rubella, mumps, or chickenpox), parasitic or bacterial infections, or hepatitis vaccination.

Immune thrombocytopenia

Antibodies of either autoimmune or isoimmune origin may produce increased destruction of platelets. An example of an autoimmune thrombocytopenia is neonatal autoimmune thrombocytopenia. This condition occurs in infants born to mothers with chronic immune thrombocytopenia following transplacental passage of maternal IgG platelet autoantibodies.

Examples of thrombocytopenias of isoimmune origin include posttransfusion purpura and isoimmune neonatal thrombocytopenia. Posttransfusion purpura is a rare form of isoimmune thrombocytopenia. Isoimmune neonatal thrombocytopenia results from the immunization of a pregnant female by a fetal platelet antigen. The antigen is inherited by the fetus from the father and is absent on maternal platelets.

Thrombocytopenia in pregnancy

Pregnant women generally have lower platelet counts than nonpregnant women. Gestational thrombocytopenia is caused by a combination of hemodilution and increased platelet activation and clearance. A decrease of approximately 10% in the platelet count is typical toward the end of the third trimester of pregnancy.

Heparin-Induced Thrombocytopenia

HIT is the most common drug-induced thrombocytopenia. HIT and antiphospholipid syndrome (APS) are two prothrombotic syndromes in which antibodies against complexes of charged molecules are of fundamental importance. In the case of APS, the antibodies are autoantibodies compared to the drug-induced antibodies of HIT. In both syndromes, IgG antibodies directed against positively charged endogenous proteins, β2 glycoprotein I (GP I) in APS and platelet factor 4 (PF4) in HIT, are of major importance.

HIT is a serious complication of heparin therapy. This condition is also called "white clot syndrome" because it poses a high risk of potentially catastrophic venous or arterial thrombosis. The mortality rate of patients with thrombosis is approximately 25%.

Thrombocytopenia and thrombosis are the predominant clinical symptoms of HIT.

Two types of HIT exist

1. Nonimmune HIT: Type I
2. Immune HIT: Type II

Nonimmune Heparin-Induced Thrombocytopenia

Nonimmune HIT is a benign disorder affecting up to 10% of patients receiving heparin anticoagulant therapy. The mechanism of action is direct interaction between heparin and platelets.

Typically, the platelet count is greater than 100.00×10^{12}/L. Although a rapid decline is observed within the first 2 days of heparin administration, the platelet count returns to normal levels within 5 days despite continued heparin use or within 2 days if heparin therapy is discontinued.

Immune Heparin-Induced Thrombocytopenia

Approximately 8% of patients who receive heparin therapy develop HIT antibody but do not experience thrombocytopenia. Another 1% to 5% of patients receiving heparin therapy do develop HIT antibody and manifest thrombocytopenia.

At least 30% of thrombocytopenic patients develop venous and/or arterial thrombosis.

The lowest platelet counts range between 20 and 150 × 10^{12}/L. The lowest count is reached at about 5 days after the onset of the declining platelet count. The platelet count begins to rise approximately 2 days after heparin therapy is discontinued and usually returns to normal within 4 to 10 days after discontinuing heparin. In rare cases, it can take up to 25 days. The heparin-induced antibody disappears within 2 to 3 months after discontinuing heparin administration.

Thrombosis occurs in most patients after the platelet count diminishes by 30% to 50% of the normal level. The risk of thrombosis persists for up to 30 days after discontinuing heparin. Rare cases of thrombosis have been reported before the platelet count declines.

A rare manifestation of delayed-onset HIT has been observed. In these cases, thrombocytopenia began at least 5 days after discontinuation of heparin therapy. Bleeding is uncommon.

Pathophysiology

Immune HIT is caused by an antibody that recognizes heparin bound to platelet factor 4 (PF4) on the platelet surface. The antibody binds to the heparin-PF4 complex, which then allows the antibody to bind the Fc receptor on the platelet. Interaction with the Fc receptor activates the platelet that results in the loss of platelets, thrombocytopenia, and platelet aggregation (thrombosis). A small number of cases of HIT may involve an antigen other than the PF4 complex.

Laboratory Data

In addition to the platelet count, three specific laboratory assays can be used in patients with HIT:

1. Enzyme-linked immunosorbent assay (ELISA)
2. Platelet aggregation
3. Serotonin release

The ELISA assay and serotonin release assay have sensitivities of more than 90%, with very high specificity for HIT antibody. Platelet aggregation is between 50% and 80% and is very specific.

Increased Utilization of Platelets

Accelerated consumption of platelets is another cause of thrombocytopenia. One of the most important and frequently encountered forms of increased consumption of platelets is **immune (idiopathic) thrombocytopenic purpura (ITP)**. This antibody-related response, which may be preceded by infection, is believed to have a devastating effect on platelet survival. ITP may complicate other antibody-associated disorders such as **systemic lupus erythematosus (SLE)**. Patients with immunological thrombocytopenic purpura usually demonstrate petechiae, bruising, menorrhagia, and bleeding after minor trauma.

Immune Thrombocytopenia

There is a new standard nomenclature, immune thrombocytopenia (ITP), to replace the term, idiopathic thrombocytopenic purpura. ITP is an acquired immune-mediated

TABLE 24.1	Characteristics of Immune Thrombocytopenia	
Characteristic	**Newly Diagnosed**	**Chronic**
Peak age	2–5 years	Adulthood (30–60 years)
History of infection	Common	Uncommon
Spontaneous remission	Common	Rare

disorder characterized by isolated thrombocytopenia (platelet count $< 100 \times 10^9$/L) and the absence of any obvious initiating and/or underlying cause of the thrombocytopenia. ITP occurs in children and adults and is characterized by a low platelet count, normal bone marrow, and the absence of other causes of thrombocytopenia. Various characteristics exist in ITP (Table 24.1).

Epidemiology

ITP is a fairly rare, generally benign illness in the pediatric population. About two thirds of children recover spontaneously. In adults, the incidence is approximately equal for both genders except in the mid-adult years (30 to 60 years), when the disorder is more prevalent in women. ITP is classified by duration into newly diagnosed, persistent (3 to 12 months duration), and chronic ($\geq$12 months).

Typically, adult ITP is a chronic disease. ITP in children is a clinically distinct disorder and is usually acute. Among adults, ITP is most common in young women (approximately 70% of patients are 10 to 40 years old). Chronic ITP is a destructive thrombocytopenia caused by an autoantibody. Approximately 80% of patients experience remissions after either corticosteroid therapy or splenectomy. Some patients respond to other therapy; in a substantial group of patients, the disease is refractory to therapy.

Clinical Signs and Symptoms

Onset is often insidious. Purpura, epistaxis, and gingival bleeding are common. Hematuria and gastrointestinal bleeding are less common, and intracerebral hemorrhage is rare. Serious bleeding does not occur in most patients.

Pathophysiology

The old concept was that thrombocytopenia resulted from antibody-mediated platelet destruction. There are two new concepts:

1. The same antibodies that mediate platelet destruction also mediate impaired platelet production by damaging megakaryocytes and/or blocking their ability to release proplatelets. T cell–mediated effects are believed to play a role
2. Ten to twenty percent of cases are not antibody mediated

In acute ITP, the mechanism of platelet destruction is suggested to be either by absorption of viral antigen onto the platelet surface followed by antibody binding or by formation of an immune complex on the surface of platelets via the platelet Fc (immunoglobulin) receptors. In chronic ITP, the target for the autoantiplatelet antibodies is platelet membrane GPs (e.g., GPIIb/IIIa, GPIb/IX, GPIa/IIa, and GPIV). The majority of platelet autoantigens are present on either GPIIb/IIIa or GPIb/IX complex. The mechanism of autoantibody formation is unknown.

Laboratory Data

Isolated thrombocytopenia is the essential abnormality. Diagnosis requires exclusion of other causes of thrombocytopenia. Antibodies to specific platelet-membrane GPs can be detected in most patients, but neither these assays nor measurements of platelet IgG, which are often erroneously referred to as antiplatelet-antibody tests, are important for the diagnosis or management.

The American Society of Hematology has established the following guidelines for the diagnosis of ITP:

1. Presence of thrombocytopenia, lack of anemia unless blood loss has occurred, and lack of white cell abnormalities
2. Absence of other causes of thrombocytopenias (e.g., collagen vascular diseases or lymphoproliferative disorders)
3. Absence of infections, particularly human immunodeficiency virus (HIV)

Treatment

Platelet transfusions are seldom indicated. Survival time of transfused platelets is short, but they are important for controlling severe hemorrhage. The efficacy of platelets may improve immediately after an infusion of intravenous immune globulin. Intravenous immune globulin is an important agent in managing acute bleeding and in preparing for procedures, such as delivery. Treatment of pregnant women with ITP is a complex problem.

Splenectomy was a well-recognized treatment for ITP for more than 30 years before glucocorticoids were introduced in 1950, and its success in achieving complete responses in two thirds of patients has been remarkably consistent for more than 60 years. A response to splenectomy typically occurs within several days; responses after 10 days are unusual. When treatment is considered for patients with more severe thrombocytopenia and symptoms, it must be with the understanding that complete and permanent correction of thrombocytopenia is infrequent with any therapy.

Thrombocytopenia

Intravascular coagulation, vascular injury or occlusion, and tissue injury can all contribute to the increased utilization of platelets. DIC rapidly consumes platelets. Trauma, obstetrical complications, and microbial sepsis are examples of disorders that can trigger the accelerated consumption of platelets. In the case of bacterial sepsis, thrombin-induced platelet aggregation in vivo contributes to the thrombocytopenia. Vascular injury (vasculitis) causes a decrease in platelets because of the direct consumption of platelets at the sites of endothelial loss without appreciable depletion of clotting factors such as fibrinogen.

Thrombotic Thrombocytopenic Purpura

Thrombotic thrombocytopenic purpura (TTP) is a clinical syndrome with a high mortality rate that is characterized by formation of microthrombi in the microvasculature.

Clinical signs and symptoms include

- Severe thrombocytopenia
- Microangiopathic hemolytic anemia
- Fever
- Neurologic symptoms, for example, headache, stroke
- Renal disease

The hematological findings of thrombocytopenia and red blood cell schistocytes are diagnostic of the disease. Coagulation testing will demonstrate normal prothrombin and activated partial thromboplastin time (aPTT) but elevated D-dimer and fibrinogen levels. TTP is in contrast to DIC that demonstrates abnormal prothrombin time (PT) and aPTT.

Three types of TTP have been identified

1. Idiopathic
2. Secondary
3. Inherited (Upshaw-Shulman)

Idiopathic TTP has an unknown etiology but has been linked to an enzyme, ADAMTS13 (A Disintegrin-like And Metalloprotease domain with ThromboSpondin-type motifs), responsible for the breakdown of large von Willebrand factor (vWF) multimers. High–molecular-weight vWF in the plasma of patients with TTP promotes the aggregation of platelets in vivo, which produces most of the clinical symptoms.

Secondary TTP is diagnosed in patients with a history of medications, for example, quinine, immunosuppressants, or some cytotoxins used in cancer therapy. This form of TTP has been seen in some conditions, for example, HIV, autoimmune disorders, and allogeneic bone marrow transplants.

Upshaw-Shulman syndrome accounts for 5% to 10% of cases. It is the result of inheritance of a deficiency of ADAMTS13. This milder form of TTP is manifested in childhood when there is increased vWF, for example, inflammation.

Another disorder, hemolytic uremic syndrome (HUS) is a clinical syndrome with presentation and manifestations similar to TTP. Unlike TTP, which has a peak age incidence in the third decade, HUS has a peak incidence between 6 months and 4 years of age. Unlike TTP, HUS is characterized by

- Association with *Escherichia coli* O 157:H7 in 80% of cases
- Renal failure and limited to the kidneys
- Small vWF multimers predominate
- Normal level of ADAMTS13 activity

Disorders of Platelet Distribution

A platelet distribution disorder can result from a pooling of platelets in the spleen, which is frequent if splenomegaly is present. This type of thrombocytopenia develops when more than a double or triple increase in platelet production is required to maintain the normal quantity of circulating platelets. Disorders that may produce splenomegaly with resultant splenic pooling or delayed intrasplenic transit include alcoholic or posthepatic cirrhosis with portal hypertension, lymphomas and leukemias, and lipid disorders such as Gaucher disease.

Thrombocytosis

Thrombocytosis is generally defined as a substantial increase in circulating platelets over the normal upper limit of 450×10^9/L. Thrombocytosis can be classified into three major categories:

1. Hereditary or familial thrombocytosis associated with germline mutations of the thrombopoietin (THPO) gene in the THPO receptor (MPL) gene
2. Thrombocytosis associated with myeloproliferative neoplasms and/or myelodysplastic disorders (clonal thrombocytosis associated with somatic mutations of JAK2[V617F], MPL, and additional currently unknown genes)
3. Reactive (secondary thrombocytosis)

Many patients with thrombocytosis have reactive thrombocytosis. Reactive thrombocytosis may be observed in a variety of disorders and conditions, including chronic blood loss, chronic inflammatory diseases, chronic infections, drugs, asplenic states and splenectomy, malignancies, rebound thrombocytosis following treatment of immunological thrombocytopenic purpura, pernicious anemia, discontinuance of myelosuppressive drugs, acute blood loss, exercise, and myelodysplastic and hemolytic anemias. After splenectomy, increases are noted because of the loss of the spleen. As the bone marrow adjusts to new requirements, platelet numbers progressively return to normal.

Because of a poorly understood mechanism of stimulation associated with the hemolytic process, thrombocytosis may also be seen in **autoimmune hemolytic anemia.**

QUALITATIVE CHARACTERISTICS OF PLATELETS: THROMBOCYTOPATHY

If platelets are normal in number but fail to perform effectively, a platelet dysfunction exists. In addition to both an individual and family medical history, laboratory tests are critical in determining a platelet dysfunctional diagnosis. Laboratory tests of platelet function include bleeding time, clot retraction, platelet aggregation, platelet adhesiveness, and antiplatelet antibody assay.

TABLE 24.2	Categories of Platelet Dysfunctions	
Type	**Etiology**	**Typical Disorders**
Acquired	Blood plasma inhibitor	Uremia, pernicious anemia, liver disease
Drug induced	Aspirin	
Hereditary	Defect of connective tissue or coagulation factors	von Willebrand disease
	Structural or biochemical defects of platelets	Bernard-Soulier syndrome, Glanzmann thrombasthenia

Types of Platelet Dysfunctions

Three separate categories of platelet dysfunctions can be identified based on etiology (Table 24.2). These include the more common acquired causes and the less frequent hereditary causes. Disorders within these categories can be identified using specific laboratory tests (Table 24.3). Hyperactive platelets associated with hypercoagulability and thrombosis make up an additional category of abnormal platelet function.

Acquired

Acquired platelet function defects can be caused by a blood plasma inhibitory substance. Examples of disorders or diseases that may exhibit this dysfunction include infused dextran, uremia, liver disease, and pernicious anemia. Laboratory testing reveals the presence of fibrinolytic degradation or split products (discussed later in this chapter).

The most common acquired platelet defects are summarized in Table 24.4. Many patients with these platelet function disorders, who are candidates for surgery, may bleed profusely as a result of surgery or from trauma.

Myeloproliferative Syndromes

Acquired platelet dysfunction is commonly seen in the myeloproliferative syndromes. Platelet aggregation patterns are often not characteristic and could represent any combination of platelet aggregation defects.

Uremia

Uremia is commonly accompanied by bleeding caused by platelet dysfunction. It is proposed that circulating guanidinosuccinic acid or hydroxy phenolic acid interferes with platelet function. Dialysis often corrects or improves platelet function. Other mechanisms of altered platelet function in uremia, including altered prostaglandin metabolism, have been proposed.

Paraprotein Disorders

Paraprotein disorders including malignant or benign paraprotein, such as multiple myeloma, Waldenström macroglobulinemia, or other monoclonal gammopathies, harbor platelet dysfunction. Dysfunction results from the paraprotein coating the platelet membranes but does not depend on the type of paraprotein present. Almost all patients with malignant paraprotein disorders will demonstrate clinically significant bleeding and abnormal platelet function by aggregation.

Cardiopulmonary Bypass and Platelet Function

These conditions demonstrate severe platelet function deficit that assumes major importance in surgical bleeding after bypass.

Miscellaneous Disorders Associated With Platelet Dysfunction

Acquired defects are seen in autoimmune disorders, such as SLE, rheumatoid arthritis (RA), ITP, and scleroderma. Fibrinogen degradation products or fibrinogen split products (FDPs or FSPs) including the later degradation products, fragments D and E, have a high affinity for the platelet membrane and produce a severe platelet function defect. Patients with severe iron, folate, or cobalamin deficiency may also have platelet function defects.

TABLE 24.3	Selected Laboratory Tests for Platelet Dysfunctions					
					Aggregation	
Disorder	**Clot Retraction**	**Bleeding Time**	**Adhesion**	**ADP**	**Ristocetin**	**Release of ADP**
von Willebrand disease	Decreased	Usually prolonged	Decreased	Normal	Decreased or normal	Normal
Glanzmann thrombasthenia	Absent	Prolonged	Decreased	Absent	Normal	Normal
Storage disease	Normal	Prolonged	Decreased	Usually normal	Normal	Decreased

ADP, adenosine diphosphate.

TABLE 24.4	Acquired Platelet Function Defects

Myeloproliferative syndromes
   Essential thrombocythemia
   Chronic myelogenous leukemia
   Polycythemia vera
   Paroxysmal nocturnal hemoglobinuria
   Myelofibrosis
   RAEB syndrome
   Sideroblastic anemia
Paraprotein disorders
   Multiple myeloma
   Waldenström macroglobulinemia
   Essential monoclonal gammopathy
Autoimmune diseases
   Collagen vascular disease
   Antiplatelet antibodies
   Immune thrombocytopenias
Fibrinogen degradation products
   Disseminated intravascular coagulation
   Primary fibrinolytic syndromes
   Liver disease
Anemia
   Severe iron deficiency
   Severe B_{12} or folate deficiency
Uremia
Drug induced

RAEB, refractory anemia with excess blasts.

TABLE 24.5	Examples of Inherited Platelet Dysfunction

Surface membrane defects
   Bernard-Soulier syndrome
   Glanzmann thrombasthenia
   Platelet-type von Willebrand disease
Defects of granule storage
   Alpha-granule deficiency
      Gray platelet syndrome
   Dense granules
      Wiskott-Aldrich syndrome
      Hermansky-Pudlak syndrome
      Chédiak-Higashi syndrome
      TAR baby syndrome

penicillin, and alcohol. In addition, prostaglandin pathways are inhibited by aspirin, ibuprofen, hydrocortisone, and cyclosporine (Sandimmune, Neural, NOVARTIS, Basel, Switzerland).

The arachidonic acid platelet aggregation assay is the only practical way to monitor the effects of aspirin therapy, now widely used to prevent stroke and heart attacks.

Hereditary

Hereditary platelet dysfunctions are caused by an inherited platelet defect that is either structural or biochemical (Table 24.5). Examples of adhesion disorders include Bernard-Soulier syndrome, a collagen receptor defect, Glanzmann thrombasthenia, and storage granule abnormalities. Secondary aggregation disorders include hereditary storage pool defect and hereditary aspirin-like defects.

Also included among hereditary disorders are defects of connective tissue, such as collagen, and failure of platelets to adhere to the subendothelium because of a decrease or defect in plasma coagulation factors. An example of a defect of platelet plug formation owing to decreased platelet adhesion to the subendothelium is von Willebrand disease (see discussion later in this chapter).

Bernard-Soulier Syndrome

Bernard-Soulier syndrome, an **autosomal** hereditary bleeding disorder, is a platelet adhesion disorder in which platelet membrane GPs Ib, V, and IX are missing. Heterozygotes are often asymptomatic. The condition is characterized by the presence of giant platelets. In this syndrome, there is mild thrombocytopenia, but the predominant abnormality is of the

Drug Induced

Many drugs can induce platelet function defects, resulting in hemorrhage. A typical example of this dysfunction is the ingestion of aspirin. One or two aspirin tablets are sufficient to extend the bleeding time to twice the normal value.

The most common mechanisms of interference involve drug interference with platelet membrane or membrane receptor sites, drug interference with prostaglandin biosynthetic pathways, and drug interference with phosphodiesterase activity.

Platelet Membrane Receptors

Platelet membrane receptors can be altered by drugs, such as chlorpromazine (Thorazine, Glaxo Smith Kline Research Triangle Park, North Carolina), cocaine, Xylocaine, cephalothin (Keflin, Eli Lilly, Indianapolis, Indiana), ampicillin,

TABLE 24.6	Laboratory Profiles of Disorders of Platelet Function

Disorder	Laboratory Profile
Bernard-Soulier syndrome	Giant platelets; borderline platelet count; abnormal adhesion; abnormal ristocetin aggregation; normal or decreased thrombin aggregation; other aggregation responses normal
Von Willebrand disease	Abnormal adhesion; abnormal ristocetin aggregation (type IIB— increased, exhibits increased sensitivity to low concentrations)
Glanzmann thrombasthenia	Clot retraction abnormal; bleeding time prolonged; primary aggregation absent with ADP, thrombin, collagen, epinephrine; PF3 abnormal; ADP primary and secondary; epinephrine primary and secondary; ristocetin not diagnostic
Storage pool defect	Bleeding time prolonged; ADP and epinephrine primary and secondary responses decreased; arachidonic acid normal or decreased; collagen decreased; thrombin and ristocetin not diagnostic
Aspirin-like disorder or aspirin ingestion; aspirin (aspirin-like disorder); deficiency of cyclooxygenase inhibitor; or thromboxane	Bleeding time prolonged; aggregation primary and secondary; ADP and epinephrine decreased; arachidonic acid decreased; collagen decreased; thrombin and ristocetin not diagnostic

ADP, adenosine diphosphate.

membrane GP Ib. This abnormal platelet membrane lacks the receptor site for vWF, which is necessary for platelets to adhere to vascular subendothelium. A blood film from a patient with Bernard-Soulier syndrome may resemble that from a patient with ITP. Platelet aggregation is normal with all agents except ristocetin. Clinical features include easy bruising, epistaxis, hypermenorrhagia, and petechiae (Table 24.6).

Glanzmann Thrombasthenia and Essential Athrombia

Glanzmann thrombasthenia and **essential athrombia** are similar, rare, primary aggregation disorders. Glanzmann thrombasthenia is an autosomal recessive disorder. Clinical features involve platelet dysfunction, easy and spontaneous bruising, subcutaneous hematomas, and petechiae. Intra-articular bleeding with hemarthrosis may occur in some patients but tends to diminish with age.

This disorder involves an abnormality of the surface membrane GP complex IIb/IIIa. On a peripheral blood film, platelets from patients with this disorder remain isolated and do not exhibit the clumping that is normally seen. Epinephrine, collagen, and thrombin fail to induce aggregation. This results in a prolonged bleeding time in the presence of a normal platelet count, decreased platelet retention in glass bead columns, and an absence of a primary wave of aggregation in response to adenosine diphosphate (ADP). Clot retraction is also decreased.

Hereditary Storage Pool Defect

Hereditary storage pool defect is a secondary aggregation disorder. Overall, hereditary storage pool disorders are more common than primary aggregation disorders of

the hereditary platelet function defects. In rare instances, storage pool defects are seen in patients with other diseases, including Wiskott-Aldrich syndrome, TAR baby syndrome, Hermansky-Pudlak syndrome, and Chédiak-Higashi syndrome. Clinical features of secondary aggregation disorders are mucocutaneous hemorrhages and hematuria, peristasis, and easy and spontaneous bruising. Petechiae are less common than in other qualitative platelet disorders.

Hereditary aspirin-like defects are a rarer form of secondary aggregation defect. Clinical features are similar to other platelet function defects.

Storage granule abnormalities, primarily an absence of the dense granules, exist in conjunction with other clinical disorders, such as Chédiak-Higashi syndrome, Wiskott-Aldrich syndrome, and Hermansky-Pudlak syndrome. In these disorders, platelet aggregation with weaker agents, such as ADP and epinephrine, is diminished.

BLEEDING DISORDERS RELATED TO BLOOD CLOTTING

Vascular response and platelet plug formation are responsible for the initial phases of hemostasis. Subsequent to these activities, the clotting factors are initiated to form the fibrin clot. Fibrin formation can occur if the activity of various factors is at least 30% to 40% of normal.

Bleeding and defective fibrin clot formation are frequently related to a coagulation factor. Disorders of the blood coagulation factors (Table 24.7) can be grouped into three categories:

TABLE 24.7	Clinical Comparison of Disorders	
Observation	Disorders of Platelets or Vessels ("Purpuric" Disorders)	Disorders of Coagulation
Petechiae	Characteristic	Rare
Deep dissecting hematomas	Rare	Characteristic
Superficial ecchymosis	Characteristic; usually small and multiple	Common; usually large and solitary
Hemarthrosis	Rare	Characteristic
Delayed bleeding	Rare	Common
Bleeding from superficial cuts and scratches	Persistent; often profuse	Minimal
Patient gender	Relatively more common in females	80%–90% of hereditary forms occur in females
Positive family history	Rare	Common
Site of bleeding	Skin, mucous membranes, gums, nose, etc.	Deep in soft tissue (e.g., joints, muscles)
Bleeding after surgery	Immediate, usually mild	Delayed (usually 1–2 days), often severe

1. Defective production
2. Excessive destruction
3. Pathological inhibition

Defective Production

Vitamin K Deficiency

A condition of defective production may be related to a deficiency of vitamin K. The synthesis of vitamin K and dependent factors can be disrupted because of disease or drug therapy (e.g., cephalosporin antibiotics). Vitamin K deficiencies are also encountered in neonates, malabsorption syndrome, biliary obstruction, and patients taking oral anticoagulants. Vitamin K depletion develops within 2 weeks if both intake and endogenous production are eliminated. Factors II, VII, IX, and X are vitamin K dependent. Factor VII has the shortest half-life and usually declines in the early stages of vitamin K depletion. A mild deficiency of vitamin K may present as an asymptomatic prolongation of a patient's PT assay.

Severe Liver Disease

Because the liver is the primary site of synthesis of coagulation factor, severe liver disease can cause defective production of coagulation factors. Severe liver disease may produce decreased plasma levels of fibrinogen, although low levels of fibrinogen rarely produce hemorrhage. In patients with liver disease, the PT is noticeably prolonged, whereas the aPTTs are variable.

Hereditary Clotting Defects

Classic hemophilia (hemophilia A) and von Willebrand disease are examples of hereditary disorders that represent functionally inactive factor VIII.

Hemophilia

Etiology

Hemophilia has been used as a paradigm for understanding the molecular pathological processes that underlie hereditary disease. The cloning of factor VIII facilitated the identification of mutations that lead to hemophilia A, an inherited deficiency of factor VIII coagulant activity that causes severe hemorrhage. Two types of mutations dominate the defects identified so far: gene deletions and point mutations. Gene deletions are associated with severe hemophilia A in which no factor VIII circulates in the blood. To date, approximately 50 deletion mutations in the gene for factor VIII have been characterized at the molecular level, and 34 independent deletion mutations in the factor IX gene have been found to be the cause of hemophilia B. Point mutations, in which a single base in DNA is mutated to another base, represent a second type of mutation that causes hemophilia.

Epidemiology

Individuals with hereditary clotting defects may be either genetically homozygous or heterozygous carriers of the trait. The level of factor activity ranges from 0% to 25% in persons homozygous for the trait and from 15% to 100% in persons heterozygous for the trait. Defects of this origin may result from the decreased production of a clotting factor, factor VIII, or the production of functionally inactive molecules of the clotting factor. Hemophilia A, a sex-linked homozygous disorder expressed in males, occurs in 1 in 10,000 males.

Pathophysiology

Classic hemophiliacs have an intact high–molecular-weight moiety and a deficient low–molecular-weight procoagulant portion. This disorder of procoagulant synthesis expresses

TABLE 24.8	Nomenclature of the Factor VIII–von Willebrand Factor Complex

Term	Description
VIII:C	Factor VIII procoagulant activity
VIII:Cag	Antigenic expression of VIII:C
vWF:Ag	Antigenic expression of vWF
Ristocetin cofactor	A property of vWF that promotes agglutination of platelets in the presence of the antibiotic ristocetin
Factor VIII–vWF complex	The form in which VIII:C and vWF usually circulate in plasma

itself by decreased factor VIII clotting activity in laboratory assay and a normal bleeding time. Conversely, severe von Willebrand disease has both a decreased high–molecular-weight portion and a decreased low–molecular-weight portion.

Plasma levels of factor VIII can be temporarily corrected and the bleeding tendency reversed in most patients following infusion of factor VIII in appropriate blood products. One would expect that correction of the hemostatic defect would place a patient at the same risk of thromboembolism as an unaffected individual, but thromboembolic events in patients with hemophilia A are distinctly uncommon.

Von Willebrand Disease

In 1926, Erik von Willebrand first described a hemorrhagic disorder characterized by a prolonged bleeding time and an autosomal inheritance pattern that distinguished the disease from classic hemophilias. In the early 1950s, an additional component of the disease was identified: a deficiency of factor VIII procoagulant activity (Table 24.8). These and other observations distinguish von Willebrand disease from classic factor VIII:C deficiency (hemophilia A). In addition, evaluation of the multimeric structures of vWF has aided in the classification of the variant forms of von Willebrand disease. Three major types of von Willebrand disease have been identified.

Etiology

von Willebrand disease may be an acquired or inherited disorder. The congenital disorder is autosomally dominant in most cases. Inherited abnormalities in von Willebrand disease are associated with a defect of the vWF gene on chromosome 12, but in some patients, the coexistence of an impaired response of plasminogen activator and telangiectasia suggests the presence of a regular defect or more extensive endothelial abnormalities. In several families, a large vWF gene deletion has been identified as the basis for von Willebrand disease.

More than 20 distinct clinical and laboratory subtypes of von Willebrand disease have been described (Table 24.9). Three broad types of von Willebrand disease are recognized. In addition, a platelet-type von Willebrand disease (pseudo–von Willebrand disease) is caused by an abnormal platelet receptor for vWF. In addition, acquired von

TABLE 24.9	Classification of von Willebrand Disease

Type	Features
IA	All vWF multimers are present in plasma in normal relative proportion
	No evidence of intrinsic functional abnormality of vWF
	Subgroups: platelet concentration and activity may be normal, low, or discordant
IB	All vWF multimers are present in plasma but the larger ones are relatively decreased
	vWF has less ristocetin cofactor activity than normal
IC	All vWF multimers are present in plasma in normal relative proportion but a structural abnormality of individual multimers is present
	vWF has less ristocetin cofactor activity than normal
Miscellaneous: I-1, I-2, I-3, I	Variable deficiencies of vWF:Ag in plasma and/or platelets, and other abnormalities

(continued)

| TABLE 24.9 | Classification of von Willebrand Disease (continued) |

New York, undesignated types

Type	Features
IIA	Large and intermediate vWF multimers are absent in plasma and platelets
	Increased proteolysis of vWF; some variability in size of multimer present; few cases show recessive inheritance
IIA-1, IIA-2, and IIA-3	Subtypes demonstrate variable concentrations of plasma and/or platelet vWF:Ag
IIB	Hyperresponsiveness to low doses of ristocetin; large vWF multimers are absent in plasma; all multimers are present in platelets
	Increased proteolysis of vWF; few cases demonstrate recessive inheritance
IIC, IID	Large vWF multimers are absent; unique structural abnormality of individual multimers
	Decreased proteolysis of vWF
IIE	Large vWF multimers are appreciably decreased; structural abnormality of individual multimers
	Recessive inheritance
	Decreased proteolysis of vWF
IIF, IIG, IIH, type B	Rare examples of a variety of abnormalities
III	Severe form of the disease; also called severe type I

vWF, von Willebrand factor.

Willebrand disease may complicate other diseases such as lymphoproliferative and autoimmune disorders, and proteolytic degradation of vWF complicates myeloproliferative disorders. Variant forms of von Willebrand disease can be identified by their patterns of genetic transmission and the vWF abnormalities in the plasma and the cellular compartment. Distinguishing between various subtypes of von Willebrand disease is important in determining appropriate therapy (Table 24.10).

Epidemiology

von Willebrand disease is recognized as one of the most common hereditary bleeding disorders in humans. The exact incidence is difficult to determine because milder forms are often not clinically recognized, but it has been estimated to have a prevalence as high as 1% in the general population.

No racial or ethnic predisposition has been determined. Both genders are affected, but there is a higher frequency of clinical manifestation in women.

Pathophysiology

von Willebrand disease is characterized by abnormal platelet function, expressed as a prolonged bleeding time. This is a consistent finding and may be accompanied by decreased factor VIII procoagulant activity.

vWF circulates in the blood in two distinct compartments, with two types of cells being responsible for vWF produc-

tion. Vascular endothelium is the primary source of the synthesis and release of plasma vWF; the other type of cell that synthesizes vWF is the megakaryocyte. Approximately 15% of circulating vWF is produced in the megakaryocyte. vWF circulates in platelets, being stored primarily in the alpha granules, in association with factor VIII procoagulant protein (VIII:Ag). Platelet vWF is released from the alpha granules by various agonists and subsequently rebinds to the GP IIb/IIIa complex. The site synthesis of VIII:Ag remains unknown, although the liver is thought to play an important role.

vWF is a large, adhesive, multimeric GP present in plasma, platelets, and subendothelium. It is synthesized as a large precursor that consists of a signal peptide, a propeptide (von Willebrand antigen II), and the vWF subunit. It has the two main functions of regulating coagulant activity (VIII:C) and aiding in adhesion of platelets to subendothelial cell walls following vessel damage. In circulating blood, vWF is part of a noncovalent bimolecular complex with the factor VIII procoagulant protein. This complex stabilizes factor VIII and protects it from rapid removal from the circulation. The vWF portion represents more than 95% of the mass of the complex and therefore controls the molecular stereochemistry. The vWF consists of repeating multimers, with the smallest circulating multimer thought to be a dimer or tetramer.

Circulating vWF undergoes proteolytic cleavage under physiological conditions; thus, it can be distinguished from platelet vWF, which is not proteolyzed. The pathogenesis of

TABLE 24.10	Characteristics of Various Types of von Willebrand Disease					
Feature	Type I	Type IIA	Type IIB	Platelet	Type IIC	Type III
Platelet count	N	N	N or ↓	Low N or ↓	N	N
Bleeding time	↑ or N	↑	↑	↑	↑	↑
Factor VIII:C	N or ↓	N or ↓	N or ↓	N or ↓	N	N
vWF:Ag	↓	N or ↓	N or ↓	N or ↓	N	
vWF:RCoF	↓	↓	N or ↓	N or ↓		
RIPA	N or ↓	↓ or absent	↑	↑	↓	Absent

vWF, von Willebrand factor; vWF:RCoF, ristocetin cofactor; RIPA, ristocetin-induced platelet aggregation; N, normal.

von Willebrand disease is based on quantitative or qualitative abnormalities, or both, of vWF. When an abnormality is present, the decreased factor VIII procoagulant activity is attributable to the reduced concentration of vWF.

vWF is essential in providing the basis for formation of a normal platelet thrombus. vWF binds to specific sites on the platelet, namely GP Ib and GP IIb/IIIa, while concurrently binding to the subendothelium of damaged vessel walls, forming a bridge. Patients with decreased levels of vWF, especially the larger multimeric forms, will lack adequate bridging action that produces prolonged bleeding times. Qualitative or quantitative abnormalities of vWF result in decreased adhesion and are responsible for the bleeding associated with von Willebrand disease.

The significance of vWF in the regulation of VIII:C remains unclear. The increase in VIII:C following infusion of purified vWF suggests a possible role of vWF in the synthesis, release, or stabilization of VIII:Ag. Therefore, decreased levels of vWF may prolong the rate of blood clotting.

Clinical Signs and Symptoms

The severity of symptoms among patients with von Willebrand disease varies greatly. Severe cases are not easily distinguishable clinically from severe hemophilia A, in which bleeding occurs into the joints and fascial planes. Characteristically, in patients with von Willebrand disease, the bleeding is mucosal in origin, with epistaxis, menorrhagia, and gastrointestinal bleeding being the most common. Bleeding associated with surgical procedures and oral surgery is a particular problem. Homozygous patients may experience severe bleeding, including hemarthrosis, or potentially lethal gastrointestinal tract or central nervous system hemorrhage.

Inherited Classification of von Willebrand Disease

Type I is the most common variant of von Willebrand disease and appears to be based on a quantitative deficiency of vWF. It is expressed as an autosomal dominant trait and is presumed to be caused by an inheritance of one normal and one deficient allele. Patients with severe type III disease

may have homozygous type I (or compound heterozygous) disease. The molecular basis for type I and type III disease is unclear but is characterized by decreased circulating levels of vWF. Factor VIII:C is decreased proportionally with respect to vWF.

Most patients with von Willebrand disease (50% or more) have quantitative abnormalities and no evidence of a functional abnormality of vWF, which corresponds to type I von Willebrand disease and its subtypes. The genetic transmission of the disease is dominant, except possibly for subtype I-3. Most patients have low plasma levels of vWF antigen (usually between 5% and 30% of normal) and correspondingly low levels of ristocetin cofactor activity (the assay reflects the property of vWF to bind to GP Ib and mediate platelet agglutination). The factor VIII procoagulant protein is also decreased in proportion to the decrease in vWF. In these cases, the bleeding is caused by insufficient levels of circulating vWF and factor VIII. Bleeding manifestations are less severe in patients who have a normal concentration of platelet vWF than in others (Table 24.11).

TABLE 24.11	von Willebrand Factor Requirements for Primary Hemostasis		
Activity	Interaction	Reaction
Plasma vWF	Subendothelial deposition interaction with GP Ib	Platelet contact
Platelet vWF	Binding to GP IIB/IIIa subendothelial surface	Platelet spreading
	Platelet-platelet interaction	Platelet aggregation

vWF, von Willebrand factor.

| TABLE 24.12 | Clinical Features of Various Types of von Willebrand Disease |

Type	Bleeding Time	Bleeding Tendency	Petechiae	Hemarthrosis[a]
I	Normal or increased	Mild	None	Uncommon
II	Increased	Moderate	Usually none	Uncommon
II	Increased	Often severe	Occasionally	Uncommon

[a]Only occurs in the most severely affected.

In all patients whose vWF shows low ristocetin cofactor activity, except for those designated as having type B disease, the vWF has an abnormal multimeric structure and there is a decrease in or absence of the large multimers.

Type II is characterized by structurally abnormal vWF. The circulating levels of vWF may be decreased or normal, and VIII:C may be affected similarly. Type IIA and type IIB are autosomally dominant, whereas type IIC is recessive.

Patients with type III, the most severe form of von Willebrand disease, are likely to have a major episode of bleeding early in life because significantly decreased amounts of vWF and VIII:C are produced. Genetically, they are thought to be homozygous or double heterozygous. These patients probably comprise a separate group because of the typically recessive modality of genetic transmission (Table 24.12).

Acquired von Willebrand Disease

von Willebrand disease is occasionally seen as an acquired condition. Associations have been made with lupus erythematosus and other autoimmune disorders as well as myeloproliferative disorders. The presence of a circulating antibody to vWF may be implicated in some cases. Another mechanism responsible for decreased amounts of vWF in acquired states is the absorption of the coagulation component onto abnormal cell surfaces. Hemorrhagic complications are generally more severe in patients with acquired von Willebrand disease. Bleeding from mucous membranes is more common and reflects the much lower levels of vWF activity in these individuals. vWF activity is typically 20% or less of normal.

Pseudo–von Willebrand Disease

This is a rare disorder in which patients resemble those with von Willebrand disease because of low levels or absence of large multimeric forms of vWF in the plasma. Patients with pseudo–von Willebrand disease have a platelet abnormality in which spontaneous platelet aggregation occurs. Low levels of larger multimers result from increased consumption during platelet aggregation.

Increased Levels of vWF

Increased levels of vWF have been associated with stress, inflammation, postsurgical states, pregnancy, renal disease, diabetes, rheumatoid disorders, scleroderma, and Raynaud phenomena. vWF may be an indicator of vascular endothelial status. Drugs such as 1-deamino-8-D-arginine vasopressin (DDAVP), steroids, and hormones may also result in elevated levels of vWF.

Laboratory Findings

The following laboratory results are typical of von Willebrand disease:

- Bleeding time: mildly to moderately prolonged
- Platelet retention: typically decreased
- Platelet agglutination: ristocetin—abnormal
- Platelet aggregation: normal with all but ristocetin
- vWF function (ristocetin cofactor activity)

Quantitation of vWF antigen (vWF:Ag) can be determined by immunoelectrophoresis. These assays measure total amounts of vWF protein, independent of its ability to function. Finally, vWF multimeric analysis is useful in distinguishing between subtypes and in determining therapeutic management. vWF multimeric analysis uses sodium dodecyl sulphate (SDS) agarose gel electrophoresis and radiolabeled antibody to visualize the different molecular weight multimers.

Other Hereditary Deficiencies

A deficiency of factor IX is known as **hemophilia B** or **Christmas disease**. This form of hemophilia is non–sex linked and occurs at a rate of 1/50,000 in the general population, with a defective molecule being the usual cause. It is clinically indistinguishable from hemophilia A and must be differentiated by laboratory testing. A deficiency of factor XI is referred to as **hemophilia C**. This genetic defect is an autosomal recessive trait that occurs almost exclusively in people of Jewish descent. It is usually a mild disorder characterized by easy bruising, epistaxis, and hemorrhage in conjunction with trauma. The laboratory results in this defect, as well as those of other hemophilias and von Willebrand disease, are presented in Table 24.13.

Hereditary fibrinogen deficiency may exist as absent or decreased levels of fibrinogen, afibrinogenemia, or hypofibrinogenemia, respectively. Production of dysfunctional molecules produces dysfibrinogenemia. Afibrinogenemia is associated with a severe bleeding tendency but is less common than hypofibrinogenemia. Patients with hypofibrinogenemia

TABLE 24.13	Laboratory Test Results in Hereditary Coagulation Defects			
Test	**Hemophilia A**	**von Willebrand Disease**	**Hemophilia B**	**Hemophilia C**
Bleeding time	Normal	Increased	Normal	Normal
Clot retraction	Normal	Normal	Normal	Normal
Platelet count	Normal	Normal	Normal	Normal
Platelet aggregation	Normal	Decreased	Normal	Normal
PT[a]	Normal	Normal	Variable	Normal
aPTT	Increased	Increased	Increased	Increased
PT consumption	Decreased	Decreased	Decreased	Decreased
Fibrinogen	Normal	Normal	Normal	Normal
Factor VIII	Decreased	Decreased		
Factor VIII:C	Decreased 2% or less	Decreased 10%–30%		
Factor VIIIC:Ag	Normal	Decreased		
Factor VIII/vWF	Normal	Decreased or absent		
Factor IX assay			Decreased	Normal
Factor XI assay			Normal	Decreased

[a]This test is normal when performed with human brain thromboplastin, but in a variant of the disease, the PT is prolonged if bovine brain thromboplastin is used. This variation is produced by a molecular abnormality of factor IX that inhibits the thromboplastin–factor VII reaction of the extrinsic pathway.
PT, prothrombin time; aPTT, activated partial thromboplastin time.

are usually asymptomatic except in situations of surgery or trauma. Patients with dysfibrinogenemia may be asymptomatic or experience a mild bleeding tendency if heterozygous for the defect, or they may have a severe bleeding tendency if homozygous for the defect.

Hereditary deficiencies of the other coagulation factors are relatively rare (Box 24.2). Examples of rare defects include **factor XII deficiency**, in which no clinical bleeding tendencies

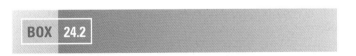

BOX 24.2

Coagulation Disorders

EXAMPLES OF BLEEDING DISORDERS RELATED TO COAGULATION FACTOR DEFICIENCIES
Factors I, II, V, VII, VIII (hemophilia A), IX (hemophilia B), X, XI, XII, XIII

CONDITIONS RELATED TO DEFICIENCIES OF MULTIPLE COAGULATION FACTORS
Hepatic disease, anticoagulant overdose (e.g., heparin or warfarin), DIC, vitamin K deficiency

are apparent, and **factor XIII deficiency**, which is associated with spontaneous abortion and poor wound healing.

Disorders of Destruction and Consumption

Enhanced fibrin deposits can result in thrombosis and damage to organs owing to impeded blood flow and ischemia. The fibrinolytic system serves as a protective mechanism against excessive fibrin deposits by lysing both fibrin and fibrinogen.

Blood coagulation factors can be destroyed in vivo by enzymatic degradation or by pathological activation of coagulation with excessive utilization of the clotting factors. Enzymatic destruction can result from bites by certain species of snakes whose venom contains an enzyme that degrades fibrinogen to a defective fibrin monomer. In vivo activation of coagulation by tissue thromboplastin–like materials can produce excessive utilization of clotting factors. Conditions associated with this consumption of coagulation factors include obstetrical complications, trauma, burns, prostatic and pelvic surgery, shock, advanced malignancy, septicemia, and intravascular hemolysis.

General Features of Fibrinolysis

Primary and secondary fibrinolysis are recognized as extreme complications of a variety of intravascular and extravascular disorders and may have life-threatening consequences.

TABLE 24.14	Selected Characteristics of Primary and Secondary Fibrinolysis	
Laboratory Test	**Primary Fibrinolysis**	**Secondary Fibrinolysis**
Platelet count	Normal	Decreased
Protamine sulfate test	Negative	Positive
Fibrin split products	Increased	Increased
Fibrinogen	Decreased	Decreased

Primary fibrinolysis is associated with conditions in which gross activation of the fibrinolytic mechanism with subsequent fibrinogen and coagulation factor consumption occurs. The important characteristic of primary fibrinolysis is that no evidence of fibrin deposition occurs. Primary fibrinolysis occurs when large amounts of plasminogen activator enter the circulatory system as a result of trauma, surgery, or malignancies.

Although the same clinical conditions may also induce secondary fibrinolysis or DIC, the distinction between the two is essentially in the demonstration of fibrin formation. In secondary fibrinolysis, excessive clotting and fibrinolytic activity occur. Increased amounts of fibrin split (degradation) products (FSPs) and fibrin monomers are detectable because of the action of thrombin on the fibrinogen molecule. This fibrinolytic process is only caused by excessive clotting; therefore, it is a secondary condition. Distinguishing between primary and secondary fibrinolysis (Table 24.14) is important in treatment.

Disseminated Intravascular Coagulation

Etiology

DIC is actually a complication or intermediary phase of many diseases and does not constitute a disorder in itself. It is also known as consumptive coagulopathy or defibrination syndrome. Triggering events that may predispose patients to DIC include alterations in the endothelium, direct activation of fibrinogen, release of thromboplastin-like substances, and erythrocyte or platelet destruction. Extravascular trauma, abruptio placentae, advanced malignancy, leukemia, and retained fetal syndrome are examples of clinical situations in which tissue thromboplastin can activate coagulation.

Infections, most commonly Gram-negative microorganisms, can trigger DIC by producing endotoxins that expose collagen. Stasis, shock, or tissue necrosis can have the same effect. Snakebites may introduce substances that initiate coagulation by direct activation of fibrinogen to form fibrin. Red blood cell or platelet injury may contribute to the consumptive coagulopathy by releasing phospholipids that accelerate coagulation. Red cell injury may be a result of intravascular hemolysis caused by malaria, incompatible transfusion products, and other clinical states. Platelet destruction also releases coagulation factors V, VIII, XII, and XIII.

Other causes can include liver disease, lymphoproliferative disorders, and renal disease. In addition, DIC can also be triggered by trauma including shock, hypothermia, and extensive tissue damage, such as in myocardial infarction and eclampsia. It has been associated with multiple surgical, obstetrical, and medical disorders. Coma and convulsions can result.

Pathophysiology

The overall DIC process involves coagulation factors, platelets, vascular endothelial cells, fibrinolysis, and plasma inhibitors. This major breakdown of the hemostatic mechanism occurs when the procoagulant factors outweigh the anticoagulant mechanisms.

Initiation of DIC can be caused by a number of factors. If vascular endothelial damage results in the exposure of collagen and basement membrane, collagen can activate factor XII. Factor XII has multiple roles in the direct or indirect activation of coagulation including

1. Initiation of the intrinsic clotting cascade resulting in thrombin formation
2. Participation as a cofactor for the conversion of prekallikrein to kallikrein
3. Initiation of fibrinolysis

Regardless of the initiating event, DIC is characterized by excess thrombin formation, conversion of fibrinogen to fibrin, and platelet consumption and deposition. Secondary fibrinolysis occurs as a result of fibrin deposition and can decrease plasma coagulation factors, leading to a hemorrhagic diathesis.

Thrombin is central to the mechanism of consumptive coagulopathy. The action of thrombin on the coagulation systems includes

1. Proteolytic cleavage of fibrinogen to fibrin monomer, releasing fibrinopeptides A and B (fibrin monomer may form soluble complexes with fibrinogen or form fibrin thrombi that entrap platelets during thrombus formation)
2. Activation of factor XIII, which stabilizes fibrin by cross-linking
3. Stimulation of platelets, resulting in decreased circulating platelets. These stimulated platelets undergo shape change, adhesion, aggregation, and secretion. The contents of the

dense alpha-granules are released, leading to an acquired storage pool deficiency. If, during perhaps a 3-hour span, platelet counts and fibrinogen levels decrease significantly in a critically ill patient, DIC should be the prime suspect as the cause of this change

4. Activation of factors V and VIII; however, thrombin activation results in unstable end products that have decreased factor V and VIII activity
5. Activation of protein C, which degrades factors V and VIII

The deposition of fibrin thrombi in the vasculature, primarily in the microvasculature, initiates fibrinolysis. This secondary fibrinolysis is responsible for the hemorrhagic complication of DIC.

When the fibrinolytic system is activated, plasminogen is converted to plasmin. Alpha-2 antiplasmin is the fibrinolytic inhibitor uniquely designed to cope with plasmin. The more plasmin generated, the more alpha-2 antiplasmin the patient consumes. This produces a vicious cycle in which increased activation leads to decreased inhibitors; this, in turn, allows more increased activation to continue. This is known as a positive feedback loop and leads to a situation incompatible with life.

Damaged tissue, especially renal cells, releases plasminogen activators that convert plasminogen to plasmin. Plasmin is a proteolytic enzyme that destroys fibrin, fibrinogen, and clotting factors V and VIII. Circulating plasmin may lead to systemic fibrinolysis, causing increased hemorrhagic events.

In the microcirculation, plasmin's action is primarily directed against fibrin. In the circulation, the breakdown of fibrin results in FSPs, labeled X, Y, D, and E, which inhibit thrombin and normal platelet function.

As fibrinogen is degraded by plasmin, FSPs form. Degradation occurs whether the plasmin comes from DIC or primary fibrinogenolysis. FSPs compete with regular fibrinogen molecules for thrombin molecules. This competitive binding makes the thrombin unavailable for the conversion of fibrinogen to fibrin. In this situation, patients with high FDP/FSP levels have a circulating anticoagulant behaving like heparin. If the FSP level is high, the thrombin clotting time is significantly prolonged and fibrinogen quantitation is low. The second effect is on platelets. These split products coat the platelet surface, blocking the receptor site needed for further platelet activation.

When pathological fibrinolysis occurs, not only are factors destroyed, but, through the destruction of fibrinogen, a profound anticlotting effect inhibits secondary hemostasis and platelets.

If the fibrinolytic system is activated, it will contribute to the consumption of many coagulation factors. Plasmin, the primary proteolytic enzyme of fibrinolysis, directly attacks and destroys them. This becomes another form of consumptive coagulopathy originating from an entirely different source with the same end result.

When systemic clotting activation begins, the body usually attempts to stop it. The two major inhibitor systems of coagulation are antithrombin and the protein C and S systems. These inhibitors are consumed in the DIC process.

Therefore, the compensatory mechanisms are often unable to stabilize the consumptive process. Coagulation factors and platelets are consumed more rapidly than they can be replaced, antithrombin III (AT-III) levels are depleted, and the impaired mononuclear phagocytic system cannot effectively remove the activated coagulation proteins.

Alternate Forms of DIC

Acute DIC presents in one of several forms in which a patient's clotting and/or fibrinolytic system is suddenly activated throughout the body. In essence, it is a systemic pathological process. Because two types of systems are involved, the clotting and/or the fibrinolytic system, several types of DIC can be identified clinically:

1. DIC: Clotting and lysis strongly activated (most common type)
2. DIC: Clotting predominates with little or no lysis (poor prognosis)
3. Primary fibrinogenolysis: Only lysis activated, but many coagulation factors consumed

In the usual form of DIC, the patient's clotting system and the fibrinolytic system are activated. Patients are systemically forming thrombin, which, in turn, converts fibrinogen to fibrin. In most instances, the simultaneous generation of plasmin will dissolve the fibrin. Both the clotting and fibrinolytic states are performing at abnormally high rates. If clot lysis does not occur, a different form of DIC exists. In this case, the prognosis is very poor. A third type is represented by a state in which the patient predominantly has fibrinolysis-disseminated intravascular fibrinogenolysis. Coagulation factors are degraded by the excess plasmin being generated.

The Role of Factor VIII

A very close relationship exists between factor VIII:C (procoagulant) and factor VIII:CAg (procoagulant antigen). In DIC, it is believed that the VIII:CAg is inactivated to a lesser extent than VIII:C by enzymes released during the process. It is known that factor VIII:C activity is destroyed by minute amounts of thrombin, plasmin, and activated protein C (aPC).

It is strongly suspected that the in vivo inactivation of VIII:C found in DIC is related to the degree of severity of DIC. Furthermore, low values of factors VIII:C and VIIIR:Ag and factors VIII:C and VIIIR:CoF found in patients with irreversible shock indicate a grave clinical outcome. Discrepancies are also known to exist between VIII:C and VIIIR:Ag in patients with thromboembolic disease. Such ratios are useful indicators for assessing the severity of DIC. Current thinking indicates that data on the factor VIII complex show that the dogma of a characteristic decrease of the factor VIII procoagulant activity in DIC formulated in the past is not generally valid.

The Role of Protein C

Protein C (PC) is a major regulatory mechanism of hemostasis. In addition, PC is now recognized as playing a crucial role in the pathogenesis of acute and chronic inflammatory diseases, for example, sepsis or asthma. When inflammation occurs, coagulation is also set in motion and actively participates in enhancing inflammation.

PC is a vitamin K–dependent serine protease that is synthesized, predominantly in the liver, as a single polypeptide chain of 461 amino acids and is a natural anticoagulant protein. The conversion of PC to activated PC (aPC) is enhanced by interaction of PC with endothelial PC receptor (EPCR) on the cell surface. Activation can also be triggered by thrombin alone at a less efficient rate and is probably not relevant in the circulation. The function of aPC as an anticoagulant is manifested by its ability to inactivate two important cofactors of the coagulation cascade: factor V/Va and factor VIII/VIIIa. These events are enhanced by the presence of Ca^{2+}, phospholipids, and cofactor protein S.

Other functions of aPC in hemostasis are in maintaining a fluid state of blood. aPC has the ability to downregulate thrombin and suppress the activation of thrombin activatable fibrinolytic inhibitor, which indirectly promotes fibrinolysis. Fibrinolysis is also stimulated because of the ability of aPC to inhibit plasminogen activator inhibitor-1 (PAI-1).

The induction of fibrinolytic activity by the protein C system may facilitate the clearance of excess thrombi and generation of FSPs. If aPC is being consumed too rapidly, the regulatory ability of the protein C system is sharply reduced, which results in uncontrollable thrombosis.

Thromboembolic complications occur in patients with hereditary deficiencies of protein C (levels 60% or less of normal). Fatal neonatal purpura develops in individuals born with a homozygous protein C deficiency. The stimuli that can induce DIC may ultimately result in abnormal levels of protein C. Both normal and abnormal levels of protein C antigen can be found, depending on the sample time relative to the onset of DIC. Plasma levels of protein C antigen and activity have been found to be decreased in patients with DIC. Whereas three fourths of DIC patients have a decrease in protein C antigen, almost all DIC patients have a decreased level of protein C activity. Monitoring patients reveals that protein C antigen and activity decrease progressively during the initial stages of DIC and remain at a low level for 24 to 48 hours before gradually returning toward normal in nonfatal cases.

The Role of Thrombin

Mechanisms involved in DIC result in the generation of thrombin in the circulating blood. Among its many feedback reactions, thrombin participates indirectly in the activation of the fibrinolytic system secondary to DIC and activates protein C. The latter reaction is accelerated by the presence of the endothelial cell cofactor, protein S.

In addition to cleaving fibrinogen and performing its other procoagulant functions, some of the excess thrombin binds to protein S on the endothelial cell surface. This event leads to increased levels of APC in the plasma. Once the generation of excess thrombin is decreased by the action of APC

and other regulatory mechanisms, the coagulation process can return to normal. This negative feedback mechanism has the potential to slow the formation of excess thrombin and to stop DIC.

Clinical Signs and Symptoms

The DIC phenomenon has varied clinical and laboratory manifestations (Table 24.15) owing to the many physiological abnormalities associated with the syndrome. DIC may be acute or subacute (chronic). Chronic DIC is more common than acute DIC but is often more difficult to diagnose. Chronic DIC can convert to acute consumption if the balance of procoagulant-anticoagulant is lost.

Either form may initially be seen with varying degrees of thrombosis and hemorrhage, but bleeding is usually the major symptom, particularly in acute cases. Both hemorrhagic and thrombotic complications may accompany DIC, often being manifested in the same patient. Thrombosis may predominate in chronic or low-grade DIC. Thrombotic complications can include deep venous thrombosis.

Acute DIC is severe and often life threatening. Its onset is rapid, and both fibrinogen and platelets may be depleted. Patients with chronic DIC may have mild manifestations of the disorder or be recognizable only by laboratory data. Hemorrhagic complications are also seen but are generally milder than in acute DIC.

Clinical manifestations of DIC include petechiae, purpura, hemorrhagic bullae, surgical wound bleeding, traumatic wound bleeding, venipuncture site bleeding, arterial line oozing, and subcutaneous hematomas.

TTP is a condition that is similar to DIC (Tables 24.16 and 24.17). In addition, pediatric respiratory distress syndrome (PRDS), adult respiratory distress syndrome (ARDS), HUS, preeclampsia or frank eclampsia, circulating immune complex, cavernous hemangiomas, and Rocky Mountain spotted fever can resemble DIC.

TABLE 24.15	Significant Laboratory Findings in Disseminated Intravascular Coagulation

Peripheral blood smear—fragmented RBC
Platelet count—decreased
Fibrinogen levels—decreased
Thrombin time—prolonged
Reptilase time—prolonged
aPTT and PT—prolonged
Fibrin split products (FSPs)—present
Ethanol gel or protamine sulfate test—positive
Other tests—euglobulin clot lysis time, antithrombin III, coagulation factor assays, and plasminogen level abnormal

TABLE 24.16	Comparative Test Results in Diagnosing Various Forms of Acute Consumptive Coagulopathy		
Test	**Clotting and Lysis**	**Clotting**	**Lysis**
Fibrinogen	Decreased	Decreased	Decreased
Platelets	Decreased	Decreased	Decreased or normal
Fibrin split products	Positive	Negative	Positive
Fibrin monomers	Positive	Positive	Negative
D-dimer	Positive	Negative	Negative

Laboratory Findings

Although the quantitative measurement of FSPs cannot distinguish between primary and secondary fibrinolysis, such measurement plays the major role in diagnosing and monitoring these conditions. Laboratory diagnosis of DIC requires the availability of tests that are rapid and simple to perform. There is no single test that confirms the diagnosis, but rather a combination of tests. Because DIC is a dynamic process, values from tests performed a single time, whether normal or abnormal, cannot be used as diagnostic indicators. Sequential testing is necessary to provide an accurate diagnosis and effectively manage therapy. The most important consideration in the treatment of DIC is the resolution of the underlying disease or triggering event.

Tests for Fibrinolysis and DIC

Because the manifestations of fibrinolysis and DIC are extremely variable, diagnosis depends on laboratory testing. Coagulation assays such as the platelet count, fibrinogen levels, FSP test, factor V assay, ethanol gelation test, and thrombin time–reptilase test can all be useful. Prekallikrein and

AT-III have also been suggested to be of prognostic value. The key feature is an elevation of circulating fibrinogen-FSPs.

Typical results in DIC include prolonged aPTT, PT, and thrombin time and an increased level of D-dimers. Fibrinogen levels and the total platelet count may vary, although thrombocytopenia and a decrease in fibrinogen are common. The platelet count decreases earlier than fibrinogen in endotoxin-induced DIC. The reverse is true when tissue factor release is responsible, such as in obstetrical accidents or trauma. Excessive fibrinolysis with the release of FSPs occurs secondary to intravascular fibrin formation. Although the presence of FSPs is characteristic, the finding is not specific for DIC and cannot be used as the sole criterion for diagnosis.

Disorders Related to Elevated Fibrin Split Products

The normal level of serum FSPs is less than 10 µg/mL. Serum values can vary owing to exercise or stress. Elevated urinary levels are always indicative of a disease state. High levels of FSPs indicate renal dysfunction. Normal urinary FSP values

TABLE 24.17	Disseminated Intravascular Coagulation Compared With Thrombotic Thrombocytopenia Purpura		
	Clinical Manifestations	**Laboratory Abnormalities**	**Micropathological Findings**
TTP	Unexplained fever; central nervous system dysfunction; renal failure in 11%	Thrombocytopenia; FDP/FSP mildly elevated in 50%; hemolytic anemia with and schistocytes fragmented red cells	Microvascular thrombosis with impaired fibrinolysis
DIC	Fever; hypotension; hemorrhage; thrombosis; shock	Thrombocytopenia; anemia; schistocytes and fragmented red cells; elevated FDP/FSP	Microvascular thrombosis; fibrin deposition; active fibrinolysis
	Wide variety of underlying illnesses; all ages		

TTP, thrombotic thrombocytopenia purpura; DIC, disseminated intravascular coagulation; FDP, fibrin degradation products; FSP, fibrin split products.

are generally less than 0.25 µg/mL but may rise to as high as 50 µg/mL in certain kidney disorders.

Elevated levels of FSPs can be found in diseases of the neonate, in sepsis, or in the DIC that these conditions may generate. In cases of pulmonary embolism, levels can exceed 100 µg/mL; however, in rare cases, values can reach more than 400 µg/mL. These excessively high levels return to near normal within 24 hours after the cessation of the disorder (e.g., sepsis). FSP levels are elevated, frequently as high as 80 µg/mL, in cases of mild chronic intravascular coagulation, which occurs when the placenta slowly releases thromboplastic substances into the circulation. The FSP test can help distinguish between eclampsia and hypertension and edema associated with pregnancy.

THE HYPERCOAGULABLE STATE

Systemic inflammation has long been recognized as being associated with hypercoagulability. It commonly occurs in patients with DIC in severe sepsis. Recently, the molecular basis of the influence of inflammation has been recognized. Most of the hypercoagulable effects of inflammation are mediated by inflammatory cytokines, including IL-1, IL-6 and tumor necrosis factor (TNF).

The processes of coagulation, thrombosis, and inflammation do not occur in isolation. There is interaction between these systems. Thrombosis and coagulation can act as triggers for inflammation, and severe or systemic inflammatory responses can trigger coagulation. A laboratory assay, high-sensitivity C-reactive protein (hsCRP), may herald an impending acute thrombotic event.

Thrombi may form because coagulation is enhanced or because protective devices such as fibrinolysis are impaired. An increase in the likelihood of blood to clot is referred to as the **hypercoagulable state**.

Thrombosis is promoted by vascular damage, by retarded blood flow, and by alterations in the blood that increase the likelihood of clotting. A variety of high- and low-incidence disorders are associated with thrombosis (Box 24.3). A number of factors may contribute to hypercoagulation.

Primary States of Hypercoagulability

Hypercoagulable states include various inherited and acquired clinical disorders characterized by an increased risk for thromboembolism. Primary hypercoagulable states (Table 24.18) include relatively rare inherited conditions that lead to disordered endothelial cell thromboregulation. These conditions include decreased thrombomodulin-dependent activation of APC, impaired heparin binding of AT-III, or downregulation of membrane-associated plasmin generation.

The major inherited inhibitor disease states include AT-III deficiency, protein C deficiency, and protein S deficiency. These conditions should be considered in patients who have recurrent, familial, or juvenile deep venous thrombo-

Thrombotic Disorders

EXAMPLES OF HIGH-INCIDENCE DISORDERS
APC resistance (factor V [Leiden] and related mutations)
Antiphospholipid antibody syndrome

EXAMPLES OF LOW-INCIDENCE DISORDERS
Antithrombin deficiency
Essential thrombocytopenia
Heparin-induced thrombocytopenia
Protein C or S deficiency
Thrombotic thrombocytopenic purpura

sis or occlusion in an unusual location such as a mesenteric, brachial, or cerebral vessel.

Secondary States of Hypercoagulability

Secondary hypercoagulation states may be seen in a number of heterogeneous disorders. In many of these conditions, endothelial activation by cytokines leads to the loss of normal vessel-wall anticoagulant surface functions, with conversion to a proinflammatory thrombogenic phenotype. Important clinical syndromes associated with substantial thromboembolic events include the APS, heparin-induced thrombopathy, myeloproliferative syndromes, and cancer.

Hypercoagulability can be associated with systemic inflammation due primarily to an increase in procoagulant functions, an inhibition of fibrinolysis, and a downregulation of the three major physiologic anticoagulant systems of protein C, AT-III, and tissue factor inhibitor.

Pregnancy-Associated Thrombosis

Normal pregnancy beginning at the time of conception is associated with increased concentrations of coagulation factors VII, VIII, and X and von Willebrand factor. In addition, a significant change in fibrinogen is noted. Free protein S, the active, unbound form, is decreased during pregnancy. Plasminogen activator inhibitor type 1 (PAI-1) levels are increased fivefold. PAI-2 produced by the placenta increases significantly during the third trimester. Thrombin generation markers, for example, prothrombin F1+2, and thrombin-antithrombin (TAT) complexes are also increased. It may take up to 8 weeks after delivery (postpartum) for the levels of the cited constituents to return to the reference range.

Pregnant women have an increased risk of thromboembolism due to hypercoagulability. The condition of hypercoagulability in pregnancy is most likely evolved to protect women

TABLE 24.18	Primary and Secondary Hypercoagulable States	
Primary Hypercoagulable States	**Secondary Hypercoagulable States**
Antithrombin II deficiency	Cancer
Protein C deficiency	Pregnancy
Protein S deficiency	Oral contraceptive use
Fibrinolytic abnormalities	Nephrotic syndrome
Hypoplasminogenemia	Myeloproliferative disorders
Dysplasminogenemia	Hyperlipidemias
Tissue plasminogen activator release deficiency	Diabetes mellitus
	Paroxysmal nocturnal hemoglobinuria
Increased levels of plasminogen	Postoperative states
activator inhibitor	Vasculitis
Dysfibrinogenemia	APS
Homocystinuria	Increased levels of factor VII and fibrinogen
Heparin cofactor II deficiency	Anticancer drugs
Increased levels of histidine-rich GP	Heparin thrombocytopenia
	Obesity

against the bleeding challenges of childbirth or miscarriage. Pregnant women are at a four- to fivefold increased risk of thromboembolism during pregnancy and the postpartum period compared to nonpregnant women. Eighty percent of the thromboembolic events in pregnancy are venous with an incidence of 0.49 to 1.72 per 1,000 pregnancies.

Risk factors for developing hypercoagulability include

- History of thrombosis
- Inherited and acquired thrombophilia
- Maternal age less than 35 years of age
- Certain medical conditions and/or complications of pregnancy and childbirth

General Features

Vascular Damage and Blood Flow

Vascular endothelial damage exposes circulating blood to subendothelial structures that initiate thrombosis. Constriction of blood vessels additionally creates stasis. Thrombosis can begin in areas of low blood flow or in situations in which the viscosity of blood is increased. In patients with a high risk of thrombosis, the concentration of fibrinogen is often elevated. High concentrations of fibrinogen may induce aggregation of circulating erythrocytes, which produces increased blood viscosity. This may encourage thrombosis by decreas-

ing the blood flow at critical sites with the accumulation of activated clotting factors.

Platelets

Stasis makes it easier for platelets to be detached from flowing blood. An increase in the number of circulating platelets may create a tendency toward thrombosis. Platelets accumulate at the site of vascular damage, where they can furnish phospholipid for the intrinsic pathway and also promote thrombin formation by adsorbing activated factor X from plasma to their surfaces. High platelet counts additionally foster thrombosis.

Another possibility is that a thrombotic tendency may be caused by qualitative alterations in platelets. These alterations may be caused by intrinsic platelet defects or by changes in the surrounding plasma. Qualitative abnormalities may result in spontaneous aggregation, enhanced sensitivity to aggregating agents, or increased adhesiveness.

Blood Clotting Factors

Congenital and acquired hypercoagulable states arise when there is an imbalance between the anticoagulant and prothrombotic activities of plasma in which the prothrombotic activities predominate.

A tendency toward thrombophilia (abnormal thrombosis) may be caused by qualitative alterations in blood clotting factors or an increased titer of activated clotting factors that can create a tendency toward thrombosis. These factors can contribute to thrombosis in that activated factors might reach critical levels in the circulating blood.

Factor V (Leiden)

The factor V gene is an autosomal, codominantly inherited gene. Factor V R506Q (Leiden) mutation is the most common underlying genetic cause of thrombophilia (e.g., venous thrombosis).

Factor V (Leiden) mutation results from a G-A point mutation that results in an Arg^{506}-Gly substitution in the protein. This mutation renders factor V resistant to the activity of APC and induces a defect in the natural anticoagulation system. The overall effect of this mutation is an alteration in the anticoagulant properties of factor V.

Factor V, like thrombin, possesses both anticoagulant and procoagulant properties. The APC-mediated cleavages, if performed on factor V, transform it into an APC cofactor (FVac). FVac acts in unison with APC and protein S to increase the rate of inactivation of factor VIII.

In contrast to other coagulopathies, factor V (Leiden) poses a lifelong risk of deep venous thrombosis with a greater frequency of occurrence of thrombi in the lower limbs than in the chest. Fortunately, everyone who has the mutation will not suffer a thrombotic event. Heterozygotes have a low (approximately 10%) lifetime risk, but homozygotes can experience a 50- to 100-fold increase in risk.

Laboratory Assessment

A panel of assays is required to assess hypercoagulability. Functional screening tests include the following:

- PT
- Activate and partial thromboplastin time (aPTT)
- Lupus anticoagulant (LA) screening
- Factor VIII and fibrinogen (factor I) assays
- APC assay
- Protein C and protein S assays
- D-dimer screening test

In addition, acute-phase reactants (e.g., C-reactive protein [CRP]) may be assayed.

Traditionally, the APC resistance assay identifies patient insensitivity to APC. The assay is based on the aPTT assay with and without reagent APC. The aPTT in the presence of APC (CaCl$_2$/APC) is divided by the unaltered (CaCl$_2$) aPTT to yield a unitless ratio. A ratio of greater than 2 (a longer clotting time) generally indicates an unaffected condition. A ratio of less than 2 (a shorter clotting time) indicates a potential factor V (Leiden) mutation and resistance to APC. Factor V–deficient plasma may be added to the test system to correct for any existing factor deficiencies. The APC resistance assay may be affected by other conditions (e.g., LA, elevated factor VIII and fibrinogen levels, oral contraceptive use, or pregnancy).

Another method of testing for the mutation is by a dilute Russell's viper venom time (DRVVT) based test. The DRWT

method avoids limitations inherent in the aPTT-based method, which requires a normal baseline aPTT and may be affected by high concentrations of factor VIII, LA, and anticoagulant therapy. The DRWT also eliminates the technical requirement of prediluted patient samples with factor V deficient plasma.

Genetic Testing

Single-nucleotide polymorphisms (SNPs) are major contributors to genetic variation, comprising approximately 80% of all known polymorphisms. Their density in the human genome is estimated to be on average 1 per 1,000 base pairs. APC-resistant patients may be confirmed for factor V (Leiden) mutation by DNA PCR amplification of a segment of the potentially affected gene. General population screening is not recommended. At this point, the recommendations for testing focus primarily on individuals younger than age 50 who have already had an idiopathic thrombotic event.

The three most common assays ordered to investigate a genetic predisposition to thrombosis are

1. Factor V (Leiden)
2. Prothrombin mutation
3. Methylenetetrahydrofolate reductase enzyme (MTHFR)

Prothrombin (factor II) mutation leads to an increased risk of cerebral vascular thrombosis. MTHFR deficiency leads to hyperhomocysteinemia that may injure the vascular endothelium. It may play a role in venous thromboembolism. These three assays can be performed simultaneously by analyzing genomic DNA in peripheral blood mononuclear cells using polymerase chain reaction (PCR).

Circulating Anticoagulants

Acquired inhibitors of clotting proteins, also known as circulating anticoagulants, inactivate or inhibit the usual procoagulant activity of coagulation factors. Inhibitors are frequently characterized as specific, those directed against a coagulation factor, or nonspecific, those directed against a complex of factors, such as the LA.

The majority of these inhibitors exhibit biochemical properties, suggesting that they are immunoglobulins. Inhibitors may arise following transfusion of blood products or in patients with no previous hemostatic disorders. Acquired inhibitors can be a significant cause of hemorrhage.

Specific inhibitors against factors II, V, VII, VIII, IX, XII, XIII, and vWF have been detected in patients with individual factor deficiencies. However, some inhibitors of factors II, V, VII, IX, XII, and vWF have been observed in patients having no deficiencies of coagulation factors. Patients with acquired specific inhibitors may exhibit hemorrhagic episodes, whereas nonspecific inhibitors are not generally associated with bleeding tendencies.

Etiology

The incidence of circulating anticoagulants has been benchmarked at 0.75% of the general population, but certain patient populations have a higher incidence of inhibitor development. Inhibitors, found in both serum and plasma, are not inactivated by heating at 56°C for 30 minutes and remain stable when stored at −20°C. Inhibitors are more stable than clotting factors and more tolerant of changes in pH and temperature. Inhibitors may remain in the circulation for months and in some instances have been found in patients years after development.

Specific Inhibitors

Antiphospholipid Antibodies (Lupus Anticoagulant and Anticardiolipin Antibodies)

The **lupus anticoagulant (LA)** occurs in approximately 30% to 40% of patients with SLE. LA is the most common coagulation inhibitor found in SLE patients, although these patients may have other acquired inhibitors as well. LA occurs in the presence of disease states other than SLE, such as acquired immunodeficiency syndrome (AIDS) and malignancy, and in procainamide, hydralazine, or chlorpromazine therapy. Although LA exhibits an anticoagulant effect, it is rarely associated with bleeding.

LA, an IgM, IgG, or IgA immunoglobulin, interferes with phospholipid-dependent coagulation reactions in laboratory assays but does not inhibit the activity of any specific coagulation factor. LA is an inhibitor that prolongs phospholipid-dependent clotting tests in vitro. LA is the most common cause of prolonged aPTT.

In 1995, the Subcommittee on Lupus Anticoagulant Standardization Committee published criteria (Box 24.4) for the diagnosis of LA. This guideline recommends at least two screening tests based on different assay principles. In addition, a mixing study for the verification of the presence of a coagulation inhibitor and a confirmation test for the documentation of phospholipids dependency should also be performed. All assays should be performed on citrate anticoagulated specimens that are platelet poor and free of underlying defects.

In comparison, anticardiolipin antibodies (ACAs), IgM, IgG, or IgA immunoglobulins, bind to the phospholipids cardiolipin in the presence of beta 2-GP 1-cardiolipin complex. It may be detected in healthy patients and in those with a variety of conditions (e.g., SLE).

LA and ACA are risk factors for thrombosis but the mechanism of action is unclear.

Antiphospholipid Syndrome

The APS is defined by the persistent presence of antiphospholipid antibodies. APS is a prothrombotic disorder with various manifestations in patients with a history of recurrent venous or arterial thromboembolism or a history of miscarriages. APS is an important cause of acquired thrombophilia. APS can occur alone or in association with other autoimmune conditions, particularly SLE. The core clinical manifestation is thrombosis. In women, it can be associated with recurrent fetal loss. Fetal morbidity and mortality may be due to factors such as placental thrombosis and placental inflammation due to complement activation.

Antiphospholipid antibodies include

- LA
- Anticardiolipin antibodies
- Anti-β2-glycoprotien-1 antibodies. In the laboratory, elevated levels of antibody are required to establish a diagnosis. The predominant antigenic targets in APS are β 2-GP I and prothrombin. Complement activation is suspected because increased complement activation products have been found in APS patients who have suffered from a cerebral ischemic event. Dysregulated platelet activation may contribute to thrombotic manifestations. Elevated levels of platelet-derived thromboxane metabolic breakdown products have been demonstrated in the urine of APS patients.

Factor VIII Inhibitor

Factor VIII inhibitors are the most common specific factor inhibitors. Inhibitors of factor VIII develop in 10% to 15% of patients with factor VIII deficiency (hemophilia A), and the majority occur in patients with severe hemophilia (those having less than 1% factor VIII activity). Inhibitors have developed in patients exposed to factor VIII after as few as 10-exposure days but may develop after several hundred days. Approximately 65% of patients with hemophilia who develop inhibitors do so before the age of 20. Nonhemophiliac women have been reported to develop factor VIII inhibitors during the postpartum period, most frequently after the birth of their first child. Patients with underlying immunological disorders such as RA, SLE, drug allergies, ulcerative colitis, and bronchial asthma also have an increased tendency to develop factor VIII inhibitors. Many patients have been observed to develop factor VIII inhibitors with no underlying disease. The majority of these patients are middle aged or older, and both genders are affected.

BOX 24.4

Criteria for the Laboratory Diagnosis of Lupus Anticoagulant

- Prolongation of a phospholipid-dependent clotting assay
- Evidence of an inhibitor demonstrated by a mixing study
- Evidence of a phospholipid-dependent inhibitor based on neutralization of the inhibitor effect with added phospholipids
- Lack of specific inhibition of any one coagulation factor

Source: Thrombosis and Haemostasis International Society on Thrombosis 74(4):1185–1190, 1995. Haemostasis (University of North Carolina, Chapel Hill, NC). Subcommittee on Lupus Anticoagulant Standardization Committee, Criteria for the Diagnosis of Lupus Anticoagulant.

Inhibitors against vWF occur in patients with von Willebrand disease, underlying diseases such as malignancy or SLE, and in previously healthy persons. A familial tendency for the development of vWF inhibitors has been noted.

Factor IX Inhibitor

Inhibitors are found in approximately 2% to 3% of factor IX–deficient (hemophilia B) patients, but the incidence of inhibitors in severe hemophilia B may be as high as 12%. Although these inhibitors are predominantly a result of transfusion of blood products, spontaneous inhibitor formation has been reported.

Factor V Inhibitor

Factor V inhibitors are rare and are not generally associated with hereditary factor V deficiency. Some patients have had exposure to streptomycin but no causal relationship has been established.

Fibrinogen, Fibrin, and Factor XIII Inhibitors

Inhibitors of fibrinogen, fibrin, and factor XIII have been reported. These inhibitors have occurred following plasma transfusions or appeared spontaneously. Some patients have a common denominator of taking isoniazid, an antituberculosis drug.

Factor II, VII, IX, and X Inhibitors

Factor II, VII, IX, and X inhibitors are rare. The causes for factor inhibitor development are varied and include congenital deficiencies, immune disorders, and amyloidosis.

Factor XI and XII Inhibitors

Inhibitors of factors XI and XII have been reported infrequently in patients with SLE, Waldenström macroglobulinemia, and other disorders, as well as with chlorpromazine administration.

Clinical Presentation

The LA is the most commonly acquired and has an interesting presentation. In the absence of other hemostatic abnormalities, the LA is rarely associated with bleeding tendencies, even with surgical procedures. Bleeding episodes in these patients are usually the result of thrombocytopenia or another anomaly. Paradoxically, patients with LA are at increased risk for arterial and venous thromboembolism. Venous thrombosis involving the leg veins, with associated pulmonary emboli, is the most frequent complication. Spontaneous abortion and intrauterine deaths are also increased in patients with LA.

The presence of a specific factor inhibitor can be suspected in patients with no history of bleeding episodes who experience hemorrhage from various sites or in hemophiliac patients not responsive to their usual dosage of blood product infusion. Bleeding episodes in hemophiliac patients with inhibitors do not appear to be any more frequent or severe than in patients without inhibitors. When hemorrhagic events do occur, treatment of a patient with inhibitor is difficult.

Nonhemophiliac patients with acquired inhibitors of factor VIII can have major bleeding requiring transfusion. Patients with inhibitors to vWF, factor XI, and factor XII do not generally exhibit a hemorrhagic tendency. However, therapy for these patients can be complicated by the presence of the inhibitor. Patients with acquired factor IX inhibitors have clinical courses similar to hemophilia A patients with inhibitors. Factor V inhibitors may cause clinical bleeding, although the degree of hemorrhage varies considerably. Inhibitors of factors XIII, II, VII, IX, and X; fibrin; or fibrinogen can result in serious hemorrhagic events.

Laboratory Findings

Prolonged PT or aPTT are classic laboratory findings. Incubation of patient's plasma with normal plasma at 37°C (mixing study) and determination of aPTT and PT may detect the presence of an inhibitor. The mixing study will be prolonged in the presence of an inhibitor. Inhibitors are more time and temperature stable than their specific clotting factors. To quantitate the levels of inhibitors, the Bethesda assay is most commonly used in the United States. One Bethesda unit is defined as the amount of antibody that will neutralize 50% of the inhibitor activity in a mixture of equal parts of normal plasma and antibody containing plasma that has been incubated for 2 hours at 37°C.

Detection of antiphospholipid antibody is based on prolongation of phospholipid-dependent coagulation assays. Antiphospholipid antibody is considered one of the most common causes of a prolonged aPTT. Assays include the Russell's viper venom time, kaolin clotting time, platelet neutralization procedure, and tissue thromboplastin inhibition test.

Impaired Fibrinolysis

Impaired fibrinolytic mechanisms have been noted to be both genetic and acquired in their origin. Impairment of fibrinolysis may predispose an individual to thrombosis. Patients with type II hyperlipoproteinemia caused by familial hypercholesterolemia demonstrate impairment of fibrinolysis. A high incidence of recurrent thrombosis has been noted in patients with hereditary deficiencies of protein C or AT-III. Protein S deficiency also joins the group of other plasma protein deficiencies associated with inherited thrombophilia (Table 24.19). Deficiencies of inhibitors to factors VIII and V have also been correlated with recurrent thrombosis.

Protein C Deficiencies

Protein C activity has been demonstrated to be related to the commonly occurring thrombotic episodes in patients with an inherited deficiency of protein C and protein S. However, the hypercoagulable state in patients with proteinuria is not caused by decreased levels of protein C. Elevated protein C levels may represent a protective mechanism to the hypercoagulable state in patients with proteinuria because the anticoagulant activities of AT-III and protein C are probably complementary.

TABLE 24.19	Prevalence of Congenital Deficiencies	
Deficient Protein	**All Patients**	**Patients With Recurrent Thrombosis**
Protein C	4%–8%	12%–18%
Protein S	2%–8%	15%–18%

Deficiencies of protein C and protein S can be acquired or congenital. Acquired deficiencies occur in DIC, severe liver disease, vitamin K deficiency, and oral anticoagulation therapy. Congenital deficiencies are transmitted in an autosomal dominant fashion. Thrombotic complications usually involve the venous system, although more recently protein S has been associated with arterial thrombosis as well.

Several types of protein C defects have been reported (Table 24.20). Type I protein C deficiency is characterized by low antigenic and functional levels of the protein. In those with type II deficiency, the antigenic level of protein C is normal, but the function of the molecule is impaired. Two subtypes of the type II defect have been described: classic type IIa, in which both chromogenic and clotting functional assays are abnormal, and type IIb, in which only the clotting functional method is abnormal. Protein C deficiencies should, accordingly, be screened by using a protein C functional assay (clot based or chromogenic), because this will detect both types I and II. Once a low level of protein C activity is determined, an immunological assay should be performed to distinguish type I from type II protein C deficiency.

Activated Protein C Resistance

APC resistance, a new discovery, has been added to the list of causes of thrombotic disease. APC resistance may be caused by an inherited deficiency of an anticoagulant factor that functions as a cofactor to APC. APC resistance appears to be inherited as an autosomal dominant trait, suggesting that a single gene is involved. It is possible that patients with severe APC resistance are homozygous for the genetic defect, whereas an APC response closer to the normal range indicates heterozygosity. The genetically determined defect in

anticoagulation characterized by resistance to APC is highly prevalent in patients with venous thrombosis. This defect appears to be at least 10 times more common in such patients than any of the other known inherited deficiencies of anticoagulant proteins. The anticoagulant cofactor that corrects inherited APC resistance is identical to unactivated factor V. APC-resistant plasma contains normal levels of factor V procoagulant, which suggests that APC resistance may be caused by a selective defect in an anticoagulant function of factor V (Fig. 24.2).

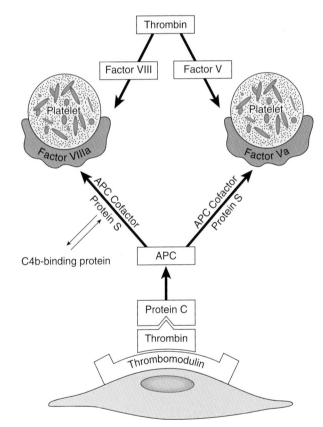

FIGURE 24.2. The protein C anticoagulant pathway. Thrombin converts factor VIII and factor V to their activated forms, factor VIIIa and factor Va. A complex of thrombin with the endothelial cell receptor thrombomodulin activates protein C. APC inactivates factor VIIIa and factor Va on the platelet surface, and this reaction is accelerated by APC cofactor and free protein S. (Adapted with permission from Bauer KA. Hypercoagulability—A new cofactor in the protein C anticoagulant pathway, *N Engl J Med*, 330(8):566, 1994. Copyright© 1994 Massachusetts Medical Society. All rights reserved.)

TABLE 24.20	Classification of Congenital Protein C Deficiency	
Classification	**Functional**	**Antigenic**
Type I	Decreased	Decreased
Type IIa	Decreased[a]	Normal
Type IIb	Normal/abnormal[b]	Normal

[a]Chromogenic and functional.
[b]Chromogenic is normal; clotting is abnormal.

TABLE 24.21	Classification of Congenital Protein S Deficiency			
Classification	Functional Clotting	Free PS Antigen	Total PS Antigen	C4b-BP
Type I	Decreased	Decreased	Decreased	—
Type II	Decreased	Normal	Normal	—
Type III	Decreased	Decreased	Normal	Normal
Acute-phase reaction	Decreased	Decreased	Normal	Increased

Protein S Deficiency

Familial studies indicate that patients with a deficiency of protein S have an increased incidence of thrombosis. Early descriptions indicate that protein S deficiency is much more common than either protein C or AT-III deficiency.

The congenital deficiency of protein S is associated with an increased risk of recurrent juvenile venous and arterial thromboembolism. The association of a thrombotic diathesis with acquired protein S deficiency is less clear cut.

Congenital Protein S Deficiency

Diagnosis of protein S deficiency differs significantly from that of vitamin K–dependent plasma proteins owing to protein S binding with C4b-BP and repartitioning between free (functional) and bound (nonfunctional) forms. The classification of congenital protein S is based on the comparison of functional and antigenic (free and total) as well as C4b-BP levels (Table 24.21). Currently, three types of congenital deficiencies have been identified: type I, low functional and antigenic protein S levels; type II, low functional protein S levels with a normal antigenic repartition (molecule dysfunctional); and type III, low functional protein S levels corresponding to a decrease in free antigenic protein S along with a normal C4b-BP. However, a decrease in free/functional protein S caused by increased synthesis of C4b-BP can occur transiently during acute-phase reactions.

A protein S functional assay should be used to screen for all types of protein S deficiencies. Antigenic levels of both free and total forms of protein, as well as C4b-BP, will then be determined to differentiate types I, II, and III.

Antithrombin III Deficiency

Hereditary defects of AT-III may be caused by quantitative or qualitative defects. Quantitative deficiency of AT-III is transmitted as an autosomal dominant disorder. Type I (quantitative) deficiencies represent the majority of cases. Familial studies reveal that severe thromboembolic problems usually begin to be manifested in late adolescence or early adulthood. Manifestations of AT-III deficiency are rare

in infancy. Women with the deficiency have a much higher incidence of thrombosis because pregnancy, delivery, and oral contraceptives are causative factors.

Defects of a qualitative nature (type II deficiency) are often characterized by decreased heparin cofactor activity. This functional manifestation of defective AT-III is not associated with a reduction in molecular concentration. More than half of patients with type II deficiency develop recurrent deep venous thrombosis.

Decreased AT-III Levels: Congenital

The relative incidence of congenital AT-III deficiency is between 1:2,000 and 1:5,000. AT-III deficiency is inherited as an autosomal dominant disorder. Homozygotes have not been reported in AT-III deficiency. Patients manifest signs and symptoms of between 10 and 30 years of age, their first thrombotic event. An initial event is spontaneous in approximately half of patients. Women frequently experience manifestations during pregnancy or because of oral contraceptive use. Decreased levels of AT-III usually correlate with the severity of venous thrombosis. Arterial thrombosis is a less common finding in AT-III deficiency.

Decreased AT-III Levels: Acquired

Acquired AT-III deficiency can be caused by decreased synthesis, increased consumption, or other disorders; it can also be drug induced. The associated disorders are

> Decreased synthesis: arteriosclerosis, cardiovascular disease, chronic hepatitis, cirrhosis, type II diabetes mellitus
> Increased consumption: DIC, homocystinuria, nephrotic syndrome, postoperative, postpartum, protein-losing enteropathy, pulmonary embolism, stroke, thrombophlebitis
> Drug induced: fibrinolysin, heparin, L-asparaginase, oral contraceptives
> Other disorders: burns, malignancies

Heparin Cofactor Deficiency

Although deficiency of AT-III is the most common, recurrent thrombotic complications have been associated with a deficiency of heparin cofactor II. The latter defect is inherited in an autosomal dominant manner. Sympathetic heterozygous patients exhibit about half the normal plasma levels of heparin cofactor II activity. This deficiency results from defective protein synthesis rather than from a qualitative abnormality. Heparin cofactor II deficiency can also be demonstrated in patients with DIC. In these situations, both AT-III and heparin cofactor II levels are diminished in parallel.

Clinical Signs and Symptoms

Clinical presentations of patients with deficiencies of naturally occurring anticoagulants are similar. Deficiencies of 50% of normal for protein C, protein S, and AT-III may lead to serious thrombotic events. Frequent presenting conditions include thrombophlebitis, deep venous thrombosis, and pulmonary emboli. The frequency of protein deficiencies correlated with recurrent thromboembolic disease is as follows:

Protein S: 5% to 10%
Protein C: 7%
AT-III: 2% to 4%

Venous Thromboembolism

Venous thromboembolism has an incidence of 300,000 episodes per year in the United States, and the complication of pulmonary embolism causes 5% to 10% of all deaths in the hospital. Venous thrombosis can result from hereditary or acquired factors or both.

Patients with venous thromboembolism can be divided into two groups. The first group includes patients with a disease such as cancer, a predisposing factor such as recent surgery, or an acquired abnormality such as the LA that is known to increase the risk of thrombosis. The pathophysiology is poorly understood (Table 24.22).

A second category consists of patients without the usual risk factors that predispose people to venous thrombosis. In some of these patients, it is possible to identify a deficiency of AT-III, protein C, or protein S, and family studies show hereditary defects. APC resistance occurs in about one third of patients. Precipitating factors for thrombosis, such as pregnancy and the use of oral contraceptives, are identified in 60% of these patients. APC resistance appears to be 5 to 10 times more common than a deficiency of AT-III, protein C, or protein S in patients with venous thrombosis.

Laboratory Assessment of Hypercoagulable States

Four major areas of clinical testing are available to evaluate a patient for hypercoagulability. These categories are

1. Natural anticoagulants—protein C deficiency, protein S deficiency, factor V (Leiden), antithrombin deficiency, and heparin cofactor II deficiency
2. Fibrinolysis—plasminogen deficiency, poor tissue plasminogen activator release, excessive plasminogen activator inhibitor, and dysfibrinogenemia

TABLE 24.22 Hypercoagulable States Associated With Venous Thrombosis

Hypercoagulable State	Comments
Mutation in factor V gene	Replaces arginine 506 with glutamine, rendering factor V resistant to inactivation by activated protein
Mutation in protein C gene	Associated with protein C deficiency
Protein S deficiency	Protein S is a cofactor for protein C
Antithrombin III deficiency	Autosomal dominant inheritance
Antiphospholipid antibodies	Encompasses ACAs and LA; associated with venous and arterial thrombosis
Elevated concentration of factor VIII	Relative risk of venous thrombosis is fivefold higher among patients with factor V concentrations greater than 1,500 IU/L
Frequency in venous thrombosis	
Protein C, 2%–4%	
Protein S, 2%–5%	
Antithrombin, 1%–3%	
Plasminogen, 0.5%–2%	

Source: Goldhaber SZ. Deep vein thrombosis and pulmonary embolism. In: *Intensive Review of Internal Medicine*, Boston, MA: Harvard University, 1995:75.

3. Antiphospholipid antibodies—ACAs, LA
4. Hyperhomocysteinemia

CHAPTER HIGHLIGHTS

Vascular Disorders

Abnormal bleeding involving the loss of red blood cells from the microcirculation expresses itself as **purpura**, which is characterized by hemorrhages into the skin, mucous membranes, and internal organs.

Purpura may be associated with a variety of vascular abnormalities including direct endothelial cell damage, an inherited disease of the connective tissue, decreased mechanical strength of the microcirculation, mechanical disruption of small venules, microthrombi (small clots), and vascular malignancy.

Abnormal Platelet Morphology

When examining a peripheral blood smear for platelets, the morphology of the platelets should be observed. Abnormal variations in size should be noted. Disorders of platelet size include Wiskott-Aldrich syndrome, May-Hegglin anomaly, Alport syndrome, and Bernard-Soulier syndrome.

Quantitative Platelet Disorders

The normal range of circulating platelets is 150×10^9/L to 450×10^9/L. When the quantity of platelets decreases to levels below this range, a condition of thrombocytopenia exists. If the quantity of platelets increases, thrombocytosis is the result.

Thrombocytopenia can result from a wide variety of conditions, such as following the use of extracorporeal circulation in cardiac bypass surgery or in alcoholic liver disease. HIT and associated thrombotic events, relatively common side effects of heparin therapy, can cause substantial morbidity and mortality. Most thrombocytopenic conditions can be classified into the major categories of disorders of production, disorders of destruction, and disorders of platelet distribution and dilution.

Decreased production of platelets may be caused by hypoproliferation of the megakaryocytic cell line or ineffective thrombopoiesis caused by acquired conditions or hereditary factors.

Thrombocytopenia caused by hypoproliferation can result from acquired damage to hematopoietic cells of the bone marrow caused by factors such as irradiation, drugs and cancer chemotherapeutic agents, chemicals, and alcohol. Hypoproliferation may also result from nonmalignant conditions, such as infections, lupus erythematosus, granulomatous disease such as **sarcoidosis**, and idiopathic causes. Ineffective thrombopoiesis may result in decreased platelet production. Thrombocytopenias of this type may be the manifestation of a nutritional disorder, such as a deficiency of vitamin B_{12} or folic acid.

Another disorder related to ineffective thrombopoiesis is iron deficiency anemia, which usually results in a decrease in megakaryocyte size and the suppression of megakaryocyte endoproliferation and size. Hereditary thrombocytopenias include Fanconi syndrome, constitutional aplastic anemia and its variants, amegakaryocytic thrombocytopenia (TAR syndrome), X-linked amegakaryocytic thrombocytopenia, Wiskott-Aldrich syndrome, May-Hegglin anomaly, and hereditary macrothrombocytopenia (e.g., Alport syndrome).

Increased destruction or utilization of platelets may result from a number of mechanisms. It can be caused by antigens, antibodies, drugs, or foreign substances. Bacterial sepsis causes increased destruction of platelets owing to the attachment of platelets to bacterial antigen-antibody immune complexes. Antibodies of either autoimmune or isoimmune origin may produce increased destruction of platelets.

Accelerated consumption of platelets is another cause of thrombocytopenia. One of the most important and frequently encountered forms of increased consumption of platelets is ITP. This antibody-related response, which may be preceded by infection, is believed to have a devastating effect on platelet survival. ITP may complicate other antibody-associated disorders such as SLE. Patients with ITP usually demonstrate petechiae, bruising, menorrhagia, and bleeding after minor trauma.

Disorders of Platelet Distribution

A platelet distribution disorder can result from a pooling of platelets in the spleen, which is frequent if splenomegaly is present. This type of thrombocytopenia develops when more than a double or triple increase in platelet production is required to maintain the normal quantity of circulating platelets.

Thrombocytosis is generally defined as a substantial increase in circulating platelets over the normal upper limit of 450×10^9/L. Thrombocytosis is usually grouped according to cause: reactive or benign etiologies versus platelet elevations linked to a specific hematological disorder.

Qualitative Platelet Disorders

If platelets are normal in number but fail to function properly, one of four separate categories of platelet dysfunction can exist. These include the more common acquired and less frequent hereditary causes. Hyperactive platelets associated with hypercoagulability and thrombosis make up an additional category of abnormal platelet function.

Acquired platelet function defects can be caused by a blood plasma inhibitory substance. In addition, acquired platelet dysfunction is commonly seen in the myeloproliferative syndromes and uremia. Miscellaneous disorders can be associated with platelet dysfunction. Many drugs can induce platelet function defects, resulting in hemorrhage.

Hereditary disorders include adhesion disorder; Bernard-Soulier syndrome; primary aggregation disorders, such as Glanzmann thrombasthenia and essential athrombia; and secondary aggregation disorders, such as hereditary storage pool defect and hereditary aspirin-like defects.

Bleeding Disorders Related to Blood Clotting

Bleeding and defective fibrin clot formation are frequently related to a coagulation factor. Disorders of the blood coagulation factors can be grouped into three categories: defective production, excessive destruction, and pathological inhibition.

A condition of defective production may be related to a deficiency of vitamin K. Severe liver disease may produce decreased plasma levels of fibrinogen, although low levels of fibrinogen rarely produce hemorrhage. Hereditary clotting defects including classic hemophilia (hemophilia A) and von Willebrand disease are examples of hereditary disorders that represent functionally inactive factor VIII.

Hemophilia has been used as a paradigm for understanding the molecular pathological processes that underlie hereditary disease. The cloning of factor VIII facilitated the identification of mutations that lead to hemophilia A, an inherited deficiency of factor VIII coagulant activity that causes severe hemorrhage. von Willebrand disease may be an acquired or inherited disorder. The congenital disorder is autosomally dominant in most cases. Three broad types of von Willebrand disease are recognized. In addition, a platelet-type von Willebrand disease (pseudo–von Willebrand disease) is caused by an abnormal platelet receptor for vWF. Acquired von Willebrand disease may complicate other diseases such as lymphoproliferative and autoimmune disorders, and proteolytic degradation of vWF complicates myeloproliferative disorders.

A deficiency of factor IX is known as **hemophilia B** or **Christmas disease**. A deficiency of factor XI is referred to as **hemophilia C. Fibrinogen deficiency** as a genetic disorder may represent a defect of production or dysfunctional molecules. Hereditary deficiencies of the other coagulation factors are relatively rare. Examples of rare defects include **factor XII deficiency**, in which no clinical bleeding tendencies are apparent, and **factor XIII deficiency**, which is associated with spontaneous abortion and poor wound healing.

Disorders of Destruction and Consumption

Blood coagulation factors can be destroyed in vivo by enzymatic degradation or by pathological activation of coagulation with excessive utilization of the clotting factors. Enzymatic destruction can result from bites by certain species of snakes whose venom contains an enzyme that degrades fibrinogen to a defective fibrin monomer. In vivo activation of coagulation by tissue thromboplastin–like materials can produce excessive utilization of clotting factors. Conditions that can cause this consumption of coagulation factors include obstetrical complications, trauma, burns, prostatic and pelvic surgery, shock, advanced malignancy, septicemia, and intravascular hemolysis.

Primary and secondary fibrinolysis are recognized as extreme complications of a variety of intravascular and extravascular disorders and may have life-threatening consequences. Primary fibrinolysis is associated with conditions in which gross activation of the fibrinolytic mechanism with subsequent fibrinogen and coagulation factor consumption occurs. The important characteristic of primary fibrinolysis is that no evidence of fibrin deposition occurs. Primary fibrinolysis occurs when large amounts of plasminogen activator enter the circulatory system as a result of trauma, surgery, or malignancies.

Although the same clinical conditions may also induce secondary fibrinolysis or DIC, the distinction between the two is essentially in the demonstration of fibrin formation. In secondary fibrinolysis, excessive clotting and fibrinolytic activity occur. Increased amounts of FSPs and fibrin monomers are detectable because of the action of thrombin on the fibrinogen molecule. This fibrinolytic process is only caused by excessive clotting; therefore, it is a secondary condition. This distinguishes between primary and secondary fibrinolysis.

The Hypercoagulable State

Thrombi may form because coagulation is enhanced or because protective devices such as fibrinolysis are impaired. An increase in the likelihood of blood to clot is referred to as the **hypercoagulable state**.

Hypercoagulable states include various inherited and acquired clinical disorders characterized by an increased risk for thromboembolism. Primary hypercoagulable states include relatively rare inherited conditions that lead to disordered endothelial cell thromboregulation. These conditions include decreased thrombomodulin-dependent activation of APC, impaired heparin binding of AT-III, or downregulation of membrane-associated plasmin generation.

The major inherited inhibitor disease states include AT-III deficiency, protein C deficiency, and protein S deficiency. Secondary hypercoagulation states may be seen in many heterogeneous disorders.

Acquired inhibitors of clotting proteins, also known as circulating anticoagulants, inactivate or inhibit the usual procoagulant activity of coagulation factors. Inhibitors are frequently characterized as specific, those directed against a coagulation factor, or nonspecific, those directed against a complex of factors, such as the LA. The majority of these inhibitors exhibit biochemical properties, suggesting they are immunoglobulins. Inhibitors may arise following transfusion of blood products or in patients with no previous hemostatic disorders. Acquired inhibitors can be a significant cause of hemorrhage.

Specific inhibitors against factors II, V, VII, VIII, IX, XII, and XIII and vWF have been detected in patients with individual factor deficiencies. However, some inhibitors of factors II, V, VII, IX, and XII and vWF have been observed in patients having no deficiencies of coagulation factors.

CASE 24.1

A 2-year-old boy fell from a backyard gym set. His shoulder and upper arm became very swollen shortly after the fall. The boy's mother took him to the emergency department a few hours after the incident because he was complaining of pain. On physical examination, the physician noted that a large hematoma had formed in the upper part of the boy's right arm. There was no history of surgery (he had not been circumcised), injury, or illness. The boy was receiving no medication.

Emergency department treatment consisted of aspirating the hematoma. Subsequent to this treatment, the boy began to bleed extensively. He was admitted to the hospital.

The following STAT laboratory tests were ordered: a hemoglobin and hematocrit, platelet count, and bleeding time. Because the bleeding continued, a type and crossmatch for two units of fresh blood were ordered on a standby basis.

Additional information from the mother revealed that the boy's cousin had a "bleeding problem."

Laboratory Data

Hemoglobin 8.0 g/L
Hematocrit 26%
Platelet count 200 × 10⁹/L (normal, 150 to 450 × 10⁹/L)
Bleeding time 5 minutes (normal, 3 to 8 minutes)

Subsequent coagulation profile tests were ordered before the transfusion of two units of fresh whole blood. The results of these tests were as follows:

PT 12 seconds (normal, 11 to 15 seconds)
aPTT 60 seconds (normal, 28 to 35 seconds)
Thrombin time–reptilase method 20 seconds (normal, 18 to 22 seconds)

Questions

1. Do the laboratory data support a diagnosis of a disorder of hemostasis?
2. What types of disorders can be preliminarily identified by the tests that were performed?
3. What confirmatory tests must be done in this case?

Discussion

1. Yes, the abnormal results of the aPTT suggest that a coagulation defect may be the cause of this child's bleeding.
2. A normal platelet count and bleeding time suggest that platelets are not the causative agent in this bleeding disorder. Because the thrombin time was normal, a decrease or abnormality of fibrinogen and the presence of a circulating anticoagulant can be excluded.

By comparing the aPTT and PT, certain blood coagulation factors can be isolated as being deficient.

aPTT	PT	DEFICIENT FACTOR(S)
Increased	Normal	VIII, IX, XI, or XII
Increased	Increased	II, V, X, or anticoagulant
Normal	Increased	VII

In this case, an increased aPTT with a normal PT suggests that the patient is deficient in any of the following factors: VIII, IX, XI, or XII.

3. Factor substitution testing might be valuable before a specific factor assay is performed. This screening test is useful in isolating either specific factors or groups of factors that are deficient in a patient's plasma. To confirm a specific factor deficiency, a factor assay must be performed. In this case, a factor VIII assay revealed that the boy was deficient in factor VIII.

DIAGNOSIS: Factor VIII Deficiency (Hemophilia type A)

CASE 24.2

A 21-year-old black prison inmate was admitted to the hospital for the repair of an abdominal hernia. His physician was concerned that strangulation of the hernia could occur. The patient was in extremely good physical condition. He did not remember having any unusual illnesses. His family history did include minor bleeding problems among some of his relatives.

Laboratory Data

On admission, the hemoglobin and hematocrit were 15.0 g/L and 44%, respectively. The PT was 13 seconds (normal, 10 to 15 seconds), and the aPTT was 55 seconds (normal, 28 to 35 seconds).

Because of the results obtained on the original and a repeat specimen of the aPTT in conjunction with a vague family history of bleeding, this patient's surgery was postponed until a bleeding disorder could be ruled out.

Questions

1. What coagulation deficiencies might be present in this patient?
2. What supplementary laboratory assays would be appropriate?
3. How could this be distinguished from other similar disorders?

Discussion

1. As in Case 1, a prolonged aPTT with a normal PT suggests the presence of a deficiency of factor VIII, IX, XI, or XII. Because deficiencies of factors XI and XII are rare, it is unlikely that they would be responsible for the

(continued)

prolonged aPTT. Either a deficiency of factor VIII or IX would be more common.
2. Factor substitution studies would be valuable. If the substitution studies reveal an abnormality, a specific factor assay should be conducted.
3. In this case, factor VIII activity was found to be decreased (patient, 30% activity; normal, 50% to 150%). This finding and the lack of a bleeding history in the patient suggest that he may not have a classic factor VIII deficiency. Further testing was performed. The results were as follows: bleeding time increased, platelet aggregation decreased, factor VIII decreased, and factor VIII/vWF decreased. Based on these findings, the diagnosis of classic hemophilia was excluded. The laboratory findings support a diagnosis of von Willebrand disease.

DIAGNOSIS: von Willebrand Disease

CASE 24.3

A 62-year-old white man with a history of abnormal bleeding was admitted to the hospital for a medical workup before dental surgery. A brother had died at age 19 of traumatic bleeding after being injured in a car accident.

The patient had his first bleeding episode at 7 years of age following a lymph node resection. He reported having significant hemorrhaging as a teenager following mild trauma. At age 30, the patient had a tooth extraction followed by 3 weeks of bleeding, at which time he received a blood transfusion. At age 31, he was given a blood transfusion before an appendectomy and on that occasion had no bleeding whatsoever. Two years before admission, the patient suffered from gastrointestinal bleeding following surgery for a hiatal hernia. At that time, he was given two units of bank blood and two units of fresh blood. Bleeding subsided and his subsequent recovery was good.

Laboratory Data

The laboratory findings were as follows:

Hemoglobin 7.0 g/L
Hematocrit 23%
Platelet count 498×10^9/L
Bleeding time (Ivy) 2 minutes (normal, less than 8 minutes)
Whole blood clotting time averaged 188 minutes (normal, less than 70 minutes)
Platelet aggregation normal
aPTT 53 seconds (control, 39 seconds)
PT 13.8 seconds (control, 13.3 seconds)

Specific assays for factors VIII and IX were performed. The level of activity of factor IX was less than 5%.

Questions

1. What is the diagnosis in this case?

2. Can this patient safely undergo surgery?
3. What is the role of the laboratory in a surgical case of this type?

Discussion

1. The diagnosis in this case is factor IX deficiency.
2. Yes, but the patient received a factor IX concentrate rather than whole or fresh blood to correct the deficiency. He did receive two units of blood because of his low red cell volume.
3. Because factor IX has a half-life of 8 to 24 hours, it is important that the patient receives appropriate amounts of concentrates. A minimum static level of 20% to 30% must be achieved before and during surgery. The level of factor activity must be sustained until healing is sufficient to prevent breakthrough bleeding. The figure below depicts how the patient was monitored preoperatively and postoperatively. Each specimen was drawn within 30 minutes of the administration of the concentrate. The solid line denotes assay values; the broken line denotes therapeutic factor IX.

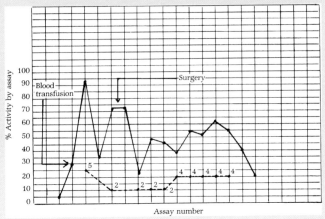

DIAGNOSIS: Hemophilia B (Christmas Disease)

CASE 24.4

A 22-year-old white woman had recently graduated from college and relocated to accept her first professional job. She was being seen for the first time by a local gynecologist because of prolonged menstrual bleeding. Her medical history included several episodes of severe nosebleeds during childhood that required cauterization to arrest. She reported that her menses lasted from 8 to 12 days. When questioned about family illnesses or disorders, she reported that her mother and two sisters also had long menstrual periods and that one of her two brothers needed several blood transfusions after an appendectomy.

Physical examination revealed an essentially normal patient. However, she appeared pale and several large bruises were noted on her extremities. The patient was

(continued)

referred to the outpatient laboratory for a hemoglobin, hematocrit, and coagulation profile.

Laboratory Data

Hemoglobin 10.0 g/L
Hematocrit 27%

Her coagulation profile results were as follows:

Bleeding time 7 minutes (normal, 1 to 3 minutes)
PT 11 seconds (control, 12.2 seconds)
aPTT 29 seconds (control, 34 seconds)
Clot retraction decreased

Questions

1. What additional tests would be suggested based on the initial laboratory results?
2. What would the Wright-stained blood film look like?
3. What is the most likely diagnosis and prognosis?

Discussion

1. A platelet count and qualitative platelet studies would be appropriate follow-up procedures in view of the prolonged bleeding time and poor clot retraction.
2. If a platelet disorder is suspected, the peripheral blood smear may be valuable. Obviously, decreases in platelets would support the quantitative assay and an abnormality in platelet size could be detected. In this case, both the distribution and morphology of the platelets appeared normal.
3. Further testing for platelet function revealed a deficiency in both platelet aggregation and adhesion. The diagnosis of Glanzmann thrombasthenia was made. This autosomal recessive disorder usually becomes less severe as a patient ages. In this woman's case, severe bleeding or future surgical interventions would need to be supported by the use of platelet concentrates.

DIAGNOSIS: Glanzmann Thrombasthenia

CASE 24.5

A woman was admitted in labor to the obstetrical unit at 11 PM. Her history and physical examination revealed no significant abnormalities. At the time of admission, she was having irregular contractions.

In the delivery room, bleeding became extensive. A STAT hemoglobin, hematocrit, type and crossmatch for four units of blood, and coagulation profile were ordered.

Laboratory Data

Hemoglobin 10.0 g/L
Hematocrit 27%
Platelet count 75×10^9/L
Bleeding time 10 minutes
aPTT 65 seconds (control, 29 seconds)
PT 19 seconds (control, 11 seconds)
Thrombin time 24 seconds (normal, 18 to 22 seconds)
Fibrinogen 90 mg/dL (normal, 200 to 400 mg/dL)
FSP screen positive
Protamine sulfate test positive

Questions

1. What is the most probable cause of the extensive bleeding in this case?
2. What is the etiology of this disorder?
3. Will the transfusion of whole or fresh blood repress the bleeding?

Discussion

1. The laboratory test results support the condition of fibrinolysis, specifically DIC. In secondary fibrinolysis as compared with primary fibrinolysis, the platelet count is decreased and the protamine sulfate test result is positive.
2. The release of placental tissue into the maternal circulation can trigger the coagulation mechanism. When this stimulation supersedes the body's natural protective mechanism, secondary bleeding occurs. In this case, the consumption of coagulation factors is evident in the laboratory findings.
3. Although transfusions may temporarily replace the blood volume lost through bleeding, they will not alleviate the problem. Overwhelming fibrinolysis can be fatal. In many cases, heparin is administered to stop the cyclical process that is in progress.

DIAGNOSIS: Disseminated Intravascular Coagulation (DIC)

REVIEW QUESTIONS

1. Which of the following is a condition associated with purpura?
   A. Direct endothelial damage
   B. Inherited disease of the connective tissue
   C. Mechanical disruption of small venules
   D. All of the above

Questions 2 through 4: Match the following platelet disorders with the appropriate morphology (use an answer only once).

2. _____ Wiskott-Aldrich syndrome
3. _____ May-Hegglin anomaly

(continued)

4. _____ Bernard-Soulier syndrome
   A. Giant platelets
   B. Smallest platelets seen
   C. Large platelets

Questions 5 through 7: Match the etiologies of these platelet dysfunctions with the appropriate associated disorder (use an answer only once).

5. _____ Acquired
6. _____ Drug induced
7. _____ Hereditary
   A. Aspirin
   B. von Willebrand disease
   C. Uremia

8. Which of the following parameters can be abnormal in classic von Willebrand disease type I?
   A. Bleeding time
   B. PT
   C. Platelet count
   D. All of the above

9. The most common form of von Willebrand disease is
   A. type I
   B. type II
   C. type III
   D. all have about the same incidence

10. Laboratory results in acute DIC reflect abnormalities in which of the following coagulation components?
   A. Platelet function
   B. Excessive clotting and fibrinolysis
   C. Accelerated thrombin formation
   D. Fibrin formation

11. Primary fibrinolysis is characterized by
   A. gross activation of the fibrinolytic mechanism
   B. consumption of fibrinogen
   C. consumption of coagulation factors
   D. all of the above

12. The hallmark of secondary fibrinolysis is the presence of
   A. fibrin split products
   B. fibrin degradation products
   C. fibrin monomers
   D. all of the above

13. DIC is characterized by
   A. microvascular thrombosis
   B. fibrin deposition
   C. active fibrinolysis
   D. all of the above

14. Which of the following factors can contribute to hypercoagulation?
   A. Vascular endothelial damage
   B. Increased blood flow
   C. Decreased platelets
   D. Decreased titers of clotting factors

Questions 15 through 19: Match the following.

15. _____ Antithrombin III deficiency
16. _____ Oral contraceptives
17. _____ Protein C deficiency
18. _____ Cancer
19. _____ Pregnancy
   A. Primary hypercoagulable state
   B. Secondary hypercoagulable state

Questions 20 through 22: Match the following terms with the appropriate description.

20. _____ Circulating anticoagulants
21. _____ LA
22. _____ Factor VIII inhibitor
   A. The most common specific factor inhibitor
   B. Acquired inhibitors of clotting proteins
   C. Also known as antiphospholipid or anticardiolipin

BIBLIOGRAPHY

Adcock DM. Is there a genetic relationship between arterial and venous thrombosis? *Clin Lab Sci*, 20(4):221–223, 2007.

Agapitov AV, Haynes WG. Role of endothelin in cardiovascular disease, *J Renin Angiotens Aldost Syst*, 3(1):1–15, 2002.

Arepally GM, Ortel TL. Heprin-induced thrombocytopenia, *N Engl Med*, 355(8):809–817, 2006.

Aster RH, Bougie DW. Drug induced immune thrombocytopenia, *N Engl Med*, 357(6):580–587, 2007.

Bates SM, Ginsberg JS. Treatment of deep-vein thrombosis, *N Engl Med*, 351(3):268–277, 2004.

Bernard GR, et al. Efficacy and safety of recombinant human activated protein C for severe sepsis, *N Engl J Med*, 344(10):699–709, 2001.

Bromberg ME. Immune thrombocytopenic purpura-the changing therapeutic landscape, *N Engl Med*, 355(16):1643–1645, 2006.

Canfield P, Perotta PL. Recognizing HIT, *Adv Lab*, 16(2):42–43, 2007.

Castellone D. A case study in coagulation, *Adv Lab*, 15(1):51–53, 2006.

Cazzola M. Molecular basis of thrombocytosis, *Haematologica*, 93(5):646–648, 2008.

Dahlbäck B. Advances in understanding pathogenic mechanisms of thrombophilic disorders, *Blood*, 112(1):19–27, 2008.

Danese S, et al. The protein C pathway in tissue inflammation and injury: pathogenic role and therapeutic implications, *Blood*, 115(6), 1121–1130, 2010.

Drygalski AV, et al. Vancomycin-induced immune thrombocytopenia, *N Engl Med*, 356(9):904–910, 2007.

Federici AB. VWF propeptide: a useful marker in VWD, *Blood*, 108(10):3229, 2006.

Fritsma GA. Managing the bleeding patient, *Clin Lab Sci*, 16(2): 107–110, 2003.

Fritsma GA, Marques MB. Top 10 problems in coagulation, *Adv Med Lab Prof*, 16(13):22–29, 2004.

Fritsma MG. Use of blood products and factor concentrates for coagulation therapy, *Clin Lab Sci*, 16(2):115–119, 2003.

Gardner J. Factor V Leiden with deep venous thrombosis, *Clin Lab Sci*, 16(1):6–9, 2003.

George JN, et al. Chronic idiopathic thrombocytopenic purpura, *N Engl J Med*, 331(18):1207–1215, 1994.

Giannakopoulos B, et al. Current comcepts on the pathogenesis of the antiphospholipid syndrome, *Blood*, 190(2):422–430, 2007.

Giannakopoulos B, et al. How we diagnose the antipholipid syndrome, *Blood*, 113(5):985–994, 2009.

Grody WW, Telatar M. Multiplex SNP analysis: Screening factor V R506Q (Leiden) mutations, *Am Biotechnol Lab*, 21(2):34–38, 2003.

Haberichter SL, et al. Assay of the von Willebrand factor (VWF) propeptide to identify patients with type 1 von Willebrand disease with decreased VWF survival, *Blood*, 108(10):3344–3351, 2006.

Hajjar KA. Factor V Leiden—An unselfish gene, *N Engl J Med*, 330(23):1585–1586, 1994.

Ingram GIC. The history of haemophilia, *J Clin Pathol*, 29(6):469–479, 1976.

Kakkar N, Gupta V. Spurious thrombocytopenia in a young male, *Labmedicine*, 39(8):463–464, 2008.

Kashyap AS, et al. Treatment of von Willebrand's disease, *N Engl J Med*, 351(22):2345, 2004.

Kasirer-Friede A, et al. Role of ADAP in shear flow-induced platelt mechanotransduction, *Blood*, 115(11), 2274–2282, 2010.

Kurtz ME. Diagnostic dilemmas of mild bleeding disorders, *Adv Lab*, 9(9):38–42, 2000.

Lambert MP. Childhood ITP:knowing when to worry? *Blood*, 114(23) 4758–4759, 2009.

Laposata M. Whom to monitor for hypercoagulability—Report of the CAP Consensus Conference on Thrombophilia Testing. Presented June 27, 2003, Cambridge, MA, *Curr Concept Clin Pathol.*

Lange RA, Hillis, LD. Concurrent antiplatelet and fibrinolytic therapy, *N Engl J Med*, 352(12):1248–1250, 2005.

Mannucci PM. Treatment of von Willebrand's diease, *N Engl J Med*, 351(7):683–694, 2004.

Marques MB. Treatment of single factor deficiencies: A case study approach, *Clin Lab Sci*, 16(2):120–122, 2003.

Martin VL, et al. D-dimer: more than just a number, Part 1, *Adv Lab*, 15(1):68, 2006.

Monahan PE, White GC. Hemophilia gene therapy: Update, *Curr Opin Hematol*, 9(5):430–436, 2002.

Moroose R, Hoyer LW. von Willebrand factor and platelet function, *Annu Rev Med*, 37:157–163, 1986.

Nachman RL, Silverstein R. Hypercoagulable states, *Ann Intern Med*, 119(8):819–827, 1993.

Passamonti F, et al. Prognostic factors for thrombosis, myelofibrosis, and leukemia in essential thrombocythemia: a study of 605 patients, *Haematologica*, 93(11):1645–1651, 2008.

Patrono C. Aspirin as an antiplatelet drug, *N Engl J Med*, 330(18): 1287–1294, 1994.

Peter K. Proteomics unravels platelet function, *Blood*, 115(20): 4008–4009, 2010.

Provan D, et al. International consensus report on the investigation and management of primary immune thrombocytopenia, *Blood*, 115(2), 168–186, 2010.

Rivera-Begeman A, et al. New-onset thrombocytopenia and anemia in a patient with a complex medical history, *Labmedicine*, 37(1): 24–27, 2006.

Refaai MA, Laposata M. A primer on bleeding and thrombotic disorders, *Adv Admin Lab* 12(4):46–55, 2003.

Refaai MA, Laposata M. Heparin-induced thrombocytopenia, *Clin Lab News*, 29(10):10–12, 2003.

Ridker PM, et al. Ethnic distribution of Factor V Leiden in 4047 men and women, *N Engl J Med*, 277(16):1305–1307, 1997.

Ridker PM, et al. Long-term, low-intensity warfarin therapy for the prevention of recurrent venous thromboembolism, *N Engl J Med*, 348(15):1425–1434, 2003.

Sadler JE. Von Willebrand factor, ADAMTS13, and thrombotic thrombocytopenic purpura, *Blood*, 112(1):11–18, 2008.

Schneider M. Thrombotic microangiopathy (TTP and HUS): advance in differentiation and diagnosis, *Clin Lab Sci*, 20(4):216–220, 2007.

Svensson PJ, Dahlback V. Resistance to activated protein C as a basis for venous thrombosis, *N Engl J Med*, 330(8):517–522, 1994.

Taylor LJ. Laboratory management of the bleeding patient, *Clin Lab Sci*, 16(2):111–114, 2003.

Thrasher AJ. New insights into the biology of Wiskott-Aldrich syndrome (WAS), *Am Soc Hematol*, Education Book, 132–136, 2009.

Triplett DA. Laboratory diagnosis of von Willebrand's disease, *Mayo Clin Proc*, 66:832–840, 1991.

Triplett DA. Coagulation and bleeding disorders: review and update, *Clin Chem*, 46(8B):1260–1269, 2000.

Van Cott EM. Heparin-induced thrombocytopenia and its management with new anticoagulants. Presented June 27, 2003, Cambridge, MA, *Curr Concept Clin Pathol.*

Wagner DD, Bonfanti R. von Willebrand factor and the endothelium, *Mayo Clin Proc*, 66:621–627, 1991.

Warkentin TE. Drug-induced immune-mediated thrombocytopenia from purpura to thrombosis, *N Engl J Med*, 356(9):891–893, 2007.

Williams JL. Introduction: new directions in hemostasis and coagulation, *Clin Lab Sci*, 20(4):215, 2007.

Williams JL. Cross talk between the inflammation and coagulation systems, *Clin Lab Sci*, 20(4):224–229, 2007.

Yarranton H, Machin SJ. Thrombotic thrombocytopenic purpura: New approaches to diagnosis and management, *Blood Ther Med*, 2(3):82–91, 2003.

PART SIX

Fundamentals of Hematological Analysis

CHAPTER **25** Body Fluid Analysis*

Introduction

■ Associate the various terms for body fluids with their respective synonyms.

Cerebrospinal fluid

■ Describe the anatomical structures involved in the circulation of cerebrospinal fluid (CSF).
■ Explain how CSF is produced.
■ Describe the collection procedure for CSF.
■ Name the appropriate type or types of testing for each of the aliquots of a specimen.
■ Compare the descriptive characteristics of CSF on gross examination and the respective associated abnormalities.
■ Describe the characteristics seen on microscopic examination and the associated disorders.
■ Name and describe cells unique to the CSF.

Pleural, peritoneal, and pericardial fluids

■ Define the term **effusion**.
■ Compare the major characteristics of transudates and exudates.
■ Identify the location of the pleura.
■ Name at least three disorders associated with the existence of pleural exudate.
■ Associate the various colors of exudate with the typical disorders.
■ Name at least two reasons for turbidity in pleural fluid.
■ Name the disorder that produces an extremely elevated total leukocyte count in pleural fluid.
■ Name the types of cells that can be encountered in pleural fluid.
■ Name the characteristics of malignant cells that can be found in a pleural effusion.
■ Discuss the cellular abnormalities encountered in pleural and peritoneal fluid.
■ Identify the location of the peritoneum.
■ Name at least three disorders or diseases that can cause a peritoneal effusion.
■ List at least two reasons for a turbid peritoneal effusion.
■ Associate a variety of conditions with various colors or appearances of peritoneal effusion.

■ Name several conditions that can produce a high total leukocyte count in peritoneal fluid.
■ List the types of cells that can be seen in peritoneal effusion and associate these cell types with a representative disorder.
■ Describe the anatomy of the pericardium.
■ Associate the various types and causes of pericardial effusion.
■ Name a cause of an increased total leukocyte count with mostly polymorphonuclear segmented neutrophils (PMNs).

Seminal fluid

■ Describe the anatomical structures and their respective cellular and/or chemical components.
■ Discuss the proper collection and handling of seminal fluid.
■ Name the normal number of sperm cells per milliliter or per liter.
■ Name the types of microscopic assays and the respective normal values.

Synovial fluid

■ Define the term **arthrocentesis**.
■ List at least three disorders that can be diagnosed definitively by synovial fluid analysis.
■ List several sites that may be aspirated.
■ Name the tests that should be included in the routine analysis of synovial fluid.
■ Name the procedures included in the gross examination of synovial fluid.
■ List and describe the types of crystals that may be observed in synovial fluid.
■ Describe the normal total cell count and differential in synovial fluid.
■ Compare the laboratory findings in noninflammatory and inflammatory arthritis.

Body fluid slide preparation

■ Compare the features of various methods of body fluid sediment preparation.
■ Differentiate the characteristics of Wright-Giemsa and Papanicolaou stains.

Amniotic fluid

■ Describe the composition of amniotic fluid and its importance to the fetus.

*Additional procedures, in CLSI format, are provided on this book's companion website at thepoint.lww.com/Turgeon5e.

INTRODUCTION

Frequently, the analysis of body fluids is assigned to the hematology laboratory. Gross physical examination, total cell count, microscopic examination, and other special tests are generally within the job responsibility of hematology technicians and technologists. Because clinical correlations of body fluid analyses are diagnostically important, clinical information is presented in each section of this chapter.

Chemical analyses and microbial and cytological examinations are generally performed in the chemistry, microbiology, and cytology departments, respectively. For this reason, specific procedures in these disciplines are not included in this chapter.

Sterile body fluid can be found in various body cavities under normal conditions. In diverse disorders and disease processes, the quantity of these fluids can increase significantly. Fluid specimens aspirated from different anatomical sites (Table 25.1) can be analyzed for the total number of cells, differentiation of cell types, chemical composition, and microbial contents. All body fluids should be handled with caution. **Standard precautions** must be practiced.

The type of examination performed on the body fluid depends on the source of the specimen. However, a portion of the examination of CSF; serous fluids from the pleural, pericardial, and peritoneal cavities; synovial fluid; and seminal fluid is frequently performed in the hematology laboratory.

CEREBROSPINAL FLUID

Anatomy and Physiology

CSF acts as a shock absorber for the brain and spinal cord, circulates nutrients, lubricates the central nervous system (CNS), and may also contribute to the nourishment of brain tissue. The CSF circulates through the ventricles and subarachnoid space that surrounds both the brain and the spinal cord. The ventricles (Fig. 25.1) consist of four hollow, fluid-filled spaces inside the brain. A lateral ventricle lies inside each hemisphere of the cerebrum. The two lateral ventricles communicate with the third ventricle through the foramen of Monro. The third ventricle, a narrow channel between the hemispheres through the area of the thalamus, communicates with the fourth ventricle, located in the pons and medulla, by means of the aqueduct of Sylvius in the midbrain portion of the brainstem. This ventricle is continuous with the central canal of the spinal cord.

Three openings in the roof of the fourth ventricle, a pair of lateral apertures (foramina of Luschka) and a median aperture (foramen of Magendie), allow CSF to flow into the basal cisterns and subarachnoid space of the spinal cord. From these basal cisterns, CSF migrates over the convexities toward the cerebral sinuses.

Production of Cerebrospinal Fluid

CSF production is primarily a function of the choroid plexus, with a smaller proportion being derived from the ependymal lining and perivascular spaces. The plexus is composed of two layers: the ependyma (the lining epithelium of the ventricle) and the pia mater. The folded projections of the highly vascularized pia lined with epithelium are referred to as the choroidal epithelium. Choroidal epithelium, blood vessels, and interstitial connective tissue form the choroid plexus. The plexuses in the lateral ventricles are the largest and produce most of the CSF. The choroid plexus epithelium and the endothelium of capillaries in contact with CSF constitute the anatomical structure of the **blood-brain barrier**. The **ependyma** is a single layer of cells with villous projections and cilia on its surface. **Tanycytes** are specialized ependymal cells without cilia, located on the floor of the third ventricle. The main portion of this cell is directed toward the ventricle, and the neck and tail portions contact the capillary wall. These cells are not believed to be involved in the production of CSF.

Specimen Collection: Lumbar Puncture

CSF is found inside all the ventricles, in the central canal of the spinal cord, and in the subarachnoid space around both the brain and the spinal cord. The subarachnoid space is the area between the arachnoid mater, the middle meningeal membrane covering the brain and spinal cord, and the pia mater, the innermost meningeal membrane. The total maximum volume of CSF in adults is about 150 mL. The maximum volume in neonates is approximately 60 mL. The rate of formation in adults is approximately 500 mL/day or 20 mL/hour and is reabsorbed at the same rate, so the volume remains constant.

Introducing a needle into the subarachnoid space makes it possible to measure CSF pressure and to obtain fluid for analysis (Table 25.2). This procedure is contraindicated when there is a skin infection at the puncture site or when

TABLE 25.1	**Body Fluids**
Fluids	**Synonyms**
Bronchoalveolar lavage	Bronchial washings
Cerebrospinal fluid	Spinal fluid Lumbar puncture fluid Ventricular fluid Meningeal fluid
Synovial fluid	Joint fluid
Peritoneal fluid	Dialysate fluid Paracentesis fluid Ascitic fluid
Pericardial fluid	Fluid from around the heart Pericardiocentesis fluid
Pleural fluid	Chest fluid Thoracic fluid Thoracentesis fluid
Seminal fluid	Semen

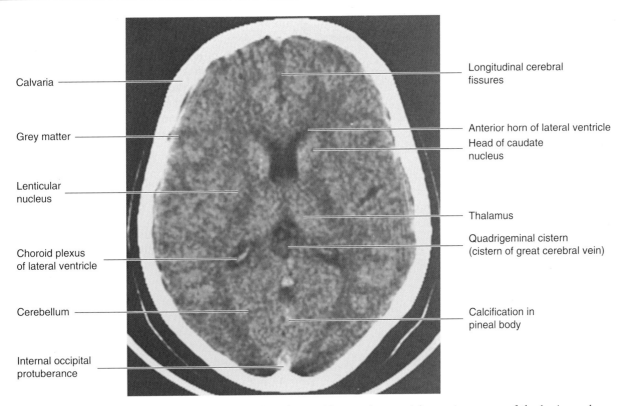

FIGURE 25.1 Transverse (axial) CT image of the brain. Observe the ventricles, various parts of the brain, and the choroid plexus of the lateral ventricle. (Reprinted with permission from Moore KL and Dalley AF II. *Clinical Oriented Anatomy*, 4th ed, Baltimore, MD: Lippincott Williams & Wilkins, 1999.)

the patient has septicemia or a general systemic infection, because of the risk of spreading the infection into the meninges.

The patient is placed in a horizontal position, and the site is thoroughly cleansed to reduce the possibility of contamination with normal skin microbial flora. A stylet needle is introduced by a physician into the intervertebral space between the L4 and L5 (lumbar) vertebrae. Up to 20 mL of fluid can be removed if the patient has a normal opening pressure. The specimen should be placed into sterile tubes. After CSF collection, the closing pressure is measured, the stylet replaced, and the needle removed. Specimens must be *promptly* delivered to the laboratory for analysis. The patient should be given appropriate aftercare because the procedure is not without risk.

Indications for spinal fluid examination are changing as other diagnostic methods are improved. Only in a few conditions, such as meningitis, is the lumbar puncture essential and often diagnostic. It may be of differential value in other cases.

Laboratory Analysis

General Principle

A specimen of CSF is examined visually and microscopically. The total number of cells can be enumerated, and the types of cells can be morphologically distinguished.

Specimen

From three to five samples of 2 to 4 mL each are collected in sterile tubes by a physician. The number of tubes and specified examination related to each tube depends on institutional protocol. Typically, tube 1 is for chemical and serological examination; tube 2 is for microbiological examination; and tube 3 is for gross examination, cell count, and morphology. Because cells disintegrate rapidly, they *must be counted within 1 hour* of specimen collection.

Caution: All CSF specimens should be handled with extreme care. These specimens could potentially harbor viruses or other infectious organisms.

TABLE 25.2	Reasons for Performance of a Lumbar Puncture and Removal of an Aliquot of CSF
Therapeutic	Relief of increased intracranial pressure
Diagnostic	Identification of conditions such as subarachnoid hemorrhage, meningeal infection (meningitis), multiple sclerosis, and neoplasms

TABLE 25.3	**Changes in CSF Following Hemorrhage**
Gross Examination	
2–12 h	Xanthochromia (pink to orange)
12–24 h	Xanthochromia (yellow color, disappears in 2–4 wk)
Microscopic Examination	
2–24 h	Erythrocytes, neutrophilic granulocytes (PMNs), monocytes, and a few lymphocytes
≥48 h	Monocytes and PMNs, erythrophagocytosis, siderophages (may persist for 2–8 wk)

Gross Physical Examination

The spinal fluid is examined visually for turbidity (cloudiness), color, and viscosity. Normal CSF is clear and colorless. Its appearance and viscosity are comparable to those of water.

Turbidity

If any turbidity exists, it should be graded using a scale of 0 to 4+. In the absence of a set of known standards for comparison, the rating scale is subjective. This scale ranges from 1+, slight cloudiness, to 4+, in which newsprint cannot be seen through the tube. Cloudiness or turbidity may be caused by pleocytosis (increased concentrations of leukocytes, erythrocytes, or microorganisms) or, less commonly, radiographic contrast media or the presence of fat globules.

Grossly bloody specimens can result from a traumatic tap or from conditions such as a bleeding subarachnoid hemorrhage or intracerebral hemorrhage. Traumatic taps more commonly occur in children because of movement during the procedure.

It is important to differentiate between specimens from a traumatic tap and those that are related to the patient's clinical condition. A freshly collected specimen should be examined *immediately*. If the reddish color diminishes between the first and the last tube, the blood in the specimen is due to a traumatic tap. In addition, clots may be observed in traumatically collected specimens because of the presence of an increased concentration of protein or blood, or in a specimen from a patient with a subarachnoid block or meningitis.

Color

Any presence of color should be noted. A yellow coloring of a specimen or the supernatant of a centrifuged specimen is referred to as **xanthochromia**. The release of hemoglobin from hemolyzed erythrocytes (red blood cells [RBCs]) in the CSF is a potential cause of xanthochromia. The lysis of RBCs in CSF begins about 2 hours after the occurrence of a subarachnoid hemorrhage (Table 25.3). Other conditions (Table 25.4) and a delay in the examination of a specimen (which can cause a false-positive result) can produce xanthochromia.

Viscosity

Normal CSF has the viscosity of water. Clotting in CSF can be caused by a variety of conditions, including increased protein or gel formation on standing due to an increased fibrinogen content.

Microscopic Examination: Cellular Enumeration

Electronic cell counters are usually used to count cells in CSF. Occasionally, total leukocyte cell counts on body fluids are performed manually.

TABLE 25.4	**Potential Causes of Xanthochromic CSF**	
Cause		**Example**
Clinical Conditions (In Vivo)		
Oxyhemoglobin from RBCs lysed "in vivo"		Recent subarachnoid hemorrhage
Bilirubin from RBCs lysed "in vivo"		Older subarachnoid hemorrhage
Increased direct bilirubin with normal blood-brain barrier		Significant jaundice
Premature infants with an underdeveloped blood-CSF barrier and hyperbilirubinemia		Hemolytic disease of the newborn
Increased CSF protein levels (>150 mg/dL)		Severe meningeal inflammation or infection
Carotenoids in CSF (uncommon)		Meningeal melanosarcoma
Technical Conditions (In Vitro)		
"In vitro" RBC lysis		Traumatic tap with detergent in needle, delay in examination
Antiseptic contamination of CSF		Merthiolate or Mercurochrome
Delayed examination of CSF specimen		Lysis of intact RBCs

CSF, cerebrospinal fluid.

TOTAL LEUKOCYTE COUNT PROCEDURE

Principle

To enumerate the number of WBCs to assist in the development of a differential diagnosis (e.g., bacterial meningitis, viral meningitis, ruptured brain abscess).

Reagents, Supplies, and Equipment

1. 10% acetic acid: Prepare by filling a 100-mL volumetric flask about half full with distilled water. Using a safety bulb, pipette 10 mL of glacial acetic acid into the flask. Add distilled water to the calibration mark and mix.
2. Wright-Giemsa or Wright stain or 1% methylene blue in methyl alcohol: Prepare by weighing 1 g of methylene blue and transferring it to a 100-mL volumetric flask. Dilute to the calibration mark with methyl alcohol. Mix.
3. Small (12 × 75-mm) test tubes, Pasteur pipettes, rubber bulb, and microscope slides
4. Neubauer hemocytometer
5. Centrifuge, microscope, and immersion oil
6. Disinfectant solution
7. Disposable gloves and safety goggles

Procedure

1. Mix the spinal fluid by inversion. With a Pasteur pipette, transfer nine drops of spinal fluid to a small test tube. Add one drop of 10% acetic acid. Mix by gently tapping the tube.
2. Allow this mixture to stand for 5 minutes. Mix again.
3. To each side of the chamber of a clean hemocytometer with a coverslip, load a small amount of the diluted spinal fluid. Allow the counting chamber to sit covered, with a moistened filter paper in half of a Petri plate, for a few minutes to allow the cells to settle and the erythrocytes to completely lyse.
4. Place the hemocytometer under the 10× microscopic objective (low power). Erythrocytes should either be absent or appear as ghost cells. The nucleus of polymorphonuclear segmented neutrophils will be bright, while the lymphocyte nucleus will be round.
5. The leukocytes in all nine squares of each side of the chamber should be counted (see Fig. 25.2). Remove the "R" from the inner five squares. If cells touch the inner or middle lines of two adjacent lines, for example, upper and left-hand side, they can be counted. Cells touching the outer lines or the opposite adjacent lines should not be counted (see Fig. 25.3).

The number of cells counted in all nine squares should not differ by more than five cells. Average the count from both sides.

6. Soak the hemocytometer in a 10% bleach solution to disinfect. Discard the capillary pipette and contaminated supplies in a biohazard bag.

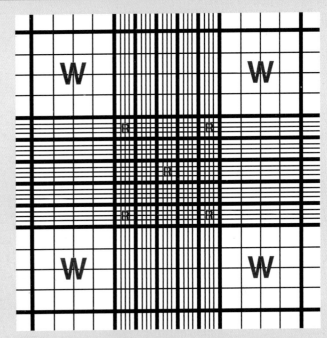

FIGURE 25.2 Neubauer counting chamber. R, red cell area; W, white cell area.

Calculations

$$9 \times \frac{10}{9} = 11 \text{ leukocytes}/\mu L$$

(These calculations may need to be adjusted if the quantity of the specimen varies.)

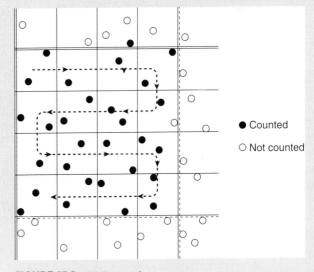

● Counted
○ Not counted

FIGURE 25.3. RBC counting square.

(continued)

TOTAL LEUKOCYTE COUNT PROCEDURE *(continued)*

Reporting Results

Normal CSF is crystal clear and colorless. No clots or RBCs should be observed. In addition, normal CSF has the viscosity of water.

Normal values: 0 to 5 cells/µL or 0 to 5×10^6/L (lymphocytes and monocytes).

Some use a reference value of 0 to 10/µL or 0 to 10×10^6/L.

Neonates have a higher normal range, 0 to 30 mononuclear cells $\times 10^6$/L.

Values in children are comparable to those in adults.

Notes:

1. A disposable, plastic hemacytometer may be used. The C-Chip DHC-N01 has a grid pattern and depth that are the same as the Neubauer hemacytometer. This all-in-one unit does not require a coverslip. Use a micropipette to load 10 µL of sample into the sample injection areas on either end of the chamber. The chamber will fill by capillary action. Be careful to prevent introduction of air bubbles. After use, dispose of the hemacytometer in a biohazard container. If a different type of disposable hemacytometer is used, follow the manufacturer's instructions and use the formula provided to calculate the cell count.
2. Clear specimens may be counted undiluted, provided no overlapping of cells is seen on microscopic examination.

When dilutions are required, calibrated automatic pipettes are used. Dilutions are made with normal saline, mixed by inversion, and loaded into the hemacytometer with a micropipette. The appropriate dilution factor must be used in the calculation.

3. Crystal violet stain can be used to facilitate the differentiation of WBCs from RBCs. Rinse a microhematocrit tube with crystal violet stain to coat the inside. Draw the fluid into the coated microhematocrit tube, mix, and charge the counting chamber.

CELLULAR ENUMERATION PROCEDURE NOTES
Sources of Error

If the specimen is not examined promptly after collection, WBC lysis will give a false impression of the number of WBCs present. If a delay is anticipated, the specimen should be refrigerated.

Clotted specimens result in a falsely low cell count because RBCs and WBCs will be trapped in the clot. In unusual circumstances, manual peripheral blood WBC or platelet counts may be needed. Unopettes for this procedure have been discontinued but Bioanalytic Gmg-H and Biomedical Polymers, Gardner, MA, www.biomedical polymers.com, manufacture substitutes.

Microscopic Examination: Cellular Differentiation

Normal CSF contains a few mononuclear cells (lymphocytes and monocytes) and rare ependymal cells. There is no general agreement as to the significance of a few neutrophilic leukocytes in a CSF specimen.

Cells observed in the CSF resemble comparable cells seen in the peripheral blood or bone marrow in terms of size and nuclear and cytoplasmic features. However, the appearance of cells in the CSF that are also seen in peripheral blood may vary in some details. A Wright-Giemsa stain is recommended for the microscopic differentiation of cells.

Cells that may be encountered in CSF include granulocytes (mature and immature neutrophils, eosinophils, and basophils), mature lymphocytes or reactive lymphocytes, mononuclear phagocytes (monocytes, histiocytes, and macrophages), plasma cells, ependymal cells and choroidal cells, leukemic blasts, and malignant cells (e.g., lymphoma cells or tumor cells). Other types of cells can include immature, nucleated erythrocytes and intracellular bacteria. Lupus erythematosus (LE) cells are rarely observed in CSF.

Lymphocytes

The features of CSF lymphocytes are similar to those of small lymphocytes in peripheral blood. Normal CSF has a few observable lymphocytes. Large lymphocytes and lymphocytes with a darker blue cytoplasm are occasionally seen in normal CSF.

Degenerative changes such as vacuolization, pyknotic nuclear changes, and variations in the staining pattern may be present. Artifactual changes can include overall cell shrinkage, a shrunken nucleus or dense clumps of very dark coloration in the nucleus, and an irregular cytoplasmic border caused by slow drying of the specimen on the slide.

An increased number of lymphocytes in the CSF is typically associated with viral infections but may be seen in a variety of disorders. These disorders include viral meningoencephalitis, aseptic meningitis syndrome (the majority of cases), fungal meningitis, syphilitic meningoencephalitis, and partially treated bacterial meningitis. Noninfectious causes of increased numbers of lymphocytes include conditions such as multiple sclerosis.

CSF specimens from patients with acute viral meningitis may contain reactive lymphocytes, which must be differentiated from lymphoblasts associated with leukemia, as well as a large number of lymphocytes. In addition, patients who have undergone chemotherapy and irradiation for conditions such as leukemia may have reactive lymphocytes in their CSF subsequent to treatment. Reactive lymphocytes are variable in shape and maturation, compared with blasts, which are uniform in shape and degree of maturation. Reactive lymphocytes are also larger, have more cytoplasm, and usually lack the large nucleoli of lymphoblasts.

Patients with disorders other than acute viral meningitis or patients who have received chemotherapy or radiation therapy can manifest reactive lymphocytes in their CSF. These conditions include subacute and chronic meningoencephalitis, tuberculous meningitis, listeriosis, cerebral phlegmona, purulent encephalitis, subacute sclerosing panencephalitis, multiple sclerosis, and bacterial meningitis (recuperative phase).

In addition, viral inclusions may be seen in patients with viral meningoencephalitis, but they are rare.

Mononuclear Phagocytes

Monocytes

The morphological appearance of CSF monocytes is similar to that of blood monocytes. These cells do, however, degenerate more rapidly than lymphocytes in vitro. Young monocytic cells have less cytoplasm than do mature cells and the cytoplasm is more basophilic. The nucleus may be rounder or more convoluted in younger cells. Activated monocytic cells are larger in overall size and nucleoli may be observed in the nucleus. The cytoplasm may be vacuolated and cytoplasmic pseudopods may be seen.

Less than 2% of the cells seen in normal CSF should be monocytes. They are more numerous, especially in degenerated and stimulated forms, in infants and small children than in adults. Disease states that can produce an increase in monocytes in CSF include tuberculous meningitis, syphilis, and viral encephalitis. In addition, meningeal irritation and subarachnoid hemorrhage can induce increased numbers of monocytes. Monocytes also may be seen in leukemic infiltration of the meninges and infectious states.

Macrophages

The morphological characteristics of macrophages (histiocytes) are described in detail in the section describing pleural fluids. Macrophages can be seen in the CSF from patients with meningitis or meningeal inflammation, infectious diseases, CNS leukemia, lymphoma, malignant melanoma, or other metastatic tumors that have spread to the meninges of the brain or spinal cord. In addition, macrophages can be seen in patients who have had hemorrhage in the CSF space or who have undergone pneumoencephalography, intrathecal chemotherapy, or irradiation therapy of the brain. Macrophages with ingested leukocytes can be observed following a surgical procedure that involves the CNS.

Polymorphonuclear Segmented Neutrophils

Very few, if any, polymorphonuclear segmented neutrophils (PMNs) should be observed in the CSF. PMNs may demonstrate rapid disintegration if the specimen is not examined promptly. The cells may appear as shadows or totally disappear in an aged specimen. In addition, the cytoplasm is usually pale staining, and azurophilic granulation may not be evident in a specimen that is a few hours old. Vacuolization of PMNs may be noted in abnormal or old specimens.

The overall size of PMNs may be enlarged if the cell is in the process of phagocytosis. The nucleus may be hyperlobulated with long and narrow filaments. Older neutrophils can exhibit pyknosis or karyorrhexis (one or more spherical, densely staining nuclear fragments) and be mistaken for nucleated RBCs.

The observation of more than an occasional PMN in the CSF classically suggests bacterial infection. However, an increase in the number of PMNs can be caused by infectious and noninfectious agents. Infectious disorders with a predominance of PMNs include acute, untreated bacterial meningitis; viral meningoencephalitis during the first few days of the infection; early tuberculosis; and mycotic meningitis. Aseptic meningitis can exist in cases in which the septic focus is adjacent to the meninges. Noninfectious causes of increased PMN numbers include a reaction to CNS hemorrhage (3 to 4 days afterward), injection of foreign substances such as lidocaine into the subarachnoid space, and leukemic infiltration.

Other Granulocytic Cells

Eosinophils and basophils are not normally seen in the CSF. Their appearance in CSF is similar to that in peripheral blood.

Eosinophils may be increased owing to causes similar to those of an increase in PMNs (e.g., bacterial infection). However, unique causes of an increase in eosinophils include systemic parasitic or fungal infections, systemic drug reaction, and idiopathic eosinophilic meningitis.

Increased basophil numbers can be observed in chronic basophilic leukemia, which involves the meninges; chronic granulocytic leukemia; purulent meningitis; inflammatory processes; and parasitic infections.

Plasma Cells

Plasma cells are normally absent in the CSF. They may be found in association with viral disorders such as herpes simplex virus infection, meningoencephalitis, syphilitic involvement of the CNS, and Hodgkin disease as well as after a subarachnoid hemorrhage.

Erythrocytes

A few erythrocytes (RBCs) may be seen. An increased concentration of RBCs may be seen in traumatic tap specimens or in CSF from patients who have conditions such as a bleeding subarachnoid hemorrhage or intracerebral hemorrhage (see the discussion of gross examination). The number of RBCs may also be increased in chronic myelogenous leukemia or leukoerythroblastic conditions.

Mesothelial Cells

Mesothelial cells are not found in normal CSF. If seen, they can resemble pia arachnoidal or ependymal cells. Both monocytes and mesothelial cells may be transformed into macrophages, and the morphological distinction is not always obvious.

Immature Cells

Immature cells can be seen in patients with leukemias or malignant lymphomas. Although a single blast is insignificant unless accompanied by clinical symptoms, the demonstration of a number of leukemic cells is strongly suggestive of involvement of the subarachnoid space in patients with leukemia or lymphoma.

Malignant Cells

The presence of even a few cells with malignant features is diagnostic of metastatic involvement of the subarachnoid space. These cells may also originate from primary tumors of the brain or spinal cord. Approximately 25% of primary tumors of the CNS shed identifiable malignant cells into the CSF.

Malignant cells are recognizable by the dyssynchrony in maturation between cells. In addition, malignant cells occur singly or in clusters. Malignant cells are usually accompanied by many histiocytes.

Medulloblastoma, a highly malignant tumor, often invades the subarachnoid space and sheds cells into the CSF. The cells of medulloblastoma are small and hyperchromatic. They can occur singly, in rosette formations, or in clumps. These malignant cells are very similar in appearance to neuroblastoma, retinoblastoma, and oat cell carcinoma cells.

Cells Unique to the Cerebrospinal Fluid

Ependymal Cells

A few ependymal cells, the cuboidal epithelial cells that cover the surface of the cerebral ventricles and the choroid plexus, may be seen in normal CSF. These cells become rounded in appearance after separating from the lining and resemble lymphocytes or monocytoid cells. Ependymal cells are medium in size and may appear in clusters or as individual cells. The nucleus is round and generally in the center of the cell. The chromatin is dense and may be slightly grainy or pyknotic. In addition, nucleoli may be seen. The nuclear-cytoplasmic ratio is 1:2 to 1:3. Cellular cytoplasm is usually abundant and stains a cloudy gray-blue or pinkish color with Wright-Giemsa stain. The cytoplasm displays indefinite borders, and fragmented projections of cytoplasm or pseudopods may be seen.

Although ependymal cells appear similar to choroidal cells on light microscopy, they differ from choroidal epithelial cells because of the absence of intracytoplasm inclusions and the border of cilia extending into the ventricular cavity.

An increased number of ependymal cells in the CSF is rare. However, they may be observed in specimens from young children and in patients with hydrocephalus, or following pneumoencephalography. Finding these cells in the CSF is of limited diagnostic value.

Choroidal Cells

Choroidal cells are medium in size (about the size of a mature lymphocyte) and usually occur in a clump of similar cells. The nucleus is round or cuboidal and eccentrically located. It has a loose chromatin structure and nucleoli are not visible. A generous amount of cytoplasm is evident and is gray or slightly basophilic.

The nucleus changes from a blue to pink-tinted color in older samples. In addition, peripheral vacuolization in the cytoplasm can be observed in an aging specimen.

PROCEDURE FOR DIFFERENTIATION OF CELLS IN SPINAL FLUID

Principle

Slide preparations are routinely performed on all CSF specimens. If the total leukocyte count exceeds the normal value, a differential count is usually performed.

Reagents, Supplies, and Equipment

1. Conical centrifuge tubes
2. Microscope slides and Pasteur pipettes
3. Centrifuge
4. Methylene blue or Wright stain

Procedure

The sediment to be examined should be prepared using a cytocentrifuge, filtration, or sedimentation technique. The cytocentrifuge is the preferred method for concentrating CSF specimens. If these methods are not available, an older alternative can be used.

Alternative Method for Sediment Preparation

1. Pour 1 to 2 mL of fresh undiluted spinal fluid into a conical centrifuge. Balance the centrifuge and centrifuge at 2,500 rpm for 10 minutes.
2. Following centrifugation, remove the supernatant fluid with a Pasteur pipette and either save at 4°C to 6°C or freeze for other analyses, if needed. Resuspend the precipitate by gently tapping the tip of the centrifuge tube against the palm of the hand.
3. Transfer a small drop of the resuspended sediment onto a glass slide and smear out as a blood smear. Air-dry thoroughly.
4. Stain with either methylene blue or Wright stain. The methylene blue stain is preferred and should be applied to the smear for approximately 12 minutes. Gently wash off the stain with distilled water.
5. Allow the smear to air-dry. Examine using the 100× (oil immersion) objective. Count the number of different cells observed on a total count of 100 leukocytes.

Reporting Results

Few mononuclear cells (lymphocytes and monocytes) and a rare ependymal cell are considered normal findings.

Procedure Notes

Sources of Error

Artifactual distortion of cells prepared with a cytocentrifuge can lead to misidentification. Specimens should be prepared with a cytocentrifuge, but these preparations may demonstrate

(continued)

artifacts. Portions of fragmented nuclei or cytoplasm can be seen. In addition, cells may assume distorted shapes, granules may become localized in the cytoplasm, and vacuoles may appear in the cytoplasm. Abnormal cells are more prone to exhibit artifactual disruptions, perhaps because of increased cellular fragility. In addition, cellular size can be distorted by cytocentrifuge preparation. Cells in the interior of a specimen may be smaller and have a denser nucleus than cells at the periphery.

Clinical Applications

Normal CSF is crystal clear and colorless. Gross blood may be observed in traumatic tap specimens or in cases of pathological bleeding caused by spontaneous subarachnoid hemorrhage or intracerebral hemorrhage.

Xanthochromia may be indicative of the pathological condition subarachnoid hemorrhage, if the erythrocytes have been present long enough to hemolyze.

Clotting can be caused by the presence of peripheral blood, increased protein, or gel formation on standing due to an increased fibrinogen content.

Turbidity is seen if at least 200 leukocytes $\times 10^6$/L, or 400 erythrocytes $\times 10^6$/L, or microorganisms are present. Increased segmented neutrophil counts classically suggest bacterial infection; however, increased PMNs can be from infectious and noninfectious agents. Infectious disorders include bacterial meningitis, viral meningoencephalitis (the first few days of infection), early tuberculosis, and mycotic meningitis. Aseptic meningitis can exist in cases in which the septic focus is adjacent to the meninges. Noninfectious causes of increases in PMNs include reaction to CNS hemorrhage (3 to 4 days afterward), injection of foreign substances such as lidocaine into the subarachnoid space, and leukemic infiltration.

Increased numbers of lymphocytes are typically associated with viral infections but may be seen in a variety of disorders. These disorders include viral meningoencephalitis, fungal meningitis, syphilitic meningoencephalitis, and partially treated bacterial meningitis. Noninfectious causes of increased lymphocyte numbers include conditions such as multiple sclerosis.

Other types of cells are rarely encountered. Plasma cells are normally absent. Eosinophils may be increased because of causes similar to those of an increase in PMNs; increased basophils can be seen in chronic basophilic leukemia, which involves the meninges; and monocytes may be seen in leukemic infiltration of the meninges and infectious states.

Associated Findings

Glucose and protein values are important to correlate with gross and microscopic findings in the CSF. In general, a decreased glucose level in the CSF in the presence of a normal blood glucose level indicates bacterial utilization of glucose. In addition, an elevated total protein concentration is also suggestive of an inflammatory reaction or a bacterial infection. A viral infection will not have a dramatic effect on CSF glucose levels and may not affect the total protein level significantly.

PLEURAL, PERITONEAL, AND PERICARDIAL FLUIDS

Effusions: Transudates and Exudates

An **effusion** is an abnormal accumulation of fluid in a particular space of the body. Effusions in the pleural, pericardial, and peritoneal cavities are divided into **transudates** and **exudates**. Transudates generally indicate that fluid has accumulated because of the presence of a systemic disease. In contrast, exudates are usually associated with disorders such as inflammation, infection, and malignant conditions involving the cells that line the surfaces of organs (e.g., lung or abdominal organs).

Transudates and exudates frequently differ in characteristics such as color and clarity and in total leukocyte cell count. Classically, transudates have been considered to differ from exudates based on the properties of specific gravity and total protein. These characteristics, however, are unreliable in consistently differentiating the two categories of effusions. For example, the mean values of total protein display considerable overlap between transudates and exudates.

A variety of physical and chemical properties need to be considered when fluids are categorized as transudates or exudates (Table 25.5).

Pleural Fluid

Anatomy of the Pleura

The lungs lie in the thoracic (chest) cavity, where they are separated by the heart in the mediastinum. Each lung is covered by a serous membrane, the visceral pleura (Fig. 25.4). The interior of the chest wall, the superior surface of the diaphragm, and the lateral portion of the mediastinum are also lined by a thin membrane, the parietal pleura. The layers of the visceral and parietal pleurae are contiguous, and the potential space between them on each side of the thorax forms the pleural cavity. However, the pleural cavity is not a true cavity. It becomes a cavity if an abnormal condition creates an excess accumulation of fluid or air in it.

The pleural cavity is lined by a single-cell layer of mesothelial cells that form the mesothelium. Mesothelial cells are supported by layers of connective tissue that contain an extensive network of lymphatic vessels and blood capillaries. Although

TABLE 25.5	Comparison of Transudates and Exudates[a]	
Characteristics	**Transudate**	**Exudate**
Physical Characteristics		
pH	7.4–7.5	7.35–7.45
Specific gravity	<1.016	>1.016
Cellular Characteristics		
Erythrocytes	Few	Variable
Leukocytes	<1,000	>1,000
Chemical Analyses		
Glucose level	Equal to serum	Possibly decreased
Protein level	<3.0 g/dL	>3.0 g/dL
Pleural fluid–serum ratio of protein	<0.5	>0.5
LDH level	<200	>200 IU/L
Pleural fluid–serum ratio of LDH[b]	<2:3 (<0.6)	>2:3 (>0.6)

[a]Variations can be observed in examples of various conditions.
[b]If nonhemolyzed, nonbloody effusion.
LDH, lactic dehydrogenase.

the function of the pleural space is obscure, the stretchable mesothelial cells that line this potential space provide the lungs and other intrathoracic organs with the flexibility to expand and retract.

Pleural fluid is normally produced by the parietal pleura and absorbed by the visceral pleura as a continuous process.

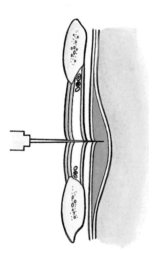

FIGURE 25.4 Thoracocentesis. Sometimes it is necessary to insert a hypodermic needle through an intercostal space into the pleural cavity—the potential space between the parietal pleura lining the pulmonary cavity and the visceral pleura covering the lung—to obtain a sample of pleural fluid, or to remove blood or pus. To avoid damage to the intercostal nerve and vessels, the needle is inserted superior to the rib, high enough to avoid the collateral branches. (Reprinted with permission from Moore KL, Agur A. *Essential Clinical Anatomy,* 2nd ed, Philadelphia, PA: Lippincott Williams & Wilkins, 2002.)

Although healthy individuals form 600 to 800 mL of fluid daily, the normal volume of fluid in each pleural space is estimated at less than 10 mL. This fluid is formed by the filtration of blood plasma through the capillary endothelium. The fluid is reabsorbed by lymphatic vessels and venules in the pleura. Transport in and out of the pleural space is dependent on the balance of hydrostatic pressure in the capillary network of the parietal and visceral pleurae and capillary permeability, plasma oncotic pressure, and lymphatic reabsorption.

Pleural Effusion

The accumulation of fluid in the pleural space is referred to as **pleural effusion**. Excess fluid accumulates if the balance of fluid formation and absorption is in disequilibrium. This may be caused by an increased production or a decreased absorption of fluid. Large quantities may need to be drained. Aspiration of pleural fluid is referred to as **thoracentesis** (Fig. 25.5). Failure to remove an increased accumulation of leukocytes or blood from the pleural space may lead to the formation of fibrothorax and a subsequent impairment of pulmonary function.

The location of a pleural effusion may be suggestive of the type of disorder involved in causing the effusion (Box 25.1). Typically, left-sided effusions are associated with conditions such as a ruptured esophagus or acute pancreatitis.

If a fluid has the general characteristics of an exudate, at a minimum, a Gram stain and culture and cytological studies need to be performed. An open lung biopsy of tissue for examination with histochemical stains and electron microscopy may be required for a diagnosis in suspected malignant conditions.

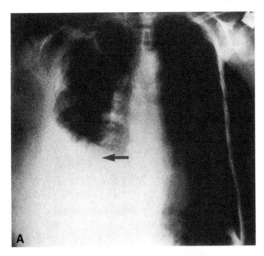

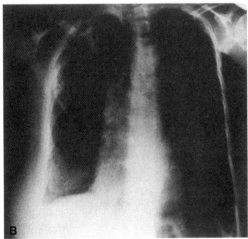

FIGURE 25.5 **A:** A substantial amount of pleural fluid has accumulated in this patient's right chest cavity (*arrow*). **B:** After draining off more than 100 mL of fluid, the patient's chest radiograph reveals a decreased amount of fluid in the right chest cavity.

Laboratory Analysis

Physical Characteristics

Transudates are usually clear, are pale yellow, and do not clot. In comparison, exudates can display a range of colors depending on the associated disorder (Table 25.6). Only 2 mL of circulating blood in 1 L of pleural fluid will produce a blood-tinged appearance. Very viscous fluids, clear or bloody, are characteristic of mesothelioma. In addition, exudates may be cloudy or purulent and frequently clot on standing because of the presence of fibrinogen.

Specimen turbidity may be caused by lipids or result from an increased number of leukocytes. A clear supernatant after centrifugation indicates the presence of an abundant number of leukocytes, but a white supernatant is caused by chylomicrons. In contrast, chyliform or pseudochylous pleural effusions resemble a chylous effect. These effusions have a milky or greenish appearance and might have a pearly opalescent sheen. This appearance results from cellular debris and cholesterol crystals.

Cell Count

Erythrocyte and leukocyte counts are of limited value in the differential diagnosis of pleural effusions. A massively bloody (hemorrhagic) effusion in the absence of trauma almost always suggests malignancy, or occasionally pulmonary infarct. Pure blood in the pleural cavity, true hemothorax, results from severe chest injuries. In these cases, a microhematocrit determination will confirm that the microhematocrit value is similar to the patient's peripheral blood packed RBC volume.

Extremely elevated total leukocyte (WBC) counts of 50.0×10^9/L or higher are consistent with a diagnosis of empyema. In general, WBC counts less than 1.0×10^9/L are associated with transudates, and WBC counts greater than $1,000 \times 10^9$/L are associated with exudates.

BOX 25.1

Clinical Correlations (Pleural Fluid)

TRANSUDATES
Congestive heart failure
Cirrhosis with ascites

EXUDATES
Infectious diseases
Empyema
Tuberculosis
Malignant neoplasms
Lymphoma
Mesothelioma
Pancreatitis
Rheumatoid arthritis

TABLE 25.6 **Representative Exudate Appearance**

Appearance	Typical Associated Disorder
Dark red-brown	Amebiasis
Greenish to greenish yellow and turbid	Classic rheumatoid effusion
Yellow and turbid	Infectious process
Milky	Chylothorax (chylous or pseudochylous)
Bloody (hemorrhagic)	Traumatic tap, malignancy, pulmonary infarction, trauma, pancreatitis, tuberculosis
Clearly visible pus (WBCs)	Empyema
Foul odor	Anaerobic bacterial infection

Use undiluted fluid to perform the cell count (refer to the spinal fluid cell count procedure). Electronic counting instruments should be used with caution, because debris may cause falsely increased counts.

Cell Differential Examination

Smears should be prepared for microscopic examination by cytocentrifugation, filter preparation (Millipore), or sedimentation methods. Following preparation of the sediment, the smears should be properly stained with Wright or Wright-Giemsa stain for differential leukocyte evaluation, or stained with Papanicolaou stain for cytological evaluation.

Cell types that can be encountered in the examination of a Wright-Giemsa–stained specimen include PMNs, eosinophils, basophils, lymphocytes, plasma cells, mononuclear phagocytes (monocytes, histiocytes, and macrophages), mesothelial cells (normal, reactive, atypical, and malignant), and metastatic tumor (malignant) cells. In addition, in vivo LE cells have also been observed in pleural fluids.

If a cytocentrifuge is used for sediment preparation, artifacts may be encountered. Cells in the interior of a specimen may be smaller in overall size with a denser nucleus than cells at the periphery. Abnormal cells in particular are more likely to be affected because of their propensity to be more fragile. In addition, nuclear-induced changes can include distorted shape and segmentation, fragmentation, or holes. Cytoplasmic artifacts can include irregular fragmentation, localization of granules, and peripheral vacuolization.

PMNs should be distinguished from mononuclear cells. It can be difficult to differentiate lymphocytes from monocytes.

Polymorphonuclear Segmented Neutrophils

PMNs in pleural fluid may appear morphologically identical to those in the circulating blood or may be difficult to recognize. Immature neutrophils are rarely seen except in chronic granulocytic leukemia or a leukoerythroblastic condition.

In long-standing effusions, signs of cellular degeneration such as vacuolization and a decreased number of granules can occur in the cytoplasm. The nuclei may appear as densely stained spherical fragments and resemble nucleated erythrocytes (RBCs). Occasionally, the cytoplasm may have a bluish color and resemble the cytoplasm of a lymphocyte.

An increase in PMNs (Table 25.7) is associated with exudates from patients with infectious diseases of a bacterial etiology.

Lymphocytes

Lymphocytes resembling small peripheral blood lymphocytes are seen in variable numbers in most body fluids. However, lymphocytes may be variable in size and have an immature appearance. The cellular nucleus can be cleaved and exhibit nucleoli that are often more prominent than those in peripheral blood lymphocytes.

Degenerative changes in aged specimens can include vacuolization, pyknotic nuclear changes, and variations in the staining pattern. Artifactual changes can include a shrunken nucleus or dense clumps of very dark coloration, overall cell shrinkage, and an irregular cytoplasmic border owing to slow drying of the specimen on the slide.

Effusions from patients with tuberculosis or malignancies frequently show a predominance of lymphocytes. Effusions from patients with non-Hodgkin lymphoma can manifest malignant lymphocytes that are generally uniform in comparison to benign conditions in which there is usually a mixture of different types of lymphocytes (small, medium, and large).

Detection of lymphocyte subsets (T and B lymphocytes) in pleural effusion may aid in the differential diagnosis. The T subset is considerably higher in fluids from patients with pulmonary tuberculosis than in their blood. The B subset is usually significantly lower in pleural fluid than in the circulating blood in patients with pulmonary tuberculosis, pulmonary malignant disorders, or nonspecific pleuritis. The presence of a monoclonal B-cell population is usually associated with malignant lymphoma.

Mononuclear Cells

Mononuclear phagocytes (monocytes, histiocytes, and macrophages) are seen in variable numbers in both benign and malignant effusions. The terms macrophage and histiocyte are used synonymously. Both monocytes and mesothelial cells may be transformed into macrophages; the morphological distinction is not always obvious.

Macrophages vary in size, with a diameter ranging from 15 to 25 µm. The cytoplasm is pale gray and frequently vacuolated. Macrophages may contain phagocytized material such as RBC particles. The nucleus is eccentrically located, with one or more observable nucleoli. **Signet ring cells** are a type of macrophage that forms when the small vacuoles of the cell fuse and form one or two large vacuoles that push the nucleus against the side of the cell membrane. The nucleus forms the stone component of the ring. Signet ring macrophages with a normal-size nucleus are commonly seen in sterile inflammatory effusions.

The degeneration and death of a macrophage are characterized by an irregular nuclear shape and pyknosis, and cytoplasmic vacuolization and inclusions, with peripheral fraying.

The number of mononuclear cells usually increases as an inflammatory process becomes chronic. Mononuclear cells predominate in early inflammatory effusions (e.g., pneumonia, pulmonary infarct, pancreatitis, and subphrenic abscess). After several days, macrophages, lymphocytes, and mesothelial cells may predominate.

Eosinophils

An increased number of eosinophils (eosinophilia) in pleural fluid is nonspecific. Eosinophilia in pleural fluid (greater than 10% of total WBCs) may signify that air or blood has been introduced into the pleural space (e.g., repeated thoracenteses, pneumothorax, and traumatic hemothorax). However, it is not diagnostically significant. Eosinophilia may also be manifested

TABLE 25.7	Examples of Cellular Abnormalities Encountered in Pleural and Peritoneal Fluids
Condition	**Cellular Characteristics**
Bacterial Inflammation	
• Acute	Many neutrophils, histiocytes, and mesothelial cells May display bacteria
• Chronic	Some neutrophils and eosinophils Many lymphocytes, plasma cells, and histiocytes Reactive mesothelial cells May display bacteria
Chronic granulomatous inflammation (e.g., tuberculosis, sarcoidosis, fungal infections, rheumatoid arthritis)	Elongated or round multinuclear giant cells Histiocytes, lymphocytes, and plasma cells Some neutrophils Many reactive mesothelial cells Amorphous background material from the center of granulomas May display fungi (special stain), if fungal inflammations May display tuberculous bacilli (special stains), if tuberculosis
Malignant mesothelioma	Abundant number of cells (single or cluster) Gland-like peculiar multinucleated cells present Clusters of cells are made of more than 4–5 cells Calcified bodies Occasional psammoma bodies
Metastatic tumors	Malignant cells (single or clusters) Cytoplasm may display intracellular vacuole, associated with mucin in adenocarcinoma, or squamous cell carcinoma Intracellular mucin appears as large paranuclear vacuole containing granular blue material Nucleus may be marginated Sarcomas have very large elongated cells with oval to rod-shaped nuclei, small nucleoli and coarse chromatin, abundant cytoplasm—elongated and finely reticular to granular Poorly differentiated sarcomas have very large tumor cells with large pleomorphic nuclei
After chemotherapy or radiation therapy	Atypical mesothelial cells Increased number of histiocytes
Viral infections	Many lymphocytes, plasma cells, histiocytes, and mesothelial cells

in parasitic or fungal diseases, pulmonary infarction, and polyarteritis nodosa.

Plasma Cells

The plasma cells resemble those encountered in the bone marrow. An increase in plasma cells accompanies an increase in lymphocytes in patients with multiple myeloma. Plasma cells may also be seen in effusions from patients with tuberculosis, rheumatoid arthritis, malignancy, Hodgkin disease, or other conditions associated with lymphocytosis.

Mesothelial Cells

Mesothelial cells (middle lining of cells) form the lining of the pleural, pericardial, and peritoneal cavities. In vivo, the cells form a single-cell layer or sheet of uniform cells.

Normally, a small number of cells are sloughed into the serous cavities.

These cells vary in appearance, frequently manifesting atypical or reactive changes, and usually cause the most difficulty during the evaluation of cell types. It is extremely difficult to distinguish between mononuclear phagocytes and intermediate forms of mesothelial cells. Therefore, they may be mistaken for malignant cells.

Mesothelial cells may appear as single cells, in clusters, or as sheets. Clustering of cells may be caused by centrifugation and may closely resemble malignant cells. Clumps of benign mesothelial cells can be differentiated from malignant cells by comparing the appearance of the cells in the clump with other more easily distinguished mesothelial cells in the same smear. In addition, a uniform, regular arrangement of cells that display fenestrations (openings or windows) between the cytoplasmic membranes of these cells usually indicates that they are benign.

Mesothelial cells have a large overall size and average from 12 to 30 μm in diameter. Benign mesothelial cells can have various appearances; some resemble large plasma cells. The nucleus or nuclei have a round to oval appearance and occupy about one third to one half of the cell's diameter. Although one to three nucleoli may be seen, cells may be multinucleated. Occasionally a cell may contain 20 or more nuclei. The nuclear contour is usually smooth and regular, with stippled and dark-purple nuclear chromatin.

The cytoplasm is abundant and varies from light gray to deep blue. Localized basophilic areas are often seen in the center of the cell. This perinuclear zone of pallor resembles a fried egg in appearance. Cytoplasmic vacuoles of various sizes are often seen. Vacuoles or clear areas at the periphery of the cytoplasm probably represent glycogen.

Degenerative mesothelial cells may show pyknosis and karyorrhexis. They may also exhibit phagocytosis and transform into macrophages. Tiny projections of microvilli may be observed extending from the periphery of the cytoplasm; this is an artifact.

Mesothelial cells are seen in variable numbers in most effusions and are increased in sterile inflammations caused by such conditions as pleurisy associated with pulmonary infarction. Few cells, if any, are seen in effusions from patients with tubercular pleurisy or when an increased number of pyogenic organisms are present in the effusion. If the number of large mesothelial cells, differing from macrophages, is more than 5%, tuberculosis is ruled out.

Cytological Examination

Most malignant effusions are caused by metastatic adenocarcinoma because of its peripheral location and high incidence. Analysis of body fluids, secretions, and tissue biopsy specimens can be valuable in the diagnosis of carcinoma. Another source for the diagnosis of pleural malignancy is sputum.

The presence of a massive bloody (hemorrhagic) effusion in the absence of trauma is highly suggestive of malignancy. The number of malignant cells varies. On microscopic examination, tumor cells frequently aggregate in clumps and sometimes show gland-like formation. Characteristics of malignant cells include the following:

1. Variation in cell sizes and shapes (pleomorphic) or similar in appearance (monomorphic)
2. Multiple, round aggregates of cells
3. High nuclear-cytoplasmic (N:C) ratio
4. Irregularity in nuclear size and shape
5. Coarseness and clumping of chromatin
6. Large, prominent, irregular nucleoli
7. Possible giant vacuoles
8. Basophilic or vacuolated (mucin-containing) cytoplasm
9. Irregular and abnormal mitosis
10. Engulfment of malignant cells by other malignant cells

Peritoneal Fluid

Anatomy of the Peritoneum

The peritoneum is a smooth membrane that covers the abdominal walls and viscera of the abdomen and pelvis (Fig. 25.6). The continuous sheet of single-cell layers of mesothelial cells supported by connective tissue forms the visceral and parietal peritonea. The potential space between the parietal and visceral layers of the peritoneum is the peritoneal cavity. The parietal peritoneum lines the entire abdominal cavity. At the posterior midline, the left and right sheets of the membrane come together to form a double membrane, the mesentery. Each of the abdominal organs is suspended by this mesentery. As the sheets separate to surround an organ, they become the visceral peritoneum of the organ. In two places within the abdominal cavity, mesenteries extend beyond the organs and form a four-layered thickness, the omenta. Omenta contain phagocytic cells that protect the abdominal cavity from infection. However, peritonitis, an inflammation of these membranes, can result from infection or chemical irritation.

A small amount of fluid, formed by the ultrafiltration of plasma, lubricates the peritoneum. The presence of this fluid, called peritoneal fluid, reduces friction between the visceral and parietal peritonea as they move against each other.

Peritoneal Effusion

An abnormal amount of fluid (an effusion) can accumulate in the peritoneal cavity if the balance between fluid formation and reabsorption is altered by a disease process. The collection of fluid in the peritoneal cavity, **ascites**, results from increased hydrostatic pressure in the systemic circulation, increased peritoneal capillary permeability, decreased plasma oncotic pressure, or decreased fluid reabsorption by the lymphatic system. The procedure for removing fluid from the peritoneal cavity is **paracentesis**.

Causes of Peritoneal Effusions

The causes of peritoneal effusions range from disorders and diseases that directly represent involvement of the peritoneum, such as bacterial peritonitis, to abdominal conditions that do not directly involve the peritoneum, such as hepatic cirrhosis, cirrhosis, congestive heart failure, Budd-Chiari syndrome, hypoalbuminemia (caused by nephrotic syndrome or protein-losing enteropathy malnutrition), and miscellaneous disorders such as myxedema, ovarian diseases, pancreatic disease, and chylous ascites.

Effusions that may conform with the definition of transudates can be associated with congestive heart failure, hepatic cirrhosis, and hypoproteinemia.

Effusions that may conform with the definition of exudates can be associated with primary or secondary peritonitis, malignant disorders, trauma, and pancreatitis.

Laboratory Analysis

The laboratory criteria for distinguishing transudates from exudates are less clearly defined for peritoneal (ascitic) fluid than for pleural fluid. Transudates are usually clear and pale

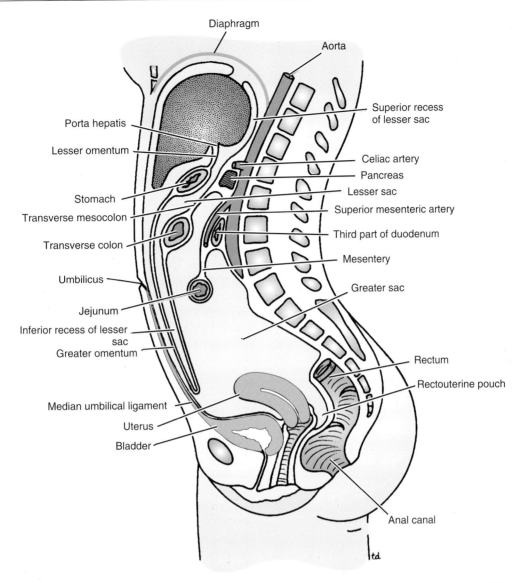

FIGURE 25.6 Sagittal section of the female abdomen showing the arrangement of the peritoneum. (Reprinted with permission from Snell RS. *Clinical Anatomy By Regions*, 8th ed, Philadelphia, PA: Lippincott Williams & Wilkins, 2008.)

yellow. Exudates are cloudy or turbid because of an increased concentration of leukocytes, elevated protein levels, and occasionally microorganisms. Exudates may be seen in peritonitis, cases of perforated or infarcted intestine, and pancreatitis. An evaluation of ascitic fluid includes gross inspection, total cell count, microscopic examination of sediment for cell differentiation, cytological studies, chemical analysis for constituents such as total protein and lactic dehydrogenase, and microbial culture.

Physical Characteristics

A variety of clinical conditions (Table 25.8) can produce a deviation from the anticipated yellow or straw-colored fluid. Grossly bloody (hemorrhagic) peritoneal fluid may be seen in trauma patients with a ruptured spleen or liver, intestinal infarction, pancreatitis, or malignancies.

Green-colored effusion results from the presence of bile. This type of discoloration may be seen in patients with perforated gallbladders or intestines, or in those with duodenal ulcers. Greenish fluid, however, may also be present in patients with cholecystitis (inflammation of the gallbladder) or acute pancreatitis. The presence of bile can be confirmed with a spot test for bilirubin.

Chylous (milky-appearing) peritoneal fluid is rare. Chylous ascites is caused by a leakage of lymphatic vessels resulting from trauma, lymphoma, tuberculosis, hepatic cirrhosis, or carcinoma. Malignant lymphoma and carcinoma are the two most common causes of chylous peritoneal fluid. In contrast, pseudochylous fluid has a milky or greenish appearance because of the presence of cellular debris and cholesterol crystals. This abnormality may be associated with chronic effusions produced by a wide variety of causes.

TABLE 25.8	Variations in Peritoneal Fluid Appearance
	Examples of Conditions
Color	
Pale yellow	Normal
Straw colored	Normal
	Congestive heart failure
	Cirrhosis
	Neoplasm
Reddish brown or bloody	Neoplasm
	Pancreatitis
	Pulmonary infarct
	Trauma
	Traumatic thoracentesis
	Tuberculous peritonitis
Appearance	
Clear	Normal
	Tuberculous peritonitis
Turbid (cloudy)	Bacterial peritonitis
	Pancreatitis
	Conditions with increased cellular components
Mucinous	Neoplasm
Chylous[a] (milky)	Obstruction of lymphatic duct (e.g., lymphoma)
	Tuberculous peritonitis
	Trauma
	Pancreatitis
Purulent	Bacterial peritonitis

[a]Supernatant is white because of chylomicrons.

Total Cell Count

Total erythrocyte (RBC) and leukocyte (WBC) counts are usually performed on ascitic fluid. Use undiluted fluid to perform the cell count (refer to the spinal fluid cell count procedure). Use electronic counting instruments with care because debris may cause falsely increased counts. Smears should be prepared for microscopic examination by cytocentrifugation, filter preparation (Millipore), or sedimentation methods.

Cell counts improve the accuracy and specificity of diagnosis by peritoneal lavage (flushing of space with Ringer lactate solution). However, the total cell count is of less accuracy in the diagnosis of penetrating trauma (gunshot and stab wounds) of the abdomen than in other conditions (Table 25.9). A positive result by lavage is indicative of laparotomy. If the test results are equivocal, another lavage may be indicated in 1 to 2 hours.

Total WBC counts are of limited value in differential diagnosis, but a total WBC count higher than 0.3×10^9/L is considered to be abnormal. More than half of patients with infected ascites have a total WBC count higher than 0.3×10^9/L, with more than 25% PMNs on the leukocyte differential smear. Leukocyte counts greater than 0.5×10^9/L are considered to be useful presumptive evidence in distinguishing between bacterial peritonitis and cirrhosis. In bacterial peritonitis, the total WBC count is higher than 0.5×10^9/L, with more than 50% PMNs.

A wide variation in the peritoneal WBC count is seen in patients with chronic liver disease because of extracellular shifts in fluid associated with ascites formation or resolution. During diuresis, the total leukocyte concentration may increase dramatically, but the concentration of PMNs usually remains low. Therefore, the variance of the total WBC count usually does not lead to confusion between cirrhosis and bacterial peritonitis.

Total WBC counts may occasionally be elevated in peritoneal fluid independently of the RBC count. This is particularly true in patients with penetrating abdominal trauma with visceral injury. If lavage is performed immediately after the injury occurs, the WBC count may not yet be elevated (Table 25.10).

Cellular Differential Examination

Following preparation of the sediment, the smears should be properly stained with Wright or Wright-Giemsa stain for differential leukocyte evaluation or with Papanicolaou stain for cytological evaluation.

A differential cell count should be performed on the Wright-Giemsa–stained smear. If a cytocentrifuge is used for sediment preparation, artifacts may be encountered (see "Pleural Fluid" for a discussion of the artifact induced by cytocentrifuge preparation).

Although the quantities of some cells in peritoneal fluid compared with pleural fluid may vary in some disorders, the cell types that can be encountered are the same as those that can be seen in pleural fluids. These cells include PMNs, eosinophils, basophils, lymphocytes, plasma cells, mononuclear phagocytes (monocytes, histiocytes, and macrophages), mesothelial cells (normal, reactive, atypical, or malignant), and metastatic tumor (malignant) cells. In addition, in vivo LE cells have also been observed.

Polymorphonuclear Segmented Neutrophils

A distribution of PMNs higher than 25% is considered abnormal. A high proportion of PMNs is suggestive of bacterial infection, although about one third of patients with alcoholic cirrhosis demonstrate a ratio of PMNs in excess of 30%.

In addition, an absolute neutrophil count may also be helpful. A count greater than 0.25×10^9/L is a fairly sensitive indicator of spontaneous or secondary bacterial peritonitis.

TABLE 25.9	Criteria for Diagnosing Blunt and Penetrating Trauma by Analysis of Peritoneal Lavage Fluid	
Diagnosis	**Gross Findings**	**Laboratory Analysis**
Positive	Blood in aspirate or lavage Lavage fluid retrieved via Foley catheter or chest tube Evidence of food, foreign particle, or bile	RBC count >0.1 × 10^{12}/L; >0.05 × 10^{12}/L in cases of penetrating trauma WBC count >0.5 × 10^9/L Amylase level >2 × serum amylase level
Indeterminate	Small amount of bloody fluid noted in dialysis catheter on insertion	RBC count 0.05–0.1 × 10^{12}/L; 0.01–0.05 × 10^{12}/L in cases of penetrating trauma WBC count 0.001–0.005 × 10^9/L Amylase levels slightly higher than serum amylase levels
Negative		RBC count <0.025 × 10^{12}/L WBC count <0.001 × 10^9/L Amylase level lower than serum amylase level

Eosinophils

Eosinophilia of the peritoneal fluid is less common than that of the pleural fluid. Eosinophilic ascites is rare, but when present, more than 50% of the cells in the peritoneal fluid are eosinophils. Eosinophilic ascites manifests in patients with eosinophilic gastroenteritis, ruptured hydatid cysts, lymphoma, or vasculitis. In addition, patients with chronic peritoneal dialysis may also exhibit eosinophilic ascites.

Lymphocytes

A predominance of lymphocytes is seen in transudates from patients with congestive heart failure, cirrhosis, or nephrotic syndrome. On differential examination, lymphocytes may represent the majority of leukocytes in chylous effusions and in patients with tuberculous peritonitis or malignancies.

TABLE 25.10	Examples of Cell Count Variations
Erythrocytes (RBCs)	
High	Neoplasm, tuberculous peritonitis
Variable	Pancreatitis
Low	Cirrhosis, bacterial peritonitis, congestive heart failure
Leukocytes (WBCs)	
High	Bacterial peritonitis (PMNs)
	Congestive heart failure (mesothelial)
	Neoplasm (>50% lymphocytes)
	Tuberculous peritonitis (>70% lymphocytes)

Mesothelial Cells

In contrast to pleural effusions, tuberculous peritoneal effusions may contain many mesothelial cells. Ascitic fluid associated with cirrhosis may contain many highly atypical mesothelial cells.

Malignant Cells

It is possible to observe malignant tumor cells in peritoneal fluids. Cytological examination should be performed if a malignancy is suspected. It is important to distinguish between malignant and mesothelial cells because the cells most difficult to differentiate from malignant cells are mesothelial cells.

Diagnosis of Ascites

Ascites is a condition in which fluid accumulates within the peritoneal space (cavity). This constitutes a peritoneal effusion. More than several hundred milliliters of peritoneal fluid must usually be present before the effusion can be detected by physical examination. Small amounts of effusion may be asymptomatic. Increasing amounts, however, cause abdominal distention and discomfort, anorexia, nausea, early satiety, heartburn, frank pain, and respiratory distress in patients.

Radiographic studies such as ultrasonography and computed tomography (CT) scans are very sensitive and allow the radiologist to observe the presence of an effusion and to distinguish it from a cystic mass. Rarely is a laparoscopy or exploratory laparotomy required.

Diagnostic abdominal paracentesis with the removal of 50 to 100 mL of fluid is essential for the establishment of a differential diagnosis. Aspiration may be combined with lavage.

Patients with abdominal pain who have chronic ascites or ascites of unknown origin, sudden onset of ascites (intraperitoneal hemorrhage, infarct, or pancreatic ascites), suspected perforation of a peptic ulcer or bowel perforation, or blunt trauma to the abdomen need to have a paracentesis performed. Two of the most common indications for paracentesis are complications of cirrhosis (e.g., spontaneous bacterial peritonitis) and suspected intra-abdominal malignancy.

The effusion specimen needs to be analyzed promptly. Laboratory assessment includes gross examination for characteristics such as color and clarity; total erythrocyte and leukocyte cell counts; differential leukocyte examination; chemical assays such as total protein, amylase, and lactic dehydrogenase; and microbial studies including Gram stain, routine cultures, anaerobic cultures, tuberculosis cultures, and cytological examination.

Pericardial Fluid

Anatomy of the Pericardium

The pericardium (Fig. 25.7) is a fibroserous sac, composed of external (fibrous) and internal (serous) layers, that encloses the heart and roots of the great blood vessels. The inner serous portion of the pericardium consists of the parietal and visceral layers. The outer parietal layer is in contact with the fibrous pericardium; the inner visceral layer, also referred to as the epicardium, is in contact with the heart and roots of the great blood vessels. The potential space between the parietal and visceral layers, which is filled with a small amount of fluid to reduce friction between the layers, is the pericardial cavity.

Pericardial Effusion

An abnormal accumulation of fluid in the cavity, a **pericardial effusion**, is most frequently caused by damage to the lining of the cavity and increased capillary permeability. In addition, in acute pericarditis, interference with pericardial venous and lymphatic drainage predisposes the patient to effusion development.

The physiological function of the normal pericardium is considered to be pericardial restraint, which tends to oppose dilatation of the heart. In many circumstances, the restraining effect of the pericardium is essentially reflected by the

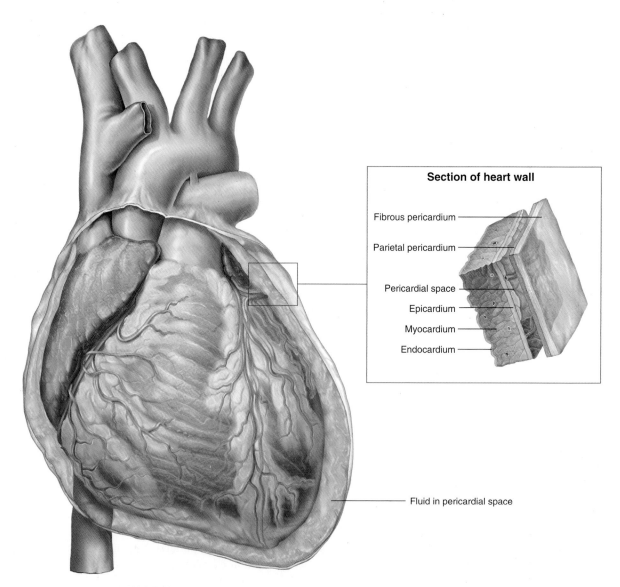

Section of heart wall

Fibrous pericardium

Parietal pericardium

Pericardial space

Epicardium

Myocardium

Endocardium

Fluid in pericardial space

FIGURE 25.7 Pericardial effusion. (Asset provided by Anatomical Chart Co.)

mean central venous pressure. The term **cardiac tamponade** is often used to indicate a critical state of cardiovascular compromise, usually with hypotension, caused by pericardial fluid under increased pressure. It is widely accepted that any elevation of central venous pressure that is caused by pericardial effusion constitutes cardiac tamponade. Therapeutic removal of pericardial fluid, pericardiocentesis, is usually indicated if the central venous pressure rises to approximately 10 mm Hg.

Pericardial effusion is usually accurately assessed by echocardiography, but there are pitfalls in the interpretation of such studies. For example, tamponade can be produced by localized pockets of pericardial effusion that may not be evident by echocardiography, particularly if the pocket is located adjacent to the right atrium laterally. CT scans and magnetic resonance imaging (MRI) are also accurate means of demonstrating pericardial effusion and are less subject to the limitations of echocardiography in localized effusions. Pericardial disease causes effusions that are left sided or bilateral; they are rarely exclusively right sided. Patients with congestive heart failure typically manifest right-sided or bilateral effusions.

Causes of Pericardial Effusion

A wide variety of diseases and disorders can produce pericardial effusion (Table 25.11). Neoplastic disease produces a significant volume of fluid in the pericardium and is one of the most common causes of pericardial effusion. Primary tumors of the pericardium (mesothelioma) are rare. However, metastatic tumors of the pericardium and heart are common in patients with advanced malignant disease from primary sites (such as the lung and breast) and in patients with leukemia or lymphoma. These types of metastases are the most common causes of malignant effusions. Therefore, one of the most important parts of the laboratory examination of pericardial fluid is cytological studies for malignant cells.

Laboratory Analysis

Gross Examination

Normal fluid is transparent and pale yellow. Hemorrhagic (bloody) effusions may result from a variety of abnormal conditions or from aspiration of intracardiac blood into the specimen. On visible examination, a hemorrhagic effusion should not form clots in a plain (nonanticoagulant) tube, but aspirated blood usually exhibits clotting. A milky-appearing effusion may be a true or pseudochylous fluid (see "Pleural Fluid" for a discussion of milky effusions).

The value of the measurement of pH is not well established. However, specimens with a pH less than 7.0 may be associated with infectious or rheumatoid disease. In addition, hemorrhagic specimens typically demonstrate a pH that is lower than the pH in circulating blood.

Cell Counts

Erythrocyte and leukocyte cell counts are of limited value in the differential diagnosis of a pericardial effusion. Erythrocyte counts or a determination of packed cell volume (microhematocrit), however, can be valuable in distinguishing a hemorrhagic effusion from aspirated blood in a specimen. The quantity of erythrocytes is usually lower in a hemorrhagic effusion than in a simultaneously assayed circulating blood specimen. In contrast, aspirated blood, if sufficient in quantity, will exhibit an erythrocyte volume that is comparable to that in the circulating blood.

Pericardial fluid is relatively acellular. An increase (more than $1 \times 10^9/L$) is suggestive of microbial infection or malignancy.

Evaluation of Smears

Sediment should be prepared for microscopic examination as previously described in the section "Pleural Fluid". The sediment should be stained and examined for leukocytic cells and malignant mesothelial cells.

Leukocyte Differential

The value of a differential leukocyte count in establishing a differential diagnosis is debatable. However, an elevated total leukocyte count in conjunction with mostly PMNs can be observed in bacterial pericarditis. In contrast, pericardial fluid may demonstrate increased lymphocytes in viral pericarditis.

Mononuclear phagocytes (monocytes, histiocytes, and macrophages) can be seen in variable numbers in pericardial effusions. In addition, in vivo LE cell formation has been observed in pericardial fluids.

TABLE 25.11	**Causes of Pericardial Effusion**
Type	**Cause**
Infectious agents	Viruses, especially Coxsackie group viruses, bacteria (e.g., tubercular, fungal)
Cardiovascular disease	Myocardial infarction, Dressler (postinfarction) syndrome, cardiac rupture, congestive heart failure, acute aortic dissection
Collagen vascular disease	Rheumatic disease
Hemorrhagic	Trauma, anticoagulant therapy, leakage of aortic aneurysm
Renal disease	Kidney failure and uremia (common), long-term dialysis
Neoplastic disease	Mesothelioma, metastatic carcinoma, leukemia, lymphoma

Cytological Examination

Smears should be closely examined for the presence of malignant mesothelial cells. The appearance of these cells was previously described in "Pleural Fluids."

Seminal Fluid

The main function of seminal fluid (semen) is to transport sperm to female cervical mucus. After deposition in the female reproductive tract, sperm remain in the seminal plasma for a short time while attempting to enter the mucus.

Anatomy and Physiology

Each of the male reproductive structures (Fig. 25.8) contributes specific components to seminal fluid. In addition to spermatozoa, this fluid has a highly varied composition (Table 25.12).

On ejaculation, sperm, which constitute only a small part of the total volume of seminal fluid, are released from the epididymal stores and combine with fluids from accessory glands to form seminal fluid. Initially, secretions are added from the prostate gland and then from the seminal vesicles. Prostatic fluid has an acidic pH and provides components (e.g., fibrinolysin for liquefaction of the clot that forms at ejaculation) to the semen. The seminal vesicle, which has an alkaline pH, contributes 70% of the seminal fluid volume and other components (e.g., enzymes for coagulum formation).

The first part of the ejaculated seminal fluid contains sperm and prostatic secretions. The second part of the seminal fluid is composed primarily of seminal vesicle secretions.

Analysis of Seminal Fluid

Principle

Seminal fluid (semen) is examined macroscopically and microscopically. These procedures are performed to determine the physical and chemical properties of the fluid, to quantitate the number of sperm cells, and to examine cellular motility and morphology. Semen analysis is the primary test for the evaluation of male infertility. Although no specific measures are diagnostic of infertility, sperm concentration, motility, and morphology can be used to classify men as subfertile, of indeterminate fertility, or fertile (Table 25.13). Semen also can be analyzed for a variety of reasons, including artificial insemination protocols, postvasectomy assessment, and evaluation of probable sexual assault.

Specimen Collection

A fresh specimen is needed. The specimen may be collected in a clean, sterile, glass or plastic container. Ideally, seminal fluid should be analyzed within 30 minutes of collection. It is mandatory that the specimen be kept at 37°C and examined within 1 hour of collection. After 60 minutes of storage in a plastic container, sperm motility is significantly reduced.

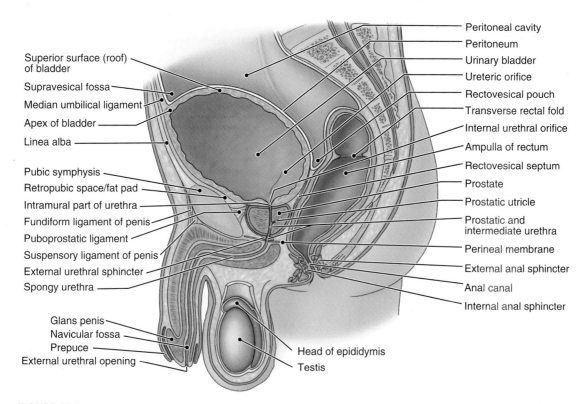

FIGURE 25.8 Sagittal section of the male pelvis. The peritoneum drapes over the relatively simple topology of the bladder and rectum. The prostate gland, which is subject to hyperplasia with advancing age, can be palpated via the rectum. (Reprinted with permission from Moore KL, Dalley AF. *Clinically Oriented Anatomy*, 5th ed, Baltimore, MD: Lippincott Williams & Wilkins, 2006; Figure 3.17A, p. 397.)

TABLE 25.12	Composition of Seminal Fluid
Structure	**Component**
Testicle	Sperm, steroids: testosterone and dihydrotestosterone
Testicle or epididymis	Androgen-binding protein
Testicle (most probable source)	Proteins (enzymes), lipids, electrolytes
Epididymis	Carnitine, acetyl carnitine, glyceryl phosphorylcholine
Seminal vesicles	Flavin, fructose, prostaglandins
Seminal vesicles and prostate	Magnesium
Prostate	Citric acid, enzymes, zine, p30 glycoprotein
Cowper glands, glands of Litter	Unknown

Most laboratories examine two specimens collected a few days apart. Collection, proper transport, and prompt examination are critical factors in the analysis of seminal fluid. Standard precautions should be adhered to when handling semen, blood, and other body fluids.

It is recommended that a 3- to 5-day period of sexual abstinence be observed before specimen collection. Two days may be sufficient; the period should not exceed 5 days. Condoms treated with spermicide or lubricants with spermicidal properties must be avoided during specimen collection. In addition, patients need to be advised to keep the specimen warm, if it is collected at home. In addition, they must be aware that it must be delivered promptly to the laboratory.

Macroscopic Examination

A fresh specimen should be examined for coagulum formation, color, pH, volume, and viscosity. *This procedure, in CLSI format, is provided on this book's companion website at thepoint.lww.com/Turgeon5e.* The results may be useful not only in the assessment of fertility, but also in the detection of other disorders.

Microscopic Examination

Several microscopic procedures may be valuable in the assessment of seminal fluid. *These procedures, in CLSI format, are provided on this book's companion website at thepoint.lww.com/Turgeon5e.* Enumeration of the number of sperm and examination of the morphological characteristics of the cells are routinely performed procedures. Other microscopic procedures include motility, viability, and agglutination studies.

Agglutination may indicate sperm-agglutinating antibodies or prostatitis. A significant increase in abnormal movements of sperm, notably immobilizing-type motion, is highly suggestive of the presence of sperm-immobilizing antibodies in the fluid. Viability and mobility studies should also be correlated.

Morphological characteristics, the commonly encountered variant forms, are presented in Table 25.14. Increases in the number of tapered spermatozoa and immature forms are frequently characteristic of patients with a varicocele and those who have been under extreme stress. Increases in both of these variants are referred to as a nonspecific stress pattern. Other variants have no direct correlation with specific disorders.

Sperm viability requires a very simple two-step staining procedure using eosin-Y as the stain and nigrosin as a

TABLE 25.13	Threshold Values of Semen
Classification[a]	**Values**
Subfertile	<13.5 × 10^6/mL sperm concentration
	<32% of sperm with motility
	<9% of sperm with normal morphologic features
Fertile	>48.0 × 10^6/mL sperm concentration
	>63% of sperm with motility
	>12% of sperm with normal morphologic features

[a]Values between subfertile and fertile are classified as indeterminate.

TABLE 25.14 Sperm Morphology (Variant Forms)	
Type	**% Normal Limits**
Immature sperm cells (spermatids)	<15
Tapered heads	<15
Poorly formed heads	<15
Double heads	<5
Large heads	<5
Small heads	<5
Double or broken tails	<5

counterstain. Using these stains, sperm that do not take up the stain are alive; dead sperm cells appear as pink cells because they do not take up the eosin stain. Additionally, a peroxidase stain, for example, Leucostain, can be used to identify peroxidase-positive leukocytes.

Additional Laboratory Procedures

Other techniques for the examination of semen may be requested in various situations. In cases of infertility, cervical mucus and sperm compatibility tests may be warranted to determine whether the sperm cells are able to penetrate the cervical mucus.

In medicolegal cases, identification and security are paramount, and the procedural protocol is determined by local jurisdiction. In cases of alleged rape or suspected sexual assault, vaginal smears may be submitted for evaluation of the presence of sperm. Sperm can be detected in the vagina for 24 to 72 hours after intercourse. However, the absence of sperm does not mean that intercourse has not taken place. Procedures for the identification of semen stains on clothing may also be requested. These procedures can include screening for A, B, or H blood group substances, the labile enzyme marker peptidase A, and phosphoglucomutase in combination with ABO typing. Other procedures can include examination for fluorescence under ultraviolet light, acid phosphatase test, and enzyme-linked immunosorbent assay for p30 male-specific semen glycoprotein of prostatic origin or an immunological precipitin test to identify semen of human origin on clothing.

Other Microscopic Features

When sperm are being examined for morphological characteristics, the presence of other cellular elements (e.g., erythrocytes, leukocytes, or bacteria) in the specimen should be observed. Debris (e.g., precipitated stain) should not be mistaken for bacteria. All specimens should be observed for *Trichomonas* parasites, particularly donor semen.

Technical Notes: If bacteria are observed, a sterile portion of the specimen should be cultured. However, the probability of a positive finding is low. Semen for artificial insemination should be tested for infectious diseases (e.g., *Neisseria gonorrhoeae*). If a man is being evaluated for infertility, the specimen should be cultured for *Mycoplasma*.

Synovial Fluid

Synovial (joint) fluid is a transparent, viscous fluid secreted by the synovial membrane. This fluid is found in joint cavities, bursae, and tendon sheaths (Fig. 25.9). Its function is to lubricate the joint space and transport nutrients to the articular cartilage. Impaired function of synovial fluid with age or disease may play a role in the development of degenerative joint disease (osteoarthritis). A variety of disorders produce changes in the number and types of cells and the chemical composition of the fluid. Analysis of synovial fluid plays a major role in the diagnosis of joint diseases.

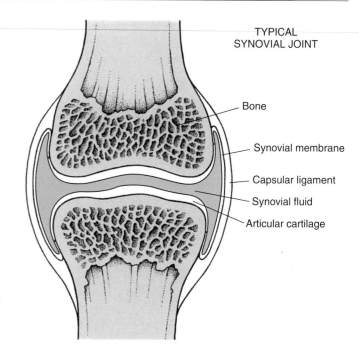

FIGURE 25.9 Synovial joint. (Reprinted with permission from Werner R, Benjamin BE. *A Massage Therapist's Guide to Pathology*, 2nd ed, Baltimore, MD: Lippincott Williams & Wilkins.)

Anatomy and Physiology of Joints

Diarthrodial joints are lined at their margins by a synovial membrane (synovium), with synovial cells lining this space. The lining cells synthesize protein and are phagocytic. Mechanical, chemical, immunological, or bacteriological damage may alter the permeability of the membrane and capillaries to produce varying degrees of inflammatory response. In addition, inflammatory joint fluids contain lytic enzymes that produce depolymerization of hyaluronic acid, which greatly impairs the lubricating ability of the fluid.

Purpose of Arthrocentesis

Arthrocentesis constitutes a liquid biopsy of the joint. It is a fundamental part of the clinical database, together with the medical history, physical examination, and plain radiographic films. Analysis of aspirated synovial fluid is essential in the evaluation of any patient with joint disease because it provides a better reflection of the events in the articular cavity compared with blood tests. For example, abnormal test results such as antinuclear antibody (ANA), increased erythrocyte sedimentation rate (ESR), elevated uric acid concentration, and rheumatoid factor can be seen in healthy individuals or in those with unrelated joint diseases.

Disorders such as gout, **calcium pyrophosphate dihydrate (CPPD)** deposition disease, and septic arthritis can be diagnosed definitively by synovial fluid analysis and may allow for consideration or exclusion of rheumatoid arthritis and systemic lupus erythematosus (SLE). Synovial fluid analysis can also support a diagnosis of diseases as disparate as amyloidosis, hypothyroidism, ochronosis, hemochromatosis, and even simple edema.

In addition, arthrocentesis may alleviate elevated intra-articular pressure. The removal of fluid will relieve symptoms and potentially decrease joint damage. Removal of the products of inflammation is an important component in the treatment of infectious arthritis and may be beneficial in other forms of arthritis.

Aspiration

Arthrocentesis is the process performed by a physician to obtain synovial fluid. Synovial fluid is readily obtained by aspiration from most joints. Frequent sites of aspiration include the knee, shoulder, elbow, wrist, interphalangeal joints, hip, and ankle.

Although aspiration was once performed in surgery, it is now considered to be a bedside procedure. As with other procedures involving potentially infectious fluids, gloves should be worn when performing an aspiration or handling the fluid. Infiltration of the site with lidocaine to decrease pain into the deeper, pain-sensitive structures of the capsule or periosteum increases the risk of injecting anesthetic into the joint space and can interfere with the results of some assays.

Laboratory Assays

Routine analysis of synovial fluid (see procedures, *in CLSI format, provided on this book's companion website at thepoint. lww.com/Turgeon5e*) should include microscopic examination of a wet preparation, crystals, Gram stain, and microbiological culture. If the fluid is very turbid, or if septic arthritis is considered for other reasons, the specimen should be sent for Gram stain and culture. A Gram stain is needed if a high likelihood of infection exists.

Gross Examination

Other observations or procedures can include volume and appearance, viscosity, mucin clot test, chemical analysis for protein and glucose.

Appearance

Synovial fluid is a plasma dialysate; however, certain molecules are preferentially excluded from the joint. Normal, noninflamed joints have small quantities of clear or transparent fluid. This fluid is viscous and slightly alkaline and, if normal, does not clot.

Inflammatory fluid can be translucent or opaque. In general, the more inflammatory the fluid is, the more opaque or purulent its appearance is, but there is no discrete gross appearance that separates infected from noninfected fluid. Cloudiness is not always the result of leukocytes. Fluids can also be opaque because of crystals or other materials (Box 25.2).

The color of synovial fluid ranges from pale yellow to straw colored depending on the amount of albumin, bilirubin, cells,

BOX 25.2

Particulate Matter Found in Synovial Fluid

Adipose tissue fragments	Immune complexes
Amyloid fibrils	Lipid
Bacteria and fungi	Metal and plastic fragments
Cartilage fragments	Parasites
Cells	Rice bodies
Collagen fibrils	Synovial fragments
Crystals	Unrecognizable junk
Fibrin strands and clumps	

and other debris present. Edema produces relatively colorless fluid because of its low protein content. The presence of a grossly bloody fluid should raise the suspicion of a number of disorders (Box 25.3).

Viscosity

The description of viscosity is a time-honored test. In fact, this property gave synovial fluid its name. If synovial fluid is allowed to drip from the aspirating needle, a long string implies high viscosity and an absent or short string implies low viscosity. An implied justification for estimating viscosity is to differentiate between noninflammatory (high-viscosity) and inflammatory (low-viscosity) fluids. Unusually, viscous fluids are obtained from ganglia, hypothyroid effusions, and patients with SLE.

BOX 25.3

Examples of Conditions Associated With Hemarthrosis

Anticoagulant therapy
Hereditary deficiency of clotting factors
    (e.g., hemophilia or von Willebrand disease)
Infection
Metallic joint prostheses
Osteoarthritis
Postsurgery or prosthesis
Preexisting arthritis
Pseudogout
Rheumatoid arthritis
Sickle cell disease (crisis)
Synovial hemangioma
Thrombocytopenia
Thrombocytosis
Trauma with or without fracture

Mucin Clot Test

The best use of the mucin clot test is to distinguish the anatomical origin of bloody or other fluids. The presence of a mucin clot implies that it is synovial fluid.

The mucin clot procedure estimates the density and friability of the precipitate that forms when synovial fluid is placed in dilute acetic acid. The addition of several drops of normal synovial fluid to a dilute (2% to 5%) acetic acid solution results in the formation of a tight, sticky, rope-like mass (polymerization of synovial fluid hyaluronate) that remains intact when shaken. A good or excellent clot implies high–molecular-weight hyaluronic acid and normal hyaluronate-protein interactions. A fair or poor clot implies inflammatory arthritis. There are, however, no standard criteria for performance of the test, and the end point is subjective.

Microscopic Examination

Wet Preparation Examination

Fresh synovial fluid should be examined under a clean coverslip by routine microscopy for cells and particulate material. Cytoplasmic inclusions within granulocytes sparkle and can appear to be light or dark. These inclusions are believed to represent distended phagosomes or droplets containing lipid. It is important to note whether crystalline material is intracellular or extracellular. In acute attacks of gout and pseudogout, crystals are engulfed by leukocytes. During intercritical periods, crystals may lie free in the fluid. Immunofluorescent studies have demonstrated that some inclusions contain immunoglobulins and complement.

Fracture or trauma to a joint can produce free lipid droplets in the synovial fluid, which can also be seen in aseptic necrosis and fat embolism. These droplets are rarely seen in inflammatory effusions. Irregular strands of fibrin or fibrillar fragments of cartilage may be observed in specimens from patients with degenerative arthritis.

Cells and other particulate matter should not be confused with crystalline materials. One basis for differentiation is that crystals have straight, parallel edges. In addition to routine light microscopy, examination with a polarized light microscope is recommended for the identification of crystals (Table 25.15).

Basic Calcium Phosphate

Basic calcium phosphate (BCP) crystals include hydroxyapatite (HA), octacalcium phosphate, and tricalcium phosphate. The size of BCP crystals is below the limits of resolution of optical microscopy. If aggregated, they are visible by light microscopy and appear as shiny, laminated, printed coins. With a polarized microscope, BCP crystals are nonbirefringent.

BCP crystals are associated with subcutaneous calcification and calcific periarthritis and tendinitis. In addition, BCP crystals can be found in both acute and chronic synovitis.

Monosodium Urate

Monosodium urate (MSU) crystals are 8 to 10 μμ in length and are needle- or rod-shaped. The crystals may be pointed and intracellular or extracellular. With a polarization microscope, MSU crystals appear as strongly birefringent rods or needles that are bright against a dark, fully polarized background. With a red compensator, they appear yellow in color when the longitudinal crystal axis is parallel (negative birefringence) to the slow component of the compensator. The crystals appear to be blue when perpendicular to the axis of the compensator.

MSU crystals are pathognomonic for gouty arthritis.

Calcium Pyrophosphate Dihydrate

Calcium pyrophosphate dihydrate (CPPD) crystals are more easily seen with a good light microscope. CPPD crystals assume multiple, three-dimensional forms: rods, rhomboids, and parallelpipeds occur simultaneously.

With a polarizing microscope, CPPD crystals are less birefringent than MSU crystals and are more difficult to identify. With a red compensator, CPPD crystals appear blue when the longitudinal axis is parallel to the slow component of the compensator. They exhibit positive birefringence. CPPD crystals are yellow when perpendicular to the axis of the compensator.

CPPD crystals are associated with CPPD deposition disease. However, they may be identified in effusions from a number of inflammatory joint diseases, particularly rheumatoid arthritis.

Cholesterol Crystals

Cholesterol crystals are usually easy to distinguish because of their large size and flat, plate-like shape. Characteristically, these rectangular plates have notched corners. They may, however, appear as long, birefringent needles or as rhomboids, resembling MSU or CPPD crystals.

The presence of cholesterol crystals is considered to be nonspecific. However, they are usually found in chronic effusions from patients with rheumatoid arthritis.

Artifacts

Artifacts can be mistaken for crystals, although crystals have sharp, clearly defined edges and straight sides. Particulate matters that can be confused with crystals include plastic joint prostheses, nail polish, dust particles, immersion oil droplets, and refractile collagen fibrils.

CPPD and MSU crystals can be confused with other birefringent materials including crystalline anticoagulants, such as calcium oxalate, ethylenediaminetetraacetic acid (EDTA), and lithium heparin; certain corticosteroid preparations; and talcum powder.

Clinical Applications

The distinction between various types of arthritis is not always easy to make based on clinical observations. Traditionally, synovial fluids have been classified into several categories (Tables 25.16 and 25.17) based on gross appearance, total leukocyte and differential cell counts, and physical and chemical examinations.

TABLE 25.15	Characteristics of Synovial Fluid Crystals		
Crystal	**Mircroscopic Appearance**	**With Polarization**	**Associated Disorders**
Monosodium urate (MSU)	Acicular	Strongly negatively birefringent	Acute gouty arthritis Tophaceous gout
Calcium pyrophosphate dihydrate (CPPD)	Polymorphic	Weakly positively birefringent	CPPD deposition disease
Calcium hydroxyapatite	Too small to identify; with electron microscopy, as small needles or rods	Not birefringent	Calcific tendinitis Apatite-associated destructive arthritis Soft tissue calcifications in the connective tissue diseases
Calcium oxalate	Polymorphic, classically bipyramidal	Variable; positively birefringent or strongly to weakly birefringent	Chronic renal disease Oxalosis
Lipid liquid	"Maltese cross"	Strongly positively birefringent	Acute and chronic arthritis
Cholesterol	Large, plate like, with punched-out corners	Strongly variably birefringent	Chronic rheumatoid effusions
Corticosteroids	Polymorphic clumps, rods, or rhomboids	Strongly variably birefringent	Iatrogenic
Talc	Varying size	Strongly positively birefringent	Contaminant

MSU, monosodium urate; CPPD, calcium pyrophosphate dihydrate.

TABLE 25.16	**Comparison of Inflammatory and Noninflammatory Synovial Fluids**

Category	Total WBC Count	% polymorpho-nuclear segmented neutrophils
Inflammatory	>2 × 10⁹/L	>75%
Noninflammatory	<2 × 10⁹/L	<75%

Body Fluid Slide Preparation

A differential cell count on a body fluid should be performed on stained smears prepared from a concentrated preparation—not in a hemocytometer. Some of the techniques of sediment preparation and staining are different for body fluids than for blood. *The procedure, in CLSI format, is provided on this book's companion website at thepoint.lww. com/Turgeon5e.*

Ordinary centrifugation can be used to concentrate cellular elements in the sediment, and slides can be prepared with the traditional push method. This method has the advantage of requiring no special equipment, but the recovery of cells is variable and a considerable amount of cellular damage is produced.

More effective methods of concentrating cells include sedimentation, cytocentrifugation, and filtration.

Staining of Body Fluid Sediment

Morphological descriptions of cells encountered in body fluids reflect their microscopic appearance with Wright or Wright-Giemsa stain. The coloration of cells with Papanicolaou stain (Table 25.18) is somewhat different. However, the Papanicolaou stain is a commonly used cytological stain. *This procedure, in CLSI format, is provided on this book's companion website at thepoint.lww.com/Turgeon5e.*

The Wright-Giemsa stain is basically a cytoplasmic stain with moderate nuclear staining ability. In contrast, the Papanicolaou stain is predominantly a nuclear stain with a modest ability for cytoplasmic differentiation. The Wright-Giemsa staining method is simpler than the Papanicolaou

TABLE 25.17	**Classification of Synovial Fluid**

Group	Description
I	Noninflammatory
II	Inflammatory
III	Infectious
IV	Crystal induced
V	Hemorrhagic

method because it requires no immediate fixation of the slide and therefore fewer steps in the staining procedure. However, a difference in cell size is evident between the two staining protocols. Cells appear larger when prepared by the air-dried, Wright-Giemsa procedure. It is most helpful, if possible, to prepare and stain specimens by both methods to gain as much information as possible. The criteria for diagnosis are exactly the same for normal or abnormal cells by either method.

Amniotic Fluid

Amniotic fluid is the nourishing and protecting liquid contained by the amnion of a pregnant woman. It consists of mostly water but also contains proteins, carbohydrates, lipids and phospholipids, urea, and electrolytes, all of which aid in the growth of the fetus. In the late stages of gestation, most of the amniotic fluid consists of fetal urine.

The volume of amniotic fluid increases until about 34 weeks of gestation, at which time the amount of amniotic fluid is about 800 mL and is reduced to about 600 mL at the time of birth (about 40 weeks).

Amniotic fluid is continually being swallowed and "inhaled" and replaced through being "exhaled." It is essential that the amniotic fluid be breathed into the lungs by the fetus in order for the lungs to develop normally.

The analysis of amniotic fluid, tapped from the mother's abdomen, is called amniocentesis. The fluid contains fetal cells that can be examined for genetic defects, and chemical analysis, e.g., fibronectin, and other assays can determine fetal lung maturity.

Fetal fibronectin (fFN) is a protein produced during pregnancy and functions as a biological glue, attaching the fetal sac to the uterine lining. fFN is performed if a woman is 26 to 34 weeks pregnant and having symptoms of premature labor. The goal then is to intervene to prevent the potentially serious health complications of a preterm baby.

A cervical or vaginal fluid sample is collected and analyzed for fFN. During the first trimester and for about half of the second trimester (up to 22 weeks of gestation), fFN is normally present in the cervicovaginal secretions of pregnant women. In most pregnancies, after 22 weeks, this protein is no longer detected until the end of the last trimester (1 to 3 weeks before labor). The presence of fFN during weeks 24 to 34 of a high-risk pregnancy, along with symptoms of labor, suggests that the "glue" may be disintegrating ahead of schedule and alerts doctors to a possibility of preterm delivery.

A negative fFN result is highly predictive that preterm delivery will not occur within the next 7 to 14 days. A negative fFN can reduce unnecessary hospitalizations and drug therapies. High levels can be due to causes other than risk of preterm delivery. The American College of Obstetrics and Gynecology currently does not recommend routine fFN screening of pregnant women, as its use has not been shown to be clinically effective in predicting preterm labor in low-risk, asymptomatic pregnancies.

TABLE 25.18 Papanicolaou-Stained Morphology		
Cell Type	**Nucleus**	**Cytoplasm**
Neutrophils (mature)	Multilobulated; hyperchromatic	Green or pink; granules not evident
Neutrophils (immature)		Green or pink; primary granules not visible; secondary granules present
Lymphocytes	Round with finely granular chromatin; no nucleolus visible	Green; absent or scanty
Lymphocytes (reactive)	Oval to cleaved; finely granular with evenly distributed chromatin; small chromocenter	Green; moderate amount
Monocyte (usually macrophages in pleural fluid)	Lacy	Some color; moderate amount; slightly vacuolated
Macrophage	Lacy chromatin pattern; irregular shape	Green; degenerating cell may be pink
Mesothelial cell	Size variable (may occupy up to 50% of the cell); round to oval; usually central; well-defined membrane; evenly distributed granular chromatin; small nucleoli may be present; multinucleated	Deep pink or green; homogeneous distribution; may be more densely stained in center of the cell and around the nucleus; pale cytoplasmic vacuoles may be seen
Ependymal cells	Round; central dense chromatin; may be grainy or possible nucleoli	Green or pink; may have "brush" borders; generous amount
Choroidal cells	Round; central, smooth, dense chromatin	Pale green; moderate amount
Plasma cells	Round to oval; eccentrically located; clumped chromatin	Dense and green; abundant; paranuclear area present; may contain small vacuoles (e.g., Russell bodies, "grape cells")
Basophils		Granules do not stain

CHAPTER HIGHLIGHTS

Sterile body fluid can be found in various body cavities under normal conditions. Specimens can be analyzed for the total number of cells, differentiation of cell types, chemical composition, and microbial contents depending on the source of the aspirate. Standard precautions must be practiced.

Cerebrospinal Fluid

CSF acts as a shock absorber for the brain and spinal cord, circulates nutrients, lubricates the CNS, and may also contribute to the nourishment of brain tissue. Clinically, the examination of spinal fluid is useful in diagnosing a variety of disorders including subarachnoid hemorrhage, meningeal infection (meningitis), multiple sclerosis, and neoplasms.

Normal CSF is crystal clear and colorless. A yellow coloring of a specimen or the supernatant of a centrifuged specimen is referred to as xanthochromia. This discoloration is caused by the release of hemoglobin from hemolyzed erythrocytes (RBCs) in the CSF. Gross blood may also be observed in traumatic tap specimens or in cases of pathological bleeding caused by spontaneous subarachnoid hemorrhage or intracerebral hemorrhage. Normal CSF has the viscosity of water. Clotting can be caused by increased protein. Gel formation on standing is caused by an increased fibrinogen content.

Total WBC counts are useful in developing a differential diagnosis. Very few leukocytes should be seen in normal CSF. Elevated WBC counts can be observed in acute, untreated, bacterial meningitis. Very high WBC counts are unusual and suggest intraventricular rupture of a brain abscess. Normal CSF contains a few mononuclear cells (lymphocytes and monocytes) and rare ependymal cells. Cells that may be encountered in CSF include granulocytic leukocytes (mature and immature neutrophils, eosinophils, and basophils), mature lymphocytes or reactive lymphocytes, mononuclear phagocytes (monocytes, histiocytes, and macrophages), plasma cells, ependymal cells and choroidal cells, leukemic blasts, and malignant cells (e.g., lymphoma cells or tumor cells). Other types of cells can include immature, nucleated erythrocytes or intracellular bacteria.

Glucose and protein values are important to correlate with gross and microscopic findings. In general, a decreased glucose level in the CSF in the presence of a normal blood glucose level indicates bacterial utilization of glucose. In addition, an elevated total protein concentration is suggestive of an inflammatory reaction or a bacterial infection. A viral infection will not have a dramatic effect on CSF glucose levels and may not affect the total protein level significantly.

Pleural, Peritoneal, and Pericardial Fluids

An **effusion** is an abnormal accumulation of fluid in a particular space of the body. Effusions in the plural, pericardial, and peritoneal cavities are divided into transudates or exudates. **Transudates** generally indicate that fluid has accumulated because of the presence of a systemic disease. In contrast, **exudates** are usually associated with disorders such as inflammation, infection, and malignant conditions involving the cells that line the surfaces of organs (e.g., lung or abdominal organs). Transudates and exudates frequently differ in characteristics such as color and clarity and total leukocyte cell count.

Pleural fluid is normally produced by the parietal pleura and absorbed by the visceral pleura, as a continuous process. Although healthy individuals form 600 to 800 mL of fluid daily, the normal volume of fluid in each pleural space is estimated to be less than 10 mL. The accumulation of fluid in the pleural space is referred to as a pleural effusion. Aspiration of pleural fluid is referred to as **thoracentesis**. The location of a pleural effusion may be suggestive of the type of disorder involved in causing the effusion. Erythrocyte and leukocyte counts are of limited value in the differential diagnosis of pleural effusions. A massively bloody (hemorrhagic) effusion in the absence of trauma almost always suggests malignancy or occasionally pulmonary infarct. Pure blood in pleural cavity, true hemothorax, results from severe chest injuries. Extremely elevated total WBC counts are consistent with a diagnosis of empyema. Cell types that can be encountered in the examination of a Wright-Giemsa–stained specimen include polymorphonuclear segmented neutrophils (PMNs), eosinophils, basophils, lymphocytes, plasma cells, mononuclear phagocytes (monocytes, histiocytes, and macrophages), mesothelial cells (normal, reactive, atypical, or malignant), and metastatic tumor (malignant) cells. In addition, in vivo LE cells have also been observed in pleural fluids.

The presence of peritoneal fluid reduces friction between the visceral and parietal peritonea as they move against each other. An abnormal amount of fluid (an effusion) can accumulate in the peritoneal cavity if the balance between fluid formation and reabsorption is altered by a disease process. The collection of fluid in the peritoneal cavity is called **ascites**. The procedure for removing fluid from the peritoneal cavity is paracentesis. The causes of peritoneal effusions range from disorders and diseases that directly represent involvement of the peritoneum, such as bacterial peritonitis, to abdominal conditions that do not directly involve the peritoneum, such as hepatic cirrhosis, cirrhosis, congestive heart failure, Budd-Chiari syndrome, hypoalbuminemia (caused by nephrotic syndrome or protein-losing enteropathy malnutrition), and miscellaneous disorders such as myxedema, ovarian diseases, pancreatic disease, and chylous ascites. A variety of clinical conditions can produce a deviation from the anticipated yellow or straw-colored fluid seen on gross examination. For example, grossly bloody (hemorrhagic) peritoneal fluid may be seen in trauma patients with a ruptured spleen or liver, intestinal infarction, pancreatitis, or malignancies. Total RBC and WBC counts are usually performed on ascitic fluid.

Smears should be prepared for microscopic examination and properly stained with Wright or Wright-Giemsa stain for differential leukocyte evaluation or stained with Papanicolaou stain for cytological evaluation.

Although the quantities of some cells in peritoneal fluid compared to pleural fluid may vary in some disorders, the cell types that can be encountered are the same as those that can be seen in pleural fluids. These cells include PMNs, eosinophils, basophils, lymphocytes, plasma cells, mononuclear phagocytes (monocytes, histiocytes, and macrophages), mesothelial cells (normal, reactive, atypical, or malignant), and metastatic tumor (malignant) cells. In addition, in vivo LE cells have also been observed.

The pericardium is filled with a small amount of fluid to reduce friction between the layers of the pericardial cavity. An abnormal accumulation of fluid in the cavity is called a **pericardial effusion**. Pericardial effusion is usually accurately assessed by echocardiography. A wide variety of diseases and disorders can produce pericardial effusion. Neoplastic disease, which produces a significant volume of fluid in the pericardium, is one of the most common causes of pericardial effusion. Normal fluid is transparent and pale yellow. Hemorrhagic (bloody) effusions may result from a variety of abnormal conditions or from aspiration of intracardiac blood into the specimen. Pericardial fluid is relatively acellular.

Seminal Fluid

The main function of seminal fluid is to transport sperm to the female cervical mucus. Seminal fluid is examined physically, chemically, and microscopically. These procedures are performed to determine the physical and chemical properties, to quantitate the number of sperm cells, and to examine cellular motility and morphology. Fresh specimens should be examined for color, pH, volume, and viscosity. Increased viscosity can be of significance if it impedes sperm motility. Several microscopic procedures may be valuable in the assessment of seminal fluid. Enumeration of the number of sperm and examination of the morphological characteristics of the cells are routinely performed procedures. Other microscopic procedures may include motility, viability, and agglutination studies. Other techniques for the examination of semen may be requested in various situations. In cases of infertility, cervical mucus–sperm compatibility tests may be warranted to determine whether the sperm cells are able to penetrate the cervical mucus.

Seminal fluid can be analyzed for a variety of reasons, including infertility studies, artificial insemination protocols, postvasectomy assessment, and evaluation of probable sexual assault. In cases of alleged rape or suspected sexual assault, vaginal smears may be submitted for evaluation of the presence of sperm.

Synovial Fluid

Synovial fluid is a transparent, viscous fluid secreted by the synovial membrane. This fluid is found in joint cavities, bursae, and tendon sheaths. Its function is to lubricate the joint space and transport nutrients to the articular cartilage. Impaired function of synovial fluid with age or disease may play a role in the development of degenerative joint disease (osteoarthritis). A variety of disorders produce changes in the number and types of cells and the chemical composition of the fluid.

Analysis of synovial fluid plays a major role in the diagnosis of joint diseases. Arthrocentesis constitutes a liquid biopsy of the joint. Analysis of aspirated synovial fluid is essential in the evaluation of any patient with joint disease because it provides a better reflection of the events in the articular cavity than do blood tests. For example, abnormal test results such as ANA, increased ESR, elevated uric acid level, and rheumatoid factor can be seen in healthy individuals or in those with unrelated joint diseases. Disorders such as gout, CPPD deposition disease, and septic arthritis can be diagnosed definitively by synovial fluid analysis and may allow for consideration or exclusion of rheumatoid arthritis and SLE. Synovial fluid analysis can also support a diagnosis of diseases as disparate as amyloidosis, hypothyroidism, ochronosis, hemochromatosis, and even simple edema. In addition, arthrocentesis may alleviate elevated intra-articular pressure.

Body Fluid Slide Preparation

A differential cell count on a body fluid should be performed on stained smears prepared from a concentrated preparation—not in a hemocytometer. Ordinary centrifugation can be used to concentrate cellular elements in the sediment, and slides can be prepared with the traditional push method. More effective methods of concentrating cells include sedimentation, cytocentrifugation, and filtration.

REVIEW QUESTIONS

Questions 1 to 5: Match each of the terms with their appropriate synonyms.
1. _____ CSF
2. _____ Synovial fluid
3. _____ Peritoneal fluid
4. _____ Pericardial fluid
5. _____ Pleural fluid
   A. Lumbar puncture fluid
   B. Joint fluid
   C. Chest fluid
   D. Ascitic fluid
   E. Fluid from around the heart

Questions 6 to 8: Match the fluids with the appropriate normal characteristics.
6. _____ CSF
7. _____ Synovial fluid
8. _____ Seminal fluid
   A. Clear and yellow
   B. Turbid and viscous
   C. Clear and colorless

Questions 9 to 11: Match the fluids and normal total leukocyte or total sperm count.
9. _____ CSF
10. _____ Synovial fluid
11. _____ Seminal fluid
    A. 0 to 10×10^6/L
    B. 60 to 150×10^9/L
    C. Less than 200/μL
12. The anatomical structures associated with the circulation of CSF are
    A. ventricles and subarachnoid spaces
    B. subarachnoid space and pia mater
    C. ependyma and pia mater
    D. arachnoid mater and pia mater

13. CSF production is associated with the
    A. arachnoid mater and pia mater
    B. choroid plexus and ependymal lining
    C. arachnoid mater and subarachnoid space
    D. subarachnoid space and pia mater
14. CSF is collected from an intervertebral space between the _____ and _____ vertebrae.
    A. T4, T5
    B. L2, L3
    C. L3, L4
    D. L4, L5

Questions 15 to 17: Match the following test tube aliquots of CSF with the typical type of testing that should be performed.
15. _____ Tube 1
16. _____ Tube 2
17. _____ Tube 3
    A. Gross examination, cell count, and morphology
    B. Microbial examination
    C. Chemical and serological examination

Questions 18 to 21: Match the following gross examination findings of CSF with the appropriate diagnosis.
18. _____ Cloudy and turbid
19. _____ Grossly bloody specimen
20. _____ Xanthochromia (yellow color)
21. _____ Gel formation
    A. Increased fibrinogen
    B. Subarachnoid hemorrhage
    C. Subarachnoid hemorrhage (more than 12 hours after the bleed)
    D. Pleocytosis

(continued)

Questions 22 to 26: Match the following microscopic findings of CSF with the associated condition.

22. _____ Intraventricular rupture of brain abscess
23. _____ Viral infection
24. _____ 0 to 5×10^6/L
25. _____ Bacterial infection
26. _____ CNS leukemia or lymphoma
   A. Lymphocytosis
   B. Increased polymorphonuclear segmented neutrophils (PMNs)
   C. Macrophages
   D. Extremely elevated leukocyte count in CSF
   E. Normal leukocyte reference range for CSF

27. Normal CSF contains
   A. lymphocytes and ependymal cells
   B. ependymal and choroidal cells
   C. mesothelial and ependymal cells
   D. erythrocytes and leukocytes

28. The cell count on a CSF specimen should be performed within _____ of collection.
   A. 30 minutes
   B. 1 hour
   C. 2 hours
   D. 12 hours
   E. 24 hours

29. Clotting in CSF may be caused by
   A. increased protein concentration
   B. increased electrolyte concentration
   C. increased glucose concentration
   D. the presence of bacteria

30. An increased total leukocyte count in a CSF specimen can be caused by
   A. bacterial meningitis
   B. viral meningoencephalitis
   C. intravascular rupture of a brain abscess
   D. both A and C

31. An increase in the number of lymphocytes in a CSF specimen can be caused by
   A. multiple sclerosis
   B. viral meningoencephalitis
   C. fungal meningitis
   D. all of the above

32. Which of the following is (are) characteristic of an effusion?
   A. Abnormal accumulation of fluid
   B. Can be a transudate
   C. Can be an exudate
   D. All of the above

33. A transudate can be described as
   A. specific gravity >1.016, low to moderate number of leukocytes, and lactic dehydrogenase <200 IU/L
   B. specific gravity <1.016, pH 7.4 to 7.5, and lactic dehydrogenase <200 IU/L

   C. pH 7.35 to 7.45 and protein concentration >3.0 g/dL
   D. lactic dehydrogenase <200 IU/L and protein concentration >3.0 g/dL

Questions 34 to 36: Match the term with the appropriate physical description.

34. _____ Pleura
35. _____ Peritoneum
36. _____ Pericardium
   A. Covers abdominal walls and viscera of the abdomen
   B. Covers the lungs
   C. A fibrous sac around the heart

37. Conditions not associated with pleural effusion include
   A. tuberculosis
   B. infectious diseases
   C. mesothelioma
   D. viral pneumonia

Questions 38 to 42: Match the representative exudate appearance with a typical associated disorder.

38. _____ Yellow and turbid
39. _____ Milky
40. _____ Bloody
41. _____ Clearly visible pus
42. _____ Foul odor
   A. Empyema
   B. Infectious process
   C. Anaerobic bacterial infection
   D. Chylothorax
   E. Malignancy in the absence of trauma

43. Pleural fluid can have a white supernatant fluid after centrifugation owing to
   A. increased concentration of leukocytes
   B. presence of lipids
   C. presence of chylomicrons
   D. both A and B

44. An extremely elevated leukocyte concentration in pleural fluid is typically associated with
   A. hemothorax
   B. malignancy
   C. empyema
   D. classic rheumatoid effusion

45. Which of the following cells can be seen in pleural fluid?
   A. LE cells
   B. Mononuclear phagocytes
   C. Mesothelial cells
   D. All of the above

46. All of the following describe the characteristics of malignant cells except
   A. multiple round aggregates of cells
   B. high N:C ratio
   C. large, irregular nucleoli
   D. smooth chromatin

(continued)

Questions 47 to 50: Match the cellular abnormality encountered in pleural and peritoneal fluids with a representative disorder (use an answer only once).

47. _____ Many neutrophils, histiocytes, and mesothelial cells
48. _____ Abundant, multinuclear cells and clusters of cells
49. _____ Many malignant cells (in clusters)
50. _____ Many lymphocytes, mesothelial cells, histiocytes, and plasma cells
 A. Viral infection
 B. Acute bacterial inflammation
 C. Metastatic adenocarcinoma
 D. Malignant mesothelioma
 E. Chronic granulomatous inflammation

Questions 51 and 52: In a pleural effusion, the percentage of (51) _____ is extremely high in pneumonia and the percentage of (52) _____ is extremely high in viral peritonitis.

51. A. polymorphonuclear segmented neutrophils
 B. eosinophils
 C. basophils
 D. monocytes
52. A. polymorphonuclear segmented neutrophils
 B. eosinophils
 C. basophils
 D. lymphocytes
53. The causes of peritoneal effusion include all of the following except
 A. bacterial peritonitis
 B. hepatic cirrhosis
 C. congestive heart failure
 D. tuberculosis
54. An abnormal-appearing peritoneal effusion can be caused by all of the following except
 A. bacterial peritonitis
 B. pancreatitis
 C. neoplasm
 D. tuberculous peritonitis

Questions 55 to 57: Match the following peritoneal effusion colors with the respective condition (use each answer once).

55. _____ Pale yellow
56. _____ Straw colored
57. _____ Bloody
 A. Normal
 B. Pulmonary infarct
 C. Congestive heart failure
58. An extremely increased leukocyte concentration in peritoneal fluid can be caused by
 A. bacterial peritonitis
 B. pancreatitis
 C. cirrhosis
 D. none of the above

Questions 59 to 61: Match an increase in the following cells in peritoneal fluid with the representative abnormality.

59. _____ Eosinophils
60. _____ Lymphocytes
61. _____ Mesothelial cells
 A. Chronic peritoneal dialysis
 B. Congestive heart failure, cirrhosis, and nephrotic syndrome
 C. Tuberculous peritonitis

Questions 62 to 64: Match the various types and respective causes of pericardial effusion.

62. _____ Infectious agents
63. _____ Collagen vascular disease
64. _____ Neoplastic disease
 A. Rheumatic disease
 B. Mesothelioma
 C. Dressler postinfarction syndrome
 D. Coxsackie group viruses
65. A cause of an increased concentration of cells in pericardial fluid is
 A. microbial infection
 B. malignancy
 C. congestive heart failure
 D. both A and B

Questions 66 to 69: Match the following male reproductive structures with their constituents.

66. _____ Testicle
67. _____ Seminal vesicles
68. _____ Prostate
69. _____ Cowper glands
 A. Fructose and prostaglandins
 B. Unknown
 C. Sperm
 D. p30 glycoprotein
70. Sperm motility can become decreased if the specimen is
 A. stored at room temperature
 B. stored in a plastic container for more than 1 hour
 C. examined after 2 hours of storage
 D. all of the above
71. The normal value of sperm cells is _____ × 10⁹/L.
 A. 15 to 30
 B. 30 to 45
 C. 30 to 60
 D. 60 to 150

Questions 72 to 76: Match the normal values or appropriate term.

72. _____ Motility (fresh specimen)
73. _____ Sperm morphology
74. _____ Viability (fresh specimen)
75. _____ Agglutination

(continued)

76. _____ Artificial insemination
   A. At least 50%
   B. 40% to 90% (mature and oval headed)
   C. Test for infectious disease
   D. Prostatitis or sperm-agglutinating antibodies
   E. Greater than 60%

77. Arthrocentesis is
   A. a bone biopsy
   B. a liquid biopsy
   C. not as accurate as blood testing
   D. a good test to monitor the effects of chemotherapy

78. Disorders that can be diagnosed definitively by synovial fluid analysis are
   A. gout, CPPD deposition disease, and rheumatoid arthritis
   B. CPPD deposit disease, rheumatoid arthritis, and SLE
   C. rheumatoid arthritis, SLE, and septic arthritis
   D. gout, CPPD deposition disease, and septic arthritis

79. Which of the following would not be an aspiration site for synovial fluid?
   A. Knee
   B. Elbow
   C. Posterior iliac crest
   D. Ankle

80. If a synovial fluid aspirate is very turbid and septic arthritis is suspected, a _____ should definitely be performed.

   A. total cell count and differential count
   B. crystal examination
   C. Gram stain and culture
   D. all of the above

81. Crystals that are in multiple three-dimensional forms are
   A. CPPD crystals
   B. BCP crystals
   C. MSU crystals
   D. cholesterol

82. An increased percentage of polymorphonuclear segmented neutrophils (PMNs) is characteristic of
   A. chronic urticaria
   B. septic arthritis
   C. rheumatoid arthritis
   D. rheumatic fever

Questions 83 to 86: Match the following crystals with an associated disorder (use each answer once).

83. _____ MSU
84. _____ Calcium oxalate
85. _____ Cholesterol
86. _____ Lipid liquid "maltese cross"
   A. Chronic renal disease
   B. Chronic rheumatoid effusions
   C. Acute and chronic arthritis
   D. Acute gouty arthritis

BIBLIOGRAPHY

Baker DJ. Performing a quality semen analysis in the clinical laboratory, *Med Lab Observ*, 32(12):20–31, 2000.

Baker DJ. Questions about semen analysis, *Med Lab Observ*, 33(4): 5,2001.

Baker DJ. Semen analysis, *Clin Lab Sci*, 20(3):172–187, 2007.

Barry E. Risk to offspring is found in male biological clock, *The Boston Globe*, (www.boston.com/dailyglobe). Retrieved December 4, 2002.

Braunwald E, et al. Ascites. In: Wilson JD (ed.). *Harrison's Principles of Internal Medicine*, 12th ed, New York, NY: McGraw-Hill, 1988:70–74.

Cannon DC, Henry JB. Seminal fluid. In: Henry JB (ed.). *Clinical Diagnosis and Management by Laboratory Methods*, 18th ed, Philadelphia, PA: Saunders, 1991:497–503.

Eastern JD. Spinal fluid examination. In: Stein JH (ed.). *Internal Medicine*, Boston, MA: Little, Brown & Co., 1990:1870–1871.

Guzick DS, et al. Sperm morphology, motility, and concentration in fertile and infertile men, *N Engl J Med*, 345(19):1388–1393, 2001.

Hoffman GS. Arthritis due to deposition of calcium crystals. In: Wilson JD (ed.). *Harrison's Principles of Internal Medicine*, 12th ed, New York, NY: McGraw-Hill, 1990:1479–1482.

Jones CD, Cornbleet PJ. Wright-Giemsa cytology of body fluids, *Lab Med*, 28(11):713–716, 1997.

Judkins SW, Cornbleet PJ. Synovial fluid crystal analysis, *Lab Med*, 28(12):774–779, 1997.

Krieg AF, Kjeldsberg CR. Cerebrospinal fluid and other body fluids. In: Henry JB (ed.). *Clinical Management and Diagnosis by Laboratory Methods*, Philadelphia, PA: Saunders, 1991:445–457, 463–469.

Lipsky PE. Rheumatoid arthritis. In: Wilson JD (ed.). *Harrison's Principles of Internal Medicine*, 12th ed, New York, NY: McGraw-Hill, 1990:1437–1471.

Lyons MK, Meyer FB. Cerebrospinal fluid physiology and the management of increased intracranial pressure, *Mayo Clin Proc*, 65: 684–707, 1990.

McCarty DJ. Arthritis associated with calcium-containing crystals. In: Stein JH (ed.). *Internal Medicine*, Boston, MA: Little, Brown & Co., 1990:1809–1813.

Nosanchuck JS, Kim CW. Lupus erythematosus cells in CSF, *JAMA*, 25:2883–2884, 1976.

Oehmichen M, et al. Origin, proliferation and fate of cerebrospinal fluid cells, *J Neurol*, 227:145–150, 1982.

Plaut D. Analysis of body fluids, *Adv Lab*, 14(11):46–52, 2005.

Pleural effusions. In: *Medical Knowledge Self-Assessment Program VIII*, *Pulmonary Medicine*, Part A, Book 6. Philadelphia, PA: American College of Physicians, 1988:231.

Rheumatology. In: *Medical Knowledge Self-Assessment Program VIII*, Part B, Book 6. Philadelphia, pA: American College of Physicians, 1988.

Rothman SA, Reese AA. Semen Analysis: the test techs love to hate, *Med Lab Observ*, 39(4):18–27, 2007.

Rotrosen D. Infectious arthritis. In: Wilson JD (ed.). *Harrison's Principles of Internal Medicine,* 12th ed, New York, NY: McGraw-Hill, 1990: 544–549.

Sampson JH, Alexander NJ. Semen analysis: A laboratory approach, *Lab Med*, 13:218–223, 1982.

Schumacher HR Jr. (ed.). Arthrocentesis and synovial fluid analysis. In: *Primer on the Rheumatic Diseases,* 9th ed, Atlanta, GA: Arthritis Foundation, 1988:55–60, 79–80.

Schumacher HR Jr. Synovial fluid analysis. In: Kelley WN, et al. (eds.). *Textbook of Rheumatology,* Philadelphia, PA: Saunders, 1985:561–568.

Schumann GB, Linker G. Cytopreparatory techniques for bronchoalveolar lavage specimens, *Lab Med*, 23(2):115–119, 1992.

Shmerling RH, et al. Synovial fluid tests—What should be ordered? *JAMA*, 264(8):1201–1203, 1990.

Strickland DM, Ziaya PR. Reduced sperm motility in plastic containers, *Lab Med,* 18(5):310–312, 1987.

Terry M. Body fluids: manual and automated urinalsys, *Adv Med Lab Prof*, 17(20):23–27, 2005.

Tunkel AR, Scheld WM. Acute meningitis. In: Stein JH (ed.). *Internal Medicine,* Boston, MA: Little, Brown & Co., 1990:1281–1290.

Vaitkus PT, et al. Treatment of malignant pericardial effusion, *JAMA*, 272(1):59–64, 1994.

Walters J. Hematology and the analysis of body fluids, *Adv Med Lab Prof*, 8(9):10–11, 18–19, 1996.

Weisman MH, Karchmer AW. Infections of the joints. In: Stein JH (ed.). *Internal Medicine,* Boston, MA: Little, Brown & Co., 1990:1780–1786.

World Health Organization *WHO Laboratory Manual for Examination of Human Semen and Semen–Cervical Mucus Interaction,* 4th ed, Cambridge, UK: Cambridge Univesity Press, 1999.

Zvaifler NJ. Synovial fluid analysis. In: Stein JH (ed.). *Internal Medicine,* Boston, MA: Little, Brown & Co., 1990:1681–1684.

CHAPTER 26

Manual Procedures in Hematology

- Describe the general principles of basic and selected specialized procedures in hematology, special stains, and coagulation procedures.
- Describe the proper type of specimen collection and handling for the stated procedure.
- Prepare the necessary reagents for the stated procedure.
- Describe the quality control steps needed for the stated procedure.
- Perform the stated procedure.
- Perform any calculations needed for reporting the results in the procedure.
- State the reference range values for the parameters measured by the procedure.
- Describe the sources of error and clinical applications of the procedure.

PROCEDURAL FORMAT

The procedures in this chapter are presented in a format that is consistent with the guidelines set forth by the CLSI. This format is

1. Procedure title and specific method
2. Test principle including type of reaction and the clinical reasons for the test
3. Specimen collection and preparation
4. Reagents, supplies, and equipment
5. Calibration of a standard curve
6. Quality control
7. Procedure
8. Calculations
9. Reporting results (normal values)
10. Procedure notes including sources of error, clinical applications, and limitations of the procedure
11. References

All specimens should be treated with caution. All blood, tissues, and blood derivatives should be considered potentially infectious. Specimen handling notes that are particularly important to coagulation studies are presented on the page immediately preceding the Coagulation Procedures section. Many of the procedures in this chapter are classic methods that are infrequently performed in the working clinical laboratory. These procedures are included for use in special circumstances such as in the student laboratory or small clinical laboratories.

HEMATOLOGY PROCEDURES

LEUKOCYTE DIFFERENTIAL COUNT

Principle

A stained smear is examined to determine the percentage of each type of leukocyte present and assess the erythrocyte and platelet morphology. Increases in any of the normal leukocyte types and the presence of immature leukocytes or erythrocytes in peripheral blood are important diagnostically in a wide variety of inflammatory disorders and leukemia. Erythrocyte abnormalities are clinically important in various anemias. Platelet size irregularities are suggestive of particular thrombocyte disorders.

Specimen

Peripheral blood, bone marrow, or body fluid sediments, such as spinal fluid, are appropriate specimens. Whole blood smears may be made from EDTA-anticoagulated blood or prepared from free-flowing capillary blood. Smears should be made within 1 hour of blood collection from EDTA specimens stored at room temperature to avoid distortion of cell morphology. Unstained smears can be stored for indefinite periods, but stained smears gradually fade.

Reagents, Supplies, and Equipment

1. A manual cell counter designed for differential counts
2. Microscope, immersion oil, and lens paper

Quality Control

Training and experience in examining immature and abnormal cell morphology are essential. A set of reference slides with established parameters should be established to assess the competence of an individual to perform differential and

(continued)

HEMATOLOGY PROCEDURES (continued)

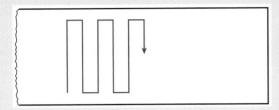

FIGURE 26.1 The method of slide examination in the leukocyte differential count.

morphological identification of leukocytes and erythrocytes. Participation in a quality assurance program continues to document the expertise of the hematologist in microscopy. Questionable or abnormal smears should be referred to a supervisor for verification.

Procedure

1. Begin the slide examination with a correctly prepared and stained smear (see Chapter 2 for specimen preparation).
2. Focus the microscope on the 10× objective (low power). Scan the smear to check for cell distribution, clumping, and abnormal cells. Add a drop of immersion oil and switch to the 100× (oil immersion) objective. Begin the count by determining a suitable area (Fig. 26.1). Extend the examination from the area where approximately half of the erythrocytes are barely overlapping to an area where the erythrocytes touch each other. *It is important to examine cellular morphology and to count leukocytes in areas that are neither too thick nor too thin.* In areas that are too thick, cellular details such as nuclear chromatin patterns are difficult to examine. In areas that are too thin, distortion of cells makes it risky to identify a cell type.
3. Count the leukocytes using a tracking pattern. Each cell identified should be immediately tallied as a neutrophil (band), neutrophil (segmented), or polymorphonuclear neutrophil (PMN); lymphocyte; monocyte; eosinophil;

or basophil. A brief leukocyte morphology reference is included (Table 26.1); however, refer to specific chapters in the text for a complete discussion of leukocyte and erythrocyte cellular morphology.

4. Abnormalities of leukocytes, erythrocytes, and platelets should be noted. Normally, 8 to 20 platelets are present in an oil immersion field in a properly prepared smear (where the RBCs barely touch each other). After examining at least 10 different fields, the average number of platelets can be multiplied by a factor of 20,000 to arrive at an approximate total circulating platelet concentration. Nucleated erythrocytes are *not* included in the total count but are noted per 100 white blood cells (WBCs). A total of at least 100 leukocytes should be counted. Express the results as a percentage of total leukocytes counted.

Reporting Results

Reference values, particularly the band neutrophil percentage, may vary. Values for children differ from adult reference values. See inside back cover for a full discussion of reference values.

Procedure Notes

A well-made and well-stained smear is essential to the accuracy of the differential count. The knowledge and ability of the cell morphologist are critical to high-quality results.

A minimum of 300 leukocytes must be within the acceptable working area, when the total leukocyte count is no less than 4×10^9/L. The neutrophils, monocytes, and lymphocytes should appear evenly distributed in the usable fields of the film. Less than 2% of the leukocytes should be disrupted or nonidentifiable forms except in certain forms associated with pathological states. If a disrupted cell is clearly identifiable, include it in the differential count. Classify nonidentifiable disrupted cells (smudges or baskets) as "other" and note them on the report if more than a few are observed.

| TABLE 26.1 | A Comparison of Normal Leukocytes in Peripheral Blood |

	Segmented Neutrophil	Band Neutrophil	Lymphocyte	Monocyte	Eosinophil	Basophil
Nuclear shape	Lobulated	Curved	Round	Indented or twisted	Lobulated	Lobulated
Chromatin	Very clumped	Moderately clumped	Smooth	Lacy	Very clumped	Very clumped
Cytoplasmic color	Pink	Blue, pink	Light blue	Gray-blue	Granulated	Granulated
Granules	Many	Many	Few or absent	Many	Many	Many
Color of granules	Pink, a few blue	Pink	Red	Dusty blue	Orange	Dark blue
Average percentage	56%	3%	34%	4%	2.7%	0.3%

(continued)

The blood smear preparation techniques described in Chapter 2 are commonly used in the laboratory for the preparation of blood smears. In certain circumstances, the preparation of a buffy coat peripheral blood smear increases the accuracy of the leukocyte differential count.

Preparation of Buffy Coat Smears

Principle

An anticoagulated specimen of whole blood is centrifuged to physically separate the blood into three layers: plasma, leukocytes and platelets, and erythrocytes. The interface layer between the plasma and erythrocytes is referred to as the buffy coat. If this layer of concentrated cells is removed by pipetting, push-wedge–type smears can subsequently be prepared and stained for microscopic examination. This technique is useful in the performance of leukocyte differential counts on patients with extremely low total leukocyte counts or in special testing procedures.

Specimen

A freshly drawn specimen of EDTA-anticoagulated whole blood is needed.

Procedure

1. Centrifuge the specimen of whole anticoagulated blood for at least 5 minutes at 2,000 to 2,500 rpm.
2. With a Pasteur pipette, remove most of the top plasma layer and discard.
3. The interface layer along with a small amount of plasma and a small volume of erythrocytes can then be removed using a Pasteur pipette.
4. A drop of this suspension can be placed on a microscope slide and a push-wedge smear prepared. Air-dry and stain.

Alternative Technique

A refinement of the classic buffy coat technique has been developed for use with automated blood smear equipment. In this technique, saline solution and 22% albumin are added to the interface layer. This enhancement produces better cell separation on the peripheral smear and minimizes the spreading artifact during centrifugation. To add this enhancement to the basic technique,

1. Proceed from step 3 above by transferring the interface layer to a disposable Wintrobe (ESR) tube. This tube is placed into a 16 × 100-mm test tube and centrifuged for a minimum of 5 minutes at 2,000 rpm.
2. After centrifugation, the top plasma layer is removed with a Pasteur pipette and discarded. Remove approximately 0.03 mL of the interface layer and a small volume of erythrocytes and transfer to a 20-mL test tube or plastic vial. Add enough isotonic (0.85%) saline solution to the test tube or vial to prepare a 1% to 2% suspension of cells.
3. Add 22% albumin to the suspension at the rate of three drops of albumin for each 10 mL of resulting cell suspen-

sion. If the amount of albumin is too great, the cells will appear too dark and may have pseudopods.
4. This preparation can then be transferred to the sample holder and treated according to the instrument manufacturer's directions.

Clinical Applications

Selected Disorders Associated with Increases in Normal Leukocyte Types

Neutrophils
Bacterial infections
Inflammation
Stress
Chronic leukemia

Lymphocytes
Viral infections
Whooping cough
Chronic leukemia

Monocytes
Tuberculosis
Rheumatoid arthritis
Fever of unknown origin

Eosinophils
Active allergies
Invasive parasites

Basophils
Ulcerative colitis
Hyperlipidemia

BIBLIOGRAPHY

Provided on this book's companion Web site at thepoint. lww.com/Turgeon5e.

PACKED CELL VOLUME OF WHOLE BLOOD: MICROHEMATOCRIT METHOD

Principle

The packed cell volume (PCV) is a measurement of the ratio of the volume occupied by the RBCs to the volume of whole blood in a sample of capillary or venous blood. Following centrifugation, this ratio is measured and expressed as a percentage or decimal fraction. Clinically, the PCV is used to detect anemia, polycythemia, hemodilution, or hemoconcentration. In conjunction with an erythrocyte count, the PCV is used to calculate the mean corpuscular volume (MCV). The PCV is also used in conjunction with the hemoglobin concentration to calculate the mean corpuscular hemoglobin concentration (MCHC).

Specimen

Venous blood anticoagulated with EDTA or capillary blood collected directly into heparinized capillary tubes can be used. Specimens should be centrifuged within 6 hours of collecting. Hemolyzed samples cannot be used for testing.

(continued)

HEMATOLOGY PROCEDURES (continued)

Reagents, Supplies, and Equipment

1. Capillary tubes (75 mm long with an ID of 1.155 mm). Blue-banded tubes contain no anticoagulant and are used with EDTA-anticoagulated blood. Red-banded tubes are heparinized for use with capillary blood.
2. Clay-type tube sealant
3. Microhematocrit centrifuge and reading device

Calibration

The calibration of the centrifuge should be checked regularly for timer accuracy, speed, and maximal packing of cells. Use a stopwatch for accuracy, a tachometer for speed, and a time-versus-constant-volume method to check packing of erythrocytes. Check the capillary tube reading device against another reader periodically.

Quality Control

Commercially available whole blood can be used to check the accuracy of normal and abnormal levels.

Procedure

1. Well-mixed anticoagulant blood should be drawn into two microhematocrit tubes by capillary action. The tubes should be filled to about three fourths of their length. Wipe off the outside of the tubes with gauze or wipes. Free-flowing capillary samples should be collected in the same manner.
2. Seal one end of each tube with a small amount of clay-like material. Place the dry end of the tube into the sealant, holding the index finger over the opposite end to prevent blood from leaking out of the tube onto the sealant.
3. Place the filled and sealed capillary tubes into the centrifuge. The sealed ends should point toward the outside of the centrifuge. The duplicate samples should be placed opposite each other to balance the centrifuge. Record the position number of each specimen.
4. Securely fasten the flat lid on top of the capillary tubes. Close the centrifuge top and secure the latch. Set the timer for 5 minutes. The fixed speed of centrifugation should be 10,000 to 15,000 rpm.
5. After the centrifuge has stopped, open the top and remove the cover plate. Promptly read the PCV on an appropriate piece of equipment or specially designed card. Measure the PCV by adjusting the top of the clay sealant to the zero mark and reading the top of the red cell column. A reader with an ocular that has cross-markings produces the most accurate reading.

Note: When taking readings, be sure that the bottom of the packed cell column is lined up correctly to the zero mark. Do not include the buffy coat in reading the packed erythrocyte column. *Do not* allow the tubes to remain in the centrifuge for more than 10 minutes because the interface between the plasma and the cells will become slanted and an inaccurate reading will result.

Reporting Results

The PCV is preferentially expressed as a decimal fraction, such as 0.45 L/L, rather than as 45%. In current practice, the percentage expression is commonly used. Reference values: males, 41.5–50.5%; females, 36.0–45.0%.

Procedure Notes

Sources of Error

Erroneous results can be caused by inclusion of the buffy coat in reading the packed column, hemolysis of the specimen, and inadequate mixing. If the centrifugation time is too short or the speed is too low, an increase in trapped plasma (1% to 3%) will occur in normal blood. Increased amounts of trapped plasma can produce errors in cases in which an erythrocyte abnormality exists, such as sickle cell anemia. Other sources of error include prolonged tourniquet stasis and excess EDTA, which cause cells to shrink and pack more tightly than they should.

Clinical Applications

The PCV is used for detecting anemia, polycythemia, hemodilution, or hemoconcentration.

BIBLIOGRAPHY

Provided on this book's companion Web site at thepoint. lww.com/Turgeon5e.

RED BLOOD CELL INDICES

The erythrocyte indices are used to mathematically define cell size and the concentration of hemoglobin within the cell. They are
1. MCV
2. Mean corpuscular hemoglobin (MCH)
3. MCHC

Mean Corpuscular Volume

Principle

The MCV expresses the average volume of an erythrocyte.

Calculations

$$MCV = \frac{Patient's\,PCV\,or\,hematocrit\,(L/L)}{Erythrocyte\,count\,(\times 10^{12}/L)} = fL$$

Example: If the patient's hematocrit is 35%, or 0.35 L/L, and the erythrocyte count is 4.0×10^{12}/L, the MCV is determined thus:

$$MCV = \frac{0.35\,(L/L)}{4.0 \times 10^{12}/L} = 87.5 \times 10^{-15}\,L = 87.5\,fL^{a}$$

(continued)

Reporting Results

Reference value: 80 to 96 fL.

Mean Corpuscular Hemoglobin

Principle

The MCH expresses the average weight (content) of hemoglobin in an average erythrocyte. It is directly proportional to the amount of hemoglobin and the size of the erythrocyte.

Calculations

$$MCV = \frac{Hemoglobin\,(\times 10\,g/dL)}{Erythrocyte\,count\,(\times 10^{12}/L)} = pg^{b}$$

Example: If the patient's hemoglobin is 14 g/dL and the erythrocyte count is $4 \times 10^{12}/L$, the MCH would equal

$$MCV = \frac{140\,g/dL}{4 \times 10^{12}/L} = 35 \times 10^{-12}\,g = 35\,pg$$

Reporting Results

Reference value: 27 to 32 pg.

Mean Corpuscular Hemoglobin Concentration

Principle

The MCHC expresses the average concentration of hemoglobin per unit volume of erythrocytes. It is also defined as the ratio of the weight of hemoglobin to the volume of erythrocytes.

Calculations

$$MCHC = \frac{Hemoglobin\,(g/dL)}{PCV\,or\,hematocrit\,(L/L)} = g/dL$$

Example: If the patient's hemoglobin is 14 g/dL and the hematocrit is 0.45 L/L, the MCHC would equal

$$MCHC = \frac{14\,g/dL}{0.45\,L/L} = 31\,g/dL = 31\,g/dL$$

^{a}One femtoliter (fL) = 10^{-15} L = 1 cubic micrometer (μm^{3})
^{b}One pictogram (pg) = 10^{-12} g = 1 micromicrogram ($\mu\mu g$)

Reporting Results

Reference value: 32% to 36%.

RETICULOCYTE COUNT: NEW METHYLENE BLUE METHOD

Principle

Supravital stains, such as new methylene blue N or brilliant cresyl blue, bind, neutralize, and cross-link RNA. These stains cause the ribosomal and residual RNA to coprecipitate with the few remaining mitochondria and ferritin masses in living young erythrocytes to form microscopically visible

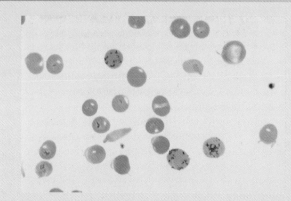

FIGURE 26.2 Peripheral blood smear with reticulocytes; staining is with new methylene blue dye. The blue granules represent precipitated, residual RNA. (Reprinted with permission from McClatchey KD. *Clinical Laboratory Medicine*, 2nd ed, Philadelphia, PA: Lippincott Williams & Wilkins, 2002.)

dark-blue clusters and filaments (reticulum). An erythrocyte still possessing RNA is referred to as a **reticulocyte** (see Fig. 26.2). The enumeration of reticulocytes is important in assessing the status of erythrocyte production in the bone marrow (erythropoiesis).

Specimen

Whole blood that is anticoagulated with either EDTA or heparin is suitable. Capillary blood drawn into heparinized tubes or immediately mixed with stain may also be used. The test should be performed promptly after blood collection. Stained smears retain their color for a prolonged period.

Reagents, Supplies, and Equipment

Reagent

New methylene blue solution: This solution is prepared as follows:

1. Weigh out 0.5 g of new methylene blue N, 1.4 g of potassium oxalate, and 0.8 g of sodium chloride. Place these chemicals in a 100-mL volumetric flask and dilute to the calibration mark with distilled water.
2. Mix well. Place in a clean brown bottle that is properly labeled with the name of the reagent, date of preparation, and name of the individual who prepared the solution.
3. *Filter* solution daily or immediately before use to remove any precipitate.

Supplies and Equipment

1. Capillary tubes
2. Glass slides
3. Wright or Wright-Giemsa stain
4. Microscope, lens paper, and immersion oil
5. Miller ocular disc (optional)

(continued)

An alternative specimen collection and processing method is *BD Unopette® Brand Test Reticulocyte Stain Kit*. See package insert for the procedure.

Procedure

1. One third of a capillary tube should be filled with well-mixed blood.
2. An equal amount of filtered stain is then drawn into the tube. The tube is rotated back and forth by hand.
3. An alternative method is to mix two drops of blood and two drops of filtered stain.
4. Allow this mixture to stand for at least 10 minutes.
5. Gently remix and expel small drops of the stain and blood mixture onto several microscope slides and prepare smears.
6. Air-dry.
7. Two or three dried slides may be counterstained with Wright stain (see procedure for staining blood smears).
8. Using the 10× microscope objective, focus the smear. Add a drop of oil to the slide and move to the oil immersion (100×) objective. The appropriate counting area is the portion of the smear where the erythrocytes are evenly distributed and not overlapping. Before beginning the count, scan the slide to check that reticulocytes can be located on that slide.
9. To count the reticulocytes, a minimum of 1,000 (both reticulin-containing and nonreticulated) erythrocytes must be counted. Normally, 500 erythrocytes will be counted on each of two slides. If the number of reticulocytes on these two slides do not agree within 20%, a third slide of 500 erythrocytes must be counted. Be sure to count all cells that contain a blue-staining filament, fragment, or granule of reticulum in the erythrocyte. The counting field can be reduced by using paper hole reinforcers or small pieces of paper cut to fit the oculars with a small hole cut out in the middle of each. This makes counting easier than viewing the entire field.

Note: A Miller ocular disc can be used to facilitate counting the number of reticulocytes and total RBCs.

Calculations

If 47 reticulocytes are found when 1,000 erythrocytes are examined (47 reticulocytes and 953 mature erythrocytes), the reticulocyte count is calculated as follows:

$$\frac{47}{1,000} \times 100 = 4.7\% \text{ reticulocytes (uncorrected)}$$

Reporting Results

Reference values: 0.5% to 1.5%; neonates, 2.5% to 6.5%. Some laboratories express the reticulocyte count in absolute rather than proportional terms (see Chapter 5). Reporting

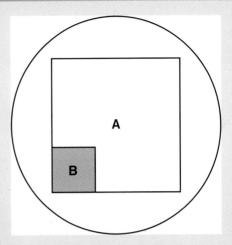

FIGURE 26.3 Miller ocular disc. Square A is nine times the area of square B. Reticulocytes are counted in square A; erythrocytes are counted in square B in successive microscopic fields until at least 300 RBCs are counted.

in absolute terms is becoming the preferred method of reporting. The correction for anemia is additionally helpful for clinical interpretation of the reticulocyte count (see Chapter 5).

Miller Ocular Disc

Principle

A Miller ocular disc inserted into the eyepiece of the microscope permits a rapid survey of erythrocytes. This disc (see Fig. 26.3) imposes two squares (one nine times the area of the other) onto the field of view

Procedure

Reticulocytes are counted in the large square and erythrocytes in the small square in successive microscopic fields until at least 300 RBCs are counted. This allows for an estimate of reticulocytes among a minimum population of 200 erythrocytes. The **absolute reticulocyte count** can be determined by multiplying the reticulocyte percentage by the RBC count.

Calculations

$$\text{Reticulocytes}_{\text{(expressed in percentage)}} = \frac{\text{No. of reticulocytes in large squares}}{\text{No. of RBCs in small squares} \times 9} \times 100$$

Example: Given that there are 50 reticulocytes in the large squares and 300 red blood cells in the small squares,

$$\text{Reticulocytes}_{\text{(expressed in percentage)}} = \frac{50}{300 \times 9} \times 100 = 1.86$$

Note: Reticulocytes may also be counted by automated methods.

HEMATOLOGY PROCEDURES *(continued)*

Decreased Reticulocytes	Increased Reticulocytes
Aplastic anemia	Blood loss
Aplastic crises of hemolytic anemia	Crisis associated with hemolytic anemia
Chemotherapeutic or radiation-induced hypoproliferation	Subsequent to treatment of pernicious anemia, folic acid deficiency, or iron deficiency
Pernicious anemia	
Decreased erythropoiesis	

Sources of Error

A refractile appearance of erythrocytes should not be confused with reticulocytes. Refractile bodies are due to poor drying owing to moisture in the air. Filtration of the stain is essential because precipitate can resemble a reticulocyte.

Erythrocyte inclusions should not be mistaken for reticulocytes. Howell-Jolly bodies appear as one or sometimes two, deep-purple, dense structures. Heinz bodies stain a light blue-green and are usually present at the edge of the erythrocyte. Pappenheimer bodies are more often confused with reticulocytes and are the most difficult to distinguish. These purple-staining iron deposits generally appear as several granules in a small cluster. If Pappenheimer bodies are suspected, stain with Wright-Giemsa to verify their presence.

Falsely decreased reticulocyte counts can result from understaining the blood with new methylene blue. High glucose levels can also cause reticulocytes to stain poorly.

Clinical Applications

Selected Disorders Associated with Abnormal Results

BIBLIOGRAPHY

Provided on this book's companion Web site at thepoint.lww.com/Turgeon5e.

SEDIMENTATION RATE OF ERYTHROCYTES: WESTERGREN METHOD

The Westergren method has been selected as the method of choice by the NCCLS.

Principle

The erythrocyte sedimentation rate (ESR), also called the sed rate, measures the rate of settling of erythrocytes in diluted human plasma. This phenomenon depends on an interrelationship of variables, such as the plasma protein composition, the concentration of erythrocytes, and the shape of the erythrocytes. The ESR value is determined by measuring the distance from the surface meniscus to the top of the erythrocyte sedimented in a special tube that is placed perpendicular in a rack for 1 hour. The clinical value of this procedure is in the diagnosis and monitoring of inflammatory or infectious states.

Specimen

Fresh anticoagulated blood collected in either sodium citrate or EDTA may be used. Sodium citrate is the preferred anticoagulant, and the specimen must fill the entire tube—if an evacuated tube is used—to achieve the correct ratio of blood to anticoagulant. The ratio is 4 vol of blood to 1 vol of sodium citrate. If EDTA anticoagulant is used, it *must* be diluted to the ratio of 4 vol of blood to 1 vol of 0.9% sodium chloride.

Blood should be at *room temperature for testing* and should be no more than 2 hours old. If anticoagulated blood is refrigerated, the test must be set up within 6 hours. Hemolyzed specimens *cannot* be used.

Reagent, Supplies, and Equipment

1. Westergren pipettes
2. Vertical rack: This special rack is equipped with a leveling bubble device to ensure that the tubes are held in a vertical position within 1°. The fittings on the rack should be clean and uncracked to prevent leakage of the diluted blood.

Procedure

1. Mix the blood citrate or blood-EDTA-saline mixture thoroughly.
2. Aspirate a bubble-free specimen into a clean and dry Westergren pipette. Fill to the zero mark. Do not pipette by mouth.
3. Place the pipette into the vertical rack at 20°C to 25°C in an area free from vibrations, drafts, and direct sunlight.
4. After 60 minutes, read the distance in millimeters from the bottom of the plasma meniscus to the top of the sedimented erythrocytes.
5. Record the value as millimeters in 1 hour.

Reporting Results

The reference value of this test varies depending on age. In persons younger than 50 years of age, the average reference values are up to 10 mm/hour in males and 13 mm/hour in females. For persons older than 50 years of age, average reference values are up to 13 mm/hour in males and up to 20 mm/hour in females.

Procedure Notes

Sources of Error

Numerous sources of error have been cited for the ESR procedure. The age of the specimen is important, the test should

(continued)

be performed at 20°C to 25°C, and the blood should be at room temperature. Other sources of error include incorrect ratios of blood and anticoagulant, bubbles in the Westergren tube, and tilting of the ESR tube. Tilting of the tube accelerates the fall of erythrocytes, and an angle of even 3° from the vertical can accelerate sedimentation by as much as 30%.

Clinical Applications

The ESR is directly proportional to the weight of the cell aggregate and inversely proportional to the surface area. Microcytes sediment more slowly than macrocytes. Erythrocytes with abnormal or irregular shapes, such as sickle cells or spherocytes, hinder rouleaux formation and lower the ESR. The removal of fibrinogen by defibrination also produces a decreased ESR.

An increased ESR value can be seen owing to various abnormal blood conditions: rouleaux, increased fibrinogen levels, a relative increase of plasma globulins caused by the loss of plasma albumin, and an absolute increase of plasma globulins. Clinical conditions associated with increased ESR values include anemia, infections, inflammation, tissue necrosis (such as myocardial infarction), pregnancy, and some types of hemolytic anemia.

BIBLIOGRAPHY

Provided on this book's companion Web site at thepoint. lww.com/Turgeon5e.

SEDIMENTATION RATE OF ERYTHROCYTES: WINTROBE METHOD

Principle

See Principle at the Westergren Method (above) for details.

Specimen

Fresh blood collected in EDTA anticoagulant may be used. A minimum of 2 mL of whole blood is needed. The specimen must be well mixed, and the procedure must be performed within 2 hours of blood collection.

Reagent, Supplies, and Equipment

1. Wintrobe Sedrate tubes: These tubes are available in either reusable glass or disposable form. Depending on the type of Wintrobe rack used, the choice of tube includes graduated or plain.
2. Wintrobe sedimentation rack (graduated or plain)
3. Pasteur pipette (long-tipped) and rubber pipette bulb

Procedure

1. Gently and thoroughly mix the anticoagulated blood.
2. Draw as much blood as possible into the Pasteur pipette with the attached pipette bulb.

3. Place the tip of the pipette (filled with blood) into the Wintrobe tube until the tip touches the bottom of the tube.
4. Gently begin to press the pipette bulb and slowly move the pipette tip up from the bottom of the tube. *Continuous pressure must be kept on the pipette bulb while the pipette tip is moved up from the bottom of the tube.* The pipette tip must be in continuous motion to avoid introducing air bubbles into the column of blood.
5. The Wintrobe tube must be filled to the zero mark.
6. Place the tube into a Wintrobe tube holder that has been adjusted to a perfectly level position.
7. Allow the tube to stand for 1 hour at room temperature in a draft-free room.
8. Read the tube from the bottom of the plasma meniscus to the top of the sedimented erythrocytes. Each line on the tube represents 1 mm.

Reporting Results

The patient's value is reported in millimeters per hour. The reference value is 0 to 20 mm/hour for women and 0 to 9 mm/hour for men.

Procedure Notes

One of the major drawbacks of this procedure is that the 100-mm tube length and the narrow bore of the tube limit readings in excess of 60 mm/hour. Care must be taken to avoid introducing air bubbles into the column and to fill the tube to the zero mark.

Sources of Error

Falsely *increased* results can be produced by
1. Positioning the tube at an incline rather than in a vertical position
2. Allowing the tube to stand for longer than 1 hour
3. A room temperature above normal

Falsely *decreased* results can be produced by
1. An improper concentration of anticoagulant–whole blood ratio
2. Anticoagulated blood that is more than 2 hours old
3. Allowing the tube to stand for less than 1 hour
4. Refrigerated blood or a decreased room temperature

Clinical Applications

Refer to the Westergren Method above.

BIBLIOGRAPHY

Provided on this book's companion Web site at thepoint. lww.com/Turgeon5e.

(continued)

ACIDIFIED SERUM LYSIS TEST: HAM METHOD

Principle

Erythrocytes are incubated with fresh and heated serum to test for hemolysis. Weak acid is used in specific serum cell mixtures to maximize hemolytic activity. The presence of hemolysis, depending on the test conditions, may be observed in cases of antibody-sensitized coated erythrocytes, sphero-cytes, or paroxysmal nocturnal hemoglobinuria (PNH).

This procedure, in CLSI format, is provided on this book's companion Web site at thepoint.lww.com/Turgeon5e.

BONE MARROW EXAMINATION

Principle

A bone marrow aspiration is performed by a physician to examine the cellular activities of the marrow. Properly pre-pared specimens are usually stained with a Wright-Giemsa stain and special stains, such as Prussian blue, and cytochem-ical stains for various enzymes. A specimen of the marrow is also examined histologically using a hematoxylin-eosin (H&E) stain.

Bone marrow examination is valuable in the diagnosis of disorders specifically involving the marrow, such as multiple myeloma, and in the study of leukemias and some types of anemia. In most cases, the bone marrow presents the early developmental events that produce the blood picture seen in peripheral blood or evidence of an underlying systemic disease.

Specimen

Refer to Chapter 2 for details on specimen collection and Wright-Giemsa staining. For details on special stains, refer to the specific staining procedure in this section. A peripheral blood smear should also be collected on the same day as the bone marrow aspiration.

Procedure

Examination of Bone Marrow Slides

1. Using the 10× objective, the smear is scanned for any apparent overall cellular abnormalities. An estimation of cellularity can also be appraised. Semiquantitative assess-ments of cellularity in aspirates can be classified into hypoplastic, normal, and hyperplastic levels. Cellularity varies with a patient's age and the site of the bone marrow aspiration. Marrow cellularity is expressed as the ratio of the volume of hematopoietic cells to the total volume of the marrow space (cells plus fat as well as other stromal elements) (see Fig. 26.4).

2. Using the 100× (oil) immersion objective, a differ-ential count of at least 200 cells is performed. Any abnormalities in distribution will be apparent by this

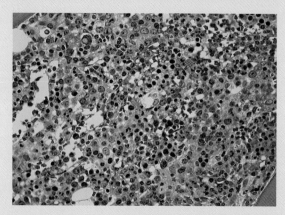

FIGURE 26.4 Bone marrow biopsy sections demonstrate normal cellularity. Virtually 100% cellular marrow from a newborn boy. (Reprinted with permission from McClatchey KD. *Clinical Labo-ratory Medicine*, 2nd ed, Philadelphia, PA: Lippincott Williams & Wilkins, 2002.)

examination. Erythrocyte maturational and morphologi-cal abnormalities and megakaryocyte morphology should be examined during cell differentiation. Nonhematopoi-etic cells of normal bone marrow may also be seen. These cells are reticulum cells (marrow macrophages), osteo-blasts and osteoclasts, and mast cells. Reticulum cells are peaceful macrophages that represent the skeletal and structural components of the marrow sinuses. Osteo-blasts and osteoclasts are uncommon in marrow aspi-rates because they are not involved in hematopoiesis. The function of osteoblasts and osteoclasts is formation and remodeling of bone. Mast cells are connective tissue cells with no defined ancestral relationship to the blood baso-phil or its precursors. Mast cells along with plasma cells are characteristic of marrow damage or depletion. Clus-ters of metastatic neoplastic cells may also be observed in bone marrow smears.

3. Using duplicate bone marrow smears, any special stains (e.g., iron) should be promptly performed and exam-ined.

4. The peripheral blood smear should be simultaneously examined.

Reporting Results

The technologist usually refers the slides and slide exami-nation report to a pathologist for comparison with the H&E preparation. The cellularity of the specimen is usu-ally determined from the histological specimen, and the myeloid-erythroid (M/E) ratio is determined from the bone marrow aspiration slides. The pathologist will then assign a diagnosis to the case and suggest supplementary tests, if necessary.

(continued)

Normal Distribution of Bone Marrow Cells in an Adult

Cell Type	Mean %
Rubricytic series	21.5
Rubriblasts	0.6
Prorubricytes	2.0
Rubricytes	12.4
Metarubricytes	6.5
Neutrophil series	56.0
Blasts	1.0
Promyelocytes	3.4
Myelocytes	11.9
Metamyelocytes	18.0
Bands	11.0
PMNs	10.7
Eosinophil series	3.2
Basophils	<0.1
Lymphocytes	15.8
Monocytes	1.8
Megakaryocytes	<0.1
Reticulum cells	0.3
Plasma cells	1.8
M/E ratio	2.5:1

BIBLIOGRAPHY

Provided on this book's companion Web site at thepoint. lww.com/Turgeon5e.

DONATH-LANDSTEINER SCREENING TEST

Principle

The Donath-Landsteiner antibody test is used to demonstrate the presence of this extremely potent hemolysin. This antibody requires cold incubation to exhibit hemolysis in the patient's serum. A positive result is diagnostic of paroxysmal cold hemoglobinuria (PCH), the rarest form of autoimmune hemolytic anemia.

This procedure, in CLSI format, is provided on this book's companion Web site at thepoint.lww.com/Turgeon5e.

GLUCOSE-6-PHOSPHATE DEHYDROGENASE ACTIVITY IN ERYTHROCYTES: VISUAL FLUORESCENT SCREENING TEST

Principle

The enzyme glucose-6-phosphate dehydrogenase (G6PD) catalyzes the following reaction:

$$\underset{\text{(not fluorescent)}}{\text{Glucose-6-phosphate} + \text{NADP}} \xrightarrow{\text{G6PD}} \underset{\text{(fluorescent)}}{\text{6-phosphogluconate} + \text{NADPH}}$$

The reaction mixture containing glucose-6-phosphate, nicotinamide adenine dinucleotide phosphate (NADP), and blood is incubated, and at timed intervals, drops of the mixture are applied to filter paper. The fluorescence of reduced nucleotides, when activated with long-wave (340 to 370 nm) ultraviolet (UV) light, is used for visual examination of G6PD activity. The observed rate of the appearance of bright fluorescence is proportional to the blood G6PD activity. G6PD deficiency is one of the most prevalent hereditary erythrocyte enzyme deficiencies. A deficiency of this enzyme can produce drug- or stress-induced hemolytic anemia in afflicted persons.

This procedure, in CLSI format, is provided on this book's companion Web site at thepoint.lww.com/Turgeon5e

HEMOGLOBIN ELECTROPHORESIS: CELLULOSE ACETATE METHOD

Principle

Electrophoresis may be defined as the movement of charged particles on various media under the influence of an electric current. Particles move at different speeds because of their weight and electric charge.

In hemoglobin electrophoresis, a hemolysate prepared from intact erythrocytes is placed on a medium such as cellulose acetate. The strips of cellulose acetate are placed in an alkaline buffer (pH 8.0 to 8.6) and electrical charge is applied. The strips are stained to see the hemoglobin fractions. A comparison of the unknown hemolysate with hemolysates from known hemoglobin types is made. Hemoglobin electrophoresis by cellulose acetate is useful in identifying and quantifying hemoglobin variants and abnormal quantities of hemoglobin fractions.

This procedure, in CLSI format, is provided on this book's companion Web site at thepoint.lww.com/Turgeon5e.

HEMOGLOBIN S SCREENING TEST: QUALITATIVE DIFFERENTIAL SOLUBILITY TEST

Principle

This is a biphasic system consisting of an upper organic phase of toluene and a lower, aqueous phase containing phosphate buffer, saponin, and reducing agents. Erythrocytes are lysed by toluene and saponin, with the released hemoglobin being reduced by sodium hydrosulfite. The resulting colors of the aqueous phase and the interface phase allow for the differentiation of hemoglobin types AA, AS, and SS.

Detection of the abnormal Hb S is diagnostic of sickle cell disease. Hb S, if inherited in the homozygous state (SS), results in sickle cell anemia. Inheritance of the heterozygous state (AS) produces a benign and asymptomatic condition,

(continued)

except under conditions of reduced oxygen levels. The detection of this heterozygous state is important to diagnose in individuals who are involved in strenuous physical sports, such as long-distance runners, or in individuals whose occupations have the potential for reduced oxygen levels, such as test pilots.

This procedure, in CLSI format, is provided on this book's companion Web site at thepoint.lww.com/Turgeon5e.

MALARIAL SMEARS

Principle

Thick and thin blood smears are prepared, stained, and examined microscopically for the presence of one of four malaria types. Detection and correct identification of the species of malaria (*Plasmodium malariae, P. vivax, P. falciparum,* or *P. ovale*) are important to ensure proper treatment.

Specimen

Smears of capillary or EDTA-anticoagulated blood are prepared as described in the section on specimen preparation in Chapter 2.

Reagents, Supplies, and Equipment

1. American Chemical Society (ACS)-grade methanol
2. ACS-grade glycerol
3. Buffer (pH 6.4 or 6.8)
Solution A: Prepare by placing 9.47 g of anhydrous secondary sodium phosphate (Na_2HPO_4) or 11.87 g of hydrated sodium phosphate ($Na_2HPO_4 \cdot 2H_2O$) into a 1-L volumetric flask. Dilute to the calibration mark with deionized water. Mix.
Solution B: Weigh and transfer 9.080 g of primary potassium phosphate (KH_2PO_4) into a 1-L volumetric flask. Dilute to the calibration mark with deionized water. Mix.
Solutions A and B can be mixed in various proportions to achieve a different pH. Buffer (6.4 pH). Mix 26.7 mL of solution A and 73.3 mL of solution B. Buffer (6.8 pH). Mix 49.6 mL of solution A and 50.4 mL of solution B. *Refrigerate all solutions to store.*
4. Giemsa stock stain: Prepare by adding 5 g of powdered Giemsa stain to 330 mL of reagent-grade glycerol. Mix. Place in a 60°C oven for 2 hours. Allow to cool. Mix. With constant stirring, slowly add 330 mL of methanol. Transfer to a stoppered brown bottle and shake for a few minutes. Label. Filter *before use.*
Working Giemsa stain: Prepare by adding 10 mL of filtered Giemsa stock stain to 90 mL of buffer solution. Mix.
5. Coplin or other type of staining jar and slide holder
6. Microscope, immersion oil, and lens paper

Quality Control

A reference slide set should be maintained to validate the ability of microscopists to identify various malarial species.

Participation in a quality assurance program, such as the College of American Pathologists program, is important in maintaining expertise in this area, particularly in laboratories that infrequently encounter positive results.

Procedure

1. Following blood smear preparation, allow the smears to air-dry for approximately 30 minutes. Fix the thin smears in methanol for a few seconds. Do not fix the thick smears.
2. Place the smears in a Coplin jar containing Giemsa staining solution for 30 minutes. Rinse the smears in running tap water and allow to air-dry.
3. Examine the smears using the oil immersion objective. The erythrocytes on the thick, unfixed smears will be destroyed, making examination easier. The thick smear is used as a screening test to establish the presence of the parasite. The thin smear, which allows for careful examination of cellular morphology, permits identification of the species of malaria.

Reporting Results

The diagnosis of malaria is based on the demonstration of the *Plasmodium* species in the blood. Refer to Fig. 26.5 for illustrations of the typical appearance of various species. A brief morphological description is given in Table 26.2. For a complete discussion of each of the *Plasmodium* species, as well as other factors related to malaria, see Chapter 6.

Procedure Notes

Sources of Error

Malarial parasites can be confused with platelets. It is important to distinguish between malarial parasites *in* the erythrocyte and platelets that are superimposed *on* the erythrocyte. Malarial parasites are never seen in the spaces between erythrocytes.

Clinical Applications

It is important to recognize and distinguish between the various types of malaria to properly treat the patient. Treatment is important because plasmodia infect and destroy erythrocytes.

Limitations

The procedure is tedious, and it is frequently very difficult to locate infected erythrocytes.

BIBLIOGRAPHY

Provided on this book's companion Web site at thepoint. lww.com/Turgeon5e.

(continued)

SPECIAL HEMATOLOGY PROCEDURES *(continued)*

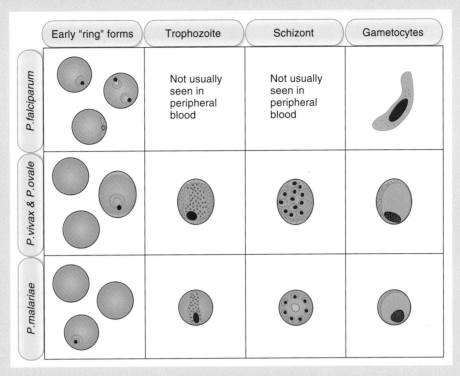

FIGURE 26.5 Malarial parasites in blood cells. This schematic drawing illustrates the most prominent morphological features that distinguish human malarial species in blood smears. The nuclear chromatid bodies of all of the malarial parasites are shaded in dark blue–gray in this diagram but actually appear red in Giemsa-stained preparations. *Plasmodium falciparum usually* appears as small, fine, ring forms, sometimes more than one per red blood cell. More-mature forms of the species are not usually seen in the peripheral blood. The gametocyte is characteristically banana shaped. *P. vivax* and *P. ovale* are distinguished by details not illustrated here. Infected cells and ring forms are larger than those of *P. falciparum*. At the trophozoite stage, red Schüffner dots are seen. The schizont contains more than a dozen merozoites before it ruptures. *P. malariae* infects smaller, senescent cells. Schüffner dots are not present. At the schizont stage, 8 to 12 merozoites are arranged peripherally around the central malarial pigment. (Reprinted with permission from Engleberg NC, Dermody T, DiRita V. *Schaecter's Mechanisms of Microbial Disease*, 4th ed, Baltimore, MD: Lippincott Williams & Wilkins, 2007.)

TABLE 26.2 | Morphological Comparison of *Plasmodium* sp

| Species | RBC Appearance | | Parasitic Appearance | |
	Size	Inclusions	Cytoplasm	Merozoites
P. vivax	Enlarged	Schüffner dots	Blue discs with red nucleus	12–24
			Accolé forms	
			Signet ring forms	
P. falciparum	Normal	Maurer dots	Minute rings	6–32
			Two chromatic dots	
			Accolé forms	
			Gametes: crescent-shaped	
P. malariae	Normal	Ziemann dots	One ring with one dot	6–12
P. ovale	Enlarged	Schüffner dots	One ring form	6–14

(continued)

MONOSPOT TEST (ORTHO DIAGNOSTICS, RARITAN, NJ)
Principle
This procedure is based on agglutination of horse erythrocytes by heterophile antibody present in infectious mononucleosis. Because horse RBCs exhibit antigens directed against both Forssman and infectious mononucleosis antibodies, a differential absorption of the patient's serum is necessary to distinguish the specific heterophile antibody from those of the Forssman type. The basic principle of the absorption steps in this procedure is comparable to that originally described by Davidsohn in his sheep agglutinin test. Serum or plasma is absorbed with both guinea pig kidney and beef erythrocyte stroma. Guinea pig kidney contains only the Forssman antigen and beef erythrocytes contain only the antigen associated with infectious mononucleosis. Guinea pig kidney will absorb only heterophile antibodies of the Forssman type, and beef erythrocytes will absorb only the heterophile antibody of infectious mononucleosis. Agglutination of horse RBCs by the absorbed patient specimen is indicative of a positive reaction for heterophile antibody.

This procedure, in CLSI format, is provided on this book's companion Web site at thepoint.lww.com/Turgeon5e.

OSMOTIC FRAGILITY OF ERYTHROCYTES: DACIE METHOD
Principle
In the osmotic fragility test, whole blood is added to varying concentrations of sodium chloride solution and allowed to incubate at room temperature. The amount of hemolysis is then determined by examining the supernatant fluid either visually or with a spectrophotometer.

If erythrocytes are placed in an isotonic solution (0.85%) of sodium chloride, water molecules will pass in and out of the membrane in equal amounts. In hypotonic solutions, erythrocytes will hemolyze because more water molecules enter into the cell than leave. This net influx of water molecules eventually ruptures the cell membrane.

The main factor in this procedure is the shape of the erythrocyte, which is dependent on the volume, surface area, and functional state of the erythrocytic membrane. A spherocytic erythrocyte ruptures much more quickly than normal erythrocytes or erythrocytes that have a large surface area per volume, such as target or sickle cells. The fragility of erythrocytes is increased when the rate of hemolysis is increased. If the rate of hemolysis is decreased, the erythrocytic fragility is considered to be decreased. The clinical value of the procedure is in differentiating various types of anemias.

This procedure, in CLSI format, is provided on this book's companion Web site at thepoint.lww.com/Turgeon5e.

SUCROSE HEMOLYSIS TEST
Principle
Erythrocytes in PNH lyse when exposed to serum solutions of low ionic strength containing complement. This test demonstrates the sensitivity of erythrocytes to the protein, complement. Normal erythrocytes under similar circumstances do not lyse.

This procedure, in CLSI format, is provided on this book's companion Web site at thepoint.lww.com/Turgeon5e.

ACID PHOSPHATASE IN LEUKOCYTES: CYTOCHEMICAL STAINING METHOD WITH AND WITHOUT TARTRATE
Principle
Peripheral blood or bone marrow smears are fixed and incubated in a solution of naphthol AS-BI phosphoric acid and fast garnet GBC salt. Naphthol AS-BI, released by enzymatic hydrolysis, couples immediately at acid pH with fast garnet GBC to form an insoluble maroon dye deposit at sites of activity. This is the reaction that occurs at the cellular sites of acid phosphatase activity.

Naphthol AS-BI phosphate-acid phosphatase → naphthol AS-BI

Naphthol AS-BI + fast garnet GBC → insoluble maroon pigment

Duplicate blood or bone marrow smears are incubated in a solution that also contains l-(+) tartrate–containing substrate. Cells containing tartaric acid–sensitive acid phosphatase do not exhibit any dye deposits, whereas those mononuclear cells containing tartaric acid–resistant acid phosphatase are not affected by such treatment.

Most leukocytes exhibit a positive acid phosphatase reaction to varying degrees. Lymphocytes display less activity than other leukocytes. Most of the acid phosphatase isoenzyme is inhibited by l-tartaric acid. The cells of hairy cell leukemia, Sézary syndrome, and some T-cell acute lymphoblastic leukemias are tartrate resistant.

This procedure, in CLSI format, is provided on this book's companion Web site at thepoint.lww.com/Turgeon5e.

(continued)

SPECIAL STAINS (continued)

ALKALINE PHOSPHATASE IN LEUKOCYTES: CYTOCHEMICAL STAINING METHOD

Principle

Peripheral blood or bone marrow smears are fixed and incubated in an alkaline-dye solution of naphthol AS-MX phosphate and fast blue RR salt or fast violet B salt. As the result of phosphatase activity, naphthol AS-MX is liberated and immediately coupled with a diazonium salt, forming an insoluble, visible pigment at the sites of phosphatase activity. The following reactions occur at cellular sites of alkaline phosphatase activity:

Naphthol AS-MX phosphate-alkaline phosphatase
→ naphthol AS-MX
Naphthol AS-MX + fast blue RR salt → blue pigment

or

Naphthol AS-MX + fast violet B salt → violet pigment

Leukocyte alkaline phosphatase (LAP) activity can be increased, normal, or decreased in a variety of conditions. This procedure is frequently used to distinguish between leukemoid reactions and chronic granulocytic (myelogenous) leukemia.

Specimen

Capillary blood is preferred to anticoagulated whole blood. If anticoagulated whole blood must be used, heparin is preferred. EDTA must be avoided. Blood smears should be stained within 8 hours after preparation. However, if this is not possible, gradual loss of alkaline phosphatase activity may be delayed by fixation and storage overnight in the freezer. Smears should be dried at least 1 hour before fixation, and 3 hours postfixation, before freezing.

Reagents, Supplies, and Equipment

Reagents: Sigma Diagnostics Kit No. 85, fast blue RR salt, fast violet B salt, naphthol AS-MX phosphate alkaline solution, and Mayer's hematoxylin solution are provided ready for use in the procedure. Store fast blue RR salt and fast violet B salt below 0°C. Store naphthol AS-MX phosphate alkaline solution at 2°C to 8°C. Reagents are stable until expiration date. Store Mayer's hematoxylin solution tightly capped at 18°C to 26°C. Do not return to original container after use in Coplin jar. Citrate concentrate is not included in the No. 85 kit.

1. Discard when the time required for a suitable stain exceeds the time recommended in the procedure by 5 minutes.

Note: Mayer's hematoxylin solution is harmful by inhalation, in contact with skin, and if swallowed.

2. Citrate concentrate: Store at room temperature. Suitable for use if no turbidity (microbial growth) is observed.

Citrate working solution: Prepare by pipetting 2 mL of citrate concentrate into a 100-mL volumetric flask. Dilute to the calibration mark with deionized water. Store at 2C° to 6°C. Suitable for use if turbidity (microbial growth) is absent.

3. Acetone (ACS- or USP-grade).
4. Fixative solution: Prepare by adding 2 vol of *room-temperature citrate working solution* to 3 vol of acetone. Stir constantly. Discard after use.
5. (Optional) Reagent: Scott's tap water substitute concentrate. Store at room temperature. If a small quantity of crystals form, they will not affect reagent performance.
6. Coplin jars or staining dishes, and slide holder
7. 100-mL Erlenmeyer flask
8. Microscope, immersion oil, and lens paper

Quality Control

A negative control can be prepared by immersing a normal fixed blood smear into boiling water for 1 minute to inactivate the enzyme. Blood from women who are either in their third trimester of pregnancy or within 2 days postpartum provides a highly positive control. A blood sample from a healthy adult provides a suitable normal control.

Procedure

Fixation of Blood Smears

1. Allow smears to dry for at least 1 hour before fixation.
2. Immerse smears in room-temperature fixative for 30 seconds.
3. Rinse thoroughly but gently for 45 seconds in deionized water. Do not allow slides to dry.

Staining and Counterstaining Procedure

1. Prepare stains *immediately* before use. Into an Erlenmeyer flask, place 48 mL of distilled water. Add the contents of a fast blue RR salt capsule or fast violet B salt capsule. Mix thoroughly. A magnetic stirrer is helpful. Add 2 mL of naphthol AS-MX phosphate alkaline solution. Mix. Use immediately and discard after use.
2. Immediately immerse slides in this fresh mixture and incubate at 23°C to 26°C for 30 minutes away from direct light.
3. Remove slides and wash gently with deionized water for 2 minutes. Do not allow slides to dry.
4. Place in Mayer's hematoxylin solution for 10 minutes to counterstain.
5. If fast blue RR salt was used, rinse counterstained slides for 3 minutes in deionized water. This produces a red-violet nuclear staining. If fast violet B salt was used, rinse slides in tap water (if alkaline) or immerse in Scott's tap water substitute for 2 minutes. This will produce a blue nuclear stain.

(continued)

SPECIAL STAINS (continued)

6. Air-dry and examine as unmounted slides. Unmounted stained slides usually remain unchanged for years.

Calculations

The deposits of blue or violet pigment viewed microscopically reflect the sites of granulocytic alkaline phosphatase activity. The granulocyte population is rated on the basis of the number of cells stained and the intensity of the pigment deposits.

Scan the smear using the oil immersion (100×) objective and select a thin area where erythrocytes are barely touching. Select 100 consecutive band and segmented neutrophilic granulocytes. Rate on a scale of 0 to 4+ on the basis of quantity and intensity of precipitated dye within the cytoplasm of cells (see Fig. 26.6) and (Table 26.3).

The percentage represents the proportion of total cytoplasmic volume occupied by the dye precipitate.

Obtaining Results

To obtain the LAP activity score, the number of cells counted in each category (0 to 4+) is multiplied by the value for that category. These scores are summed for the cumulative total. *Example:*

50 cells with a 4+ rating = 200

30 cells with a 3+ rating = 90

20 cells with a 2+ rating = 40

Total 100 cells   330 LAP score

Reporting Results

The normal range depends on the type of azo dye used. If fast blue RR is used, the normal range is 32 to 182. If fast violet B is used, the normal range is 12 to 180.

Procedure Notes

Sources of Error

Certain drugs and the age of the specimen are known to influence circulating alkaline phosphatase activity. Oral contraceptives,

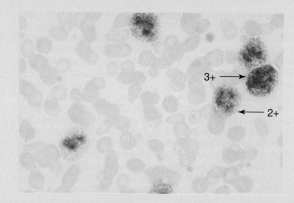

FIGURE 26.6 Leukocyte alkaline phosphatase (LAP) stain. *Cell Type:* Granulocytes; distinguishes leukemoid reaction from chronic myelogenous leukemia. *Description:* LAP is an enzyme associated with the specific granules; presence of activity indicates intracellular metabolic activity; positivity is indicated by either a ruby red color or a blue-purple color; positivity is quantitated; 100 consecutive bands or segmented neutrophils are scored using the following criteria: 0 = Colorless; 1 = Diffuse positivity, occasional granules; 2 = Diffuse positivity, moderate numbers of granules; 3 = Strong positivity, numerous granules; 4 = Very strong positivity, dark, confluent granules. The scores of the 100 cells are summed. *Clinical Conditions:* Increased: Leukemoid reaction Polycythemia vera Pregnancy Infections CML blast crisis Myelofibrosis Decreased: Chronic myelogenous leukemia Paroxysmal nocturnal hemoglobinuria Some myelodysplastic syndromes Idiopathic thrombocytopenic purpura. (Reprinted with permission from Anderson SC. *Anderson's Atlas of Hematology*, Philadelphia, PA: Wolters Kluwer Health/Lippincott Williams & Wilkins, Copyright 2003.)

cortisol, and stress may result in elevated LAP scores. Occasionally, weak staining lymphocytes may be observed. Bone marrow osteoblasts and endothelial cells stain strongly.

Clinical Applications

This test is clinically most useful in differentiating chronic myelogenous leukemia from leukemoid reactions. Leukemoid

TABLE 26.3	LAP Cytochemical Stain Scoring Characteristics		
Cell Rating	**Amount (%)[a]**	**Size of Granule**	**Stain Intensity**
0	None	—	None
1+	50	Small	Faint to moderate
2+	50–80	Small	Moderate to strong
3+	80–100	Medium to large	Strong
4+	100	Medium to large	Brilliant

[a]*Percent volume of cytoplasm occupied by dye precipitate.*

(continued)

reactions may result from infections, toxic conditions, and neoplasms as well as miscellaneous conditions such as the treatment of megaloblastic anemia, acute hemorrhage, and acute hemolysis.

Alkaline phosphatase activity can be associated with various conditions and disorders. Postsurgical patients experience a rise in activity with a peak 2 to 3 days postoperatively and a gradual return to normal values within 1 week. Persisting elevation of the LAP score is strong evidence of an active inflammatory process. LAP scores are useful in diagnosing ectopic pregnancy and an anovulatory menstrual cycle. The LAP score is also useful in differentiating choriocarcinoma from hydatidiform mole because the test score is normal in choriocarcinoma and high in cases of hydatidiform mole.

Limitations

This procedure depends on the subjective rating of stained cells. This can result in a wide variation of ratings.

LAP Scores and Some Related Conditions

Increased	Usually Normal	Usually Decreased
Leukemoid reactions	Infectious mononucleosis	Chronic myelogenous leukemia
Bacterial infections		
Chronic and acute lymphatic hemoglobinuria leukemia	Viral hepatitis	
Relative polycythemia	Paroxysmal nocturnal	
Hereditary hypophosphatasia		
Multiple myeloma		
Polycythemia vera		
Hodgkin disease		
Lymphoma		
Pregnancy and immediately postpartum		
Trisomy 21 (Down syndrome)		

BIBLIOGRAPHY

Provided on this book's companion Web site at thepoint. lww.com/Turgeon5e.

ESTERASE (ALPHA-NAPHTHYL ACETATE ESTERASE) IN LEUKOCYTES: CYTOCHEMICAL STAINING METHOD

Principle

Esterases are ubiquitous in nature and encompass a variety of different enzymes acting on selective substrates. In this procedure, blood or bone marrow smears or touch preparations are incubated with alpha-naphthyl acetate in the presence of a stable diazonium salt. Enzymatic hydrolysis of ester linkages liberates free naphthol compounds. These naphthol compounds then couple with diazonium salt, forming highly colored deposits at the sites of enzyme activity (see Fig. 26.7). Under defined conditions, this method provides a means to distinguish cells of the granulocytic series from cells of the monocytic series. This is particularly useful in the differentiation of leukemias.

This procedure, in CLSI format, is provided on this book's companion Web site at thepoint.lww.com/Turgeon5e.

ALPHA-NAPHTHYL ACETATE ESTERASE WITH FLUORIDE INHIBITION

To differentiate positive reacting cells conclusively from monocytes, sodium fluoride is incorporated with the incubation system. The monocyte enzyme is inactivated in the presence of this compound.

This procedure, in CLSI format, is provided on this book's companion Web site at thepoint.lww.com/Turgeon5e.

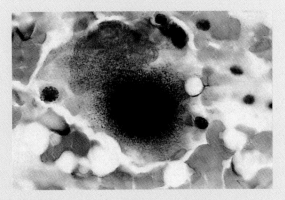

FIGURE 26.7 Strong α-naphthyl acetate esterase activity in a normal megakaryocyte. (Reprinted with permission from Mills SE. *Histology For Pathologists*, 3rd ed, Philadelphia, PA: Lippincott Williams & Wilkins, 2007.)

(continued)

ESTERASE (NAPHTHOL AS-D CHLOROACETATE ESTERASE) IN LEUKOCYTES: CYTOCHEMICAL STAINING METHOD

Principle

(See Alpha-Naphthyl Acetate Esterase.)

In this procedure, blood or bone marrow smears are incubated with naphthol AS-D chloroacetate in the presence of a stable diazonium salt. Naphthol compounds are coupled with diazonium salt, forming highly colored deposits at the sites of enzyme activity.

This procedure, in CLSI format, is provided on this book's companion Web site at thepoint.lww.com/Turgeon5e.

HEINZ BODIES

Principle

Whole blood is mixed with crystal violet stain and allowed to incubate. Moist preparations of the blood and stain mixture are examined for the presence of Heinz bodies in the erythrocytes. Heinz bodies represent unstable types of hemoglobin, which are denatured by dyes, such as crystal violet or brilliant cresyl blue, and appear as intraerythrocytic stained bodies (see Fig. 26.8).

Specimen

Whole blood collected in EDTA or heparin anticoagulants.

Reagents, Supplies, and Equipment

1. 0.85% sodium chloride (NaCl)
2. 1% brilliant cresyl blue

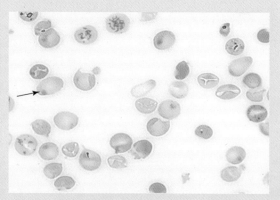

FIGURE 26.8 Heinz bodies. *Cell Type*: Young and mature red blood cells. *Description*: Round, refractile inclusions found on the periphery of the cell when stained with a supravital dye; consists of denatured globin produced by the destruction of hemoglobin; they may occur in multiple numbers. *Clinical Conditions*: Drug-induced anemias Thalassemia G-6-PD deficiency and other red blood cell enzymopathies. Unstable hemoglobinopathies. (Reprinted with permission from Anderson SC. *Anderson's Atlas of Hematology*, Philadelphia, PA: Wolters Kluwer Health/Lippincott Williams & Wilkins, Copyright 2003.)

Working solution: Weigh out 1.0 g of dye. Transfer to a 100-mL volumetric flask and dilute to the calibration mark with 100 mL of NaCl. Mix and filter the stain through No. 42 Whatman paper before use.

3. Test tubes (12 × 75 mm)

Quality Control

A normal control blood must be run simultaneously with the patient's blood. The control must demonstrate a low percentage of Heinz bodies.

Procedure

1. Place 1.0 mL of well-mixed whole blood into a test tube.
2. Add 0.5 mL of the brilliant cresyl blue solution.
3. Mix and allow to incubate at 37°C for a maximum of 2 hours.
4. At intervals of 30 minutes, 1 hour, and 2 hours, prepare specimens for examination. This procedure consists of remixing the blood and stain solution and placing a small drop of the mixture onto a glass slide. Place a coverslip over this preparation.
5. Examine the unstained slides immediately after preparation, using the oil immersion (100×) objective.

Reporting Results

Heinz bodies appear as blue, refractile, intracytoplasmic inclusions. They are irregularly shaped bodies of varying sizes, up to 2 μm in diameter, and are found close to the cellular membrane. There may be more than one Heinz body present in an erythrocyte. The test detects in vivo precipitated Heinz bodies.

Procedure Notes

Heinz bodies are detectable in wet preparations and by using supravital stains such as brilliant cresyl blue, new methylene blue N, methyl violet, and crystal violet. Heinz bodies are *not* seen when stained with Wright or Wright-Giemsa stain. In patients whose erythrocytes have defective reducing systems, many (45% to 92%) of the erythrocytes may contain five or more Heinz bodies.

Clinical Applications

Heinz bodies are formed when the glycolytic enzymes in the erythrocytes are unable to prevent the oxidation of hemoglobin. As a result, the hemoglobin is eventually denatured and precipitated to form Heinz bodies. Erythrocytic enzyme systems decrease as the cell ages; therefore, occasional Heinz bodies will be observed in normal blood.

Increased numbers of Heinz bodies represent unstable forms of hemoglobin that are present in a number of hemolytic disorders. Heinz bodies occur in disorders such as G6PD or glutathione deficiencies, secondary to the action of certain oxidant drugs and in the presence of unstable hemoglobins such as Hb Zurich and Hb H.

Caution: Refer to Material Safety Data Sheets.

(continued)

SPECIAL STAINS (continued)

BIBLIOGRAPHY

Provided on this book's companion Web site at thepoint. lww.com/Turgeon5e.

HEMOGLOBIN F DETERMINATION BY ACID ELUTION: KLEIHAUER AND BETKE METHOD MODIFIED BY SHEPARD, WEATHERALL, AND CONLEY

Principle

After blood smears are fixed with ethyl alcohol, a citric acid–phosphate buffer solution removes (*elutes*) hemoglobin other than Hb F from erythrocytes. The Hb F (fetal hemoglobin)–containing erythrocytes are visibly identifiable on microscopic examination when appropriately stained (see Fig. 26.9). Shortly after birth, the amount of Hb F in humans decreases to low levels. Increased amounts of Hb F are found in various hemoglobinopathies such as hereditary persistence of fetal hemoglobin, sickle cell anemia, and the thalassemias.

This procedure, in CLSI format, is provided on this book's companion Web site at thepoint.lww.com/Turgeon5e.

PERIODIC ACID–SCHIFF (PAS) IN LEUKOCYTES: CYTOCHEMICAL OR HISTOCHEMICAL STAINING METHOD

Principle

When treated with periodic acid, glycols are oxidized to aldehydes. After reaction with Schiff's reagent (a mixture of pararosanilin and sodium metabisulfite), a pararosaniline adduct is released that stains the glyco-containing cellular elements (see Fig. 26.10). Clinically, the PAS stain is helpful in recognizing some cases of erythroleukemia and acute lymphoblastic leukemia.

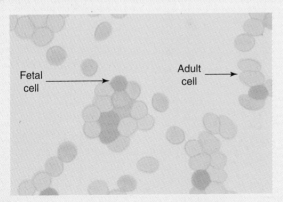

FIGURE 26.9 Acid elution or Kleihauer-Betke stain. *Cell Type*: Red blood cell. *Description*: Cells containing hemoglobin F will appear pink to red; cells containing no hemoglobin F will only have their outer membrane visible (ghost cells). *Clinical Conditions*: Hereditary persistence of fetal hemoglobin MDS Some leukemias. (Reprinted with permission from Anderson SC. *Anderson's Atlas of Hematology*, Philadelphia, PA: Wolters Kluwer Health/Lippincott Williams & Wilkins, Copyright 2003.)

This procedure, in CLSI format, is provided on this book's companion Web site at thepoint.lww.com/Turgeon5e.

PEROXIDASE (MYELOPEROXIDASE) IN LEUKOCYTES: CYTOCHEMICAL STAINING METHOD

Principle

Myeloperoxidase (MP) is detected by means of the enzyme's interaction with diaminobenzidine (DAB), a benzidine substitute. The brown reaction product is first intensified with copper salts followed by Gill's modified Papanicolaou stain, which results in intense gray-black granules at sites of neutrophil and monocyte myeloperoxidase activity (see Fig. 26.11). The reaction can be illustrated as:

$$DAB + H_2O_2 - MP \rightarrow \text{oxidized DAB (light brown pigment)}$$
$$\text{Oxidized DAB} + Cu(NO_3)_2 \rightarrow \text{gray-black pigment}$$

This procedure differentiates cells of lymphoid origin from granulocytes and their precursors and monocytes.

This procedure, in CLSI format, is provided on this book's companion Web site at thepoint.lww.com/Turgeon5e.

SIDEROCYTE STAIN: PRUSSIAN BLUE STAINING METHOD

Principle

The Prussian blue reaction precipitates free iron into small blue or blue-green granules in erythrocytes. Free iron is not identifiable on Wright- or Wright-Giemsa–stained blood smears. An immature or mature erythrocyte containing free iron is referred to as a sideroblast or siderocyte, respectively. Increased numbers of siderocytes are seen in disorders such as thalassemia major or in patients after a splenectomy. If the iron granules encircle the nucleus of the erythrocyte, it is referred to as a **ringed sideroblast.** Although alcoholism is the most common cause of ringed sideroblasts, they may also be seen in cases of lead poisoning or anemia.

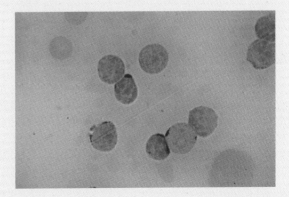

FIGURE 26.10 Periodic acid-Schiff stain of acute lymphoblastic leukemia L1. (Reprinted with permission from McClatchey KD. *Clinical Laboratory Medicine*, 2nd ed, Philadelphia, PA: Lippincott Williams & Wilkins, 2002.)

(continued)

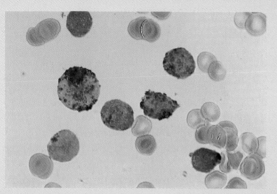

FIGURE 26.11 Myeloperoxidase stain of acute myelogenous leukemia M2. (Reprinted with permission from McClatchey KD. *Clinical Laboratory Medicine*, 2nd ed, Philadelphia, PA: Lippincott Williams & Wilkins, 2002.)

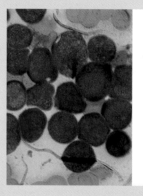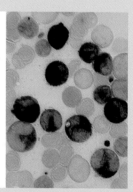

FIGURE 26.12 Sudan black B (**left**) stain of acute myelogenous leukemia M4. (Reprinted with permission from McClatchey KD. *Clinical Laboratory Medicine*, 2nd ed, Philadelphia, PA: Lippincott Williams & Wilkins, 2002.)

This procedure, in CLSI format, is provided on this book's companion Web site at thepoint.lww.com/Turgeon5e.

SUDAN BLACK B STAIN: CYTOCHEMICAL STAINING METHOD

Principle

Following fixation, blood or bone marrow films are immersed in a buffered Sudan black B solution. After rinsing, slides are counterstained with Mayer hematoxylin. Cells are examined microscopically for the presence of blue-black discrete granulation (see Fig. 26.12). Cells committed to the lymphoid pathway display negative staining reactions, whereas myeloid and monocytoid forms display characteristic positive reactions. The Sudan black B staining pattern usually parallels the myeloperoxidase stain and is useful in the identification of myelogenous and myelomonocytic leukemias.

This procedure, in CLSI format, is provided on this book's companion Web site at thepoint.lww.com/Turgeon5e.

TERMINAL DEOXYNUCLEOTIDYL TRANSFERASE TEST

Principle

Terminal deoxynucleotidyl transferase (TdT) is a non–template-directed DNA polymerase that catalyzes the irreversible addition of deoxynucleotides to the 3′-hydroxy groups on the end of DNA. The primary methods of detection are immunofluorescence and immunoperoxidase using a monoclonal antibody.

TdT is a cell marker found on immature and neoplastic cells frequently seen in leukemic states.

This procedure, in CLSI format, is provided on this book's companion Web site at thepoint.lww.com/Turgeon5e.

COAGULATION PROCEDURES

In coagulation testing, replicate analysis is frequently performed. However, in a study of replicate testing, it was concluded that repeat testing does *not* enhance the precision or the accuracy of coagulation tests. Accuracy and precision are controlled by quality assurance procedures, such as frequent calibration checks and multilevel commercial controls, as well as the practices described below.

Specimen Quality

All coagulation testing critically depends on the quality of the specimen. Minimum tissue trauma and the avoidance of hemolysis are essential. Proper phlebotomy techniques described in Chapter 2 must be strictly followed.

Special Collection Techniques

To reduce the possibility of introducing tissue thromboplastin into a whole blood sample and the subsequent utilization of certain factors with clot formation, certain techniques should be followed. Specimens collected for coagulation studies are not normally drawn initially, if multiple samples are collected. If a single sample is collected using an evacuated tube, a small amount of blood should be allowed to enter the plastic needle holder before collecting blood in the tube. Nonwettable evacuated tubes should be used to prevent activation of factors XII and VII by the glass walls of the container.

If a sample is collected using the syringe technique, two syringes are used. Approximately 1 mL of venous blood is collected in the first tube, and this syringe is disconnected from the needle hub. Immediately, a second syringe is connected to the hub of the needle and the specimen is collected in this syringe.

Anticoagulants

Sodium citrate (3.2%) is the anticoagulant of choice (see Chapter 2). The 3.2% citrate concentration has several advantages:

1. It has a closer osmolality to plasma and produces more accurate activated partial thromboplastin time (APTT) results when patients are being treated with heparin.
2. This citrate concentration is used as the mean of the normal range in the calculation of the international normalized ratio. Other anticoagulants (e.g., heparin, EDTA, or oxalate) should not be used.

The introduction of plastic tubes for safety reasons requires that new reference ranges for all coagulation assays be established. At least 10 female and 10 male patients who are in the laboratory's patient population and who are not receiving anticoagulation therapy should be tested to establish a reference range.

Because of the importance of the ratio of blood to anticoagulant, the proper vacuum in an evacuated tube must be maintained. The expiration date on the tube container needs to be monitored. If tubes are stored in sealed metal containers, precautions should be taken to monitor the premature loss of the tubes' vacuum. Tubes are stored best in open containers in an upright position.

The ratio of 9:1 in a specimen anticoagulated with sodium citrate is achieved with a properly collected specimen if a patient's PCV is between 0.20 and 0.60 L/L. However, in polycythemic or grossly anemic patients, a correction in the amount of anticoagulant or the amount of blood drawn must be made.

To determine the *amount of anticoagulant* in extreme cases, the following correction formula is used:

$$0.00185 \times \text{volume of blood (mL)}$$
$$\times (100 - \text{patient's packed cell volume})$$

To determine the *amount of whole blood* needed,

$$\frac{60}{100 - \text{patient's packed cell volume}} \times 4.5$$

Specimen Handling

Once a sample is in vitro, changes begin to occur and labile factors, such as factor VIII, begin to deteriorate quickly. It is strongly recommends that testing for prothrombin time (PT) should be completed within 24 hours and APTT should be completed within 4 hours. Samples should only be held for a maximum of 2 hours at 4°C, if testing cannot be performed immediately.

If testing is not conducted, plasma should be separated from the cells by centrifugation to produce a platelet-poor plasma (platelet count $<10 \times 10^9$/L). This is prepared by centrifuging the whole blood specimen for a minimum of 20 minutes at 2,500 rpm.

Specimens can be stored at -20°C for up to 2 months or -70°C for up to 6 months. Frost-free freezers should not be used for storage of specimens. Storage in a frost-free freezer or at temperatures higher than -20°C can compromise specimen quality (e.g., prolonged clotting time of a lupus anticoagulant screening assay).

To use a frozen specimen, it should be rapidly thawed at 37°C while being gently inverted to prevent denaturation of fibrinogen. Testing should be conducted immediately. If a thawed sample cannot be tested immediately, the sample may be held for a maximum of 2 hours at 4°C until tested.

For other assays (e.g., lupus anticoagulant), the capped specimens should be centrifuged at 1,500g for no less than 15 minutes at room temperature, and the plasma removed and then centrifuged again.

Specimen Preparation

Specialized testing for coagulation factors may require *adsorbed plasma* or *aged serum*. Plasma can be adsorbed using either barium sulfate or aluminum hydroxide. After adsorption, the resulting adsorbed plasma contains factors I, V, VIII, XI, and XII. Aged serum contains factors VII, IX, XI, and XII. Refer to the factor substitution studies procedure in this section for the technique.

Barium sulfate adsorption: To 1 mL of plasma, add 50 mg of barium sulfate. Incubate at 37°C for 15 minutes with frequent mixing. Centrifuge at 2,000 rpm to obtain a clear supernatant fluid. Use immediately after preparation.

Aluminum hydroxide adsorption: An aluminum hydroxide suspension is prepared by adding 1 g of aluminum hydroxide to 4 mL of distilled water. Add 1 vol of the suspension to 9 vol of citrated plasma. Mix well and incubate for 5 minutes at 37°C. Centrifuge at 2,500 rpm to obtain a clear supernatant.

Aged serum: A specimen of nonanticoagulated whole blood should be allowed to clot. This specimen should be incubated at 37°C for 3 hours. Add 0.1 M sodium citrate in the ratio of 1 vol of 0.1 M sodium citrate to 9 vol of whole blood to the specimen tube. Allow the tube to incubate at 37°C for an additional 2 hours. Centrifuge for 10 minutes and remove the serum. Serum should be used immediately or stored at -20°C. Before to use, dilute the aged serum with 0.85% sodium chloride using a ratio of 1 vol of serum to 4 vol of sodium chloride.

General Sources of Error

Glassware must be clean. Disposable glassware is preferred to reusable equipment because detergent residues and scratched glassware can produce erroneous results. All procedural directions must be strictly followed because variations in pH, reagent concentration, and temperature are major sources of error.

Quality Control

Water baths and heat blocks must be monitored continually for accurate temperatures. Refrigerators and freezers should also be monitored to ensure the stability of specimens and test reagents. Reagents must not be beyond their stated expiration date. Procedural technique must be consistent and appropriate.

BIBLIOGRAPHY

Provided on this book's companion website at thepoint.lww.com/ Turgeon5e.

COAGULATION PROCEDURES

ACTIVATED PARTIAL THROMBOPLASTIN TIME

Principle

The APTT procedure measures the time required to generate thrombin and fibrin polymers via the intrinsic pathway. Although a partial thromboplastin time test can be performed, contact factors can be activated more thoroughly by the addition of substances such as kaolin in the activated form of this assay.

In the APTT, calcium ions and phospholipids that substitute for platelet phospholipids are added to blood plasma. The generation of fibrin is the end point. Clinically, the APTT is used to identify and quantitate deficiencies in the intrinsic clotting system and to control anticoagulant therapy.

Specimen

Fresh plasma from citrated whole blood is needed. Centrifuge unopened whole blood specimens at 2,500 rpm for 20 minutes. Promptly transfer the plasma to a labeled plastic tube and place in an ice bath until tested. Specimens should be tested within 2 hours of collection.

Reagents, Supplies, and Equipment

1. Partial thromboplastin substrate containing an activator (such as Platelin Plus Activator or automated APTT from Organon Teknika Corp. or equivalent)
2. 0.025 M calcium chloride
3. Ice bath
4. (If manually performed) Stopwatch, 12×75-mm test tubes, nichrome loop, 0.1-mL pipettes, and a 37°C water bath or heat block

Quality Control

The routine testing of control materials is essential. Both normal and abnormal controls should be tested simultaneously with patient specimens. Results within and outside the normal range are equally important to monitor.

Commercial normal and abnormal control plasmas should be used for a comprehensive quality control program. To prepare these controls, reconstitute normal and abnormal plasma with the *exact* amount of reagent-grade water specified on the label. Allow to stand for 30 minutes at room temperature. Swirl gently to ensure complete rehydration. Mix gently before use. Store rehydrated vials at 2°C to 8°C and use within 24 hours. Unopened vials should be stored at 2°C to 8°C and used before the expiration date on the label.

Procedure

1. Place an aliquot of 0.025 M calcium chloride in a test tube and incubate at 37°C for a minimum of 5 minutes and a maximum of 60 minutes.
2. Pipette 0.1 mL of the partial thromboplastin substrate into a test tube and incubate for 2 minutes.
3. Pipette 0.1 mL of patient or control plasma into the substrate. Shake briskly to mix. Begin timing for *exactly 5 minutes*.
4. After 5 minutes of activation, transfer 0.1 mL of prewarmed calcium chloride to the mixture. *Immediately* begin to time with a stopwatch. Insert nichrome loop and sweep it across the bottom of the tube at the rate of 2 times per second.
5. At the first appearance of fibrin, stop the stopwatch. Record the number of seconds. Repeat this procedure (steps 2 through 5) for each assay.

Note: Performance of this test by automated methods is described in Chapter 25.

Reporting Results

Reference values are dependent on the activator and phospholipid reagents used; however, 20 to 35 seconds is typically normal. In some laboratories, ranges may be from 28 to 42 seconds, with 42 to 46 seconds being marginal.

Procedure Notes

Sources of Error

Various sources of error include poor specimen collection or storage, improper reconstitution and storage of reagents, reaction temperature, timing, and clot detection.

Clinical Applications

The APTT is widely advocated as the test of choice for the control of heparin therapy. It is also important in the screening profile of prekallikrein; high-molecular-weight kininogen; factors XII, XI, IX, VIII, X, V, II, and I; and inhibitors against these factors.

(continued)

BIBLIOGRAPHY

Provided on this book's companion Web site at thepoint. lww.com/Turgeon5e.

ANTITHROMBIN III: CLOTTING ASSAY METHOD

Principle

In the presence of heparin, thrombin is neutralized at a rate that is proportional to the antithrombin (AT III) concentration. Following defibrination, plasma is assayed in a two-stage procedure that utilizes standardized amounts of heparin, fibrinogen, and thrombin. The resulting clotting time is interpreted using a calibration curve. Clinically, the AT III assay is useful prior to and subsequent to treatment with heparin in cases of disseminated intravascular coagulation (DIC).

This procedure, in CLSI format, is provided on this book's companion Web site at thepoint.lww.com/Turgeon5e.

BLEEDING TIME: STANDARDIZED IVY METHOD

Principle

The bleeding time test is an in vivo measurement of platelet adhesion and aggregation on locally injured vascular sub-endothelium. This test provides an estimate of the integrity of the platelet plug and thereby measures the interaction between the capillaries and platelets. The bleeding time reflects this aspect of platelet function by measuring the length of time two standardized punctures of the ventral forearm take to stop bleeding. Clinically, the bleeding time is prolonged in thrombocytopenia, qualitative platelet disorders such as von Willebrand disease, aspirin ingestion, or the presence of vascular problems.

This procedure, in CLSI format, is provided on this book's companion Web site at thepoint.lww.com/Turgeon5e.

CIRCULATING ANTICOAGULANTS

Principle

Some coagulation deficiencies are caused by inhibitors to specific factors rather than the lack of a factor. These inhibitors are sometimes referred to as circulating anticoagulants. To detect a circulating anticoagulant, the APTT and the PT that were originally abnormal are repeated using various dilutions of patient plasma and normal plasma. The dilutions are incubated at 37°C and tested after 10, 30, 60, and 120 minutes of incubation. If the abnormality is a deficiency, 10% normal plasma will correct the test result to close to the normal range, as will the addition of 50% normal plasma. If the abnormality is caused by a circulating anticoagulant, more correction will usually be shown as the ratio of normal plasma increases in the mixture. The detection of an inhibitor may show up immediately or may require incubation

Patient Plasma	Normal Plasma
9 parts	1 part
5 parts	5 parts
1 part	9 parts

of the normal plasma in the presence of the inhibitor. Differentiation between a coagulation factor deficiency and a circulating anticoagulant is important in the correct treatment of a patient.

Specimen

Refer to the APTT procedure for treatment of the original specimen.

Reagents, Supplies, and Equipment

Refer to the APTT procedure.

Quality Control

A normal patient plasma should be tested at the same time as that of the unknown patient.

Procedure

1. Using fresh plasma, prepare the following dilutions:
2. Incubate the control and patient specimens and mixtures at 37°C and perform an APTT or PT assay on each plasma, control, and plasma-control mixture after 10, 30, and 60 minutes.

Reporting Results

If the abnormality is that of a deficiency, a normal plasma sample will correct the assay results to a reference value. If the abnormality is caused by a circulating anticoagulant (inhibitor), a greater correction is demonstrated as the ratio of normal plasma increases in the mixture.

Patient	Normal	Deficiency	Inhibitor
9 parts	1 part	Significant correction	No significant correction
5 parts	5 parts	Significant correction	Some correction
1 part	9 parts	Significant correction	More correction

Note: It is important to incubate the test specimens for 60 minutes because some inhibitors act progressively, and it may take time for the APTT and/or PT results of the patient plasma and patient plasma–normal control mixtures to show the effects of the inhibitor (a prolonged clotting time). To interpret the results, the end point of the normal control has to be compared to the patient-normal plasma mixtures. As the specimens incubate, a slight increase in the end points will be observed because of the loss of labile clotting factors. The degree of prolongation in the patient and patient-control mixtures must be greater than the normal control plasma.

(continued)

Factor	Disorder
II	Myeloma, systemic lupus erythematosus (SLE)
V	Streptomycin administration, idiopathic
VIII	SLE, rheumatoid arthritis, drug reaction, asthma, inflammatory bowel disease, postpartum
VIII, IX	Following replacement therapy for hereditary deficiency
IX	SLE—rare
X	Amyloidosis
X, V	SLE—common
XI	SLE—very rare
XIII	Isoniazid administration, idiopathic

Clinical Applications

Various types of anticoagulants may interfere with coagulation at different stages, especially factor VIII, heparin-like activity, and antithromboplastins. Most acquired anticoagulants are autoantibodies (usually IgG, sometimes IgM) directed against specific coagulation factors. Below is a list of circulating anticoagulants associated with clinical disorders.

Approximately 5% to 10% of patients with SLE, many patients on phenothiazine therapy, patients taking a variety of medications, and patients with lymphoproliferative disorders may demonstrate inhibitors known as **lupus-like anticoagulants.**

In addition to testing for circulating anticoagulants to specific coagulation factors, the platelet neutralization procedure (PNP) and the tissue thromboplastin inhibition test (TTIT) may be valuable. The PNP test separates lupus-like inhibitors from factor VIII, X, and V inhibitors but does not distinguish the presence of heparin from an acquired inhibitor. The TTIT procedure is less specific than the PNP but screens for lupus-like anticoagulant with inhibitory activity against tissue thromboplastin. Details of the PNP and TTIT procedures can be found in works of Lenahan and Smith.

BIBLIOGRAPHY

Provided on this book's companion Web site at thepoint. lww.com/Turgeon5e.

D-DIMER ASSAY

Principle

The fundamental principle of the D-dimer assay has remained largely unchanged: recognition of the unique neo-epitope in D-dimer by specific antisera. D-dimer contains a neo-epitope

Commercially Available D-dimer Assays

Method	Vendor
Microplate ELISA	Asserachrom Ddi (Stago), Enzygnost (Dade-Behring)
ELISA and Fluorescence (ELFA)	Vidas DD (bioMerieux), Stratus D-dimer (Dade-Behring)
ELISA and Chemiluminescence	Pathfast (Mitsubishi), Immulite (Siemens)
Immunofiltration and Sandwich-type	NycoCard (Nycomed), Cardiac D-dimer (Roche)
Semiquantitative Latex Agglutination	Dimertest latex (IL), Fibrinosticon (bioMerieux)
Manual, Whole-Blood Agglutination	SimpliRED (Agen), Clearview Simplify D-dimer (Agen)
Second-Generation Latex Agglutination (immunoturbidimetric)	TinaQuant (Roche), Liatest (Stago), MDA D-dimer (bioMerieux)

Source: Adapted from Righini M, Perrier A, De Moerloose P, Bounameaux H. D-dimer for venous thromboembolism diagnosis: 20 years later, *J Thromb Haemost*, 6:1059–1071, 2008.

that is formed following the cross-linking of adjacent D domains by factor XIIIa. It is this epitope that is recognized by specific antisera used in clinical assays.

The classic microplate ELISA was considered the gold standard for measuring D-dimer. Today, more than 30 different D-dimer assays are commercially available. These assays represent a wide range of techniques.

EUGLOBULIN LYSIS TIME

Principle

The euglobulin fraction of plasma contains plasminogen, fibrinogen, and activators with the potential for transforming plasminogen to plasmin. This fraction is precipitated with 1% acetic acid and resuspended in a borate solution. The euglobulins are then clotted by the addition of thrombin. The clot is incubated and the time of lysis is reported. Clinically, the euglobulin lysis test is a screening procedure for fibrinolytic activity.

This procedure, in CLSI format, is provided on this book's companion Web site at thepoint.lww.com/Turgeon5e.

SUBSTITUTION STUDIES AND FACTOR ASSAYS

Substitution Studies

Substitution studies and factor assays can be used to identify specific coagulation factor deficiencies.

(continued)

COAGULATION PROCEDURES *(continued)*

Principle

Substitution studies may be performed using adsorbed plasma and aged serum with the APTT to identify deficiencies of blood coagulation. Substitution studies may also be performed using adsorbed plasma with the PT to identify a factor VII deficiency.

Specific Factor Assays

Principle

Factor assays are based on the ability of the plasma in question to correct a factor-deficient substrate, such as factor VIII. The actual assay is the same as the APTT with the exception of the factor-deficient substrate. Identification of specific factor deficiencies is valuable in both the diagnosis and the treatment of patients.

This procedure, in CLSI format, is provided on this book's companion Web site at thepoint.lww.com/Turgeon5e.

FIBRIN SPLIT PRODUCTS: THROMBO-WELLCOTEST METHOD

Principle

Whole blood is added to thrombin (to ensure complete clotting) and soya bean enzyme inhibitors (to prevent any breakdown of fibrin). After incubation, the patient's serum is diluted and mixed with latex particles that have been coated with anti–fibrin split products. If fibrin split products are present, agglutination will occur. If these products are present in increased amounts with normal hepatic and renal function, it is assumed that a recent fibrinolytic event has taken place or is taking place. Clinically, elevated results demonstrate that the activation of plasmin has occurred or is occurring, such as in primary fibrinolysis and DIC with secondary fibrinolysis.

This procedure, in CLSI format, is provided on this book's companion Web site at thepoint.lww.com/Turgeon5e.

FIBRINOGEN ASSAY: METHOD CLOTTING ASSAY

Principle

Fibrogen — thrombin factor II → fibrin

When plasma is diluted and clotted with excess thrombin, the fibrinogen concentration is inversely proportional to the clotting time, yielding a linear relationship when plotted on log-log paper. Fibrinogen assays are useful in detecting deficiencies of fibrinogen and in detecting an alteration in the conversion of fibrinogen to fibrin.

This procedure, in CLSI format, is provided on this book's companion Web site at thepoint.lww.com/Turgeon5e.

PLATELET AGGREGATION

See Chapter 27.

PROTAMINE SULFATE ASSAY

Principle

Protamine is used to neutralize the effects of heparin. If protamine is administered in excess therapeutically, it is capable of interfering with factor IX activity and thromboplastin generation. A positive result indicates the inappropriate presence of intravascular fibrin monomers. (See Chapter 25 for more information on platelet aggregation.)

This procedure, in CLSI format, is provided on this book's companion Web site at thepoint.lww.com/Turgeon5e.

PROTHROMBIN TIME

Principle

This basic procedure involves adding plasma to an excess of extrinsic thromboplastin-calcium substrate. Thromboplastin is derived from tissues that supply phospholipoprotein, such as animal brain. The length of time required to form a fibrin clot is measured in seconds.

Clinically, this procedure is used to monitor oral anticoagulant therapy, as a screening test in the diagnosis of coagulation deficiencies, and as a component of a liver profile assessment. Prolonged results can indicate a deficiency of one or more factors in the extrinsic pathway: factors VII, X, and V, and factor II or I. The presence of an inhibitor will also produce prolonged values.

Specimen

Fresh plasma from citrated whole blood is preferred, although oxalated plasma may be used. The sample should be centrifuged promptly after collection, with the plasma removed from the erythrocytes. Plasma may be stored for several hours at 2°C to 6°C before testing.

Reagents, Supplies, and Equipment

1. Thromboplastin
2. 12 × 75-mm test tubes
3. Pipettes: 0.1 mL (100 μL)
4. 37°C water bath or heat block
5. Stopwatch
6. Nichrome loop

Quality Control

Normal and abnormal citrated or oxalated test plasma should be run with each patient assay or test batch.

Procedure

This procedure is commonly performed using automated equipment. However, in some cases a manual procedure may be desired.

1. Prewarm plasma at 37°C for a minimum of 2 minutes and a maximum of 10 minutes.
2. Prewarm thromboplastin at 37°C for a minimum of 2 minutes and a maximum of 60 minutes.

(continued)

COAGULATION PROCEDURES *(continued)*

TABLE 26.4	**Probable Coagulation Deficiencies Based on APTT and PT Test Results**					
	Deficient Factor					
Test	**V**	**VII**	**VIII**	**IX**	**X**	**XI or XII**
PT	Abnormal	Abnormal	Normal	Normal	Abnormal	Normal
APTT	Abnormal	Normal	Abnormal	Abnormal	Abnormal	Abnormal
Adsorbed plasma	Corrects	No change	Corrects	No change	No change	Corrects
Aged serum	No change	Corrects	No change	Corrects	Corrects	Corrects

PT, Prothrombin time; APTT, activated partial thromboplastin time.

3. Add 0.1 mL of plasma to 0.2 mL of thromboplastin. If performing this procedure manually, pipette quickly. Start a stopwatch simultaneously.
4. Using the nichrome loop technique, the loop is swept through the mixture at 2 sweeps per second until the first strand of fibrin appears. The tube may also be tilted using a magnifier to observe clot formation.
5. Repeat this procedure in duplicate for all specimens, including controls. The duplicate results should be within 1 second of one another.

Reporting Results

Reference values range from 10 to 15 seconds. Report both the patient and control specimens in seconds. An older alternative method of reporting is to express the percentage of patient activity. This is calculated as

$$\frac{\text{Control time (seconds)}}{\text{Patient's time (seconds)}} \times 100 = \% \text{ activity of patient}$$

Clinical Applications

This test depends on the activity of factors VII, V, X, II, and I. A deficiency of any of these may produce a 3- to 4-second prolongation in the test (Table 26.4).

BIBLIOGRAPHY

Provided on this book's companion Web site at thepoint.lww.com/Turgeon5e.

THROMBIN TIME

Principle

The thrombin time test determines the rate of thrombin-induced cleavage of fibrinogen to fibrin monomers and the subsequent polymerization of hydrogen-bonded fibrin polymers. Clinically, extremely low fibrinogen levels, abnormal fibrinogen thrombin inhibitors, and high concentrations of immunoglobulin (e.g., myeloma proteins) will produce abnormal results. The presence of heparin and high concentrations of fibrin-fibrinogen degradation products will also prolong the time. This procedure is particularly useful if other parameters, such as the APTT and PT, are prolonged.

This procedure, in CLSI format, is provided on this book's companion Web site at thepoint.lww.com/Turgeon5e.

Refer to the reference values on the inside back cover as well as additional procedures at thepoint.lww.com/Turgeon5e.

REVIEW QUESTIONS

1. What is the appropriate reagent for the reticulocyte count?
   A. New methylene blue
   B. Phyloxine B
   C. Solution lyses erythrocytes and darkens the cells to be counted
2. What is the appropriate procedure and characteristic for the Westergren method

A. The diluting solution lyses erythrocytes with propylene glycol and contains sodium carbonate and water.
B. The procedure measures the rate of erythrocyte settling.
C. Ferrous ions are oxidized to the ferric state.
D. The diluting solution is either 1% hydrochloric acid or 2% acetic acid.

(continued)

3. What source of error will have greatest effect on PCV (hematocrit)
   A. Incorrect dilution of blood and diluent
   B. Hemolysis of whole blood specimen
   C. Excessive anticoagulant will produce shrinkage of cells

Questions 4 and 5: Match the procedure and the source of error that will have the greatest effect on the test result.
4. _____ Platelet count
5. _____ Reticulocyte count
   A. Refractile bodies can produce a false-positive observation.
   B. Specimens stored at room temperature for more than 5 hours will produce inaccurate results.

Questions 6 through 8: Match the procedure and correct reference value.
6. _____ Erythrocyte count (adult male)
7. _____ Hemoglobin assay (adult female)
8. _____ Lymphocytes (adult)
   A. 0.15 to 0.3 × 10^9/L
   B. 12.0 to 16.0 g/dL
   C. 4.5 to 5.9 × 10^{12}/L
   D. 22 to 40%

Questions 9 through 13: Match the procedure and reference value.
9. _____ Total leukocyte count
10. _____ PCV (adult, female)
11. _____ Direct platelet count
12. _____ Reticulocyte count (newborn infant)
13. _____ Westergren ESR method (adult male age 65 years)
   A. Up to 13 mm/hour
   B. 2.5 to 6.0%
   C. 150 to 450 × 10^9/L
   D. 36 to 45%
   E. 4.4 to 11.3 × 10^9/L

14. What clinical or specimen condition will produce an increased total leukocyte count.
   A. Active allergies
   B. Immediate hypersensitivity reactions
   C. Inflammation
   D. A lipemic blood specimen

Questions 15 through 17: Match the following procedures with a clinical or specimen condition that will produce an increased test result.
15. _____ PCV
16. _____ Reticulocyte count
17. _____ Westergren ESR method
   A. Splenectomy
   B. Rouleaux formation
   C. Polycythemia
   D. Crisis associated with hemolytic anemia

Questions 18 through 21: Match the following leukocyte types with a clinical condition that will produce an increased value.
18. _____ Neutrophils
19. _____ Lymphocytes
20. _____ Monocytes
21. _____ Eosinophils
   A. Invasive parasites
   B. Bacterial infections
   C. Viral infections
   D. Tuberculosis

Questions 22 and 23: Match the following procedure with a clinical condition that will produce a decreased value.
22. _____ Reticulocyte count
23. _____ Westergren ESR
   A. Polycythemia vera
   B. Acute leukemias
   C. Megaloblastic anemia

24. A normal blood smear should have no more than approximately _____ (maximum) number of platelets per oil immersion field in an area where the erythrocytes are just touching each other.
   A. 10
   B. 15
   C. 20
   D. 25

25. The PCV procedure can be affected by the
   A. speed of the centrifuge
   B. length of time of centrifugation
   C. ratio of anticoagulant to whole blood
   D. all of the above

26. Which of the following erythrocytic inclusions contain RNA and can be observed by staining with new methylene blue?
   A. Howell-Jolly bodies
   B. Heinz bodies
   C. Pappenheimer bodies
   D. Reticulocytes

27. The sedimentation rate of erythrocytes can be affected by the
   A. ratio of anticoagulant to whole blood
   B. position of the tube
   C. temperature of the specimen or laboratory
   D. all of the above

Questions 28 through 31: Match the following procedures with the specific stains (use an answer only once).
28. _____ Acidified serum lysis test (Ham test)
29. _____ Donath-Landsteiner test
30. _____ Alpha-naphthyl acetate esterase
31. _____ Naphthol AS-D chloroacetate esterase
   A. Positive in monocytes
   B. Measures an extremely potent hemolysin at 4°C

(continued)

C. Positive in cell of granulocytic lineage

D. Measures hemolysis

Questions 32 through 35: Match the following procedures with the appropriate test reactions (use an answer only once).

32. _____ G6PD activity

33. _____ Heinz bodies

34. _____ Kleihauer-Betke test

35. _____ Hemoglobin S screening test

A. Erythrocytes lysed by toluene and saponin with the released product being reduced by sodium hydrosulfite

B. Fetal hemoglobin is not eluted

C. Denatured by crystal violet

D. Screens for one of the most prevalent hereditary enzyme deficiencies

Questions 36 through 39: Match the following procedures with the appropriate test reactions.

36. _____ Osmotic fragility

37. _____ Periodic acid–Schiff

38. _____ Peroxidase stain

39. _____ Prussian blue stain

A. Precipitates free iron into blue or blue-green granules

B. Observation of hemolysis in varying sodium chloride dilutions

C. Lymphocytes stain negative

D. Intense cytoplasmic granular staining in erythroleukemia

Questions 40 through 43: Match the procedure with a possible source of error.

40. _____ Acidified serum lysis test (Ham test)

41. _____ Donath-Landsteiner test

42. _____ G6PD assay

43. _____ Hemoglobin electrophoresis

A. Identical mobilities

B. Use of ABO-incompatible test serum

C. Quenched by PCVs greater than 0.50 L/L

D. Hemolyzed specimen

Questions 44 through 47: Match the procedure with a possible source of error.

44. _____ Hemoglobin S screening test

45. _____ Malaria preparation

46. _____ Sickle cell screening

47. _____ Sudan black B

A. Superimposed platelets may produce a false-positive result.

B. Blood specimen from a recently transfused patient may produce a false-negative result.

C. Old blood specimen will produce a false-negative result.

D. Test reagent more than 1 day old will produce a false-negative result.

Questions 48 through 51: Match the procedure with the appropriate reference value or positive test result.

48. _____ Acidified serum lysis test (Ham test)

49. _____ Leukocyte alkaline phosphatase

50. _____ G6PD assay

51. _____ Kleihauer-Betke test

A. Normal range: 32 to 182 with fast blue RR dye

B. Positive test: 10% to 50% hemolysis

C. Normal: less than 1% Hb F in adults

D. Zero time control should not fluoresce or fluoresce only slightly

Questions 52 through 54: Match the procedure with the appropriate reference value or positive test result.

52. _____ Alkaline denaturation

53. _____ Prussian blue stain

54. _____ Sucrose hemolysis test (sugar water test)

A. Negative: less than 10%

B. Newborn normal: 70% to 90%

C. Normal: 0% to 1% of mature erythrocytes

Questions 55 through 57: Match the procedure with the disorder that can be recognized through the use of the test.

55. _____ Acid serum lysis test (Ham test)

56. _____ Leukocyte alkaline phosphatase stain

57. _____ Donath-Landsteiner test

A. Positive in PCH

B. Diagnostic for paroxysmal nocturnal hemoglobinuria

C. Increased in hereditary spherocytosis

D. Increased in a leukemoid reaction

Questions 58 through 60: Match the procedure with the disorder that can be recognized through the use of the test.

58. _____ Heinz bodies

59. _____ Kleihauer-Betke test

60. _____ Osmotic fragility test

A. Detects physical alterations in the erythrocyte membrane

B. Positive result if unstable hemoglobins are present

C. Increased in cord blood samples

61. Which of the following procedures is used to detect the complement-sensitive cells in paroxysmal nocturnal hemoglobinuria?

A. Sucrose lysis test

B. Donath-Landsteiner test

C. Acidified serum lysis (Ham test)

D. Both A and C

62. Leukocytes that demonstrate a positive reaction in the tartratic acid-resistant acid phosphatase cytochemical stain are the lymphocytes seen in

A. infectious lymphocytosis

B. malignant lymphoma

C. acute lymphoblastic leukemia (non-T type)

D. hairy cell leukemia

(continued)

63. A decreased leukocyte alkaline phosphatase (LAP) score is seen in
   A. polycythemia vera
   B. chronic myelogenous leukemia
   C. leukemoid reactions
   D. acute myelogenous leukemia

Questions 64 through 66: Steps in leukocyte alkaline phosphatase scoring, in sequence, are (64) _____, (65) _____, and (66) _____.
   A. adding the scores for the 100 neutrophils counted
   B. grading the neutrophils using a 0 to 4 pt scale
   C. averaging the scores for all neutrophils counted
   D. multiplying the number of neutrophils in each category by their respective scores

67. In the leukocyte alkaline phosphatase procedure, blood smears should be stained
   A. within 8 hours of specimen collection
   B. within 48 hours of specimen collection
   C. within 72 hours of specimen collection
   D. within 5 days of specimen collection

Questions 68 and 69: The alpha-naphthyl acetate esterase stain is detected primarily in (68) _____ and is almost absent in (69) _____.
   A. megakaryocytes
   B. monocytes
   C. granulocytes
   D. erythrocytes

70. If many dense and dark-staining cells are seen in the Kleihauer-Betke test, the specimen could be from a patient with
   A. beta-thalassemia
   B. hereditary persistence of fetal hemoglobin
   C. sickle cell anemia
   D. all of the above

71. The reagent used in the traditional sickle cell screening test is
   A. sodium chloride
   B. sodium citrate
   C. sodium metabisulphite
   D. sodium-potassium oxalate

72. Which of the following is a nucleated erythrocyte with diffuse iron in the cytoplasm?
   A. Ring sideroblast
   B. Sideroblast
   C. Pappenheimer bodies
   D. Siderocyte

73. An increased number of siderocytes can be seen
   A. in chronic lymphocytic leukemia
   B. in lead poisoning
   C. after splenectomy
   D. both B and C

Coagulation Procedures

Questions 74 through 77: Match the following procedures with the appropriate principle or description of the test.
74. _____ Activated partial thromboplastin time (APTT)
75. _____ Antithrombin III assay
76. _____ Bleeding time
77. _____ Circulating anticoagulant assay
   A. In the presence of heparin, thrombin is neutralized
   B. Measures the time required to generate thrombin and fibrin polymers via the intrinsic pathway
   C. Measures inhibitors of specific factors
   D. An in vivo measurement of platelet adhesion and aggregation on locally injured vascular subendothelium

Questions 78 through 82: Match the following procedures with the appropriate reference value or diagnostic characteristic.
78. _____ APTT
79. _____ Antithrombin III
80. _____ Ivy bleeding time
81. _____ Aspirin tolerance test
82. _____ Circulating anticoagulant
   A. Positive result: increased ratio of normal plasma to patient plasma
   B. Normal: 2 to 8 minutes
   C. Normal: 20 to 35 seconds (28 to 42 seconds), the range depending on the activator and phospholipid reagents
   D. Increased twofold in 92% to 95% of patients after ingesting two tablets of salicylate
   E. Normal: 80% to 100% (range, 107 ± 19%)

Questions 83 through 86: Match the following procedures with the appropriate reference value.
83. _____ Factor VIII assay
84. _____ Fibrin split products
85. _____ Fibrin-stabilizing factor
86. _____ Fibrinogen assay
   A. Normal: no dissolution of the clot at 24 hours
   B. Normal: less than 8 to 10 μg/mL
   C. Normal: 50% to 150%
   D. Normal: 200 to 400 mg/dL or a titer of 1:123 to 1:256

Instrumental principles

- Describe the basic theory of the electrical impedance principle of cell counting and sizing.
- Describe the basic theory of the optical detection principle of cell counting and sizing.
- Explain the fundamental concepts of laser technology.
- Describe the principles of flow-cell cytometry and two basic uses of this technology in hematology.

Whole blood cell analysis

- Define the terms **parameter** and **sample.**
- List the parameters measured by basic bench-top hematology analyzers.
- Describe the methods used to measure the parameters named in the preceding objective.
- Name the parameters measured by total cell counting systems.
- Define the abbreviation **RDW**.
- Describe the process and output of total cell and histogram electrical impedance systems.
- Describe the process and output of a laser scatter technology system.
- Compare the process and output of the continuous flow system to the other two types of total cell and differential cell counters.
- Describe the general characteristics of histograms.

Analysis of instrumental data output

- Describe the appearance of microcytic and macrocytic erythrocytes on a histogram.
- Name two conditions that would contribute to a bimodal cellular distribution on an erythrocyte histogram.
- Explain how the red cell distribution width (RDW) is calculated and give the normal range.
- Describe the relationship of the RDW to the mean corpuscular volume (MCV).
- Name the six classifications of erythrocytes based on the RDW and MCV.
- Explain how the red cell mean index (RCMI) is calculated and give the normal value.
- Describe the appearance of a leukocyte histogram generated by the electrical impedance method.
- Describe the appearance of a leukocyte histogram generated by the optical detection method.
- Describe the construction of a platelet histogram.

- Explain how the mean platelet volume (MPV) is calculated.
- Compare the relationship between MPV and the platelet count.
- Name at least four disorders in which the MPV is abnormal.
- Explain the purpose of the platelet distribution width (PDW) and its normal value.

Laser technology

- Describe the generation, by laser technology, of a histogram for red blood cells (RBCs).
- Explain how a platelet histogram is generated.
- Describe the analysis and interpretation of the peroxidase analysis.
- Explain the output of the basophil/lobularity channel.
- Describe the process of lymphocyte subtyping.

Applications of flow cytometry

- Describe the general functions that flow cytometry analysis can provide.
- Name the three factors that have contributed to the rapid advance of the technology of flow cytometry.
- Name and discuss three hematological applications of flow cytometry.
- Name and discuss three other cellular applications of flow cytometry.

Digital Microscopy

- Describe the function of artificial neural networks.
- Explain the benefits and advantages of digital microscopy.

Single-purpose instrumentation

- Explain the principles of a pattern recognition leukocyte differential analyzer.

Instruments in coagulation studies

- Describe the two most common types of instruments used in the clinical laboratory for the detection of fibrin clots.
- Explain the principles of electromechanical and optical detection systems.
- Describe the methodological principle of platelet aggregation.

Case studies

- Analyze and discuss the significance of the erythrocyte and leukocyte histograms and the nomogram presented in the six case studies.

*Additional procedures, in CLSI format, are provided on this book's companion website at thepoint.lww.com/Turgeon5e.

INSTRUMENTAL PRINCIPLES

Instrumentation and the automation of procedures continue to increase in the clinical hematology laboratory. Since the first Coulter Cell Counter Model A was introduced in the 1950s, the types of automated equipment and instrumental capabilities of instrumentation have become more diverse and sophisticated. Cell counting and automated differential analysis are now routinely found in most laboratories. Microprocessor applications have increased instrument programming capabilities and data output in ways that were unimagined a decade ago.

The counting of the cellular elements of the blood (erythrocytes, leukocytes, and platelets) can be based on one of two classic methods:

1. Electrical impedance
2. Optical detection

The Electrical Impedance Principle

This method of cell counting was originally developed by Coulter Electronics and is referred to as the Coulter principle. Cell counting and sizing are based on the detection and measurement of changes in electrical impedance (resistance) produced by a particle as it passes through a small aperture. Particles such as blood cells are nonconductive but are suspended in an electrically conductive diluent. As a dilute suspension of cells is drawn through the aperture, the passage of each individual cell momentarily increases the impedance (resistance) of the electrical path between two submerged electrodes that are located on each side of the aperture (Fig. 27.1). The number of pulses generated during a specific period is proportional to the number of particles or cells. The amplitude (magnitude) of the electrical pulse produced indicates the cell's volume (Fig. 27.2). The output histogram is a display of the distribution of cell volume and frequency. Each pulse on the x-axis represents size in femtoliters (fL); the y-axis represents the relative number of cells.

The Optical Detection Principle

In the optical or hydrodynamic focusing method of cell counting and cell sizing, laser light is used. A diluted blood specimen passes in a steady stream through which a beam of laser light is focused. As each cell passes through the sensing zone of the flow cell, it scatters the focused light. Scattered light is detected by a photodetector and converted into an electrical pulse. The number of pulses generated is directly proportional to the number of cells passing through the sensing zone in a specific period.

The application of light scatter means that as a single cell passes across a laser light beam, the light will be reflected and scattered. The patterns of scatter are measured at various angles (forward scatter 180°, and right angle 90°). Scattered light provides information about cell structure, shape, and reflectivity. These characteristics can be used to differentiate the various types of white blood cells (WBCs) and to produce scatter plots with a five-part differential.

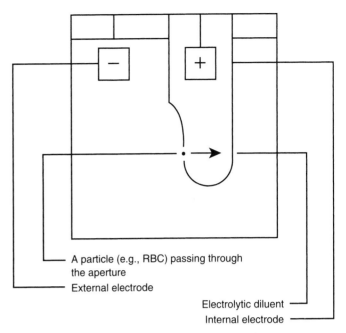

FIGURE 27.1 Coulter aperture: electronic impedance principle. When the aperture of an electronic particle counter is immersed in a dilution of whole blood in an electrolyte solution, changes in electrical resistance can be measured. The passage of each cell increases the resistance of the electrical path between two electrodes that are located on each side of the aperture. (Adapted with permission from Pierre R. *Significant Advances in Hematology*. Hialeah, FL: Coulter Electronics, 1985:6.)

Characteristics of Light Scatter

Optical Light Scatter

In this category, light amplification is generated by stimulated emission of radiation. Three independent processes are operational. These are

1. Diffraction and the bending of light around corners with the use of small angles
2. Refraction and the bending of light because of a change in speed with the use of intermediate angles
3. Reflection and light rays turned back by the surface or an obstruction with the use of large angles

Angles of Light Scatter

Various angles of light scatter can aid in cellular analysis. These are

1. Forward light scatter 0°. This is diffracted light, which relates to the volume of the cell.
2. Forward low-angle light scatter 2° to 3°. This characteristic can relate to size or volume.
3. Forward high angle 5° to 15°. This type of measurement allows for description of the refractive index of cellular components.
4. Orthogonal light scatter 90°. The result of this application of light scatter is the production of data based on reflection and refraction of internal components, which correlates with internal complexity.

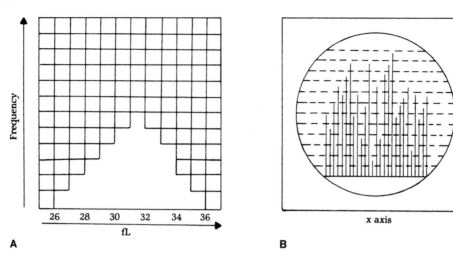

FIGURE 27.2 Cell counting: impedance principles. The number of pulses on the oscilloscope screen indicates the number of particles passing through the aperture. The height (amplitude) of each pulse reflects the volume of each cell. **A:** Histogram distribution of normal erythrocytes. **B:** Oscilloscope appearance as erythrocytes pass through the cell counting aperture and produce an electrical resistance. (Adapted with permission from Pierre R. *Seminars and Case Studies: The Automated Differential,* Hialeah, FL: Coulter Electronics, 1985:4.)

Radio Frequency

In this newer application, high-voltage electromagnetic current is used to detect cell size, based on the cellular density. The radio frequency (RF) pulse is directly proportional to the nuclear size and density of a cell. RF or conductivity is related to the nuclear-cytoplasmic ratio, nuclear density, and cytoplasmic granulation.

Fundamentals of Laser Technology

In 1917, Albert Einstein speculated that under certain conditions atoms or molecules could absorb light or other radiation and then be stimulated to shed this gained energy. In the 1950s, physicists theorized how this borrowed energy could be multiplied and emitted in high quantities. A decade later, new lasers were developed and used in medical and industrial applications.

The electromagnetic spectrum ranges from long radio waves to short, powerful gamma rays (Fig. 27.3). Within this spectrum is a narrow band of visible or white light, which is composed of red, orange, yellow, green, blue, and violet light. *Light amplified by stimulated emission of radiation* (laser) light ranges from the ultraviolet and infrared spectrum through all the colors of the rainbow.

In contrast to other diffuse forms of radiation, laser light is concentrated. Laser light is almost exclusively of one wavelength or color and its parallel waves travel in one direction.

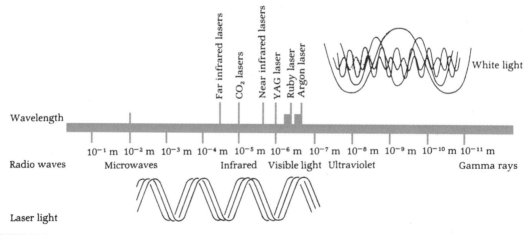

FIGURE 27.3 The electromagnetic spectrum ranges from long radio waves (10^{-1} m) to short gamma rays (10^{-1} m). The narrow band of the electromagnetic spectrum that constitutes white or visible light is composed of red, orange, yellow, green, blue, and violet light. A comparison of white light and laser light demonstrates that visible or white light and all radiation waves are diffused and jumbled. Laser light by comparison is organized and concentrated. YAG, yttrium, aluminum, garnet.

Through the use of fluorescent dyes, laser light can occur in numerous wavelengths. The types of lasers include glass-filled tubes of helium and neon lasers; the *y*ttrium, *a*luminum, *gar*-net (YAG) type, an imitation diamond; argon; or krypton.

Lasers sort the energy in atoms and molecules, concentrate it, and release it in powerful waves. In most lasers, a medium of gas, liquid, or crystal is energized by high-intensity light, an electrical discharge, or even nuclear radiation. When an atom extends beyond the orbits of its electrons or when a molecule vibrates or changes its shape, they instantly snap back, shedding energy in the form of a **photon.** The photon is the basic unit of all radiation. When a photon reaches an atom of the medium, the energy exchange stimulates the emission of another photon in the same wavelength and direction. This process continues until a cascade of growing energy sweeps through the medium.

Photons travel the length of the laser and bounce off mirrors. First a few and eventually countless photons synchronize themselves, until an avalanche of light streaks between the mirrors. In some gas lasers, transparent discs, referred to as Brewster windows, are slanted at a precise angle, which polarizes the laser's light. The photons, which are reflected back and forth, finally gain so much energy that they exit as a powerful beam. The power of lasers to pass on energy and information is measured in watts.

Principles of Flow Cytometry

Laser light is the most common light source used in flow cytometers because of the properties of intensity, stability, and monochromatism. Flow cytometry is defined as the simultaneous measurement of multiple physical characteristics of a single cell as the cell flows in suspension through a measuring device. Flow cytometry combines the technologies of fluid dynamics, optics, lasers, computers, and fluorochrome-conjugated monoclonal antibodies that rapidly classify groups of cells with heterogeneous mixtures.

The principle of flow cytometry is based on the fact that cells are stained in suspension. Flow cytometry has specifically come to denote the use of fluorescence measurement, usually with a laser light source. In laser flow cytometers, light scatter is used to measure the intrinsic size and granularity of the cell. In addition, fluorescence can be used to measure extrinsic features (e.g., specific protein expression and nucleic acid content) by adding reagents (e.g., fluorescent stains and antibodies). Virtually all flow cytometric assays use fluorescent stains. Fluorescent dyes used in flow cytometry must bind or react specifically with the cellular component of interest (e.g., reticulocytes, peroxidase enzyme, or DNA content). Fluorescent dyes include acridine orange, thioflavin T, pyronin Y, fluorescein isothiocyanate (FITC), and phycoerythrin (PE). FITC and PE are used when dual color analysis is desired.

Many flow cytometric assays use direct immunofluorescence staining with fluorochrome-conjugated monoclonal antibodies to identify cells expressing specific antigens. Fluorochromes are molecules that absorb light of one wavelength and emit light of a higher wavelength. Fluorochromes are covalently bonded to monoclonal antibody molecules. This provides a mechanism that allows for the determination by the flow cytometer if a labeled antibody has bound to the cell surface.

An argon laser, which produces blue light, is the most commonly used laser. Some instruments add a red helium-neon laser and occasionally a mercury arc lamp is substituted.

Each fluorochrome has a maximal excitation wavelength at or near the wavelength of the laser and has a characteristic emission spectrum. The fluorochrome, excited by the laser light, will fluoresce at a longer wavelength. Fluorescein emits a green fluorescence, PE emits orange, and peridinin chlorophyll protein or PE coupled to cyanin 5 emits a red fluorescence.

Some flow cytometers have a second laser that can excite other fluorochromes. Like the side-scattered blue light, all of these fluorescent signals pass through the objective set at 90° to the incident laser light. The number of colors in flow cytometry output refers to the number of individual fluorochrome-labeled antibodies used simultaneously in a given reaction tube. For example, mixing a cell suspension with a combination of antibodies labeled with two fluorochromes is referred to two-color flow cytometry.

A suspension of stained cells is pressurized using gas and transported through plastic tubing to a quarts flow chamber (Fig. 27.4) within the instrument. In the flow chamber, the specimen is injected through a needle into a stream of physiological saline solution called the sheath. The sheath and specimen both exit the flow chamber through a 75-μm orifice. This laminar flow design confines the cells to the very center of the saline sheath with the cells moving in single file.

The stained cells next pass through the laser beam. The laser activates the dye and the cell fluoresces. The interaction between each cell and the laser beam provides the following two types of information:

1. The amount of light scattered by each cell hit by the laser beam
2. The intensity of the fluorescence emitted by labeled antibodies bound to antigens on the different types of suspended cells

Although the fluorescence is emitted throughout a 360° circle, it is usually collected via optical sensors located at 90° relative to the laser beam. The fluorescence information is then transmitted to a computer. Flow cytometry performs fluorescence analysis on single cells at rates up to 50,000 cells/minutes. The computer is the heart of the instrument; it controls all decisions regarding data collection, analysis, and cell sorting.

The Basis of Cellular Identification

One of the major advantages of flow cytometry is that more than one measurement can be made on every cell during the few milliseconds that the cell spends passing through the laser beam. Each cell can be optically measured for the intensity of scattered light.

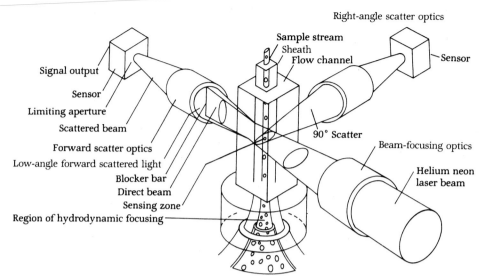

FIGURE 27.4 Laser flow cytometry. The optical detection of forward- and right-angle light scatter using a laser light source is accomplished by using a sensor as the cells pass through the beam under conditions of laminar flow. (Courtesy of Ortho Diagnostic Systems, Westwood, MA, 1985.)

The cellular light scatter patterns can be used to identify cells. Both intrinsic and extrinsic properties of cells can be analyzed by flow cytometry. Intrinsic properties include forward- and right-angle light scatter, which correlate with size and granularity of a cell, respectively. This data output does not require addition of dyes or stains for detection. In contrast, extrinsic properties rely on the binding of various probes to the cells. The scattered light passes through a variety of filters and lenses and is then measured by photomultiplier tubes, which convert the light signals into electronic signals for computer analysis. Light scattered along the axis of the laser beam is "forward scatter," and light scattered perpendicular to the axis is "side scatter" or "orthogonal scatter." Forward scatter is roughly proportional to cell size; side scatter to cytoplasmic granularity. Granulocytes have a much larger side-scattered light signal than do lymphocytes.

Data Analysis

Data are plotted on histograms. Populations of similar cells form discrete and characteristic two-dimensional "clusters" of scatter when the forward and side scatters are plotted against each other.

Most hematological samples contain multiple cell populations. It is necessary to first identify the population of interest for further analysis. Whole blood is commonly used for platelet and erythrocyte assays. Data collected by the flow cytometer can be displayed as a 1-parameter histogram or as 2-parameter plots. A 1-parameter histogram is described as either the percentage of cells within a set of markers or as the mean fluorescent intensity of a population. A 2-parameter plot is usually divided into four quadrants, each containing a percentage of the total population. This is used to distinguish between fluorescent and nonfluorescent cells. It also defines the expression and nonexpression of a cell molecule marked by a fluorescent antibody or other fluorochrome.

It is often necessary to analyze a single population within several populations and debris.

Electronic gating allows isolation of a specific cluster of cells for analysis. Gating is a software feature used to restrict analysis to a particular population. A gate is created by drawing a graphic boundary (Fig. 27.5) around a population of cells.

Quadrant markers divide 2-parameter plots into four sections called quadrants. The quadrants are used to distinguish negative, single-positive, and double-positive populations

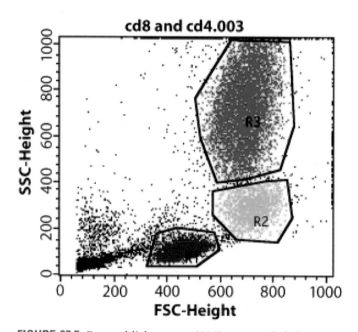

FIGURE 27.5 Forward light scatter (FSC) versus side light scatter (SSC) of normal peripheral blood. Electronic regions (gates) have been set to identify lymphocytes (R1), monocytes (R2), and granulocytes (R3). (Reprinted with permission from McCoy JP. Flow cytometry, *Am Assoc Clin Chem Clin Lab News*, 29(9):8–10, 2003.)

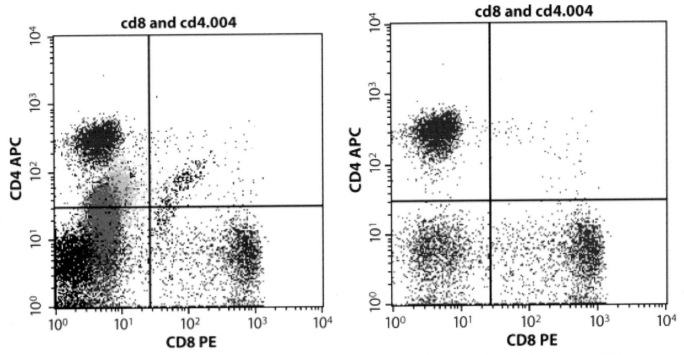

FIGURE 27.6 A: The peripheral blood in Figure 27.8A was stained with phycoerythrin (PE)-conjugated CD8 antibodies (*X*-axis) and allophycocyanin (APC)-conjugated CD4 antibodies (*Y*-axis) in a two-color immunophenotyping procedure. This figure is ungated and illustrates the difficulty in analyzing ungated data from heterogeneous specimens. **B:** This histogram illustrates the CD4 and CD8 staining on only the gated lymphocytes in the peripheral blood from Figure 27.7. By eliminating monocytes and granulocytes from the analysis, interpretation of staining is made much easier. (Reprinted with permission from McCoy JP. Flow cytometry, *Am Assoc Clin Chem Clin Lab News,* 29(9):8–10, 2003.)

from one another (Fig. 27.6). A negative population is located in the lower left (LL) quadrant.

WHOLE BLOOD CELL ANALYSIS

Clinical laboratory automation has been evolving rapidly during the past 40 years. A significant innovation is automated front-end (preanalytical [preexamination]) instrumentation/robotics and total work cells linked by a track or conveyor. Because specimen processing is perhaps the most labor-intensive portion of the testing process, automating this preanalytical (preexamination) process is one option for streamlining procedures to reach maximum efficiency and to improve customer service. The critical workload volume to reach to invest in front-end automation is between 1,500 and 2,000 specimens per day.

Automated analyzers now form the backbone of clinical laboratories both large and small. Smaller analyzers are commonly used in STAT labs, freestanding clinics, physicians' offices, and small hospital laboratories. Larger and more complex systems are used in larger clinical and research laboratories.

The degree of instrumental sophistication is frequently described by the number of parameters that the instrument generates. The term **parameter** is a statistical term that refers to any numerical value that describes an entire population. Parameter should be clearly distinguished from the term **sample**, which is a subset of a population. Any numerical value describing a sample is called a **statistic.**

The smaller hematology instruments measure erythrocytes (RBCs), leukocytes (WBCs), and platelets. Entry-level hematology instruments generate eight measured or calculated parameters (WBC, RBC, hemoglobin [Hgb], hematocrit [Hct], MCV, mean corpuscular hemoglobin [MCH], mean corpuscular hemoglobin concentration [MCHC], and platelets). Computerized systems generally flag high or low patient results. These systems are automated from sample aspiration through result printout (Fig. 27.7). Additional basic parameters include erythrocyte morphology information expressed as RDW, MPV, or leukocyte histogram differential. Other calculated output is expressed differently, depending on the manufacturer (Table 27.1).

Technology continues to deliver new automation capabilities in hematology. For example, automated reticulocyte counting was a leading edge technology a few years ago but is a routinely measured parameter in many clinical laboratories today. Some of the latest instruments prepare and stain peripheral blood smears and automatically correct for leukocyte (WBC) interference. Newly developed instrumental capabilities continue to be developed. Some of the innovations include

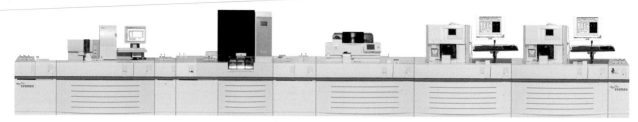

FIGURE 27.7 Sysmex lavender top hematology and diabetes testing solution. (Courtesy of Sysmex America, Inc.)

- Quantitation of nucleated erythrocyte (NRBC) counts
- A channel for enumeration of immature granulocytes (IGs)
- Random access CD4 lymphocyte counting
- Analysis for CD34, CD38, and CD61 cell markers
- Measurement of reticulocyte hemoglobin
- Enumeration of hematopoietic progenitor cells (HPCs)
- Counting of IGs

Types of Automated Cell Counting Instruments

Major types of automation are representative of the ways that blood cells can be counted, leukocytes differentiated, and other components (e.g., MCH and MCHC) calculated. Hemoglobin is measured by the traditional cyanmethemoglobin flow-cell method at 525 and 546 nm, depending on the instrument manufacturer. A summary of currently marketed automated instruments is shown in Tables 27.2 to 27.4. Models and features of instrumentation change rapidly. The reader is advised to refer to the respective manufacturers' Web sites for any updates.

Examples of Automated Instruments

Cell-Dyn Series (http://www.abbott.com)

The basic system uses multiangle polarized scatter separation (MAPSS) flow cytometry with hydrodynamic focusing of the cell stream is universal to Abbott five-part differential analyzers. The CELL-DYN Sapphire is the most advanced of the CELL-DYN analyzers. These analyzers feature dual leukocyte counting methods. The leukocyte differential without the use of a stain is accomplished with light scatter with 0°, 90°, 10°, and 90° (depolarized) as well as nuclear optical count by light scatter at 0° and 10°. In addition, the CELL-DYN Sapphire uses three color fluorescence measurements made on cells that are stained with fluorochromes dyes: FL1 (green, 515 to 545 nm), FL2 (yellow, 565 to 595 nm), and FL3 (red, 615 to 645 nm). The CELL-DYN Ruby does not employ fluorescence analysis. This mode uses a more economical, red (632.8 nm) wavelength laser for MAPSS analysis.

Erythrocytes and platelets are counted by light scatter at 0° and 10°. Red cell indices (MCV, MCH, MCHC) are generated. Mature reticulocytes and immature reticulocyte fraction (IRF) are measured and reported.

A unique feature is cyanide-free hemoglobinometry. Rapid cell lysis followed by the formation of an imidazole-hemoglobin complex is measured. The HB Flow Cell is illuminated by a light-emitting diode (LED) and a photodetector measures transmitted light at 540 nm.

In addition, the Cell-Dyn 4000 incorporates the technologies used in the basic model and features three independent measurements and focused flow impedance. A hydrodynamically focused impedance method is employed for primary erythrocyte counts, secondary platelet counts, and erythrocyte and platelet size distribution analysis.

Multidimensional light scatter and fluorescent detection are used as well. DNA and RNA fluorescence are used to distinguish NRBCs from viable and nonviable leukocytes (WBCs). RNA fluorescence can measure reticulocytes and the IRF.

Horiba ABX Diagnostics, Inc. (http://www.adx.com)

The Pentra 60C+ is a small bench-top instrument. It reports 20 parameters and RBC, platelets (PLT), and basophil (BASO) histograms. Two patented methodologies are used.

TABLE 27.1	Calculated Output		
Type	**Hematocrit**	**RDW**	**MCV**
Beckman-Coulter	RBC × MCV	CV% of RBC histogram	Mean of RBC size distribution histogram
Abbott	RBC × MCV	Relative value to CV	Mean of RBC size distribution histogram
Sysmex	Mean pulse	RDW-SD (fL)	HCT/RBC
Bayer	RBC × MCV	CV%	Mean of RBC volume histogram

RDW, red cell distribution width; MCV, mean corpuscular volume; RBC, red blood cell; CV, coefficient of variation; RDW-SD, red cell distribution width based on standard deviation; HCT, hematocrit.

TABLE 27.2	Summary of Automated Instruments		
Name of Hematology Analyzer	**First Year Sold in the United States**	**Manufacturer**	**Test Menu**	**Unique Tests**
CELL-DYN 3200	1997	Abbott Diagnostics www.abbott.com	WBC, RBC, Hb, Hct, MCV, MCH, MCHC Platelets Number and percent, neut, lymphs, mono, eos, baso RDW, MPV	Three-dimensional optical RBC analysis with advanced MCV measurement
CELL-DYN 3700	1999		WBC, RBC, Hct, MCV, MCH, MCHC Platelets Number and percent, segs, lymphs, mono, eos, baso RDW, MPV Retic number and percent, IRF	IRF
CELL-DYN Ruby			WBC, RBC, Hb, Hct, MCV, MCH, MCHC Platelets percent and number, neut, mono, lymp, eos, baso RDW, MPV RETIC percent and number	
CELL-DYN Sapphire			WBC, RBC, Hb, Hct, MCV, MCH, MCHC Platelets percent and number, neut, mono, lymp, eos, baso RDW, MPV RETIC percent and number, IRF NRBC percent and number, CD61, CD3T percent and number, CD4T percent and number, CD8T percent and number 4/8	
CELL-DYN Emerald			WBC, RBC, Hb, Hct, MCV, MCH, MCHC Platelets, mono, lymp percent and number, gran percent and number, mid percent and number RDW, MPV	
Coulter HmX	1999	Beckman Coulter Inc. www.beckmancoulter.com	WBC, RBC, Hct, MCV, MCH, MCHC Platelets Number and percent segs, lymphs, mono, eos, baso RDW, MPV Retic number and percent, IRF, MPV, graded RBC morph	None

(continued)

TABLE 27.2   Summary of Automated Instruments *(Continued)*

Name of Hematology Analyzer	First Year Sold in the United States	Manufacturer	Test Menu	Unique Tests
Coulter LH 500	2003		WBC, RBC, Hct, MCV, MCH, MCHC Platelets Number and percent segs, lymphs, mono, eos, baso RDW, MPV Retic number and %, IRF, graded RBC, morph NRBC percent and number TNC and RBC on CSF synovial and serous fluids	
Coulter LH 780/785	2006/2007		WBC, RBC, Hb, Hct, MCV, MCH, MCHC Platelets Number and percent, neut, mono, lymph, eos, baso RDW, RDW-SD, MPV Retic number and percent, IRF, MPV, graded RBC, morph NRBC number and percent TNC and RBC on CSF synovial and serous fluids	
Coulter LH 750/755	2001		WBC, RBC, Hb, Hct, MCV, MCH, MCHC Platelets Number and percent, neut, mono, lymph, eos, baso RDW, MPV Retic number and percent, IRF, MPV, graded RBC, morph NRBC number and percent TNC and RBC on CSF synovial and serous fluids	
Coulter AcT diff Family	2001		WBC, RBC, Hct, MCV, MCH, MCHC Platelets Number and percent segs, lymphs, mono, eos, baso RDW, MPV	
Coulter LH 1500	2002/2003		WBC, RBC, Hb, Hct, MCV, MCH, MCHC Platelets Number and percent, neut, lymphs, mono, eos, baso RDW, MPV Retic percent and number, IRF, graded RBC, morph NRBC percent and number TNC and RBC on CSF, synovial and serous fluids	

(continued)

Instrument	Year	Manufacturer	Parameters
Pentra 60c+	2000	Horiba ABX Diagnostics, Inc. www.abx.com	WBC, RBC, Hct, MCV, MCH, MCHC Platelets Percent segs, lymphs, mono, eos, baso + ALY & LIC (percent and number) RDW, MPV
Pentra DY 120			WBC, RBC, Hct, MCV, MCH, MCHC Platelets Number and percent segs, lymphs, mono, eos, baso RDW, MPV, reticulocytes proportional, absolute, and corrected reticulocyte counts; proportional immature reticulocytes; mean reticulocyte volume; and mean fluorescence index Reticulocyte RNA content IRF
Pentra XL80	2004		WBC, RBC, Hct, MCV, MCH, MCHC Platelets Number and percent segs, lymphs, mono, eos, baso RDW, MPV Automatic dilution of overrange results, customized dilution ratio (all parameters), atypical lymphs, atypical lymphs percent, LIC, LIC percent
Pentra XL120	2005/2004		WBC, RBC, Hct, MCV, MCH, MCHC Platelets Number and percent, neut, lymphs, mono, eos, baso NRBCs, reticulocytes, IRF, MRV
Advia 120	1998	Siemens	WBC, RBC, Hct, MCV, MCH, MCHC Platelets Number and percent segs, lymphs, mono, eos, baso CHCM, MPV, RDW, HDW, LUC number and % Retic % and number, CHR, CHCMr, MCVr CSF:WBC, RBC, PMN, MN, neutron, lymph, mono
Advia 2120i	2008		WBC, RBC, Hb, Hct, MCV, MCH, MCHC Platelets percent and number, neut, mono, lymph, eos, baso CHCM, MPV, RDW, HDW LUC percent and number Retic percent and number, CHr, CHCMr, cellular Hgb, MCVr; CSF:WBC, RBC, PMN, MN, neut, lymph, mono
Sysmex XE-2100	2000	Sysmex Sysmex.com/usa	WBC, RBC, Hct, MCV, MCH, MCHC Platelets Number and percent segs, lymphs, mono, eos, baso NRBC number and percent Retic number and percent, RDW-SD, RDW-CV, IRF, Plt-O, HPC number, MPV

TABLE 27.2 Summary of Automated Instruments *(Continued)*

Name of Hematology Analyzer	Manufacturer	First Year Sold in the United States	Test Menu	Unique Tests
Sysmex XE-2100		2001	WBC, RBC, Hct, MCV, MCH, MCHC Platelets Number and percent segs, lymphs, mono, eos, baso NRBC number and percent Retic number and percent, RDW-SD, RDW-CV, IRF, Plt-O, HPC number, MPV	
Sysmex XE-2100L		2001	WBC, RBC, Hct, MCV, MCH, MCHC Platelets Number and percent segs, lymphs, mono, eos, baso NRBC number and percent, RDW-SD, RDW-CV, HPC number, MPV	
Sysmex XE-5000		2008/2007	WBC, RBC, Hb, Hct, MCV, MCH, MCHC Platelets percent and number, neut, mono, lymph, eos, baso NRBC percent and number Retic percent and number, RDW-SD, RDW-CV, IRF, Plt-O, HPC#, MPV, IG percent, RET-He, IPF	
Sysmex XE-Alpha N/HST-N		2000	WBC, RBC, Hb, Hct, MCV, MCH, MCHC Platelets percent and number, neut, mono, lymph, eos, baso RDW-SE, RDW-CV, IG percent, IG number NRBG percent, NRBC number, retic percent and number, IRF, Plt-O, HPC#, MPV, RET-He, IPF, HPC	
Sysmex XT-2000i		2002	WBC, RBC, Hct, MCV, MCH, MCHC Number and percent segs, lymphs, mono, eos, baso Retic number and percent, IRF, Plt-O, RDW-SD, RDW-CV, MPV	
Sysmex XT-1800i		2002	WBC, RBC, Hct, MCV, MCH, MCHC Platelets Number and percent segs, lymphs, mono, eos, baso RDW-SD, RDW-CV, MPV	

ALY, atypical lymphocytes (for informational use only); CBC, complete blood count; CHCM, cellular hemoglobin concentration mean; CHCM, reticulocyte hemoglobin concentration mean; CHR, reticulocyte hemoglobin content/platelet count; CSF, cerebrospinal fluid; Hct, hematocrit; HDW, hemoglobin distribution width; HLS, high light scatter (reticulocytes)—for research use only, not for use in diagnostic procedures; HPC, hematopoietic progenitor cell; IG, immunoglobulin; IPF, immature platelet fraction; IRF, immature reticulocyte fraction; LIC, large immature cells (for informational use only); LUC, large unstained cell; MAPSS, multiangle polarized scatter separation; MCH, mean corpuscular hemoglobin; MCHC, mean corpuscular hemoglobin concentration; MCV, mean corpuscular volume; MCVr, reticulocyte mean corpuscular volume; MPV, mean platelet volume; MRV, mean reticulocyte volume; NRBC, nucleated erythrocyte; PCT, PDW, platelet distribution width; Plt-O, fluorescent optical platelets; PMN, polymorphonuclear neutrophil; QC, quality control; RBC, red blood cell; RDW, red cell distribution width; RET-He, reticulocyte Hgb equivalent; Retic, reticulocyte; RF/DC; VCS, volume, conductivity, and scatter; WBC, white blood cell; WVF, white cell viability fraction.

TABLE 27.3 | Automated Leukocyte Differential Methods

Instrument	Manufacturer	Leukocyte Differential Method Used	Scattergram Display: Cell Specific Color/Histogram Display: Color With Threshold
CELL-DYN 3200	Abbott www.abbottdiagnostics.com	Multi-Angle Polarized Scatter Separation (MAPSS)	Yes/yes
CELL-DYN 3700		MAPSS	Yes/yes
CELL-DYN Ruby		MAPSS	Yes/yes
CELL-DYN Sapphire		Optical scatter and three-color fluorescent	Yes/yes
CELL-DYN Emerald		Impedance counting	No/no
Coulter HmX	Beckman Coulter, Inc. www.beckmancoulter.com	Coulter's 3D VCS technology	Four colors/cell types. Colors without thresholds
Coulter LH 500		Coulter's 3D biophysical flow cytometry with AccuGate 500, Reaction Manager technologies	Yes/yes
Coulter LH 780/785		Coulter's 3D VCS biophysical flow cytometry with IntelliKinetics, AccuGate and AccuFlex technologies	Yes/yes
Coulter LH 750/755		Coulter's 3D VCS biophysical flow cytometry with IntelliKinetics, AccuGate and AccuFlex technologies	Yes/yes
Coulter AcT Diff Family		AcT technology combining cytochemistry, focused flow impedance, and light absorbance principles of measurement	No/yes
Coulter LH 1500		Coulter's 3D VCS biophysical flow cytometry with IntelliKinetics, AccuGate and AccuFlex technologies	Yes/yes
Pentra 60c+	Horiba ABX Diagnostics Inc. www.abx.com	Double Hydrodynamic Sequential System (DHSS) and Multi-Distribution Sampling System (MDSS) technology combining cytochemistry, focused flow impedance, and light absorbance principles of measurement	Yes/yes
Pentra DX120		Cytochemistry (chlorazol black E) and absorbance	Yes/yes
Pentra XL80		DHSS technology combining cytochemistry, focused flow impedance, and light absorbance	Yes/yes

(continued)

TABLE 27.3   Automated Leukocyte Differential Methods *(Continued)*

Instrument	Manufacturer	Leukocyte Differential Method Used	Scattergram Display: Cell Specific Color/Histogram Display: Color With Threshold
Advia 120	Siemens Healthcare Diagnostics www.siemens.com/diagnostics	Peroxidase-cytochemistry staining with light scatter and absorption; baso-cytochemistry stripping with two-angle laser light scatter	Yes/yes
Advia 2120i		Peroxidase WBC—peroxidase cytochemistry staining with light scatter and absorption; baso-cytochemistry stripping with two-angle laser light scatter	Yes/yes
Sysmex XE-Alpha N/HST-N	Sysmex America Inc. www.sysmex.com	Fluorescent flow cytometry, RF/DC detecting method	Yes/yes
Sysmex XE-2100		Fluorescent flow cytometry, RF/DC detecting method	Yes/yes
Sysmex XE-2100D		Fluorescent flow cytometry	Yes/yes
Sysmex XE-2100L		Fluorescent flow cytometry, RF/DC detecting method	Yes/yes
Sysmex XE-5000		Fluorescent flow cytometry, RF/DC detection method	Yes/yes
Sysmex XT-2000i		Fluorescent flow cytometry	Yes/yes
Sysmex XT-1800i		Fluorescent flow cytometry	Yes/yes
Sysmex XS-1000I and XS-1000i Autoloader		Fluorescent flow cytometry	Yes/yes

TABLE 27.4	Automated Instruments	
Analyzer	**Manufacturer**	**Summary of Distinguishing Features / Distinguishing Features**
CELL-DYN 3200	Abbott Diagnostics www.abbottdiagnostics.com	MAPSS cell-by-cell analysis provides a better differential analysis; focused flow 2D optical RBC and platelet analysis provides better separation between microcytic RBCs and large platelets; uses only three reagents; 3D MCV
CELL-DYN 3700		MAPSS cell-by-cell analysis provides a better differential analysis; reticulocyte with reportable IRF; 60-species veterinary package
CELL-DYN Ruby		Touch-sensitive screen, all optical technology; onboard maintenance videos; lyse-resistant RBC mode; rules-based result annotations
CELL-DYN Sapphire		Four optical and three fluorescent detectors providing multiple scatterplot analysis; 2D optical platelets that avoid interferences; fluorescent analysis of reticulocytes, NRBCs, and three-color monoclonal analysis on a routine hematology analyzer; OpenFlow MAb test selections
CELL-DYN Emerald		Small: simple size, reagent volumes used, and physical size; reliable: system averages one service call per year; easy to use: system has touch-screen software with intuitive icons and minimal layers
Coulter HmX	Beckman Coulter Inc. www.beckmancoulter.com	VCS technology; lowest review rate in class; no routine daily maintenance; triplicate counting; aperture burn circuit; sweepflow; SmartStart system; autoloader and single sample models
Coulter LH 500		Extensive decision support, extended linearity for WBC and platelet, lowest review rate in class, small footprint, superior reliability, ProService, electronic IQAP
Coulter LH 780/785		Extensive onboard user-defined decision support, extended linearity for WBC and Plt using AccuCount technology; enumeration of NRBCs with every differential; random access/automation ready; integrated slidemaker/slidestainer options; proservice; electronic IQAP; expanded QC module; RUO: WBC research population data
Coulter LH 750/755		Extensive decision support; enumeration of NRBCs with every differential; random access; automation ready; extended linearity for WBC and platelet; RUO: WBC RPD
Coulter Ac. Tdiff Family		Quantitative five-part WBC differential; aspirate only 30 µL of sample; requires small space footprint and runs quietly; AL has auto repeat based on decision rules
Coulter LH 1500		System automatically loads and unloads cassettes, performs reflex and repeat testing, sorts tubes for off-line tests, stores tubes with availability for retrieval for any type of test; multiple configurations available; RUO: WBC research population data
Pentra 60c+	Horiba ABX Diagnostics, Inc. www.abx.com	Reliable five-part WBC differential technology-MTBF over 200 d; small footprint; small sample size of 53 µL; Hemalink Data Manager
Pentra DX 120		High-throughput cell counter with integrated reticulocyte methodology and slidemaker/slidestainer; fluorescent NRBC counting, auto rerun and reflex testing, autovalidation
Pentra XL80		Compact five-part differential instrument with autoloader and autodilution capability, autorun feature, autovalidation
Advia 120	Siemens Healthcare Diagnostics www.siemens.com/diagnostics	Unique laser technology provides cellular hemoglobin for RBCs and retics; 2D platelet analysis that eliminates interference from RBC fragments and inclusion of large platelets; dual WBC counts with linearity of up to 400,000; CSF assay
Advia 2120i		Unique laser technology provides cellular hemoglobin for RBCs and retics; 2D platelet analysis eliminates interference from RBC fragments and inclusion of large platelets; dual WBC counts with linearity of up to 400,000; CSF assay

(continued)

TABLE 27.4 Automated Instruments (Continued)

Analyzer	Manufacturer	Summary of Distinguishing Features
Sysmex XE-Alpha N/HST-N	Sysmex America Inc. www.sysmex.com	High throughput, flexible, scalable configurations available (>125 standard configurations); platelet linearity—5 million; new parameters for platelet monitoring—IPF and retic Hb measurement and RET He, HPC analysis, lavender top management, standardized technology, reagents, controls and operations
Sysmex XE-2100 1999		Throughput of 150 CBCs per hour; random access; discrete testing; online QC; remote diagnostics, body fluid analysis; platelet linearity to 5 million, hematocrit linear to 75%; HPC testing, IG enumeration; immature platelet fraction; reticulocyte hemoglobin equivalent; standardized reagents, controls and operations with other Sysmex X-series analyzers
Sysmex XE-2100D		150 CBC/hr; platelet linearity—5 million, hematocrit extended to 75%; standardized technology, reagents, controls and operations; ISBT compliant
Sysmex XE-2100L		Remote diagnostics; online QC; random access; HPC testing; 150 CBCs per hour throughput; discrete testing; NRBC enumeration, IG enumeration
Sysmex XE-5000		Low-end linearity for all body fluids; two-part differential (mononuclear % + # and polymorphonuclear % + H) or body fluid; reticulocyte hemoglobin content; immature platelet fractions; throughput of 150 CBCs per hour; random access; discrete testing; online QC; remote diagnostics, body fluid analysis; platelet linearity to 5 million, hematocrit nonlinear to 75%; HPC testing; IG enumeration; immature platelet fraction; reticulocyte hemoglobin equivalent; standardized reagents, controls and operations with other Sysmex X-series analyzers
Sysmex XT-2000i		High throughput, remote diagnostics; online QC; random access; fluorescent optical platelets; discrete testing; reagent monitoring; customized chartable report formats; XT-V unit for use in toxicology and research and veterinary reference labs; body fluids now FDA cleared, standardized technology, reagents, controls and operations with other X-series analyzers
Sysmex XT-1800i		Remote diagnostics; online QC; random access; discrete testing; reagent monitoring; chartable report formats; XT-V unit for use in toxicology and research and veterinary reference labs; unique specimen-gating software is FDA Part II compliant; body fluids now FDA cleared, standardized technology, reagents, controls and operations with other X-series analyzers
Sysmex XS-1000I and XS-1000i Autoloader		Standardized technology, reagents, controls and operations with other X-series analyzers; small sample volume requirements for CBC + five-part diff.; remote diagnostics; online QC; discrete analysis; reagent monitoring; chartable report; remote calibration verification

ALY, atypical lymphocytes (for informational use only); CBC, complete blood count; CHCM, cellular hemoglobin concentration mean; CHCMr, reticulocyte hemoglobin content/platelet count; CSF, cerebrospinal fluid; Hct, hematocrit; HDW, hemoglobin distribution width; HLS, high light scatter (reticulocytes)—for research use only, not for use in diagnostic procedures; HPC, hematopoietic progenitor cells; IG, immunoglobulin; IRF, immature reticulocyte fraction; LIC, large immature cells (for informational use only); LUC, large unstained cell; MAPSS, multiangle polarized scatter separation; MCH, mean corpuscular hemoglobin; MCHC, mean corpuscular hemoglobin concentration; MCV, mean corpuscular volume; MCVr, reticulocyte mean corpuscular volume; MPV, mean platelet volume; MRV, mean reticulocyte volume; NRBC, nucleated erythrocyte; PCT, PDW, platelet distribution width; PMN, polymorphonuclear neutrophil; QC, quality control; RBC, red blood cell; RDW, red cell distribution width; Retic, reticulocyte; RF/DC; VCS, volume, conductivity, and scatter; WBC, white blood cell; WVF, white cell viability fraction.

Siemens Healthcare Diagnostics (http:www/medical.siemens.com)

The ADVIA series uses two separate and independent flow cytometers to count and identify cells. This technology uses unifluidics, a darkfield optical method. Once a specimen is aspirated, it is delivered into a ceramic shear valve, where it is divided into separate aliquots for analysis in various reaction chambers. Dual leukocyte methods of peroxidase staining and basophil lobularity are used. Erythrocytes and platelets are counted in the RBC reaction chamber by flow cytometry. Hemoglobin has dual readings and colorimetric or cyanmethemoglobin and corpuscular hemoglobin concentration mean.

Reticulocyte enumeration using oxazine 750 stain is determined by low-angle light scatter, high-angle light scatter, and absorption measurements as the aliquot of specimen travels through the reticulocyte reaction chamber. The low-angle scatter and high-angle scatter are proportional to cell size and hemoglobin concentration. The light absorption measurement is proportional to ribonucleic acid (RNA) content because stained reticulocytes absorb more light than mature erythrocytes. The output of these three parameters is plotted on a reticulocyte volume histogram, on a hemoglobin concentration histogram, and on the reticulocyte hemoglobin content histogram. The reticulocyte hemoglobin content (CHr) demonstrates the functional state of erythropoiesis. CHr is an important indicator of asymptomatic anemia, which is particularly important in children under the age of 2 years and pregnant women. The reference range is 0 to 200 fL.

Two separate methods are used by the ADVIA 120/2120 system to analyze WBCs. The total WBC count is measured from two reaction chambers: the peroxidase chamber and the lobularity/nuclear density chamber. In the peroxidase chamber, WBCs are fixed and peroxidase reagent is used. This chamber is heated to a high temperature to lyse RBCs and platelets and to fix the WBCs. The WBC size is measured by forward angle laser light scatter. Peroxidase activity is measured by tungsten light optics. Myeloperoxidase is a granulocyte enzyme marker. Data are displated on a PEROX cytogram with light absorption depicted on the *x*-axis and forward scatter on the *y*-axis. In the lobularity/nuclear density reaction chamber, an aliquot of whole blood is introduced into an acid buffer that selectively lyses the cytoplasm of all cells, except basophils. Samples flow through a laser light path, where low-angle scatter and high-angle scatter are measured. Basophils are not lysed and appear larger, scatter more light, and appear higher on the vertical axis of a scattergram compared to the bare nuclei of other WBCs. A primary WBC count and basophil count are generated from this channel.

Data generated by the ADVIA system indicate relative percentages and absolute values for granulocytes (neutrophils, eosinophils, basophils), lymphocytes, and monocytes. In addition, interpretative data to signal the presence of abnormalities in the sample are generated as well as the percentage of large unstained cells (LUCs). An increased number of LUCs suggests the presence of variant lymphocytes or blast cells.

Body fluid analysis, for example, cerebrospinal fluid (CSF) can be analyzed for RBCs and WBCs. Cells are counted and differentiated on three optical measurements: low angle scatter, high angle scatter, and absorbance. These data points, and the percentage and absolute values for mononuclear cells PMNs, lymphocytes, and monocytes are generated.

Beckman-Coulter (http://www.beckmancoulter.com)

The latest generation of Beckman Coulter (the LH Series) is a fully automated complete blood count (CBC) and differential analyzer. The use of the Beckman Coulter AccuCount technologies, the Coulter Principle, and VCS (see Box 27.1) technologies delivers expanded productivity and advances in cellular flow analysis of individual cells. These applications allow for nucleated red blood cells (NRBCs) counts with a corrected total leukocyte (WBC) count, correction for WBC interference, and the ability to analyze body fluids, for example, CSF. If the analyzer and work cells are combined, many of the pre-evaluation and post-evaluation steps are automated.

A second Beckman Coulter technology, AccuGate, uses a gating method to separate WBCs or RBCS and reticulocytes by using contour gates around cell populations. Leukocyte analysis is performed in three dimensions and is displayed as a 3D cube. Individual cells are represented as points on a scatterplot reflecting cell volume, conductivity, and laser light scatter characteristics. Reticulocytes is conducted by combining traditional supravital staining with new methylene blue stain and flow cytometry using VCS technology. NRBC is performed using the proprietary VCS technology.

A third technology, AccuFlex, allows end-users to optimize the levels of individual flags for improved data point performance. Contour discriminators examine areas between different cell populations. Flagging messages identify the type of cell population (e.g., WBC), the suspected variation (e.g., variant lymphocytes), and cell date of related condition (e.g., abnormal WBC population). A definitive condition, for example, leucopenia or leukocytosis, is also generated.

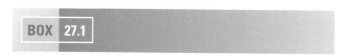

BOX 27.1

VCS Technology

Volume (V): using direct current impedance, the volume of each cell is measured.

Conductivity (C): radiofrequency penetrate the cell which generates the data points of cell size and cell internal structure.

Scatter (S): mid-angle scatter detected by a beam of laser light which generates data about cellular granularity and cell surface structure.

VCS: single channel that analyzes approximately 8,000 cells in a near-native condition.

Sysmex (http://www.sysmex.com)

In the Sysmex X series, there are four modes of sample introduction:

1. Sampler mode
2. Manual mode
3. Manual closed mode
4. Capillary mode

The Sampler mode is the primary mode of peration. This mode automatically mixes, aspirates, and analyzes samples with removing the rubber stopper of an evacuated tube filled with anticoagulated blood. In Manual mode, the most commonly used method for STAT assay, the rubber stopper of an evacuated tube filled with anticoagulated blood, is manually removed, and the individual blood sample is aspirated with a pipet. Using the Manual closed mode, the sampler is used to aspirate a specimen of anticoagulated whole blood without removing the rubber stopper of an evacuated tube. The Manual closed mode is essentially the same as the Sampler mode, but mixing and continuous analysis cannot be performed automatically. The Capillary mode is used to analyze a very small sample of whole blood that has been diluted 1:5.

The XS series of Sysmex instruments are automated hematology systems consisting of two units: the Main Unit that aspirates, dilutes, mixes, and analyzes anticoagulated whole blood specimens and the IPU that processes data from the Main Unit and provides an operator interface. Flags and error messages alert laboratory personnel to specimen abnormalities.

Red cell distribution width, an expression of anisocytosis, is reported as RDW-SD and RDW-CV. The RDW-SD is an actual measurement of the width of the RBC histogram The RDW-CV, by comparison, is a mathematically derived parameter. The RDW-CV is dependent on the average size of the RBCs or the MCV. Some models produce nucleated RBC and reticulocyte counts. Reticulocytes are enumerated by fluorescent flow cytometry using laser light and a nucleic acid fluorescent dye. Results are reported as RBC-O (optical) and reticulocyte number (RET#), and reticulocytes percent (RET%). Reticulocyte maturation can be assessed. The RET-He or reticulocyte hemoglobin equivalent is used to monitor the availability of iron in RBCs. Hemoglobin is measured using sodium lauryl sulfate (SLS-hemoglobin method), a noncyanide compound. In the Sysmex series, erythrocytes and platelets are analyzed by

■ Hydrodynamic focusing
■ Direct current (DC)
■ Automatic discrimination

The leukocyte count is analyzed by the DC detection method and automatic discrimination. A five-part differential is produced for leukocytes by a differential detector channel (analyzed by RF and DC). A differential scattergram and an immature myeloid information (IMI) scattergram are produced by fluorescent flow cytometry. Each cell is measured by forward-scatter laser light, lateral-scatter laser light, and lateral fluorescent light.

Three additional parameters can be performed on the XE-2100 analyzer. These are IG, immature platelet fraction (IPF), and hematopoietic progenitor cell (HPC).

RBC and WBC cell counts can be performed on body fluids, including CSF, serous fluid, and synovial fluid.

Instrument Data Output

Flags or messages are generated if abnormal results are generated. Different cell types are distinguished electronically by impedance by the pulses they generate. The pulses that are generated are sorted according to size. These individual pulses appear on the oscilloscope and are categorized by the computer. From the WBC histogram, the percent and absolute number of lymphocytes, mononuclear cells, and granulocytes are determined. Each channel on the x-axis represents size increasing by 1 fL (1 fL = 1 μm^3) from left to right. Each division on the y-axis represents one in that channel, providing the relative number of cells (Fig. 27.8).

Quality Control of Output Data

The Joint Commission, College of American Pathologists (ISO 15189 CAP), and the Clinical laboratory Improvement Amendments require a quality assurance/quality control system. A variety of quality control methods are available via computerized programming. These include instrument checks that ensure that the background is acceptably low and confirm the calibration stability of the electronic system. Control specimen data can be monitored with the generation of a Levey-Jennings graph for each parameter.

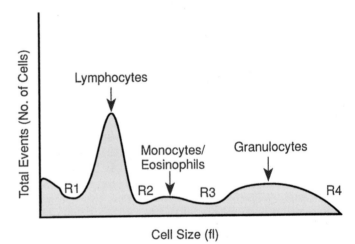

FIGURE 27.8 Blood cell histograms (Coulter STKS). Example of a WBC count differential histogram based on volumetric studies. The various components of the WBC are shown on the graph. R1 to R4 correspond to flags generated by the instrument representing distribution abnormalities warranting manual observation. R1, nucleated RBCs, platelet clumps, large platelets, cryoglobulin, small lymphocytes, unlysed RBCs; R2, reactive lymphocytes, lymphoblasts, basophils, clotted sample; R3, eosinophilia, monocytosis, blasts, clotted sample; R4, granulocytosis. (Reprinted with permission from McClatchey KD. *Clinical Laboratory Medicine*, 2nd ed, Philadelphia, PA: Lippincott Williams & Wilkins, 2002.)

Patient results can be monitored with continuous *X*B analysis (weighted moving averages), which uses the patient's own data to monitor population values and instrument performance. Batches of 20 samples are used to track MCV, MCH, and MCHC values. This method can be used to detect changes in sample handling, reagents, or instrument performance.

Delta checks are another quality control method for comparing a patient's own leukocyte, hemoglobin, MCV, and platelet values with previous results. If the difference between the two is greater than laboratory-set limits, the current result is immediately flagged for review.

General Histogram Characteristics

Histograms are graphic representations of cell frequencies versus sizes. In a homogeneous cell population, the curve assumes a symmetrical bell-shaped or **Gaussian distribution.** A wide or more flattened curve is seen when the standard deviation (SD) from the mean is increased. Histograms not only provide information about erythrocyte, leukocyte, and platelet frequency and their distribution about the mean, but also depict the presence of subpopulations.

Histograms provide a means of comparing the sizes of a patient's cells with those of normal population's. Shifts in one direction or the other can be of diagnostic importance. The position of the curve on the *x*-axis reflects the cell size. In the Coulter system, the size (volume in femtoliters) is represented on the *x*-axis.

ANALYSIS OF INSTRUMENTAL DATA OUTPUT

The Erythrocyte Histogram

The erythrocyte histogram reflects the native size of erythrocytes or any other particles in the erythrocyte size range. The erythrocyte histogram in the Coulter system displays cells as small as 24 fL, but only those greater than 36 fL are counted as erythrocytes. The extension of the lower end of the scale from 36 to 24 fL allows for the detection of erythrocyte fragments, leukocyte fragments, and large platelets.

Although normal quantities of leukocytes are present in the erythrocyte bath and are included in the erythrocyte count, they are *not* significant in the histogram. The system can be calibrated to compensate for 7.5×10^9/L leukocytes. If the leukocyte count is significantly elevated, the histogram will be affected.

If the cells are larger than normal, the histogram curve will be more to the right, as in the megaloblastic anemias. If the cells are smaller than normal, the curve will be more to the left (Fig. 27.9), as in untreated iron deficiency anemia. After appropriate treatment of the underlying cause of an anemia, the curve should move toward the normal range.

If the normal unimodal distribution is altered, the early stages of an underlying disorder may be revealed. A histogram distribution that is bimodal can be seen in various situations, including cold agglutinin disease, after the trans-

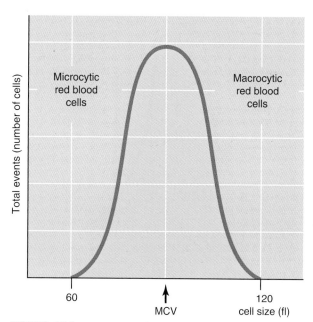

FIGURE 27.9 Histogram illustrating normal RBC size distribution with smaller than normal RBCs to the left; larger than normal RBCs to the right.

fusion of normal erythrocytes into a person with abnormally sized erythrocytes, in the presence of erythrocyte fragments, or with agglutination.

Quantitative Descriptors of Erythrocytes

An expression of erythrocyte size is the RDW in the Coulter series. This term refers to variation in erythrocyte size. Correlations between the RDW and the MCV exist for various types of anemias. A classification of erythrocyte populations has been proposed based on the similarities or dissimilarities in the erythrocyte population and in the RDW and MCV.

Red Cell Distribution Width

A new parameter, the RDW, expresses the coefficient of variation of the erythrocyte volume distribution. It is calculated directly from the histogram. A portion of the curve (Fig. 27.10) at the extreme ends is excluded from the computation to exclude clumps of platelets, large platelets, or electrical interference on the left side of the curve. The portion of the right side of the curve that is excluded represents grouped or clumped erythrocytes.

The RDW is calculated by dividing the SD by the mean of the red cell size distribution.

$$RDW = \frac{SD}{Mean\,size} \times 100$$

The RDW is expressed numerically as the coefficient of variation percentage. The normal range is 11.5% to 14.5%. Abnormalities can be observed on the high side

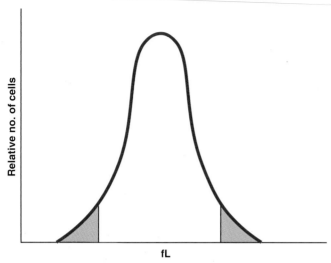

FIGURE 27.10 Red cell distribution width (RDW) calculation. The RDW is an expression of the coefficient of variation of the red cell volume distribution. Both the MCV and RDW are calculated from the erythrocyte (RBC) histogram. The MCV is calculated from the entire area under the curve, but the RDW is calculated *only* on the basis of the trimmed histogram (*middle area*). (Adapted with permission from Pierre R. *Seminars and Case Studies: The Automated Differential,* Hialeah, FL: Coulter Electronics, 1985:39.)

but no abnormalities have been noted on the low side. The RDW is increased above the normal limits in iron deficiency, vitamin B_{12} deficiency, and folic acid deficiency. In the hemoglobinopathies, the RDW is increased in proportion to the degree of anemia that accompanies the hemoglobin disorder.

Relationship of RDW and MCV

Quantitative descriptors of erythrocyte size include both the RDW and the conventional erythrocyte index, the MCV. The RDW is independent of high, low, or normal MCV and is an earlier sign of nutritional deficiency than the MCV. The relationship of the RDW and MCV can characterize various erythrocytic abnormalities (Table 27.5).

The MCV of a specimen is calculated using the entire area under the erythrocyte curve. Because the RDW is a mathematical ratio, patients with an increased MCV may have a wide or heterogeneous distribution curve and a normal RDW. Patients with a low MCV may have a distribution curve with a normal (homogeneous) width, which produces a high RDW. A particularly valuable distinction based on the RDW is one between iron deficiency anemia (high RDW and either low or normal MCV) and anemia of chronic disease (normal RDW and normal or low MCV).

Classification of Erythrocytes Based on MCV and RDW

As long as the red cell volume distribution histogram is unimodal, erythrocyte size is described efficiently by the mean (MCV) and coefficient of variation (RDW). An increased RDW may occur with a low MCV even when the width of the curve is normal.

Erythrocytes with a normal RDW are homogeneous in character and exhibit very little anisocytosis on a peripheral blood smear. Erythrocytes with an increased RDW are referred to as heterogeneous and exhibit a high degree of anisocytosis on a peripheral blood smear. A classification of erythrocytes that includes the homogeneity or heterogeneity of the erythrocytes in addition to the MCV and RDW values has been proposed (Table 27.6).

The Leukocyte Histogram

Size-referenced leukocyte histograms display the classification of leukocytes according to size following lysis. It does *not* display the native cell size. The lytic reagent causes a cytochemical reaction. As a result of the reaction, the cytoplasm collapses around the nucleus, producing differential shrinkage. Therefore, the histogram of leukocyte subpopulations reflects the sorting of these cells by their relative size, which is primarily related to their nuclear size.

The Coulter models system classifies approximately 20,000 particles when the leukocyte count is at the 10.0×10^3 cells/μL level. As the leukocytes pass through the aperture in the

TABLE 27.5	**Examples of the Relationship of Mean Corpuscular Volume and Red Cell Distribution Width**		
		MCV	
RDW	**High**	**Normal**	**Low**
High	Megaloblastic anemias	Normocytic anemias	Iron deficiency anemia
Normal	Aplastic anemia in adults	Reticulocytosis[a]	Heterozygous thalassemias Anemias of chronic inflammation or disorders

MCV, mean corpuscular volume; RDW, red cell distribution width.
[a]The MCV and RDW are normal because the reticulocytes are only slightly larger than the cells into which they will mature in compensated hemolytic anemia.

TABLE 27.6	Classification of Anemias Based on Red Cell Distribution Width and Mean Corpuscular Volume		
	MCV		
RDW	**High**	**Normal**	**Low**
High	Macrocytic	Normocytic	Microcytic
Normal	Macrocytic	Normocytic	Microcytic

RDW, red cell distribution width; MCV, mean corpuscular volume.

electrical impedance system, they displace their volume in a conductive fluid, which causes a change in electrical resistance as each cell passes through the aperture. This change is proportional to the cell volume. The histogram generated by the Coulter principle provides size information.

Although the Coulter leukocyte histogram displays all cells as small as 30 fL, only those greater than 35 fL are counted as leukocytes. The histogram differentiates lymphocytes, mononuclear cells, and granulocytes (Fig. 27.11). Mononuclear cells include blasts or other immature cells, such as promyelocytes and myelocytes, as well as monocytes; however, in a normal specimen, monocytes represent the mononuclear cells.

On the x-axis of the histogram, four regions are noted at approximately 35, 90, 160, and 450 fL. There are certain expected characteristics of the curves at these locations. A valley or depression should be seen between the lymphocytes and mononuclear cells and between the mononuclear cells and granulocytes.

The computer program uses these locations to determine the three populations; however, each differential analysis is individualized to determine the position of the populations in each specimen. Leukocytes normally occur at 35 fL or above; the region below 35 fL should be clear. Particles such as clumped or giant platelets, NRBCs, and nonlysed erythrocytes might produce interference at or below 35 fL.

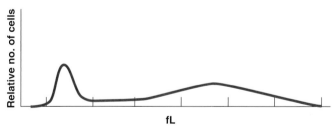

FIGURE 27.11 Electrical impedance leukocyte histogram. Three different cell types can be identified using the impedance principle. Because the lytic agent acts on the cellular membrane and cytoplasm and produces cellular shrinkage, these populations can be distinguished from one another. The cellular population on the extreme left represents lymphocytes, the middle population represents mononuclear cells, and the population of cells on the extreme right side represents granulocytes. (Adapted with permission from Pierre R. *Seminars and Case Studies: The Automated Differential,* Hialeah, FL: Coulter Electronics, 1985:39.)

The instrument detects abnormal patterns. The types of alert signals include

1. Cells below 35 fL.
2. Cells between the lymphocyte and mononuclear cell region. Lymphocytes that are larger than normal, such as variant lymphocytes, certain blast forms, plasma cells, or, in some cases, eosinophilia and basophilia, can trigger an alert.
3. Cells between the mononuclear and granulocyte populations; an increase in IGs or other abnormal cell populations, such as certain types of blasts and eosinophils.
4. Cells to the far right region of the curve, usually a high absolute granulocyte count.
5. An abnormality detected at exactly the 35-fL threshold.
6. A significant increase in the mononuclear population.
7. A multiple alert, when more than one of these regions is affected.

In A^{c}V differential technology, there is a correlation of signals to DiffPlot populations (Figs. 27.12 and 27.13). Lymphocytes are typically small with a regular shape. They are smaller in volume and lower in absorbance than the other cells and are positioned in the lower part of the DiffPlot. Neutrophils will absorb light depending on the presence of cytoplasmic granules and segmented nuclei.

Platelet Histograms

Platelet counting and sizing in both the electrical impedance and optical systems reflect the native cell size. In the electrical impedance method, counting and sizing take place in

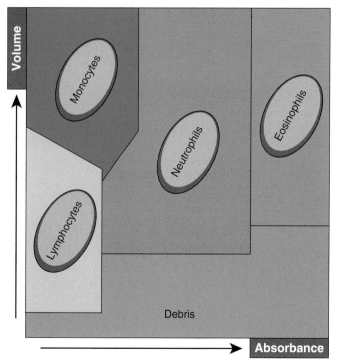

FIGURE 27.12 Correlations of signals to DiffPlot populations in Coulter AcT. (Reproduced with kind permission of Beckman-Coulter, Inc.)

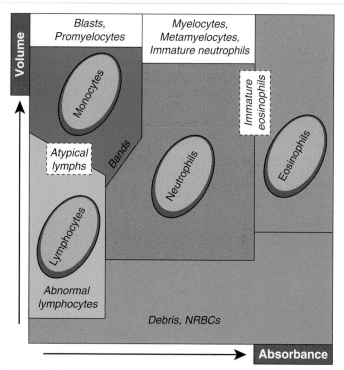

FIGURE 27.13 DiffPlot normal and abnormal cell populations with Coulter AcT. (Reproduced with kind permission of Beckman-Coulter, Inc.)

the RBC aperture. In the optical system, forward light scatter pattern discrimination between erythrocytes and platelets in the flow cell determines the platelet count and frequency distribution.

In the electrical impedance system, the analyzer's computer classifies particles that are greater than 2 fL or less than 20 fL as platelets. In optical systems, the cell pulse area is determined. The raw data from either the RBC aperture or forward light scatter are sorted. These raw data histograms are then smoothed and tested against mathematical criteria that eliminate nonplatelet particles and are finally fitted to a log-normal distribution curve in the impedance method. This distribution curve has a range of 0 to 70 fL. The final platelet count is derived from the integrated area under this best-fit log-normal curve (Fig. 27.14).

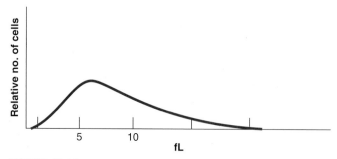

FIGURE 27.14 Platelet histogram. Platelet counting and sizing in both electrical impedance and optical systems reflect the native cell size. (Adapted with permission from Pierre R. *Seminars and Case Studies: The Automated Differential*, Hialeah, FL: Coulter Electronics, 1985.)

The expected cell coincidence error (more than one cell passing through the aperture at the same time) is corrected based on mathematical probability. In the Coulter models, a minimum of 400 particles per aperture must be detected and evaluated. If an insufficient number of particles are present in the 2- to 20-fL range, a no-fit condition is reported. The data for the size distribution histogram are taken from three sensing channels in this system. This method additionally creates three curves and compares the counts. All three must agree statistically. If any inconsistency exists, an alert results. An alert is also generated if the results are not within the range of 3 to 15 fL.

Particles within the platelet size range can interfere with the platelet count and histogram. Small particles, such as bubbles or dust, can overlap at the low end of the histogram. Microcytic erythrocytes can interfere at the upper end. However, the curve-fitting process attempts to eliminate interference at the upper and lower ends to obtain a correct platelet count. If the histogram does not return to the baseline at both the right and the left of the peak, either there is severe thrombocytopenia or nonplatelets are being counted. Either erythrocyte or leukocyte fragments may be responsible. In such cases, the platelet count and derived parameters of MPV and PDW are not reliable.

Derived Platelet Parameters

Platelet size has been measured for more than a decade by either micrometry or flow cytometry methods. However, sizing information from data obtained from whole blood specimens and the application of computer technology now make it possible for additional parameters to be generated instrumentally. The Coulter models systems yield the additional parameters of MPV and PDW. These parameters are derived from the platelet histogram and allow for a size comparison between a patient's specimen and the normal population's. Size comparisons are useful as an indicator of certain disorders.

Mean Platelet Volume Calculation

The MPV is a measure of the average volume of platelets in a sample. The MPV is analogous to the erythrocytic MCV. It is derived from the same data as the platelet count. In ethylenediaminetetraacetic acid (EDTA)–anti-coagulated blood, platelets undergo a change in shape. This alteration (swelling) causes the MPV to increase approximately 20% during the first hour. After this time, the size is stable for at least 12 hours; however, MPV values should be based on specimens that are between 1 and 4 hours old.

In healthy patients, there is an inverse relationship between platelet count and size (Fig. 27.15). The volume increases as the platelet count decreases. Because of this inverse relationship, the MPV and the platelet count must be considered together. This relationship between the platelet count and MPV is illustrated as a graph, the **MPV nomogram**, and is used to determine whether a patient's MPV is normal. The distribution of platelet size is generally a right-skewed, single peak.

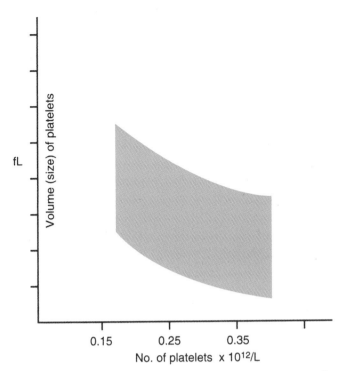

FIGURE 27.15 Mean platelet volume (MPV) nomogram. An inverse relationship between platelet size and platelet count exists and is expressed as the MPV nomogram. (Adapted with permission from Pierre R. *Seminars and Case Studies: The Automated Differential,* Hialeah, FL: Coulter Electronics, 1985.)

No single normal range exists. Patients with a lower platelet count normally have a higher MPV, and patients with a higher platelet count have a lower MPV. Analysis of a nomogram demonstrates that an MPV between 9.0 and 9.8 fL is in the normal range, if the platelet count is normal. MPVs from 7.8 to 8.9 fL or from 9.9 to 12.0 fL may be in the normal range, depending on the platelet count.

Disorders of Mean Platelet Volume

Various disorders are associated with altered MPV values (Table 27.7). The MPV is often decreased in aplastic anemia, in megaloblastic anemia, or as the result of chemotherapy. Hypersplenism is associated with an MPV that is inappropriately low for the platelet count. In septic thrombocytopenia, the nomogram varies as thrombocytopenia develops, with the MPV rising as the platelet count falls. Platelet destruction associated with disseminated intravascular coagulation causes an increase in the MPV proportional to the severity of thrombocytopenia. The MPV is often increased in patients with myeloproliferative disorders or heterozygous thalassemia.

Platelet Distribution Width

The PDW is a measure of the uniformity of platelet size in a blood specimen. This parameter serves as a validity check and monitors false results. A normal PDW is less than 20%.

The PDW can be increased in aplastic and megaloblastic anemias, in chronic myelogenous leukemia, and as the result

TABLE 27.7	Mean Platelet Volume in Selected Disorders
Decreased MPV	**Increased MPV**
Aplastic anemia	Idiopathic thrombocytopenic purpura
Megaloblastic anemia	After splenectomy
Wiskott-Aldrich syndrome	Sickle cell anemia
After chemotherapy	

MPV, mean platelet volume.

of antileukemic chemotherapy. The causes of increased PDW are not known but are probably related to dysfunctional megakaryocytic development. Falsely elevated results can be caused by extraneous particles, such as erythrocyte fragments, which broaden the platelet volume distribution beyond that of actual platelet's.

LASER TECHNOLOGY

Some systems use the principle of flow cytometry based on differential light scattering and cytochemistry. Three distinct steps are involved in its function:

1. Cytochemical reactions prepare the blood cells for analysis.
2. A cytometer measures specific cell properties.
3. Algorithms convert these measurements into familiar results for cell classification, cell count, cell size, and hemoglobinization.

The instrument's sampling mechanism divides blood samples into aliquots that are treated in four separate reaction chambers:

1. Hemoglobin
2. Red cell/platelet
3. Peroxidase
4. Basophil/lobularity or nuclear channel

Red Blood Cells/Platelets

The RBC/platelet channel uses a laser-based optical assembly that is shared with the basophil/lobularity channel. A buffered reagent isovolumetrically spheres and fixes RBCs and platelets. The light scattered at low and high angles simultaneously measures RBC volume (size) and optical density (hemoglobin concentration) of each cell. The signal pairs are transformed by a computer into a cytogram and two histograms (Fig. 27.16).

Additional parameters (see Chapter 5 for a full discussion of RBC parameters) obtained from the histograms are MCV and the RDW (reference range, 10.2% to 11.8%). Based

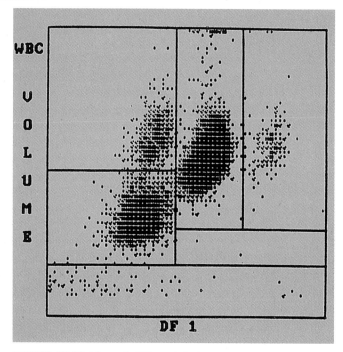

FIGURE 27.16 Normal differential. (Reprinted with permission from McClatchey KD. *Clinical Laboratory Medicine*, 2nd ed, Philadelphia, PA: Lippincott Williams & Wilkins, 2002.)

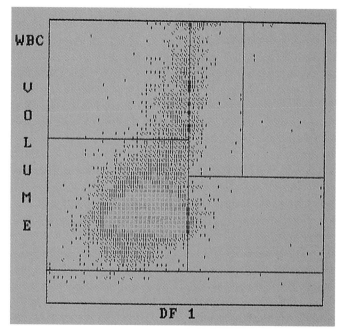

FIGURE 27.17 Histogram—chronic lymphocytic leukemia. (Reprinted with permission from McClatchey KD. *Clinical Laboratory Medicine*, 2nd ed, Philadelphia, PA: Lippincott Williams & Wilkins, 2002.)

on the hemoglobin concentration of each cell, the cellular hemoglobin concentration mean (CHCM) is determined. The hemoglobin distribution width (HDW) is determined. The HDW is the SD of the hemoglobin concentration histogram. Hematocrit, MCH, and MCHC are calculated from the measured hemoglobin, RBC count, and MCV. The red cell cytogram enables simultaneous observation of cell volume and hemoglobin concentration.

The platelet histogram (Fig. 27.17) is derived from measurements made with the high-angle detector. The MPV is the mode of the measured platelet volumes.

Peroxidase

In this tungsten light–based optics channel, RBCs are lysed and WBCs are fixed and then stained. A dark precipitate forms in the primary granules of leukocytes containing peroxidase when a chromogen is added with hydrogen peroxide as the substrate. Eosinophils and neutrophils are strongly positive and monocytes are weakly positive. Peroxidase is not present in basophils, lymphocytes, blasts, or LUCs.

Thousands of cells are characterized by a combination of their size (scatter) and peroxidase activity (absorbance) (Fig. 27.18). Scatter is plotted on the *y*-axis and absorption on the *x*-axis. Each cell is represented by a dot. The position of the dot is dependent on the combination of the light scattered and absorbed by each cell.

The clusters of dots that are generated are defined and analyzed, the number of cells in each is counted, and the cells are classified based on information stored in the computer. This information is used to generate the total WBC count

and differential count, except for basophils. The relative percentages and absolute values of leukocytes are included. The parameter **mean peroxidase index** (MPXI), the index of the mean peroxidase activity of neutrophils as measured by their stain intensity, is generated. Increased myeloperoxidase

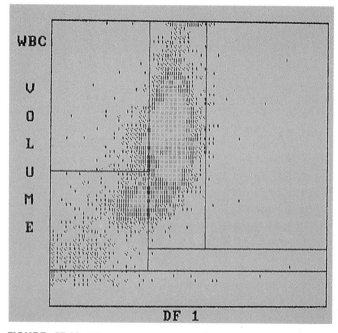

FIGURE 27.18 Histogram—acute myelogenous leukemia (Reprinted with permission from McClatchey KD. *Clinical Laboratory Medicine*, 2nd ed, Philadelphia, PA: Lippincott Williams & Wilkins, 2002.)

activity may be associated with megaloblastic anemia, hyperproliferative granulopoiesis, or reactive states. Increased numbers of LUCs may indicate the presence of blasts or abnormal lymphocytes. The reference ranges of 0% to 3.7% for LUCs and 0% to 5.4% for HPX have been established.

Basophil/Lobularity (Nuclear) Channel

The nuclear channel is used to measure the conformation of the nucleus of WBCs. The principle of the reaction in this channel is that when white blood cells are exposed to a surfactant at a low pH, the membranes and cytoplasm of specific leukocytes, neutrophils, eosinophils, lymphocytes, and monocytes disintegrate and only the bare nuclei remain.

The nuclear channel cytometer distinguishes leukocytes by differences in nuclear shape and counts basophils. This laser-based cytometer measures light scattering at two different angles, low (0° to 5°) and high (5° to 15°). Low-angle scatter measures size, and the low-angle scatter of intact basophils is much greater than the bare nuclei of other leukocytes. A fixed horizontal threshold separates basophils from the nuclei of other leukocytes (Fig. 27.18). High-angle scatter is responsive to the lobularity of nuclei. The more lobulated the nuclei, the larger the high-angle signal.

On the cytogram, polymorphonuclear neutrophil (PMN) appear on the right and mononuclear nuclei (MN) appear on the left with a valley between them. A vertical threshold separates the two clusters. The ratio of PMN:MN, the lobularity index (LI), is an index of the degree of PMN nuclear segmentation; a low value suggests a left shift. Blast cells appear to the left of the normal mononuclear cells on the x-axis and are counted for flagging purposes. (A system of flags for abnormal morphology alerts the instrument operator that additional work, such as microscopic examination of the blood, may be required.) Nucleated RBCs, if present, appear within the PMN cluster.

Lymphocyte Subtyping

An immunoperoxidase reaction is used for lymphocyte subtyping (Fig. 27.19). A specific monoclonal antibody is first reacted with whole blood. A second biotinylated antibody, which binds only to the monoclonal antibody, is added, followed by an avidin-peroxidase reagent. Peroxidase is used as a stain, using a similar method to that of the peroxidase channel. Lymphocytes, which have been labeled by the immunoperoxidase reaction, appear between the unlabeled lymphocyte population and the monocytes. Cells with endogenous peroxidase such as neutrophils stain intensely and appear far to the right.

APPLICATIONS OF FLOW CYTOMETRY

The introduction of the flow cytometer into the clinical laboratory is a major technological advance. Flow cytometry is a field that has evolved rapidly during the past three decades. Instruments based on the flow cytometry principle were initially designed to count and size cells. Later modifications were designed to perform differential leukocyte counts by identifying specific cytochemical reactions in the cells. The current types of flow cytometry instruments can analyze

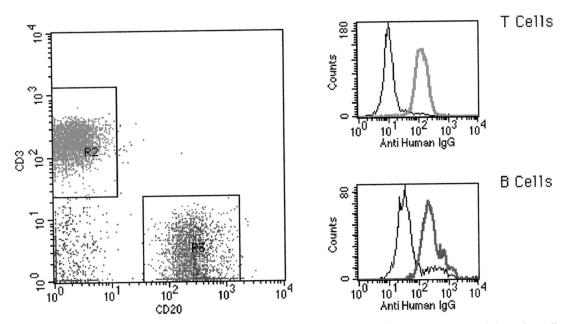

FIGURE 27.19 Three-color flow cytometric crossmatch. **Left:** Dot-plot displaying CD-20 PE staining of B cells (x-axis) versus CD3-PerCP staining of T cells (y-axis). **Right:** single parameter histogram of T and B cells. Staining fluorescence with the normal human serum control is shown in *black*; staining fluorescence observed with a positive serum sample is shown in *green* and *red* color for T and B cells, respectively.

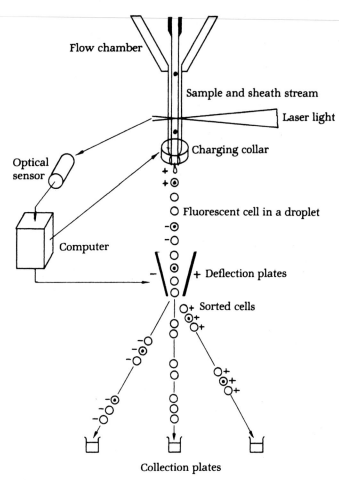

FIGURE 27.20 Laser and cell-sorting schematic. In a flow cytometry system, stained cells flow through a sample tube. As the cells and a stream of saline solution leave the flow chamber, they move like a string of beads in the center of the sheath. The fluorescence of the cells is detected by a sensor. Cells can be appropriately charged as they move through a charging collar or deflection plates. Sorting of the cells is accomplished by deflecting charged cells depending on the charge (either positive or negative).

cells for many constituents and sort cells into subpopulations (Fig. 27.20).

General Properties of Flow Cytometry

Most flow-cell instruments can simultaneously analyze multiple parameters at the rate of 5,000 to 10,000 cells/seconds. The cellular analysis yields quantitative data about the chemical and physical properties of individual cells, and after analysis, cells can be physically separated into subpopulations for further study at the rate of 5,000 cells/seconds. The major advances in this technology are owing to several factors:

1. The ability to produce monoclonal antibodies resulted in the subsequent development of specific surface markers for various subpopulations of cells.
2. The development of new fluorescent probes for DNA, RNA, and other cellular components increased the variety of possible applications at the molecular and cellular level.

3. The expansion of computer applications has improved the instrumentation technology, making it easier to operate and more practical for use in clinical as well as research laboratories.

Hematological Applications

Flow cytometry can be applied practically to several techniques in the clinical hematology laboratory. These applications include automated leukocyte differentiation and reticulocyte enumeration.

Automated Differentials

Automated differentials can be based on a variety of principles. These include determination of cell volume by electrical impedance or forward light scatter, cytochemistry or peroxidase staining, and VCS technology. Evaluation of internal cellular organelles and nuclear characteristics can be by

■ 90° laser scatter
■ Polarizing laser light
■ RF

Separate measurements can be made of individual measurements of volume, conductivity, and light scatter. An additional method is to integrate the three in VCS technology into a three-dimensional (3D) leukocyte analysis. The volume aspect is by volumetric sizing by impedance and RF opacity for internal composition. In addition, helium-neon laser light scatter is applied so that laser light can produce scattering characteristics of each cell at different angles for granularity and nuclear structure.

In addition, different reagents can be used to lyse certain cells. Different types of technologies are used by instrument manufacturers to produce an automated leukocyte differential. These include

Beckman-Coulter: VCS
Abbott: MAPPS—0°, 90°, 10°, 90° depolarized
Roche (Sysmex): RF, DC
Siemens Healthcare Diagnostics (formerly Bayer and Technicon): peroxidase staining; optical scatter and absorption; basophils: differential lysis laser scatter high and low

Clinical Applications of Flow Cytometry

Because single-cell suspensions of peripheral blood and bone marrow are easy to obtain, most clinical applications of flow cytometry are in the specialties of hematology and immunology. A number of instruments are currently manufactured for various uses (Table 27.8).

Counting Reticulocytes and Platelets

Reticulocytes

Manual counting of reticulocytes has been conducted since the 1940s. It is tedious and time-consuming and analyzes fewer erythrocytes than do flow cytometry systems. Enumeration of reticulocytes by flow cytometry is more

TABLE 27.8	Hematology Analyzers With a Reticulocyte Enumeration Feature
Manufacturer	**Instrument**
Abbott Diagnostics	CELL-DYN 3700 CELL-DYN Ruby CELL-DYN Sapphire
Beckman Coulter Inc. Horiba	HmX, LH 500, LH 700/750, LH 785, LH 1500, LH 7801
ABX Diagnostics	Pentra DX 120
Siemens Diagnostics Healthcare	Advia 120, Advia 2120, Advia 2120i
Sysmex	XE 2100, XE 5000, XE-alpha N, XT-2000i

accurate, precise, and cost-effective than manual counting. Flow cytometry also provides additional reticulocyte parameters of the IRF, or reticulocyte maturity index (RMI), and the measurement of reticulocyte maturity.

Reticulocytes can be counted by using a stain for residual RNA in erythrocytes (e.g., new methylene blue, thiazole orange, and oxazine 750); proprietary fluorescent dye CD4K530 is used by one manufacturer. The Coulter system uses neomethylene blue and sulfuric acid as reagents.

In addition, fully automated flow cytometers specifically designed for reticulocyte enumeration by optical light scatter have been incorporated into existing hematology analyzers (see Table 27.8).

Platelets

Measurement of platelets provides an estimate of young, reticulated platelets by counting platelets that stain with an RNA dye (e.g., thiazole orange or coriphosphine-O). Platelets in whole blood are also labeled with PE-conjugated CD41 antibody to distinguish them from other small particles. CD-41–positive platelets are evaluated for RNA content. The finding of elevated reticulated platelets indicates "stress" platelets from increased bone marrow production and is consistent with a diagnosis of immune thrombocytopenic purpura.

Other platelet assays include platelet surface receptor quantitation and distribution for the diagnosis of congenital platelet function disorders, platelet-associated immunoglobulin G (IgG) quantitation for the diagnosis of immune thrombocytopenias, and platelet cross-matching for transfusion. Other assays include fibrinogen receptor occupancy studies for monitoring the clinical efficacy of platelet-directed anticoagulation in thrombosis. Detection of activated platelet surface markers, cytoplasmic calcium ion measurements, and platelet microparticles for the assessment of hypercoagulable states can be performed.

Other Cellular Applications

Flow cytometry applications are extended to various areas of specialized study.

Immunophenotyping

Monoclonal antibodies, identified by a cluster designation (CD), are used in most flow cytometry immunophenotyping (Fig. 27.21; Table 27.9). Cell surface molecules recognized by monoclonal antibodies are called antigens because antibodies can be produced against them or markers because they identify and discriminate between ("mark") different cell populations. Markers can be grouped into several categories. Some are specific for cells of a particular lineage (e.g., CD4+ lymphocytes) or maturational pathway (e.g., CD34+ progenitor stem cells), and the expression of others varies according to the state of activation or differentiation of the same cells.

Measuring T Cells for Acquired Immunodeficiency Syndrome Analysis

The quantitation of T and B cells using monoclonal surface markers can be performed using flow cytometry. With the flow cytometer, 10,000 cells can be assayed into subsets in 1 minute with multiparameter analysis. Through the use of monoclonal antibodies, T- and B-cell populations can be divided into subpopulations with specific functions. For example, T cells are divided into two functional subpopulations, T-helper (TH) and T-suppressor (TS) cells. Normal individuals have a TH/TS ratio of 2 to 3:1. This ratio is inverted in certain disorders and diseases. These conditions include the acute phase of cytomegalovirus mononucleosis, subsequent to bone marrow transplantation, and acquired immunodeficiency syndrome (AIDS).

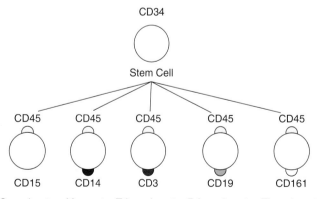

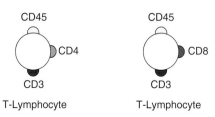

FIGURE 27.21 CD membrane markers.

TABLE 27.9	Examples of Commonly Used Monoclonal Antibodies in Flow Cytometry

CD Designation	Target Cell
CD3	T lymphocytes
CD4	T lymphocytes (helper cells), monocytes (dimly expressed)
CD8	T lymphocytes (cytotoxic), macrophages
CD19	B lymphocytes
CD34	Progenitor (hematopoietic stem cells)

The CD4 (helper subset) T-lymphocyte cell count is one of the standard measures for diagnosing AIDS and the management of disease progress in patients with human immunodeficiency virus (HIV) disease. The analysis of the T cell and B cell ratio is clinically useful in evaluating the immune system status of patients who may be at an increased risk of opportunistic infections. In addition, the absolute number of CD4+ lymphocytes is reflective of the degree of immune deficiency in HIV-infected individuals and may be used as a guide for timing the institution of antiretroviral therapy as well as monitoring the level of immune reconstitution following initiation of therapy.

In these cases, two cell-surface antigens—CD3, which is present on mature T lymphocytes, and CD4, which is only present on the helper subset of T lymphocytes—are used. The percentage of CD4 lymphocytes is determined by using a fluorochrome-conjugated CD3 antibody (e.g., FITC-CD3) together with a CD4 antibody conjugated to a second fluorochrome (e.g., PE-CD4). The absolute CD4 count can be determined by a single-platform method, which uses a sample spiked with a predetermined number of beads per unit volume to index the CD4 count comparatively. A second approach is a dual-platform method. The absolute count of CD4-bearing lymphocytes is calculated by multiplying the percentage of CD4-bearing lymphocytes by the absolute lymphocyte count (calculated independently from the total leukocyte count and percent of lymphocytes in a peripheral blood smear differential).

The absolute number of CD4 lymphocytes is reflective of the degree of immune deficiency in HIV-infected patients and may be used as a guide for timing the administration of antiretroviral therapy as well as monitoring the level of immune reconstitution following initiation of therapy.

Basic Lymphocyte Screening Panel

A basic immune screening panel typically consists of detection and quantitation of CD3, CD4, CD8, CD19, and CD16/56. Anti-CD45/CD14 is included to assist in distinguishing lymphocytes from monocytes. This panel reveals the frequency of T cells (CD3+), B cells (CD19+), and natural killer cells (CD3−, CD16+, CD56+). It also provides the frequency of TH-inducer cells (CD3+, CD4+) and T-suppressor/cytotoxic cells (CD3+, CD8+).

Typical ranges for lymphocyte subset percentages in adult donors are CD3, 56% to 86%; CD4, 33% to 58%; CD8, 13% to 39%; CD16+ CD56, 5% to 26%; and CD19, 5% to 22%.

It does not provide information on cell activation or signaling pathway receptors, frequency of T subsets (e.g., Th_1 or Th_2), stem or blast cells, B lymphocytes (e.g., immunoblasts or plasma cells), or nonlymphoid elements.

Hematological Malignancy

Flow cytometry has become an important tool in the diagnosis and classification of hematologic neoplasia by immunophenotyping. Numerous, well-characterized antibodies and their various combinations used in flow cytometry allow for rapid, reliable identification and characterization of these neoplasms.

Intracellular staining is most often used to aid in the diagnosis of acute leukemias and lymphomas as an adjunct to surface antigen detection. For these assays, multiple cell-surface and intracellular antigens may be studied simultaneously. Three or four antibodies are used simultaneously; each one is conjugated to a unique fluorochrome to characterize the cells in each tube. This technique is referred to as three-color or four-color immunophenotyping. Examples of commonly used antibodies in hematopathology (Table 27.10) are CD3, CD13, CD22, myeloperoxidase (MPO), terminal deoxynucleotidyl transferase (TdT), and cytoplasmic immunoglobulins (kappa and lambda light chains, M heavy chain).

Research applications of immunocytochemistry (IC) immunophenotyping include IC cytokine expression to examine functional subtypes of lymphocytes in acquired and primary immunodeficiencies and to measure engraftment success after a transplant procedure. Detection of cancer-related markers in tumors as prognostic indicators (e.g., estrogen and progesterone receptors, oncoproteins, p53) is an additional application.

DNA Ploidy and Cell Cycling

One of the earliest clinical applications of flow cytometry was the detection of aneuploidy and cell cycling status of solid tumors, particularly selected breast tumors. Since 1996, the use of DNA analysis has significantly decreased. It is now most often performed in patients with node-negative breast cancer and other tumors in which the clinical correlation prognostic significance is strongest. Recent technological innovations may lead to a revival of interest in clinical DNA analysis.

Because approximately a 2-week lag exists between bone marrow activity and its resultant expression in the peripheral blood, it is important to assess the current status of the bone marrow cells under certain conditions (i.e., cell cycle

TABLE 27.10	Relationship Among Representative Membrane Antigens, Hematopoietic Cells, and Malignancies	
IC Antigen	Cellular Distribution	Hematologic Malignancy
CD3	T lymphocytes	T-acute lymphoblastic leukemia
CD 13	Granulocytes	Acute myelogenous leukemia
CD22	B lymphocytes	B-acute lymphoblastic leukemia
TdT	Usually immature lymphocytes	Acute lymphoblastic leukemia

kinetics). Flow cytometry allows for analysis of the bone marrow cell cycle parameters with no time lag.

Flow cytometry techniques with bone marrow cells are applicable to DNA cell cycle analysis, which quantitates the number of cells in various phases of the cell cycle (Fig. 27.22). The cell cycle stage is important in drug therapy. Antineoplastic drugs exhibit specificity for different phases of the cell cycle. Inhibitors of microtubule function affect cells in M phase; glucocorticoids inhibit cells in G1; antimetabolites and folate pathway inhibitors inhibit cells in S phase; antitumor antibiotics inhibit cells in G2; topoisomerase inhibitors inhibit cells in S phase and G2. Alkylating agents and platinum complexes affect cell function in all phases and are therefore cell cycle nonspecific. Different cell cycle specificities allow various drug classes to be used in combination to target different populations of cells. Specific drugs can be administered to target actively replicating neoplastic cells, and nonspecific agents can be used to target nonreplicating neoplastic cells.

Solid Organ Transplantation

Flow cytometric cross-matching uses fluorochrome-conjugated antihuman IgG to detect the binding of alloantibodies to donor lymphocytes in allogeneic organ transplantation. CD3 and CD19 coupled with anti-IgG in a three-color assay can distinguish T-lymphocyte and B-lymphocyte mismatches. Patient serum can be screened against known HLA antigens for the detection of corresponding antibodies.

Stem Cell Transplantation

Flow cytometry is widely used to enumerate the CD34-positive implanted stem cells. In some cases, CD45 and nucleic acid stains are also detected. In bone marrow transplantation, flow cytometry applications can include pretransplantation determinations of the efficacy of ex vivo T cell graft depletion, posttransplantation evaluation of immune recovery, graft rejection, graft versus host disease, and the graft versus leukemia effect.

Monitoring Monoclonal Antibody Therapy

In conjunction with IC and molecular techniques, flow cytometry has been essential for measuring the expression of cell surface and intracellular markers of multiple drug resistance (MDR) in cancer patients, assessing the intracellular accumulation and efflux of chemotherapeutic

drugs and studying the other mechanisms leading to MDR. Ligand, antigen, or molecule-targeted biologic therapy using monoclonal antigens (e.g., myelotarg [CD33] and rituximab [CD20] for some leukemias) is the most rapidly growing area of pharmacology. In some cases, these agents work by directly disrupting cell proliferation and antiapoptosis by clocking the cell membrane receptors and circulating ligands associated with signal transduction. Others serve as the targeting system for other cytotoxic products. The first of this new class of pharmaceutical agents was anti-CD3.

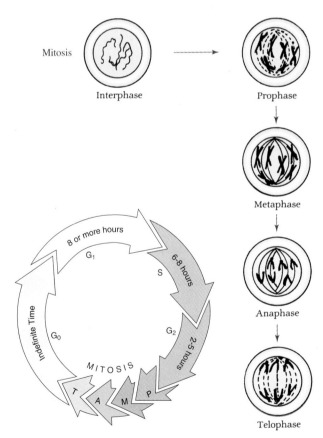

FIGURE 27.22 Cell cycle. G0, nondividing cell; G1, cell growth; S, DNA replication; G2, protein synthesis; M, mitosis, which lasts for 1 to 3 hours and is followed by cytokinesis or cell division. (telophase [T], anaphase [A], mitosis [M], prophase [P]). (Adapted with permission from Porth CM. Pathophysiology Concepts of Altered Health States, 7th ed. Philadelphia, PA: Lippincott Williams & Wilkins, 2005.)

More recently, monoclonal antibodies directed against CD20, CD25, CD33, CD45, and CD52 have been developed. Before treatment, flow-cell analysis is critical for confirming that the antigen is expressed by the offending cells. During and after treatment, flow cytometry is used to verify binding of the antibody and to monitor the efficacy of tumor cell eradication.

Paroxysmal Nocturnal Hemoglobinemia Testing

The detection of paroxysmal nocturnal hemoglobinemia (PNH) by the traditional methods of Ham's (acid hemolysis) and the sucrose lysis test has been replaced in many clinical laboratories by flow cytometry analysis. The glycosyl phosphatidyl inositol (GPI)-linked proteins, CD55 and CD59, are examined to determine if a deficiency or absence of these cell surface markers exists. If a deficiency or absence of CD55 and CD59 is established, the condition is diagnostic of PNH.

Fetal Hemoglobin

Detection of fetal hemoglobin and F cells by flow cytometry is becoming common. The assay uses monoclonal antibodies to hemoglobin F. This analysis allows for the detection of a variety of diseases including sickle cell disease and fetal-maternal hemorrhage. In addition, this methodology allows for quantitation of fetal hemoglobin.

Blood Parasites

Malarial parasites can be screened by flow cytometry methods. If erythrocytes are stained with acridine orange, the mature erythrocytes containing no DNA do not fluoresce with this stain. However, malarial erythrocytes contain DNA and thus will fluoresce.

Cell Functioning Analysis

Every event that occurs during the process of lymphocyte activation can be measured by flow cytometry. The measurements with the greatest clinical significance include tyrosine phosphorylation, calcium flux, oxidative metabolism, neoantigen expression, and cellular proliferation.

Flow cytometry measurement of the oxidative burst in neutrophils has been used as a screening test for chronic granulomatous disease (CGD).

Chromosomal Analysis

Flow cytometry can be used for karyotyping analysis. A chromosomal histogram consists of seven peaks that represent the different groups of chromosomes. By evaluating the peaks, various disorders can be diagnosed.

Cell Sorting

Some flow cytometers have additional hardware that allows them to act as cell sorters. After quickly making the appropriate measurements, the computer makes the decision to sort or isolate a single cell by applying a charge to that cell just as it leaves the flow cell. The cell is electrostatically deflected into a test tube. Any cell type can be sterilely sorted and recovered alive based on any combination of light scatter and fluorescence measurements. The cell type of interest can be separated from a complex mixture of cell types even though it may be an extremely rare or minor subpopulation.

DIGITAL MICROSCOPY

Recent advances in artificial neural networks (ANNs), image analysis, and slide handling have combined to produce instruments that automate manual differentials in new ways. This new technology, referred to as *automated digital cell morphology* (Fig. 27.23), provides an unprecedented level of efficiency and consistency. In its simplest form, automated digital cell morphology is a process where blood cells are automatically located and preclassified into categories of blood cells. Images of these cells are retained for confirmation by a technologist and can be shared electronically and stored as digital images. This adaptability allows for future review and comparisons by laboratory professionals and physicians.

Artificial Neural Networks

An ANN is an information-processing model that simulates the way the human brain processes information. ANN emulates the neural structure of the brain, which is composed of a large number of highly interconnected processing elements (neurons) working together to solve specific problems. ANNs have been around since the 1940s, but it was not until the mid-1980s that algorithms became sophisticated enough and computers powerful enough for general applications to develop.

Digital Cell Morphology

New hardware and the development of databases have aided in developing image analysis systems that can finally meet the demands of the hematology laboratory. The most dramatic change in microscopy over the last three decades is

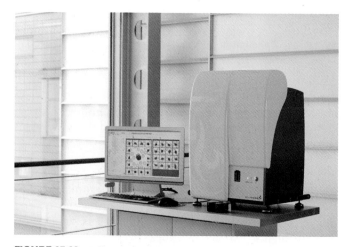

FIGURE 27.23 Cellavision DM-1200. (Courtesy of Cellavision, Inc.)

the ability to digitize image specimens and transmit these images electronically for remote analysis. This capability is now called *virtual microscopy*.

In 2000, CellaVision (Lund, Sweden) launched the DiffMaster Octavia. The system consists of an automated microscope with a 100× objective; a stepper motor and light control unit; and a progressive three-chip CCD color camera connected to a computer with software for localization, segmentation, and classification of white and RBCs. The system processes eight slides per batch, utilizing a slide holder. It allows for remote review of a smear and storage of up to 20,000 slides with images in a database.

In comparison with earlier attempts by other manufacturers, the DiffMaster Octavia handles wedged smears stained according to the Wright, Wright-Giemsa, or May Grünwald–Giemsa staining protocols and uses ANNs trained on a large database of cells. It was the first image analysis system to locate and preclassify cells into 15 different categories and automatically precharacterize six RBC morphologic characteristics. The platelet estimates and erythrocyte precharacterization are performed in an overview image corresponding to eight high-power fields (100×). Review and release of results can be done remotely.

INSTRUMENTS IN COAGULATION STUDIES

In 2003, seven different manufacturers produced 33 laboratory-based coagulation analyzers, many of which are capable of performing clottable, immunoassay, and chromogenic assays (Table 27.11). The difficulty with some instruments is that many of them are unable to transmit an industry-standard test identifier (LOINC code) to the host laboratory information system (LIS).

Various models are available in a wide range of prices designed for different size laboratories. Each instrument offers unique advantages (e.g., high throughput, reduced reagent volume, integral bar-code reader, cap piercing, or automatic sample predilution). Many instruments offer user-programmable methods and preprogrammed methods.

Suggested screening panels include thrombotic hemostasis panel (Box 27.2) and a fibrinolytic hemostasis panel (Box 27.3).

Electromechanical Methods

The earliest instruments to detect blood clotting were developed between 1920 and 1940. These instruments were based primarily on detection of the formation of a fibrin clot and replaced visual observation of the formation of a fibrin clot in a test tube. By the mid-1960s, electromechanical instruments were in widespread use. In the 1970s, photo-optical methods replaced electromechanical devices in most laboratories, except student laboratories or as a backup method in routine laboratories.

The principle of electromechanical methodology is the measurement of conduction or impedance of an electrical current by the formation of fibrin. An example of such a

semiautomated instrument is the fibrometer. This system consists of a 37°C heat block, an automatic pipette, and a mechanical mixer and timer block.

After the appropriate containers are filled and plasma samples and thromboplastin substrate are incubated, plasma is added to the substrate to initiate the timing mechanism. This timing mechanism triggers a digital readout time and the probe unit. The probe arm holds two electrodes. When in operation, it drops down and allows the electrodes to fall into place within the reaction well containing the plasma-thromboplastin mixture. The stationary probe *does not* move when the instrument is in operation but functions in conjunction with the moving electrode. This stationary electrode is responsible for creating an electrical potential between it and the moving electrode. The moving electrode is located in front of the stationary electrode in the probe arm. When a test is being performed, this electrode cycles through the plasma-thromboplastin mixture every half second until a clot forms. A detection circuit is activated when a fibrin strand is formed between the two electrodes, thus completing the circuit. Circuit activation stops the timer and prevents further movement of the moving electrode. Electromechanical methods, such as the fibrometer, can be used for various coagulation assays. These include activated partial thromboplastin time (APTT), prothrombin time (PT), and factor assays.

A new generation of PT point-of-care testing is the HEMOSENSE INRatio (Milpitas, CA). This handheld instrument (Fig. 27.24) provides the PT and corresponding international normalized ratio (INR) value by measuring the electrical impedance using fresh capillary whole blood. The INR system performs a modified version of the one-stage PT test. The clot formed in the reaction is detected as a change in the electrical impedance of the blood sample that occurs when fibrinogen is converted into fibrin. The test strip itself consists of layers of transparent plastic, one of which is an electrode layer (Fig. 27.25).

Photo-Optical Methods

The principle of photo-optical measurement is that a change in light transmission measured as optical density (absorbance) versus time can be used to quantitatively determine the activity of various coagulation stages or factors. Photo-optical clot detection systems can be used for the determination of a wide variety of assays (e.g., APTT, PT, fibrinogen levels, and thrombin time). Quantitative factor assays based on the APTT (factors VIII, IX, XI, and XII) and quantitative factor assays based on the PT (factors V, VII, and X) are examples of available assays.

These microprocessor-controlled instruments have separate detector cells with their own red light–emitting diode (LED) light source, which is driven by a constant current regulator to give each a noise-free light beam. The light beam passes through a cuvette, where it is altered by fibrin clot formation. The light beam then passes through a diffuser and falls on the sensor, which instantly converts the transmitted light into an electrical signal. An amplified

TABLE 27.11 Examples of Coagulation Analyzers

Manufacturer	First Year Sold	Model Name		
		Optical Clot Detection[a]	Chromogenic[a]	Immunologic[a]
American Labor/Lab A.C.M. Inc.	CD2000 1986	PT, PTT, fibrinogen, any citrated plasma clot-based assay	None	None
American Labor/Lab A.C.M. Inc.	CoaLab/1991	Any clot-based detection, PT, APTT, TT, PT-based fibrinogen, Clauss fibrinogen factor assays, protein C, protein S, LAC screen, LAC confirm, APCR-V		
Diagnostica Stago Inc.	STA-R Evolution Hemostasis System 2005	PT, APTT, TT, fibrinogen, reptilase, intrinsic and extrinsic factors, proteins C and S, lupus anticoagulant DRVV, screen and confirm	Heparin (UFH and LMWH), protein C, AT, plasminogen, antiplasmin	D-dimer, VWF, total and free protein S, AT antigen
Diagnostica Stago Inc.	STA Satellite 2009	PT, APTT, fibrinogen	Heparin (UFH, LMWH), AT	D-dimer
Diagnostica Stago Inc.	STA Compact CT 2001	PT, APTT, TT, fibrinogen, reptilase, intrinsic and extrinsic factors, proteins C and S, lupus anticoagulant, DRVV		
Diagnostica Stago Inc.	STA Compact Hemostasis System 1996	PT, APTT, TT, fibrinogen, reptilase, factors, proteins C and S, lupus anticoagulant, DRVV screen and confirm	Unfractionated heparin (UFH and LMWH), LMWH, protein C, AT, plasminogen and antiplasmin	D-dimer, VWF, total and free protein S, AT antigen
Diagnostica Stago Inc.	Start 4 1998	PT, APTT, TT, fibrinogen, reptilase, intrinsic and extrinsic factors, proteins C and S, lupus anticoagulant	None	None
Helena Laboratories	Cascade M 1991	PT, APTT, fibrinogen, TCT, factor assay II, V, VII-XII	None	None
Helena Laboratories	Cascade M-4 1992	PT, APTT, fibrinogen, TCT, factor assay II, V, VII-XII	None	None
Instrument Laboratory/Beckman Coulter, Inc.	ACL TOP 500 CTS 2008	PT, APTT, fibrinogen (Clauss & PT based), TT, intrinsic and extrinsic factors, lupus (SCT & dRVVT), proteins C/S, APCR factor V leiden	Heparin Xa, protein C, AT, plasminogen, plasmin inhibitor	D-dimer, D-dimer HS, vWF (Act. and Ag.), free protein S, factor XIII Ag., homocysteine
Instrument Laboratory/Beckman Coulter, Inc.	ACL TOP Series 2004	PT, APTT, fibrinogen (Clauss and PT based), TT, factors, lupus (SCT & DRVVT), proteins C/S, APCR-V	Heparin Xa, protein C, AT, plasminogen, plasmin inhibitor	D-dimer, D-dimer HS, vWF (Act. and Ag.), free protein S, factor XIII Ag., homocysteine

Manufacturer	Instrument	Tests	Chromogenic/other assays	D-dimer
Instrument Laboratory/ Beckman Coulter, Inc.	ACL Classic Series 1997	PT, APTT, fibrinogen (Clauss and PT based), TT, factors, lupus (SCT and drVVT), proteins C/S, APCR-V	Heparin Xa, protein C, AT, plasminogen, plasmin inhibitor	—
Dade Behring, Inc. Siemens Healthcare	BFT II 1999	PT, APTT, fibrinogen	None	None
Dade Behring, Inc. Siemens Healthcare	Sysmex CA-530 2006	PT, APTT, fibrinogen, TT, factor assays, reptilase time, protein C clot	ATIII, protein C chromo, heparin	None
Dade Behring, Inc. Siemens Healthcare	Sysmex CA-560 2003	PT, APTT, fibrinogen, TT, factor assays, reptilase time, protein C clot	ATIII, protein C chromo, heparin	Advanced D-dimer, Innovance D-dimer
Dade Behring, Inc. Siemens Healthcare	Sysmex CA-1500 1999 worldwide, 2000 US	PT, APTT, fibrinogen, factor assays, reptilase time, TT, dRVVT screen and confirm, factor V leiden, protein C clot, protein S activity	ATIII, plasminogen, factor VIII chromo, alpha-2 antiplasmin, protein C chromo, heparin	Advanced D-dimer, Innovance D-dimer
Dade Behring, Inc. Siemens Healthcare	BCS XP 2006	PT, APTT, fibrinogen, factor assays, reptilase time, TT, dRVVT, screen and confirm, factor V leiden, protein C clot, protein S activity	ATIII, factor VIII chromo, alpha-2 antiplasmin, plasminogen, protein C chromo, heparin	Advanced D-dimer, Innovance D-dimer
Dade Behring, Inc. Siemens Healthcare	Sysmex CA-7000 2002	PT, APTT, TT, reptilase time, factor assays, dRVVT screen and confirm, factor V leiden, protein C clot, protein S activity	ATIII, plasminogen, factor VIII chromo, alpha-2 antiplasmin, protein C chromo, heparin	Advanced D-dimer, Innovance D-dimer
Trinity Biotech	KC1 2001	PT, APTT, fibrinogen.	n/a	n/a
Trinity Biotech	KC4 2001	PT, APTT, fibrinogen, TT, intrinsic and extrinsic factors	n/a	n/a
Trinity Biotech	AMAX Destiny			
Trinity Biotech	Destiny Plus 2005	PT, APTT, fibrinogen, TT, atroxin, factors II, V, VII, VIII, IX, X, XI, and XII	AT, heparin Xa	D-dimer

[a]Food and Drug Administration (FDA) cleared.

APCR, activated protein C resistance; APTT, activated partial thromboplastin time; dRVVT, dilute Russell Viper Venom Time; ISI, international sensitivity index; LAC, lupus anticoagulant; LMWH; lowmolecular weight heparin; n/a, not applicable; PT, prothrombin time; TCT, thrombin clotting time; TT, thrombin time; vWF, von Willebrand factor.

Thrombotic Hemostasis Panel Assays
Antithrombin
Factor VIII:C
Heparin
Lupus anticoagulant
Protein C
Protein S and free protein S

signal is converted to a digital value for further processing. The computer-processed results are subsequently sent to the visual display monitor and printer.

A system is ready for operation when the temperature indicator reads 37 ± 1°C. Preprogrammed modes select the test parameters for each test method, which determines the proper volumes of specimen and reagents. The appropriate amounts of reagents are placed in the specific reagent storage wells. Pressing the start button initiates the test cycle. The optical density (absorbance) of the reaction mixture is then monitored until the rate of change exceeds a predetermined level for a defined period, indicating the presence of a fibrin clot end point. The time (in seconds) of the end point is stored and may be printed or displayed on demand at the end of each series of determinations.

Quality control in these systems includes automatic self-checking of the optical system and the storage of standard and assay curves. A coefficient of determination can be used to check precision.

In addition to routine clot testing, newer instruments offer chromogenic channel models to automate the growing range of specialized diagnostic tests in coagulation.

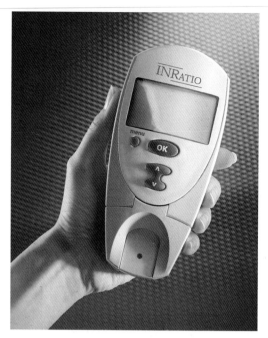

FIGURE 27.24 HEMOSENSE INRatio. (Courtesy of HEMOSENSE Milpitas, CA.)

Viscosity-based Detection System

Viscosity is defined as the resistance that a material has to a change in its form. If this principle is used as a mechanism for clot detection, the natural thickening (viscosity) is monitored by the motion (amplitude of an oscillating steel ball in a specially designed cuvette) as a change in form takes place. The final result is accurate and is insensitive to colored plasma, lipemic plasmas, bilirubin, or turbid reagents and reliable

Fibrinolytic Hemostasis Panel Assays
α-2-Antiplasmin
Plasminogen
Plasminogen activator inhibitor
Tissue plasminogen activator

Solution	Container No.	Time
Fixative	2	30 s
Wright stain	3	3 min
Stain-buffer	4	6 min
Deionized water	5	1.5 min
Drying stage	6	3 min

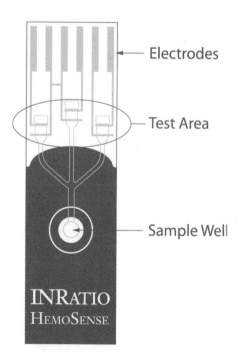

FIGURE 27.25 INRatio test strip. (Courtesy of HEMOSENSE Milpitas, CA.)

measurement for the hemostasis laboratory. Diagnostica Stago manufactures an instrument based on this principle. The steps in the viscosity-based detection system (VDS) are

1. Movement of the steel ball is triggered by two activating coils, working alternately to induce and maintain a natural oscillation.
2. When the start reagent is added, the detection starts immediately.
3. When the ball starts oscillating left and right, a chronometer (clock) begins to time the clotting of the sample.
4. As the ball oscillates left and right, the amplitude or motion is also measured. A peak is formed when the ball is detected in the center of cuvette.
5. Amplitude is monitored during the entire clotting process.
6. As the clot appears, the viscosity increases, and the amplitude decreases.
7. Based on different algorithms, the chronometer is stopped even if the clot is peak, and/or the ball is still in motion.

Platelet Agglutination

The ristocetin cofactor assay measures the ability of a patient's plasma to agglutinate formalin-fixed platelets in the presence of ristocetin. The rate of ristocetin-induced agglutination is related to the concentration of von Willebrand factor, and the percent normal activity can be obtained from the standard curve. Patient values are determined by comparison to a standard curve, allowing quantitation of percent ristocetin cofactor activity.

Platelet Aggregation

Most platelet aggregation procedures are based on some variation of Born method. Agents such as adenosine diphosphate (ADP), collagen, epinephrine, snake venom, thrombin, and ristocetin can also be used to aggregate platelets.

The principle of the test is that platelet-rich plasma is treated with a known aggregating agent. If aggregated, cloudiness or turbidity patterns are determined by photometrically comparing the light transmitted through a suspension of aggregated platelets with that of a suspension of nonaggregated platelets using an aggregometer. The curve that is obtained can be used to assess platelet function.

Primary Response

Primary response is the reversible aggregation of platelets by the aggregating agent. The appearance of a biphasic reaction, showing both primary and secondary response, can occur for some agonists at low concentrations.

Secondary Response

Secondary response is the result of enhancement of the initial aggregation process caused by the release of endogenous ADP and the formation of thromboxane A_2. The secondary response is irreversible.

New Automation

The PFA-100 (Siemens Healthcare Diagnostics) is an automated system that incorporates a high shear flow system to simulate the in vivo hemodynamic conditions of platelet adhesion and aggregation as encountered at a vascular lesion. The system evaluates the ability of platelets to occlude an aperture in a biochemically active membrane. Results are reported as closure time (CT). This instrument offers several advantages over traditional aggregometry because it assesses multiple facets of primary hemostasis—adherence, activation, and aggregation.

SUMMARY

Instrumental Principles

Various principles of cell counting are used in instrumentation. The impedance principle is based on the detection and measurement of changes in electrical resistance produced by a particle as it passes through a small aperture. In the optical principle, the degree of scatter and the amount of light reaching the sensor depend on the volume of the cell. The volume of each cell is proportional to the intensity of the forward scatter of light. In both systems, the number of pulses generated is directly proportional to the number of cells passing through the sensing zone in a specific period.

Based on the original ideas of Einstein and physical theories in the 1950s, laser light was applied to medical and scientific instrumentation. Lasers are able to sort the energy in atoms and molecules, concentrate it, and release it in powerful waves.

Flow-cell cytometry is another method that is applied in the study of cells. The principle of flow cytometry is based on the fact that cells can be stained specifically with a fluorescent dye to identify exact cell types. Laser light is combined with this method in state-of-the-art instrumentation for cell identification and sorting.

Automated instruments that count and/or identify blood cells range from small bench-top units to large sophisticated instruments. The values that an instrument generates are referred to as parameters. The simplest units count erythrocytes, leukocytes, and platelets. The most sophisticated instruments generate many additional parameters. Some instruments are based on a variety of principles including the electrical impedance principle and the optical principle of laser scatter technology. In addition to numerical outputs, the larger instruments are capable of generating graphic displays of the frequency distributions of erythrocytes, leukocytes, platelets, and histograms. Quality control systems, such as Levey-Jennings charts, are also generated by the larger instruments.

Analysis of Electrical Impedance Instrumental Data Output

Erythrocyte histograms are valuable in determining the similarity of the population of RBCs being tested. Quantitative parameters that express variation in the erythrocyte population are either the RDW or the RCMI. The RDW and MCV can be correlated and classified in various disease categories.

The graphic display of leukocytes, the WBC histogram, classifies them into three categories: lymphocytes, mononuclear cells or monocytes, and granulocytes. Computer programming allows for the differentiation of leukocytes graphically, in terms of percentage and absolute values.

Platelet histograms, the MPV, and the DPW can be generated by computer-assisted instruments in addition to the platelet count. The MPV is an expression of the measure of the average volume of the platelets in the sample. No single normal value exists for the MPV; however, an inverse relationship exists between the MPV and the platelet count. This relationship is expressed graphically in a nomogram. The PDW is a measure of the uniformity of platelet size. A normal PDW is less than 20%. Increased or decreased values are associated with various categories of disease.

Laser Technology

Some systems are based on the principle of differential light-scattering cytochemistry. Cytochemical reactions prepare the blood cells for analysis, a cytometer measures specific cell properties, and algorithms convert these measurements into cell classification, cell count, cell size, and hemoglobinization.

Applications of Flow Cytometry

Instruments based on the flow-cell cytometry principle were initially designed to count and size cells; later modifications included leukocyte differential analysis. Today, the applications of the technology are highly diverse and include both cellular component identification and cell-sorting capabilities.

Monoclonal antibodies and fluorescent probes have had a major effect on advances in flow cytometry applications. In the hematology laboratory, in addition to leukocyte differentiation, applications can include reticulocyte counting and screening for malarial parasites. Other cellular applications include analysis of the ratio of T cells to B cells in immunodeficiency states such as AIDS, the study of DNA in cell cycle kinetics, and the investigation of chromosomes.

Instruments in Coagulation Studies

Manual methods have been replaced in the clinical hematology laboratory by electromechanical and optical systems. In the electromechanical system, two electrodes work in conjunction with one another. When a fibrin strand forms in the plasma-thromboplastin mixture between these two electrodes, a complete circuit is formed. Completion of the circuit automatically stops the timer and the length of the reaction time is displayed.

In the optical system, a change in light transmission through the reaction mixture of plasma-thromboplastin is measured as optical density versus time. Formation of a fibrin clot alters the light path, and after the data are processed by the onboard microprocessor, the time in seconds that the reaction took is displayed or printed.

Both methods can measure APTT, PT, factor levels, and various other parameters. The optical systems offer the advantage of internal quality control features. Chromogenic capabilities are also available.

Platelet aggregation procedures are used to test the qualitative response of platelets to various aggregating agents, such as collagen, thrombin, and ristocetin. Turbidity patterns are determined photometrically by comparing the patient's platelet activity with nonaggregated suspension and normal platelets. A curve is generated using a recording spectrophotometer.

Case Studies

Because the relationship between histogram and nomogram information is important to understanding the data output capabilities of modern instrumentation, specific examples become important in establishing a diagnosis and monitoring treatment of a patient. A knowledge and understanding of these newer sources of patient information is important to the clinical laboratory scientist. Each of the cases presented in this chapter represents a fairly typical example of a specific type of disorder.

CASE STUDIES

CASE 27.1

■ **Laboratory Data**
A 28-year-old white woman had the following erythrocyte results:
RBC count 3.2×10^{12}/L
Hemoglobin 8.7 g/dL
Hematocrit 26%
MCV 81 fL
MCH 19 pg
MCHC 27.2 g/dL
RCMI 13.2

Her RBC histogram appears below. All other parameters were within normal ranges.

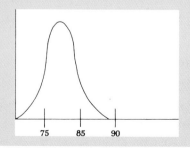

(continued)

CASE STUDIES *(continued)*

■ Questions
1. Do the histogram or other erythrocyte results demonstrate any abnormalities?
2. What type of disorder, if any, is suggested by the RBC results and histogram?
3. What further laboratory testing should be considered?

■ Discussion
1. The histogram demonstrates a nongaussian distribution and is shifted to the left. The hemoglobin, hematocrit, MCV, MCH, and RCMI are not within their respective normal ranges.
2. The data generated suggest a microcytic anemia of unknown cause.
3. A peripheral blood smear should be examined to further describe the morphology of the erythrocytes. Other tests could include serum iron and total iron-binding capacity because microcytic anemias are frequently caused by iron deficiency. See Chapter 10 for a full discussion of anemias. In this case, further testing led to the diagnosis.

DIAGNOSIS: Iron Deficiency Anemia

CASE 27.2

■ Laboratory Data
A 48-year-old black woman had the following RBC results:
RBC 2.36×10^{12}/L
Hemoglobin 8.6 g/dL
Hematocrit 27%
MCV 114 fL
MCH 36.4 pg
MCHC 32 g/dL
RDW 28%
Her RBC histogram appears below. All additional parameters were within normal ranges.

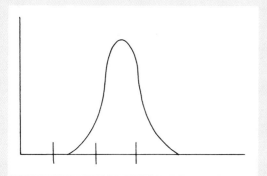

■ Questions
1. Do the histogram or other erythrocyte results demonstrate any abnormalities?

2. What type of disorder, if any, is suggested by the RBC results and histogram?
3. What further laboratory testing should be considered?

■ Discussion
1. All the erythrocyte parameters, except the MCHC, are abnormal.
2. The RDW is indicative of a substantial amount of anisocytosis in this patient's specimen. The MCV and erythrocyte histogram demonstrate that the variation in cell size is in the macrocytic direction.
3. A peripheral blood smear should be examined to further evaluate the morphology of the erythrocytes. Macrocytic erythrocytes frequently reflect a deficiency of vitamin B_{12} or folic acid. Additional tests should include assays for vitamin B_{12} and folic acid. See Chapter 11 for a full discussion of anemias. In this case, further testing led to the diagnosis.

DIAGNOSIS: Megaloblastic Anemia (Pernicious Anemia)

CASE 27.3

■ Laboratory Data
A 57-year-old white man with a total leukocyte count of 15×10^9/L had a three-part leukocyte differential:
Lymphocytes 68%
Mononuclear cells 4%
Granulocytes 28%
Absolute lymphocyte value 10.2×10^9/L
Absolute granulocyte value 4.2×10^9/L
The WBC histogram appears below. All other parameters were within normal ranges.

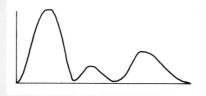

■ Questions
1. Do the histogram or other leukocyte results demonstrate any abnormalities?
2. What type of disorder, if any, is suggested by the WBC results and histogram?
3. What further laboratory testing should be considered?

■ Discussion
1. The WBC histogram demonstrates a reversal in the normal adult proportions of lymphocytes and granulocytes. Additionally, the percentage and absolute values for the

(continued)

CASE STUDIES *(continued)*

lymphocytes are increased, whereas the percentage and absolute values for the granulocytes are decreased.

2. A condition of lymphocytosis is demonstrated by the data presented.

3. A peripheral blood smear should be examined to further evaluate the morphology of the lymphocytes. Other laboratory tests need to be conducted to determine the cause of this disorder and to establish a definitive diagnosis. In this case, additional testing confirmed a diagnosis of chronic lymphocytic leukemia.

DIAGNOSIS: Chronic Lymphocytic Leukemia

CASE 27.4

■ Laboratory Data

A 14-year-old white girl with a total leukocyte count of 29×10^9/L had the following histogram results:

Lymphocytes 15%
Mononuclear cells 48%
Granulocytes 37%

Her WBC histogram appears below. The platelet count was decreased. All erythrocytic parameters were within normal ranges; however, the values tended to be in the low ends of the ranges.

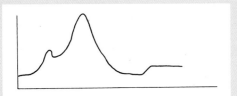

■ Questions

1. Do the histogram or other leukocyte results demonstrate any abnormalities?
2. What type of disorder, if any, is suggested by the WBC results and histogram?
3. What further laboratory testing should be considered?

■ Discussion

1. The histogram and percentage of mononuclear cells far exceed the normal distribution for this type of cell.
2. A variety of disorders may be revealed by this type of cellular distribution. Increases in mononuclear cells may result from the presence of immature cells or monocytes.
3. A peripheral blood smear should be examined to further evaluate the morphology of the mononuclear cells. Other laboratory tests need to be conducted to determine the nature of this disorder and to establish a definitive diagnosis. In this case, additional testing confirmed a diagnosis of acute myelogenous leukemia.

DIAGNOSIS: Acute Myelogenous Leukemia (FAB M1)

CASE 27.5

■ Laboratory Data

A 12-year-old black boy had a total leukocyte count of 55.0×10^9/L. His histogram appears below.

His platelet count was low, as were his erythrocyte parameters. Additionally, his platelet histogram was abnormal.

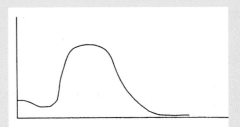

■ Questions

1. Do the histogram or other leukocyte results demonstrate any abnormalities?
2. What type of disorder, if any, is suggested by the WBC results and histogram?
3. What further laboratory testing should be considered?

■ Discussion

1. Although his total WBC count was extremely elevated, the histogram failed to separate the leukocyte subpopulations. From the appearance of the histogram, an excessive number of mononuclear cells may be interfering with discrimination of the adjacent subpopulations.
2. The total WBC count reflects an extreme leukocytosis; however, the nature of the increase cannot be determined.
3. A peripheral blood smear should be reviewed to further evaluate the morphology of the leukocytes. Other laboratory tests need to be conducted to determine the nature of this disorder and to establish a definitive diagnosis. In this case, additional testing confirmed a diagnosis of acute lymphoblastic leukemia.

DIAGNOSIS: Acute Lymphoblastic Leukemia

CASE 27.6

■ Laboratory Data

A 28-year-old white woman underwent a chemotherapeutic regimen for the treatment of leukemia. Her initial platelet count and MPV as well as successive platelet counts and MPVs, beginning on the 7th day after the termination of treatment, were assayed every other day and charted by the laboratory.

(continued)

CASE STUDIES *(continued)*

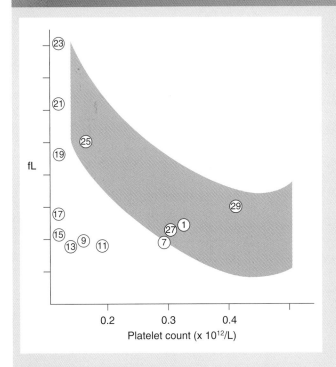

Platelet count (x 10¹²/L)

Questions

1. Did the patient have an initial abnormality?
2. Did the patient develop any abnormalities following treatment?
3. Did the patient's values return to normal?

Discussion

1. Initially, the patient's platelet count and MPV were within the normal range as demonstrated on the nomogram.
2. Subsequent to treatment, the patient's platelet count and MPV were decreased. As the recovery period began, the MPV began to rise before the total platelet count. The nomogram demonstrates that the relationship between the platelet count and MPV is not within the normal range.
3. On the 27th day after treatment, both the platelet count and MPV returned to normal. The results remained within the normal range on the 29th day after treatment.

DIAGNOSIS: Posttherapeutic Platelet Response in a Case of Acute Leukemia

CASE 27.7

■ History and Physical

M.W., a 50-year-old male clinical laboratory scientist, saw his primary care provider for an examination prior to a 6-month international volunteer assignment. He felt well and had no symptoms of any abnormalities.

A urinalysis and CBC were ordered.

■ Laboratory Data

Urinalysis: All results within reference ranges.

■ Hematology Laboratory

Measurement	Patient data	Reference range[a]
RBC	5.03 × 10⁶/μL	4.00–6.20
HGB	15.2 g/dL	11.0–18.8
HCT	45%	35.0–55.0
WBC	5.1 × 10³/μL	6.0–11.0
PLT	175 × 10³/μL	150.0–400.0
MCV	89 fL	80.0–100.0
MCH	30 pg	26.0–34.0
MCHC	34 g/dL	31.0–35.0
RDW	18%	10.0–20.0
MPV	9.1 fL	6.0–10.0

fL, femtoliters; pg, pictogram.
[a]published for Beckman Coulter A^CT ™.

■ Leukocyte Differential Examination

Cell type	%
Neutrophils (band neutrophils + polymorphonuclear segmented neutrophils [PMNs])	58
Lymphocytes	35
Monocytes	4
Eosinophils	2
Basophils	1
Total	100

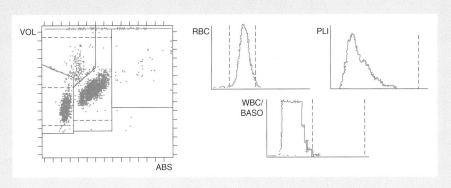

(continued)

CASE STUDIES *(continued)*

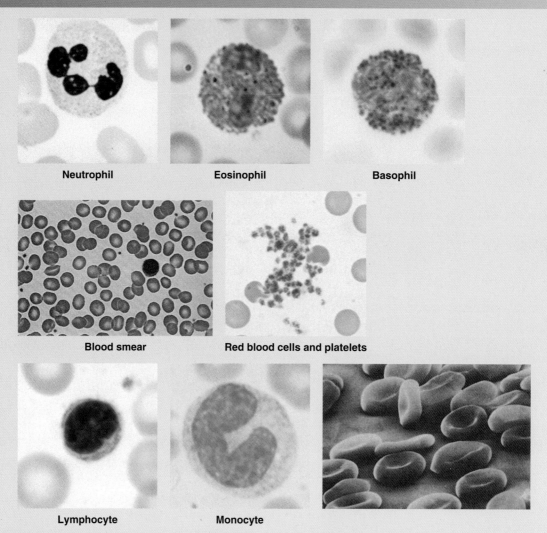

Neutrophil   Eosinophil   Basophil

Blood smear   Red blood cells and platelets

Lymphocyte   Monocyte

Reprinted with permission from Cohen BJ, Wood DL. *Memmler's The Human Body in Health and Disease,* 9th ed, Philadelphia, PA: Lippincott Williams & Wilkins, 2000.

■ **Absolute Cell Counts**

	Units	Patient value	Reference range
Neutrophils	$10^3/\mu L$	2.96	2.0–8.0
Lymphocytes	$10^3/\mu L$	1.79	1.0–5.0

■ **Questions**
1. Are any of the laboratory values abnormal?
2. Why are the absolute cell counts important data?
3. Should additional laboratory assays be ordered?

■ **Discussion**
1. All of the values and histograms are within the reference ranges and display no abnormalities.

2. Absolute cell counts are important in partially assessing the adequacy of cellular body defenses, for example, phagocytosis, antigen recognition, and antibody production.
3. No further laboratory assays need to be ordered.

DIAGNOSIS: Normal (Adult)

CASE 27.8

■ **History and Physical**
S.S., a 10-year-old white female, came to the pediatrician complaining of a cold and cough with pain in the neck and chest. She had an elevated temperature and a slight cough. Physical examination revealed enlarged lymph nodes, wheezing, and an elevated temperature.

(continued)

CASE STUDIES *(continued)*

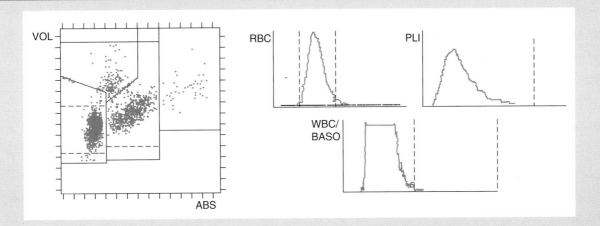

A urinalysis, CBC, and throat culture were ordered.

Laboratory Data

Urinalysis: all results within reference ranges.

Complete Blood Count

Measurement	Units	Reference range[a]
RBC	$5.14 \times 10^6/\mu L$	4.00–6.20
HGB	13.8 g/dL	11.0–18.8
HCT	41%	35.0–55.0
WBC	$35 \times 10^3/\mu L$	6.0–11.0
PLT	$200 \times 10^3/\mu L$	150.0–400.0
MCV	81 fL	80.0–100.0
MCH	27 pg	26.0–34.0
MCHC	32 g/dL	31.0–35.0
RDW	15%	10.0–20.0
MPV	9.0 fL	6.0–10.0

fL, femtoliters; pg, pictogram.
[a]*Published for Beckman Coulter A^cT™.*

Leukocyte differential	%
Band neutrophils	0
Polymorphonuclear segmented neutrophils (PMNs)	30
Lymphocytes	62
Monocytes	5
Eosinophils	2
Basophils	1
Total	100

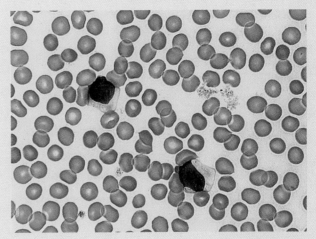

Reprinted with permission from McClatchey KD. *Clinical Laboratory Medicine,* 2nd ed, Philadelphia, PA: Lippincott Williams & Wilkins, 2002.

Absolute Cell Counts

	Units	Patient value	Reference range
Neutrophils	$10^3/\mu L$	1.11	2.0–8.0
Lymphocytes	$10^3/\mu L$	22	1.0–5.0

Questions

1. Are any of the laboratory values abnormal?
2. Why are the absolute cell counts important data?
3. Should additional laboratory assays be ordered?

Discussion

1. Yes. Several laboratory measurements are abnormal. The lymphocyte region of the histogram shows an increase in the density of lymphocytes. The leukocyte differential count shows an increase in lymphocytes. The average lymphocyte values in peripheral blood for a 10-year-old is 38%. The term for this is lymphocytosis.

(continued)

2. The absolute lymphocyte cell count is extremely elevated and the absolute neutrophil cell count is below the reference range. The term for this condition is neutropenia. In this case, it demonstrates the relationship of the percentage of neutrophils to lymphocytes.

The total leukocyte and lymphocyte values are major laboratory findings and may be present before symptoms intensify.

3. A throat culture was ordered. The results demonstrated the presence of *Bordetella pertussis*.

DIAGNOSIS: Lymphocytosis Secondary to *Bordetella pertussis* Infection

CASE 27.9

■ **History and Physical**

K.C., a 70-year-old nurse, suffered from degenerative arthritis. She visited her rheumatologist because of increasing pain in her knees.

A CBC and erythrocyte sedimentation rate (ESR) were ordered. Synovial fluid was removed from one knee for examination.

■ **Laboratory Data**

Measurement	Units	Reference range[a]
RBC	$3.41 \times 10^6/\mu L$	4.00–6.20
HGB	11.0 g/dL	11.0–18.8
HCT	31%	35.0–55.0
WBC	$18 \times 10^3/\mu L$	6.0–11.0
PLT	$210 \times 10^3/\mu L$	150.0–400.0
MCV	92 fL	80.0–100.0
MCH	32 pg	26.0–34.0
MCHC	35 g/dL	31.0–35.0
RDW	12%	10.0–20.0
MPV	9 fL	6.0–10.0

fL, femtoliters; pg, pictogram.
[a]Published for Beckman Coulter A^{C}T™.

Leukocyte differential	%
Band neutrophils	5
Polymorphonuclear segmented neutrophils (PMNs)	65
Lymphocytes	8
Monocytes	20
Eosinophils	1
Basophils	1
Total	100

■ **Absolute Cell Counts**

	Units	Patient value	Reference range
Neutrophils	$10^3/\mu L$	13	2.0–8.0
Lymphocytes	$10^3/\mu L$	1.44	1.0–5.0
Monocytes	$10^3/\mu L$	3.6	0.1–1.0

■ **Questions**

1. Are any of the laboratory values abnormal?
2. Why are the absolute cell counts important data?
3. Should additional laboratory assays be ordered?

■ **Discussion**

1. Yes. The manual white blood cell differential demonstrated an increase in monocytes. The appearance of the monocytes showed increased granulation and vacuolization. The white blood cell histogram reveals a population of monocytes that extends into the upper monocyte and neutrophil range.

   Her synovial fluid exhibited an increase in total leukocytes.

2. Absolute cell count values are of the greatest importance in assessing neutrophils and lymphocytes. An increase in monocytes suggests an inflammatory state but is not diagnostic.

3. A culture of the synovial fluid to rule out a bacterial infection would be of value. Otherwise, no additional laboratory assays would be of value at this time.

DIAGNOSIS: Monocytosis Secondary to Chronic Inflammation and Potential Infection

CASE 27.10

■ **History and Physical**

MT, a 45-year-old white female, began to experience abdominal pain over the last several days. She went to a primary care clinic for help.

A CBC was ordered.

Measurement	Units	Reference range[a]
RBC	$5.1 \times 10^6/\mu L$	4.00–6.20
HGB	13.0g/dL	11.0–18.8
HCT	37%	35.0–55.0
WBC	$23.0 \times 10^3/\mu L$	6.0–11.0
PLT	$450 \times 10^3/\mu L$	150.0–400.0
MCV	72 fL	80.0–100.0
MCH	25 pg	26.0–34.0
MCHC	35 g/dL	31.0–35.0
RDW	17%	10.0–20.0
MPV	8.0 fL	6.0–10.0

fL, femtoliters; pg, pictogram.
[a]Published for Beckman Coulter A^{C}T™.

(continued)

CASE STUDIES (continued)

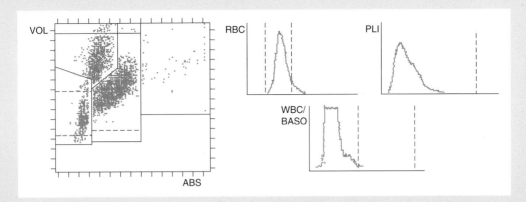

Laboratory Data

Leukocyte differential	%
Band neutrophils	10
Polymorphonuclear segmented neutrophils (PMNs)	80
Lymphocytes	7
Monocytes	1
Eosinophils	1
Basophils	1
Total	100

RBC morphology: 3+ microcytosis, 3+ hypochromia, 1+ anisocytosis.

Absolute Cell Counts

Neutrophils	$10^3/\mu L$	20.7	2.0–8.0
Lymphocytes	$10^3/\mu L$	1.6	1.0–5.0

Questions

1. Are any of the laboratory values abnormal?
2. Why are the absolute cell counts important data?
3. Should additional laboratory assays be ordered?

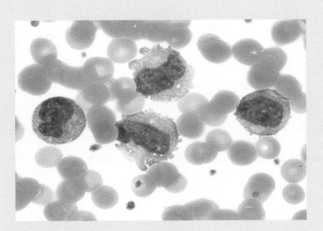

Reprinted with permission from Anderson SC. *Anderson's Atlas of Hematology*, Philadelphia, PA: Wolters Kluwer Health/Lippincott Williams & Wilkins, Copyright 2003.

Discussion

1. Yes. The MCV and MCH are below the reference range. The total leukocyte count is elevated. Platelets are increased. A small population of cells in the lower lymphocyte region of the histogram suggest possible platelet aggregates.
2. The total leukocyte count, differential ratio of leukocyte, and absolute cell counts support neutrophilia.
3. Additional testing should investigate the etiology of the leukocytosis—possibly an acute infection or acute inflammation. The patient's hemoglobin and hematocrit, and red blood cell indices should be monitored as well.

DIAGNOSIS: Leukocytosis Etiology Unknown
Microcytic Anemia Etiology Unknown

CASE 27.11

History and Physical

A.C. is a 27-year-old white male. On New Year's day, he discovered swollen lymph nodes in his arm pits. He had been becoming progressively tired and weak over the last several weeks but thought that he had the flu.

He went to the Emergency Department where a stat

Measurement	Units	Reference range[a]
RBC	$4.0 \times 10^6/\mu L$	4.00–6.20
HGB	11 g/dL	11.0–18.8
HCT	34%	35.0–55.0
WBC	$9.0 \times 10^3/\mu L$	6.0–11.0
PLT	$20.0 \times 10^3/\mu L$	150.0–400.0
MCV	85 fL	80.0–100.0
MCH	28 pg	26.0–34.0
MCHC	33g/dL	31.0–35.0
RDW	15%	10.0–20.0
MPV	9.0fL	6.0–10.0

fL, femtoliters; pg, pictogram.
[a]Published for Beckman Coulter A^{c}T™.

(continued)

CASE STUDIES (continued)

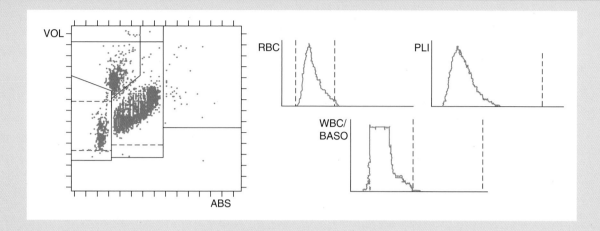

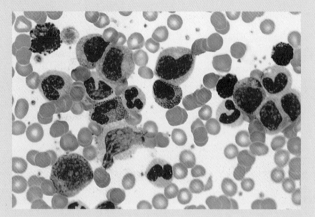

Reprinted with permission from McClatchey KD. *Clinical Laboratory Medicine,* 2nd ed, Philadelphia, PA: Lippincott Williams & Wilkins, 2002.

CBC was ordered.

■ **Laboratory Data**

Leukocyte differential	%
Blasts	7
Metamyelocytes	2
Band neutrophils	10
Polymorphonuclear segmented neutrophils (PMNs)	14
Lymphocytes	50
Monocytes	14
Eosinophils	0
Basophils	3
Total	100

■ **Absolute Cell Counts**

Neutrophils	10³/µL	23.4	2.0–8.0
Lymphocytes	10³/µL	4.5	1.0–5.0

■ **Questions**

1. Are any of the laboratory values abnormal?

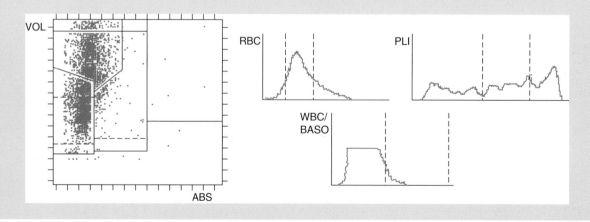

(continued)

CASE STUDIES *(continued)*

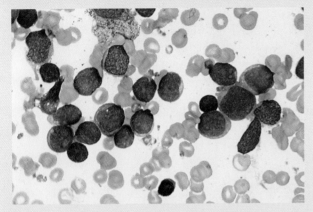

Reprinted with permission from McClatchey KD. *Clinical Laboratory Medicine*, 2nd ed, Philadelphia, PA: Lippincott Williams & Wilkins, 2002.

2. Is the histogram abnormal?
3. Should additional laboratory assays be ordered?

■ **Discussion**

1. Yes. The peripheral blood differential revealed immature white blood cells and decreased platelets. The only measured component that was abnormal was the decreased platelet count.
2. The histogram is also abnormal. It demonstrates a huge population of cells in the lymphocyte region extending through the regions of lymphocytes, variant lymphocytes, monocytes, and the upper monocyte region. Cells associated with this region include blasts, large monocytes, promyelocytes, and myelocytes.
3. Yes. A further workup is needed to establish the thrombocytopenia in the presence of red and white blood cells within the reference range. The presence of blasts and many mononuclear cells believed to be lymphocytes needs to be investigated. Either special staining or flow cytometry should be used to further identify the hematologic abnormality in peripheral blood and/or bone marrow.

DIAGNOSIS: **Thrombocytopenia Etiology Unknown with Increased Number of Mononuclear Peripheral Blood Cells**

REVIEW QUESTIONS

1. Which of the following is not a benefit of laboratory instrumentation to the hematology laboratory?
   A. Produces faster results from specimens
   B. Reduced cost on rarely performed procedures
   C. Less variation in technique from technologist to technologist
   D. Increased accuracy because data are collected on more cells counted or analyzed

Questions 2 and 3: Match the following principles of cell counting instrumentation.

2. _____ Electrical impedance principle
3. _____ Optical detection principle
   A. The volume of each cell is proportional to the degree of light scatter
   B. Each cell momentarily increases resistance

4. The abbreviation laser stands for
   A. light-associated simulated emission of radiation
   B. largely amplified by simulated emission of radiation
   C. light amplified by stimulated emission of radiation
   D. liquid amplified by stimulated emission of radiation

5. A photon is
   A. a diffuse form of energy
   B. a piece of equipment in a laser assembly
   C. the basic unit of all radiation
   D. equivalent to an atom

6. The major application of flow-cell cytometry is
   A. determining cell size and granularity
   B. sorting of cells and cellular identification using monoclonal antibodies
   C. treating cancer cells and identifying specific virus types
   D. counting leukocytes and platelets

7. The term parameter means
   A. a subset of a population
   B. the mean value of a sample
   C. two SDs on either side of the mean value
   D. any numerical value that describes an entire population

8. Data output from three-part differential counters includes
   A. an erythrocyte histogram
   B. a leukocyte histogram
   C. a platelet histogram
   D. all of the above

9. Which parameters are calculated rather than directly measured?
   A. Hematocrit and erythrocyte distribution width
   B. Erythrocyte count and leukocyte count
   C. Leukocyte count and hematocrit
   D. Platelet count and platelet volume

(continued)

10. The delta check method of quality control
    A. uses the patient's own data to monitor population values
    B. uses batches of 20 samples to track MCV, MCH, and MCHC values
    C. compares the patient's leukocyte and platelet counts with his or her previous results
    D. monitors the patient's values within two SDs of the mean

11. Applying the optical principle of laser scatter technology to cell counting and analysis, discrimination between erythrocytes and platelets depends on the
    A. cellular volume
    B. cellular refractive index
    C. time of flight through the sensing zone
    D. all of the above

12. In an erythrocyte histogram, the erythrocytes that are larger than normal will be to the _____ of the normal distribution curve.
    A. right
    B. left
    C. in the middle

13. A bimodal histogram distribution is suggestive of
    A. cold agglutinin disease
    B. posttransfusion of normal red cells to a person with abnormally sized red cells
    C. the presence of RBC fragments
    D. all of the above

Questions 14 and 15: Match the appropriate formulas.

14. _____ RDW
15. _____ Red cell measurement index

$$A. \quad \frac{\text{Patient RBC variaton} - \text{average normal RBC variation}}{\text{SD of average normal RBC variation}}$$

$$B. \quad \frac{\text{SD}}{\text{Mean}} \times 100$$

16. The RDW and MCV are both quantitative descriptors of erythrocyte size. If both are increased, the most probable erythrocytic abnormality would be
    A. iron deficiency anemia
    B. acquired aplastic anemia
    C. megaloblastic anemia
    D. hemoglobinopathy

17. If the RBC distribution on a histogram demonstrates a homogeneous pattern and a small SD, the peripheral blood smear would probably exhibit
    A. extreme anisocytosis
    B. very little anisocytosis
    C. a single population of spherocytes
    D. a single population of macrocytes

18. The _____ can be determined from a WBC histogram.
    A. percent of lymphocytes
    B. absolute number of lymphocytes
    C. frequency distribution of granulocytes
    D. all of the above

Questions 19 and 20: The sorting of leukocyte subpopulations in the WBC histogram determined by electrical impedance reflects the (19) _____, which is primarily related to their (20) _____.

19.
    A. overall size
    B. relative size
    C. nuclear size
    D. chromatin pattern

20.
    A. cytoplasmic size
    B. nuclear size
    C. concentration of granules
    D. cytoplasmic color

21. The mononuclear cells in a WBC histogram can include
    A. blast cells
    B. promyelocytes
    C. monocytes
    D. all of the above

22. A combined scatter histogram measures
    A. overall size versus nuclear size
    B. cytoplasm-to-nucleus ratio
    C. cell size and granularity
    D. cell shape and cytoplasmic color

23. The MPV is
    A. analogous to the MCHC
    B. a direct measure of the platelet count
    C. a measurement of the average volume of platelets
    D. a comparison of the patient's value to the normal value

24. The MPV is often decreased
    A. in sickle cell anemia
    B. in megaloblastic anemia
    C. in idiopathic thrombocytopenic purpura
    D. after splenectomy

25. A normal PDW is
    A. less than 5%
    B. less than 10%
    C. less than 15%
    D. less than 20%

26. Which of the following can be an application of flow-cell cytometry?
    A. Screening erythrocytes for malaria
    B. Counting of reticulocytes
    C. Quantitation of T and B cells
    D. All of the above

(continued)

REVIEW QUESTIONS (continued)

27. Major systems in a flow cytometer include all of the following except
   A. fluidics
   B. optics
   C. computerized electronics
   D. gating

28. The restriction of data analysis to one cell population is accomplished by
   A. amplification
   B. gating
   C. compensatory monitoring
   D. data limitation

29. Which cell surface membrane marker is used for enumeration of HPC enumeration?
   A. CD4
   B. CD8
   C. CD34
   D. CD45

30. Reticulocytes can be detected by using _____ stain.
   A. new methylene blue
   B. thiazole orange
   C. propidium iodide
   D. both A and B

31. The newer clinical instruments for measuring blood clotting are based on
   A. clot elasticity
   B. fibrin adhesion
   C. conduction of impedance of an electrical current by fibrin
   D. changes in optical density

32. The fibrometer relies on the principle of
   A. clot elasticity
   B. fibrin adhesion
   C. conduction or impedance of an electrical current by fibrin
   D. changes in optical density

33. In the photo-optical method, the change in light transmission versus the _____ is used to determine the activity of coagulation factors or stages.
   A. amount of patient's plasma
   B. amount of test reagent
   C. time
   D. temperature

34. In measuring platelet aggregation, platelet-rich plasma can be treated with _____ to aggregate platelets.
   A. saline
   B. collagen
   C. epinephrine
   D. both B and C

35. With a particle-counting instrument, a high background count can be due to
   A. a partial obstruction of the aperture
   B. an electrical line interference
   C. contaminated diluent
   D. bubbles in the diluent

36. A source of error when using the fibrometer in coagulation studies can be
   A. improper reaction temperature
   B. overincubation of the substrate reagent
   C. overincubation of the test plasmas
   D. all of the above

BIBLIOGRAPHY

Aller R (ed.). Coagulation analyzers, *CAP TODAY*, 1:19–34, 2009.

Bakke AC. ASCP Tech Sample Hematology No. H-6, 287–235, 2002.

Bakke AC. The principles of flow cytometry, *Lab Med*, 32(4):207–211, 2001.

Boraiko AA. A splendid light—lasers, *Nat Geo*, 1984:335–341.

Coulter Electronics, Inc. *Calibrating and Caring for Semiautomated Models of the Coulter Counter,* Hialeah, FL: Coulter Electronics, 1982.

Coulter Electronics, Inc. *Platelet Counting in the '80s,* Hialeah, FL: Coulter Electronics, 1982.

Coulter Electronics, Inc. *Expanding Information,* Hialeah, FL: Coulter Electronics, 1983.

Coulter Electronics, Inc. *Significant Advances in Hematology,* Hialeah, FL: Coulter Electronics, 1983 (slide-tape program).

Coulter Electronics, Inc. *Improved Classification of Anemias,* Hialeah, FL: Coulter Electronics, 1985 (slide-tape program).

Dadoun R. Implementing preanalytical automation, *Med Lab Observ,* 32(1):32–36, 2000.

DeRitis S, Smith T. Next-generation hematology, *Adv Admin Lab,* 11(11):18–25, 2002.

Dunphy CH. Applications of flow cytometry to diagnostic hematopathology, *Adv Med Lab Prof,* 15(3):19–21, 2003.

Ford A. High-Volume hematology analyzers, *TODAY,* 17(12):33–49, 2003.

Gonder J, Mell LD. Everything you wanted to know about automated instrument selection, but were afraid to ask, *Adv Med Lab Prof,* 14(21):17–20, 2002.

HemoSense Product Literature (www.hemosense.com), 2009.

Jamieson B. The continued climb of hematology automation, *Adv Admin Lab,* 12(4):56–60, 2003.

Jones AR. *Evaluation of the Coulter Histogram Differential: A Review of the Literature,* Hialeah, FL: Coulter Electronics, 1986.

Kelliher AS, et al. Multiparameter flow cytometry in the clinical lab: Present capacities & future projections, *Adv Med Lab Prof,* 13(17):9–12, 2001.

Kottke-Marchant K, Aller RD. Towards multi-functional analyzers, *CAP TODAY,* 17(1):18, 2003.

LaPorta AD. Advance in hematology, *Adv Med Lab Prof,* 14(25):14–16, 2002.

McCoy JP. Flow cytometry applications in diagnostic pathology, *Clin Lab News,* 29(9):8–10, 2003.

Orsulak PJ. Automation of pre-analytical processing in the clinical laboratory, *Adv Admin Lab,* 12(1):46–49, 2003.

Pierre R. *Seminar and Case Studies: The Automated Differential,* Hialeah, FL: Coulter Electronics, 1985.

Riley RS, Mahin EJ, Ross W. The value of flow cytometry, *Adv Admin Lab,* 11(7):101–106, 2002.

Schmitz JL. Theory, clinical applications of flow cytometry, *Adv Admin Lab,* 12(1):32–36, 2003.

Tamul KR. Looking inside the cell: Intracellular flow cytometry, *Adv Med Lab Prof,* 14(9):18–20, 2002.

Thomas J. Flow cytometry: Not just cells anymore, *Adv Med Lab Prof,* 11(8):12–16, 1999.

A   Answers to Review Questions

CHAPTER 1

1. D
2. A
3. C
4. B
5. A
6. A
7. D
8. D
9. B
10. B
11. D
12. B
13. B
14. C
15. B
16. C
17. B
18. D
19. A
20. A
21. B
22. C
23. B
24. C
25. A
26. D
27. B
28. C
29. A
30. C
31. A
32. D
33. D
34. B

CHAPTER 2

1. B
2. B
3. D
4. B
5. D
6. C
7. A
8. E
9. B
10. A
11. D
12. C
13. A
14. C
15. B
16. D
17. D
18. D
19. D
20. D
21. D
22. D
23. B
24. D
25. D
26. C
27. A
28. B
29. A
30. A
31. A
32. B
33. C

CHAPTER 3

1. B
2. B
3. B
4. D
5. D
6. E
7. A
8. C
9. B
10. D
11. C
12. A
13. B
14. C
15. D
16. A
17. B
18. D
19. D
20. B
21. E
22. A
23. C
24. B
25. E
26. A
27. D
28. B
29. C
30. D
31. D
32. D
33. C
34. D
35. C
36. D
37. D
38. A
39. D
40. B
41. D
42. A
43. D

CHAPTER 4

1. C
2. C
3. D
4. B
5. B
6. B
7. A
8. A
9. B
10. E
11. D
12. C
13. B
14. A

CHAPTER 5

1. B
2. D
3. A
4. A
5. D
6. D
7. C
8. A
9. C
10. D
11. C
12. C
13. C
14. D
15. C
16. D
17. B
18. A
19. C
20. B
21. D
22. D
23. B
24. D
25. B
26. B
27. B
28. B
29. D
30. D
31. B
32. C
33. C
34. A
35. B
36. C
37. A
38. D
39. B
40. C
41. D
42. D
43. C
44. D
45. D
46. D
47. B
48. B
49. B
50. D

51. A
52. A
53. D
54. D
55. D
56. D
57. D
58. A
59. C
60. B
61. C
62. B
63. A

CHAPTER 6

1. C
2. B
3. C
4. A
5. D
6. D
7. A
8. C
9. B
10. A
11. C
12. B
13. D
14. C
15. A
16. D
17. B
18. D
19. C
20. A
21. D
22. B
23. D
24. C
25. A
26. B
27. D
28. A
29. B
30. C
31. D
32. D
33. A
34. B
35. C
36. B
37. D
38. A
39. C
40. C
41. A

CHAPTER 7

1. D
2. D
3. A
4. C
5. D

CHAPTER 8

1. B
2. A
3. A
4. B
5. B
6. C
7. D

CHAPTER 9

1. D
2. B
3. D
4. D
5. D
6. A
7. C
8. B
9. D
10. A

CHAPTER 10

1. D
2. D
3. E
4. A
5. B
6. D
7. C
8. C
9. C
10. D
11. A
12. B
13. D
14. B
15. A
16. A
17. D
18. D
19. C
20. D
21. D
22. D

23. A
24. A
25. D
26. D

CHAPTER 11

1. D
2. D
3. D
4. D
5. A
6. C
7. D
8. C
9. A
10. A
11. B
12. C
13. C
14. D
15. C

CHAPTER 12

1. A
2. B
3. A
4. B
5. B
6. A
7. C
8. B
9. C
10. A
11. E
12. D
13. B
14. A
15. B
16. A
17. B
18. A
19. C
20. D
21. B
22. B
23. A
24. C
25. C
26. D
27. C
28. C
29. C
30. A

CHAPTER 13

1. C
2. D
3. A
4. A
5. D
6. B
7. B
8. B
9. B
10. C
11. A
12. C
13. D
14. C
15. A
16. A
17. A
18. D
19. A
20. D

CHAPTER 14

1. A
2. C
3. A
4. B
5. B
6. C
7. C
8. B
9. B
10. D
11. D
12. D
13. D
14. A
15. D
16. A
17. B
18. D
19. D
20. A
21. B
22. D
23. D
24. D
25. A
26. D
27. C
28. A
29. A
30. B

CHAPTER 15

1. D
2. D
3. D
4. D
5. D
6. B
7. A
8. D
9. C
10. C
11. A
12. B
13. B
14. D
15. C
16. A
17. B
18. B
19. A
20. A
21. A
22. D
23. B
24. D

CHAPTER 16

1. B
2. C
3. B
4. A
5. A
6. B
7. D
8. A
9. C
10. D
11. B
12. B
13. C
14. A
15. B
16. B
17. A
18. B
19. A
20. B
21. A
22. C
23. D
24. D
25. A
26. C
27. D
28. A
29. D

CHAPTER 17

1. D
2. B
3. B
4. A
5. B
6. A
7. B
8. A
9. A
10. A
11. C
12. A
13. C
14. D
15. B

CHAPTER 18

1. D
2. B
3. B
4. D
5. C
6. D
7. A

CHAPTER 19

1. D
2. B
3. C
4. A
5. D
6. C
7. D
8. C
9. E
10. B
11. A
12. D
13. D
14. B
15. C
16. A
17. A
18. B
19. A
20. C
21. C
22. B
23. A
24. A
25. C
26. A
27. A
28. A
29. D
30. D

CHAPTER 20

1. B
2. C
3. B
4. C
5. D
6. D
7. B
8. C
9. D
10. B
11. D

CHAPTER 21

1. C
2. A
3. B
4. A
5. C
6. B
7. B
8. D
9. C
10. C
11. D
12. D
13. C
14. D
15. B
16. D
17. D
18. D
19. A
20. D
21. A
22. D
23. B
24. D
25. C
26. C
27. C
28. D
29. D
30. A
31. C

CHAPTER 22

1. B
2. D
3. C
4. C
5. D
6. D
7. D
8. B
9. B
10. A
11. C
12. B

CHAPTER 23

1. B
2. E
3. B
4. A
5. D
6. C
7. B
8. A
9. B
10. A
11. D
12. D
13. D
14. D
15. A
16. B
17. D
18. D
19. D
20. B
21. A
22. B
23. D
24. C
25. D
26. A
27. B
28. B
29. B
30. A
31. C
32. D
33. D
34. C
35. D

36. A
37. C
38. B
39. C
40. B
41. D
42. A
43. B
44. C
45. A
46. B
47. B
48. B
49. D
50. C
51. D
52. A
53. C
54. D
55. B
56. D
57. A
58. C
59. D
60. B
61. D
62. D
63. A
64. D

CHAPTER 24

1. D
2. B
3. C
4. A
5. C
6. A
7. B
8. A
9. A
10. B
11. D
12. D
13. D
14. A
15. A
16. B
17. A
18. B
19. B
20. B
21. C
22. A

CHAPTER 25

1. A
2. B
3. D
4. E
5. C
6. C
7. A
8. B
9. A
10. C
11. B
12. A
13. B
14. D
15. C
16. B
17. A
18. D
19. B
20. C
21. A
22. D
23. A
24. E
25. B
26. C
27. A
28. B
29. A
30. D
31. D
32. D
33. B
34. B
35. A
36. C
37. D
38. B
39. D
40. E
41. A
42. C
43. C
44. C
45. D
46. D
47. B
48. C
49. D
50. A
51. A
52. D
53. D
54. D
55. A

56. C
57. B
58. A
59. A
60. B
61. C
62. D
63. A
64. B
65. D
66. C
67. A
68. D
69. B
70. D
71. D
72. E
73. B
74. A
75. D
76. C
77. B
78. D
79. C
80. C
81. A
82. B
83. D
84. A
85. B
86. C

CHAPTER 26

1. A
2. B
3. C
4. B
5. A
6. C
7. B
8. A
9. E
10. D
11. C
12. B
13. A
14. C
15. C
16. D
17. B
18. B
19. C
20. D
21. A
22. C

23. A
24. C
25. D
26. D
27. D
28. D
29. B
30. A
31. C
32. A
33. C
34. B
35. D
36. B
37. D
38. C
39. A
40. D
41. B
42. C
43. A
44. B
45. A
46. D
47. C
48. B
49. A
50. D
51. C
52. B
53. C
54. A
55. B
56. D
57. A
58. B
59. C
60. A
61. D
62. D
63. B
64. B
65. D
66. A
67. A
68. B
69. C
70. D
71. C
72. A
73. D
74. B
75. A
76. D
77. C
78. C
79. E

80. B
81. D
82. A
83. C
84. B
85. A
86. D

CHAPTER 27

1. B
2. B
3. A

4. C
5. C
6. B
7. D
8. D
9. A
10. A
11. D
12. A
13. D
14. B
15. A
16. C
17. B

18. D
19. B
20. B
21. D
22. C
23. C
24. B
25. D
26. D
27. D

28. B
29. C
30. D
31. D
32. C
33. C
34. D
35. C
36. D

Medical terminology encompasses many of the words used in the biological sciences; however, terms that are unique to medical applications are also included. Latin and Greek terms form the basis of many of these words. The Romance languages (French, Spanish, Portuguese, and Italian) continue to reflect their Latin origins. Many terms are encountered in modern English.

The reader should be able to

- Name the three basic components of a medical term
- Define the listed prefixes, root terms, and suffixes

A medical term is ideally composed of three principal parts: a **prefix**, a **stem** or **root term**, and a **suffix.** A prefix is located at the beginning of the term. The root term, which commonly refers to a body part or anatomical structure, is found in the middle of the term. The suffix is located at the end of the term.

The word **thrombocytopenia** is an example of a hematological term. This term can be divided into three basic components: **thrombo-** (the prefix), **-cyto-** (the root), and **-penia** (the suffix). By combining the meanings of each of these components, the definition of the word emerges.

Thrombo- means clot, **-cyto-** means cell, and **-penia** means a severe decrease. Hence, the term **thrombocytopenia** is defined as a severe decrease in the cells that are associated with clotting (platelets).

Prefixes may also serve as coupling forms. In this case, a term may have only two components: a prefix and a suffix. An example of this is the word **anemia.** The two components are **an-** and **-emia. An-** means no, not, or without, and **-emia** means blood. Literally translated, the term **anemia** means "without blood." Two-part terms may also be composed of a root term and a suffix such as the word **appendectomy.** The root term, **-appendico-**, refers to the appendix and the suffix, **-ectomy**, refers to surgical removal. Therefore, an appendectomy is the surgical removal of the appendix.

Many new terms are introduced within the text of this book. Some of these terms describe conditions such as leukocytosis, whereas other terms relate to an overall patient diagnosis such as aplastic anemia. Definitions of newly introduced terms are included either within the text or in the Glossary; however, a basic working knowledge of commonly used prefixes, roots, and suffixes is essential. The following short list of prefixes and suffixes should be mastered.

PREFIXES

a-, an-, no, not, without
ab-, away from
acantho-, spiny
aniso, unequal
ante-, before
anti-, against
auto-, self
baso-, basic
bi-, two
bili-, bile
blast-, germ cell
chromo-, color
crena-, wrinkled
cryo-, extreme cold
di-, two
dys-, difficult, painful
eosin-, orange-red
erythro-, red
gen-, precursor, producer
granulo-, granular
hema-, hemato-, blood
hyper-, increased

hypo-, decreased
intra-, within
iso-, equal
leuk-, white
macro-, large
megalo-, extremely large
micro-, small
mono-, one, single
morpho-, appearance
multi-, many
neo-, new
neutro-, neutral
ortho-, normal
pan-, all
para-, next to
path-, disease
peri-, around
phago-, to eat
poikilo-, irregular
poly-, many
post-, after
pre-, before

pro-, before
pykno-, dense
reticulo-, netlike
rubri-, red
sidero-, iron
sphero-, round
thrombo-, clot
trans-, across

-ectomy, incision and removal
-emia, blood
-itis, an inflammation
-logy, the study of
-lysis, to break up
-oma, a tumor
-osis, a condition
-penia, a severe decrease
-phil, love of
-plasia, growth
-poiesis, cell growth
-rhage, -rhagia, to flow
-rhea, discharge, to flow
-scopy, to visually examine
-tomy, to cut
-uria, urine

SUFFIXES

-algia, pain along a nerve
-ase, an enzyme
-cide, the killer of
-crit, to separate
-cyte, a cell

MEDICAL TERM QUIZ

Match the prefix with the term.

1. Endo-
2. Card-
3. Ex-
4. Hemo-
5. A-, an-
6. Hypo-
7. Mal-
8. Path-
9. Phleb-
10. Trans-

A. Heart
B. No, not
C. Disease
D. Inner
E. Vein
F. Out of
G. Decreased
H. Bad, growing worse
I. Across
J. Blood
K. Increased

Explain these general terms:

1. Hematoma
2. Hematuria
3. Erythrocyte
4. Cardiogram
5. Dyspnea
6. Cytoscopy
7. Pathology
8. Calculus
9. Dermatitis
10. Thrombophlebitis

Match the suffix with the term.

1. -algia
2. -ectomy
3. -otomy
4. -oscopy
5. -ostomy

A. Incision and formation of an opening
B. To examine visually
C. Respiration
D. Incision
E. Pain
F. To remove

SI Units

SI units have been recommended for the standardization of clinical laboratory data. This system is based on an international system of units (Système International) proposed in 1967 and is supported by the International Committee for Standardization in Hematology. It is expected that these units will be adopted worldwide for reporting clinical laboratory data.

The SI units consist of seven dimensionally independent base units:

Quantity	Name	Symbol
Length	Meter	m
Mass	Kilogram	kg
Time	Second	s
Electrical current	Ampere	A
Temperature	Kelvin	K
Luminous intensity	Candela	cd

There are two kinds of derived units: coherent units, which are derived directly from base units without the use of conversion factors, and noncoherent units, which are constructed from the base units and which contain a numerical factor to make the numbers more convenient to use.

Examples of prefixes to denote fractions of multiple bases and derived SI units are as follows: deci 10^{-1}, centi 10^{-2}, milli 10^{-3}, micro 10^{-6}, nano 10^{-9}, pico 10^{-12}, and femto 10^{-15}.

The expression of SI units in hematology is usually straightforward, for example:

	Conventional Units	Factor	SI Units
Erythrocytes	$4.6 \times 10^{12}/\mu L$	10^6	$4.6 \times 10^{12}/L$

However, occasionally the conversion will result in a new appearing value, as in the following:

	Conventional Units	Factor	SI Units
Hemoglobin	13.5 gm/dL	0.155	2.09 mmol/L

English-Spanish Medical Phrases for the Phlebotomist

English (inglés)	Spanish (español)
Common Terms and Phrases	
Hello	¡Hola!
Good morning	Buenos días
Good afternoon	Buenas tardes
Good evening	Buenas noches
Please, come in	Por favor, pase usted
Do you speak English?	¿Habla usted inglés?
Do you speak Spanish?	¿Hablas español?
My name is	Me llamo es _____.
Who is the patient?	¿Quién es el (la) paciente?
What is your name?	¿Cómo se llama usted?
It is nice to meet you.	Mucho gusto en conocerle.
How are you?	¿Cómo está usted?
I need for you to sign this form.	Necesito que usted firme este formulario.
Please	Por favor
Thank you	Gracias
Yes	Sí
No	No
Did you come alone?	¿Vivo usted solo(a)?
Who brought you?	¿Quién le trajo?
Where were you born?	¿Dónde nació usted?
Where do you live?	¿Dónde vive usted?
What is your address?	¿Cuál es su dirección?
Specimen Collection	
I'm going to take a blood sample.	La presión sanguinea
I need to prick your finger to obtain a specimen	Necesito pincharle el dedo para obtener una muestra.
Are you comfortable?	¿Está usted confortable?
I need to apply a tourniquet around your arm.	Tengo que ponerle un torniquete alrededor del brazo.
You're going to feel a needlestick	Usted va a sentir un piquete de aguja.
This glucometer is used to measure your blood sugar.	Este glucómetro se usa para medir el azúcar en la sangre.
You need to provide a urine specimen.	Tiene usted que darnos un espécimen de orina.
Phlebotomy Complications	
Please, bend over forward.	Por favor, inclínese usted hacia atrás.
Please, lean forward	Por favor, inclínese usted hacia atrás.
Please, lie down.	Por favor, acuéstese usted.
Please, lie on your back.	Por favor, acuéstese usted boca arriba.
Do you need a blanket?	¿Necesita usted una manta (cobija)?
You can use the emesis basin if you need to vomit.	Usted puede usar esta cubeta si tiene que vomitar.

Source: McElroy OH, Grabb LL. *Spanish-English, English-Spanish Medical Dictionary*, 3rd ed, Baltimore, MD: Lippincott Williams & Wilkins, 2005; *English & Spanish Medical Words & Phrases*, 3rd ed, Springhouse, PA: Lippincott Williams & Wilkins, 2004.

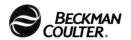

MATERIAL SAFETY DATA SHEET
Doc. ID: 628017-75 AC
Revised (year/month/day) 2008/12/03

Section 1 Company and Product Identification

Product Name	Coulter® DxH Diluent
Part Number	628017
Product Use	For In Vitro Diagnostic Use. See product literature for details.
Manufacturer	Beckman Coulter, Inc. 4300 Harbor Blvd. Fullerton, CA 92835-3100, U.S.A.
EC REP Address	Beckman Coulter Ireland Inc. Mervue Business Park Mervue, Galway, Ireland 353 91 774068
Distributor and Emergency Phone No.	Refer to attached list, Document ID: 472050, for local distributor and emergency phone numbers.

Section 2 Hazards Identification

Emergency Overview	**Colorless; Clear; Liquid; Odorless** **Nonflammable aqueous solution.** **Does not meet EU, OSHA or WHMIS criteria for hazardous materials.**
Physical Hazards	No physical hazards were determined from a review of available literature.
Potential Health Effects Summary	This product does not meet EU, OSHA or WHMIS criteria for hazardous materials.
Potential Environmental Effects	None identified.

Product Hazard Classifications	**Meets Hazardous Criteria for Preparation/Mixture**		
	EU: Not applicable	**WHMIS:** Not applicable	**US OSHA:** Not applicable

Section 3 Composition and Information on Ingredients

Hazardous Ingredients:	None

Section 4 First Aid Measures

Inhalation	If product is inhaled, move exposed individual to fresh air. If individual is not breathing, begin artificial respiration immediately and obtain medical attention.

Section 4 First Aid Measures (Continued)

Eye Contact	If product enters eyes, wash eyes gently under running water for 15 minutes or longer, making sure that the eyelids are held open. If pain or irritation occur, obtain medical attention.
Skin Contact	In case of skin contact, flush with copious amounts of water for at least 15 minutes. If pain or irritation occur, obtain medical attention.
Ingestion	If ingested, wash mouth out with water. If irritation or discomfort occurs, seek medical attention.

Section 5 Fire Fighting Measures

Flammable Properties	Nonflammable aqueous solution.
Extinguishing Media	Use extinguishing media suitable for surrounding fire.
Special Fire and Explosion Hazards	None identified.
Hazardous Combustion Products	No combustion products posing significant hazards are expected from this product (a dilute aqueous solution).
Protective Equipment for Firefighters	Self-contained breathing apparatus is recommended for firefighters in all chemical fire situations.

Section 6 Accidental Release Measures

Personal Precautions	No special precautions are necessary. Use good laboratory procedures.
Spill and Leak Procedures	Absorb spilled material with an appropriate inert, non-flammable absorbent and dispose according to local regulations.
Environmental Precautions	Contain spill to prevent migration.

Section 7 Handling and Storage

Handling Precautions	No special precautions are necessary; use good laboratory procedures.
Recommended Storage Conditions	Keep away from incompatible material (see Section 10). To maintain efficacy, store according to the instructions in the product labeling.

Section 8 Exposure Controls and Personal Protection

Exposure Limits

US OSHA:	None established
ACGIH:	None established
DFG MAK:	None established
NIOSH	None established

Section 8 Exposure Controls and Personal Protection (Continued)

Japan	None established
Engineering Controls	No special engineering controls are required. Use with good general ventilation.
Respiratory Protection	Under normal conditions, the use of this product should not require respiratory protection.
Eye Protection	Safety glasses or chemical goggles should be worn to prevent eye contact.
Skin Protection	Impervious gloves, such as Nitrile or equivalent, should be worn to prevent skin contact.

Section 9 Physical and Chemical Properties

Physical State	Liquid
Color	Colorless
Transparency	Clear
Odor	Odorless
Odor Threshold	Not applicable
pH	7.0 - 7.2
Freezing Point	Not available
Boiling Point	Not available
Flash Point	Not applicable
Evaporation Rate	Not available
Flammability (Solid, Gas)	Not applicable
Flammable Limits	Not applicable
Vapor Pressure	Not available
Vapor Density	Not available
Specific Gravity	≈ 1.02 @20°C
Solubility	
Water	Miscible
Organic	Not available
Coefficient of Water/Oil Distribution	Not available
Autoignition Temp.	Not applicable
Decomposition Temperature	Not available
Percent Volatiles	Not applicable

Section 10 Stability and Reactivity

Stability	Stable under normal temperatures and pressures.
Hazardous Incompatibilities	Strong acids Strong bases Strong oxidizers
Hazardous Decomposition Products	No decomposition products posing significant hazards would be expected from this product (a dilute aqueous solution).
Conditions to Avoid	Avoid contact with incompatible materials.

Section 11 Toxicological Information

Toxicity Data for Hazardous Ingredients	Not applicable
Primary Routes of Exposure	Eye contact, ingestion, inhalation, and skin contact.
Potential Effects of Acute Exposure	None identified.
Potential Effects of Chronic Exposure	None identified.
Symptoms of Overexposure	None identified.
Carcinogenicity	No ingredients in this product are listed as carcinogens by ACGIH, IARC, NTP, OSHA or 67/548/EEC Annex I.
Other Effects	None identified.
Conditions Aggravated by Exposure	None identified.

Section 12 Ecological Information

Ecotoxicity	No information available.
Biodegradability	No information available.
Bioaccumulation	No information available.
Mobility	No information available.
Other Adverse Effects	No information available.

Section 13 Disposal Considerations

Waste Disposal	Dispose of waste product, unused product and contaminated packaging in compliance with federal, state and local regulations. If unsure of the applicable requirements, contact the authorities for information.

Section 14 Transport Information

Transportation of this product is not regulated under ICAO, IMDG, US DOT, European ADR or Canadian TDG.

Section 15 Regulatory Information

US Federal and State Regulations

SARA 313	Magnesium Nitrate is subject to reporting requirements of Section 313, Title III of SARA.
CERCLA RG's, 40 CFR 302.4	No ingredients listed.
California Proposition 65	No ingredients listed.
Massachusetts MSL	Trisodium Nitrilotriacetate is listed. Sodium Sulfate is listed. Magnesium Nitrate is listed.
New Jersey Dept. of Health RTK List	Magnesium Nitrate is listed.
Pennsylvania RTK	Sodium Sulfate is listed. Magnesium Nitrate is listed.

EU Labeling Classification

Preparation not classified.

Canada

This product does not meet WHMIS criteria for hazardous materials.

PIN:	Not applicable
Ingredients on Ingredient Disclosure List:	None
Ingredients with unknown toxicological properties:	None

Some hazardous ingredients listed in Section 15 are below OSHAs and WHMIS' 1.0% w/w (0.1% for carcinogens) or EU's ingredient specific concentrations required for reporting in Section 3.

Section 16 Other Information		
Beckman Coulter Safety Rating	**Flammability (Section V): 0** **Health (Section XI): 1** **Reactivity with Water (Section X): 0** **Contact (Section VIII): 1**	Code 0=none 1=slight 2=caution 3=severe
Revision Changes	None	
For further information, please contact your local Beckman Coulter representative.		

WHILE BECKMAN COULTER, INC. BELIEVES THE INFORMATION CONTAINED HEREIN IS VALID AND ACCURATE, BECKMAN COULTER MAKES NO WARRANTY OR REPRESENTATION AS TO ITS VALIDITY, ACCURACY, OR CURRENCY. BECKMAN COULTER SHALL NOT BE LIABLE OR OTHERWISE RESPONSIBLE IN ANY WAY FOR USE OF EITHER THIS INFORMATION OR MATERIALS TO WHICH IT APPLIES. DISPOSAL OF HAZARDOUS MATERIALS MAY BE SUBJECT TO LOCAL LAWS OR REGULATIONS.

Printed in U.S.A.

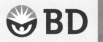

BD Vacutainer® Venous Blood Collection
Tube Guide

For the full array of BD Vacutainer® Blood Collection Tubes, visit www.bd.com/vacutainer.
Many are available in a variety of sizes and draw volumes (for pediatric applications). Refer to our website for full descriptions.

BD Vacutainer® Tubes with BD Hemogard™ Closure	BD Vacutainer® Tubes with Conventional Stopper	Additive	Inversions at Blood Collection*	Laboratory Use	Your Lab's Draw Volume/Remarks
Gold	Red/Gray	• Clot activator and gel for serum separation	5	For serum determinations in chemistry. May be used for routine blood donor screening and diagnostic testing of serum for infectious disease.** Tube inversions ensure mixing of clot activator with blood. Blood clotting time: 30 minutes.	
Light Green	Green/Gray	• Lithium heparin and gel for plasma separation	8	For plasma determinations in chemistry. Tube inversions ensure mixing of anticoagulant (heparin) with blood to prevent clotting.	
Red	Red	• Silicone coated (glass) • Clot activator, Silicone coated (plastic)	0 5	For serum determinations in chemistry. May be used for routine blood donor screening and diagnostic testing of serum for infectious disease.** Tube inversions ensure mixing of clot activator with blood. Blood clotting time: 60 minutes.	
	Orange	• BD Vacutainer® Rapid Serum Tube • Thrombin-based clot activator	5 to 6	For stat serum determinations in chemistry. Tube inversions ensure mixing of clot activator with blood. Blood clotting time: 5 minutes.	
Orange		• Thrombin-based clot activator	8	For stat serum determinations in chemistry. Tube inversions ensure mixing of clot activator with blood. Blood clotting time: 5 minutes.	
Royal Blue		• Clot activator (plastic serum) • K_2EDTA (plastic)	8 8	For trace-element, toxicology, and nutritional-chemistry determinations. Special stopper formulation provides low levels of trace elements (see package insert). Tube inversions ensure mixing of either clot activator or anticoagulant (EDTA) with blood.	
Green	Green	• Sodium heparin • Lithium heparin	8 8	For plasma determinations in chemistry. Tube inversions ensure mixing of anticoagulant (heparin) with blood to prevent clotting.	
Gray	Gray	• Potassium oxalate/sodium fluoride • Sodium fluoride/Na_2 EDTA • Sodium fluoride (serum tube)	8 8 8	For glucose determinations. Oxalate and EDTA anticoagulants will give plasma samples. Sodium fluoride is the antiglycolytic agent. Tube inversions ensure proper mixing of additive with blood.	
Tan		• K_2EDTA (plastic)	8	For lead determinations. This tube is certified to contain less than .01 µg/mL(ppm) lead. Tube inversions prevent clotting.	
	Yellow	• Sodium polyanethol sulfonate (SPS) • Acid citrate dextrose additives (ACD): **Solution A -** 22.0 g/L trisodium citrate, 8.0 g/L citric acid, 24.5 g/L dextrose **Solution B -** 13.2 g/L trisodium citrate, 4.8 g/L citric acid, 14.7 g/L dextrose	8 8 8	SPS for blood culture specimen collections in microbiology. ACD for use in blood bank studies, HLA phenotyping, and DNA and paternity testing. Tube inversions ensure mixing of anticoagulant with blood to prevent clotting.	

(continued)

BD Vacutainer® Tubes with BD Hemogard™ Closure	BD Vacutainer® Tubes with Conventional Stopper	Additive	Inversions at Blood Collection*	Laboratory Use	Your Lab's Draw Volume/Remarks
Lavender	Lavender	• Liquid K_3EDTA (glass) • Spray-coated K_2EDTA (plastic)	8 8	K_2EDTA and K_3EDTA for whole blood hematology determinations. K_2EDTA may be used for routine immunohematology testing, and blood donor screening.*** Tube inversions ensure mixing of anticoagulant (EDTA) with blood to prevent clotting.	
White		• BD Vacutainer® PPT™ Tube • K_2EDTA with gel	8	For use in molecular diagnostic test methods (such as, but not limited to, polymerase chain reaction [PCR] and/or branched DNA [bDNA] amplification techniques.) Tube inversions ensure mixing of anticoagulant (EDTA) with blood to prevent clotting.	
Pink	Pink	• Spray-coated K_2EDTA (plastic)	8	For whole blood hematology determinations. May be used for routine immunohematology testing and blood donor screening.*** Designed with special cross-match label for patient information required by the AABB. Tube inversions prevent clotting.	
Light Blue / Clear	Light Blue	• Buffered sodium citrate 0.105 M (≈3.2%) glass 0.109 M (3.2%) plastic • Citrate, theophylline, adenosine, dipyridamole (CTAD)	3-4 3-4	For coagulation determinations. CTAD for selected platelet function assays and routine coagulation determination. Tube inversions ensure mixing of anticoagulant (citrate) to prevent clotting.	
Clear	Red/ Light Gray (New)	• None (plastic)	0	For use as a discard tube or secondary specimen tube.	

Note: BD Vacutainer® Tubes for pediatric and partial draw applications can be found on our website.

BD Diagnostics
Preanalytical Systems
1 Becton Drive
Franklin Lakes, NJ 07417 USA

BD Global Technical Services: 1.800.631.0174
BD Customer Service: 1.888.237.2762
www.bd.com/vacutainer

* Invert gently, do not shake
** The performance characteristics of these tubes have not been established for infectious disease testing in general; therefore, users must validate the use of these tubes for their specific assay-instrument/reagent system combinations and specimen storage conditions.
*** The performance characteristics of these tubes have not been established for immunohematology testing in general; therefore, users must validate the use of these tubes for their specific assay-instrument/reagent system combinations and specimen storage conditions.

Printed in USA   1/10   VS5229-11

(Courtesy and © Becton, Dickinson and Company.)

ADH	antidiuretic hormone	HMWK	high-molecular-weight kininogen
AGT	antiglobulin test	IAT	indirect antiglobulin test
AHG	antihuman globulin	IF	intrinsic factor
AIDS	acquired immune deficiency syndrome	Ig	immunoglobulin
ANA	antinuclear antibody	IL	interleukin
APTT	activated partial thromboplastin time	IM	infectious mononucleosis
ASCLS	American Society for Clinical Laboratory Science	IU	international unit
ASCP	American Society of Clinical Pathologists	IV	intravenous
ASO	antistreptolysin O	JCH	The Joint Commission
CAP	College of American Pathologists	L	liter
CBC	complete blood count	LAP	leukocyte alkaline phosphatase
CDC	Centers for Disease Control and Prevention	M	meter
CFU	colony-forming unit	MCH	mean cell hemoglobin
CLIA '88	Clinical Laboratory Improvement Amendments of 1988	MCHC	mean cell hemoglobin concentration
		MCV	mean cell volume
CLT	clinical laboratory technician	MPV	mean platelet volume
COLA	Commission on Office Laboratory Accreditation	MSDS	material safety data sheets
CSF	colony stimulating factor; cerebrospinal fluid	MT	medical technologist
DAT	direct antihuman globulin test	NAD	nicotinamide adnine dinucleotide, oxidized form
DIC	disseminated intravascular coagulation	NADH	nicotinamide adenine dinucleotide, reduced form
DNA	deoxyribonucleic acid	OSHA	Occupational Safety and Health Administration
EA	early antigen	PCV	packed cell volume
EBV	Epstein-Barr virus	PEP	post-exposure prophylaxis
EDTA	ethylenediaminetetraacetic acid	PKK	plasma prekallikrein
EIA	enzyme immunoassay	PMN	polymorphonuclear neutrophil
ELISA	enzyme-linked immunosorbent assay; enzyme-labeled immunosorbent assay	PT	prothrombin time
		PTT	partial thromboplastin time
ESR	erythrocyte sedimentation rate	QA	quality assurance
FIA	fluorescence immunoassay	QC	quality control
FISH	fluorescent iin situ hybridization	RBC	red blood cell
HBV	hepatitis B virus	RDW	red cell distribution width
Hct (or Ht)	hematocrit	SI	International System of Units
HCV	hepatitis C virus; previously called non-A, non-B hepatitis virus	SLE	systemic lupus erythematosus
		SPIA	solid-phase immunosorbent assay
HDN	hemolytic disease of newborn	TLC	thin-layer chromatography
Hgb	hemoglobin	TT	thrombin time
HHS	Department of Health and Human Services	vWD	von Willebrandís disease
HIV	human immunodeficiency virus	vWF	von Willebrandís factor
HLA	human leukocyte antigen	WBC	white blood cell

GLOSSARY

A

absolute lymphocytosis – an increase in the total number of lymphocytes in the circulating blood. Seen in viral infections such as infectious mononucleosis and rubella (German measles)

absolute polycythemia – see *secondary polycythemia*

absolute reticulocyte count – see *corrected reticulocyte count*

absorbance – optical density

accuracy – describes how close a test result is to the true value

actomyosin (thrombosthenin) – a contractile protein found in platelets

acute – severe and of short duration

adenopathy – swelling of the lymph nodes

adhesiveness – in coagulation, the process of platelets sticking to the blood vessel wall

ADP – adenosine diphosphate

agammaglobulinemia – the absence or severe decrease of the gamma globulin protein fraction in the blood

agglutination – clumping of cells

agglutinin – an antibody produced in response to a specific antigen (foreign substance)

aggregation – in blood coagulation, the process in which platelets stick or clump together

Alder-Reilly inclusions – abnormal purple-red particles representing precipitated mucopolysaccharides thatare seen primarily in neutrophilic, eosinophilic, and basophilic leukocytes

aleukemic leukemia – a form of leukemia in which little change is seen in the total leukocyte count or cellular maturity in the peripheral blood. An increased number of immature cells can be found in the bone marrow

alkaline – a basic solution (pH 7.1 to 14.0) with the ability to neutralize acids

ALL – acute lymphoblastic leukemia

allele – one of two or more genes that occur at the same locus on homologous chromosomes

alpha granule – a type of storage granule found in the mature platelet

amplitude – height or magnitude

amyloidosis – the abnormal deposition of amyloid, a protein, in various tissues

anaphase – a stage in cellular division (mitosis)

anaphylaxis – a severe and often life-threatening reaction to a foreign protein

anaplasia – highly pleomorphic and bizarre cytologic features associated with malignant tumors that are poorly differentiated

anemia – a condition of decreased or dysfunctional erythrocytes

anemia of chronic inflammation – a term used to describe anemia associated with inflammation, chronic infection, malignancy, or various systemic diseases. Also known as anemia of chronic diseases (ACD)

angina – any condition characterized by spasmodic feelings of suffocation

anisochromia – variation of the color of erythrocytes caused by unequal hemoglobin concentration

anisocytosis – a general term used to denote an increased variation in cell size

ANLL – acute nonlymphoblastic leukemia

anomaly – a significant deviation from normal

anorexia – loss of appetite

anoxia – without oxygen. The reduction of oxygen in the tissues below physiological levels

antibody – an immunoglobulin produced in response to an antigen

antihemophilic factor – factor VIII

anti–human globulin test (AHG) – previously referred to as the Coombs' test. May be either a direct or an indirect test to detect the presence of antibodies on erythrocytes (direct test) or the presence of antibodies capable of coating erythrocytes (indirect test)

antithrombin III – an alpha-2 globulin that circulates in the plasma

apoferritin – a protein that combines with iron to form ferritin

appendicular skeleton – the bones of the limbs of the body

APTT – activated partial thromboplastin time

argon – an inert gas used in lasers

arteries – distributing blood vessels that leave the heart

arterioles – microscopic continuations of arteries that give off branches called metarterioles, which in turn join the capillaries

arthritide – an eruption of the skin caused by gout

arthrocentesis – entry into a joint cavity to aspirate fluid

arthrography – radiographic (x-ray) study of a joint

artifact – any artificial particles seen in stained preparations, diluting fluids, etc

aspirate – the process of physically removing, usually with a syringe, fluid from a body cavity or space

assay – the determination of the purity of a substance or the amount of a particular substance in a mixture or compound

ATP – adenosine triphosphate

atrophy – a decrease in the number or size of cells that produces a reduction in the size of a normal organ or tissue

atypical antibody – an antibody not usually found in the blood plasma. Also referred to as an alloantibody

Auer rods or Auer bodies – these cellular inclusions are aggregates of cytoplasmic granules that appear as red, elongated structures. They may occur alone or in groups in myeloblasts and occasionally monoblasts

autoantibody – antibodies capable of reacting with one's own cells. In autoimmune hemolytic anemia, patients develop antibodies that produce hemolysis of the patient's own cells

autosomal dominant – a genetic trait that expresses itself, if present, and is carried on one of the chromosome pairs 1 through 22

axial skeleton – the bones of the head and trunk of the body

azurophilic granules – granules that stain red due to azure dyes

B

B cell disease – disorders associated with B-type lymphocytes such as CLL

B cells or B lymphocytes – the primary source of cells responsible for antibody responses

bacteremia – a bacterial infection of the blood

base pair – a nucleotide (either adenine, guanine, cytosine, thymidine, or uracil) and its complementary base on the opposite strand

basic calcium phosphate (BCP) – a type of crystal that can be seen in joint (synovial) fluid

basophilia – an abnormal increase in the number of erythrocytes with a blue appearance. The presence of fine, evenly distributed basophilic granules is referred to as polychromatophilia in Wright-stained blood smears

basophilic granules – blue-staining granules

BCP – see *basic calcium phosphate*

Bence Jones protein – the abnormal protein frequently found in the urine of patients with multiple myeloma. It precipitates at 50°C, disappears at 100°C, and reappears on cooling to room temperature

benign – nonmalignant or noncancerous

Bernard-Soulier syndrome – a disorder characterized by the largest platelets seen in a platelet disorder

beta-thalassemia – a form of anemia in which beta chain synthesis is impaired

bilirubin – a breakdown product of heme from hemoglobin

biliverdin – a breakdown product arising from the oxidation of bilirubin

bit map – a polygonal figure with as many as 16 sides drawn around the cells to be analyzed or sorted in flow-cell cytometry

blast – the most immature form of a cell

blast crisis – the dominance of immature blood cells in the blood or bone marrow of patients with a treated leukemia previously in remission

Blood–brain barrier – walls of blood vessels of the central nervous system that prevent or delay the entry of certain blood substances into the brain tissue

blotting – transfer or fixation of nucleic acids onto a solid matrix, such as nitrocellulose, so that they may be hybridized with a probe

bone marrow – the material in the cavities of bones. Red marrow is the site of hematopoiesis

buffer solution – a solution that will resist sudden changes in acidity or alkalinity

buffy coat – the interface layer in a tube of anticoagulated blood between the plasma and erythrocytes. This layer contains leukocytes and thrombocytes

burst-forming unit-erythroid – the most primitive identifiable unipotent erythroid stem cell in primitive fetal cells

C

Cabot rings – ring-shaped, figure-eight, or loop-shaped inclusions seen in stained erythrocytes

calcium pyrophosphate dihydrate – an abnormal crystal found in joint (synovial) fluid

calibration – the comparison of an instrument measurement or reading to a known physical constant

CAP – College of American Pathologists

capillaries – a unit of the microcirculation that functions as the link between the arterial and venous blood circulation

capillary blood – blood obtained from the capillaries of sites such as the fingertip, toe, or heel

catecholamines – biologically active amines such as epinephrine that are derived from the amino acid tyrosine

CDC – Centers for Disease Control and Prevention

cDNA – complementary DNA, produced from mRNA using reverse transcriptase

celiac disease – an uncommon malabsorption syndrome (also known as nontropical sprue) characterized by an inability to digest and utilize fats, starches, and sugars

cell coincidence error – more than one cell passing through the aperture of an impedance cell-counting instrument at the same time

centrioles – a pair of central spots inside the centrosome

centrosome – the area of the cell where the cytoplasm is homogeneous, where there are no mitochondria, and where there are two tiny spots at the center

cerebrospinal fluid – a fluid formed continuously in the choroid plexus of the cerebral ventricles. It is found in the subarachnoid space, four ventricles of the brain, and the central canal of the spinal cord

CFU-E – colony-forming units-erythroid

CFU-GEMM – colony-forming-unit-granulocytes-erythrocyte-macrophage-megakaryocyte

CFU-GM – colony-forming-unit-granulocyte-macrophage

CH – constant region of the immunoglobulin heavy chain gene locus

channel analyzer – a device in which individual pulses are categorized into specific-sized channels forming a histogram, with size on the x-axis and frequency on the y-axis

Charcot-Leyden crystals – colorless, hexagonal, needle-like crystals derived from disintegrating eosinophils. Found in sputum, bronchial secretions, and feces

Chédiak-Higashi anomaly – a rare inherited autosomal recessive trait that is characterized by the presence of large granules and inclusion bodies in the cytoplasm of leukocytes. The leukocytic neutrophils display impaired chemotaxis and delayed killing of ingested bacteria

chemotaxis – the release of substances that attract phagocytic cells as the result of traumatic or microbial damage

chloroma – a malignant tumor arising from myeloid tissue

chromatid – half of a chromosome pair bound together in duplicate during cell division

chromatin – the network of small fibers in the nucleus of a cell

chromoprotein – a conjugated protein having respiratory functions (e.g., hemoglobin)

chromosomes – structures consisting of DNA wrapped around a protein core that are visible in the nucleus of a cell during cell division

chronic – gradual or of long duration

chronic granulomatous disease – a sex-linked autosomal recessive genetic disorder that produces defective phagocytosis because the cells are unable to destroy previously engulfed bacteria

circulating anticoagulants – abnormal substances that can produce bleeding

CLL – chronic lymphocytic leukemia

clone – daughter cells descended from the same single cell, all having identical phenotypes and growth characteristics as the original precursor cell

coefficient of variation – a statistical term denoting the precision of results

coincidence – in automated impedance cell counting, if more than one cell is within the boundaries of the aperture at the same time, only a single pulse is counted

cold agglutinins – antibodies in the plasma that react best at 0° to 20°C

collagen – a protein found in skin, tendons, bone, and cartilage

collagen disease – diseases of the skin, tendons, bone, and cartilage, such as systemic lupus erythematosus and rheumatoid arthritis

colony-stimulating growth factor – a soluble substance that promotes cell growth

combined scatter histogram – a type of histogram that includes both forward- and right-angle scatter information

constitutional aplastic anemia – a congenital or genetic predisposition to bone marrow failure

contact group – blood coagulation factors XI and XII, prekallikrein (Fletcher factor), and high-molecular-weight kininogen (Fitzgerald factor)

control (n.) – a specimen for which the value is known that is used for comparison with the unknown specimen

control (v.) – to keep within limits

Cooley's anemia – thalassemia major is usually equivalent to beta thalassemia in a homozygous form and is sometimes called Cooley's anemia

Coombs' test – see anti–human globulin test

coproporphyrin – a porphyrin formed in the intestine from bilirubin. Abnormal amounts may be found in the urine in some forms of anemia

cord blood – blood obtained from the umbilical vessels at birth

corrected reticulocyte count – a mathematical adjustment of the reticulocyte count to account for variations caused by erythrocyte quantity

Coulter principle – a method of cell counting and volumetric sizing based on the detection and measurement of changes in electrical resistance produced by a particle, suspended in a conductive liquid, traversing a small aperture

counterstain – a stain used to enhance a previously applied primary stain

CPPD – see calcium pyrophosphate dihydrate

cryoglobulin – a serum globulin that precipitates, gels, or crystallizes spontaneously at low temperatures. May be found in multiple myeloma and collagen disease

crystalline inclusions – rod-shaped deposits of IgG

CSF – (A) refers to colony-stimulating factor, a specific glycoprotein macromolecule that stimulates the growth of granulocytes and macrophage cells; (B) an abbreviation for cerebrospinal fluid

curve-fitting – in computerized automated instruments, the instrument's computer process of fitting a log-normal curve to the platelet raw data

cytochemical stains – staining reactions that produce a colored precipitate from a specific insoluble compound in a cell

cytochemistry – the identification of specific types of molecules in a cell

cytogenetics – the branch of genetics concerned with the cellular elements of heredity

cytokinesis – cytoplasmic division during cellular division (mitosis)

cytological – refers to cells

cytology – the study of cells

cytomegalovirus infection – a herpes-family virus that can cause congenital infections in the newborn and a clinical syndrome resembling infectious mononucleosis

D

degranulation – the loss of granules such as in the basophil when an antigen binds to two adjacent IgE antibody molecules located on the surface of mast cells

deletion – a chromosomal aberration in which a segment of a chromosome is lost

delta granule – a type of storage granule found in the mature platelet

de novo – a newly presented, primary case of a disorder or disease

denaturation – the process of treating a protein with agents such as heat or acid and causing it to lose its native properties because of disruption of secondary and tertiary bonding such as hydrogen bonds

denatured DNA – double-stranded helix separates into two single strands, breaking hydrogen bonds; caused by changes in temperature, pH, or nonphysiological concentrations of salt, detergents, or organic solvents

deoxyhemoglobin – reduced hemoglobin

deoxyribonucleic acid – DNA

DH – diversity region of the immunoglobulin heavy chain gene locus

diabetes mellitus – a disorder of carbohydrate metabolism caused by an insufficiency of insulin

diagnosis – determination of the nature of a disorder or disease

dialysate – the soluble materials and fluids (e.g., water) that pass through a semipermeable membrane

diapedesis – ameboid movement of cells

DIC – this is a serious coagulation disorder that consumes platelets and blood coagulation factors. It is an example of a major breakdown of the hemostatic mechanism that occurs when the procoagulant factors outweigh the anticoagulant system

Disseminated intravascular coagulation – this is a serious coagulation disorder that consumes platelets and blood coagulation factors. It is an example of a major breakdown of the hemostatic mechanism that occurs when the procoagulant factors outweigh the anticoagulant system

diverticulitis – inflammation of the small blind pouches that form in the lining or wall of the colon

DNA – deoxyribonucleic acid

Döhle bodies (Amato bodies) – abnormal inclusion bodies that appear as light-blue–staining vacuoles predominantly in neutrophils in viral diseases and other toxic conditions

Down syndrome – a chromosomal abnormality. Previously referred to as mongolism

Downey cells – an early classification system of certain forms of variant lymphocytes. Downey I types have many vacuoles in the cytoplasm; Downey II types resemble plasma cells; Downey III types are an immature form of lymphocyte

DPG – diphosphoglycerate (2,3-DPG) combines with the beta chains of deoxyhemoglobin and diminishes the molecule's affinity for oxygen

drumsticks – an appendage of nuclear material attached to the nucleus of a segmented neutrophil. May be seen in some cells in women

DsDNA – double-stranded DNA

dyscrasia – an abnormal or pathological condition of the blood

dyserythropoiesis – defective red blood cell maturation

dysgranulopoiesis – defective white blood cell maturation

dysmegapoiesis karyocyte – defective platelet maturation

dysplasia – (adj. dysplastic) abnormal development (e.g., defective cellular development). Abnormal cytological features and tissue organization, often is a premalignant change

dyspnea – difficulty in breathing

dyspoiesis – an abnormality in the development of blood cells

dyspoietic syndrome – a combination of defective and disrupted cell line development

E

EAC – erythrocyte-antibody-complement rosette test

eclampsia – a toxic condition of pregnancy

edema – an abnormal accumulation of fluid in the body's intercellular spaces

EDTA (K3 EDTA) – tripotassium ethylenediaminetetraacetate. A commonly used anticoagulant in blood collection

electrical impedance principle – a method of cell counting and sizing based on the detection and measurement of changes in electrical resistance

elution – Removal of antibodies from the erythrocytes that they are coating or bound to

Embden-Meyerhof glycolytic pathway – the major, anaerobic, energy-yielding pathway associated with the breakdown of glucose in erythrocytes (glycolysis)

embryonic hemoglobin – primitive hemoglobins such as Gower I, Gower II, and Portland that are formed in the yolk sac

endocarditis – an inflammation of the lining membrane of the heart

endocytosis – the process in which specialized cells engulf particles and molecules, with the subsequent formation of membrane-bound vacuoles within the cytoplasm

endoplasmic reticulum (ER) – an extensive, lacelike network composed of pairs of membranes enclosing interconnecting cavities or cisternae

endoreduplication (endomitosis) – the process that occurs in the megakaryocyte during early maturation. In this process, chromosomal materials (DNA) and the other events of mitosis occur without subsequent division of the cytoplasmic membrane into identical daughter cells

endothelial cells or endothelium – simple squamous epithelium that lines blood and lymphatic vessels and the heart

endothelial dysfunction – nonadaptive changes in endothelial structure and function provoked by pathophysiological stimuli

enzyme-linked immunosorbent assay (ELISA) – technique in which an enzyme is complexed to an antigen or antibody and a substrate added that generates a color proportional to the amount of binding

enzymopathy – a pathological enzyme deficiency

eosin – an acidic stain that stains some cytoplasmic structures of the cell an orange-red color. The red-staining structures are acidophilic or eosinophilic substances

eosinophilic granules – orange-staining granules found in a specific leukocyte type

ependyma – the membrane lining the cerebral ventricles and the central canal of the spinal cord

epidemiology – the study of infectious diseases or conditions in many individuals in the same geographical location at the same time

epinephrine – a hormone produced by the adrenal medulla that acts as a vasoconstrictor

EPO – erythropoietin

Epstein-Barr virus – the virus associated with the development of infectious mononucleosis in western countries and Burkitt's lymphoma in Africa

erythrocyte – refers to red blood cells

erythroleukemia – a form of leukemia that is usually acute and represents the overproliferation of both immature granulocytic and erythrocytic cell types

erythropoiesis – the process of red blood cell (erythrocyte) production

erythropoietin – a glycoprotein hormone (mol wt 46,000) that stimulates erythropoiesis. It is produced mainly by the kidneys in response to tissue hypoxia

ESR – erythrocyte sedimentation rate. Also referred to as sed rate

etiology – the study of the cause(s) of disease

euchromatin – chromatin that is rich in nucleic acid, is genetically active, and stains lightly. It is considered to be partially or fully uncoiled

extramedullary hematopoiesis – the formation and development of blood cells outside the bone marrow in sites such as the liver and spleen

extravascular destruction – the destruction of an erythrocyte through phagocytosis and digestion by macrophages of the mononuclear phagocyte system

extrinsic pathway – the initiation of blood clotting begins with either the extrinsic or the intrinsic pathway. The extrinsic pathway is activated by the entry into the blood of phospholipoproteins and organelle membranes from disrupted tissue cells

F

FAB – French-American-British classification

familial polycythemia – an unusual genetic disorder that produces a defect in the regulation of erythropoietin production

ferritin – a storage form of iron

fibrin – a meshy protein clot formed by the action of thrombin on fibrinogen

fibrinogen – blood coagulation factor I

fibrinogen group – factors I, V, VIII, and XIII; clotting factors

fibrinolysis – the dissolution of a fibrin clot

fibrin-stabilizing factor – factor XIII

filamin – a contractile protein found in platelets

Fitzgerald factor – high-molecular-weight kininogen

fixed macrophages – macrophages that line the endothelium of capillaries, the bone marrow, and the sinuses of the spleen and lymph nodes

Fletcher factor – prekallikrein

folic acid – one of the vitamins of the B complex

folic acid antagonists – substances that inhibit the synthesis of folic acid

French-American-British classification – FAB classification

frequency distribution – the grouping of data in classes and determination of the number of observations that fall in each of the classes

G

G phase – the gap period in cellular division referred to as a part of interphase (e.g., G_1, G_2, G_0)

gastric mucosa – the lining membrane of the stomach

Gaucher's disease – a monocytic disorder that represents a deficiency of the enzyme beta-glucosidase, which normally splits glucose from its parent sphingolipid, glucosylceramide

gaussian distribution – a symmetrical bell-shaped curve

gene – the functional unit of the chromosome that is usually responsible for the structure of a single protein or polypeptide

genetics – the study of the transmission of inherited characteristics

genotype – the total genetic composition of an individual

Giemsa stain – a Romanowsky-type blood stain

gingival hyperplasia – excessive proliferation of gum tissue, often producing a white appearance

Glanzmann's thrombasthenia – a blood coagulation disorder characterized by a failure of platelets to aggregate in response to all aggregating agents

glial cells – certain cells of the brain

glycocalyx – a fluffy outer coat that surrounds the platelet's cellular membrane

glycogen – a long-chain polysaccharide composed of repeating units of glucose

glycosylated hemoglobin – a subfraction of normal hemoglobin that is formed during the maturation of the erythrocyte

Golgi apparatus – a horseshoe-shaped or hook-shaped cellular organelle with an associated stock of vesicles or sacs

gout – a form of arthritis characterized by excessive quantities of uric acid in the blood, with possible deposition in the joints and other tissues

granulocytes – segmented neutrophils, band neutrophils, metamyelocytes, basophils, and eosinophils

granulocytic kinetics – the collective term for the development, distribution, and destruction of neutrophils, eosinophils, and basophils

grape cell (Mott's cell) – a plasma cell whose cytoplasm contains inclusions that are transparent blue sacs or crystal-like in nature

H

Hageman factor – factor XII

haptoglobin – a plasma globulin that binds with the alpha-beta dimers of hemoglobin

Hb – hemoglobin

Hct – hematocrit or packed cell volume (PCV)

Heinz bodies – an accumulation in the erythrocyte of oxidized glutathione that forms an insoluble complex with hemoglobin because of the absence of NADPH

hemachromatosis – a condition acquired or hereditary, of iron overload and excessive accumulation in various tissues and organs

hemagglutination inhibition – the prevention of erythrocyte clumping

hematology – the study of blood

hematoma – accumulation of blood in the tissues or space in the body

hematopoiesis – (adj. hematopoietic) The formation and development of blood cells, chiefly in the bone marrow

hematopoietic dysplasia – see *myelodysplastic syndrome*

hematuria – blood in the urine

heme – an iron-bearing compound that is the nonprotein pigment portion of the hemoglobin molecule. It is responsible for oxygen and carbon dioxide transport

hemochromatosis – a disorder of iron metabolism characterized by the deposition of excessive iron in the tissues

hemoglobin A – the major form of normal adult hemoglobin

hemoglobin electrophoresis – a separation method of hemoglobin fractions based on the principle that hemoglobin molecules in an alkaline solution have a net negative charge and move toward the anode in an electrophoretic system

hemoglobin F – fetal hemoglobin. The predominant hemoglobin variety in the fetus and neonate

hemoglobin S – sickle-type hemoglobin found in sickle cell anemia and/or sickle cell trait

hemoglobinemia – the presence of free hemoglobin (not membrane-enclosed) in the blood plasma

hemoglobinopathies – inherited (genetic) defects related to hemoglobin. These defects may result in an abnormal structure of the hemoglobin molecule or a deficiency in the synthesis of normal adult hemoglobin

hemoglobinuria – free hemoglobin in the urine

hemolysin – a substance that liberates hemoglobin from erythrocytes

hemolytic disease of the newborn – a disorder seen in unborn and newborn infants if maternal antibodies that correspond to fetal erythrocytes pass through the placental barrier

hemophilia A – classic hemophilia. A hereditary disorder that produces factor VIII deficiency

hemophilia B – Christmas disease. A hereditary disorder that produces factor IX deficiency

hemophilia C – a hereditary disease that produces factor XI deficiency

hemosiderin – granular, iron-rich, brown pigment found in body tissues

hemosiderinuria – the presence of granular, iron-rich, brown pigment in the urine

hemostasis – the stoppage of bleeding from a blood vessel

heparin – an anticoagulant that acts as an antithrombin

hepatomegaly – excessive enlargement of the liver

hepatosplenomegaly – an enlarged liver and spleen

Hermansky-Pudlak syndrome – a blood coagulation disorder characterized by storage granule abnormalities of the platelets (thrombocytes)

heterochromatin – a type of chromatin that is tightly coiled, assumes a dark stain, and is genetically inactive

heterogeneous – dissimilar

heterozygous – in genetics, possessing the alternate characteristics on a pair of homologous chromosomes

hexose monophosphate shunt – this ancillary energy-yielding system is also referred to as the oxidative pathway. The system couples oxidative metabolism with pyridine nucleotide and glutathione reduction

high-molecular-weight kininogen – Fitzgerald factor

histogram – a pictorial display of frequency and class limits of a sample

Hodgkin's disease – a major form of malignant lymphoma

hof – the area of the cell cytoplasm encircled by the concavity of the nucleus

homeostasis – the tendency of a biological system to maintain equilibrium or balance

homogeneous – uniform or same

homozygous – in genetics, when the genes for a trait on homologous chromosomes are the same

Howell-Jolly bodies – very coarse, round, solid-staining dark-blue to purple DNA remnants seen in abnormal erythrocytes

HTLV (human T cell leukemia virus) – this virus family is associated with T cell leukemia, hairy cell leukemia, and acquired immune deficiency syndrome (AIDS)

hybridization – interaction between two single-stranded nucleic acid molecules to form a double-stranded molecule

hydrophilic – water-attracting

hydrophobic – water-repelling

hypercoagulable state – an increase in the likelihood of blood to clot in vivo

hyperplasia – excessive tissue growth or cellular multiplication

hypersegmentation – an abnormal condition in which more than five nuclear segments are observed in segmented neutrophils

hypertension – increased blood pressure

hypertrophy – increase in the size of cells that produces an enlargement of tissue mass or organ size

hypervolemia – an increased total blood volume

hypochromia – when the central pallor of erythrocytes exceeds one third of the cell's diameter

hypolobulation – a condition of neutrophils in which normal segmentation fails to occur

hypoproliferative disorders – a term that may be substituted for the reduced growth or production of cells, particularly erythrocytes

hypothyroidism – decreased thyroid activity

hypoxia – a decrease of oxygen in the body tissues

I

idiopathic – a disorder or disease without an identifiable external etiology, or self-originated

immune deficiency disease – a defect in the ability to detect antigens and/or to produce antibodies against foreign antigens

immunity – the process of being protected against foreign antigens

immunocompetent – the ability to recognize and respond to a foreign antigen

immunodeficiency – a dysfunction in the body defense mechanism that detects foreign antigens and produces antibodies against them

immunoglobulin – a protein belonging to the gamma globulin fraction. Immunoglobulins are divided into five classes, with IgG being the most abundant

immunological dysfunction – refers to immune deficiency disease

incidence – the frequency of an occurrence, for example, a disease

infarct – an area of necrosis in a tissue due to obstruction of the blood circulation

infectious mononucleosis – a benign lymphoproliferative disorder

inflammation – tissue reaction to injury caused by physical or chemical agents, including microorganisms. Symptoms include redness, tenderness, pain, and swelling

interleukins – soluble protein molecules that work with hematopoietic growth factors to stimulate proliferation and differentiation of specific blood cell lines

intravascular destruction – an alternate pathway for erythrocyte breakdown that normally accounts for less than 10% of red cell destruction

intrinsic factor (IF) – substance secreted by the parietal cells of the mucosa in the fundus region of the stomach

intrinsic pathway – the initiation of blood clotting begins with either the intrinsic or the extrinsic pathway. In the intrinsic pathway, coagulation begins with the activation of factor XII to XIIa

in vitro – in the test tube or outside the body

in vivo – within the living organism

iso – equal. Isotonic saline solution has a concentration of 0.85%, which is equal to the concentration of sodium chloride in cellular cytoplasm

isoimmune – possessing antibodies to antigens of the same system

isolation technique – precautions used to prevent the transmission of disease either to or from a patient or patient specimen

J

jaundice – a yellow appearance of the skin, sclerae, and body excretions

JCAHO – The Joint Commission on Accreditation of Healthcare Organizations

JH – joining region of the immunoglobulin heavy chain gene locus

K

kallikrein – activated Fletcher factor

karyokinesis – the division of the nuclear membrane during cellular division

karyorrhexis – a stage of cellular degeneration when chromatin is distributed irregularly throughout the cytoplasm

karyotype – the full complement of chromosomes in an organism

kb – kilobase pairs, 1,000 bases

kinins – small biologically active peptides

Kleihauer-Betke test – a semiquantitative test for fetal hemoglobin

krypton – an inert gas used in lasers

Kupffer's cells – cells in the liver that have the ability to engulf or phagocytize foreign particles as part of the mononuclear phagocytic system

kwashiorkor – a severe protein deficiency seen in infants and children

L

labile – unstable

lambda – equivalent to microliter (μL) or 1/1,000 of a milliliter (mL)

LAP – leukocyte alkaline phosphatase cytochemical stain

laparotomy – incision in the abdomen

Laser – *l*ight *a*mplification by *s*timulated *e*mission of *r*adiation

LDH – lactic dehydrogenase

leukemia – a neoplastic proliferative disease characterized by an overproduction of immature or mature cells of various leukocyte types in the bone marrow or peripheral blood

leukemoid reaction – an assay used to differentiate chronic myelogenous leukemia from a severe infection or inflammation that resembles leukemia

leukocyte – white blood cell

leukocytosis – a significant increase in the total white cell count

leukopenia – a severe decrease in the total white cell count

leukotrienes – a newly identified class of compounds that mediate the inflammatory functions of leukocytes

Levy-Jennings chart – a quality control chart used to graphically display the assay values of controls versus time

LIF – leukocytosis-inducing factor. A regulator that influences the release of neutrophils from the bone marrow into the circulatory system

lipids – one of the three major biochemical classes. This class includes the fatty acids and steroids

lipophilic dyes – stains with an affinity for fatty substances

liquefaction – the process of conversion into liquid form

Luebering-Rapaport pathway – an important oxygen-carrying pathway of erythrocytes that permits the accumulation of 2,3-DPG

lymphadenopathy – disease of the lymph nodes

lymphoblastic leukemia – a major form of leukemia characterized by the presence of increased numbers of immature lymphocytes in the peripheral blood, bone marrow, and lymph nodes

lymphocyte recirculation – the free movement of lymphocytes between the blood and lymphoid tissue

lymphocytes – a type of leukocyte

lymphocytopenia – a severe decrease in the total number of lymphocytes in the peripheral blood

lymphocytosis – a significant increase in the total number of lymphocytes in the peripheral blood

lymphoma – solid, malignant tumors of the lymph nodes and associated tissues or bone marrow

lymphoproliferative disorders – a group of diseases characterized by the proliferation of lymphoid tissues and/or lymphocytes

lymphosarcoma – malignant neoplastic disorders of the lymphoid tissues, excluding Hodgkin's disease

lyse – to break apart or dissolve

lysosomes – cytoplasmic organelles that contain lytic enzymes

M

M phase – the phase of cellular division in which the cell actually divides

macroglobulin – a high-molecular-weight protein of the globulin type

macrophage – a large mononuclear phagocytic cell of the tissues that exists either as a fixed type that lines the capillaries and sinuses of organs such as the bone marrow, spleen, and lymph nodes, or as a wandering type

malabsorption syndrome – impaired absorption of nutrients in the intestine

malaise – a general feeling of tiredness or discomfort

malignant – cancerous

manifestation – the display of symptoms of a disease or disorder

marginating pool – the granulocytes that adhere to the vascular endothelium

marrow reserve – the segmented neutrophils in the maturation-storage compartment

mast cells – tissue basophils

maturation-storage compartment – the stage following the proliferative stage. The site where metamyelocytes, band neutrophils, and a portion of segmented neutrophils are stored

Maurer's dots – red dots seen in stained erythrocytes infected with the malaria parasite *Plasmodium falciparum*

May-Hegglin anomaly – an abnormal genetic condition characterized by the presence of Döhle body–like inclusions in neutrophils, eosinophils, and monocytes. Abnormally large platelets and thrombocytopenia frequently coexist in this condition

MCH – mean corpuscular hemoglobin of an erythrocyte

MCHC – mean corpuscular hemoglobin concentration of an erythrocyte

MCV – mean corpuscular volume of an erythrocyte

MDS – see *myelodysplastic syndrome*

mean – the arithmetic average

median – the middle value of a set of numbers arranged according to size

megakaryocytes – the largest cell found in bone marrow which produce platelets

megaloblastic dyspoiesis – uneven development of the nucleus and cytoplasm during erythrocyte maturation

megalocyte – an extremely large erythrocyte with a diameter exceeding 12 μm. This cell is larger than a macrocyte

meiosis – the process in which ova or sperm with half the normal number of chromosomes (1n) are produced

mesenteric thrombosis – a condition of clotting in the membranous tissues attaching the small intestine to the posterior abdominal wall

metaphase – a period in cellular division (mitosis)

metaplasia – change from one adult cell type to another (e.g., glandular epithelium to squamous epithelium metaplasia)

metarubricyte – normoblasts (acidophilic) or nucleated red blood cells

metastatic carcinoma – a malignancy that has spread from its original focal point

metastatic disease – see *metastatic carcinoma*

methemoglobin reductase pathway – an erythrocytic metabolic pathway that functions to prevent the oxidation of heme iron

methylene blue – a basic stain that stains the nucleus and some cytoplasmic structures of a cell a blue color. The blue-stained structures are basophilic substances

microfilaments – cellular ultrastructures consisting of the protein actin

microhematocrit – packed cell volume

microtubules – small, hollow cellular ultrastructures composed of polymerized, macromolecular protein subunits, tubulin

mitochondria – cellular ultrastructures composed of an outer, smooth membrane and an inner, folded membrane, the cristae. These organelles are associated with cellular energy-yielding activities

mitogen – a substance that stimulates cell division (mitosis)

mitosis – the process of body cellular division

mode – the number of values that occur with the greatest frequency

monoclonal antibodies – immune globulins directed against antigens derived from a single cell line

monocyte – a large mononuclear type of leukocyte

mononuclear cells – cells with a single large nucleus such as monocytes, promyelocytes, myelocytes, and blasts

mononuclear phagocyte system – the body defense system that consists of a variety of types of cells that have the ability to engulf or phagocytize substances such as foreign particles

monosodium urate – an abnormal crystal that may be observed in synovial fluid

morphology – the visual appearance, form, and shape of a cell

motility – movement

Mott cells – see *Grape cells*

MPD – myeloproliferative disorders

MPV – mean platelet volume. A measure of the average volume of the platelet population contained within the platelet curve

mRNA – messenger RNA; final processed transcript of the structural gene, present in the cytoplasm, from which a protein is produced

MSU – monosodium urate

mtDNA – mitochondrial DNA

multiple myeloma – a malignant disorder of plasma cells that is also known as plasma cell myeloma

multipotential hematopoietic stem cell – the progenitor of all blood cells. Also called hematopoietic progenitor cells (HPCs)

myeloblastic – a major form of leukemia characterized by large numbers of immature or mature granulocytes or related cells such as monocytes in the peripheral blood and/or bone marrow

myelodysplastic syndrome (MDS) – a group of disorders associated with abnormalities of erythrocytes, platelets, granulocytes, and monocytes

myelogenous – refers to the myeloid or granulocytic type cell line

myocardial infarction – necrosis of the muscular tissue of the heart

myosin – a contractile protein

N

NCCLS – National Committee for Clinical Laboratory Standards

Neisseria gonorrhoeae – a Gram-negative bacteria that causes gonorrhea

neoplasm – a new growth

nephropathy – a disease of the kidneys

neutropenia – a severe decrease in the number of neutrophilic granulocytes in the peripheral blood

neutrophilia – a significant increase in the number of neutrophilic granulocytes in the peripheral blood

neutrophilic reaction – when both the basic and the acidic stains stain the cytoplasmic structures, a pink or lilac color develops

Niemann-Pick disease – a monocytic disorder that represents the deficiency of an enzyme that normally cleaves phosphorylcholine from its sphingolipid, sphingomyelin

Northern blot – hybridization technique similar to the Southern blot, using RNA instead of DNA as a target

NRBC/100 WBC – the number of nucleated erythrocytes counted during a 100-cell leukocyte differential count

NRF – neutrophil-releasing factor. A regulator that influences the release of neutrophils from the bone marrow into the circulatory system

nuclear:cytoplasmic ratio – the amount of space occupied by the nucleus in the relationship to the space occupied by the cytoplasm

nucleated red blood cells – NRBCs

nucleoli – the region of the nucleus rich in RNA

nucleotide – basic building block of nucleic acids, consisting of a nitrogenous base, a pentose sugar, and phosphoric acid

null cells – a type of lymphocyte without either T or B cell surface markers

O

ochronosis – a peculiar discoloration of body tissue

oncogenes – transforming genes of cellular origin that are contained in retroviruses and associated with acute leukemias. Altered version of normal genes

operational iron – iron used for oxygen binding and biochemical reactions

opportunistic infections – microbial diseases that infect a debilitated host

opsonization – the process of coating a particle with immunoglobulin and/or complement which enhances phagocytosis

organelles – small cellular ultrastructures that are the functional units of a cell

OSHA – Occupational Safety and Health Administration

osmotic fragility – the ability or flexibility of the cellular membrane to withstand pressure

osteoarthritis – degenerative joint disease characterized by degeneration of the articular cartilage

osteoarthropathy – any disease of the joints and bones

oxidant stress – a decrease in the level of oxygen available to the tissues caused by agents such as drugs

oxidative pathway – see *hexose monophosphate shunt*

oxyhemoglobin – oxygenated hemoglobin

P

pallor – paleness of the skin and mucous membranes

pancytopenia – a severe decrease in all of the blood cells

Papanicolaou stain – a cytological stain used most commonly to detect uterine and cervical cancer

Pappenheimer bodies (siderotic granules) – abnormal basophilic iron-containing granules seen in erythrocytes

parameter – any numerical value that describes an entire population

PAS stain – the periodic acid–Schiff stain reaction for cellular carbohydrates

pathogenesis – the origin of disease

PDW – platelet distribution width

Pelger-Huët anomaly – an autosomal dominant genetic disorder that produces hyposegmentation of neutrophils

pericardial fluid – watery liquid in the sac surrounding the heart

peripheral blood – blood in the extremities (e.g., capillary blood)

peritoneal fluid – watery liquid in the abdominal cavity

pernicious anemia – an erythrocytic disorder associated with defective vitamin B_{12} uptake

petechiae – small purple hemorrhagic spots on the skin or mucous membranes

pH – a numerical value expressing acid, neutral, or alkaline (basic) conditions of a solution. A pH of 7.0 is neutral. Values from 0 to 6.9 are acidic, and values from 7.1 to 14.0 are alkaline

phagocyte – any cell that is capable of engulfing and destroying foreign particles such as bacteria

phagocytosis – a form of endocytosis. This important body defense mechanism is the process by which specialized cells engulf and destroy foreign particles

phagosome – an isolated vacuole formed in phagocytosis

pharyngitis – an inflammation of the throat

phenotype – the outward or physical expression of an inherited characteristic

Philadelphia chromosome – the Philadelphia chromosome (Ph^1) is a translocation involving chromosomes 22 and 9. This translocation is present in the precursors and megakaryocytes of patients with chronic myelogenous leukemia

phlebotomy – the collection of venous blood or venipuncture

photon – a basic unit of radiation

pia mater – the innermost of the three meninges covering the brain and spinal cord

pinocytosis – a form of endocytosis. This is the process in which specialized cells engulf fluids

plasma – the straw-colored fluid component of blood

plasmacyte – a mature plasma cell that is not normally found in the circulating blood

plasma thromboplastin antecedent – factor XI

plasma thromboplastin component – factor IX

plasmid – small, circular, self-replicating molecule of DNA in bacteria; foreign genetic material can be introduced into the plasmid and amplified as the plasmid replicates; a cloning vector

plasmin – a proteolytic enzyme with the ability to dissolve formed fibrin clots

plasminogen – the inactive precursor of plasmin that is converted to plasmin by the action of substances such as urokinase

plasminogen activators – the kinase enzymes

platelets – also called thrombocytes

platelet plug – the meshing together of platelets into a solid mass

pleocytosis – the presence of a greater-than-normal number of cells

pleural fluid – watery liquid in the chest cavity

PLT – platelet count

PNH – paroxysmal nocturnal hemoglobinuria. A rare, acquired chronic hemolytic anemia

poikilocytosis – alterations or variations in the shape of erythrocytes

point mutation – a change that affects a single base in DNA

polychromasia – see *polychromatophilia*

polychromatophilia – fine, evenly distributed basophilic (blue) granules that impart a blue color to Wright-stained erythrocytes

polycythemia – an increase in erythrocytes in the circulatory blood

polycythemia vera – a blood dyscrasia in which the erythrocytes, leukocytes, and thrombocytes are all increased above normal

polymerase chain reaction (PCR) – method for synthetically amplifying known DNA sequences in vitro using many cycles of denaturation and polymerization with synthetic oligonucleotide primer extension employing Taq polymerase

polysaccharide – a carbohydrate containing 10 or more monosaccharides

porphyrin – any of a group of iron- or magnesium-free cyclic tetrapyrrole derivatives which form the basis of the respiratory pigments of animals and plants. Porphyrins in combination with iron form *hemes*

precision – the closeness of test results when repeated analyses of the same material are performed

prefix – the beginning portion of a medical term

prekallikrein – Fletcher factor

preleukemia – an older term for a condition preceding acute leukemia

primary lymphoid tissues – the bone marrow and thymus gland are classified as primary or central lymphoid tissue

primer – short nucleic acid sequence that pairs with ssDNA and provides a free 3′-OH end to "prime," or begin, polymerase synthesis of a complimentary polynucleotide chain

proaccelerin – factor V

probe – a known, labeled sequence of DNA or RNA used to detect complementary sequences in target polynucleotides by hybridization

proconvertin – factor VII

prognosis – a forecast of the probable outcome of a condition, disorder, or disease

prophase – the first stage in cellular division (mitosis)

prorubricyte – basophilic normoblast

prostaglandins – naturally occurring fatty acids that stimulate the contraction of uterine and other smooth muscle tissues

prostatitis – inflammation of the male gland, the prostate

prostatovesiculitis – inflammation of the prostate and seminal vesicle

proteases – enzymes that digest proteins

protein C – a plasma protein that functions as a potent natural anticoagulant

protein S – a plasma protein that functions as a potent natural anticoagulant

prothrombin – factor II

prothrombin group – blood coagulation factors II, VII, IX, and X

proto-oncogenes – antecedents of oncogenes that act as central regulators of growth in normal cells

pseudo–Pelger-Huët anomaly – a false form of this anomaly. See *Pelger-Huët anomaly*

pseudopods – cytoplasmic extrusions that resemble false feet

PT – prothrombin time

purines – an organic family that forms the nucleic acid bases

purpura – extensive areas of red or dark-purple discoloration of the skin

pyknosis – contraction of a cell's nucleus that produces a dark, dense appearance

pyrimidine analog – a compound that can be substituted for a pyrimidine base to interrupt protein synthesis in actively mitotic cells

pyrimidines – an organic family that forms the nucleic acid bases

Q

qualitative – a difference in type rather than quantity

quality control – a process that monitors the accuracy and reproducibility of patient results through the use of control specimens

R

RA – see *rheumatoid arthritis*

ragocytes – cells of the body fluid

range – the difference between the highest and lowest measurements in a series

RCMI – red cell morphology index. Derived from a comparison of the patient's measured red cell volume distribution with a distribution representing the average patient population served by the laboratory. The calculation of RCMI relates to a statistical function called z, which measures the difference between a random variable and the mean under the curve. If the RCMI is outside the –2.0 to +2.0 range, this indicates a significant number of abnormal red cells

RDW – red cell distribution width. An index of the variation in red cell size. It is computed from the red cell histogram by dividing the standard deviation by the mean and multiplying by 100

reactive eosinophilia – an increase in eosinophils caused by inflammation or allergic reaction

refractive index – a measurement of the passage of light

refractory anemia – a deficiency of red blood cells that does not readily yield to treatment

regimen – a schedule of treatment

Reiter's disease – a disease of males characterized in part by migratory polyarthritis

relative polycythemia – increases in erythrocytes results from conditions not related to increased erythropoietin production

remission – a period in which the signs and symptoms of a disease, such as leukemia, subside.

restriction endonuclease – bacterial enzyme that recognizes short palindromic sequences of DNA and cleaves the DNA near this "restriction site"; each enzyme is named for the bacteria from which it has been isolated

restriction fragment length polymorphism (RFLP) – alteration in DNA fragment size caused by a change such as a deletion; relatively stable and can be detected with nucleic acid probes; if close on the chromosome to a disease-producing gene, it can be used as a marker for this disease

reticulocyte – the last stage of the immature erythrocyte. This cell lacks a nucleus and is found in both the bone marrow and peripheral blood

reticuloendothelial system (RES) – see *mononuclear phagocyte system*

reticuloendotheliosis – increased growth and development (hyperplasia) of the reticuloendothelial system

retrovirus – reverse the normal process of converting DNA to RNA

rheumatoid arthritis – a form of arthritis most commonly seen in young adults

ribonucleic acid – RNA

ribosomes – cellular organelles that occur both on the surface of the rough endoplasmic reticulum and free in the cytoplasm. They are associated with cellular protein synthesis

Rieder cells – cells that are similar to lymphocytes

ringed sideroblasts – iron deposits encircling immature erythrocytes, particularly metarubricytes (normoblasts)

RNA – ribonucleic acid

Romanowsky stain – any stain containing methylene blue and/or its products of oxidation, and a halogenated fluorescein dye, usually eosin B or eosin Y

root term – the part of a medical term that usually refers to an anatomical structure

rouleaux formation – the appearance of erythrocytes that resembles a stack of coins

RPI – reticulocyte production index. A measurement of erythropoietic activity when "stress" reticulocytes are present

R proteins – one of the binding proteins capable of binding cobalamin (vitamin B_{12})

rRNA – ribosomal RNA; component of ribosomes that serve as scaffolding for polypeptide synthesis

rubriblast – the earliest specific red blood cell precursor. Also referred to as pronormoblast

rubricyte – polychromatophilic normoblast

Russell bodies – round, glassy, transparent bodies that may be seen in plasma cells

S

S phase – the period during the cellular division cycle in which DNA is replicated

sample – a subset of a population

Schilling list – an assay to determine the cause of vitamin B_{12} (cobalamin) deficiency

Schüffner's dots – red particles seen in erythrocytes containing malarial (*Plasmodium vivax*) parasites

scleroderma – a chronic disorder characterized by progressive collagenous fibrosis of many organs and systems

secondary lymphoid tissue – lymph nodes, spleen, and Peyer's patches in the intestine

secondary polycythemia – an increased concentration of erythrocytes in the blood

sed rate – erythrocyte sedimentation rate

seminal fluid – liquid produced by the male reproductive system

sepsis – an infection-induced syndrome defined as the presence of two or more of the following features of systemic inflammation: fever or hypothermia, leukocytosis or leukopenia, tachycardia and tachypnea, or supranormal minute ventilation

septic arthritis – joint inflammation caused by microorganisms

septicemia – the presence of pathogenic microorganisms in the blood

serotonin – a vasoconstrictor produced from tryptophan that stimulates smooth muscle

serous fluid – producing or containing serum

serum – straw-colored fluid that is present after blood clots.

serum electrophoresis – separation of serum proteins by electrical methods

Sézary cell – a large lymphocyte with a nucleus that occupies most of the cell

sickle cell disease – results from the substitution of a valine for glutamic acid at the sixth position on the beta chain of the hemoglobin molecule. In homozygous form (SS), causes sickle cell anemia

sideroblastic anemia – a disorder of iron utilization in which the body has adequate iron but is unable to incorporate it in hemoglobin synthesis

siderotic granules – Pappenheimer bodies

Singer and Nicholson's fluid mosaic model – this model explains the arrangement of the components of the cell membrane into a bilaminar layer of phospholipids, with protein molecules interspersed as either integral or peripheral units

sinusoids – specialized capillaries found in locations such as the bone marrow, spleen, and liver

size distribution histogram – a display of the distribution of cell volume and frequency. Each channel on the x-axis represents size in fetoliter (fL). The y-axis represents the relative number of cells

SLE – abbreviation for systemic lupus erythematosus

Small-bowel stricture – a narrowing of the intestine

Smoldering leukemia – see *MPD*

smudge cells – a natural artifact seen on peripheral blood smears that represents the bare nuclei of leukocytes (e.g., lymphocytes). Increased numbers are seen in CLL

sodium citrate – a blood anticoagulant that is frequently used in a concentration of 3.2% for coagulation studies

soluble transferrin receptor – an indicator of iron deficiency

Southern blot – hybridization technique invented by E. M. Southern in which DNA is digested with restriction enzymes, separated by electrophoresis, transferred to a solid matrix, and hybridized to a labeled probe

spermatozoa – male reproductive cells, sperm

splenic infarction – tissue necrosis of the spleen

splenomegaly – an extremely enlarged spleen

sprue – a chronic form of malabsorption syndrome

ssDNA – single-stranded DNA

standard – a highly purified substance of a known composition

standard deviation – the square root of the variance

stasis – stopping of bleeding

stat – immediately

statistic – any numerical value describing a sample

stem term – root term

stenosis – the narrowing of a vessel. In a blood vessel, the lumen decreases the flow of blood if stenosis exists

stercobilinogen – fecal urobilinogen

sterile body fluid – watery fluids in the body that lack microorganisms

stroma – the structural protein of an erythrocyte. Remains after the erythrocyte has been washed free of hemoglobin and appears as a ghost cell or shadow when viewed under the microscope

Stuart factor – factor X

subacute leukemia – see *MPD*

subarachnoid space – the space between the arachnoid and pia mater layers of the meninges of the brain

subsets – subgroups of a sample

sudanophilic – having an affinity for Sudan stain

suffix – the ending of a medical term

supernatant – the fluid above the solid portion in a centrifuged or settled mixture

symptomatic – a deviation from usual function or appearance

syndrome – a set or group of symptoms that occur together

synovial fluid – joint fluid

systemic circulation – blood circulation throughout the body

systemic lupus erythematosus (SLE) – a multisymptom disorder that can affect practically every organ of the body

systemic rheumatic disorders – a name commonly used for disorders of the joints, connective tissues, and collagen-vascular disorders, e.g., systemic lupus erythematosus (SLE)

T

T lymphocytes or T cells – cells responsible for the cellular immune response and involved in the regulation of antibody reactions

tanycytes – body fluid cells

Taq DNA polymerase – thermostable DNA polymerase used to polymerize new DNA strands; used in the PCR procedure

telophase – the final stage in cellular division (mitosis)

thoracentesis – piercing of the thorax (chest cavity) for the purpose of removing fluid

thrombin – a blood coagulation factor (factor IIa) that is the activated form of prothrombin

thrombocytes – blood platelets

thrombocytopenia – a severe decrease in circulating platelets

thrombocytosis – an increase in the number of circulating platelets (thrombocytes)

thromboplastin – blood coagulation factor III

thrombopoietin – a hormone believed to be of renal origin that is secreted in response to the need for platelets

thrombosis – clotting or the presence of a clot

thrombosthenin – actomyosin

thromboxane A2 – a short-lived substance that facilitates the release of platelet granular contents, induces other platelets to aggregate, and stimulates vasoconstriction

thrombus – a clot

TIBC – total iron-binding capacity

titer – the strength or concentration of a solution

toxic granulation – abnormally dark granulation seen in band and segmented neutrophils or monocytes

transcobalamin – a specific globulin protein that is involved in the physiological mechanism of vitamin B_{12}

transferrin – a beta globulin glycoprotein that binds iron and transports it back to the bone marrow for hemoglobin synthesis

transcription – process in which mRNA translates DNA into RNA nucleotide sequences

translocation – a kind of chromosomal aberration in which a segment of one chromosome breaks away from its normal location and attaches to another, nonhomologous, chromosome

trisomy – a chromosomal alteration in which a third chromosome exists with a homologous pair of chromosomes

tRNA – transfer RNA; small RNA molecules that interact with amino acids and mediate their correct insertion into a growing polypeptide chain

trophoblasts – the peripheral cells of the blastocyst

tunica adventitia – the layer of a blood vessel that consists of fibrous connective tissue innervated with automatic nerve endings

tunica intima – the smooth surface of endothelium in a blood vessel

tunica media – the thickest layer of a blood vessel. It is composed of smooth muscle and elastic fibers

turbidity – cloudiness

U

ultrastructure – cellular organelles that can be viewed with electron microscopy

unconjugated bilirubin – bilirubin not bound to protein

V

vacuolated lymphocytes – vacuolation may be seen in variant lymphocytes or as a reaction to radiation and chemotherapy

variance – the position of each observation (test) in relationship to the mean

variant lymphocytes – atypical lymphocytes. Downey cells, reactive or transformed lymphocytes, lymphocytoid or plasmacytoid lymphocytes, and virocytes. These cells may be found in infectious mononucleosis, viral pneumonia, and viral hepatitis

vasa vasorum – small networks of blood vessels that supply nutrients to the tissues of the wall of a blood vessel

vascular integrity – the resistance to vessel disruption

vasoconstriction – contraction of the blood vessel wall

VCS – volume, conductivity, scatter

veins – collecting vessels that return blood to the heart

ventricles – cerebral ventricles are hollow spaces in the brain

venules – microscopically sized veins

VH – variable region of the immunoglobulin heavy chain gene locus

viscosity – thickness

Vitamin B_{12} – cobalamin

von Willebrand's disease – a genetic disorder producing a deficiency and defect of blood coagulation factor VII and defective platelet function

W

Waldenström's primary macroglobulinemia – neoplastic proliferation of the lymphocyte plasma cell system

western blot – hybridization technique similar to the Southern blot in which the electrophoresed sample is protein and the detector is immunoglobulin

Wiskott-Aldrich syndrome – a blood coagulation disorder characterized by extremely small platelets (thrombocytes)

Wright stain – a Romanowsky-type blood stain

X

xanthochromia – yellow color

Note: Page numbers in *italics* indicate figure; Page numbers followed by b indicate box; those followed by t indicate table.

QUICK CALCULATION REFERENCES

Absolute Leukocyte Cell Count

Absolute cell value = total leukocyte count × % of WBC type on differential smear evaluation

Absolute reticulocyte count = % reticulocytes × RBC count

Total Leukocyte Count Corrected for Nucleated Erythrocytes

$$\text{Corrected Total WBC} = \frac{\text{Average total leukocyte count} \times 100}{100 + \text{number of nucleated RBCs/100 WBC in the differential count}}$$

Erythrocyte Measurements

$$\text{Mean Corpuscular Volume (MCV)} = \frac{\text{Hematocrit (PCV) L/L}}{\text{RBC count } (\times 10^{12}/\text{L})} = \text{fL}^a$$

$$\text{Mean Corpuscular Hemoglobin (MCH)} = \frac{\text{Hemoglobin } (\times 10 \text{ gm/dL})}{\text{RBC count } (\times 10^{12}/\text{L})} = \text{pg}^b$$

$$\text{Mean Corpuscular Hemoglobin Concentration (MCHC)} = \frac{\text{Hemoglobin (gm/dL)}}{\text{Hematocrit (PCV) L/L}} = \text{g/dL}$$

^{a} femtoliters
^{b} picograms

Red Cell Distribution Width (RDW) — Derived from RBC histogram

$$\text{CV of RBC distribution} = \frac{(\text{SD} \times 100)}{\text{mean}}$$

Manual Cell Counts
Body Fluids

Number of leukocytes (WBCs) =
average total of WBCs in four large squares × dilution factor × volume correction factor = WBCs × 10^9/L

Low Blood Platelet Counts

Number of platelets =
average total of platelets in five squares × dilution factor × volume correction factor = Platelets × 10^9/L

Reticulocytes

Corrected reticulocyte count (%) =

$$\text{Reticulocyte count} \times \frac{\text{Hematocrit (PCV)}}{\text{Normal PCV based on age and gender}} = \% \text{ (corrected)}$$

Reticulocyte Production Index (RPI)

$$\text{RPI (\%)} = \frac{\text{Corrected reticulocyte count (\%)}}{\text{Maturation time in days}}$$

Maturation Time Correction Factor

Hematocrit (L/L)	Maturation time
0.45	1.0
0.35	1.5
0.25	2.0
0.15	2.5

Miller Ocular Disc Calculation for Reticulocytes

$$\text{Reticulocyte} = \frac{\text{Number of reticulocytes (large square)}}{\text{Number of erythrocytes (small square)} \times 9} \times 100 = \% \text{ uncorrected}$$

International Normalized Ratio (INR)

INR = (patient PT/control)^{ISI}

BODY FLUIDS

Cerebrospinal Fluid

Total Cell Count

Adults 0–5 mononnuclear cells/μL, O RBCs/μL
Neonates 0–30 mononuclear cells/μL, O RBCs/μL

Differential Cell Count

Adults

Segmented polymorphonuclear neutrophils	0%–5%
Lymphocytes	28%–96%
Mononuclear cells	16%–56%
Ependymal cells	rare
Histiocytes	rare

Neonates

Segmented polymorphonuclear neutrophils	0%–5%
Lymphocytes	2%–38%
Mononuclear cells	50%–94%
Ependymal cells	rare
Histiocytes	1%–6%

Pleural Fluid

Total Cell Count
≤ 1000 WBCs/μL, O RBCs/μL
Differential PMN ≤ 25%, Mononuclear 0–75%

Seminal Fluid

Total volume: 1.5–5.0 mL
Total cell count 20–160 million/mL

Synovial Fluid

Total cell count
200–600 WBCs cells/μL, O RBCs/μL
Differential PMN 0%–25%, mononuclear cells 0%–75%